The Future of Pharmaceuticals

The Future of Pharmaceuticals

A Nonlinear Analysis

Sarfaraz K. Niazi, Ph.D.
University of Illinois
Chicago, IL, USA

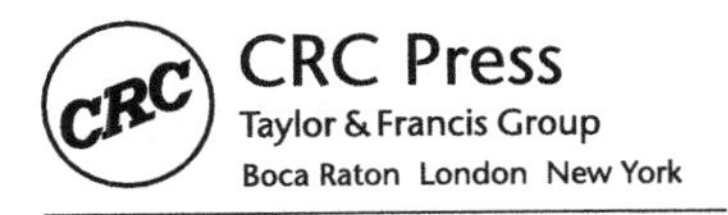

CRC Press is an imprint of the
Taylor & Francis Group, an **informa** business

First edition published 2022
by CRC Press
6000 Broken Sound Parkway NW, Suite 300, Boca Raton, FL 33487-2742

and by CRC Press
2 Park Square, Milton Park, Abingdon, Oxon, OX14 4RN

Library of Congress Cataloging in Publication Data

Names: Niazi, Sarfaraz, 1949- author.
Title: The future of pharmaceuticals : a nonlinear analysis / Sarfaraz K. Niazi.
Description: First edition. | Boca Raton : CRC Press, 2022. | Includes bibliographical references and index.
Identifiers: LCCN 2021021801 (print) | LCCN 2021021802 (ebook) | ISBN 9780367701390 (paperback) | ISBN 9780367701390 (hardback) | ISBN 9781003146933 (ebook)
Subjects: LCSH: Drugs--Research. | Pharmaceutical industry. | Pharmaceutical policy.
Classification: LCC RS122 .N53 2022 (print) | LCC RS122 (ebook) | DDC 615.1072--dc23
LC record available at https://lccn.loc.gov/2021021801
LC ebook record available at https://lccn.loc.gov/2021021802

ISBN: 978-0-367-70564-0 (hbk)
ISBN: 978-0-367-70139-0 (pbk)
ISBN: 978-1-003-14693-3 (ebk)

DOI: 10.1201/9781003146933

Typeset in Times
by Deanta Global Publishing Services, Chennai, India

To my friend, Vice President Kamala Devi Harris for breaking three nonlinear barriers.

Contents

Preface xix
Acknowledgments xxvii
Author xxix
List of Important Terminology xxxi

1 Understanding Nonlinearity 1
1.1 Background 1
1.2 Predictions 3
1.2.1 Examples 5
1.3 Modeling Systems 8
1.3.1 Bayes' Theorem 10
1.3.1.1 Phases of Paradigm Shift 14
1.3.2 Future Shifts 17
1.4 Conclusion 20
Additional Reading 20

2 The Evolution of Pharmaceuticals 23
2.1 Background 23
2.2 The Pre-Historical Era 24
2.3 The New World Era 25
2.4 The Regulatory Era 26
2.5 The Legal Era 28
2.6 The Gene Era 29
2.6.1 The Biological Medicine Era 29
2.6.2 Nobel Prizes 31
2.7 The Future Era 31
2.8 New Entities 38
2.8.1 A Special Case 39
2.9 Conclusion 41
2.10 Appendix: New Molecular Entities Approved by the FDA 2011–2020 41
Additional Reading 56

3 Artificial Intelligence 69
3.1 Background 69
3.2 Bioinformatics 71
3.3 Artificial Intelligence 73
3.4 Deep Learning Architecture 73
3.4.1 Graph Representation Learning 74
3.5 Repurposing 74
3.6 Data and Model Harmonization 75
3.7 Drug Discovery and Development 76
3.7.1 Stepwise Approach 78
3.7.2 Application Types 79
3.7.3 An Example of AI Application 82
3.8 AI Tools 83
3.9 Conclusion 86
Additional Reading 89

4 Drug Discovery Trends ... 91
4.1 Background ... 91
4.2 High-Throughput Screening (HTS) ... 91
4.2.1 Phenotypic Screening ... 94
4.2.2 Modeling ... 94
4.2.3 Screening Using Fragments (FBS) ... 95
4.2.4 Ligandomics ... 95
4.2.5 Gene-Based Testing ... 95
4.2.6 Target Identification ... 97
4.2.6.1 Hit Identification ... 98
4.2.6.2 Hit to Lead ... 109
4.2.6.3 Target Validation and Efficacy ... 109
4.2.6.4 Cell-Based Models ... 110
4.2.6.5 In Vivo Testing ... 111
4.3 Structural Biology ... 112
4.4 Hit Optimization ... 114
4.4.1 PK–PD Relationship ... 115
4.5 Chemistry and Formulation ... 118
4.5.1 Lipinski's Rule of Five (RO5) ... 119
4.6 Safety Testing ... 121
4.6.1 Animal Models ... 122
4.6.2 Replacing Animal Testing ... 123
4.7 Synthetic Biology ... 124
4.8 Libraries ... 125
4.8.1 DNA Libraries ... 126
4.9 Microphysiometry ... 128
4.9.1 Microfluidics ... 129
4.9.2 Organs-on-a-Chip (OOC) ... 129
4.9.3 Brain-on-a-Chip ... 129
4.9.4 Lung-on-a-Chip ... 130
4.9.5 Heart-on-a-Chip ... 130
4.9.6 Kidney-on-a-Chip ... 130
4.9.7 Nephron-on-a-Chip ... 130
4.9.8 Vessel-on-a-Chip ... 131
4.9.9 Skin-on-a-Chip ... 131
4.9.10 Human-on-a-Chip ... 131
4.10 Clinical Trials ... 132
4.10.1 Biomarkers ... 133
4.10.1.1 BEST ... 136
4.11 Exploratory IND ... 137
4.12 Repurposing ... 139
4.13 Orphan Drugs ... 140
4.14 Conclusion ... 141
Additional Reading ... 141

5 Drug Development Assays ... 143
5.1 Background ... 143
5.1.1 Assay Optimization ... 143
5.2 Assay Development and Validation ... 144
5.2.1 Pre-Study Validation ... 145
5.2.2 In-Study Validation ... 146
5.2.3 Cross-Validation ... 146
5.2.4 Critical Path ... 146

5.3 Receptor Binding Assays in HTS 147
5.3.1 Scintillation Proximity Assays (SPA) 147
5.3.2 Filtration Assays 149
5.4 In Vitro Biochemical Assays 150
5.4.1 Definitions.... 150
5.4.2 Signs of Enzymatic Contamination 151
5.4.3 Solutions for Enzymatic Contamination....152
5.4.4 Batch Testing....152
5.4.4.1 Identity and Mass Purity 152
5.4.4.2 Methods for Confirming Identity and Mass Purity....152
5.4.4.3 Protein Stain of SDS-PAGE 153
5.4.4.4 Western Blot with the Specific Antibody 153
5.4.4.5 Analytical Gel Filtration....153
5.4.4.6 Reversed-Phase HPLC 153
5.4.4.7 Mass Spectrometry....153
5.4.4.8 Whole Mass for Protein....153
5.4.4.9 Peptide Mass Finger Printing 154
5.4.4.10 Edman Sequencing.... 154
5.4.4.11 Crude Enzyme Preparations.... 154
5.4.4.12 Commercial Enzymes 154
5.4.4.13 Co-Purification of Contaminating Enzymes.... 154
5.4.4.14 Mock Parallel Purification.... 154
5.4.4.15 Reversal of Enzyme Activity....155
5.4.5 Detecting Enzyme Impurities....155
5.4.5.1 Consequences of Substrate Selectivity 155
5.4.5.2 Substrate Km 155
5.4.5.3 Enzyme Concentration 156
5.4.5.4 Format Selection.... 156
5.4.6 Validating Enzymatic Purity 156
5.4.6.1 Inhibitor-Based Studies 156
5.4.6.2 IC50 Value.... 157
5.4.6.3 Hill slope 157
5.4.7 Substrate-Based Studies.... 159
5.4.7.1 Substrate Km Determination.... 159
5.4.7.2 Substrate Selectivity Studies 159
5.4.7.3 Comparison Studies.... 160
5.4.7.4 Enzyme Source.... 160
5.4.7.5 Format Comparison.... 160
5.5 Enzymatic Assays for HTS....161
5.5.1 Basic Concept....161
5.5.1.1 Initial Velocity 161
5.5.2 Reagents and Method Development 162
5.5.2.1 Detection System Linearity....162
5.5.2.2 Enzyme Reaction Progress Curve....163
5.5.2.3 Measuring the Initial Velocity of an Enzyme Reaction....163
5.5.2.4 Measurement of Km and Vmax 163
5.5.2.5 What Does the Km Mean? 163
5.5.2.6 How to Measure Km 164
5.5.2.7 Determination of IC50 for Inhibitors 165
5.5.2.8 Optimization Experiments 166
5.6 ELISA-Type Assays 167
5.6.1 Basic Concept....167

5.6.2 General Considerations 167
5.6.2.1 Assay Design and Development 168
5.6.3 Fluorescence Polarization/Anisotropy 169
5.6.3.1 Assay Design 170
5.6.4 Fluorescent/Förster Resonance Energy Transfer and Time-Resolved (TR) FRET 172
5.6.5 AlphaScreen Format 173
5.6.5.1 Optical Biosensors 175
5.6.5.2 Nuclear Magnetic Resonance (NMR) 175
5.6.5.3 Isothermal Calorimetry (ITC) 175
5.6.5.4 Sedimentation Analysis (SA; Analytical Ultracentrifugation) 176
5.6.5.5 X-Ray Crystallography 176
5.7 In Vitro Toxicity and Drug Efficacy Testing 177
5.8 In Vivo Assay Validation 178
5.8.1 General Concepts 179
5.8.1.1 Pre-Study Validation 179
5.8.1.2 In-Study Validation 179
5.8.1.3 Cross-Validation 179
5.8.1.4 Resources 179
5.8.2 Assay Validation Procedures 180
5.8.2.1 Pre-Study Validation 181
5.9 Pharmacokinetics and Drug Metabolism 182
5.9.1 In Vitro Analysis 183
5.9.1.1 Lipophilicity 183
5.9.1.2 Solubility 184
5.9.1.3 Hepatic Microsome Stability 184
5.9.1.4 Plasma Stability 185
5.9.1.5 Plasma Protein Binding 185
5.9.1.6 Screening Cytotoxicity and Hepatotoxicity Test 186
5.9.1.7 CYP450 Inhibition Profiling 187
5.9.1.8 Permeability 188
5.10 Conclusion 189
Additional Reading 189

6 Nanomedicine 195
6.1 Background 195
6.2 Delivery Routes 197
6.3 Liposomes 199
6.4 Dendrimers 200
6.5 Polymers 200
6.6 Metal Particles 203
6.7 Quantum Dots 203
6.8 Fullerenes 204
6.9 Theranostics 204
6.10 Diagnostics 206
6.11 Specific Diseases 207
6.11.1 IBD 207
6.11.2 Diabetes 207
6.11.3 Cancer 207
6.12 Regulatory 211
Additional Reading 211

7 Antimicrobials 231
7.1 Background 231
7.2 Eradicable Diseases 232
7.2.1 Polio 232
7.2.2 Guinea Worm Disease (Dracunculiasis) 232
7.2.3 Lymphatic Filariasis 232
7.2.4 Measles, Mumps, and Rubella 232
7.2.5 Cysticercosis 233
7.2.6 Yaws 233
7.2.7 Trachoma 233
7.2.8 Onchocerciasis 233
7.2.9 Malaria 234
7.3 Vaccines 234
7.3.1 Live-Attenuated Vaccines 234
7.3.2 Inactivated Vaccines 234
7.3.3 Subunit, Recombinant, Polysaccharide, and Conjugate Vaccines 234
7.3.4 Toxoid Vaccines 234
7.3.5 Nucleic Acid Vaccines 234
7.4 Antibiotics 235
7.4.1 Antibiotic Discovery 235
7.4.1.1 Semi-Synthetic 236
7.4.1.2 Synthetic 236
7.4.1.3 Genomic Approaches 238
7.4.2 Reverse Genomics: Revival of Cell-Based Screening 240
7.4.3 Post-Genomics 241
7.4.3.1 Transcriptomics, Proteomics, and Lipidomics 241
7.4.3.2 Metabolomics to Meta-Omics 242
7.5 Phage Therapy 244
7.6 Microbiome 246
7.6.1 Impact on Health 246
7.6.2 Drug Metabolism 247
7.6.3 Drug Toxicity 247
7.6.4 Biomarkers 248
7.7 Conclusion 248
Additional Reading 248

8 Therapeutic Proteins 251
8.1 Background 251
8.2 Protein Structure and Properties 251
8.2.1 Primary Structure 252
8.2.2 Secondary Structure 255
8.2.2.1 Alpha Helix 256
8.2.2.2 Beta-Sheet 256
8.2.3 Tertiary Structure 256
8.2.4 Quaternary Structure 257
8.2.5 Post-Translational Modification (PTM) 257
8.2.6 Association and Aggregation 261
8.3 Non-Antibody Therapeutic Proteins 261
8.3.1 Hormone Peptide Drugs 262
8.3.2 Human Hematopoietic Factor 263
8.3.3 Human Cytokines 263

8.3.4 Human Plasma Protein Factor ... 263
8.3.5 Human Bone Formation Protein ... 264
8.3.6 Enzymes ... 264
8.4 Antibody Therapeutic Proteins ... 264
8.4.1 Mode of Action ... 266
8.4.2 Types of Antibodies ... 267
8.4.2.1 Recombinant Antibodies ... 267
8.4.2.2 Synthetic Antibodies ... 268
8.4.2.3 Affimer Proteins ... 268
8.4.2.4 Structural Protein Scaffolds ... 268
8.4.2.5 Bispecific Antibodies (BsAbs) ... 269
8.4.2.6 Multi-Specific Antibodies (MsAbs) ... 270
8.4.2.7 Fab Fragments and Single-Chain Antibodies ... 270
8.4.2.8 Humanized and Chimeric mAbs ... 270
8.4.2.9 Affinity Maturation ... 271
8.4.2.10 Antigenized Antibodies ... 272
8.4.2.11 IgG1 Fusion Proteins ... 272
8.4.2.12 Drug or Toxin Conjugation ... 272
8.4.2.13 Future Antibodies ... 273
8.4.3 Development of Antibodies ... 275
8.4.4 Exogenous Methods ... 277
8.4.4.1 Mouse Hybridoma ... 278
8.4.4.2 Transgenic Mice ... 280
8.4.5 Surface Display Libraries ... 280
8.4.5.1 Phage Display ... 281
8.4.5.2 Yeast Display ... 283
8.4.5.3 Ribosome Display ... 285
8.4.5.4 mRNA Display ... 285
8.4.6 Recombinant Expression ... 286
8.5 Immunogenicity ... 287
8.5.1 Protein Immunogenicity ... 288
8.5.2 Immunogenicity Testing ... 289
8.5.3 Innate System ... 290
8.5.4 Adaptive System ... 290
8.6 Pharmacokinetics of Therapeutic Proteins ... 291
8.6.1 Absorption ... 293
8.6.2 Distribution ... 295
8.6.3 Elimination ... 295
8.6.4 Pharmacokinetic Manipulations ... 297
8.6.4.1 Protein Modification to Increase Duration of Action ... 297
8.6.4.2 Protein Pegylation ... 298
8.6.4.3 Unnatural Construction ... 298
8.7 Conclusion ... 299
Additional Reading ... 301

9 Manufacturing Trends ... 307
9.1 Background ... 307
9.2 Process Optimizations ... 307
9.2.1 Cell Line Development ... 307
9.2.2 Media ... 308
9.2.3 High Cell Density Cryopreservation ... 309
9.2.4 Cell Culture Operations ... 309
9.2.5 Bioreactor Cycle ... 311

9.3 Single-Use Technology (SUT) 312
9.3.1 Containers and Mixing Systems 313
9.3.2 Drums, Containers, and Tank Liners 313
9.3.2.1 2D Bags 314
9.3.2.2 3D Bags 314
9.3.3 Advantages 315
9.3.4 Single-Use Bioreactors (SUBS) 315
9.3.5 Other Components 318
9.3.5.1 Optical Sensors 319
9.3.5.2 Biomass Sensors 320
9.3.5.3 Electrochemical Sensors 320
9.3.5.4 Pressure Sensors 320
9.3.5.5 Sampling Systems 321
9.3.5.6 Connectors 322
9.3.5.7 Tubing 323
9.3.5.8 Pumps 323
9.3.5.9 Tube Welder and Sealers 324
9.3.6 Sampling 324
9.3.7 Downstream Processing 325
9.3.7.1 Cell Harvest 325
9.3.7.2 Purification 326
9.3.7.3 Virus Removal 327
9.3.7.4 Filtration—UF/DF and TFF 328
9.3.7.5 General Filtration Applications 328
9.3.8 Fill Finish Operations 329
9.3.9 Safety 329
9.3.9.1 Polymers and Additives 330
9.3.9.2 Material Selection 331
9.3.9.3 Testing 331
9.3.9.4 Regulatory 332
9.4 Online Monitoring 333
9.5 Continuous Manufacturing 333
9.5.1 Continuous Chromatography Operations 336
9.5.1.1 Straight Through Processing (STP) 336
9.5.1.2 Periodic Countercurrent Chromatography (PCC) 337
9.5.1.3 Simulated Moving Bed (SMB) Chromatography 337
9.6 Conclusion 337
Appendix: Databases Relevant to Antibodies 337
Additional Reading 338

10 Therapeutic Protein Delivery Systems 345
10.1 Background 345
10.2 Route Selection 346
10.2.1 Selection 346
10.2.2 Excipients and Properties 347
10.2.2.1 pH 349
10.2.2.2 Surface Tension 350
10.2.2.3 Tonicity 350
10.2.2.4 Protectants 350
10.2.2.5 Stabilizers 351
10.2.3 Liquid Formulations 351
10.2.4 Lyophilized Formulations 352
10.3 Delivery Routes 353

10.3.1 Intravenous....353
10.3.2 Subcutaneous....353
10.3.3 Oral....355
10.3.4 Nasal....356
10.3.5 Transdermal....356
10.3.6 Pulmonary....357
10.3.7 Ocular....358
10.3.8 Rectal....359
10.4 Formulation Technologies....359
10.4.1 Hydrogels and In Situ Forming Gels....359
10.4.2 Nanoparticles....360
10.4.3 Liposome....360
10.4.4 Higher Concentration Formulations....361
10.5 Examples of Formulation....363
10.5.1 Oprelvekin Injection (Interleukin IL-11)....363
10.5.2 Interleukin Injection (IL-2)....363
10.5.3 Interferon Alfa-2a Injection....363
10.5.4 Interferon Beta-1b....364
10.5.5 Interferon Beta-1a Injection....364
10.5.6 Interferon Alfa-n3 Injection....364
10.5.7 Interferon Alfacon-1 Injection....364
10.5.8 Interferon Gamma-1b Injection....365
10.5.9 Infliximab for Injection....365
10.5.10 Daclizumab for Injection....365
10.5.11 Coagulation Factor VIIa (Recombinant) Injection....365
10.5.12 Reteplase Recombinant for Injection....366
10.5.13 Alteplase Recombinant Injection....366
10.6 Conclusion....366
Appendix 10.1: Physicochemical Properties of Proteins and Peptides Approved by the FDA....367
Additional Reading....375

11 Gene and Cell Therapy....381
11.1 Background....381
11.2 Gene Therapy....385
11.2.1 Viral Vector Manufacturing....386
11.2.2 Downstream Manufacturing....388
11.2.3 Risks of Gene Therapy....391
11.2.4 Gene Editing....392
11.2.5 Techniques....393
11.2.6 Gene Editing Technologies....395
11.2.7 CRISPR....395
11.2.8 DNA-Based Therapeutics....398
11.2.9 Gene Transfer Technologies....398
11.2.9.1 Mechanical and Electrical Techniques....398
11.2.9.2 Vector-Assisted Delivery Systems....398
11.2.10 Approved Products....399
11.3 Cell Therapy....399
11.3.1 Types of Cell Therapies....401
11.3.2 CAR-T Therapy....402
11.3.3 Allogenic Cell Therapy....403
11.4 Regulatory Considerations....404
11.4.1 Development and Characterization of Cell Populations for Administration....405
11.4.1.1 Collection of Cells....405

11.4.1.2 Tissue Typing ... 406
11.4.1.3 Procedures ... 406
11.4.2 Characterization and Release Testing of Cellular Gene Therapy Products ... 408
11.4.2.1 Cell Identity ... 408
11.4.2.2 Potency ... 408
11.4.2.3 Viability ... 408
11.4.2.4 Adventitious Agent Testing ... 408
11.4.2.5 Purity ... 408
11.4.2.6 General Safety Test ... 408
11.4.2.7 Frozen Cell Banks ... 409
11.4.3 Additional Applications: Addition of Radioisotopes or Toxins to Cell Preparations ... 409
11.4.4 Production, Characterization, and Release Testing of Vectors for Gene Therapy ... 409
11.4.4.1 Vector Construction and Characterization ... 409
11.4.4.2 Vector Production System ... 409
11.4.4.3 Master Viral Banks ... 409
11.4.4.4 Lot-to-Lot Release Testing and Specifications for Vectors ... 410
11.4.4.5 Adventitious Agents ... 410
11.4.5 Issues Related to Particular Classes of Vectors for Gene Therapy ... 411
11.4.5.1 Additional Considerations for the Use of Plasmid Vector Products ... 411
11.4.5.2 Additional Considerations for the Use of Retroviral Vector Products ... 411
11.4.5.3 Additional Considerations for the Use of Adenoviral Vectors ... 412
11.4.6 Modifications in Vector Preparations ... 413
11.4.7 Preclinical Evaluation of Cellular and Gene Therapies ... 414
11.4.7.1 General Principles ... 414
11.4.7.2 Animal Species Selection and Use of Alternative Animal Models ... 415
11.4.7.3 Somatic Cell and Gene-Modified Cellular Therapies ... 415
11.4.7.4 Direct Administration of Vectors In Vivo ... 415
11.4.7.5 Expression of Gene Product and Induction of Immune Responses ... 416
11.4.7.6 Vector Localization to Reproductive Organs ... 416
11.5 Conclusion ... 417
Additional Reading ... 417

12 Nucleic Acid Vaccines ... 421
12.1 Background ... 421
12.2 mRNA Vaccine ... 421
12.2.1 Development Cycle ... 427
12.2.2 Formulation and Delivery ... 429
12.2.3 COVID-19 Vaccine ... 432
12.3 DNA Vaccine ... 433
12.3.1 Delivery ... 435
12.3.2 Antibody Response ... 436
Additional Reading ... 437

13 Botanical Products ... 439
13.1 Overview ... 439
13.2 Complimentary Medicines ... 439
13.2.1 History ... 440
13.2.2 Development Innovations ... 441
13.2.3 Technologies ... 442

13.2.4 Genomics and Biomarkers 442
13.2.5 Proteomics 444
13.2.6 Target Identification of Label-Free Botanical Products 445
13.2.7 Metabolomics and Metabonomics 445
13.3 Regulatory Plan 446
13.3.1 Background 446
13.3.2 Chemistry 448
13.3.3 Specifications 452
13.3.4 Standardization 453
13.3.5 Efficacy and Safety 454
13.3.6 Prior Human Use 454
13.3.7 CMC 455
13.3.7.1 Starting Material 456
13.3.7.2 Control of Botanical Substances and Preparations 457
13.3.7.3 Control of Vitamins and Minerals (If Applicable) 457
13.3.7.4 Control of Excipients 457
13.3.7.5 Stability Testing 458
13.3.7.6 Testing Criteria 458
13.3.7.7 Botanical Substances 458
13.3.7.8 Botanical Product 461
13.4 Conclusion 462
Additional Reading 462

14 Regulatory Optimization 469
14.1 Background 469
14.2 Scope 470
14.2.1 Assumptions 470
14.2.2 Definitions 471
14.3 New Chemical Entities 472
14.3.1 Decision Stage #1—Target Identification 472
14.3.2 Decision Stage #2—Target Validation 472
14.3.3 Decision Stage #3—Identification of Actives 474
14.3.4 Decision Stage #4—Confirmation of Hits 474
14.3.5 Decision Stage #5—Identification of Chemical Lead 476
14.3.6 Decision Stage #6—Selection of Optimized Chemical Lead 479
14.3.7 Decision Stage #7—Selection of a Development Candidate 479
14.3.8 Decision Stage #8—Pre-IND Meeting with the FDA 482
14.3.9 Decision Stage #9—Preparation and Submission of an IND Application 482
14.3.10 Decision Stage #10—Human Proof of Concept 483
14.3.11 Decision Stage #11—Clinical Proof of Concept 483
14.4 Repurposing of Marketed Drugs 485
14.4.1 Decision Stage #1: Identification of Actives 485
14.4.2 Decision Stage #2: Confirmation of Hits 485
14.4.3 Decision Stage #3: Gap Analysis/Development Plan 485
14.4.4 Decision Stage #4: Clinical Formulation Development 490
14.4.5 Decision Stage #5: Preclinical Safety Data Package 490
14.4.6 Decision Stage #6: Clinical Supplies Manufacture 490
14.4.7 Decision Stage #7: IND Preparation and Submission 495
14.4.8 Decision Stage #8: Human Proof of Concept 495
14.5 Drug Delivery Platform Technology 495
14.5.1 Decision Stage #1: Clinical Formulation Development 495
14.5.2 Decision Stage #2: Development Plan 499
14.5.3 Decision Stage #3: Clinical Supplies Manufacture 499

14.5.4 Decision Stage #4: Preclinical Safety Package 499
14.5.5 Decision Stage #5: IND Preparation and Submission 500
14.5.6 Decision Stage #6: Human Proof of Concept 500
14.5.7 Decision Stage #7: Clinical Proof of Concept 503
14.6 Biological Products 503
14.6.1 Batch 506
14.6.2 Upstream 507
14.6.3 Downstream 508
14.6.4 Facility 509
14.6.5 Equipment 510
14.6.6 Validation 510
14.6.7 Testing 511
14.6.8 Quality 512
14.6.9 Fill 513
14.6.10 Water 513
14.6.11 Facility Design 513
14.6.12 Cleaning 515
14.6.13 Filling and Finishing 516
14.7 Testing 517
14.8 Documentation Process 522
14.8.1 Process Analytical Technology (PAT) 523
14.8.2 Automation 524
14.9 Predictions 525
14.10 Conclusion 526
Additional Reading 526

15 Intellectual Property 531
15.1 Background 531
15.2 About Patents 531
15.3 Patent Landscape 532
15.4 Patent Laws 532
15.4.1 Pharmaceutical Patenting Practices 537
15.5 Types of Patents 538
15.5.1 Utility Model in the EU 538
15.5.2 Provisional Application 539
15.6 Nonobviousness 540
15.7 Patent Management 543
15.7.1 Broad Coverage 543
15.7.2 Submarine Patents 543
15.7.3 System Expression Patents 544
15.7.4 Process Patents of Originator 544
15.7.5 Third-Party Process Patents 544
15.7.6 Formulation Composition 544
15.7.7 Lifecycle Formulation Projections 544
15.7.8 Alternate Offering 544
15.7.9 Delivery Devices 545
15.7.10 Unpatentable Inventions 545
15.7.11 Software Patents 546
15.7.12 Medical Method Patents 546
15.8 Patent Classification 546
15.8.1 Class 435 546
15.8.2 Class 424 547
15.8.3 Class 801 549

15.9 Biological Patents 550
15.9.1 Biological Products 551
15.9.2 Monoclonal Antibody Technology 552
15.9.3 Antisense Technology 552
15.9.4 Transgenic Plants 553
15.10 Freedom to Operate 553
15.11 Conclusion 555
Additional Reading 555

Index 557

Preface

If you can think of it, then it is a nonlinear thought.

—Sarfaraz K. Niazi

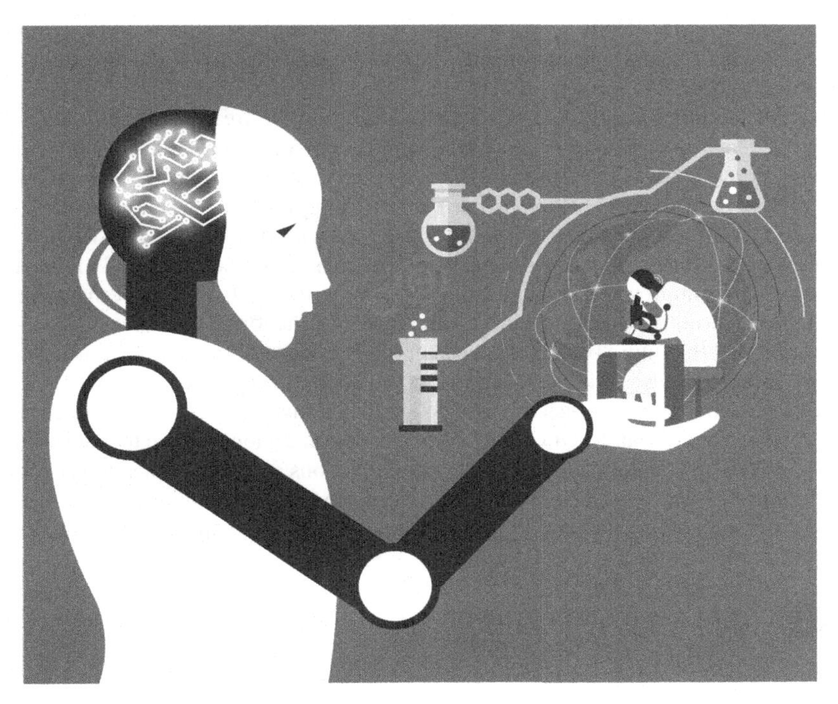

(www.scientificamerican.com/custom-media/usp-science-of-quality/as-medicine-evolves-so-too-must-those-who-assure-its-quality/)

The Future of Pharmaceuticals: A Nonlinear Analysis is a book on the history, philosophy, science, technology, and art of predicting the future. The pharmaceuticals in the near and far future will be various. Still, today, we may not expect what they would be like as derived from the nonlinear analysis that teaches us that it is impossible to focus on anything beyond 25–50 years. However, with the fast-changing pace, it may well be a decade now.

This book analyzes how far we can push our understanding of the "nonlinear," a term poorly understood and wastefully used in the literature. If you can predict it accurately, then it is not nonlinear—the very definition defies the solution. This failure comes from our abilities built upon our prior experience and belief in how the universe operates. An excellent example of this failure in projections is our evolution.

The history of human development is an excellent example of a nonlinear event that could not possibly have been envisioned by anyone living a million years ago. Scientists estimate that humans and Neanderthals (*Homo neanderthalensis*) shared a common ancestor that lived 800,000 years ago in Africa. Our lineage split from that of Neanderthals and Denisovans about 600,000 years ago.

Denisovans, who split off from Neanderthals 400,000 years ago and lived for thousands of generations in Asia. Neanderthals lived throughout Europe and parts of Asia from about 400,000 until about 40,000 years ago, but why Neanderthals went extinct abound continues to puzzle scientists who study human evolution.

So far, the earliest finds of modern *Homo sapiens* skeletons come from Africa. They date to nearly 200,000 years ago on that continent. They appear in Southwest Asia around 100,000 years ago and elsewhere in the Old World by 40,000–60,000years ago. Humans began to exhibit behavioral modernity evidence at least by about 75,000–150,000 years ago and possibly earlier. Though most human existence has been sustained by hunting and gathering in band societies, many human societies transitioned to sedentary agriculture approximately 10,000 years ago, domesticating plants and animals, thus enabling civilization's growth after the Ice Age ended. The rapid advancement of scientific and medical understanding in the 19th and 20th centuries permitted more efficient medical tools and healthier lifestyles, resulting in increased lifespans and causing the human population to rise exponentially. The global human population is about 7.8 billion in 2021.

The future pharmaceuticals, the topic of this book, can only be treated correctly if we first define the prospective patients, the diseases of the future, and the science and technology of drug discovery. The world population is expected to flatten by the end of the 21st century due to continuously dropping growth rates; we will have about 11 billion people take care of by the end of the 21st century (Figure P.1). The life expectancy will reach about 100 years (Figure P.2), with the average age skewing towards the right. The causes of death (Figure P.3) will change due to changes in the quality of life measures, environmental changes, and improved healthcare. However, we will be safe to project that while infectious diseases will reduce, cardiovascular and cancer will remain on the top of the list.

Our ability to predict the future based on the past has never worked. Despite the innate wisdom, there has never been a successful description of the future, notwithstanding random poesy like the Nostradamus predictions, a spontaneous and nonsensical construction that seems to fit many happenings because these predictions can be twisted infinitely. Our claim that we have come a long way in technological advances, so we should be able to make qualified and intelligent projections and predictions, falls back on the very basis of the confidence—the past. However, it does not mean that we cannot safely predict and project the near future, notwithstanding the paradigm shifts—the like of what happened once COVID-19 took a

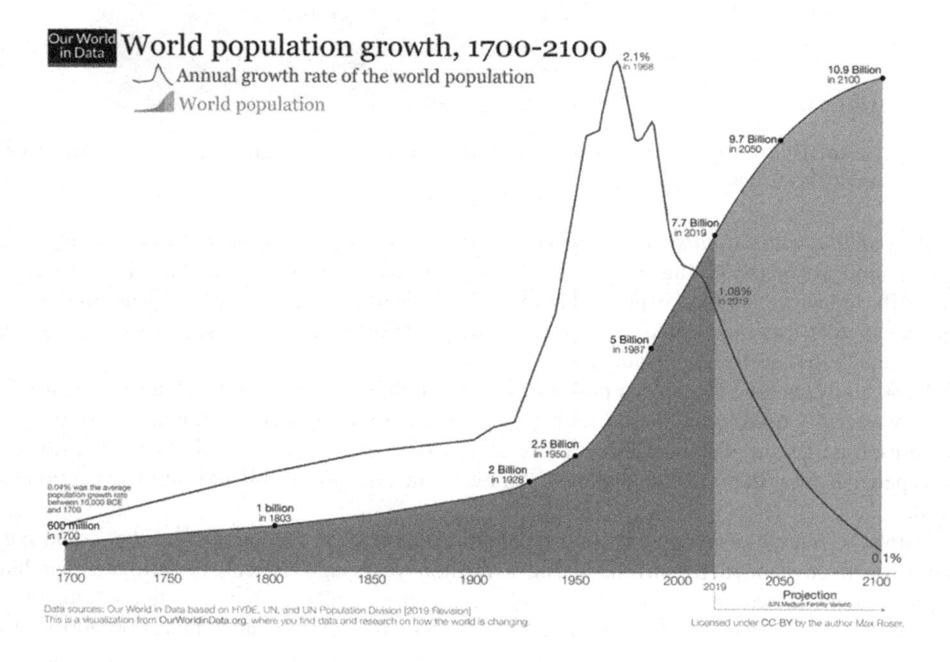

FIGURE P.1 World population growth projections.

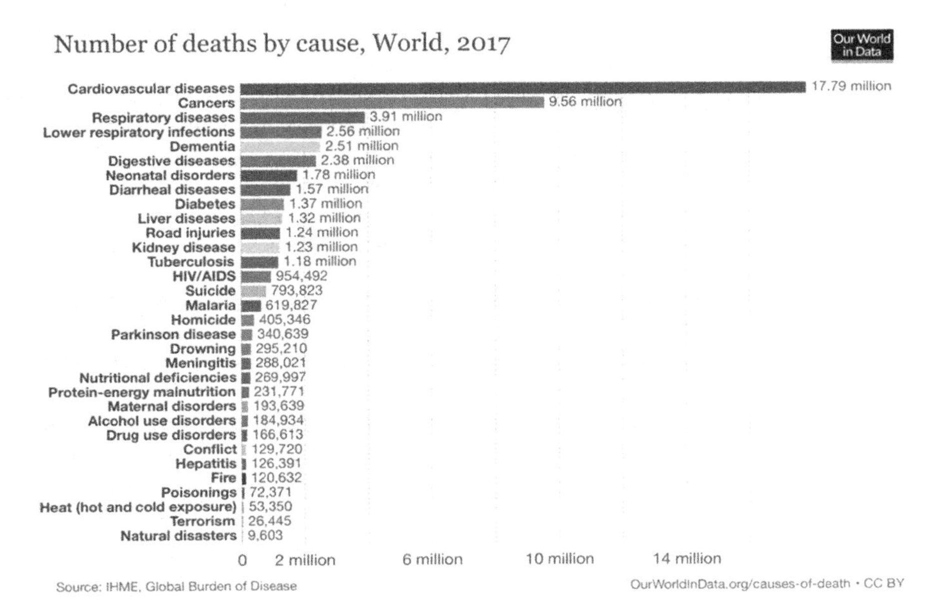

FIGURE P.2 Life expectancy.

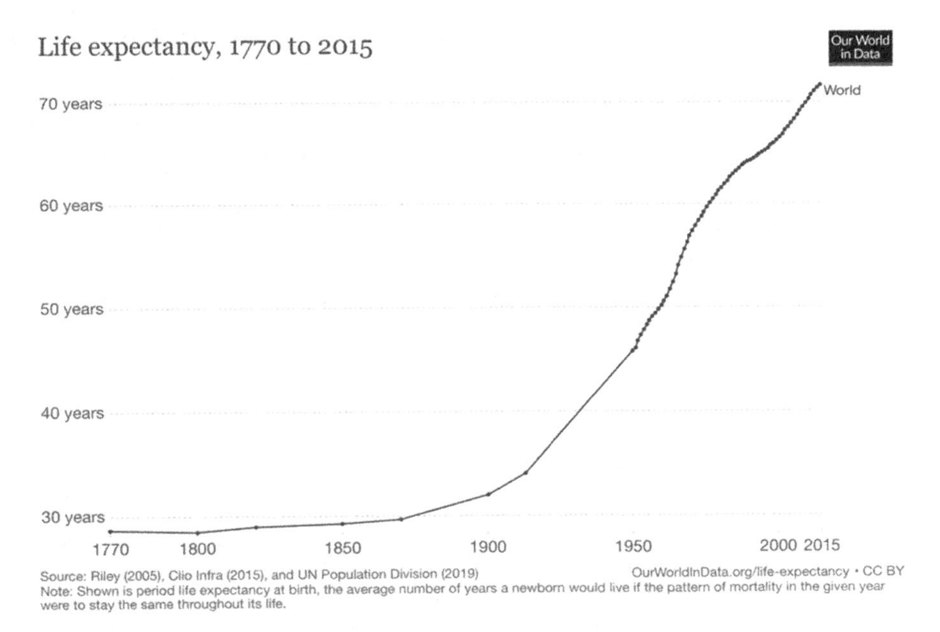

FIGURE P.3 Causes of deaths in 2017.

foothold. We were able to develop and distribute an mRNA vaccine within months that would have taken years, perhaps decades otherwise—Kuhn's paradigm shift came to the rescue.

The theme of this book is to look into the future with enhanced optimism, look into what is considered impossible today that can be made plausible and what we have accepted to be the hard facts, to soften them. Another focus of this book is to enable developers to hasten the timeline to market with reduced cost. Entering into finding solutions to diseases like autoimmune disorders, resistant microbes, genetic manipulations, and catching up with the inevitable shift to biological drugs is widely discussed in this book.

Before proceeding further, I would like to bring another clarification to my readers.

According to the FDA, a drug is defined as "A substance recognized by an official pharmacopeia or formulary. A substance intended for use in the diagnosis, cure, mitigation, treatment, or prevention of disease. A substance (other than food) intended to affect the structure or any function of the body" (https://www.fda.gov/industry/regulated-products/human-drugs#drug). According to the EMA, a medicine product is defined as "a substance or combination of substances that is intended to treat, prevent or diagnose a disease, or to restore, correct or modify physiological functions by exerting a pharmacological, immunological or metabolic action" (https://www.ema.europa.eu/en/glossary/medicinal-product). In pharmacology, a drug is a chemical substance, typically of known structure, which produces a biological effect when administered to a living organism.

When used as nouns, medicine means a substance that promotes explicitly healing when ingested or consumed in some way, whereas pharmaceutical means a pharmaceutical or pharmacological preparation or product. Medicine is also a verb with the meaning: to treat with medicine. Pharmaceutical is also adjective with the definition: of, or relating to pharmacy or pharmacists.

A pharmaceutical drug, also called a medication or medicine, is a chemical substance used to treat, cure, prevent, or diagnose a disease or promote wellbeing. Often "drug" also means chemicals that are addictive. In this book, I have chosen "future of pharmaceuticals" instead of "future of drugs or medicines" purposefully to refer to chemical substances with a desirable pharmacological response that is *purposefully developed and manufactured.* However, the term "drug discovery" is more frequently used in place of "medicine or pharmaceutical discovery." So, in describing the history, the medicines were serendipitously discovered and pharmaceutically manufactured.

The nonlinear analysis is the heart of this work—what we can expect to see in the future that is not visible to us with clarity today. Let me share examples of what has been nonlinear in the past—Nicolaus Copernicus telling that earth goes round the sun, not otherwise; Einstein explaining relativity; and Stephen Hawking suggesting that there doesn't have to be a beginning. But when it comes to pharmaceuticals' future, the serendipitous discovery of DNA in 1869 by Swiss researcher Friedrich Miescher will create the nonlinear path. I am predicting that we will eventually turn back to our genome being the solution to all ailments; we will be able to fix its mutational defects, repair damages that cause aging, and provide protection for all diseases caused by external or internal elements. For this reason, this book is heavily focused on biological products; for this reason, I am including details of the technology and science of developing biological drugs, genomic, and otherwise.

Below is an overview of the chapters and how they are sewn together to form a reliable string.

Summary of Chapters

Chapter 1: Understanding Nonlinearity

Nonlinear projections or paradigm shifts have altered humanity's course over thousands of years, from the wheel's discovery to mRNA vaccines. A paradigm shift comes only when there is a crisis, and the current technology cannot address it. The human mind is programmed towards linear thinking, so if one can claim a future prediction, we can be sure that it is nonlinear thinking. This chapter is about the philosophy, mathematics, and statistics of thinking now. We can force paradigm shifts at will, if not predict the outcome of the model. Medicines have come a long way, from anecdotal findings by the foragers to high throughput screening and antigen libraries to produce new drugs. These discoveries have saved billions of lives over time. In the 21st century, we are about to bring significant healthcare changes based on our linear thinking and nonlinear approaches. This chapter prepares you to understand the most speculative yet most likely outcome of research in the field of new medicines.

Chapter 2: The Evolution of Pharmaceuticals

To see the future, we must always look in our rearview mirror. This may not provide us with strong nonlinear leads, but it certainly provides us a back view of how serendipity has always played out in drug discovery. Modern science expedites the development of new drugs, but the subtle element of serendipity always surprises us. How humanity began drug discovery is a story that we need to remember to enable us to do better in the future. From the pre-history to the modern era and now entering the age of genes, there are many teachings that we need to learn. In this chapter, we review the history of the development of medicines and related discoveries that changed the life and saved the life. I will examine regulatory authorities' role and intellectual property laws that control new drugs' entry into the market. The best way to identify a trend is to examine its history, as we present all new drugs approved over the past decade. This chapter makes a good segue into modalities of new drug discoveries, particularly those that will qualify as nonlinear discoveries.

Chapter 3: Artificial Intelligence

This chapter is a primer on AI for scientists who are not routinely involved in digital technology. The theme of this book is to apply technology to view a nonlinear perspective. A quip in Tesler's theorem says, "Intelligence is whatever machines haven't done yet" (http://www.nomodes.com/Larry_Tesler_Consulting/Adages_and_Coinages.html). Much of the AI becomes a norm and is removed from the definition of AI, leaving researchers to seek higher targets in AI applications. If we are to create medicines with unpredictable benefits, we will need to rely on AI as the promising solution to this paradigm. The AI field draws upon computer science, information engineering, mathematics, psychology, linguistics, philosophy, and many other fields.

Chapter 4: Drug Discovery Trends

From anecdotal trial and error discovery of new drugs over thousands of years to today's age of artificial intelligence and genomics, new drugs are still discovered by the trial and error models, except we now have a much better success rate. With the analytical technology and understanding of molecular biology expanding, we can design new molecules, find mechanisms of action and identify drug–target combinations. The central theme is to point to the future direction of drug discovery, and that can come only from first understanding and appreciating the trends evolving in discovering new drugs. This chapter provides an overview of emerging technologies and established technologies that are now merging with the latest drug discovery approaches, from high throughput screening to mRNA vaccines.

Chapter 5: Drug Development Assays

An assay is an analytical measurement procedure defined by a set of reagents that produces a detectable signal, allowing a quantification process. In general, the quality of an assay is defined by the robustness and reproducibility of this signal in the absence of any test compounds or the presence of inactive compounds. Assay quality depends on the type of signal measured (absorbance, fluorescence, luminescence, radioactivity, etc.), reagents, reaction conditions, analytical and automation instrumentation, and statistical models for the data analysis. Subsequently, the quality of a high-throughput screen is defined by the behavior of a given assay utilized to screen a collection of compounds. In practice, assays developed for HTS (high throughput screening) and SAR (structure–activity relationship) measurements are roughly characterized as cell-free (biochemical) or cell-based procedures. The choice of either a biochemical or cell-based assay along with the particular assay format is ultimately a balancing act. There is a need to ensure that the measured signal can provide data that is biologically relevant. On the other side is the requirement for an assay to yield robust data in microtiter plate formats where typically 105 to 106 samples are screened during an HTS operation. Future discoveries will depend heavily on the emergence of new assay techniques, making this science highly relevant to drug discovery.

Chapter 6: Nanomedicine

The size of a particle, solid or liquid, brings many opportunities for new drug delivery systems, new therapies, new combinations of diagnostic and treatment, and most important, the ability to expose the body, particularly to toxic drugs selectively. The past two decades' developments have created many scientific breakthroughs, including the most recent delivery of lipid nanoparticles containing mRNA vaccines. The regulatory agencies and research support in developing nanomedicine are now opening wide to understand better the assessment of safety and efficacy of these new classes of drugs. This chapter lists nanotechnology under nanomedicine since the concept of pharmaceuticals is limited to manufactured drugs, while nanotechnology is widely used in diagnostics.

Chapter 7: Antimicrobials

Microbes that are pathogenic hold a symbiosis with humans and constitute the seventh most prominent cause of human suffering and death worldwide. Until recently, drugs that appear effective against microbes, antibiotics, were discovered serendipitously. While the discovery has taken a sharp turn in making it more targeted, anecdotal antimicrobials remain a potent category. Since microbes frequently become resistant to drugs, there is a growing need to develop antimicrobials to control infections. This chapter a detailed view of both therapeutic and preventive approaches to managing infections and points to the current era of genomics that is now applied heavily in developing antimicrobials. The newer mRNA vaccines now present a novel opportunity to prevent infections and many autoimmune disorders.

Chapter 8: Therapeutic Proteins

Compared to chemical drugs, biological drugs are derived from biological sources and engines, such as fermentation or recombinantly engineered microbes. In this chapter, we present the class of therapeutic proteins that are produced by biological sources. Unlike chemical drugs, biological drugs have a larger and variable structure making it not feasible to synthesize them chemically and replicate their variability. The primary drug of interest is the antibodies, hormones, and other cytokines produced by humans that often need replacement when the body fails to make them. Driven by genetic engineering sciences, therapeutic proteins now present the fastest-growing category of new drugs. Engaging with therapeutic proteins requires a detailed understanding of protein structure, how it changes between replicate manufacturing, and the modulation of their immunogenicity.

Chapter 9: Manufacturing Trends

The manufacturing of therapeutic proteins and preventive therapy products is complex due to multiple steps that must integrate well within meeting cGMP compliance requirements. This chapter provides an overview of the manufacturing system's evolution for manufacturing therapeutic proteins and advises developers on how to streamline their systems for future changes to reduce their COGS, CAPEX, and OPEX, and, most importantly, how these changes can make the regulatory approval process faster.

Chapter 10: Therapeutic Protein Delivery Systems

Delivery of biological medicinal products is a complex exercise due to their chemical structural instability, rapid physical degradation, and complex chemical interactions with excipients; besides being inherently immunogenic, their degradation can enhance immunogenicity and raise other safety issues. This chapter introduces the structural elements of therapeutic proteins that lead to chemical interactions and degradation and suggests methods to stabilize the formulated products; commercial formulations are also presented. While the current methodology for the delivery of therapeutic proteins remains parenteral, a large number of delivery forms are emerging, including oral, nasal, transdermal, pulmonary, ocular products in polymer-based, hydrogels, lipid-based emulsions, liposomes, and nanoparticle systems, which are also discussed with their future perspective.

Chapter 11: Gene and Cell Therapy

Gene therapy involves the transfer of genetic material, usually in a carrier or vector, and the gene's uptake into the appropriate cells of the body. Cell therapy involves the transfer of cells with the relevant function into the patient. Some protocols utilize both gene therapy and cell therapy. Gene and cell therapy constitute the most recent advances in the field of biological medicinal products. An overview of the diseases and risks in the use of treatment modalities, including development and ethical issues, are introduced in this chapter. Details of approved products are also provided. Gene therapy and cell therapy, including the DNA and mRNA vaccines and CAR-T techniques, are discussed in detail. Gene editing technologies, with their methodologies and their relative advantages, are also discussed. Upstream and downstream technologies for gene and cell therapy products and other allogenic products are described, including understanding regulatory controls, characterization of the cell population, release testing, and radioisotope tagging. Issues related to vectors and vector preparation are provided. Preclinical evaluation methods and challenges in the commercialization of gene and cell therapy products are pointed out.

Chapter 12: Nucleic Acid Vaccines

Traditional vaccines take years and often decades to develop; an extension of gene therapy is the use of nucleic acid vaccines, the mRNA and DNA vaccines that force the body cells to produce a targeted antigen, rather than putting the antigen in the body, as practiced in the use of traditional vaccines. Besides the development speed, nucleic acid vaccines have a much better safety profile, particularly the mRNA vaccine. Over the last decade, the fast development made it possible to manufacture and formulate an experimental mRNA vaccine because of its pressure during the COVID-19 pandemic. For the first time, the FDA and EMA have approved these vaccines to open up a broad road to discoveries. A unique application of nucleic acid vaccines involves preventing or treating autoimmune disorders that will speed up developing preventive measures for diseases like type 1 diabetes, Alzheimer's and Parkinson's diseases, etc. The use of DNA vaccines in cancer treatment is also growing fast. However, as of date, no DNA vaccine has been approved. This chapter describes the technology for these vaccines and how the regulatory guidance is evolving to develop these therapeutic possibilities.

Chapter 13: Botanical Products

Botanical products have the most prolonged use by humankind, and the discoveries from botanical sources continue to provide novel solutions to treating diseases. The emergency of chemical drugs that allowed a more focused understanding of the mechanism of action, toxicity, and clinical efficacy had put the botanical medicines backstage. Still, now that the FDA and EMA have recognized these products' value by providing appropriate regulatory guidelines to develop these products, there will be many new opportunities to find solutions to diseases. There are no current therapies available for an autoimmune disorder. A better understanding of metabolomics and metabonomics, genomics, and biomarkers allows faster development of botanical products.

Chapter 14: Regulatory Optimization

This chapter guides adopting novel approaches for the faster development of products in the regulatory pathways. It contains guidelines to develop therapeutic hypotheses, target and pathway validation, proof of concept criteria, and generalized cost analyses at various early drug discovery stages. Different decision stages in creating a new chemical entity (NCE), description of the exploratory investigational new drug (IND) and orphan drug designation, drug repurposing, and drug delivery technologies are also described and geared toward those who intend to develop new drug discovery and development programs. The data are derived from the NIH public domain report.

Chapter 15: Intellectual Property

Intellectual property, more specifically, the patents, form the core of drug discovery that enables companies to invest billions of dollars invested. Scientists must work closely with the legal teams to ensure that the discovery process includes elements and steps that can be challenged for infringement and create a new intellectual property as the development process proceeds. The laws behind patenting are complex and subject to litigation and challenges. This chapter introduces the basic concept of patenting process, the types of patents, and how the patents can expedite drug discovery and protect the inventors' long-term income.

Glossary

An accumulation of topics that define this book's scope, a reminder, and a direction of the future is provided in alphabetical order to help hone the skills of developing the future of pharmaceuticals.

Acknowledgments

I am thankful to many of my scientific and professional colleagues, particularly those whom I came to know through the landmark literature in the field but never met. I may have quoted their work thinking that this is in the public domain, erroneously; I hope they would excuse me for taking this liberty. An elaborate bibliography does not necessarily replace this obligation that I have to acknowledge their work correctly.

Finally, I would like to admit my mistakes, and I couldn't find a better statement than that which appeared in the first edition of *Encyclopedia Britannica* (1786):

> With regard to errors, in general, whether falling under the denomination of mental, typographical, or accidental, we are conscious of being able to point out a greater number than any critic whatever. Men who are acquainted with the innumerable difficulties attending the execution of a work of such an extensive nature will make proper allowances. To these, we appeal and shall rest satisfied with the judgment they pronounce.

I will appreciate receiving your comments to improve this treatise in the future, and most kindly, if you find mistakes.

Sarfaraz K. Niazi
Deerfield, IL

Author

Sarfaraz K. Niazi, Ph.D., is an Adjunct Professor at the University of Illinois and University of Houston; he has authored 60+ major books, 100+ research papers, and 100+ patents, mainly in the field of bioprocessing, drug discovery, mRNA vaccines, drug formulations, thermodynamic systems, alcohol aging, nutraceuticals and treatment of autoimmune diseases. He has established multiple biotechnology projects, from concept to market. He also serves as an advisor to major pharmaceutical and biopharmaceutical companies, regulatory agencies, the FDA, the US Congress, and several heads of state. He is also a patent law practitioner.

List of Important Terminology

21st-Century Cures implementation guidance

The FDA intends to issue new draft guidance with draft interpretations of several of the medical software provisions in the 21st-Century Cures Act, explaining their effect on pre-existing FDA policy, including policy on mobile medical applications; medical device data systems, used for the electronic transfer, storage, display, or conversion of medical device data; medical image storage devices, used to store or retrieve medical images electronically; medical image communications devices, used to transfer medical image data electronically between medical devices; low-risk general wellness products; and laboratory workflow.

3D printing

3D-printed teeth and prosthetics are already commonly used in the health industry to assist patients. However, there is a distinct lack of approved 3D-printed pharmaceutical products in the US marketplace. Medicines can be produced through 3D printing. This has interesting benefits, including unique tailoring to a specific patient's needs. In 2015, the US Food and Drug Administration (FDA) approved the first medicine that had been produced by 3D printing. The precision of the machine allowed manufacturers to create a pill with a high drug load. In one dose, patients were able to receive 1,000 mg of levetiracetam. This was a revolutionary treatment for sufferers of epileptic seizures. However, since then, there has been limited progress due to the high cost of this method. The need for precision medicine is also making pharmaceutical companies rethink the manufacturing process. A lot of research is underway for making advanced 3D printers that print tissues or cells. 3D printing of human tissues has great applications in drug development, organ engineering, and regenerative medicine. This allows the development of age or physiology-dependent medical formulations, as well as precision pills. Bioprinters also help in pushing innovation in bio-inks, tissue engineering, and microfluidics. 3D printing can create patient-specific medical devices such as implants, surgical guides, or anatomic models. Similarly, 3D-printed solid drug products can be made in various shapes, strengths, and distributions of active and inactive ingredients. Tissue-engineered 3D-printed constructs are also being researched to advance regenerative medicine. This approach provides a unique opportunity to produce medical products tailored to the individual needs of patients. The capabilities and portability of 3D printing processes also enable distributed manufacturing of complex and advanced medical products in remote or austere conditions.

Additive manufacturing

While having a 3D printer in your local pharmacy is a futuristic concept, the idea of additive pharmaceutical manufacturing is driving the industry towards a future where everyone's ailments can be individually tackled. The FDA's Additive Manufacturing of Medical Products (AMMP) core research facility is a multi-center collaboration. It augments center-specific resources and houses high-end, industry-grade 3D printing equipment, software, and expertise that can be used across the agency to perform cutting-edge regulatory research with this advanced technology. The AMMP Lab will establish a scientific foundation to assist the agency with its assessment of advanced manufacturing and provide the critical infrastructure the FDA will need to meet the future's regulatory demands. The FDA's in-house 3D printing facilities enable the FDA scientists to develop standards and metrics for the use of 3D printing for medical products; conduct research to determine how the 3D printing of drugs impacts active and inactive drug components, and identify critical quality processes and controls that affect the safety and performance of drugs and devices. The development of a compact factory that uses continuous manufacturing technology to produce drugs on demand is the future. The real-time release uses to process or other manufacturing data to ensure the quality of a product rather than, for example, testing the end product. An integrated continuous manufacturing solution that takes raw material creates the desired API, purifies the API, and produces the final dosage form in a single system that can operate fully automatically 24 hours each day, seven days per week. Part of the system is a solvent-recovery station that purifies, separates, and reuses solvents used in the production process in a closed-loop indoor system. No intermediate or API is isolated from the integrated system, but various spectroscopic techniques are located at strategic points to monitor the process to ensure product quality. A technology platform in which different modules or unit operations can be interchanged and combined; that is, the system is not designed to produce only one specific product but can manufacture various products.

Adjuvant

An additive to vaccines that modulates and/or boosts the immune response's potency, often allowing lower doses of antigen to be used effectively. Adjuvants may be based on pathogen-associated molecular patterns (PAMPs) or on other molecules that activate innate immune sensors.

Advanced manufacturing

Advanced manufacturing is a collective term for new medical product manufacturing technologies that can improve drug quality, address shortages of medicines, and speed up time to market. Every field has a different set of production techniques that are considered advanced. They often integrate novel technological approaches, Use established techniques in a new or innovative way, or apply production methods in a new domain where there are no defined best practices or experience. Innovations in manufacturing technology will help rapidly scale manufacturing capabilities for vaccines and other medical countermeasures (MCMs) to respond faster to emerging threats and other public health emergencies, such as pandemic influenza; shorten supply chains and increase manufacturing resilience to disruption by emerging threats or public health emergencies, such as natural disasters, by creating a distributed network of small manufacturing sites that can provide reserve capacity for centralized manufacturing facilities; accelerate therapy development for orphan diseases by improving the cost-efficiency of small-scale manufacturing processes; speed availability of emerging therapies by enabling manufacturing process and standards development, including for cell and gene-therapies, supporting goals of the 21st-Century Cures Act (Cures Act); provide new tools to address drug shortages and other challenges, including pharmaceutical quality; and collaborate to help facilitate next-generation influenza vaccines.

All-in-one

Space is a precious commodity. Many pharmaceutical machinery manufacturers have designed equipment to perform multiple functions or combine various machines with area conservation in mind. As an example, an in-line drying system removed the need for tumble dryers and drying tunnels. It is one machine that can effectively perform the same job as two.

Analytics

Analytical technologies for characterizing and monitoring therapeutic proteins, primarily monoclonal antibodies (mAbs), have evolved from low to high resolution that can provide foundational knowledge on critical quality attributes (CQAs) that can be monitored to ensure the safety and efficacy of biopharmaceuticals. Many technologies are available. The goal is to replace some of the older technologies with newer ones to increase product knowledge, decrease cost, and increase drug development speed. First, there is a multi-attribute-method consortium in which mass spectrometry is used to evaluate industry-wide new peak (peptide) detection performance metrics providing a sensitive impurity test and false positives false negatives that can be mitigated with proper controls. Second, an interlaboratory comparison in which protein structural dynamics are measured by hydrogen-deuterium exchange mass spectrometry (HDX-MS). Various technologies can be used to evaluate conformational ensembles. Protein therapeutics do not have a static structure, and that understanding their dynamic structure might shed light on how it influences, for example, stability, interactions, or dangerous immune responses.

Artificial intelligence and machine learning

Artificial intelligence (AI) is a branch of computer science that involves machines having the ability to perform tasks and demonstrate behaviors commonly associated with human beings. This subject is covered at length in Chapter 3. In general manufacturing, it can collate data and calculate the most efficient processes to create products and optimize the entire process. Companies are exploring the use of these technologies to introduce automation and optimization of the manufacturing processes and design effective marketing and post-launch strategies.

Automation

Automation is becoming a norm for most industries, but the regulatory constraints make such modifications of adoption cumbersome and expensive. Automation has played a large part in manufacturing for almost a century. For example, in-vehicle manufacturing, automation is used to reduce costs and better perform intricate tasks. Now, pharma businesses are looking to do just the same. Previously, scientists have become curbed by the manual task of individual genome testing. However, automation allows manufacturers to access a vast amount of data, enabling them to create unique molecular profiles of their customers and provide them with personalized care.

Bayes' theorem

One of the key ideas in Bayesian statistics is that knowledge about anything unknown can be expressed probabilistically. Bayes' theorem is a way of finding a probability when we know certain other probabilities. Briefly, the ratio of the two independent probabilities multiplied by one conditional outcome probability to get the probability of another outcome; the two outcomes' ratio is the same as the independent probabilities. We cannot apply Bayes' theorem to COVID-19 because the prior probability is not established, and it keeps changing depending on your surroundings.

Big data and analytics

The advancement in analytical techniques is turning historical and real-time data available with pharmaceutical companies into valuable assets for predictive, diagnostic, prescriptive, and descriptive analytics.

Biocatalyst

Biocatalysis offers the possibility of using multiple enzymes to synthesize an API from starting materials in a single vessel, but this "cascade" biocatalysis entails several technical challenges, such as complexity of the reaction network, characterization of evolved enzymes, and process control, characterization, and robustness of the cascades. Complex molecules, such as oligonucleotides and peptides, involve new regulatory challenges, including various issues associated with impurities and the use of analytical methods different from those used to characterize traditional small molecules. Co-processed APIs and the question, from a regulatory standpoint, of whether to treat them as drug substances or as drug-product intermediates remains to be resolved. (A co-processed API is a drug substance that contains the API and at least one noncovalently bonded nonactive component that changes the API's physical properties to improve or enable drug product manufacturing.)

Bioinformatics

Bioinformatics is the science of organizing, managing, and analyzing large sets of data. In HTS labs, bioinformatics is critical in properly storing and analyzing all aspects of compound heredity through screening results. Incorporating computer science and biology, bioinformatics allows scientists to store and access large amounts of data. Bioinformatics allows data mining, a computational process of discovering patterns in large data sets. Pharmaceutical companies have implemented programs to allow for rational and systematic screening of drug-like compounds against biological targets. Using data, scientists can determine which biological targets should be studied and what drug-like compounds would most likely affect this target. This process requires efficient technology and an organized data source but will become increasingly important as new screening techniques gather more data.

Biological manufacturing

Changes are expected within five to ten years at various stages, including upstream processing. The focus will be on improving productivity, for example, by using high-volume cell banks, high-density inoculations, and concentrated media and reducing cell perfusion rates and impurities. There will be a direct link between the reactor and the first downstream purification step; the centrifuge will become obsolete. There will be improvements in product capture in downstream processing, for example, by using affinity membranes and better connections and simplifications in product purification so that intermediate storage capacity is not needed. As a result, the facility footprint will shrink. On-demand buffer preparation will likely be integrated into the system; this will eliminate the need for buffer storage, again shrinking the facility footprint. In analytics and control, continuous operations will trigger the development of more CQA-relevant in-process analytics, and real-time release will require better in-process analytics and models. There will be more single-use technology with advanced control features, "plug-and-play" unit operations in modular facilities, benchtop-scale operations for many small-market therapeutics, and closed processing for hygienic operation on a small scale. The need for storage to support operations will mostly disappear. The importance of controlling impurities produced by cells in culture to avoid them later in the process and the importance of matching the increased upstream productivity with improved downstream technology to purify the product. To achieve integrated and continuous protein processing, an ecosystem would emerge in which companies could obtain off-the-shelf systems. Enabling continuous harvest also results in a small downstream flow. A benefit of the continuous process is that it results in healthier cells. The next-generation manufacturing framework will include a "common denominator" for equipment and facility design and a stepwise implementation strategy for companies that want to adopt continuous and integrated processing. The first step is to install an alternating tangential-flow filtration system that enables continuous harvest from the bioreactor. The second step is to install at least two columns for downstream processing.

The columns can be run in parallel or series; running in series changes the operation only slightly but might require a new virus-removal validation. The third step is to have sensors at the column outlets; sensors at the inlets to allow real-time modeling to assure that the system is operating as intended. Mechanistic and machine-learning models will be needed because next-generation manufacturing will generate substantially more data than batch manufacturing, which human operators cannot analyze. The last step is to install in-line conditioning for buffer preparation; this must be implemented for operation on a commercial scale. The bioburden control strategy may include downstream membrane absorbers and countercurrent and high-performance tangential-flow filtration, which could be seen in six years. Continuous manufacturing may not decrease the cost of goods radically but will substantially change capital costs given the much lower costs of building a manufacturing facility. Other benefits of continuous manufacturing are that it allows companies to right-size manufacturing capacity and provides the ability to make a variety of molecules. The importance of having plug-and-play capabilities with automated systems so that the process does not have to be redesigned for every new product. The manufacture of biologics differs from small-molecule manufacture in that the process is valued as intellectual property requiring continued exploration of alternative hosts or methods for producing biologics.

Blockchain

Blockchain technology is very significant for the pharmaceutical industry in every stage of the production and distribution of drugs. The stakeholders in the pharma industry are, in general, extremely secretive about their data due to the sensitive nature of the data. Blockchain technology is also being explored to tackle the use of counterfeit medicines and substandard drugs that enter into the pharmaceutical supply chain and kill thousands of patients every year. The digitalization of transactions makes blockchain a promising solution for tracking and securing the pharma transaction ecosystem.

Capacity building

As innovator pipelines are continuing to diversify with new modalities being added on, manufacturers must increase their existing capacities in addition to their current portfolio. With the focus today shifting to a small patient population and adding products in immunology and oncology, particularly with cell and gene therapy, complex biomolecules, antibody-drug, and conjugates, process efficiency is key to biological medicine production. The output capacity depends on three major factors speed, machine production capacity, and hours of operation. With efficiency in mind, pharmaceutical machinery manufacturers have created faster equipment than ever before, with an even greater hourly production capacity. The COVID-19 pandemic in 2020 has proliferated research into immunology to find both active and passive treatments. Large scale and fast manufacturing as required in producing a vaccine for COVID-19 have forced tested many technologies of the future.

CAR-T therapy

Chimeric antigen receptor T cells (also known as CAR-T cells) are the T cells genetically engineered to produce an artificial T cell receptor for immunotherapy use. Chimeric liposomes (fluid sacs surrounded by a fatty membrane) are more easily absorbed by cells than naked DNA/RNA. Various types of liposomes are used to bind preferentially to specific tissues. A subtype of membrane vesicles formed and endogenously released by cells (extracellular vesicles or "exosomes") has been used to carry small RNA sequences into specific tissues.

Cell therapy

Cell therapy transfers intact, live cells into a patient to help lessen or cure a disease. The cells may originate from the patient (autologous cells) or a donor (allogeneic cells). The cells used in cell therapy can be classified by their potential to transform into different cell types. Pluripotent cells can transform into any cell type in the body, and multipotent cells can transform into other cell types. Still, their repertoire is more limited than that of pluripotent cells. Differentiated or primary cells are of a fixed type. The type of cells administered depends on the treatment.

Continuous manufacturing

CM initiates a cascade of transformational advances in technology. It allows process intensification, enabling the miniaturization of systems with small footprints and reduced energy consumption. Miniaturization makes modularity and, ultimately, portability possible. Focusing on portable, continuous, miniature, and modular technology transforms how to develop, manufacture and distribute drug products. Continuous, direct compression in the manufacture of several solid oral drug products considers process-feed concerns, sensor limitations, content uniformity concerns, and challenges related to blending properties. To convert powders to film-coated tablets in minutes and accelerate approval or registration of some products to reduce or simplify the elements in continuous feeding and mixing operations so that cleaning processes can be accelerated. Computational process modeling, digital design, the transformation of big data into insight, and multi-particulate dosage forms provide flexibility in bringing medicines to diverse patient populations.

Continuous manufacturing

Continuous manufacturing is a version of highly intensified processing with brief downtimes compared to the typical time used for traditional batch production. Process intensification, therefore, becomes a prerequisite to continuous manufacturing technologies that can increase tier, manage high media volumes, buffers, and in general, intensify the process to extract more from the entire production process. The advantages of intensification and continuous processing are mostly concerned with increasing productivity, reduced need to invest in conventional, highly costly manufacturing facilities, mainly because businesses can synergistically use single-use and intensification facilities that lead to reduced facility footprints and costs. Continuous manufacturing is a crucial step in promoting drug quality and enhancing production efficiency, resulting in lower drug prices. Continuous manufacturing provides a quicker, more reliable way to make pharmaceuticals. The FDA is helping bring this method into widespread use. Continuous manufacturing integrates traditional step-wise manufacturing processes into a single system based on modern process monitoring and controls. In a CM process, a product is made over time, so a drug manufacturer can easily control the number of products being made to match demand. These efficient, integrated continuous systems also require smaller footprints to operate.

Controls

In using models, data analytics, and machine learning in process development, including strategies to advance process development: 1) increase understanding and optimization of unit operations to enable process intensification, 2) automate high-throughput technology to accelerate research and development, 3) develop plug-and-play modules that have integrated control and monitoring to facilitate deployment, 4) develop dynamic models for unit operations that enable automated plantwide simulation and control design, and 5) exploit data analytics and machine learning. There are many applications of pharmaceutical manufacturing strategies, such as an automated molecular synthesizer to produce, purify, and characterize a product by using flowsheet models, process intensification, optimized plug-and-play fluidic modules, and feedback control. All strategies depend heavily on models, and model development is not a linear process of making assumptions based on process knowledge and then building a model by using process data. Instead, it is an iterative process in which models are refined until a satisfactory success measure is achieved. Selecting the best data analytics tool is complex and requires substantial expertise. There are many tools, and users typically apply the tools they know, which can have suboptimal results. However, a systematic approach to tool selection allows a user to focus on objectives rather than on methods. There are two approaches to managing data and tool selection. One is to run various models and then select the best one by minimizing observed cross-validation error. Evaluating too many models can be problematic, and that the key is to choose a few that are known to be suitable for the data and the type of application. The second approach is to select the best model based on the problem type and data characteristics, assess the nonlinearity, multicollinearity, and dynamics of the data, and then select the best-based model for the characteristics. There will be advances in methods that combine data analytics and machine learning with first-principles models, increased use of tensorial data streams, and a broadening of the scope of data analytics and machine learning in pharmaceutical applications. The industry will automatically archive data for process modeling and analysis and improve monitoring and control, use plantwide data to optimize operational models, use all available data to ensure that product quality specifications are met, and ultimately use ecosystem data to connect customer needs manufacturing data.

CRISPR

The CRISPR-Cas system is a prokaryotic immune system that protects foreign genetic elements such as those found in plasmids and phages that provide a source of immunity gained. RNA harboring the spacer gene allows us to recognize and split foreign pathogenic DNA by the proteins Cas (CRISPR-associated). Specific Cas proteins that are directed by RNA break international RNA. CRISPR is present in about 50% of sequenced bacterial genomes and almost 90% of sequenced archaea. Cas9 (or CRISPR-associated protein 9) is an enzyme that uses CRISPR sequences as a tool for identifying and cleaving specific DNA strands complementing the CRISPR gene. With CRISPR sequences, Cas9 enzymes form the basis of a technology known as CRISPR-Cas9, which is used to modify genes within humans. This editing process has a wide range of applications from basic biological research, biomedical product development, and disease treatment.

Data harmonization

Data harmonization is the process of standardizing and integrating information from disparate sources to form a unified database. Data harmonization is a crucial step for guaranteeing that the developed machine-learning-based models are widely applicable in different scenarios. Establishing a high-quality data model (which is a prerequisite for organizing and standardizing the data) is the foundation for the harmonization process. In addition to data harmonization, model harmonization, which defines a unified standard for storing the computational models, is also an important aspect to enhance the generalizability and utility of the computational drug repurposing tools. The open neural network exchange (ONNX) is an example of such efforts aiming to build model exchanging standards that are interoperable. ONNX defines implemented models as an extensible acyclic graph model. Each node on the graph is a call to built-in operators with inputs and outputs defined using standard data types.

Deep learning architecture

Deep learning is a subfield of machine learning that refers to the paradigm of exploring the data with layers of linear and non-linear transformations organized hierarchically. The most widely used deep learning model is artificial neural networks. The basic building block is an artificial neuron that non-linearly transforms the weighted sum of input feature variables. A fully connected feedforward neural network (FNN) is an architecture where the artificial neurons are connected layer-by-layer from input features to output targets. A weight is associated with each connection and optimized by minimizing the output targets' prediction loss through backpropagation on training samples. FNNs are typically used for data samples represented as vectors. In the case of images being the input where each pixel is a feature variable, FNNs become infeasible as the number of weights becomes far too large. However, a convolutional neural network (CNN; panel) is particularly suitable for image processing. Instead of fully connecting neurons in adjacent layers, CNN uses filters (small matrices of weights) that apply a convolution operation on local patches of the images, which greatly reduces the weights. CNN has been used to analyze chemical images to obtain insight into therapeutic drug functions. For example, AtomNet predicts small molecules' binding affinity to proteins based on the structural information extracted by CNN.

Dendrimers

Nanoparticles made from natural biodegradable polymers can target specific organs and tissues in the body, carry DNA for gene therapy, and deliver larger molecules such as proteins, peptides, and even genes. The drug molecules are first dissolved and then encapsulated or attached to a polymer nanoparticle matrix to manufacture these polymeric nanoparticles. Three different structures can then be obtained from this process; nanoparticles, nanocapsules (in which the drug is encapsulated and surrounded by the polymer matrix), and nanospheres (in which the drug is dispersed throughout the polymeric matrix in a spherical form).

Digital clinical trials

Clinical trial processes are still weighed down by "clipboard culture," which will change digital tracking. The FDA has established a Digital Center of Excellence and issued several guidelines (www.fda.gov/medical-devices/digital-health-center-excellence/guidances-digital-health-content) that allow clinical outcome assessments to be conducted remotely or via telehealth. Many more aspects of clinical trial design and execution will be streamlined by software, including screening, consent, data capture, and patient engagement.

Digital control

Pharmaceutical machinery suppliers have taken this digital technology and incorporated it into pharmaceutical machinery. As such, soft gel machines are now being equipped with digital control systems. These systems allow manufacturers to stop, start, and control various equipment features on their machines. This is just one way digital technology is revolutionizing the pharmaceutical industry and making manufacturers' lives that much easier. New remote bioreactor sensors can be used to monitor analytes, oxygen, and carbon dioxide in small-scale systems in real-time. The sensors provide better monitoring and better process information, and that they are being evaluated on different scales and in various reactor types. The application of the sensors in the medical field, for example, as transdermal sensors to monitor premature babies, patients in clinical trials, or simply people who take drugs to treat various conditions. The development of new remote bioreactor sensors that can be used to monitor analytes, oxygen, and carbon dioxide in small-scale systems in real-time. The sensors provide better monitoring and better process information, and that they are being evaluated on different scales and in various reactor types. The application of the sensors in the medical field, for example, as transdermal sensors to monitor premature babies, patients in clinical trials, or simply people who take drugs to treat various conditions.

Digital health

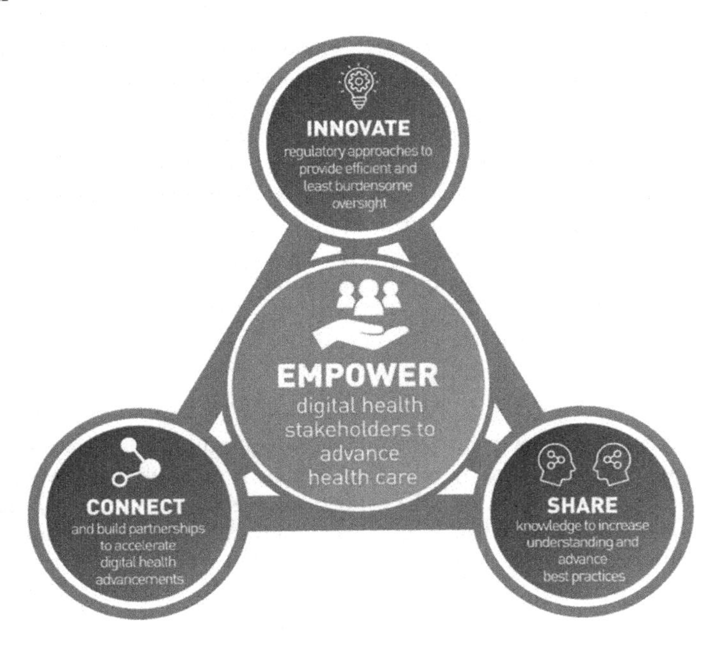

The broad scope of digital health includes mobile health (mHealth), health information technology (IT), wearable devices, telehealth and telemedicine, and personalized medicine. Digital health tools have the vast potential to improve our ability to diagnose and treat disease accurately and enhance healthcare delivery for the individual. Digital health technologies use computing platforms, connectivity, software, and sensors for health care and related uses. These technologies span a wide range of uses, from applications in general wellness to applications as medical devices. They include technologies intended for use as a medical product, in a medical product, as companion diagnostics, or as an adjunct to other medical products (devices, drugs, and biologics). They may also be used to develop or study medical products. The DHCoE is part of the US Food and Drug Administration (FDA), based in the Center for Devices and Radiological Health (CDRH). The Digital Health Center of Excellence empowers digital health stakeholders to advance health care by fostering responsible and high-quality digital health innovation.

Extended reality (XR)

Mixed reality (MR), virtual reality (VR), and augmented reality (AR) are enabling visualizations like never before. Pharma startups are exploring the possibilities of these technologies in the pharmaceutical research and manufacturing spheres. Extended reality tools enable data-rich and meaningful real-time location-agonistic interaction among research teams. Startups are making human augmentation in pharma a reality through extended reality wearables and tools.

Flexible production

The pharma industry is exploring new manufacturing methods due to the changing market dynamics, such as small batches for precision medicine. Single-use technology is gaining popularity as it reduces downtime and increases productivity by eliminating complex steps like cleaning and validation between separate production stages. New types of bioreactor systems and continuous manufacturing processes address the increasing focus on biopharmaceuticals. In addition to eliminating downtime, continuous manufacturing has low energy needs, achieves high productivity, and minimizes waste. We all know pharmaceutical cleaning equipment is essential, but sometimes it can be an absolute nightmare. In recent years, pharmaceutical machinery manufacturers have recognized this problem and created a solution—quick-disconnect features. Quick-disconnect features allow pharmaceutical manufacturers to clean their equipment with less hassle than before. It's a quick and easy way to get the job done without halting your production process for extended periods at a time. As a new pharmaceutical manufacturer, wouldn't it be easy if your production facilities came planned, equipped, and ready to use? With turnkey solutions, you can acquire tested and proven plant layouts with the corresponding high-tech equipment, saving you a ton of time and money from having to set up your operations. It is that easy.

Gene therapy

Gene therapy is a modification of a patient's genetic code to treat a disease; the transferred genetic material controls how proteins are produced by cells. Cell therapy is administering live cells into a patient to treat wherein the cells can originate from the patient (autologous cells) or a donor (allogeneic cells). When pluripotent, these transferred cells can give rise to any cell type and the multipotent cells into other cell types with limitations.

Genome sequencing power

Derived from technologies like Illumina (www.illumina.com) that provide complete DNA sequencing for less than $1,000, we can now explore new biology aspects. We already know that proteins, metabolites, DNA, RNA, and many other cell components all interact in complex, dynamic, and even spatially regulated ways. We also know that they become dysregulated in disease. New research tools will allow us to study biology at higher precision comprehensively and at a lower cost, making them valuable for fundamental R&D and better diagnosing, modulating, and intervening upon disease.

Genomic biomarkers

The quality, precise identification, and reliability of the plant species from which the natural product is obtained are important for successful innovations. The use of an incorrect plant species will likely affect the therapeutic properties due to unrelated compounds in the species. Genomic methods are essential in establishing an accurate identification method for plants and natural product species. Genomic techniques such as DNA barcoding rely on sequence diversity in short and standard DNA regions (400–800 bp) for species-level identification. DNA barcoding utilizing genomics will provide a more robust and precise identification than traditional morphological identification and local conventional (vernacular) names. DNA barcoding of botanical products has been applied in biodiversity inventories and authentication of botanical products.

High-throughput screening

Target-based drug discovery has enabled a great expansion of chemotypes and pharmacophores available for the medicinal chemist during the past three decades. New techniques like high-throughput screening (HTS), fragment-based screening (FBS), crystallography in combination with molecular modeling, and combinatorial and parallel chemistry has created a considerable diversity of chemical lead structures well beyond the known natural products and ligands used as chemical starting points for drug discovery in the past. Moreover, this wealth of chemotypes can now be used as a source for tool compounds to study unexplored biological space and find new drug targets or phenotypic screening using systems-based approaches to identify drug candidates in a target-agnostic manner.

Human interactome

The set of physical protein–protein interactions (the interactome) in human cells.

Industrial biotech

A new generation of industrialized bio platforms is now poised to enable "plug-and-play" medicines, or new therapies that leverage a common foundation and reuse programmable components. Boosted by the mRNA vaccine approvals, a long list of other therapies will benefit from the same underlying innovation. As platform biotech companies like these continue to reach maturity, they will have an outsized impact on drug discovery timelines. This will be true in essentially all biotech small molecule discovery areas, protein engineering, genome editing, gene delivery, cell therapy, and more.

Lessons learned

Regardless of the technological progress, the role of serendipitous discoveries shall remain alive. We survived as human species for long before any medicine or treatment was discovered, all because of the pharmacy inside our body—this shall continue to be the main focus of new drug discoveries, stimulated by the COVID-19 pandemic that emphasized us the value of our immune system. A new class of vaccines, mRNA or DNA, will come to the forefront, replacing the adenovirus or attenuated live virus technology, allowing ready and quick access to all future infections. This technology will also open up new venues in gene and cell therapy, including mRNA vaccines revised for all infections to make them more affordable and mRNA vaccines for autoimmune diseases and diabetes.

Libraries

Today, large and diverse compound libraries, combined with great advances in cell and organoid culture technologies, make phenotypic screening an exciting approach for target and medicine discovery. Genetic disease genes are considered a promising source of medicine targets. Most diseases are caused by more than one pathogenic factor; thus, it is reasonable to consider that chemical agents targeting multiple disease genes are more likely to have desired activities. This is supported by a comprehensive analysis of the relationships between agent activity and target genetic characteristics. The therapeutic potential of agents increases steadily with the increasing number of targeted disease genes and can be further enhanced by strengthened genetic links between targets and diseases. Data libraries and drug and disease modeling approaches have the potential of unlocking knowledge about patterns that cannot be seen today—patterns in product efficacy and failures, in product-related safety signals, and in relationships between animal and human test results. The findings from in silico testing (computer simulation, rather than laboratory or animal testing) could reduce the risk and cost of human testing by helping product sponsors make more informed decisions on how to proceed with product testing and when to remove a product from further development.

Ligandomics

In contrast to conventional approaches of discovering one ligand at a time, the emerging technology of ligandomics systematically maps disease-selective cellular ligands in the absence of molecular probes.

Biologics targeting these ligands with disease selectivity have the advantages of high efficacy, minimal adverse effects, wide therapeutic indices, and low safety-related attrition rates. Therefore, ligandomics represents a paradigm shift to address the bottleneck of target discovery for biologics development.

Lipinski's rule of five

Lipinski's rule of five, also known as Pfizer's rule of five or simply the rule of five (RO5), is a rule of thumb to evaluate drug-likeness or determine if a chemical compound with a certain pharmacological or biological activity has chemical properties and physical properties that would make it a likely orally active drug in humans. The rule was formulated by Christopher A. Lipinski in 1997, based on the observation that most orally administered drugs are relatively small and moderately lipophilic molecules. The rule describes molecular properties important for a drug's pharmacokinetics in the human body, including their absorption, distribution, metabolism, and excretion ("ADME"). However, the rule does not predict if a compound is pharmacologically active. The rule is important to keep in mind during drug discovery when a pharmacologically active lead structure is optimized step-wise to increase the activity and selectivity of the compound and ensure drug-like physicochemical properties are maintained as described by Lipinski's rule. Candidate drugs that conform to the RO5 tend to have lower attrition rates during clinical trials and have an increased chance of reaching the market.

Liposomes

Liposomes are composed of vesicular bilayers, lamellae, made of biocompatible and biodegradable lipids such as sphingomyelin, phosphatidylcholine, and glycerophospholipids. Cholesterol, a type of lipid, is also often incorporated in the lipid-nanoparticle formulation. Cholesterol can increase stability of a liposome and prevent leakage of a bilayer because its hydroxyl group can interact with the polar heads of the bilayer phospholipids. Liposomes can protect the drug from degradation, target sites for action, and reduce toxicity and adverse effects. Lipid nanoparticles can be manufactured by high-pressure homogenization, a current method used to produce parenteral emulsions.

Lyosphere

One advance in drug product production has been the development of lyosphere technology in which a dried drug product—a vaccine or biologic—is produced as a consistent bead. The approach is advantageous because it reduces the space needed for storage, allows various products to be combined easily, enables titration of doses, and allows flexible packaging to be used. The product can be improved using high-disaccharide formulations; for example, using these formulations can significantly improve product stability. Lyospheres are also targeted for oral delivery by adding a coating that resists disintegration until it reaches the target site.

Mesoscience

The traditional approaches based on coarse-graining and reductionism will change to structural and systematic consideration—a mesoscience concept. Both natural and artificial worlds are likely to be multilevel, and each level is multiscale, containing the element scale, the system scale, and the in-between mesoscale. The system scale at the lower level corresponds to the element scale at the upper level for adjacent levels. Complexity usually emerges at the mesoscale when the system is operated in the mesoregime where at least two dominant mechanisms exist. They compromise with each other in the competition to realize their respective extremal tendencies. Therefore, in tackling complex issues, it is desirable to identify the involved levels first. It is then necessary to identify its element scale, system scale, and mesoscale at each level. Subsequently, the mesoregime should be determined, where complex structures prevail (featuring spatiotemporal heterogeneity). Next comes the critical step resolving the multiple dominant mechanisms coexisting in the mesoregime under the specified internal and external conditions.

Metabolomics and metabonomics

Metabolomics is the large-scale study of small molecules, commonly known as metabolites, within cells, biofluids, tissues, or organisms. Collectively, these small molecules and their interactions within a biological system are known as the metabolome. Metabonomics is a subset of metabolomics and is defined as the quantitative measurement of the multiparametric metabolic responses of living systems to pathophysiological stimuli or genetic modification, emphasizing the elucidation of differences in population groups due to genetic modification. Metabolomics provides a more in-depth view of the biological reality governing microbial metabolism, using complex analytical methods like NMR and chromatographic techniques associated with MS, alongside advanced data analysis algorithms. Since bacterial responses to antibiotics begin rapidly and encompass various pathways, metabolomics is well suited to elucidating the MOA. Additionally, it is possible to construct metabolic networks that aggregate catalytic activity (i.e., enzymes) alongside its coding and expression (i.e., genes and their transcriptional and translational control).

MHC class I and II

MHC class I is a polymorphic set of proteins expressed on the surface of all nucleated cells that present antigen to CD8+ (including cytotoxic) T cells in the form of proteolytically processed peptides, typically 8–11 amino acids in length. MHC class II is a polymorphic set of proteins expressed on professional antigen-presenting cells and certain other cell types, which present antigen to CD4+ (helper) T cells in the form of proteolytically processed peptides, typically 11–30 amino acids in length.

Microbiome

The microbiome is a characteristic microbial community occupying a reasonably well-defined habitat that has distinct physio-chemical properties. The microbiome refers to the microorganisms involved and encompasses their theatre of activity, which results in the formation of specific ecological niches. The microbiome, which forms a dynamic and interactive micro-ecosystem prone to change in time and scale, is integrated into macro-ecosystems, including eukaryotic hosts, and here crucial for their functioning and health. The microbiome trend is rapidly growing and can become one of the major game-changers in the biopharmaceutical industry. Microbiota is the ecosystem of more than 100 trillion microorganisms living inside our body or on the skin, coexisting naturally with human organisms and performing vital functions such as synthesis of vitamins, digestion, and taking part in the immune system development. The versatility of genes of the microbiota -microbiome -attracts the increasing interest of the research community and biotech companies as they try to develop new therapies or even find novel antibiotics using the understanding of how our bacteria contribute to diseases, immune responses, and the overall organism condition.

Microfluidics

Microfluidics has generated significant interest in the drug discovery and development domain. Microfluidics offers the distinct advantage of system miniaturization. By modulating the movement of minute quantities of fluids, microfluidics helps miniaturize assays and increase experimental throughput. The past few years have witnessed a rapid rise in the use of microfluidic technologies, such as 3D cell culture systems, organ-on-a-chip and lab-on-a-chip technologies, and droplet techniques. The microfluidic device volume is minimal, and many functions can be integrated on a single chip. The chip's internal dimensions range from micrometers to millimeters; this allows the handling of samples and reagents even in the picoliter range. Microfluidic chips, coupled with multichannel and array designs, allow a high-throughput process to be achieved, increasing the speed at which you can screen. Apart from rapid screening and analysis, microfluidics lowers reagent consumption and costs by its miniaturized devices.

Microphysiometry

Microphysiometry is the in vitro measurement of the functions and activities of life or living matter (as organs, tissues, or cells) and the physical and chemical phenomena involved on a small (micrometer) scale. The primary parameters assessed in microphysiometry comprise pH and the concentration of dissolved oxygen, glucose, and lactic acid, emphasizing the first two. Measuring these parameters experimentally combined with a fluidic system for cell culture maintenance and a defined application of drugs or toxins provides the quantitative output parameters extracellular acidification rates (EAR), oxygen consumption rates (OUR), and rates of glucose consumption or lactate release to characterize the metabolic situation. Due to sensor-based measurements' label-free nature, dynamic monitoring of cells or tissues for several days or even longer is feasible. On an extended timescale, a dynamic analysis of a cell's metabolic response to an experimental treatment can distinguish acute effects (e.g., one hour after treatment), early effects (e.g., at 24 hours), and delayed, chronic responses (e.g., at 96 hours).

Microwave

A significant advance in microwave vacuum drying achieves dehydration at lower temperatures, allowing faster drying than lyophilization because heat transfer occurs by radiation rather than conduction. Advantages include: 1) faster-drying technology enables semicontinuous manufacturing, 2) the technology is compatible with multiple delivery devices, 3) one can achieve enhanced thermostability by using high-disaccharide formulations, and 4) the technology has a smaller footprint and lower operating costs than current lyophilization processes. The reduction in drying time with this technology—typically from days to hours.

mRNA vaccine

An mRNA vaccine provides acquired immunity through an mRNA containing vectors, such as lipid nanoparticles, wherein the mRNA sequence codes for antigens and identical proteins resembling those of the pathogen. Upon delivering the vaccine into the body, this sequence is translated by the host cells to produce the encoded antigens, which then stimulate the body's adaptive immune system to produce antibodies against the pathogen.

Nanomedicine

Nanomedicine, the application of nanotechnology in medicine, draws on the natural scale of biological phenomena to produce precise disease prevention, diagnosis, and treatment solutions. The integration of nanomaterials with biology has provided many diagnostic devices, contrast agents, analytical tools, physical therapy applications, and drug delivery vehicles.

Nanoparticles

Nanoparticles are small, versatile, and can be designed to be multifunctional. Several nanoparticles have been approved, and several more are in clinical trials. "Old" drugs have also been reformulated with nanotechnology to improve safety, although none is more effective than the original product. Significant challenges in using nanoparticles are associated with their complexity. There are multiple engineered components, various disciplines are needed for their design and development, their manufacture will probably be expensive, and their performance will depend on "hitting the target" precisely. A better understanding of cellular mechanisms and barriers should enable a more deliberate design of functionalized nanoparticles. There is an opportunity to engineer small-scale processes for an early study that can be scaled up, for example, by using microfluidic approaches.

Furthermore, imaging technologies and tools can help to determine whether nanoparticles are going where intended. The Nanotechnology Characterization Laboratory of the National Cancer Institute serves as a significant resource in developing new nanotherapeutics. Nanoparticles are materials whose surfaces affect behavior and performance, and that their characterization has implications for design and manufacture. The challenges in the delivery of biologics require refrigeration. They typically have poor physical stability and poor oral bioavailability, their portability often requires a temperature-controlled supply chain from production to delivery, and most are administered parenterally. However, drug delivery via microparticles has shown great promise for addressing many of those challenges. One way to create microparticles is by using spray drying and noted that low-density, spray-dried microparticles are ideal for pulmonary delivery. Inhaled antibiotics in powder form are more efficacious and safer than intravenous delivery and can be delivered in lower doses and faster than nebulized-solution inhalation. Porous microparticles can also be designed to be effective carriers of crystalline active pharmaceutical ingredients (APIs). Co-suspensions have been shown to be more robust, consistent, and reliable than crystal-only suspensions. Spray-dried microparticles have characteristics that make them ideal for pulmonary delivery, and that proteins in the form of dry amorphous powders are stable at room temperature for more than two years. Another advantage is that the process is scalable, that is, from bench to commercial production. Other techniques for producing microparticles include a microfabrication ("molding") technique and a crystallization–freeze-drying process. Many innovative products for delivery of proteins and peptides are in the pipeline for topical applications, nasal delivery of various products, and oral delivery of proteins and peptides pose a substantial challenge because of the harsh environment gastrointestinal tract.

Network medicine

A discipline that seeks to redefine disease and therapeutics from an integrated perspective using systems biology and network science methodologies, offering critical applications to drug design.

Network proximity

Measures the distances between two modules, such as drug–target and disease–gene modules. Several proximity measures have been defined, such as shortest, closest, separation, kernel, and center measures.

Neurological diseases

The slow entry of NMEs as neurological drugs comes despite many advances in basic neuroscience research that identify the genetic, molecular, cellular, and neurocircuitry aspects governing behavior. Today, we can probe brain activity in humans and experimental animals with a degree of sophistication that could not be envisioned a decade ago. Current treatments and recent approvals are still large variations on previously identified mechanisms and pathophysiologic hypotheses, which for the most part were identified serendipitously.

Nonlinearity

For linear systems of equations, a small change in the magnitude of a variable is guaranteed to yield a proportional change in the model's output. However, both of these basic approaches to confirming models encounter serious difficulties when applied to nonlinear models, where the principle of linear superposition no longer holds. In the first approach, successive small refinements in nonlinear models' initial data are not guaranteed to lead to any convergence between model behavior and target system behavior. In the second approach, keeping the data fixed but making successive refinements in nonlinear models is also not guaranteed to lead to any convergence between model behavior and target system behavior. To turn to a Bayesian framework for confirmation does not resolve the projections of nonlinear models. The best example of a nonlinear system is the living universe in network patterns that can self-organize without any central command, creating a whole that is greater than the sum of its parts. Putting it all together, all of the spirit and intelligence contained in humans, dogs, mosquitoes, Venus, and the Milky Way Galaxy provide a nonlinear network of intelligence and spirit greater than a simple addition of each element's intelligence and spirit.

Nonobviousness

The expression "inventive step" is predominantly used in Europe, while the expression "non-obviousness" is predominantly used in United States patent law. The inventive step and non-obviousness reflect a general patentability requirement present in most patent laws, according to which an invention should be sufficiently inventive—i.e., non-obvious—to be patented. In other words, "[the] non-obviousness principle asks whether the invention is an adequate distance beyond or above state of the art." The purpose of the inventive step, or non-obviousness, the requirement is to avoid granting patents for inventions that only follow from "normal product design and development," to achieve a proper balance between the incentive provided by the patent system, namely encouraging innovation, and its social cost, namely conferring temporary monopolies. The non-obviousness bar is thus a measure of what society accepts as a valuable discovery.

Nucleoside modification

The incorporation of chemically modified nucleosides, such as pseudouridine, 1-methylpseudouridine, 5-methylcytidine, and others, into mRNA transcripts, usually suppresses innate immune sensing and/or to improve the translation.

Organs-on-a-chip

An OOAC is a multi-channel 3D microfluidic cell culture chip that simulates the activities, mechanics, and physiological response of entire organs and organ systems, a type of artificial organ. It constitutes the subject matter of significant biomedical engineering research, more precisely in bio-MEMS. (Bio-MEMS is an abbreviation for biomedical [or biological] microelectromechanical systems. Bio-MEMS have considerable overlap and are sometimes considered synonymous, with lab-on-a-chip [LOC] and total microanalysis systems [μTAS].) The convergence of labs-on-chips and cell biology has permitted the study of human physiology in an organ-specific context, introducing a novel model of in vitro multicellular human organisms. One day, they will perhaps abolish the need for animals in drug development and toxin testing.

Orthogonal assay

An assay performed following (or in parallel to) the primary assay to differentiate between compounds that generate false positives from those genuinely active against the target.

Outsourced biotech R&D

The idea of fully integrated biotechnology facilities costing billions of dollars is now obsolete. Research cGMP manufacturing of products can now be outsourced at a much lower CAPEX, motivating small agile companies to take the lead.

Packaging

Packaging has become an innovative subcategory of the pharmaceutical manufacturing industry. Pharmaceutical machinery manufacturers have been quick to create machines that meet the growing need for various packaging of different types of pharmaceuticals. There is no shortage of innovative packaging introduced annually to the pharmaceutical sector from pouches to bubble packaging.

Paradigm shift

Thomas Kuhn argued that science does not evolve gradually towards truth. Science has a paradigm that remains constant before going through a paradigm shift when current theories can't explain some phenomenon, and someone proposes a new theory. A scientific revolution occurs when 1) the new paradigm better explains the observations and offers a model that is closer to the objective, external reality, and 2) the new paradigm is incommensurate with the old.

Passive immunization

In contrast to traditional (active) vaccines, these therapies do not generate de novo immune responses but can provide immune-mediated protection through the delivery of antibodies or antibody-encoding genes. Passive vaccination offers the advantage of immediate action but at the disadvantage of the high cost.

Process analytical technology (PAT)

The FDA defines process analytical technology as "a system for designing, analyzing, and controlling manufacturing through timely measurement…of critical quality and performance attributes of raw and in-process materials and processes, to ensure final product quality." Real-time data to models so that need corrections can be made quickly. Many vendors sell sensors that can provide direct, chemical-specific, quantitative measurement of product attributes. However, she said that the technology is not as mature in the biologics space and discussed how valuable advanced sensors could be in monitoring a bioreactor. The specific properties monitored in a bioreactor are temperature, pH, carbon dioxide, and dissolved oxygen; however, monitoring the feed or the product is extremely valuable, and sensors to do so are available. Mass spectrometry was an option but favored other spectroscopic techniques, such as Raman, given their lower cost and ability to provide a unique fingerprint with no sample pretreatment.

Pathogen-associated molecular pattern (PAMP)

The conserved molecular structure is produced by microorganisms and recognized as an inflammatory danger signal by various innate immune receptors.

Personal genomics

The human genome was sequenced 20 years ago, but most patients today still have never taken a genetic test to guide their medical care. That's because genetic tests are used in relatively limited settings today, such as tumor sequencing, hereditary cancer predisposition testing, non-invasive prenatal testing, and rare disease diagnosis. For most common diseases—like diabetes, heart disease, or common forms of breast cancer—many small changes in a person's genetic sequence act in combination to influence the risk of disease. This is where polygenic risk scores (PRS) have recently come in to provide risk stratification based on thousands of different genomic variants. A PRS score might identify a woman with breast cancer risk equivalent to that of a BRCA mutation carrier (suggesting early screening), or PRS scores could identify candidates for intensive lipid-lowering or lifestyle changes. It has taken time, but more and more physicians are becoming familiar with genetic tests (~60% of PCPs nationally have now ordered one). And unlike the first go-around (driven largely by consumer curiosity), we now see a willingness on the part of health systems, payors/employers, and pharma companies to invest in population genomics programs to keep patients healthier.

Phage therapy

Phage therapy, viral phage therapy, or phagotherapy is the therapeutic use of bacteriophages to treat pathogenic bacterial infections. Bacteriophages, known as phages, are a form of viruses. Phages attach to bacterial cells and inject a viral genome into the cell. The viral genome effectively replaces the bacterial genome, halting the bacterial infection. The bacterial cell causing the infection is unable to reproduce and instead produces additional phages. Phages are very selective in the strains of bacteria they are effective against. Advantages include reduced side-effects and reduced risk of the bacterium's developing resistance. Disadvantages include the difficulty of finding an effective phage for a particular infection. However, virulent phages can be isolated much more quickly than other compounds and natural products because they can be isolated from the environment with ease. In addition to this, the development of standardized manufacturing processes would make lab to clinic delivery of phages much quicker.

Point of use manufacturing

The Advanced Research Projects Agency uses this to develop compact, robust, automated systems for manufacturing biologics at the point of care within a few hours. One system uses a cell-free approach to produce proteins. His system's advantage is that it uses a lyophilized formulation that can be activated by adding buffer and DNA. RNA is then synthesized and translated into protein. The technology is consistent and can produce products rapidly, for example, in two hours. The system's potential by synthesizing purified envelope protein from the Zika virus in less than 24 hours and producing the monoclonal-antibody drug Humira (adalimumab) are some examples.

Process data analytics

Collecting, managing, and analyzing data are becoming more challenging as the industry moves from merely describing what is happening to predicting and controlling what will happen. There are barriers to leveraging process data to improve operations—physical barriers that involve capabilities to measure, access, and organize data and organizational obstacles that involve questions of trust and the desire to analyze and act on the data. The manufacturing data are not the same as data from a designed experiment, and one has to be careful not to equate correlation with causality. Furthermore, the sources of variation are often not contained in the data. Also, biological processes are nonlinear and time-variant, and the industry needs to move away from multivariate analyses.

Process intensification

The upstream and downstream processes can deliver sustainable gains that can assure an uninterrupted product supply, lower cost of goods, and more flexibility. Process intensification has been used successfully in the chemical industry, and the biomanufacturing industry is similarly seeing a great deal of interest in recent years. While it could be claimed that the bioprocessing industry has been using existing technologies effectively and efficiently over the past couple of decades, given the emerging scenarios such as smaller patient population, digital medicine, and other new entities, the depreciation of capital investments, increase in the cost of goods is anticipated to grow dramatically in the next few years. A greater emphasis is required in identifying areas where the efficiency is low and uses innovative technology to maximize output from current and new infrastructure and capital spending.

Proteomics

Complimentary to genomic and transcriptomic approaches to quality control and sample variation is the use of proteomic platforms in describing the mechanism of action of many botanical products. Proteomic approaches to innovative drug discovery from botanical products can elucidate the protein expression, protein function, metabolic and biosynthetic pathways based on therapeutic effects translating to consistency in quality and profile of the product. Approaches such as mass-spectrometry utilizing isotope tags and two-dimensional electrophoresis will give insight into quantitative protein profiling, which generates quantitative data on a scale and sensitivity comparable to what is generated at the genomic level. Proteomics application has been successfully used to identify Chinese botanical medicine species, *Panax ginseng* versus *Panax quinquefolium*. The therapeutic effects of botanical products can be elucidated using proteomics and imaging techniques to study the metabolism of botanical products and their compounds successfully. Proteomics is an effective way to explain the multi-target effects of complex natural product preparations and discover multiple compounds and fractions, characterization of botanical products, and ultimately a molecular diagnostic platform.

Quantum dots

Quantum dots (QDs) are semiconductor particles a few nanometers in size, having optical and electronic properties that differ from larger particles due to quantum mechanics. They are a central topic in nanotechnology. When the quantum dots are illuminated by UV light, an electron in the quantum dot can be excited to a state of higher energy. In the case of a semiconducting quantum dot, this process corresponds to an electron's transition from the valence band to the conductance band. The excited electron can drop back into the valence band, releasing its energy by light-emitting light. This light emission (photoluminescence) is illustrated in the figure on the right. The color of that light depends on the energy difference between the conductance band and the valence band.

Rapid scale-up

Rapidly scale manufacturing capabilities for vaccines and other medical countermeasures (MCMs) to respond faster to emerging threats and other public health emergencies, such as pandemic influenza, shorten supply chains and increase manufacturing resilience to disruption by emerging threats or public health emergencies, such as natural disasters, by creating a distributed network of small manufacturing sites that can provide reserve capacity for centralized manufacturing facilities; accelerate therapy development for orphan diseases by improving the cost-efficiency of small-scale manufacturing processes; speed availability of emerging therapies by enabling manufacturing process and standards development, including for cell and gene-therapies, supporting goals of the 21st-Century Cures Act (Cures Act).

Rare diseases

Interest in rare disease therapeutics since the precise genetic causes of thousands of rare diseases are now known due to the genomics revolution. Many biotech and pharma companies are increasingly turning their attention to rare diseases or rare, early-onset forms of common diseases. And because there is a high unmet need, a relatively small clinical trial may provide a meaningful readout. These programs are viewed as attractive ways to de-risk platform technologies before applying them to more common, complex diseases.

Repurposing

A classic way to repurpose drugs is through network medicine, which includes the construction of medical knowledge graphs containing relationships between different kinds of medical entities (e.g., diseases, drugs, and proteins) and predicts new links between existing approved drugs and diseases (e.g., COVID-19). Based on graph embedding, methods have been gaining attention for link prediction in graphs that represent nodes and edges as low-dimensional feature vectors. Using the feature vectors of drugs and diseases, we can easily measure their similarities and identify effective drugs for a given disease. One challenge for the graph embedding method is scalability. Real-world (knowledge) graphs are usually large. The number of entities in a medical knowledge graph could be as many as several million. Existing machine learning systems such as TensorFlow and PyTorch are mainly designed for regular structures but not for large-scale graphs. Therefore, several systems that are specifically designed for learning representations from large-scale graphs have been developed. A high-performance system named GraphVite is useful for drug repurposing as it can efficiently process tens or even hundreds of millions of nodes.

Structural biology

Structural biology is a vital tool in the drug discovery pipeline. Proteins are the targets for most marketed drugs, and so uncovering the molecular structure of the biological target to high resolution, interactions of the target with ligands and compounds provide vital information to structure-based drug design. Highly expressed proteins can often be readily obtained from natural sources; however, proteins produced in small quantities within cells are required to be generated recombinantly. This often involves making a synthetic, codon-optimized gene for the protein of interest, cloning it into a plasmid expression vector, and then transfecting it into cultured cells to express the recombinant protein. Common expression systems include *E. coli*, baculovirus/insect cells, or mammalian cells, each with its advantages and disadvantages.

Synthetic biology

Synthetic biology has now progressed to a stage where we can readily synthesize genes of any size and even commercially manufacture DNA using PCRs and other in vitro methods; I see significant progress in this field to make synthetic biology a cost-competitive modality to plasmid DNA production. Having a synthetic platform will reduce the risk of contamination and lower the cost of DNA and RNA vaccines and many novel antibodies.

Systems pharmacology

An inter-discipline that applies systems biology principles and data science techniques in pharmacology.

Targeted delivery

One of the key hurdles to implementing gene therapy in the clinic is safely and effectively delivering the genetic payloads (like siRNA or CRISPR editors) into the correct disease cells. The time-tested bur archaic adenovirus-associated-vectors will be replaced with like lipid nanoparticles or other antibody or peptide-based targeting approaches, in turn spurring further interest in new delivery modalities. Ultimately, there will be delivery vehicles that can target payloads to specific cells and tissue types all over the body. And all these delivery modalities need to be safe and easy to manufacture (just like the cargo itself).

Theranostics

Theranostics is a combination of the terms therapeutics and diagnostics. Theranostics is the term used to describe the combination of using one radioactive drug to identify (diagnose) and a second radioactive drug to deliver therapy to treat the main tumor and any metastatic tumors. Nanotheranostics integrates nanomaterials with theranostics, the simultaneous integration of diagnosis and therapy to enable disease diagnosis, therapy, and real-time monitoring of treatment progress and efficacy. In theranostic nanocarriers of 10–1,000 nm size, the diagnostic and therapeutic agents are adsorbed, conjugated, entrapped, and encapsulated in nanomaterials for diagnosis and treatment simultaneously at the cellular and molecular level.

1

Understanding Nonlinearity

1.1 Background

Predicting the future has always been the most favorite indulgence of thinkers and writers. Yuval Noah Harari's book *Homo Deus: A Brief History of Tomorrow* makes the following predictions:

1. Humans will ascend to the status of gods. *Homo sapiens* (smart people) are turning into *Homo deus* (god humans), with god-like control over our surroundings and the ability to create and destroy life.
2. Wellness and wellbeing will take center stage. Humans will increasingly focus on god-like goals of immortality (health) and enduring happiness as the challenges of human existence (pandemics, starvation, and war) are solved (wellbeing). Calico, a Google spinoff, has a modest goal of solving the challenge of immortality (www.calicolabs.com/).
3. The "useless class" will ascend. The expense of improving the human condition will be prohibitively high, and only a few elites will afford it. Meanwhile, people will see jobs evaporate as technology improves and becomes more productive and efficient. The new "useless class" will be unable to sell their labor, unlike the lumpenproletariat (the unorganized and unpolitical lower orders of society who are not interested in revolutionary advancement) of the past.
4. Humanism is on its way out—humanism meaning human intelligence, the human experience of emotions, thoughts, and sensations, and the celebration of humans. The human sciences will specifically attack humanism's implied human superiority and exceptionalism and the lofty beliefs in the uniqueness of human feelings, reason, and free will. We are nothing more than animals with a god complex.
5. We will witness techno-ascension. Humans will utilize biological (genetic) engineering, cyborg (bionic) engineering, and computer (AI) engineering to update themselves in their search for immortality and happiness.
6. AI sapience will defeat human sentience. Sentience is the ability to feel, and sapience is the ability to reason; the two will be decoupled, resulting in AI that is smarter and more intelligent than humans. Because nonconscious but incredibly intelligent algorithms will know us better than we know ourselves, we will increasingly rely on AI algorithms to advise and lead us in life, love, and work.
7. Humans will understand AI as a set of algorithms (formulae) for predicting and explaining behavior, just as AI does. Individuals will be perceived as divisible "dividuals" made up of constellations of "if this, then that"–style algorithmic code for personality, passions, and profile, rather than irreducible and indivisible selves.
8. Dataism will rise to the status of the new religion. As we move away from a homo-centric worldview toward a data-centric worldview, the religion of humanism will be supplanted by a new religion called "dataism." Dataism, which already has adherents in Silicon Valley, praises life as data processing, individuals and organizations appearing as mere algorithms, and the value of human life as the ability to convert experience into data.

DOI: 10.1201/9781003146933-1

9. The Everything Internet (AKA the Matrix) will take over. If humanity is a single data-processing system, our output will create a new, even more efficient data-processing system known as the Internet-of-All-Things. *Homo sapiens* will vanish once this mission is completed.
10. Humanity is on the verge of extinction. However, humans will eventually advance from semi-evolved simians into pure information and break free from their carbon-based biological chains in the next level in evolution.

These predictions may seem out of line with what most would think or predict for tomorrow; that is the beginning of nonlinear thinking, not the end. But, classically, if you can think of it, then it is not nonlinear.

The source of the word "linear" is "line." On the other hand, "nonlinear" has a slew of unrelated concepts that somehow connect; these thoughts lead to conclusions that might not have been obvious otherwise, with the implication that the conclusions are more profound and insightful. Our thinking style determines how we interpret the world around us. Our course of action is also determined by it. We'll show you how to think in two different ways: linear and nonlinear thinking (Figure 1.1).

In the process of learning, processing, and integrating knowledge, thinking is critical. Our approach to solving an issue or putting a plan or strategy into action starts with our thought process. While our left brain helps us link things together, it is the right brain that is responsible for nonlinear thinking; often, what starts from the right brain ends up in the left brain to conclude. The best example is the theory of relativity. There was no definitive motivation to think as Einstein did, but once the concepts sprouted, he took them to his left brain and made them a hard fact.

In a nonlinear model, if you can imagine it clearly, then it is not nonlinear. Today, we are developing many new drugs, using many novel testing and manufacturing approaches, but none of these are nonlinear; these are just extensions of a linear process in the hands of a good left brain. This book is about the right brain and creating thinking out of line with trends or norms.

As we see in Figure 1.2, technology evolution has always been linear for thousands of years; in the mid-19th century, we began to turn the tide once the world population exceeded the billion mark. However,

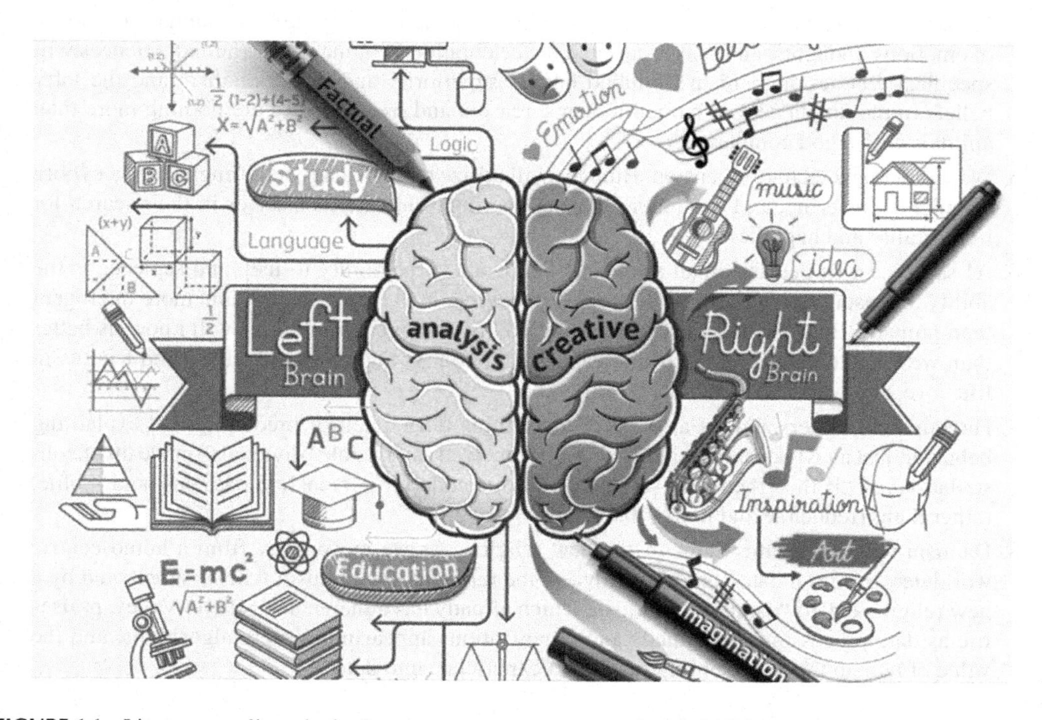

FIGURE 1.1 Linear vs. nonlinear brain. Source: www.entrepreneur.com/article/295294.

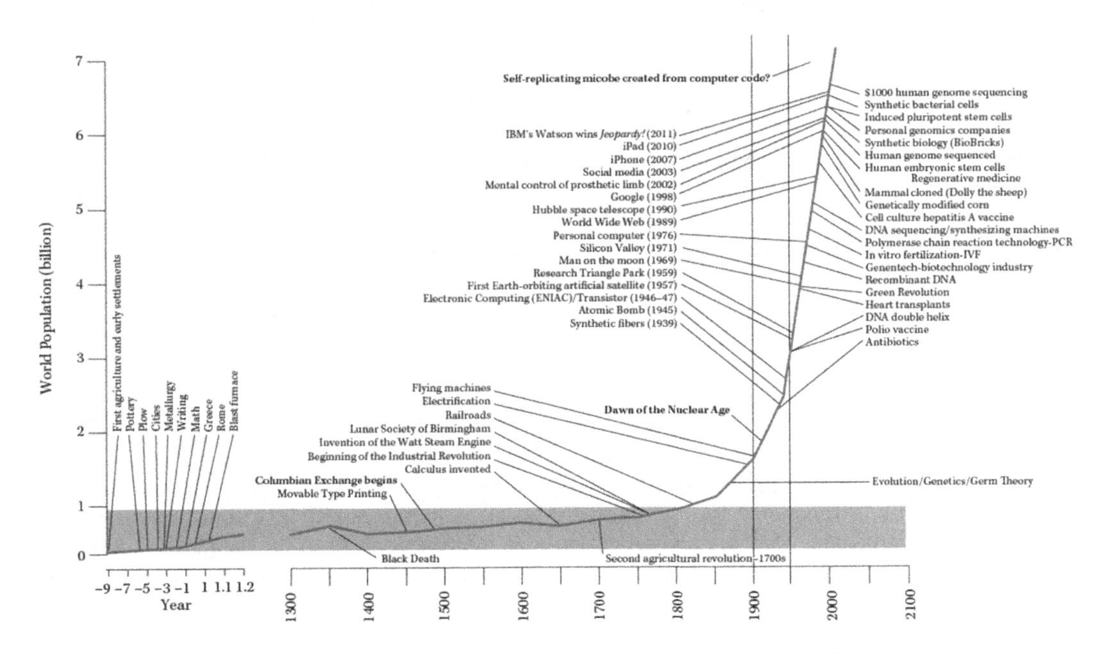

FIGURE 1.2 The growth of the world population and some major events in the history of technology. Source: based on Fogel, Robert, W. 1999. "Catching up with the Economy." *American Economic Review*, 89 (1): 1–21.

when our scientific knowledge became more common, resources to create technology became available. But the nonlinear shift occurred only when a crisis was solved; the two major wars are just one example. Thus, a need arose to create technology not based on previous knowledge.

Medical discoveries were responsible for dramatic changes in life expectancy, which shifted by almost 50 years to sustain 80% of the population over the past century.

1.2 Predictions

A prediction, often known as a forecast, is an assertion about what will occur in the future. They are frequently, but not always, founded on experience or expertise. Unfortunately, there is no universal agreement on the precise distinction between "estimate" and "prediction." The phrases have varied connotations for different writers and fields.

It is difficult to provide guaranteed precise knowledge about the future since future events are fundamentally uncertain. However, prediction can be useful in assisting with future event preparation. In a non-statistical sense, the phrase "prediction" refers to an educated guess or judgment. To make a prediction like this, abductive reasoning, inductive reasoning, deductive reasoning, and experience can all be used. It may be useful if the forecasting is done by someone knowledgeable about the subject.

The Delphi method is a regulated method for gathering expert judgment-based forecasts. In the sense that, at the very least, the "data" being used is the forecasting expert's cognitive experiences generating an intuitive "probability curve," this style of prophecy might be seen as consistent with statistical procedures.

Prediction is a type of statistical inference in statistics. Predictive inference is one method for making such inferences. However, the forecast can be made using any of the various statistical inference methods. Indeed, one way to describe statistics is that it allows you to transmit knowledge about a population sample to the entire population and other related populations, which isn't the same as forecasting across time. Forecasting is the process of transferring information across time, frequently to precise points in time. Forecasting normally necessitates the use of time series approaches, whereas prediction is frequently made with cross-sectional data.

Regression analysis and its several subcategories, such as linear regression and generalized linear models, are statistical approaches used for prediction (logistic regression, Poisson regression, probit regression). In addition, autoregressive moving average models and vector autoregression models can be used to forecast. The phrase predictive analytics is used when these and other related generalized regression or machine learning methods are employed in business settings.

It is possible to estimate the models that create the observations in various applications, such as time series analysis. Smoothed, filtered, and forecasted data estimates could be generated if models can be described as transfer functions or in terms of state-space parameters. If the underlying generating models are linear, a minimum-variance Kalman filter plus a minimum-variance smoother can be used to recover data of interest from noisy observations. These strategies employ one-step-ahead predictions (which minimize the variance of the prediction error). When the generating models are nonlinear, stepwise linearization can be applied in an extended Kalman filter and smoother recursions. In nonlinear situations, however, optimal minimum-variance performance guarantees are no longer valid.

To use regression analysis for prediction, data must be collected on the variable to be predicted, referred to as the dependent variable or response variable, and on one or more variables whose values are hypothesized to influence it, referred to as independent variables or explanatory variables. For the assumed causal link, a functional form, commonly linear, is hypothesized. The function parameters are estimated from the data; they are chosen to optimize the function's fit to the data after it has been parameterized. This concludes the estimating phase. To create predictions for the dependent variable, explanatory variable values deemed important to future (or current but not yet seen) values of the dependent variable are fed into the parameterized function.

The solar cycle predictions made by NASA in 2004 were incorrect (predicting that cycle 24 would begin in 2007 and be larger than cycle 23). However, the updated predictions made in 2012 showed that cycle 24 began in 2010 and was relatively small.

A prediction is a rigorous, often quantitative, statement in science that forecasts what would be observed under specific conditions; for example, if an apple fell from a tree, it would be seen moving towards the center of the Earth with a specified and constant acceleration, according to theories of gravity. The scientific method is based on putting propositions to the test that follow logically from scientific hypotheses. Repeatable experiments or observational studies are used to accomplish this.

- If observations and evidence contradict the predictions of a scientific hypothesis, the theory will be abandoned. Thus, it is easier to defend or deny new ideas that generate many new predictions (see predictive power). Concepts that make no testable predictions are frequently dubbed protoscience or nescience until testable predictions can be made.
- Mathematical equations and models and computer models are regularly used to characterize a process's past and future behavior within the limits of a model—in some cases, such as in quantum physics, predicting the likelihood of an outcome rather than the exact outcome is possible.
- Branch prediction allows microprocessors to avoid pipeline overflowing during branch instructions.
- Possible failure modes are predicted and avoided in engineering by rectifying the failure mechanism that caused the failure.
- In some fields, such as natural disasters, pandemics, demography, population dynamics, and meteorology, accurate prediction and forecasting are difficult. It is feasible to predict solar cycles, for example, but pinpointing their exact date and size is far more difficult.
- A mathematical model can also be used to predict the lifetime of materials in materials engineering.

In mathematics, a prime number is a number bigger than one with only two factors: itself and one. A prime number cannot be divided by another prime number without a remainder. The number 13 is an example of a prime number. It can only be divided by 1 and 13. Since Euclid established that the number of primes is unlimited over 2,300 years ago, two questions arise. First, let x be greater than zero. Second, how many prime numbers are there that are less than x? With all the computing power, we are not able to ascertain how many prime numbers there are? When expressed in base ten, the highest known prime number (as of December 2020) contains 24,862,048 digits. It was discovered in 2018 thanks to a machine donated by Patrick Laroche of the Great Internet Mersenne Prime Search (GIMPS). One would think that we should predict a pattern, a specific number, or a trend; while many theories have been adduced, we remain in this nonlinear observation.

1.2.1 Examples

New theories make predictions that can be tested in the real world. Predicting crystal structure at the atomic level, for example, is a current scientific challenge. In the early 20th century, the scientific consensus was that there was an absolute reference frame known as luminiferous ether. This absolute frame was believed to maintain consistency with the widely held belief that light travels at a constant speed. The famous Michelson–Morley experiment revealed that predictions derived from this idea did not hold in reality, proving the hypothesis of an absolute frame of reference false. Einstein proposed the special theory of relativity to explain the seeming conflict between the constancy of the speed of light and the lack of a preferred or absolute frame of reference.

Because it did not produce any consequences observable on a terrestrial scale, Albert Einstein's theory of general relativity was difficult to test. However, one of the earliest tests of general relativity predicted that enormous masses such as stars would bend light, which was observed in a 1919 eclipse, contradicting the conventional theory.

Predictions have been made utilizing paranormal or supernatural means such as prophecy or seeing omens from antiquity to the present. For millennia, methods such as water divining, astrology, numerology, fortune-telling, dream interpretation, and many more divination forms have been employed to predict the future. However, these methods of prediction have not been proven in scientific research.

Vision and prophecy are literary elements employed to illustrate a possible timeline of future occurrences in literature. They can be distinguished by their vision, which refers to what a person observes. As a literary device, the New Testament book of Revelation (in the Bible) employs vision. However, it can also be a prophecy, or prophetic literature told in a sermon or other public forum by an individual.

Divination uses an occultic standardized method or ritual to acquire insight into an issue or situation. It has been utilized in various forms for thousands of years and is a vital aspect of witchcraft. Diviners obtain their interpretations of how a querent should continue by reading signs, occurrences, or omens, or by supposed contact with a supernatural agency, most commonly portrayed as an angel or god, but considered a fallen angel or demon by Christians and Jews.

While the nonlinearity concept is treated as an oxymoron, the creativity of the human mind is not. Here are a few examples of fiction in which the authors have created a story point that appears to foreshadow a real-world event. Some of the prophecies in these novels come true with such spooky accuracy that you might wonder if fiction is truly imaginary.

Aldous Huxley's 1932 science fiction novel *Brave New World* is set in a future with chemical birth control, mood stabilizers, genetic engineering, videoconferencing, and television. All came to fruition.

The dystopian novel *1984* by George Orwell foreshadowed so many future features that it has become a catchphrase for any circumstance in which technology threatens to govern society's various parts. The novel gave rise to the term "Big Brother," which refers to government power abuse, particularly when it comes to monitoring. Even though Orwell's book was released in 1949, it described many technology developments already available in some form. His science fiction concepts are astonishingly similar to modern technology in two ways. The "telescreen," for example, is a huge television that is used to monitor people's private lives and identify them based on their facial expressions and pulse rate—to put it another way, face recognition software. The second example is the "Versificator," a system that can compose music and write on its own, akin to some of today's artificial intelligence technology.

A Song for a New Day by Sarah Pinsker is set in a society dealing with domestic terrorism and a deadly pandemic, prompting the government to outlaw gatherings larger than a certain size and radically alter the economy, forcing nearly everyone to work full-time from home and wear protective gear at all times when away from home. One of the two characters is a singer/songwriter who cannot perform as she was born to do because her livelihood depends on live audiences. Another character is a little girl who was a child during the pandemic and was scared of other people and public places. Right now, this one is a little too close to home. Here are 20 ways in which city life could change forever as a result of the coronavirus.

Tom Clancy, the perennial bestselling author of military and spy thrillers, has made many accurate predictions in *Debt of Honor* during his career. The plot climaxes (spoiler alert) with a hijacked 747 crashing into the Capitol building in this edition of his popular Jack Ryan series. Even though the novel is about a fantasized confrontation between the United States and Japan, the inclusion of a weaponized commercial airliner thrust Clancy and his book into the public eye in the aftermath of 9/11.

Earth, a novel by science fiction author David Brin published in 1990, was full of predictions about 2038. Email inboxes are being bombarded with what looks to be spam; a nuclear power plant in Japan has melted down; the globe is warming. For example, Brin stated, "Three million residents of the Republic of Bangladesh watched as early monsoons burst their hand-built levees, turning fragments of the crippled state into a realm of swampy shoals covered by the swelling Bay of Bengal." Brin admitted in the afterword that he "overstated the amount to which greenhouse warming may cause sea levels to rise by the year 2040." Still, some simulations suggest he wasn't so far off the mark after all.

When Ray Bradbury's novel *Fahrenheit 451* was published in 1953, television had already established itself as a popular source of entertainment in the United States. The majority of the programming consisted of scripted comedies and mysteries, game shows, news programs, and variety shows. However, the narrative contained elements that sounded eerily similar to present reality television.

The first true lunar explorers splashed down in the Pacific more than 100 years after Jules Verne penned *From the Earth to the Moon*, a story about three men traveling to the Moon from the United States (albeit in the sequel, *Around the Moon*). Though blasting them from a massive space gun would have destroyed the astronauts' bones, Verne got their take-off point in Florida spot on. John Paul Stapp accelerated a rocket sled from 0 to 632 mph in five seconds in the 1950s, encountering up to 20 Gs (hitting 46.2 when slowing down). Verne's cannon, if fired, would yield 23,413 Gs, according to modern estimations.

In Morgan Robertson's novel *Futility*, a giant ocean liner, dubbed "the largest craft afloat," is speeding through the North Atlantic when a watchman yells out, "Iceberg." The ship, however, collides with the ice and begins to sink. When the ship sinks, many of the passengers drown due to a lack of lifeboats. Although the story seems similar, this ship was not the *Titanic*; instead, it was the *Titan*. Robertson wrote his story 14 years before the *Titanic* set sail on its fateful maiden voyage—and those aren't the only parallels between the *Titanic* and Robertson's *Titan*. The story—now titled *The Wreck of the Titan; or, Futility*—was serialized in newspapers just a week after the *Titanic* sank as "an astonishing prophecy."

Gulliver's Travels, Jonathan Swift's biting 1726 satire, mocked many facets of British life, including scientists and their abstruse study. He claimed that the Laputans detected two moons orbiting Mars with relatively short orbital periods 150 years before two similar moons were identified. Swift got more than the moons right: the moons' "strange behavior matched quite well with Swift's description," according to SH Gould in *Journal of the History of Ideas*. Several craters on Mars's moon Phobos have been named after characters from Swift's novels.

It Can't Happen Here, by Sinclair Lewis, is an 84-year-old novel that has resurfaced due to certain parallels with the Trump administration in the United States. Set during the period it was written, the book envisages the birth of a populist character named Buzz Windrip, who rallies to defeat FDR in the 1936 election. "Like Trump, Windrip presents himself as the champion of 'Forgotten Men,' dedicated to restoring dignity and prosperity to America's white working class," according to a recent *New York Times* piece. Windrip enjoys large, emotional gatherings and rails against the mainstream media's "falsehoods."

Michel de Nostredame (1503–1566) was a French astrologer, physician, and alleged seer best known for his work *Les Prophéties*, a compilation of 942 poetic quatrains allegedly foretelling future events. *Les Prophéties*, published in 1555, was met with mixed reviews at first since it drew significantly on historical and literary precedent. Most academic sources deny that Nostradamus has any true supernatural prophetic ability, claiming that the connections between global events and Nostradamus' quatrains result from misinterpretations and mistranslations (sometimes deliberate). According to these scholars, Nostradamus' prophecies are notoriously imprecise, meaning that they might be applied to nearly anything, making them unhelpful in determining whether or not the author held actual prophetic powers.

They also point out that his quatrains' English translations are almost always of poor quality, based on later manuscripts written by authors with little knowledge of 16th-century French, and frequently mistranslated to fit whatever events the translator thought the prophecies were supposed to predict.

In Edgar Allan Poe's lone novel, *Narrative of Arthur Gordon Pym of Nantucket*, published in 1838, sailors are stranded and hungry in the ocean after a storm hits their whaling vessel. Desperate, they draw lots to determine who will be sacrificed, and Richard Parker is the one who will be eaten. After the ship *Mignonette* collapsed in a storm nearly 50 years after Poe wrote his tale of cannibalism, a real-life Richard Parker was killed and eaten by his hungry shipmates.

John Brunner's *Stand on Zanzibar*, written in the late 1960s and set in 2010, foresaw a popular leader named Obama as the President of Benin, random mass killings, a European Union, and individuals connecting to an encyclopedia over the phone. But, unfortunately, Brunner never published a book about the lotto numbers for the next week.

Isaac Asimov's *Foundation Trilogy*, first published in the early 1950s, anticipated the development of science known as "psychohistory." The future could be foretold by precisely gauging current advances and patterns in human behavior and life. Although statistics as a means of evaluating public opinion existed at the time, they were primitive compared to today's surveys and statistics.

EM Forster foresaw a future in which individuals only live and work in their rooms, connecting totally through electronic methods, in his 1909 book *The Machine Stops*. The characters in the book form and maintain their "friendships," "groups," or "teams" completely through electronic interactions, and they gradually become fearful of leaving their rooms or meeting other people in person. While the telephone was in use at the time, the radio was almost unheard of, and television had not yet been conceived. No one would have considered Forster's novella prophetic before the Internet and social media.

Octavia E. Butler, a science fiction writer who died before finishing the third book in the trilogy, imagined a bleak future with the rise of a populist demagogue in her books *Parable of the Sower* (1993) and *Parable of the Talents* (1998). While the books were well-received when first published, they have recently reappeared due to certain striking parallels between Butler's civilization and current events, such as global warming, powerful companies, and societal injustice. However, the strangest parallel she found was in *Parable of the Talents*, where she wrote about a conservative preacher running for president with the slogan "Make America Great Again."

Rokeya Sakhawat Hossain, a Muslim female social reformer from Bengal, described a region named "Ladyland" in her 1905 book *Sultana's Dream*. Men were imprisoned away so women could get things done without being distracted by things like violence and war. Hussain predicts a range of technical breakthroughs, including solar power and video chats, even if that aspect hasn't happened yet. Due to the lack of men, Ladyland's ladies have more time on their hands to invent other beneficial things, such as flying cars, weather control, and labor-free farming. Not that you needed another reminder, but here are a few of the reasons why women in today's culture are still not treated similarly to males.

Science-fiction writer HG Wells had a knack for predicting the future of warfare—including the atom bomb—in his 1914 novel. He prophesied that the difficulty of getting energy from the atom would be solved in 1933, and Leo Szilard did come up with the idea of a nuclear chain reaction in that year. However, that wasn't the only foreshadowing in *The World Set Free*: Wells also predicted how radioactive elements might be employed in "atomic bombs," which would render battlefields radioactive for years. Furthermore, in his 1899 story *When the Sleeper Wakes*, Wells's tendency of foreseeing the future of armed conflict extends to his views of the usage and importance of airpower in combat. This was a ground-breaking achievement that came 12 years before the first military airborne surveillance operation (Italians over Turkey in 1911) and four years before the Wright brothers flew a manned, heavier-than-air plane off the ground.

Predictions are frequently achieved in fantasy fiction by magic or prophecy, sometimes relating to old traditions. Many of the characters in JRR Tolkien's *The Lord of the Rings*, for example, are aware of events that will occur in the future, sometimes as prophecies, sometimes as more-or-less hazy predictions. Galadriel also employs a water "mirror" to show images, sometimes of possible future events.

In *United States of Banana* by Giannina Braschi, the character Segismundo is enslaved in prison beneath the Statue of Liberty due to a prophecy that he would bring havoc to his father, the King of the United States of Banana. Predictions in the novel include that the United States president, overly indebted to China, will sell Puerto Rico. Other predictions include natural disasters, a revolution in Puerto Rico, and the United States' disintegration into regions.

In some of Philip K Dick's books, mutant humans known as precogs can look into the future (ranging from days to years). For example, an exceptional mutant can anticipate the future to an endless range (probably up to his death) in the novella *The Golden Man*.

Frank Herbert's protagonists deal with the ramifications of seeing possible futures and choosing among them in the sequels of his 1965 novel *Dune*. This is seen by Herbert as a stagnation trap, and his protagonists take the so-called "Golden Path" out of it.

In Ursula K Le Guin's novel *The Left Hand of Darkness*, the humanoid inhabitants of planet Gethen have mastered the art of prophecy. Due to demand, they frequently create data on past, current, and future events. This was a minor plot device in this story.

Nonlinear narrative, also known as disjointed narrative or disrupted narrative, is a narrative technique used in literature, film, hypertext websites, and other narratives in which events are depicted in ways that do not follow the events' direct causality pattern, such as distinct parallel plotlines, dream immersion, and so on. It is frequently used to simulate the organization of and recall human memory, but it has also been utilized for other purposes. It dates back to antiquity and was established as an epic poetry convention with Homer's *Iliad* in the 8th century BC. The approach of delivering most of the story in flashback can also be traced back to the 5th-century BC Indian epic *Mahabharata*. Nonlinear narratives were used in several medieval *Arabian Nights* tales, including "Sinbad the Sailor," "The City of Brass," and "The Three Apples," which were inspired by Indian tales like *Panchatantra*. Modernist novelists such as Joseph Conrad, Virginia Woolf, Ford Madox Ford, Marcel Proust, and William Faulkner experimented with narrative chronology and abandoned linear order in the late 19th and early 20th centuries.

Several of Michael Moorcock's novels, especially those in the Jerry Cornelius series, are notable for extending the nonlinear narrative form to explore the complex nature of identity within a multiverse universe, particularly *The English Assassin: A Romance of Entropy* (1972) and *The Condition of Muzak* (1977).

In his book *Understanding Comics*, Scott McCloud argues that comic book narration is nonlinear because it is dependent on the reader's choices and interactions.

Prediction, prophecy, and poetry were all entwined for the ancients. Prophecies were delivered in verse, and the poet was referred to as "vates," or "prophet" in Latin. Poets and prophets both claimed to be inspired by forces beyond their control. Theological revelation and poetry are often considered separate, if not antagonistic, in contemporary civilizations. However, in their origins, goals, and objectives, the two are still frequently viewed as symbiotic.

1.3 Modeling Systems

Modeling finds its roots in the philosophical literature based on piecemeal improvement. The first step focuses on successive refinements of the model's data's accuracy without changing the model. The second step is bringing in consecutive refinements of the model while keeping the initial data fixed. The model is disproved if monotonic convergence to the intended system behavior cannot be found using one of these basic approaches (Figure 1.3).

A modest change in the magnitude of a variable in a linear system of equations will always result in a corresponding change in the model's output. However, when applied to nonlinear models, where the idea of linear superposition no longer holds, both of these basic ways of validating models face major issues. The first strategy does not guarantee that subsequent incremental modifications in nonlinear models' beginning data will result in a convergence between model behavior and target system behavior. Keeping the data unchanged while performing consecutive modifications in nonlinear models is not guaranteed to result in convergence between model behavior and target system behavior in the second approach. The projections of nonlinear models are not resolved by using a Bayesian framework for confirmation.

The living cosmos in network patterns is the best example of a nonlinear system because it may self-organize without any central command, resulting in a whole that is greater than the sum of its parts. For example, when all of the intellect and spirit in humans, dogs, mosquitoes, Venus, and the Milky Way

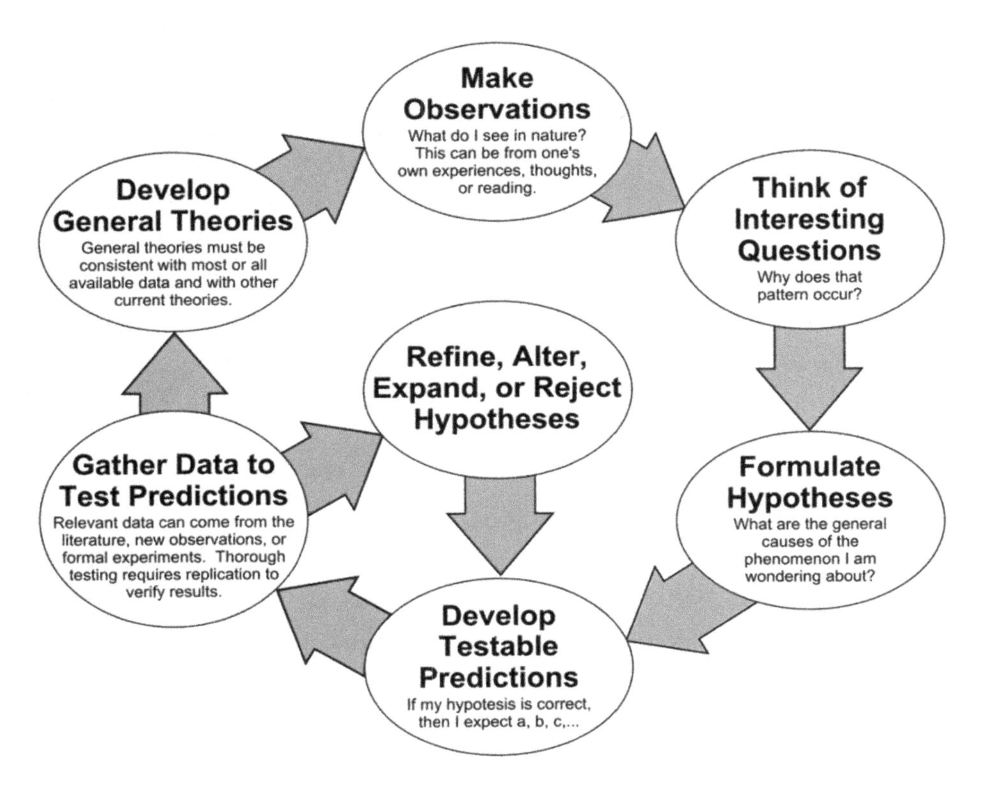

FIGURE 1.3 Scientific approach to modeling. Source: http://jpellegrino.com/teaching/scientificmethod.html.

Galaxy are added together, a nonlinear network of intelligence and spirit is created greater than the sum of each element's intelligence and spirit.

The digital age brings exponential changes to our actions and belief systems, making our existing participation in this fast-changing environment difficult due to our rigid, linear view. Therefore, to limit the danger of failure, our default behavior is to reject change and stress what has already been proven correct.

A nonlinear system in mathematics and science is one in which the output change is not proportional to the input change. Because most systems are intrinsically nonlinear, engineers, biologists, physicists, mathematicians, and other sciences are interested in nonlinear problems. In contrast to simpler linear systems, nonlinear dynamical systems, which describe changes in variables over time, might appear chaotic, unpredictable, or paradoxical. A nonlinear system of equations is a set of parallel equations in which the unknowns (or unknown functions in the case of differential equations) appear as variables in a polynomial of a degree larger than one or in the argument of a function that is not a polynomial of a degree greater than one. To put it another way, the equation(s) to be solved in a nonlinear system of equations cannot be expressed as a linear combination of the unknown variables or functions that appear in them.

Whether or not known linear functions occur in the equations, systems can be described as nonlinear. A differential equation is linear if it is linear in terms of the unknown function and its derivatives, even if it is nonlinear in terms of the other variables (Figure 1.4).

As nonlinear dynamical equations are challenging to solve, nonlinear systems are commonly approximated by linear equations (linearization). This works to a degree of accuracy and range for the input values, but linearization hides several intriguing phenomena like solitons, chaos, and singularities. As a result, some parts of a nonlinear system's dynamic behavior can appear counterintuitive, unpredictable, or even chaotic. Even though such chaotic behavior appears to be random, it is not. Some components of the weather, for example, are chaotic, with modest adjustments in one section of the system causing

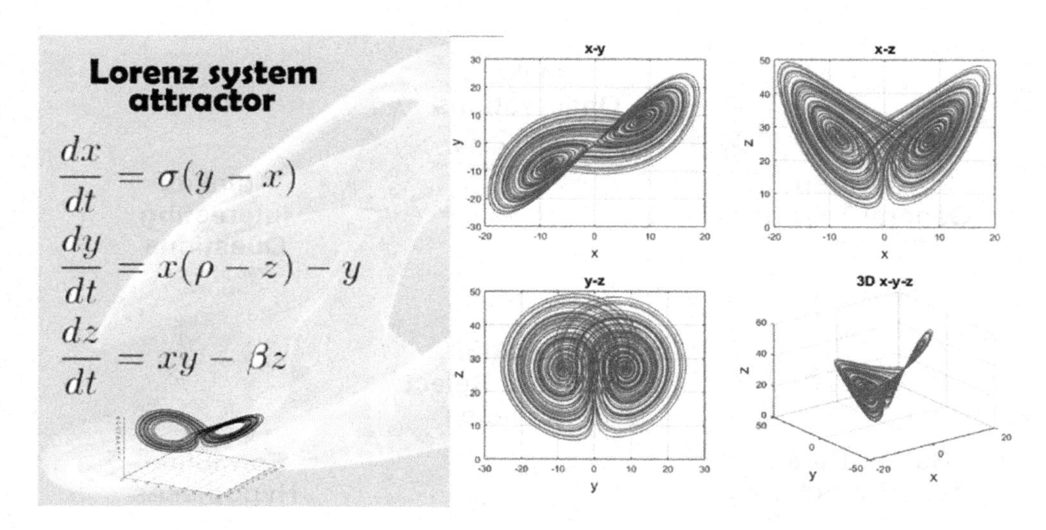

FIGURE 1.4 Theory of chaos and the butterfly effect—Lorenz attractor. Source: www.lrscom.com/2019/11/theory-of-chaos-and-butterfly-effect.html.

complicated impacts. This nonlinearity is one of the reasons that current technology makes accurate long-term forecasting impossible.

A double pendulum is a pendulum with another pendulum attached to its end in dynamical systems in physics and mathematics. It's a straightforward physical system with complex, dynamic behavior and high sensitivity to initial conditions. A double pendulum motion is governed by a set of coupled ordinary differential equations and is chaotic. The double pendulum's variants may be considered; the two limbs may be equal or unequal lengths and masses. They may be simple pendulums or compound pendulums (also called complex pendulums), and the motion may be in three dimensions or restricted to the vertical plane. The double pendulum undergoes chaotic motion and shows a sensitive dependence on initial conditions (Figure 1.4).

The Lorenz attractor has been a classic icon of modern nonlinear dynamics for about 50 years. With its interesting double-lobed structure and chaotic dynamics, the Lorenz attractor has come to symbolize order amid chaos (Figure 1.4). Mathematicians have lacked rigorous proof that the Lorenz equations' exact solutions will resemble the shape generated on a computer by numerical approximations. They were also unable to demonstrate that its dynamics are truly chaotic. Perhaps the calculations revealed something that appeared to be chaos but was only a numerical illusion. The Lorenz system is a set of ordinary differential equations with chaotic solutions for particular parameter values and initial circumstances. The Lorenz attractor, in particular, is a collection of chaotic Lorenz system solutions. The "butterfly effect," as it is known in popular culture, is based on the real-world implications of the Lorenz attractor, which states that in the absence of perfect knowledge of the initial conditions (even the tiniest disturbance of the air caused by a butterfly flapping its wings), our ability to predict the future course of any physical system will always fail. This underscores that physical systems can be completely deterministic and inherently unpredictable even without quantum effects. Despite today's technology, we cannot predict the weather for more than four to five days accurately since minute differences in the initial conditions take time to diverge.

1.3.1 Bayes' Theorem

What is the probability that you have cancer, given a positive test result? First, to solve this probability, identify the hypothesis, H, the datum, D, the probabilities of the hypothesis before the test, and the test's hit rate and false alarm rates.

- H stands for hypothesis, and in this example, H stands for the hypothesis that you have cancer, while H' stands for the hypothesis that you don't.

- D stands for datum, and in this context, D stands for a positive test result.
- Given the problem as 0.03, P(H) is the prior probability that you have cancer.
- P(D|H) is the chance of getting a positive test result *if* you have cancer. This is also known as the *hit rate*, and it was provided as 0.80 in the problem.
- P(D|H') is the chance of getting a positive test result *if* you don't have cancer. This is also known as the *false alarm* rate, which was set to 0.10. (Attention: there is no link between hit rate and false alarm, even though they sometimes appear to sum up to one.) (See Figure 1.5.)

Bayes' theorem states that the probability of having cancer [P(H|D)] when you are tested positive is given by:

$$P(H|D) = \left[P(D|H) * P(H)\right] / \left[P(D|H') * P(H)\right] + \left[P(D|H) * (1 - P(H)\right].$$

$$= \left[0.8 * 0.03\right] / \left[(0.8 * 0.03)\right] + \left[0.10 * 0.97)\right] = 0.1983 \text{ or } 19.83 \text{ percent.}$$

If new information becomes available, it will change the posterior probability, for example, if the more recent tests are more reliable or the spread of cancer has increased or decreased. Thus, the data (or information) will update the knowledge about the proposition. In most statistical problems, it is not merely the probability of a proposition of interest but the more general problem of learning about an unknown parameter or any unobserved quantity. Bayes' theorem provides a method of calculating the updated knowledge about the unknown parameter or quantity, as represented probabilistically, after observing any relevant data or information. Multiple data numbers can be analyzed, such as adding an age group, race, any prior health condition, etc., to calculate posterior probability. Bayes' theorem is the heart of artificial intelligence and machine learning and planning clinical studies among the thousands of applications that form the core of predicting the future. Since the prior probability keeps changing as newer data arrives, Bayes' theorem provides a dynamic linear view construed as nonlinear except where a paradigm shift is involved, as discussed in Figure 1.6.

One of the key ideas in Bayesian statistics is that knowledge about anything unknown can be expressed probabilistically. When we know certain other probabilities, we can use Bayes' theorem to find a probability. Briefly, the ratio of the two independent probabilities is multiplied by one conditional outcome probability to get the probability of another outcome; the two outcomes' ratio is the same as the independent probabilities. Unfortunately, we cannot apply Bayes' theorem to COVID-19 because the prior probability is not established, and it keeps changing depending on your surroundings (Figure 1.7).

In his celebrated book on *The Aim and Structure of Physical Theory* (1906), Pierre Duhem developed the methodological insight that logic and experience alone are insufficient for assessing the cognitive credentials or the hypothesis's epistemic credibility. Instead, additional criteria are required, which can only be of the non-empirical variety. This Duhemian insight provides the foundation for one of Thomas Kuhn's most significant arguments, which deals with the nature and significance of the non-empirical criteria used to assess the reliability of hypotheses theories.

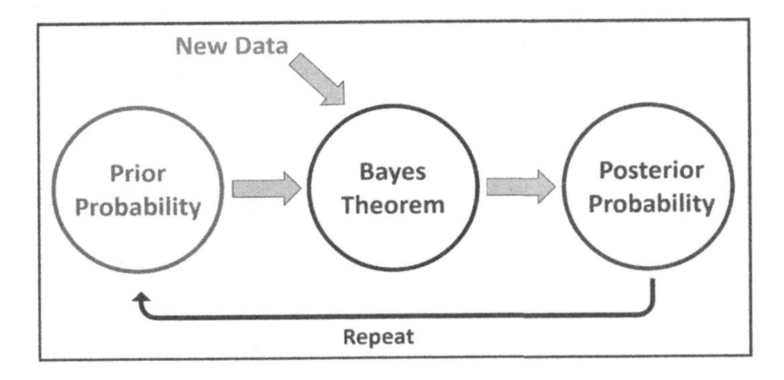

FIGURE 1.5 The Bayes Theorem.

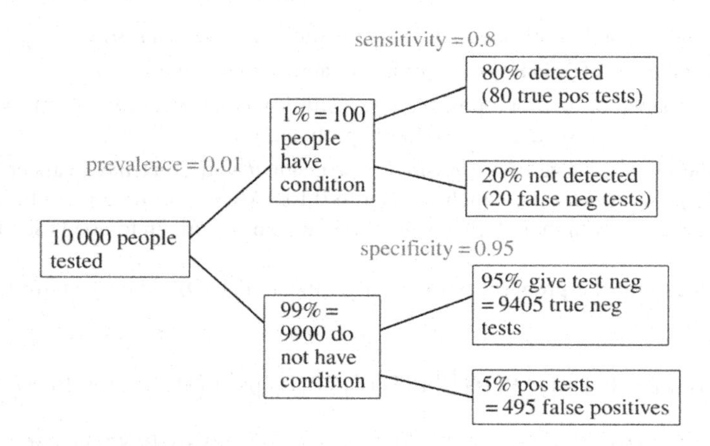

FIGURE 1.6 A Bayesian system calculation.

Kuhn claims that the process of evaluating ideas inherently and properly allows for individual preferences. Consequently, criteria with an epistemic bearing that are neutral regarding the substantive commitments involved are insufficient for determining theory choice unambiguously. According to Kuhn's analytical framework, the necessity to compare the merits of competing theories is most prevalent during crises. An established paradigm is shattered by a series of puzzle-solving failures throughout these times. To replace the accepted viewpoint, a challenger (or several) is advanced. Under these circumstances, relying just on the empirical record to assess relative success is insufficient.

On the one hand, the aging paradigm has numerous flaws; otherwise, there would have been no issue in the first place. On the other hand, the new rival strategy was devised very lately and pursued quickly. As a result, it is certain to have flaws and unresolved concerns that must be weighed when comparing relative benefits. As a result, both competing strategies are likely to have empirical flaws. On the other hand, both methods are reinforced by some effective explanations; otherwise, they would have faded from view and never been highlighted as competing ideas in a crisis. As a result, the empirical situation must be complex and confusing, preventing an unambiguous rating. Logic and experience are insufficient as a basis for theory selection, according to Kuhn's methodological ideas. Kuhn's technique turns Duhem's claim into a theorem.

Kuhn claimed that scientific fields undergo periodic "paradigm shifts" rather than progressing linearly and continuously. These paradigm shifts open new approaches to understanding what scientists would never have considered valid before; that scientific truth cannot be established at any given moment. Competing paradigms are frequently incompatible; that is, they are contradictory descriptions of reality. As a result, we can never rely solely on "objectivity" to understand science. Because all scientific results are ultimately based on researchers' and participants' subjective conditioning/worldview, science must account for subjective perspectives (Figure 1.8).

Thomas Kuhn contended that science does not linearly progress towards truth. When present theories fail to explain a phenomenon, and someone suggests a new theory, science has a paradigm that remains constant before going through a paradigm shift. A scientific revolution occurs when (i) the new paradigm better explains the findings and provides a model that is closer to objective, external reality, and (ii) the new paradigm is incompatible with the old.

In general, science can be divided into three stages (Figure 1.8). Pre-science comes first because it lacks a central paradigm. Then comes "regular science," in which scientists try to "puzzle-solve" their way out of the dominant paradigm. Normal science is extremely productive when guided by the paradigm: When the paradigm succeeds, the profession will have addressed issues that its members could scarcely have envisaged and would never have tackled without devotion to the paradigm.

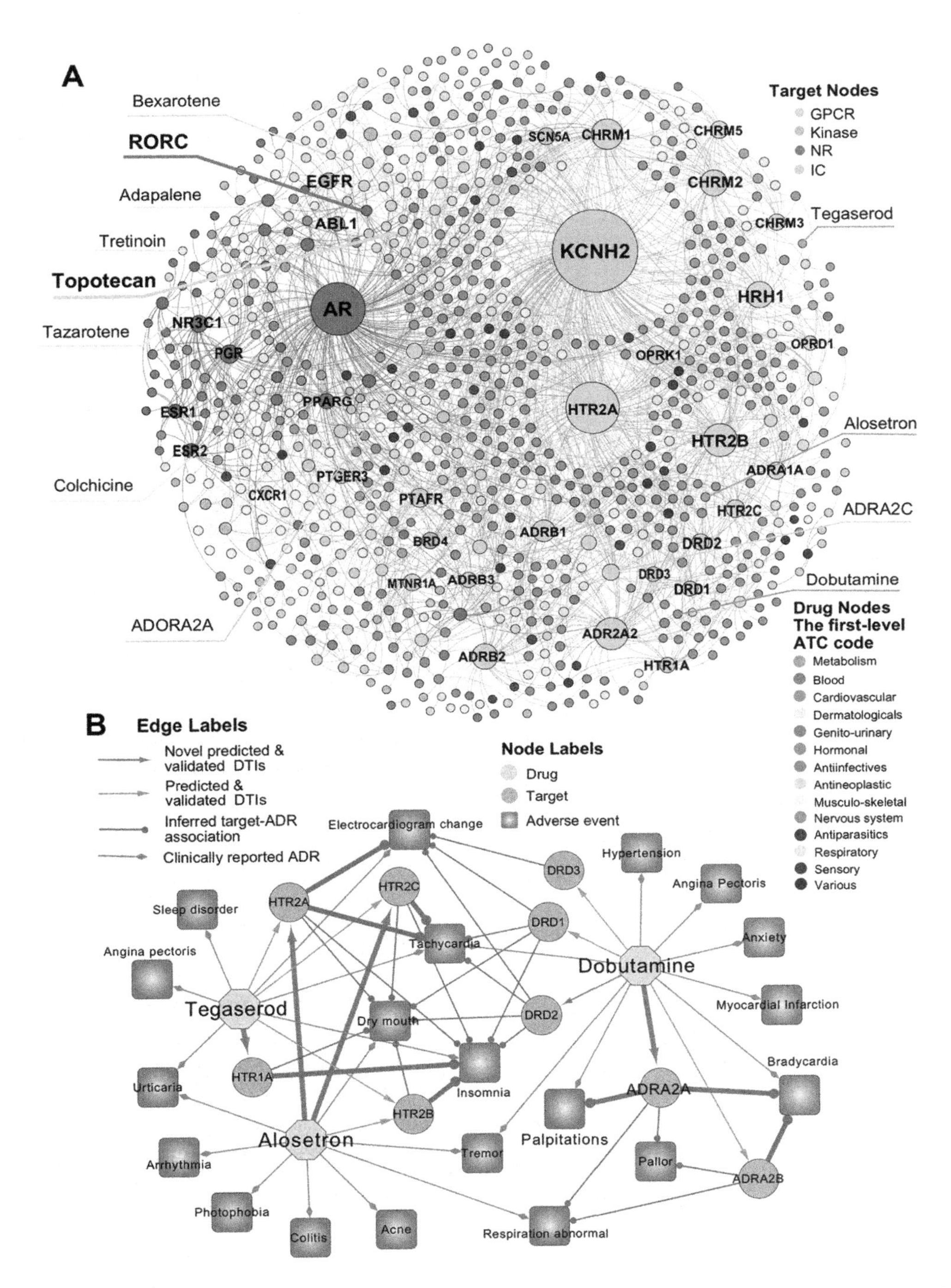

FIGURE 1.7 An example of Bayes' theorem applied to drug discovery. An illustration of the mechanisms of action of the deepDTnet-predicted GPCRs for three approved drugs validated by a high-throughput screening assay for characterizing the mechanisms of action of their clinically reported adverse events. (A) Computationally predicted drug-target networks for four well-known drug target families: G-protein-coupled receptors (GPCRs), kinases, nuclear receptors (NRs), and ion channels (ICs). Drugs are grouped by the first-level Anatomical Therapeutic Chemical classification system (ATC) codes (www.whocc.no/atc/). Drug targets comprise four groups: GPCRs, kinases, NRs, and ICs. (B) Paradigm shift.

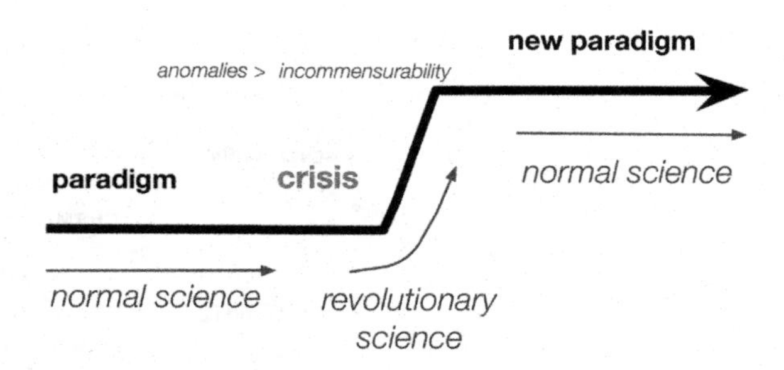

FIGURE 1.8 Paradigm shift theory of Kuhn.

1.3.1.1 Phases of Paradigm Shift

1.3.1.1.1 Phase 1: Pre-Science

- A period before a scientific consensus is reached, referred to as the pre-paradigmatic state.
- When activities are diverse and disorganized.
- There is a never-ending discussion over the fundamentals.
- There are as many theories as theorists.
- There is no widely recognized observational basis for this. Instead, the opposing hypotheses are each made up of a set of theory-dependent observations.

1.3.1.1.2 Phase 2: Normal Science

- Contrary to Popper's falsifiability criteria, the lack of a result to adhere to the paradigm is considered the researcher's error rather than a refutation of the paradigm. As a result of the accumulation of anomalous results, science reaches a point of crisis. At this point, a new paradigm is accepted, which incorporates both the old and anomalous data into a single framework. Revolutionary science is the word for this type of research.
- The grounds for acceptable work within the discipline are laid by establishing a paradigm. The articulation of the paradigm in answering the puzzles that it generates is thus considered scientific work.
- A paradigm is a common research foundation that establishes a precedent.
- Anomalies are puzzles that refuse to be solved.
- Abnormalities are allowed and do not lead to the rejection of a theory since scientists are certain that these anomalies can be explained multiple times.
- Scientists spend a significant amount of time in the model drift step battling anomalies that have arisen. They might or might not be aware of it or acknowledge it.
- Normal science requires a lack of critical thinking. For example, no detailed study would ever get done if all scientists were critical of a hypothesis and spent time trying to disprove it.
- Normal science is founded on the assumption that the scientific community has a good comprehension of the world. Much of the enterprise's success is due to the community's willingness to protect that notion, even if it means paying a high price. Normal science, for example, frequently hides important advances because they are inherently subversive of its core commitments.

1.3.1.1.3 Phase 3: Crisis

This is where the paradigm shift occurs.

- If the anomalies undercut the paradigm's underlying assumptions and attempts to remove them regularly fail, the anomalies become serious, and a crisis emerges.
- The rules for applying the paradigm become more relaxed in these cases—the development of ideas that question the established paradigm.

- There will be "exceptional science" in a crisis, with multiple competing explanations.
- The situation will be gone once the anomalies are rectified, and normal science will continue. If not, there will be a scientific revolution involving a paradigm shift.

1.3.1.1.4 Phase 4: Revolution

Eventually, a new paradigm will be established, but not because of any logically compelling justification.

- The motivations for choosing a paradigm are essentially psychological and sociological.
- The new paradigm explains the observations more clearly and is more in line with the objective, external reality.
- Different paradigms are incompatible; the laws of the old paradigm cannot be used to prove or disprove the new paradigm, and vice versa.
- There is no natural scale or measure for comparing and contrasting paradigms.

"The operations and measurements that a scientist does in the laboratory are not 'the given' of experience but rather 'the collected with difficulty,'" Kuhn (1996) says of experimentation and data-gathering to address issues through a commitment to a paradigm.

> They aren't visible to the scientist, at least not until his research is well advanced and focused. Instead, they serve as actual indicators of the content of more basic perceptions. They are chosen for normal research solely because they offer the possibility of a constructive elaboration of a recognized paradigm. Operations and measurements are paradigm-determined far more explicitly than the immediate experience from which they arise in part. Science does not deal with all types of laboratory experiments. Rather, it chooses those pertinent to the juxtaposition of a paradigm with the immediate experience that the paradigm has partially dictated. As a result, scientists from various paradigms perform various concrete laboratory manipulations.

Kuhn further claims that rival paradigms are incommensurable, meaning that one paradigm cannot be understood through the conceptual framework and terminology of another. In the social sciences, *The Structure of Scientific Revolutions* (1962) is Kuhn's most often cited book. The huge importance of Kuhn's work can be gauged by the alterations he made to the terminology of science philosophy: besides "paradigm shift," Kuhn popularized the term "paradigm" from a term used in certain forms of linguistics and Georg Lichtenberg's work to its current broader meaning, coined the term "normal science" to refer to the relatively routine, day-to-day work of scientists working within a paradigm, and was primarily responsible for the use of the term "scientific revolutions" in the plural, taking place at widely dissenting times. The common use of the term "paradigm shift" has made scientists more aware of paradigm shifts and, in many situations, more receptive to them. Kuhn's analysis of the evolution of scientific viewpoints has had an impact on that evolution.

Kuhn reiterates five criteria that determine (or help determine, more appropriately) theory choice:

- Accurate: empirically adequate with experimentation and observation
- Consistent: internally consistent, but also externally consistent with other theories
- Broad Scope: a theory's consequences should extend beyond that which it was initially designed to explain
- Simple: the simplest explanation, principally like Occam's razor
- Fruitful: a theory should disclose new phenomena or new relationships among phenomena

The paradigm choice was sustained by logical processes but not ultimately determined by them, according to Kuhn. According to Kuhn, it represented the scientific community's consensus. Accepting or rejecting a paradigm, he believed, is a social as well as a cognitive activity.

As a result, Kuhn has been labeled a relativist. Is it possible that all of the theories are equally valid? Why should we trust today's science if it could be proven wrong in the future? Kuhn vehemently disagreed, stating that scientific revolutions have always resulted in new, more precise ideas and constitute actual progress.

The paradigms that follow each other are incompatible. A later paradigm, according to Kuhn, may be a superior tool for solving puzzles than an earlier one. If each paradigm creates its puzzles, one puzzle may be meaningless to another. So, why is it progress if one paradigm is replaced with another that solves puzzles that the prior paradigm ignores? Kuhn's incommensurability argument was used to refute the idea that paradigm shifts are objective. The paradigm determines the truth.

It takes time for science to shift its perspective. Younger scientists are pioneering a new paradigm. "A new scientific fact does not triumph by persuading its opponents and making them see the light," as Kuhn (1996) put it, "but rather by its opponents dying and a new generation growing up familiar with it."

Thomas Kuhn demonstrated that current philosophers could not ignore science's history or the social environment in which it occurs. The society in which science is practiced is a product of the culture in which it is done.

Examples of a few "classical cases" of Kuhnian paradigm shifts include:

- 1473: Copernicus came up with the idea of a heliocentric universe and wrote a book about it. Still, no one believed him because it was badly written, and even the Church ignored his propositions because they needed him to design a calendar for them to use.
- 1543: The transition in cosmology advanced from a Ptolemaic cosmology to a Copernican one.
- 1543: The approval of Andreas Vesalius' work *De humani corporis fabrica*, which addressed various faults in Galen's earlier method.
- 1687: The transition in mechanics from Aristotelian mechanics to classical mechanics.
- 1783: The acceptance of Lavoisier's theory of chemical reactions and combustion in place of phlogiston theory, known as the chemical revolution.
- 1800: The transition in optics from geometrical optics to physical optics with Augustin-Jean Fresnel's wave theory.
- 1826: The discovery of hyperbolic geometry.
- 1859: The revolution in the evolution from goal-directed change to Charles Darwin's natural selection.
- 1880: The germ theory of disease overtook Galen's miasma theory.
- 1905: The development of quantum mechanics, which replaced classical mechanics at microscopic scales.
- 1887–1905: The transition from the luminiferous ether present in space to electromagnetic radiation in spacetime.
- 1919: The transition between the worldview of Newtonian gravity and general relativity.
- 1936: The Keynesian revolution brought a significant shift in macroeconomics.
- 1946: Willard Libby proposed radiocarbon dating measure carbon-14 as an objective age estimate for carbon-based objects originating from living organisms.
- 1950–1960: The cognitive revolution replaced behaviorism and psychoanalysis as the primary approach in psychology.
- 1960–1970: The LIDAR discovery for remote geospatial imaging of cultural landscapes, and the shift from processual to post-processual archaeology.
- 1964: In cosmology, cosmic microwave background radiation discovery led to the acceptance of the big bang theory over the steady-state theory.
- 1965: The acceptance of plate tectonics as the explanation for large-scale geologic changes.
- 1974: The November revolution began with discovering the J/psi meson and the acceptance of quarks, and the Standard Model of particle physics.
- 1960–1985: The acceptance of the ubiquity of nonlinear dynamical systems was promoted by chaos theory instead of a Laplacian worldview of deterministic predictability.
- 1996: The transition from "clinical judgment" to "evidence-based medicine" by Sackett et al.

- 2004: The transition from the Rational Paradigm to the Empirical Paradigm.
- 2020: COVID-19 necessitated remote working including digital healthcare, as well as the first approval of mRNA vaccines.

The paradigm shifts in the healthcare industry are abundant. Examples include chlorine in water, penicillin, Salk's polio vaccine, small molecule drugs, monoclonal antibodies, stem cell drugs, and microbial drugs. There was no antiparasitic treatment for a long time; cardiomyopathy was associated with immune disorders and denervation, and now it is a parasitic postulate; and gastric ulcers are attributed to pylori bacteria (Table 1.1).

The year 2020 saw a global crisis; COVID-19 forced the practice of many models such as remote learning, working, and telemedicine, which became an accepted routine; the crisis forced a paradigm shift even though it was not nonlinear; the nonlinear part was the acceptance of the practice. However, the pandemic also shifted interest in developing new drugs and vaccines that may not have been a primary focus in the absence of the pandemic. This is not a real nonlinear paradigm shift, except the understanding that forced the shift. The advent of mRNA vaccines is probably the best example of the paradigm shift in preventive therapy that will transform the future of pandemics, disease prevention, and global suffering; all of this will significantly improve the quality of life (Table 1.2).

The Green Revolution (also known as the "Third Agricultural Revolution"), toilets, synthetic fertilizers, blood transfusions, and vaccines are all believed to have saved one billion lives. Pasteurization, chlorination of water, antibiotics, antimalarial medications, and the bifurcated needle have saved hundreds of millions of lives. Even the ability to forecast natural disasters using satellites has saved 250,000 lives. Nuclear energy is the least deadly form of energy per kilowatt generated. The digital technologies trending in the 2020s—artificial intelligence, machine learning, robotic processes, edge computing, virtual reality and augmented reality, cybersecurity, blockchain, and the Internet of Things (IoT)—significantly impact the future of medicines.

We will be able to modify our biology thanks to the genetics revolution. We will be able to modify matter at the molecular and atomic level thanks to the nanotechnology revolution. Finally, the robotics revolution will enable us to build non-biological intelligence that is superior to human intelligence. While genetics, nanotechnology, and robots will all peak at different times over the next few decades, we already see all three in some form. Each is powerful in its own right, but their coming together will be even more so. These and other technologies will most certainly converge and have an unpredictable impact on our lives. Still, each technology will potentially bring tremendous good or enormous harm, as with all great innovations. The extent to which we can use their power to enhance people's lives will be determined by the conversations we have today and our actions.

1.3.2 Future Shifts

While the driving factors of paradigm shift remain, as does the COVID-19 pandemic, the future approaches will require research contents extended from equilibrium static states to dynamic structures and from local phenomena to system behavior. Also, research methods have gradually shifted from

TABLE 1.1

Paradigm Shift in the Science of Genetics

Observations	Genetics (Old)	Genomics (New)
Association findings	A contribution to disease is suggested even by a marginally significant association in a small cohort.	Most association findings are false positives. Thus, to believe in results, genome-wide significance and independent replication are required.
Rare variants	Rare variants that are not found in controls are likely to contribute to disease.	Rare genetic variation is frequent in patients and controls; thus, stringent testing is required.
De novo mutations	All de novo mutations and de novo deletions are pathogenic.	Every individual affected or unaffected carries 1–2 exonic de novo mutations.

TABLE 1.2

Paradigm Shifts That Had the Most Impact (Lives Saved)

1764: Bayes' theorem: 100 million
1850: Anesthesia: 50 million
1875: Toilets: 1 billion
1890: Pasteurization: 250 million
1909: Synthetic fertilizer: 1 billion
1913: Blood transfusion: 1 billion
1919: Water chlorination: 175 million
1922: Insulin: 15 million
1928: Antibiotics: 200 million
1930: Mammogram: 2 million
1935: Antimalarial drugs: 50 million
1936: Sunscreen: 10 million
1941: Cervical cancer screening: 6 million
1945: Pesticides: 25 million
1945: Third Agricultural Revolution: 1 billion
1950: Air conditioning: 2 million
1955: Vaccines: 1 billion
1957: CPR: 5 million
1960: Seat belt, airbag: 3 million
1960: Pacemakers: 8 million
1964: Bypass surgery: 3 million
1964: Anti-smoking campaign: 8 million
1965: Bifurcated needle: 130 million
1968: Oral rehydration: 50 million
1970: Higher education: 10 million
1970: Radiology: 25 million
1975: Nuclear power: 2 million
1976: Angioplasty: 15 million
1985: HIV treatment: 15 million
2000: Satellites: 0.25 million
2000: Robotic surgery: 1 million/yr
2003: Nanotechnology: inestimable
2004: Big Data: 0.05 million
2010: Medication management apps: 0.25 million/yr
2010: Online open courses: 1 million/yr
2010: Artificial intelligence: inestimable
2011: 3D printing: 0.1 million/yr
2011: Artificial organ transplant: 0.15 million/yr
2012: Wearable devices: 2 million/yr
2013: Global crowdsourced medical data: 0.5 million/yr
2013: Brain mapping: 4 million/yr
2013: Genetic mapping: 5 million/yr
2014: Self-driving cars: 1.5 million/yr
2015: IoT (in prevention of hospital errors): 1 million/yr
2016: Drones: 0.1 million/yr
2016: Renewable energy: 0.5 million/yr
2016: Desalination: 1 million/yr
2017: ATOM (Accelerating Therapeutics for Opportunities in Medicine): inestimable
2018: Ligandomics: inestimable
2019: Complex system resolution: inestimable
2020: mRNA vaccine: inestimable

qualitative analysis to quantitative prediction, from single-discipline-based to trans-discipline-oriented, and from data processing to artificial intelligence. Additionally, research domains will move from fragmented knowledge to integrated knowledge systems, from traditional theories to complexity sciences, from detail-focused to multiscale-associated, and from multilevel discipline-based study to the pursuit of universal principles. It will be essential for scientists to deduce common knowledge, even common principles, from disciplinary case studies in application-driven research. The traditional approaches based on coarse-graining and reductionism will change to structural and systematic consideration—a mesoscience concept (Figure 1.9).

Both natural and artificial worlds are likely to be multilevel, and each level is multiscale, containing the element scale, the system scale, and the in-between mesoscale. The system scale at the lower level corresponds to the element scale at the upper level for adjacent levels. Complexity usually emerges at the mesoscale when the system is operated in the mesoregime where at least two dominant mechanisms exist. They compromise with each other in the competition to realize their respective extremal tendencies. Therefore, in tackling complex issues, it is desirable to identify the involved levels first. It is then necessary to identify its element scale, system scale, and mesoscale at each level. Subsequently, the mesoregime should be determined where complex structures prevail (featuring spatiotemporal heterogeneity). Next comes the critical step: resolving the multiple dominant mechanisms coexisting in the mesoregime under the specified internal and external conditions.

Meanwhile, regime transitions can be defined by analyzing the specified conditions and their influence on the system. The final step is to solve the multi-objective (variational or optimization) problem. Additionally, when multiple levels are involved, it is necessary to realize their correlations.

Apart from genetic information, life systems share the same multilevel characteristics and similar dynamic evolution laws with material systems. The dynamic changes of small molecules, biomacromolecules, cells, organs, and organisms at other levels in specific in vivo environments are greatly significant to life and health. In particular, the structural and functional changes caused by the interaction of different levels and in vivo environmental changes should be the core of life systems. Issues to be considered include how to correctly identify different levels, whether immune mechanisms and metabolic processes

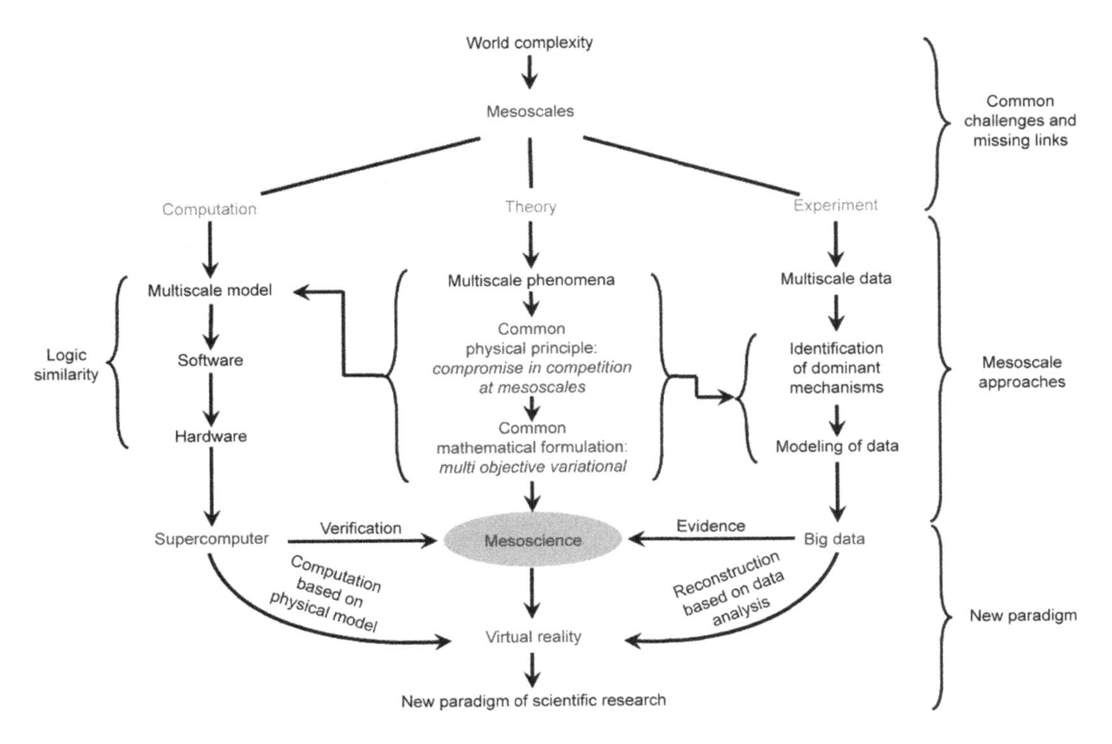

FIGURE 1.9 Mesoscales: the path to transdisciplinarity. Source: www.sciencedirect.com/science/article/abs/pii/S1385894715006233?via%3Dihub.

can be explained from this mesoscience perspective, whether a spatiotemporal alternation between normality and lesions during the transition from normal cells to cancerous cells does exist, and how to regulate the in vivo environment to make the alternating pattern return to the normal state. The principles of the first three categories of issues may apply equally to this category.

The interaction of neurology, brain science, and information science will contribute to the advent of the age of intelligence. The peripheral nervous system acts as a perceptual system, and the brain acts as the primary central system for analyzing perceptual information. The relationship between the two parts is similar to that of a computing system's input, calculation, and output functions. Therefore, revealing the multilevel features, especially the mechanisms at each level in processing signals and how different levels relate to each other and transmit information, is the key to cognitive science (related to life science but focuses on information). How to make a "yes" or "no" decision based on countless perceptual information after processing at multiple levels is the core issue. The impact of external conditions on this process and the consequent changes of modes are certainly the factors that must be considered from the perspective of a complex system, as mesoscales are the paths to breakthroughs. The process might also show three regime features, namely, "yes," "no," and the in-between "yes–no alternation."

All of the above possibilities belong to the domain of complex systems. When these problems are solved, empirical evidence will be generated for the common principles of complex systems. In the meantime, the implicit law of big data in engineering is also derived from the complex systems involved. The revelation of this law will provide physical logic for the development of artificial intelligence. The convergence of these aspects will greatly expand human knowledge systems. In other words, the development of artificial intelligence should focus on the mechanisms of human intelligent activities and the logic underlying complex systems (data) with emphasis on the possible commonalities between these two aspects. Breakthroughs in these fields may lay the scientific foundation for a new generation of artificial intelligence and play an important role in exploring future information technologies such as network, computation, and information security of the next generation.

The logic of computational science will comply with the laws of cognitive science. The key is that a common logic—the logic of complex systems—should be adopted. Establishing a computing system based on the computed objects' common logic should be an important direction for future development. Furthermore, the high efficiency of computing systems should be pursued through multilevel and multiscale physical logic and human cognitive laws.

Developing effective mathematical methods to describe all complex systems is a very important research direction. For example, how to formulate the dynamic changes of complex systems governed by multiple dominant mechanisms, most likely in the form of multi-objective variational problems, is a challenging mathematical issue worthy of great attention. The most difficult step in solving this issue is transforming the multiple objectives into a single objective, either in physical ways or in mathematical ways, to reach an inherently identical solution.

1.4 Conclusion

History transits in a nonlinear pattern; basically, if you can predict it, then it is not nonlinear. From the Lorenz theorem to the Bayesian approach to Kuhn's paradigm shift, we have the tools that teach us why we cannot predict the future unless given enough data. We may be on the right path to the future of pharmaceuticals. The history of mankind is a classic example of nonlinearity. Still, when it comes to adapting these observations for drug discovery, we have bright hope to find a future filled with pharmaceuticals that will exponentially reduce human suffering.

ADDITIONAL READING

Adams S. Information sources on post-grant actions to pharmaceutical patents. *J Chem Inf Comput Sci.* 2002;42(3):467–472.

Bollok M, Resina D, Valero F, Ferrer P. Recent patents on the *Pichia pastoris* expression system: expanding the toolbox for recombinant protein production. *Recent Pat Biotechnol.* 2009;3(3):192–201.

Brasil S, Pascoal C, Francisco R, Dos Reis Ferreira V, Videira PA, Valadão AG. Artificial intelligence (AI) in rare diseases: is the future brighter? *Genes (Basel)*. 2019;10(12):978.

Chan HCS, Shan H, Dahoun T, Vogel H, Yuan S. Advancing drug discovery via artificial intelligence. *Trends Pharmacol Sci*. 2019;40(8):592–604.

Chan HCS, Shan H, Dahoun T, Vogel H, Yuan S. Advancing drug discovery via artificial intelligence. *Trends Pharmacol Sci*. 2019;40(10):801.

Chen H, Engkvist O. Has drug design augmented by Artificial Intelligence become a reality? *Trends Pharmacol Sci*. 2019;40(11):806–809.

Chen X, Chen HY, Chen ZD, Gong JN, Chen CY. A novel artificial intelligence protocol for finding potential inhibitors of acute myeloid leukemia. *J Mater Chem B*. 2020;8(10):2063–2081.

Cockburn I, Long G. The importance of patents to innovation: updated cross-industry comparisons with biological medicines. *Expert Opin Ther Pat*. 2015;25(7):739–742.

Duhem P. *Essays in the History and Philosophy of Science*. Indianapolis: Hackett Pub. Co., 1996.

Duhem PMM. *The Aim and Structure of Physical Theory*, Translated by Philip P. Wiener. Princeton: Princeton University Press, 1991.

Faggella D. AI in pharma and biomedicine: analysis of the top 5 global drug companies. *Emerj*. 2020. Retrieved 4 April 2020, from https://emerj.com/ai-sector-overviews/ai-in-pharma-and-biomedicine/

German Patent Law of 16 December 1980 as amended by Laws of 16 July and 6 August 1998, section 16(1).

Gilvary C, Madhukar N, Elkhader J, Elemento O. The missing pieces of artificial intelligence in medicine. *Trends Pharmacol Sci*. 2019;40(8):555–564.

Green CP, Engkvist O, Pairaudeau G. The convergence of artificial intelligence and chemistry for improved drug discovery. *Future Med Chem*. 2018;10(22):2573–2576.

Khozin S, Pazdur R, Shah, A. INFORMED: an incubator at the US FDA for driving innovations in data science and agile technology. *Nat Rev Drug Discov* 2018;17:529–530.

Koromina M, Pandi MT, Patrinos GP. Rethinking drug repositioning and development with artificial intelligence, machine learning, and omics. *OMICS*. 2019;23(11):539–548.

Kuhn T. *The Structure of Scientific Revolutions*. Chicago: University of Chicago Press, 1962.

Kuhn TS. The function of dogma in scientific research. pp. 347–69 in A. C. Crombie (ed.). *Scientific Change (Symposium on the History of Science, University of Oxford, July 9–15, 1961)*. New York: Basic Books and Heineman, 1963.

Kuhn TS. *The Structure of Scientific Revolutions*. 3rd ed. Chicago: University of Chicago Press, 1996.

Murhammer DW. Review and patents and literature. The use of insect cell cultures for recombinant protein synthesis: engineering aspects. *Appl Biochem Biotechnol*. 1991;31(3):283–310.

Nagarajan N, Yapp EKY, Le NQK, Kamaraj B, Al-Subaie AM, Yeh HY. Application of computational biology and artificial intelligence technologies in cancer precision drug discovery. *Biomed Res Int*. 2019;2019:8427042.

National Academies of Sciences, Engineering, and Medicine. *Artificial Intelligence and Machine Learning to Accelerate Translational Research: Proceedings of a Workshop—in Brief*. Washington, DC: The National Academies Press, 2018. doi: 10.17226/25197.

Niazi S. *Filing Patents Online*. Boca Raton: CRC Press, 2003.

Picanco-Castro V, de Freitas MC, Bomfim AeS, de Sousa Russo EM. Patents in therapeutic recombinant protein production using mammalian cells. *Recent Pat Biotechnol*. 2014;8(2):165–171.

Price E, Gesquiere AJ. An in vitro assay and artificial intelligence approach to determine rate constants of nanomaterial-cell interactions. *Sci Rep*. 2019;9(1):13943.

Rashid MBMA. Artificial intelligence effecting a paradigm shift in drug development. *SLAS Technol*. 2020:2472630320956931.

Tirrell M. FDA moves to encourage A.I. in medicine, drug development. 2018. Retrieved 4 April 2020, from https://www.cnbc.com/2018/04/26/fda-moves-to-encourage-a-i-in-medicine-drug-development.html

United Kingdom Public and General Acts, 35 & 36 Eliz. 2 ch. 37, Patents Act 1977, s.25(1).

Vijayan V, Rouillard AD, Rajpal DK, Agarwal P. Could advances in representation learning in artificial intelligence provide the new paradigm for data integration in drug discovery? *Expert Opin Drug Discov*. 2019;14(3):191–194.

Wallis C. How artificial intelligence will change medicine. *Nature*. 2019;576(7787):S48.

Weinstein JN, Myers T, Buolamwini J, et al. Predictive statistics and artificial intelligence in the U.S. National Cancer Institute's Drug Discovery Program for Cancer and AIDS. *Stem Cells*. 1994;12(1):13–22.

World Trade Organization. Agreement on trade-related aspects of intellectual property rights. Article 33; April 1994, www.wto.org/english/docs_e/legal_e/27-trips_01_e.htm.

Wouters OJ, McKee M, Luyten J. Estimated research and development investment needed to bring a new medicine to market, 2009–2018. *JAMA*. 2020;323(9):844–853.

Wu Z, Lei T, Shen C, Wang Z, Cao D, Hou T. ADMET evaluation in drug discovery. 19. reliable prediction of human cytochrome P450 inhibition using artificial intelligence approaches. *J Chem Inf Model*. 2019;59(11):4587–4601.

Young D. FDA chief seeks to spur the use of AI, digital health tools to speed new therapies. 2018. Retrieved 5 April 2020, from https://www.spglobal.com/marketintelligence/en/news-insights/latest-news-headlines/44369790

2

The Evolution of Pharmaceuticals

2.1 Background

The discovery of drugs has been serendipitous since the beginning of human civilization. It has been lucky trial and error intended to find new foods as the foragers migrated once they ran out of edible things around their abodes. Today, we know a lot about physiology and pharmacology, yet luck and trial and error remain major determinants in sourcing new drugs. Drugs derived from natural sources were the only source in the beginning. Despite the advances in chemistry in the 19th century, we continue to rely on naturally derived materials and substances. In 2007, the FDA established a new Complementary and Alternative Medicines division and issued a guideline that encourages the development of naturally derived products and other treatment modes without the need to identify an active ingredient. Despite all the advances made in the chemical sciences and our ability to look deep into molecules, sometimes it is the synergy of a composition that proves its value without the need or ability to deconstruct the product.

Pharmacological studies of both natural and synthetic chemicals were conducted throughout the first part of the 20th century; from 1980 onwards, drug discovery was rationalized thanks to the exponential growth of molecular biology on the one side and computer technology on the other. The development of approaches for specialized receptor-directed and enzyme-directed drug discovery has resulted from gene cloning. Human hormones and other endogenous biomolecules can now be used as novel medications thanks to advances in recombinant DNA and transgenic technologies. We may be able to use biofeedback training to voluntarily restrict the release of neurotransmitters, hormones, and other molecules involved in the regulation of various physiological processes in health and disease as we learn more about the coordinating and regulating powers of the cerebral cortex, particularly the frontal lobe, over the next century.

Serendipity continues to play a significant role in drug discovery, as it has for thousands of years. COVID-19 will be remembered for a long time, a crisis that created many paradigm shifts. It also provided us with an example of how serendipity remains a critical factor in drug discovery. The AstraZeneca-Oxford University vaccine, the first of the COVID-19 vaccines based on adenovirus, had a glitch in its testing—a dose-calculation error that resulted in some participants getting half the dose, which was not discovered until they were ready for the second dose; it was fixed, and they received the total dose. The rest of the participants got two full doses. They found that the vaccine had an efficacy of about 60% in those who received two maximum doses and 90% in those errant participants who got the first dose as half a dose. There was no way to anticipate this outcome, and it would have been argued against and never tried. This is what Lorenz calls the "butterfly effect." A small change in the starting point leads to a significant outcome in the end. A reverse observation was made when the CureVac COVID-19 mRNA vaccine failed the efficacy test because the developers thought it will be better to use a wild-type or unmodified mRNA, against the common wisdom, in an effort to create new wisdom.

A broad understanding and appreciation of the history of pharmaceuticals teach us that the human body is no less complex than the universe's structure. Trillions of cells continuously spewing out proteins, fighting out non-self proteins, and creating new cells that target the disease is not possible to model, at least for now and likely in the near future. The reason for this pessimism comes from realizing that it has taken billions of years for life to start and transform. We know how our genetic code determines our attributes but we do not know why. A simpler example is the protein folding (Levinthal's) paradox

DOI: 10.1201/9781003146933-2

that it would not be possible in a physically meaningful time for a protein to reach the native (functional) conformation by a random search of the enormously large number of possible structures as it is produced in the ribosome translated from an mRNA. Autoimmune disorders work on the principle of randomness, where the B-cells express receptors that cannot be predicted. Aristotle (d. 322 BC) famously wrote, "The more you know, the more you realize you don't know," and this is the eternal teaching.

This chapter will take you through the rollercoaster of drug discovery, its success, and its failure and show you what I believe is the bright shining light at the end of this tunnel.

2.2 The Pre-Historical Era

Drug discovery and development have a long and illustrious history dating back to the dawn of civilization. Drugs were utilized for bodily ailments in ancient times but they were also associated with religious and spiritual healing. Sages or religious leaders frequently administered drugs. The first medications were made with plant components, which were then supplemented with animal substances and minerals. These drugs were most likely discovered through a combination of trial-and-error testing and observation of human and animal reactions to similar substances. If the experimenters did not live to tell the tale, many failed trials could not be documented.

The evolution of humanity owes much to the resilience of *Homo sapiens* against the challenges of nature by changing its lifestyle as knowledge became widespread. Because of the absence of travel, knowledge did not spread during ancient times, which occurred between the use of the first stone tools by hominins c. 3.3 million years ago and the invention of writing systems c. 5,300 years ago. It took thousands of years for writing to become universally accepted, and it was not employed in some human societies until the 19th century, or even now.

In different parts of the world, the end of the prehistoric era occurred at different times. Still, because it arrived earlier in the regions where medicines were developed, such as Mesopotamia, the Indus River Valley, and Egypt, we can assume that many people suffered from osteoarthritis, which was most likely caused by lifting heavy objects, which was a daily and necessary task in their societies. There is also evidence of rickets, which is caused by a deficiency in vitamin D.

Plant materials (herbs and substances derived from natural sources) were among the earliest treatments for diseases in prehistoric cultures. Earths and clays may have offered some of the first medicines to prehistoric peoples. Moving from prehistoric times to ancient civilizations, the Egyptian Imhotep describes the diagnosis and treatment of 200 diseases in 2600 BC. Hippocrates' birth in 460 BC created much of the concept of medicine, and Galen brought much to the science of medicine in 130 AD. Pedanius Dioscorides wrote *De Materia Medica* in around 60 AD. Vaccination against viral diseases occupies a large portion of the treatment history, starting with Persian physician Rhazes, who identified smallpox in 910 (but Pylarini gave the first smallpox inoculations 1701). Avicenna wrote *The Book of Healing* and *The Canon of Medicine* in 1010; Anton van Leeuwenhoek observed bacteria in 1683. Still, it was not until 1857 that Louis Pasteur identified germs as the cause of disease and developed vaccines for anthrax, rabies, and TB. Many vaccines followed. Today, we stand at the cornerstone of another dramatic era of vaccines—mRNA vaccines, as I will explain.

Although these folk medicines originated independently in different civilizations, there are several similarities, for example, in using the same herbs for treating similar diseases. This is likely to be a contribution by ancient traders, who might have assisted the spread of medical knowledge in their travels.

- Traditional Chinese medicine (TCM): This is thought to have begun in 3500 BC, during the reign of the legendary emperor Sheng Nong. The TCM texts of old China have been preserved thanks to the dynasty system and scrupulous documentation. Some notable medical literature is *Shang Han Lun* (*Discussion of Fevers*), *Huang Di Nei Jing* (*The Internal Book of Emperor Huang*), and *Sheng Nong Ben Cao Jing* (*The Pharmacopoeia of Sheng Nong*—a mythological emperor). Some active compounds from Chinese herbs have been employed in Western medications, such as Rauwouofia's reserpine for antihypertensive and emotional and mental regulation and Mahuang's alkaloid ephedrine for asthma treatment.

- Egyptian medicine: Written records of early Egyptian medical expertise were preserved on ancient papyrus. The Ebers papyrus (about 3000 BC) had 877 prescriptions and recipes for internal medicine, ophthalmology, and gynecology. Another document from circa 1800 BC, the Kahun Papyrus, provided therapies for gynecological issues. Herbal ingredients like myrrh, frankincense, castor oil, fennel, sienna, thyme, linseed, aloe, and garlic were used to make medicines.
- Indian medicine: Ayurvedic medicine, also known as Indian folk medicine, dates back 3,000–5,000 years and was practiced by ancient Brahmin sages. The therapies were outlined in religious texts known as Vedas. The materia medica is vast, and the majority of it is based on herbal mixtures. Some of the herbs, like cardamom and cinnamon, have been used in Western medicine. Susruta, a 4th-century AD physician, documented the use of henbane as antivenom for snakebites.
- Greek medicine: The Egyptians, Babylonians, and even the Chinese and Indians influenced Greek medical theories. Linseed or flaxseed was used as a calming emollient, laxative, and antitussive, whereas castor oil was used as a laxative. The fennel plant was used to cure intestinal colic and gas, and asafetida gum resin was used as an antispasmodic. Perhaps the greatest gift of the Greeks to medicine was the ability to cure ailments supposedly caused by supernatural causes or spells. Diseases were caused by natural causes, according to the Greeks. Hippocrates, the father of medicine, is credited with establishing medical ethics around 400 BC. The methods of preparing and compounding drugs to improve their absorption are discussed in the galenic formulation. Claudius Galen, a 2nd-century AD Greek physician who codified medications utilizing various ingredients, is the inspiration for the galenic formulation.
- Roman medicine: As great administrators, the Romans established hospitals primarily employed to serve the military. Organized medical treatment was made available as a result of this endeavor. The Romans significantly extended the Greek pharmaceutical practice. The *Materia Medica* of Dioscorides offers descriptions of therapies based on 80% plant, 10% animal, and 10% mineral materials. The collapse of Roman influence occurred during the Middle Ages, from roughly ad 400 to 1500 AD. In addition, epidemics ravaged numerous parts of Europe at this time. Bubonic plague, leprosy, smallpox, TB, and scabies were all common diseases. These diseases claimed the lives of millions of people.
- The early Christian Church: Herbs are mentioned in the Bible and the early Church. The Church's significant contribution to medicine, on the other hand, is the preservation and transcription of Greek medical writings and treatises. This allowed ancient knowledge to be continued and later applied throughout the Renaissance period.
- Arabian medicine (Arabic medicine): The Arabians learned and expanded their medical expertise through commerce with many other areas. Although the skills were most likely drawn from alchemists' practices, their main contribution may be their knowledge of medical preparations and distillation technologies. Around the years 900–1000 AD, Avicenna compiled a large encyclopedia of medical diagnosis and treatment. Rhazes was another well-known physician who accurately characterized measles and smallpox.

2.3 The New World Era

- Edward Jenner successfully experimented with smallpox vaccinations in 1796 paving the way for the use of vaccination to prevent the spread of many infectious diseases.
- William Withering introduced digitalis, an extract from the plant foxglove, to treat heart issues in the late 1700s.
- According to John Hunter (1768), scurvy is caused by a shortage of vitamin C. To treat scurvy, he recommended drinking lemon juice.
- Louis Pasteur (1864) established that germs caused diseases and developed a rabies vaccination. An attenuated rabies virus was used to do this.

- Quinine was initially used to cure malaria and is derived from the bark of the Cinchona tree.
- Ipecacuanha was used to treat diarrhea and was extracted from the bark or root of the Cephaelis plant.
- Aspirin is a pain medication derived from willow tree bark. It was initially used to cure fevers.
- The element mercury was once used to treat syphilis.
- Paul Ehrlich used arsphenamine, an arsenic compound, to cure syphilis.
- Gerhard Domagh discovered that the red dye Prontosil was efficient against streptococcal germs. Later, French scientists identified the active chemical as sulfanilamide, resulting in the development of a new class of sulfa medications to combat bacteria hosts.

The Renaissance created the groundwork for scientific approaches to pharmaceutical formulations and therapies. Many advances were made in anatomy, physiology, surgery, and medical treatments, including public health care, hygiene, and sanitation. Despite the advances made in the 1800s, only a few drugs were available for treating diseases at the beginning of the 1900s.

Drug research began in the early 1930s with screening natural products and the isolation of active components for treating ailments. In most cases, the active compounds are synthetic versions of natural products. New chemical entities (NCEs) are the synthetic versions. And since then, millions of new molecules have been synthesized. A large number is ending up as effective medicines treating just about every type of ailment, from modulating immune systems to inactivating viruses. To ensure that these synthetic versions, known as new chemical entities (NCEs) or new molecular entities (NMEs), are safe, potent, and effective, they must go through several iterations and tests.

Since then, large-scale production units have found, tested, and synthesized an increasing number of pharmaceuticals instead of small-batch extraction of medicinal compounds from natural sources. The modern pharmaceutical business arose after World War I, and medication discovery and development based on scientific principles became firmly entrenched. The concentration of the pharmaceutical industry in Switzerland owes to Switzerland's laws that did not recognize the patents of the thriving German chemical industry, giving incentive for Germans and others to settle in Switzerland and capitalize on German intellectual property.

2.4 The Regulatory Era

Except for the short-lived Vaccine Act of 1813, few federal rules were governing the contents and sale of domestically manufactured food and medications until the 20th century. A patchwork of state laws offered various degrees of protection against unethical sales activities such as misrepresenting the composition of food or therapeutic drugs. The FDA's origins can be traced back to the United States Department of Agriculture's Division of Chemistry in the late 1800s (later Bureau of Chemistry). The Division began undertaking research into the adulteration and misbranding of food and drugs on the American market under Harvey Washington Wiley, appointed chief chemist in 1883. Although they had no regulatory authority, the Division published its results in a ten-part series called *Foods and Food Adulterants* from 1887 to 1902. Wiley used his results and connections with state regulators, the General Federation of Women's Clubs, and national organizations of physicians and pharmacists to campaign for a new federal statute that would establish uniform food and medication standards for interstate commerce. After diphtheria antitoxin was recovered from a horse named Jim, who acquired tetanus and died, the 1902 Biologics Control Act was enacted.

The Food and Drug Act, sometimes known as the "Wiley Act" after its principal backer, was signed into law by President Theodore Roosevelt in June 1906. The Act made it illegal to transport "adulterated" food across state lines, with that term referring to the addition of fillers of lower "quality or strength," coloring to conceal "damage or inferiority," formulation with "health-harming" additives, or the use of "filthy, decomposed, or putrid" substances. Similar sanctions were imposed on the interstate sale of "adulterated" pharmaceuticals. (An interesting carryover of the restrictions on the interstate transport of drugs is spelled out in the IND [Investigational New Drug Application] which is required to test a new drug in humans and allows interstate transport of an experimental drug.) The active ingredient's "standard of strength, quality, or purity" was not stated on the label, and it was not listed in the United States Pharmacopeia or the National Formulary. The ordinance also made "misbranding" of food and drugs illegal. Wiley's USDA Bureau of Chemistry was responsible for "adulteration" or "misbranding" in foods and medicines.

Wiley used his new regulatory powers to wage a ferocious campaign against food makers who utilize chemical additives. Nonetheless, judicial rulings and introducing the Board of Food and Drug Inspection and the Referee Board of Consulting Scientific Experts as independent bodies under the USDA in 1907 and 1908, respectively, limited the Chemistry Bureau's jurisdiction. In response to a 1911 Supreme Court ruling that the 1906 act did not extend to false claims of medicinal efficacy, a 1912 amendment added "false and fraudulent" claims of "curative or therapeutic effect" to the legislation's definition of "misbranded." However, the courts proceeded to define these powers narrowly, imposing high criteria for proving fraudulent intent. The Bureau of Chemistry's regulatory functions were reorganized in 1927 under the Food, Drug, and Insecticide organization, a new USDA department. Three years later, the name was shortened to the Food and Drug Administration (FDA).

By the 1930s, a list of harmful products that had been ruled permissible under the 1906 law, including radioactive beverages, the mascara Lash Lure, which caused blindness, and worthless "cures" for diabetes and tuberculosis, had been made public by muckraking journalists, consumer protection organizations, and federal regulators. For five years, the resulting draft bill failed to pass the United States Congress. However, after the public uproar over the 1937 Elixir Sulfanilamide catastrophe, it was quickly enacted into law. Over 100 people died after taking a medicine that contained a deadly, untested solvent. A misbranding problem allowed the FDA to confiscate the product: an "Elixir" was defined as a drug dissolved in ethanol, not the diethylene glycol used in Elixir Sulfanilamide. It is suggested that if it had been branded a "solution" instead, the agency would have been powerless to track down and seize any remaining drug in the public's possession.

On June 24, 1938, President Franklin D. Roosevelt signed the new Food, Drug, and Cosmetic Act (FD&C Act) into law. By demanding a premarket study of all new drugs' safety and prohibiting misleading therapeutic claims in drug labeling without requiring the FDA to prove fraudulent intent, the new law greatly enhanced federal regulatory authority over drugs. In addition, the law authorized factory inspections and expanded enforcement authorities, established new food regulatory requirements, and brought cosmetics and medicinal devices under federal regulation. Despite numerous amendments throughout the years, this law remains the cornerstone of FDA regulatory authority to this day.

Following the passing of the 1938 Act, the FDA began designating certain medications as safe for use only under the supervision of a medical expert. The Durham-Humphrey Amendment of 1951 firmly established the category of "prescription-only" medications. While premarket drug efficacy testing was not permitted under the 1938 FD&C Act, subsequent modifications such as the Insulin Amendment and the Penicillin Amendment did require potency testing for select lifesaving pharmaceutical formulations. The FDA started using its new powers against drug companies that couldn't back up their efficacy claims. In *Alberty Food Products Co. v. United States* (1950), the United States Court of Appeals for the Ninth Circuit held that drug producers could not avoid the 1938 act's "false therapeutic claims" requirement by simply deleting the medicine's intended use from the label. These developments confirmed the FDA's broad authority to order ineffective pharmaceuticals to be recalled after being on the market. During this time, the FDA focused much of its regulatory attention on the abuse of amphetamines and barbiturates, but it also reviewed over 13,000 new drug applications between 1938 and 1962. While toxicology was still in its infancy, FDA regulators and others made rapid improvements in experimental assays for food additive and medication safety testing during this time.

Senator Estes Kefauver began organizing congressional hearings in 1959 to address concerns about pharmaceutical industry practices, such as the perceived high cost and unproven efficacy of many treatments pushed by companies. However, suggestions for a new law extending the FDA's authority were met with strong opposition. (Incidentally, the subject of drug costs in the United States is still being pursued in 2021 with no results.) The thalidomide catastrophe drastically altered the climate. Thousands of European babies were born with deformities due to their mothers taking medicine that was advertised to ease nausea during pregnancy. Due to concerns raised by FDA reviewer Frances Oldham Kelsey about thyroid damage, thalidomide was not approved for usage in the United States. Thousands of "trial samples" were given to American doctors during the drug's development's "clinical investigation" phase, which was unregulated by the FDA at the time. Individual members of Congress have mentioned the thalidomide tragedy as a reason for supporting FDA jurisdiction expansion.

The FDA's regulatory authority was revolutionized by the Kefauver-Harris Amendment to the FD&C Act in 1962. The most notable modification was adding "strong evidence" of the medicine's efficacy for a commercial indication to the existing criterion for pre-marketing demonstration of safety in all new drug applications. This was the beginning of the FDA's modern approval process. Between 1938 and 1962, all drugs licensed by the FDA were subject to an efficacy review and possible withdrawal from the market. The 1962 changes also included clauses requiring drug companies to use the "established" or "generic" name of a drug in addition to the trade name, limiting drug advertising to FDA-approved indications, and expanding FDA authorities to monitor drug manufacturing facilities.

The Controlled Substances Act of 1970 makes the use and possession of cannabis unlawful in the United States for any reason. Cannabis is classed as a Schedule I substance under the CSA, meaning it has a high potential for abuse and no recognized medicinal benefit, making even medical usage of the drug illegal. State rules on medical and recreational cannabis, on the other hand, vary widely, and in many cases, they are in direct opposition to federal law. As of early 2021, medicinal cannabis usage is allowed in 35 states, four of the five permanently inhabited US territories, and the District of Columbia, with a doctor's recommendation. Thirteen other states have passed legislation limiting THC concentration to provide cannabis products high in cannabidiol (CBD), a non-psychoactive component. Although cannabis remains a Schedule I substance, the Rohrabacher–Farr amendment shields anyone who obeys state medicinal cannabis laws from federal prosecution. Cannabis is allowed for recreational use in 15 states, the District of Columbia, the Northern Mariana Islands, and Guam. It is now permitted in 16 other states, as well as the United States Virgin Islands. Commercial cannabis distribution is lawful in all areas that have legalized cannabis, except in dispensaries.

In the 1990s and 2000s, there was a second wave of medical marijuana. Though Virginia approved a statute with limited effect in 1979, California started a more widespread trend in 1996. The Obama Administration de-emphasized federal law enforcement against patients who used the medicine under state law in 2009, but this stance was changed in 2011.

Recombinant DNA products based on cellular and molecular biology first appeared in the late 1970s. The biotechnology industry grew into existence.

Copies of approved (licensed in US) could not be marketed under the generic drug laws because the chemical structure of the active pharmaceutical ingredient (API) was not fixed and the generic drug laws required that a product should be chemically equivalent. To overcome this limitation, a new class of products were identified as biosimilars; these products have high biological and chemical similarity but are not identical. The BPCIA (Biological Price Competition and Innovation Act) allowed biosimilars to enter the market in 2009. In the EU and the US, there are now over 100 biosimilar products.

2.5 The Legal Era

For FDA examination, certain drugs are categorized as novel molecular entities (NMEs). Whether as a single ingredient medicine or as part of a combination product, many of these goods contain active moieties that have never been approved by the FDA before; these items frequently provide vital new medicines for patients. Some drugs are classified as NMEs for administrative purposes, yet they contain active moieties closely similar to active moieties in FDA-approved products. CDER, for example, identifies biological items submitted in an application under section 351(a) of the Public Health Service Act as NMEs for FDA evaluation to see if the Agency has already approved a comparable active component in another product. The FDA's judgment of whether a medicine product is a "new chemical entity" or "NCE" within the meaning of the Federal Food, Medicine, and Cosmetic Act differs from its designation of medicine as an "NME" for review purposes.

Medicine development is a complex and expensive process. The typical cost of developing a new pharmaceutical has been a point of contention, with current estimates ranging from $314 million to $2.8 billion and a regulatory clearance time of 15 years. To support the return on investment, the research companies have embarked on extensive intellectual property protection that goes well beyond protein

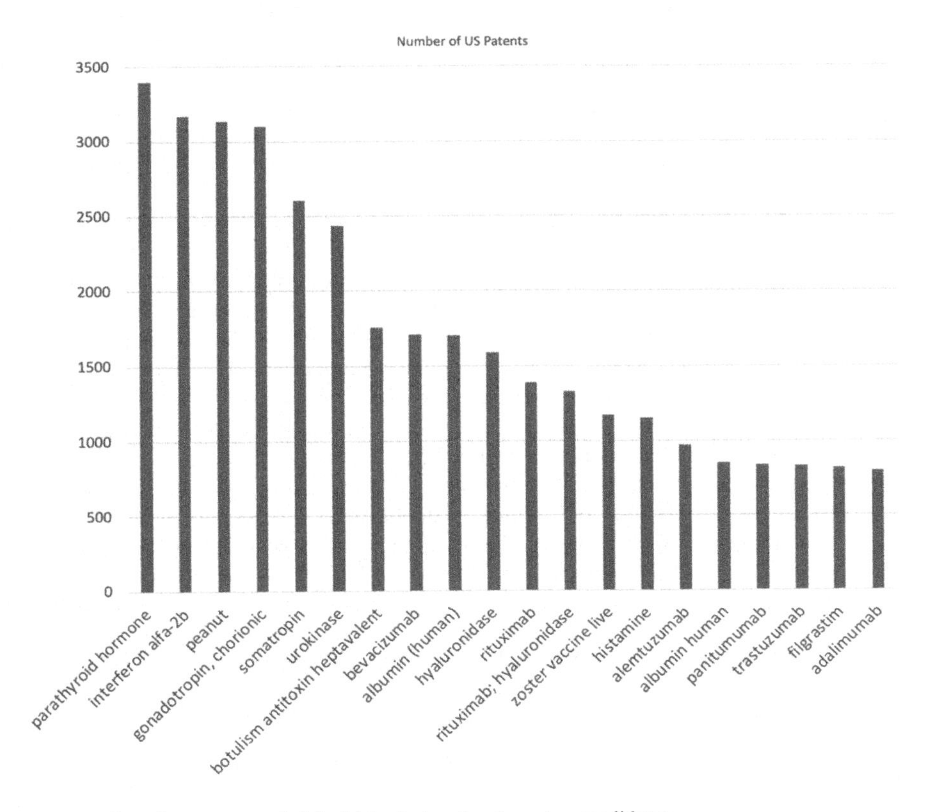

FIGURE 2.1 Number of patents awarded for biological molecules—top candidates.

identity and gene sequence to express; the patents now include protection of formulations, manufacturing process, cell lines, indications, delivery devices, and many more. Figure 2.1 shows the top 20 biomedicines and their associated patents.

2.6 The Gene Era

The past hundreds of years have seen a dramatic transformation of medicines as the scientific understanding about medicines and technology to produce them has changed; the regulatory requirements imposed further forced the industry to create new technologies and processes to make safe and effective medicines. The advancement of new technologies, genomics, biotechnology, and proteomics now offer the potential for significant change in therapeutics.

In conjunction with advances in gene therapy and understanding of disease mechanisms, the pharmaceutical industry, as well as research findings from the Human Genome Project, has opened up a plethora of opportunities and enabled the development and use of drugs that specifically target disease-causing sites.

The Human Genome Initiative is an international scientific research initiative focused on finding and mapping all of the human genome's genes, both physically and functionally, and determining the base pairs that make up human DNA. It is still the largest collaborative biological effort in the world. After the US government picked up the idea in 1984, planning began. The project began in 1990 and was officially completed on April 14, 2003.

2.6.1 The Biological Medicine Era

Humans have done well utilizing other life forms to their advantage. From the taming of the cattle and crops to making recombinant therapeutic proteins using yeast, bacteria, mammalian cells, plants, and viruses, the history of humans interacting with nature is full of great and exciting surprises, exemplified by genius exploitation and pursuit of solutions to the problems of humanity in the resources available in their surroundings.

Alexander Fleming found that *Penicillium* mold might kill staphylococcus germs in 1928. When Ernst Chain collaborated with Howard Florey ten years later, he rediscovered this truth. By 1944, large-scale production of penicillin was achievable because of Howard Florey and Ernst Chain's efforts. This technique foreshadowed the birth of biotechnology, which involves using bacteria to produce therapeutic chemicals. Insulin's discovery in 1922 revolutionized biological medicine; it was also the first biomedical medicine to be made using recombinant technology. Streptomycin was first introduced by Waksman in 1928.

The selective use of individual enzymatic transformation stages with microorganisms in chemical production pathways, particularly by biotransformation of steroids in 1950, expanded the field of biotechnological production of medicines. The increasing knowledge in regulating the biosynthesis of primary and secondary metabolites, the growing experience in the use of microorganisms as biocatalysts and sources of valuable enzymes, and the development of new economic, technical procedures raised the number and volume of medicines prepared by microbial biosynthesis and biotransformation.

The first vaccine for flu and typhus was developed in 1937. Rosalind Franklin used x-ray diffraction to study DNA structure, and Watson and Crick defined its double helix. The technology for propagating and expressing recombinant genes was invented by Stanley Cohen and Herbert Boyer in 1973.

The technological and scientific breakthrough came in the late 1970s and 1980s when the new technology related to cell culture, fusion, bioprocessing, and genetic engineering took roots in the industry. Today, prokaryotes, eukaryotes, algae, glycophytes, and halophytes are likely to contribute to future products. The techniques of DNA manipulation, monoclonal antibody preparation, tissue culture, protoplast fusion, protein engineering, immobilized enzymes, cell catalysis, antisense DNA, mRNA vaccination, etc. are the leading technologies helping humanity find solutions to their problems—a process that began with a glass of brewed grape juice that made a person feel good.

The first vaccine to target a cause of cancer came in 2006. The first mRNA vaccine was approved in 2020 against coronavirus to prevent the spread of COVID-19, a major milestone that will open the door to many new and novel biomedicine products.

Medicine discovery and development are now principally influenced by the information age, as a change in every other industry; industries that will not adopt the digital era will eventually fail. Besides the mechanical approaches to medical discovery, the functional classification of medicine has also changed exponentially, from gene-driven therapies to artificial intelligence-based treatment modalities. We are now in an era that was impossible to visualize even two decades ago.

Modern molecular biology tools have also permitted the design, manufacture, and development of biologic molecules as medicines, expanding the medicine space beyond standard synthetic tiny molecular-weight drugs.

Since 1982, hundreds of millions of people have been helped by about 400 biotechnology medicines and vaccines. Many more in the pipeline treating diseases just a couple of decades ago were considered untreatable, from AIDS to Alzheimer's disease to stroke prevention. Prevention of diseases like cancer appears possible within a short time. Many enzymes used to make food products are likely to be produced by recombinant techniques, as are the most processed foods.

Biomedicines are largely biotechnologically produced therapeutic recombinant proteins. Although various expression systems, such as mammalian cell lines, insects, and plants, can be used, new technical improvements are constantly being made to increase biomedicine's microbe production. This progression is made possible by the well-characterized genomes, plasmid vectors' versatility, availability of different host strains, and cost-effectiveness compared with other expression systems. Biomedicines are expected to account for up to 50% of all pharmaceuticals in development within the next five to ten years.

The total number of biomedicine entities approved by the FDA is 218, with multiple BLAs for some, as of early 2021. The highest number of BLAs assigned was for somatropin, followed by albumin that was also the first BLA approved. Trend analysis shows that the new biological entity approvals are rising, albeit more slowly (Figure 2.2).

Furthermore, while injections were the primary mode of delivery for the first biomedicines, future products are expected to be delivered via oral, dermatological, and inhaled formulations based on a

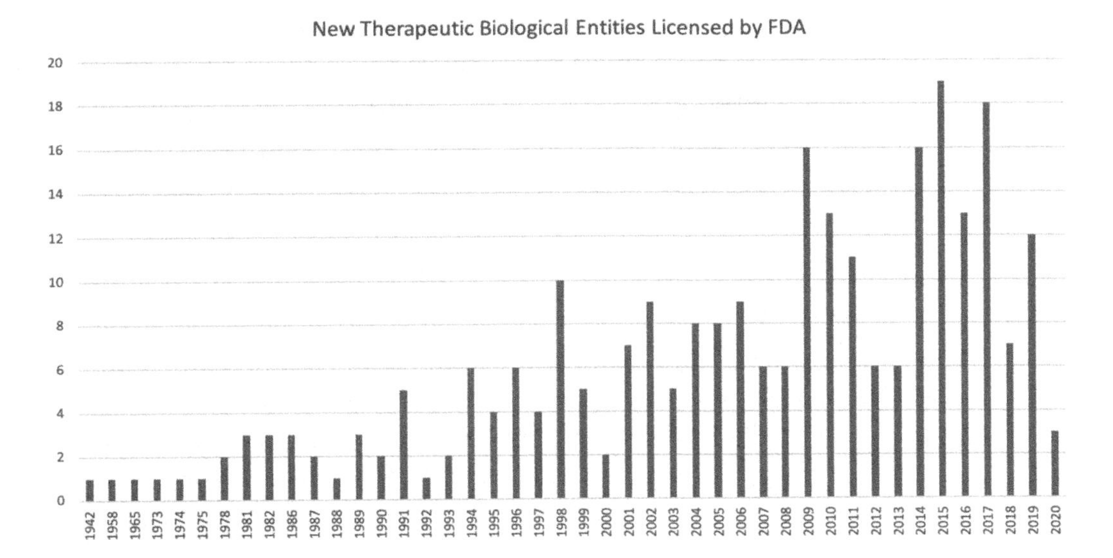

FIGURE 2.2 The FDA-licensed BLAs from 1942 to March 2020. Source: FDA Purple Book, www.fda.gov/medicines/therapeutic-biologics-applications-bla/purple-book-lists-licensed-biological-products-reference-product-exclusivity-and-biosimilarity-or.

variety of encapsulation approaches aimed at minimizing biologic instability caused by protein aggregation and denaturation as a result of physicochemical modifications such as deamination.

Another spinoff of biological medicines is the specialty medicines, a recent classification of medicines for advanced therapy medicinal products (ATMPs) that are "based on genes, cells, or tissue engineering," including gene therapy medicines, somatic-cell therapy medicines, tissue-engineered medicines, and combinations thereof. Within EMA contexts, the term "advanced therapies" refers specifically to ATMPs, although that term is relatively nonspecific outside those contexts. Gene-based and cellular biologics, for example, often are at the forefront of biomedical research and may be used to treat various medical conditions for which no other treatments are available. The DNA and RNA vaccines will fall in gene therapy, as described in this book.

The FDA has approved several cellular and gene therapy products as of early 2021. Cancer, genetic problems, and infectious diseases are among the conditions for which gene therapy products are being researched. Plasmid DNA, for example, is one sort of gene therapy product. Therapeutic genes can be genetically built into circular DNA molecules and delivered to human cells. Only "hematopoietic stem cell transplantation" operations, which are performed in patients with hematopoietic (blood-forming) system abnormalities, are allowed for use using cord blood products. Cord blood contains blood-forming stem cells that can be used to treat blood malignancies like leukemia and lymphomas and blood and immune system illnesses like sickle cell disease and Wiskott-Aldrich syndrome.

2.6.2 Nobel Prizes

We get a good understanding when we examine the Nobel Prizes awarded to discoveries and works relating to developing new therapies that belong to biomedicines (Table 2.1).

2.7 The Future Era

Drug discovery goes through periods of technological evolution (Figure 2.3). It is not always possible to predict what the future will bring to us, but we can undoubtedly conjecture that it will be a bulk of paradigm shifts (Figure 2.3).

TABLE 2.1

Noble Prizes Awarded for Work-Related Drug Discovery

Acquired immunological tolerance
Activation of innate immunity
Anaphylaxis
Antibacterial effects of prontosil
Antineurotic vitamin
Autophagy
Bacterium helicobacter pylori
Base sequence of nucleic acids
Biochemistry of nucleic acid regarding DNA
Biological synthesis of ribonucleic acid and deoxyribonucleic acid
Biosynthesis of carbohydrates
Cancer therapy by inhibition of negative immune regulation
Carbohydrates and vitamin C
Catalytic properties of RNA
Cell-free fermentation
Cell-mediated immune defense
Cellular origin of retroviral oncogenes
Chemical bonds in complex substances
Chemical nature of vitamin K
Chemical structure of antibodies
Chemical synthesis on a solid matrix
Chemical transmission of nerve impulses
Chemiosmotic theory
Cholesterol and fatty acid metabolism
Cholesterol metabolism
Chromosome in heredity
Chromosomes protection by telomeres and the enzyme telomerase
Citric acid cycle
Co-enzyme a and its importance for intermediary metabolism
Constitution of bile acid
Crystallographic electron microscopy
Dendritic cell and its role in adaptive immunity
Design and synthesis of molecular machines
Directed evolution of enzymes
Electrophoresis, adsorption—serum proteins
Enzymatic mechanism of ATP
Enzyme crystallization
Essential principles for drug treatment
Eukaryotic transcription
Function of single ion channels in cells
Gene modifications by embryonic stem cells
Genes regulating definite chemical events
Genetic code and protein synthesis
Genetic control of early embryonic development
Genetic control of enzyme and virus synthesis
Genetic principle for generation of antibody diversity
Genetic recombination and the organization of the genetic material of bacteria
Genetically determined structures on the cell surface that regulate immunological reactions
Genome editing

(*Continued*)

TABLE 2.1 (CONTINUED)

Noble Prizes Awarded for Work-Related Drug Discovery

Globular proteins
G-protein coupled receptors
G-proteins in signal transduction in cells
Growth factors
Growth-stimulating vitamins
Hepatitis C virus
Hormonal treatment of prostatic cancer
Hormones of the adrenal cortex
Human immunodeficiency virus
Human papillomaviruses causing cervical cancer
Humoral transmitters in the nerve terminals
Immune system producing monoclonal antibodies
Immunity
Insulin
Interaction between tumor viruses and the genetic material of the cell
Ion channels
Ionic mechanisms in the nerve cell membrane
Leucotomy (lobotomy) in certain psychoses
Liver therapy in anemia
Macromolecules
Malaria
Malaria and dementia paralytica
Mature cells reprogramming to pluripotent
Mechanism of DNA repair
Mechanisms of the action of hormones
Microanalysis of organics
Mobile genetic elements
Molecular mechanisms controlling the circadian rhythm
Molecular structure of nucleic acids
Mutations by x-ray irradiation
Nitric oxide and the cardiovascular system
NMR spectroscopy
Nucleotides and co-enzymes
Organ and cell transplantation in the treatment of human disease
Organic dyes
Origin and dissemination of infectious diseases
Osmotic pressure
Oxidation enzymes
Partition chromatography
PCR
Penicillin
Peptide hormone in the brain
Phage display of peptides and antibodies
Poliomyelitis virus
Prions
Prostaglandins
Proteins signaling
Purified enzyme and virus proteins
Radioactive elements

(Continued)

TABLE 2.1 (CONTINUED)

Noble Prizes Awarded for Work-Related Drug Discovery

Radioimmunoassay of peptide hormones
Regulators of the cell cycle
Replication of viruses
Respiratory enzyme
Restriction enzymes in molecular genetics
Reversible protein phosphorylation mechanism
Ribonuclease
RNA interference—gene silencing by double-stranded RNA
Roundworm parasites
Serum therapy in diphtheria
Signal transduction in the nervous system
Sinus and aortic mechanisms in respiration
Soft desorption ionization method for MS of macromolecules
Split genes
Stereochemistry
Sterols—vitamin connection
Streptomycin
Structural and functional organization of the cell
Structure and function of the ribosome
Sugar and purine synthesis
Sugar fermentation
Surface chemistry
Synthesis of hemin
Synthesis of a polypeptide hormone
Tuberculosis
Tumor-inducing viruses
Typhus
Ubiquitin-mediated degradation
Vitamins A and B2
Vitamin C and fumaric acid catalysis
Vitamin K
X-ray diffraction
Yellow fever

We have experienced several distinct waves of development (Figure 2.4); we have begun to see the new wave of an amalgamation of artificial intelligence and biotechnology.

The health of the future that we foresee in 2040 will be nothing like what we have now. We may reasonably expect digital transformation—enabled by fundamentally interoperable data, AI, and open, secure platforms—to drive much of this shift based on emerging technology. We believe that, unlike today, care will be organized around the consumer rather than the institutions that currently drive our healthcare system (Figure 2.4).

Big health data streaming, along with data from numerous other relevant sources, will most likely merge by 2040 (and possibly much before) to generate a complex and highly tailored picture of each consumer's wellbeing. Many digital health companies are already incorporating always-on biosensors and software into data-generating, data-gathering, and data-sharing devices. Advanced cognitive technologies could be created to assess many parameters and provide individualized health information to consumers. Data availability and personalized AI can enable precision wellbeing and real-time micro-interventions, allowing us to stay ahead of sickness and catastrophic disease. By 2040, health will almost certainly revolve around preventing many more diseases than curing them. Long-term diseases with a persistent need for medication to alleviate symptoms would affect far fewer people.

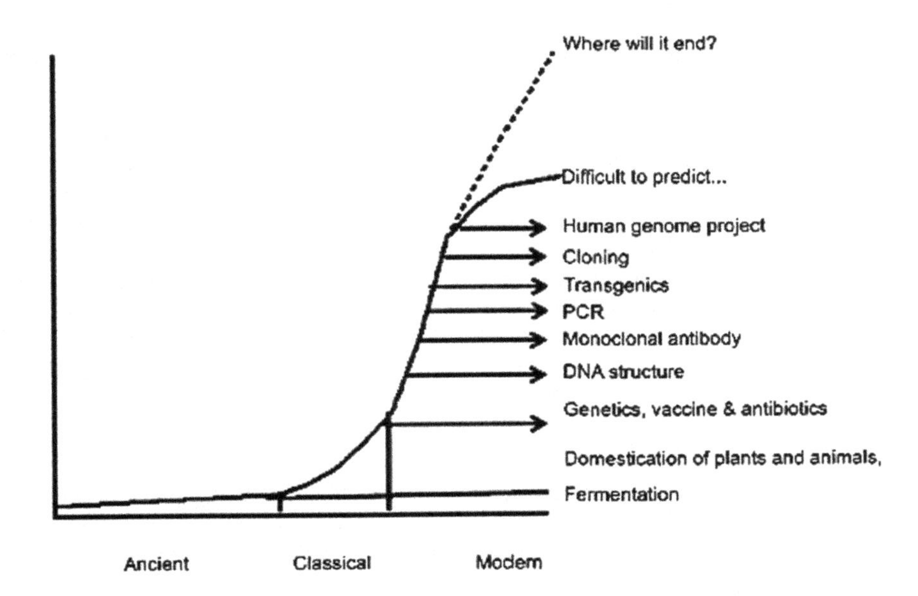

FIGURE 2.3 An exponential rise of new technologies.

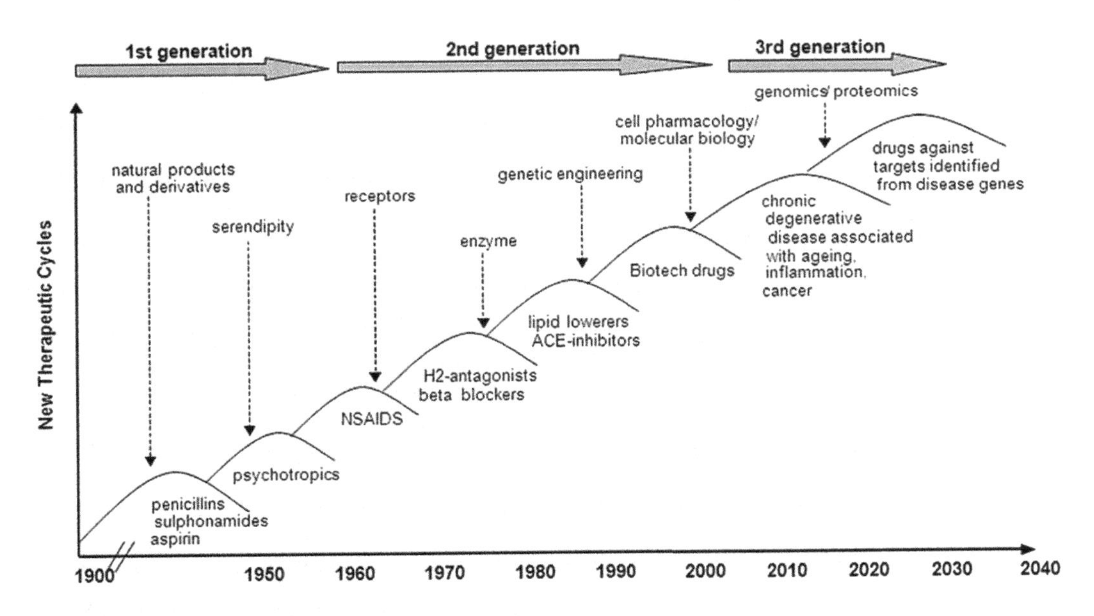

FIGURE 2.4 140 years of drug discoveries.

In the future, the era of blockbuster drugs that treat large populations will likely wane as they will be replaced with hyper-tailored therapies to cure or prevent disease rather than treat symptoms. A significant projection states that the world population will begin to dwindle within 45 years, shifting the focus to late age diseases and smaller patient populations. This reverse trend in population growth, for the first time since we began counting, is driven by the economic capping and peaking of resource consumers versus the resource producers. No planning for the medicines of the future should ignore this projection.

Personalized medications based on various patient features, such as genomes, metabolome, microbiome, and other clinical data, could be made or compounded just in time by additive manufacturing

20 years from now, rather than picking up a prescription at the pharmacy. The critical driving elements can be summarized as:

- Early detection and prediction: A major pillar of thinking on the future of health is disease prevention and a shift to wellness. Over the next 20 years, we will detect and prevent some diseases from progressing, maybe even before symptoms appear. Clinicians can now detect the early stages of melanoma far sooner than in the past, and the illness can be cured with the initial treatment. They are not waiting to intervene until it has spread to the point of causing difficulties and costly therapies. Other types of cancer could be detected earlier, reducing or eliminating the need for future treatments. Chronic disorders like Alzheimer's, diabetes, and rheumatoid arthritis may be more efficiently treated if detected early. Early discovery of a disease, or knowledge that a disease may be preventable, may encourage people to live better lifestyles. Emerging technologies have the potential to significantly increase our ability to diagnose disease in its early stages.
- Instant monitoring: A smart toilet, for example, tests nitrites, glucose, protein, and pH for suspected illnesses or disorders using always-on sensors. Biomarkers that signal a future change in health state could be detected using AI before symptoms manifest. A mole could be distinguished from a melanoma using technology implanted in a bathroom mirror. We've already made strides in our ability to diagnose cancer in its early stages. Whole-genome sequencing is a revolutionary and powerful tool. Early diagnosis of a disease, or the ability to recognize who is genetically prone to disease, could allow for the cure or prevention of an ailment in its early stages. As gene sequencing, our ability to interpret data, and gene-editing tools progress, we anticipate seeing an increase in early detection and preventative or curative therapies.
- Vaccines: In 2006, the US Food and Drug Administration (FDA) approved the first vaccine to prevent cervical cancer caused by the human papillomavirus (HPV). Other virally transfused cancers include the human T-lymphotropic virus type 3 (HTLV-3) and the hepatitis B and C viruses, which cause liver cancer. Various vaccinations to prevent more types of cancer could be developed in the next 20 years. By utilizing the patient's immunity against self-antigens generated in tumor cells, the industry is beginning to think differently about the impact vaccinations could have on various types of cancer. While these are vaccines, they have nothing in common with vaccines that protect against infectious agents. Vaccine distribution may shift away from the usual syringe in the coming years, such as giving influenza vaccine through a bandage strip laced with a patch of painless microneedles just long enough to penetrate the skin. The needles disintegrate within minutes of the vaccination being administered, and the bandage can be discarded. Such patches might be distributed directly to patients who could administer the vaccination themselves in the future, enhancing access and adoption. The most significant development in vaccination history occurred in 2020 when the FDA allowed emergency use authorization of two mRNA vaccines to combat the spread of COVID-19. This approval opens the door to a plethora of low-cost vaccinations that may be developed swiftly to prevent pandemics and various difficult diseases such as cancer and autoimmune disorders.
- Vaccines to prevent autoimmune diseases: While vaccines are typically used to prevent infections in which an antigen (e.g., an attenuated virus) is introduced into the body and antibodies against that virus are produced to prevent real-time infection, the recent approval of mRNA vaccines opens up a new venue for vaccines to prevent autoimmune disorders. A universal vaccination will have a mixture of a protein antigen that causes autoimmune disease or epitope peptides of that protein antigen and a recombinant eukaryotic vector inserted into polyclonal sites by an autoantigen or epitope peptides of that autoantigen. Examples include: insulin, glutamic acid decarboxylase, or heat shock protein, two myelin antigens, zona pellucida 3, myoglobulin, type II collagen, thyroglobulin, cell membrane surface antigen, type II colloid antigen, acetylcholine receptor, thyroid cell surface antigen, salivary gland duct antigen, thyroglobulin, superantigen, or interphotoreceptor retina. This vaccine will successfully prevent and cure autoimmune disorders by inhibiting the growth of T cells in immunological animals

and people, inducing immune suppression, and preventing and treating autoimmune diseases. A disease-focused vaccination, such as an mRNA vaccine, produced proteins against antibodies responsible for pancreatic beta-cell death, where endogenous antibodies are recognized as antigens. The mRNA protein encodes an antibody against the endogenous antibodies.

- Microbiome and nutrition: Researchers are only beginning to comprehend the relationship between these small creatures and how they influence mental and physical health because everyone has a distinct microbiome. Our body's estimated 38 trillion microbes can have an impact on our physical and emotional wellbeing, giving new meaning to the term "you are what you eat." A greater understanding of the microbiome may pave the path for more effective disease prevention. Microbes discovered in the stomachs of children, for example, may be linked to childhood disorders like type 1 diabetes. The microbiome may influence a patient's susceptibility to specific types of cancer or how well they respond to immunotherapy.
- Individualized treatment: Every person expresses disease and uniquely responds to treatment. Because we don't yet know how to stratify patient groups adequately, the great majority of patients may not obtain the full potential benefit of the pharmaceuticals they are treated with. A therapy that works for one patient might not work for another and never reach the ideal active concentration. Giving each patient a customized dose or the best treatment combination could improve their outcomes. Personalized treatment is defined as a single therapy or a combination of selected, adapted, or invented therapies used to treat a specific person. This necessitates the use of data to determine the optimal medication treatment option (single or combination therapy), the proper dosing, and even tailoring treatment for a specific patient. Researchers will require a lot of data to reach this level of personalization, either through real-world evidence (RWE) to target or repurpose current drugs effectively or from new clinical trial paradigms to find high responders and optimal doses. I believe that the earliest breakthroughs in personalized medicines will be observed with generic and late–life cycle pharmaceuticals, which have a lot of RWE available to inform illness classification, tailored doses, and tailored regimens due to data requirements.
- Disease stratification for targeting: Researchers have been able to identify subpopulations within broader illness categories thanks to advances in biomarkers and genetic markers. Parkinson's disease, for example, is divided into many genetic subtypes and mutations. Parkinson's disease is a collection of distinct disorders, and certain forms of the disease seem different than others. We will most likely identify even smaller subsets of patients in the future based on genetic abnormalities, protein expression variations, and the microbiome. Predictive analytics and the ability to evaluate longitudinal and integrated data sets for a variety of patient groups could aid biopharmaceutical companies in determining the best dose amounts for patients, as well as who is most likely to respond and under what circumstances. These data could aid companies in developing tailored treatment regimens for specific patient groups. Data on how a patient metabolizes a medicine could be utilized to ensure precise dosing, maximizing efficacy while minimizing toxicity. Clinicians in the future may be able to look at various biomarkers and genetic data, as well as clinical and behavioral digital health data, to select the best medicine combinations for a patient. This might work in the same way that doctors can sequence tumors, find mutations, and match cancer patients to the right treatment. In the late 1970s, my invention exemplified target focus by coating the gut with a fluorocarbon liquid to inhibit calorie absorption as an interventional therapy for weight loss (US Patent No. 6235796).
- Manufacturing of pharmaceuticals: Drug delivery could be revolutionized as a result of additive drug production. At the point of treatment, active pharmaceutical ingredients (APIs) might be blended to provide personalized therapies. Rather than giving them multiple medications, we will give them just one. Spritam was the first 3D-printed medicine approved by the FDA in 2015, and it was used to treat epilepsy. Furthermore, companies like FabRX are using 3D printing to create tailored pharmaceuticals. Printlets, FabRX's exclusive technology, allows for customizable dosages, polypills, chewable medications, and fast-acting tablets. Manufacturers and clinicians could use 3D printing to build highly customized, low-cost medical technology

items tailored to each patient's unique physiology. Prosthetics, skin for burn patients, organs, and implants (dental and orthopedic) can be made using 3D printing. The 3D printing of airway splints for babies with tracheobronchomalacia is a rare application. Tissue engineering, in combination with additive manufacturing, could be utilized to repair injured tissues. We could repair it, regenerate tissue, or produce substitutes, perhaps through xenotransplantation, which could cure chronic diseases and eliminate the need for long-term medication. To keep up with the growing demand for this production mode, recombinant manufacturing will expand to higher species, such as animals and plants, where larger quantities may be expressed at a low cost with fewer variances in the molecular structure.

- Healing therapies: Time-limited treatments that eliminate symptoms of a disease by correcting the underlying issue permanently (or semi-permanently) have the potential to lessen the incidence and prevalence of many diseases. Diseases caused by single genetic mutations (for example, certain malignancies, sickle cell anemia, and several rare disorders) would be among the first to receive curative treatments. In the United States, the first gene treatment was approved in 2019, and many more are in the works. For disorders including cystic fibrosis, sickle cell disease, fragile X syndrome, muscular dystrophy, and Huntington's disease, most of these medicines target a single or a few genetic abnormalities.

2.8 New Entities

An Appendix to the chapter lists the NMEs that the FDA has approved in the past decade, bringing the total new drugs to around 1,600, a relatively small size considering the opportunities to treat that remain unattended. Table 2.2 lists the frequency of drug approvals of a specific class or indication.

Some drugs are classified as new molecular entities ("NMEs") for purposes of regulatory classification. Many of these products, either as a single-ingredient medicine or as part of a combination product, contain active moieties that have never been licensed or approved by regulatory agencies before; these products frequently provide vital new therapies for patients. The NMEs may include active moieties that are closely linked to functional moieties in products that regulatory agencies have already approved. The FDA classifies biological products submitted in an application under section 351(a) of the Public Health Service Act as NMEs, regardless of whether the FDA has previously approved a comparable active component in a different product. The FDA's classification of medicine as a "new chemical entity," or "NCE," under the Federal Food, Drug, and Cosmetic Act differs from the FDA's classification of a drug as a "new medicinal entity," or "NME," for review purposes.

Of the 1600 NMEs and NCEs approved by the FDA, over 20% were biologics, and the percentage of new drugs coming as biologics is increasing rapidly (Figure 2.4). A review of the types of drugs approved over the past decade helps to understand drug discovery trends. Biological medicines, soluble receptor constructions, immunoglobulin fusion proteins, and the release of naturally occurring proteins are all dominated by antibodies. The anti-TNF alpha-blocking antibodies (infliximab, adalimumab) and the soluble TNF receptor fusion protein (etanercept) for the treatment of rheumatoid arthritis, the anti-CD20 antibody rituximab for Hodgkin's non-lymphoma, the anti-vascular endothelial growth factor A (VEGF-A) antibody bevacizumab for color

Beyond these "traditional" medications, the biologics market has exploded in recent years. This tendency will accelerate in the following years, for example, by introducing antibody small molecular weight drug conjugates or bispecific antibodies (Figure 2.2). Although biologics are now only accessible for secreted or cell surface targets, they have a high affinity for and specificity for their targets. Better procedures for selecting patients and measuring their reactions during a clinical trial, for example, can transfer immediately into improved diagnostic and monitoring approaches in the clinic.

Modernizing the medical product development sciences will also create new opportunities to improve product safety. Other areas of science, particularly genomics, proteomics, and related disciplines and bioinformatics hold great promise for better scientific understanding and prevention of safety problems. The premarket safety evaluation needs to change from a passive, empirical (i.e., trial and error), patient-exposure-based assessment of adverse events for a predictive evaluation based on a robust body of

TABLE 2.2

Frequency of Class of Drugs or Diseases Indicated for Drugs Approved in the Past Decade

Drug Class/Disease	# NMEs
Fusion protein (mab)	89
Cancer	76
Inhibitors (nib)	55
Infection	44
Antibiotics (cin)	34
Leukemia	18
Imaging	15
Antivirus	14
Tumors	14
Diagnostic	12
Multiple myeloma	12
Skin	11
Fibrosis	10
Chemotherapy	9
Sarcoma	9
Kidney disease	9
Hypertension	8
Multiple sclerosis	8
Psoriasis	8
Asthma	7
Diabetes	7
Liver	7
MAB (cept)	7
Pain	7
Schizophrenia	7
Radioactive	6
Arthritis	5
Hormone	3
Bipolar	2
Crohn's disease	2
Psychosis	2

prior knowledge about the molecular/or physical mechanisms product. Like markers that predict which patients are likely to respond positively to a product, the use of new safety biomarkers can translate rapidly from the experimental setting to the clinic.

2.8.1 A Special Case

Neurological disorders are common. For example, in the United States, a brain disability affects 6.5% to 7.9% of adults. According to the CDC, there are 5.3 million cases of Alzheimer's disease, 30,000 cases of ALS, 30,000 cases of Huntington's disease, and 2.3 million cases of epilepsy. In the United States, there are one million cases of Parkinson's disease, 28 million cases of migraines, 40 million cases of anxiety disorders, and 350,000 cases of multiple sclerosis.

The data on ClinicalTrials.gov is an excellent source of trend analysis; for instance, AML, the trend for studies retrieved from CT, has been flat since 2005, whereas schizophrenia has a negative direction, implying that targets associated with this disease are less researched (and therefore have dropped in interest). It could mean those previous efforts to learn specific targets were unsuccessful and would be

TABLE 2.3
Neurological Disorder NMEs Approved by the FDA over the Past Decade

Date	Brand	Generic Name	Indication
12/20/19	Caplyta	Lumateperone tosylate	To treat schizophrenia
3/19/19	Zulresso	Brexanolone	To treat postpartum depression (PPD) in adult women
10/5/18	Tegsedi	Inotersen	In adults, to treat polyneuropathy caused by inherited transthyretin-mediated amyloidosis
9/27/18	Emgality	Galcanezumab-gnlm	Adults suffering from migraines should take this medication as a preventative measure
9/14/18	Ajovy	Fremanezumab-vfrm	Adults suffering from migraines should take this medication as a preventative measure
8/20/18	Diacomit	Stiripentol	This drug is used to treat seizures in children aged two and up who have Dravet syndrome
8/10/18	Onpattro	Patisiran	In adult patients with inherited transthyretin-mediated amyloidosis, to treat the polyneuropathy
6/25/18	Epidioloex	Cannabidiol	To treat rare, severe forms of epilepsy
5/17/18	Aimovig	Erenumab-aooe	For the preventive treatment for migraine
10/5/15	Aristada	Aripiprazole lauroxil	To treat adults with schizophrenia
9/17/15	Vraylar	Cariprazine	Adults with schizophrenia and bipolar disorder are treated with this medication
7/10/15	Rexulti	Brexpiprazole	For the treatment of schizophrenia and as a supplement to an antidepressant to treat major depressive disorder

unwise to devote additional resources to them. The decrease in CT reports linked to schizophrenia suggests a reduction in interest in the disease.

The FDA has approved over 250 new molecular entities over the last decade with the fewest drugs for neurological disorders (Table 2.3).

The slow entry of NMEs as neurological drugs comes despite many advances in basic neuroscience research that allowed identifying the genetic, molecular, cellular, and neurocircuitry aspects governing behavior. Today, we can probe brain activity in humans and experimental animals with a degree of sophistication that could not be envisioned a decade ago. Current treatments and recent approvals are still large variations on previously identified mechanisms and pathophysiologic hypotheses, which for the most part, were identified serendipitously.

The FDA published many advice documents on clinical trials for Duchenne muscular dystrophy and migraines, as well as draft guidance documents for Alzheimer's illness, ALS, and pediatric seizures. Several novel drug approvals followed the FDA's guidance documents for the treatment or management of several neurologic conditions. Aimovig is the first FDA-approved preventive migraine medication in a new family of pharmaceuticals called calcitonin gene-related peptide inhibitors. This chemical is responsible for migraine attacks. Epidiolex is the first cannabinoid drug to receive FDA approval for the treatment of Dravet and Lennox-Gastaut syndromes. Onpattro is the first FDA-approved treatment for hATTR-related polyneuropathy, a rare, severe, and frequently deadly genetic condition marked by aberrant amyloid protein buildup in peripheral nerves, the heart, and other organs. Onpattro is the first FDA-approved medication for a new type of minor interfering ribonucleic acid.

Advances in understanding biomarkers and genetic markers have helped researchers identify subpopulations within broader disease categories. Parkinson's disease, for example, has several distinct genetic subsets and various mutations. It's a set of discrete conditions and some variations of Parkinson's look different than others. Improving the chances of drug discovery for neurological disorders will require:

- Increased use of patient selection and stratification biomarkers, along with the RDoC approach.
- Increased focus on human genetics-defined targets ("reverse translation").

- Adopt human neurobiology-informed approaches for novel target identification based on pathophysiology hypotheses and clinical observations.
- Increased use of translatable biomarkers linked to behavioral assessments and clinical endpoints.
- Adopt animal models that capture specific domains of pathophysiology instead of pretending to fully reproduce complex disorders in preclinical species ("reverse translation").
- Increased use of objective biomarker-based endpoints.
- Digitally captured endpoints that allow for repeated testing, increasing statistical power.
- Increased use of imaging and electrophysiological biomarkers to show target engagement and central pharmacodynamic activity.
- Consider mRNA therapeutics—nucleic acid–based therapeutics, including the use of messenger RNA (mRNA) as a drug molecule. Cationic liposomal formulation of mRNA delivered by intranasal delivery to the brain can stably express proteins. Luciferase mRNA encapsulated in cationic liposomes can quantify mRNA expression distribution in the brain, mainly in the cortex, striatum, and midbrain regions. There is a high possibility to demonstrate the feasibility of brain-specific, nonviral mRNA delivery to treat various neurological disorders.

The search may likely return to holistic therapies for neurological disorders, including botanicals and food supplements that might enhance the pharmacology of the drugs currently used.

2.9 Conclusion

Human instinct drove us to experiment with our surroundings to deliver solutions to our ailments, as the foragers moved around; today, we are using AI to create molecules that will target our bodies' receptors—the emphasis has returned to prevention over curing. Looking from hindsight, where we stand today represents a true nonlinear trend in technology adoption made possible by a better understanding of diseases. We may not be able to prevent death, and if we could, this would exemplify what I am defining as a nonlinear event, but we will certainly see a remarkable extension of life, better lived. We are shifting from pure chemicals to abstract biological therapies, we are shifting from diagnosis through symptoms to genetic screening, and we will eventually be able to eradicate the diseases that are currently our biggest challenge such as cancer and autoimmune disorders. It is in our genes to progress.

2.10 Appendix: New Molecular Entities Approved by the FDA 2011–2020

12/23/2020: Gemtesa (viberon): To treat overactive bladder

12/21/2020: Ebanga (ansuvimab-zykl): To treat ebola

12/18/2020: Orgovyx relugolix: To treat advanced prostate cancer

12/16/2020: Margenza margetuximab (anti-HER2 mAb): To treat HER2+ breast cancer

12/14/2020: Klisyri tirbanibulin: To treat actinic keratosis of the face or scalp

12/4/2020: Orladeyo berotralstat: To treat patients with hereditary angioedema

12/1/20: Gallium 68 PSMA-11: For detection and localization of prostate cancer

11/28/20: Firdapse (amifampridine): To treat Lambert-Eaton myasthenic syndrome (LEMS) in adults

11/25/20: Danyelza (naxitamab-gqgk): To treat high-risk refractory or relapsed neuroblastoma

11/25/20: Imcivree (setmelanotide): To treat obesity and the control of hunger associated with pro-opiomelanocortin deficiency, a rare disorder that causes severe obesity that begins at an early age

11/23/20: Oxlumo (lumasiran): To treat hyperoxaluria type 1

11/20/20: Zokinvy (lonafarnib): To treat rare conditions related to premature aging

10/22/20: Veklury (remdesivir): To treat COVID-19

10/14/20: Inmazeb (atoltivimab, maftivimab, and odesivimab-ebgn): To treat ebola virus

9/4/20: Gavreto (pralsetinib): To treat non-small lung cancer

9/3/20: Detectnet (copper Cu 64 dotatate injection): To help detect certain types of neuroendocrine tumors

8/28/20: Sogroya (somapacitan-beco): Growth hormone

8/26/20: Winlevi (clascoterone): To treat acne

8/14/20: Enspryng (satralizumab-mwge): To treat neuromyelitis optica spectrum disorder

8/12/20: Viltepso (viltolarsen): To treat Duchenne muscular dystrophy

8/7/20: Olinvyk (oliceridine): To manage acute pain in certain adults

8/7/20: Evrysdi (risdiplam): To treat spinal muscular atrophy

8/6/20: Lampit (nifurtimox): To treat Chagas disease in certain pediatric patients younger than age 18

8/5/20: Blenrep (belantamab mafodotin-blmf): To treat multiple myeloma

7/31/20: Monjuvi (tafasitamab-cxix): To treat relapsed or refractory diffuse large B-cell lymphoma

7/24/20: Xeglyze (abametapir): To treat head lice

7/7/20: Inqovi (decitabine and cedazuridine): To treat adult patients with myelodysplastic syndromes

7/2/20: Rukobia (fostemsavir): To treat HIV

7/2/20: Byfavo (remimazolam): For sedation

6/30/20: Dojolvi (triheptanoin): To treat molecularly long-chain fatty acid oxidation disorders

6/15/20: Zepzelca (lurbinectedin): To treat metastatic small cell lung cancer

6/11/20: Uplizna (inebilizumab-cdon): To treat neuromyelitis optica spectrum disorder

5/28/20: Tauvid (flortaucipir F18): Diagnostic agent for patients with Alzheimer's disease

5/26/20: Artesunate (artesunate): To treat severe malaria

5/20/20: Cerianna (fluoroestrdiol F18): Diagnostic imaging agent for certain patients with breast cancer

5/15/20: Qinlock (ripretinib): To treat advanced gastrointestinal-stromal tumors

5/8/20: Retevmo (selpercatinib): To treat lung and thyroid cancers

5/6/20: Tabrecta (capmatinib): To treat patients with non-small cell lung cancer

4/24/20: Ongentys (opicapone): To treat patients with Parkinson's disease experiencing "off" episodes

4/22/20: Trodelvy (sacituzumab govitecan-hziy): To treat adult patients with metastatic triple-negative breast cancer who received at least two prior therapies for metastatic disease

4/17/20: Pemazyre (pemigatinib): To treat certain patients with cholangiocarcinoma, a rare form of cancer that forms in bile ducts

4/17/20: Tukysa (tucatinib): To treat advanced unresectable or metastatic HER2-positive breast cancer

4/10/20: Koselugo (selumetinib): To treat neurofibromatosis type 1, a genetic disorder of the nervous system causing tumors to grow on nerves

3/25/20: Zeposia (ozanimod): To treat relapsing forms of multiple sclerosis

3/6/20: Isturisa (osilodrostat): To treat adults with Cushing's disease who either cannot undergo pituitary gland surgery or have undergone the surgery but still have the disease

3/2/20: Sarclisa (isatuximab): To treat multiple myeloma

2/27/20: Nurtec ODT (rimegepant): To treat migraine

2/26/20: Barhemsys (amisulpride): To help prevent nausea and vomiting after surgery

2/21/20: Vyepti (eptinezumab-jjmr): For the preventive treatment of migraine in adults

2/21/20: Nexletol (bempedoic acid): To treat adults with heterozygous familial hypercholesterolemia or established atherosclerotic cardiovascular disease who require additional lowering of LDL-C

2/12/20: Pizensy (lactitol): To treat chronic idiopathic constipation (CIC) in adults

1/23/20: Tazverik (tazemetostat): To treat epithelioid sarcoma

1/21/20: Tepezza (teprotumumab-trbw): To treat thyroid eye disease

1/9/20: Ayvakit (avapritinib): To treat adults with unresectable or metastatic gastrointestinal stromal tumor (GIST)

12/23/19: Ubrelvy (ubrogepant): to treat acute treatment of migraine with or without aura in adults

12/20/19: Enhertu (fam-trastuzumab deruxtecan-nxki): To treat metastatic breast cancer

12/20/19: Dayvigo (lemborexant): To treat insomnia

12/20/19: Caplyta (lumateperone tosylate): To treat schizophrenia

12/20/19: TissueBlue (Brilliant Blue G Ophthalmic Solution): Dye used in eye surgery

12/18/19: Padcev (enfortumab vedotin-ejfv): To treat refractory bladder cancer

12/12/19: Vyondys 53 (golodirsen): To treat certain patients with Duchenne muscular dystrophy

11/25/19: Oxbryta (voxelotor): To treat sickle cell disease

11/21/19: Xcopri (cenobamate): To treat partial onset seizures

11/20/19: Givlaari (givosiran): To treat acute hepatic porphyria, a rare blood disorder

11/15/19: Adakveo (crizanlizumab-tmca): To treat patients with painful complication of sickle cell disease

11/14/19: Fetroja (cefiderocol): To treat patients with complicated urinary tract infections who have limited or no alternative treatment options

11/14/19: Brukinsa (zanubrutinib): To treat certain patients with mantle cell lymphoma, a form of blood cancer

11/8/19: Reblozyl (luspatercept–aamt): For the treatment of anemia in adult patients with beta thalassemia who require regular red blood cell transfusions

11/7/19: ExEm Foam (air polymer-type A): A diagnostic agent used to assess fallopian tube patency (openness) in women with known or suspected infertility

10/21/19: Trikafta (elexacaftor/ivacaftor/tezacaftor): To treat patients 12 years of age and older with the most common gene mutation that causes cystic fibrosis

10/11/19: Reyvow (lasmiditan): For the acute treatment of migraine with or without aura, in adults

10/10/19: Fluorodopa F 18: A diagnostic agent for use in positron emission tomography (PET) to help diagnose adult patients with suspected Parkinsonian syndromes (PS)

10/8/19: Scenesse (afamelanotide): To increase pain-free light exposure in adult patients with a history of phototoxic reactions (damage to skin) from erythropoietic protoporphyria

10/7/19: Beovu (brolucizumab–dbll): Treatment of wet age-related macular degeneration

10/4/19: Aklief (trifarotene): For the topical treatment of acne vulgaris in patients nine years of age and older

9/12/19: Ibsrela (tenapanor): To treat irritable bowel syndrome with constipation in adults

8/27/19: Nourianz (istradefylline): To treat adult patients with Parkinson's disease experiencing "off" episodes

8/21/19: Ga-68-DOTATOC: For use with positron emission tomography (PET) for localization of somatostatin receptor positive neuroendocrine tumors (NETs)

8/19/19: Xenleta (lefamulin): To treat adults with community-acquired bacterial pneumonia

8/16/19: Rinvoq (upadacitinib): To treat adults with moderately to severely active rheumatoid arthritis

8/16/19: Inrebic (fedratinib): To treat adult patients with intermediate-2 or high-risk primary or secondary myelofibrosis

8/15/19: Rozlytrek (entrectinib): To treat adult patients with metastatic non-small cell lung cancer (NSCLC) whose tumors are ROS1-positive

8/14/19: Wakix (pitolisant): To treat excessive daytime sleepiness (EDS) in adult patients with narcolepsy

8/14/19: Pretomanid (PA-824): For treatment-resistant forms of tuberculosis that affects the lungs

8/2/19: Turalio (pexidartinib): To treat adult patients with symptomatic tenosynovial giant cell tumor

7/30/19: Nubeqa (darolutamide): To treat adult patients with non-metastatic castration resistant prostate cancer

7/25/19: Accrufer (ferric maltol): To treat iron deficiency anemia in adults

7/16/19: Recarbrio (imipenem, cilastatin, and relebactam): To treat complicated urinary tract and complicated intra-abdominal infections

7/3/19: Xpovio (selinexor): To treat adult patients with relapsed or refractory multiple myeloma (RRMM)

6/10/19: Polivy (polatuzumab vedotin-piiq): To treat adult patients with relapsed or refractory diffuse large B-cell lymphoma

5/24/19: Piqray (alpelisib): To treat breast cancer

5/3/19: Vyndaqel (tafamidis meglumine): To treat heart disease (cardiomyopathy) caused by transthyretin mediated amyloidosis (ATTR-CM) in adults

4/23/19: Skyrizi (risankizumab-rzaa): To treat moderate-to-severe plaque psoriasis in adults who are candidates for systemic therapy or phototherapy

4/12/19: Balversa (erdafitinib): To treat adult patients with locally advanced or metastatic bladder cancer

4/9/19: Evenity (romosozumab-aqqg): To treat osteoporosis in postmenopausal women at high risk of fracture

3/26/19: Mayzent (siponimod): To treat adults with relapsing forms of multiple sclerosis

3/20/19: Sunosi (solriamfetol): To treat excessive sleepiness in adult patients with narcolepsy or obstructive sleep apnea

3/19/19: Zulresso (brexanolone): To treat postpartum depression (PPD) in adult women

2/13/19: Egaten (triclabendazole): To treat fascioliasis, a parasitic infestation caused by two species of flatworms or trematodes that mainly the affect the liver, sometimes referred to as "liver flukes"

2/6/19: Cablivi (caplacizumab-yhdp): To treat adult patients with acquired thrombotic thrombocytopenic purpura (aTTP)

2/1/2019: Jeuveau (prabotulinumtoxinA-xvfs): For the temporary improvement in the appearance of moderate to severe glabellar lines associated with corrugator and/or procerus muscle activity in adult patients

12/21/18: Ultomiris (ravulizumab): To treat paroxysmal nocturnal hemoglobinuria (PNH)

12/21/18: Elzonris (tagraxofusp-erzs): To treat blastic plasmacytoid dendritic cell neoplasm (BPDCN)

12/20/18: Asparlas (calaspargase pegol-mknl): To treat acute lymphoblastic leukemia (ALL) in pediatric and young adult patients age one month to 21 years

12/14/18: Motegrity (prucalopride): To treat chronic idiopathic constipation

11/28/18: Xospata (gilteritinib): To treat patients who have relapsed or refractory acute myeloid leukemia (AML)

11/26/18: Vitrakvi (larotrectinib): To treat patients whose cancers have a specific genetic feature (biomarker)

11/21/18: Daurismo (glasdegib): To treat newly-diagnosed acute myeloid leukemia (AML) in adult patients

11/20/18: Gamifant (emapalumab-lzsgemapalumab-lzsg): To treat primary hemophagocytic lymphohistiocytosis (HLH)

11/16/18: Aemcolo (rifamycin): To treat travelers' diarrhea

11/9/18: Yupelri (revefenacin): To treat patients with chronic obstructive pulmonary disease (COPD)

11/2/18: Lorbrena (lorlatinib): To treat patients with anaplastic lymphoma kinase (ALK)-positive metastatic non-small cell lung cancer

10/24/18: Xofluza (baloxavir marboxil): To treat acute uncomplicated influenza in patients who have been symptomatic for no more than 48 hours

10/16/18: Talzenna (talazoparib): To treat locally advanced or metastatic breast cancer patients with a germline BRCA mutation

10/5/18: Tegsedi (inotersen): To treat polyneuropathy of hereditary transthyretin-mediated amyloidosis in adults

10/5/18: Revcovi (elapegademase-lvlr): To treat adenosine deaminase-severe combined immunodeficiency (ADA-SCID)

10/2/18: Nuzyra (omadacycline): To treat community-acquired bacterial pneumonia and acute bacterial skin and skin structure infections

10/1/18: Seysara (sarecycline): To treat inflammatory lesions of non-nodular moderate to severe acne vulgaris in patients nine years of age and older

9/28/18: Libtayo (cemiplimab-rwlc): To treat cutaneous squamous cell carcinoma (CSCC)

9/27/18: Vizimpro (dacomitinib): To treat metastatic non-small-cell lung cancer

9/27/18: Emgality (galcanezumab-gnlm): For the preventive treatment of migraine in adults

9/24/18: Copiktra (duvelisib): To treat relapsed or refractory chronic lymphocytic leukemia, small lymphocytic lymphoma, and follicular lymphoma

9/14/18: Ajovy (fremanezumab-vfrm): For the preventive treatment of migraine in adults

9/13/18: Lumoxiti (moxetumomab pasudotox-tdfk): To treat hairy cell leukemia

8/30/18: Pifeltro (doravirine): To treat HIV-1 infection in adult patients

8/27/18: Xerava (eravacycline): To treat complicated intra-abdominal infections in patients 18 years of age and older

8/23/18: Takhzyro (lanadelumab): To treat types I and II hereditary angioedema

8/22/18: Oxervate (cenegermin-bkbj): To treat neurotrophic keratitis

8/20/18: Diacomit (stiripentol): To treat seizures associated with Dravet syndrome in patients two years of age and older taking clobazam

8/10/18: Galafold (migalastat): To treat treat adults with Fabry disease

8/10/18: Annovera (segesterone acetate and ethinyl estradiol vaginal system): New vaginal ring used to prevent pregnancy for an entire year

8/10/18: Onpattro (patisiran): To treat the polyneuropathy of hereditary transthyretin-mediated amyloidosis in adult patients

8/8/18: Poteligeo (mogamulizumab-kpkc): To treat two rare types of non-Hodgkin lymphoma

7/31/18: Mulpleta (lusutrombopag): To treat thrombocytopenia in adult patients with chronic liver disease who are scheduled to undergo a procedure

7/27/18: Omegaven (fish oil triglycerides): As a source of calories and fatty acids in pediatric patients with parenteral nutrition-associated cholestasis

7/23/18: Orilissa (elagolix sodium): For the management of moderate to severe pain associated with endometriosis

7/20/18: Krintafel (tafenoquine): For the radical cure (prevention of relapse) of *Plasmodium vivax* malaria

7/20/18: Tibsovo (ivosidenib): To treat patients with relapsed or refractory acute myeloid leukemia

7/13/18: TPOXX (tecovirimat): To treat smallpox

6/27/18: Braftovi (encorafenib): To treat unresectable or metastatic melanoma

6/27/18: Mektovi (binimetinib): To treat unresectable or metastatic melanoma

6/25/18: Zemdri (plazomicin): To treat adults with complicated urinary tract infections

6/25/18: Epidioloex (cannabidiol): To treat rare, severe forms of epilepsy

6/21/18: Vyleesi (bremelanotide): To treat hypoactive sexual desire disorder in premenopausal women

6/13/18: Moxidectin (moxidectin): To treat onchocerciasis due to *Onchocerca volvulus* in patients aged 12 years and older

5/31/18: Olumiant (baricitinib): To treat moderately to severely active rheumatoid arthritis

5/24/18: Palynziq (pegvaliase-pqpz): To treat adults with a rare and serious genetic disease known as phenylketonuria (PKU)

5/21/18: Doptelet (avatrombopag): To treat low blood platelet count (thrombocytopenia) in adults with chronic liver disease who are scheduled to undergo a medical or dental procedure

5/18/18: Lokelma (sodium zirconium cyclosilicate): To treat hyperkalemia

5/17/18: Aimovig (erenumab-aooe): For the preventive treatment for migraine

5/16/18: Lucemyra (lofexidine hydrochloride): For the non-opioid treatment for management of opioid withdrawal symptoms in adults

4/19/18: Akynzeo (fosnetupitant and palonosetron): To prevent acute and delayed nausea and vomiting associated with initial and repeat courses of highly emetogenic cancer chemotherapy

4/17/18: Crysvita (burosumab-twza): To treat adults and children ages one year and older with x-linked hypophosphatemia (XLH), a rare, inherited form of rickets

4/17/18: Tavalisse (fostamatinib): To treat thrombocytopenia in adult patients with persistent or chronic immune thrombocytopenia (ITP)

3/20/18: Ilumya (tildrakizumab): To treat adults with moderate-to-severe plaque psoriasis who are candidates for systemic therapy or phototherapy

3/6/18: Trogarzo (ibalizumab-uiyk): To treat HIV patients who have limited treatment options

2/14/18: Erleada (apalutamide): To treat a certain type of prostate cancer using novel clinical trial endpoint

2/12/18: Symdeko (tezacaftor; ivacaftor): To treat cystic fibrosis in patients age 12 years and older

2/7/18: Biktarvy (bictegravir, embitcitabine, tenofovir alafenamide): To treat infection in adults who have no antiretroviral treatment history or to replace the current antiretroviral regimen

1/26/18: Lutathera (lutetium Lu 177 dotatate): To treat a type of cancer that affects the pancreas or gastrointestinal tract called gastroenteropancreatic neuroendocrine tumors (GEP-NETs)

12/21/17: Giapreza (angiotensin II): To increase blood pressure in adults with septic or other distributive shock

12/20/17: Macrilen (macimorelin acetate): For the diagnosis of adult growth hormone deficiency

12/19/17: Steglatro (ertugliflozin): To improve glycemic control in adults with type 2 diabetes mellitus

12/18/17: Rhopressa (netarsudil): To treat glaucoma or ocular hypertension

12/11/17: Xepi (ozenoxacin): To treat impetigo

12/5/17: Ozempic (semaglutide): To improve glycemic control in adults with type 2 diabetes mellitus

11/16/17: Hemlibra (emicizumab): To prevent or reduce the frequency of bleeding episodes in adult and pediatric patients with hemophilia A who have developed antibodies called Factor VIII (FVIII) inhibitors

11/15/17: Mepsevii (vestronidase alfa-vjbk): To treat pediatric and adult patients with an inherited metabolic condition called mucopolysaccharidosis type VII (MPS VII), also known as Sly syndrome

11/14/17: Fasenra (benralizumab): For add-on maintenance treatment of patients with severe asthma aged 12 years and older, and with an eosinophilic phenotype

11/8/17: Prevymis (letermovir): To prevent infection after bone marrow transplant

11/2/17: Vyzulta (latanoprostene bunod ophthalmic solution): To treat intraocular pressure in patients with open-angle glaucoma or ocular hypertension

10/31/17: Calquence (acalabrutinib): To treat adults with mantle cell lymphoma

9/28/17: Verzenio (abemaciclib): To treat certain advanced or metastatic breast cancers

9/15/17: Solosec (secnidazole): To treat bacterial vaginosis

9/14/17: Aliqopa (copanlisib): To treat adults with relapsed follicular lymphoma

8/29/17: Benznidazole): To treat children ages two to 12 years old with Chagas disease

8/29/17: Vabomere (meropenem and vaborbactam): To treat adults with complicated urinary tract infections

8/17/17: Besponsa (inotuzumab ozogamicin): To treat adults with relapsed or refractory acute lymphoblastic leukemia

8/3/17: Mavyret (glecaprevir and pibrentasvir): To treat adults with chronic hepatitis C virus

8/1/17: Idhifa (enasidenib): To treat relapsed or refractory acute myeloid leukemia

7/18/17: Vosevi (sofosbuvir, velpatasvir and voxilaprevir): To treat adults with chronic hepatitis C virus

7/17/17: Nerlynx (neratinib maleate): To reduce the risk of breast cancer returning

7/13/17: Tremfya (guselkumab): For the treatment of adult patients with moderate-to-severe plaque psoriasis

6/23/17: Bevyxxa (betrixaban): For the prophylaxis of venous thromboembolism (VTE) in adult patients hospitalized for an acute medical illness

6/19/17: Baxdela (delafloxacin): To treat patients with acute bacterial skin infections

5/22/17: Kevzara (sarilumab): To treat adult rheumatoid arthritis

5/5/17: Radicava (edaravone): To treat patients with amyotrophic lateral sclerosis (ALS)

5/1/17: Imfinzi (durvalumab): To treat patients with locally advanced or metastatic urothelial carcinoma

4/28/17: Tymlos (abaloparatide): To treat osteoporosis in postmenopausal women at high risk of fracture or those who have failed other therapies

4/28/17: Rydapt (midostaurin): To treat acute myeloid leukemia, advanced systemic mastocytosis

4/28/17: Alunbrig (brigatinib): To treat patients with anaplastic lymphoma kinase (ALK)-positive metastatic non-small cell lung cancer (NSCLC) who have progressed on or are intolerant to crizotinib

4/27/17: Brineura (cerliponase alfa): To treat a specific form of Batten disease

4/11/17: Ingrezza (valbenazine): To treat adults with tardive dyskinesia

4/3/17: Austedo (deutetrabenazine): For the treatment of chorea associated with Huntington's disease

3/28/17: Ocrevus (ocrelizumab): To treat patients with relapsing and primary progressive forms of multiple sclerosis

3/28/17: Dupixent (dupilumab): To treat adults with moderate-to-severe eczema (atopic dermatitis)

3/27/17: Zejula (niraparib): For the maintenance treatment for recurrent epithelial ovarian, fallopian tube or primary peritoneal cancers

3/23/17: Symproic (naldemedine): For the treatment of opioid-induced constipation

3/23/17: Bavencio (avelumab): To treat metastatic Merkel cell carcinoma

3/21/17: Xadago (safinamide): To treat Parkinson's disease

3/13/17: Kisqali (ribociclib): To treat postmenopausal women with a type of advanced breast cancer

2/28/17: Xermelo (telotristat ethyl): To treat carcinoid syndrome diarrhea

2/15/17: Siliq (brodalumab): To treat adults with moderate-to-severe plaque psoriasis

2/9/17: Emflaza (deflazacort): To treat patients age five years and older with Duchenne muscular dystrophy (DMD)

2/7/17: Parsabiv (etelcalcetide): To treat secondary hyperparathyroidism in adult patients with chronic kidney disease undergoing dialysis

1/19/17: Trulance (plecanatide): To treat chronic idiopathic constipation (CIC) in adult patients.

12/23/16: Spinraza (nusinersen): To treat children and adults with spinal muscular atrophy (SMA)

12/19/16: Rubraca (rucaparib): To treat women with a certain type of ovarian cancer

12/14/16: Eucrisa (crisaborole): To treat mild to moderate eczema (atopic dermatitis) in patients two years of age and older

10/21/16: Zinplava (bezlotoxumab): To reduce the recurrence of Clostridium difficile infection in patients aged 18 years or older

10/19/16: Lartruvo (olaratumab): To treat adults with certain types of soft tissue sarcoma

9/19/16: Exondys 51 (eteplirsen): To treat patients with Duchenne muscular dystrophy

7/27/16: Adlyxin (lixisenatide): To improve glycemic control (blood sugar levels)

7/11/16: Xiidra (lifitegrast ophthalmic solution): To treat the signs and symptoms of dry eye disease

6/28/16: Epclusa (sofosbuvir and velpatasvir): To treat all six major forms of hepatitis C virus

6/1/16: NETSPOT (gallium Ga 68 dotatate): A diagnostic imaging agent to detect rare neuroendocrine tumors

5/27/16: Axumin (fluciclovine F 18): A new diagnostic imaging agent to detect recurrent prostate cancer

5/27/16: Ocaliva (obeticholic acid): To treat rare, chronic liver disease

5/27/16: Zinbryta (daclizumab): To treat multiple sclerosis

5/18/16: Tecentriq (atezolizumab): To treat urothelial carcinoma, the most common type of bladder cancer

4/29/16: Nuplazid (pimavanserin): To treat hallucinations and delusions associated with psychosis experienced by some people with Parkinson's disease

4/11/16: Venclexta (venetoclax): For chronic lymphocytic leukemia in patients with a specific chromosomal abnormality

3/30/16: Defitelio (defibrotide sodium): To treat adults and children who develop hepatic veno-occlusive disease with additional kidney or lung abnormalities after they receive a stem cell transplant from blood or bone marrow called hematopoietic stem cell transplantation

3/23/16: Cinqair (reslizumab): To treat severe asthma

3/22/16: Taltz (ixekizumab): To treat adults with moderate-to-severe plaque psoriasis

3/18/16: Anthim (obiltoxaximab): To treat inhalational anthrax in combination with appropriate antibacterial drugs

2/18/16: Briviact (brivaracetam): To treat partial onset seizures in patients age 16 years and older with epilepsy

1/28/16: Zepatier (elbasvir and grazoprevir): To treat patients with chronic hepatitis C virus (HCV) genotypes 1 and 4 infections in adult patients

12/22/15: Zurampic (lesinurad): To treat high blood uric acid levels associated with gout

12/21/15: Uptravi (selexipag): To treat pulmonary arterial hypertension

12/15/15: Bridion (sugammadex): To reverse effects of neuromuscular blocking drugs used during surgery

12/11/15: Alecensa (alectinib): To treat ALK-positive lung cancer

12/8/15: Kanuma (sebelipase alfa): To treat patients with a rare disease known as lysosomal acid lipase (LAL) deficiency

11/30/15: Empliciti (elotuzumab): To treat people with multiple myeloma who have received one to three prior medications

11/24/15: Portrazza (necitumumab): To treat patients with advanced (metastatic) squamous non-small cell lung cancer (NSCLC) who have not previously received medication specifically for treating their advanced lung cancer

11/20/15: Ninlaro (ixazomib): To treat people with multiple myeloma who have received at least one prior therapy

11/16/15: Darzalex (daratumumab): To treat patients with multiple myeloma who have received at least three prior treatments

11/13/15: Tagrisso (osimertinib): To treat certain patients with non-small cell lung cancer

11/10/15: Cotellic (cobimetinib): To be used in combination with vemurafenib to treat advanced melanoma that has spread to other parts of the body or can't be removed by surgery, and that has a certain type of abnormal gene (BRAF V600E or V600K mutation)

11/5/15: Genvoya (a fixed-dose combination tablet containing elvitegravir, cobicistat, emtricitabine, and tenofovir alafenamide): For use as a complete regimen for the treatment of HIV-1 infection in adults and pediatric patients 12 years of age and older

11/4/15: Nucala (mepolizumab): For use with other asthma medicines for the maintenance treatment of asthma in patients age 12 years and older

10/23/15: Strensiq (asfotase alfa): To treat perinatal, infantile, and juvenile-onset hypophosphatasia (HPP)

10/23/15: Yondelis (trabectedin): To treat specific soft tissue sarcomas (STS)—liposarcoma and leiomyosarcoma—that cannot be removed by surgery (unresectable) or is advanced (metastatic)

10/21/15: Veltassa (patiromer for oral suspension): To treat hyperkalemia, a serious condition in which the amount of potassium in the blood is too high

10/16/15: Praxbind (idarucizumab): For use in patients who are taking the anticoagulant Pradaxa (dabigatran) during emergency situations when there is a need to reverse Pradaxa's blood-thinning effects

10/5/15: Aristada (aripiprazole lauroxil): To treat adults with schizophrenia

9/25/15: Tresiba (insulin degludec injection): To improve blood sugar (glucose) control in adults with diabetes mellitus

9/22/15: Lonsurf (trifluridine and tipiracil): To treat patients with an advanced form of colorectal cancer who are no longer responding to other therapies

9/17/15: Vraylar (cariprazine): To treat schizophrenia and bipolar disorder in adults

9/4/15: Xuriden (uridine triacetate): To treat patients with hereditary orotic aciduria

9/1/15: Varubi (rolapitant): To prevent delayed phase chemotherapy-induced nausea and vomiting (emesis)

8/27/15: Repatha (evolocumab): To treat certain patients with high cholesterol

8/18/15: Addyi (flibanserin): To treat acquired, generalized hypoactive sexual desire disorder (HSDD) in premenopausal women

7/24/15: Daklinza (daclatasvir): To treat chronic hepatitis C virus (HCV) genotype 3 infections

7/24/15: Odomzo (sonidegib): To treat patients with locally advanced basal cell carcinoma that has recurred following surgery or radiation therapy, or who are not candidates for surgery or radiation therapy

7/24/15: Praluent (alirocumab): To treat certain patients with high cholesterol

7/10/15: Rexulti (brexpiprazole): To treat schizophrenia and as an add on to an antidepressant to treat major depressive disorder

7/7/15: Entresto (sacubitril/valsartan): To treat heart failure

7/2/15: Orkambi (lumacaftor 200 mg/ivacaftor 125 mg): To treat cystic fibrosis

6/22/15: Kengreal (cangrelor): To prevent the formation of harmful blood clots in the coronary arteries for adult patients undergoing percutaneous coronary intervention

5/27/15: Viberzi (eluxadoline): To treat irritable bowel syndrome with diarrhea (IBS-D) in adult men and women.

4/29/15: Kybella (deoxycholic acid): To treat adults with moderate-to-severe fat below the chin, known as submental fat

4/15/15: Corlanor (ivabradine): To reduce hospitalization from worsening heart failure

3/17/15: Cholbam (cholic acid): To treat pediatric and adult patients with bile acid synthesis disorders due to single enzyme defects, and for patients with peroxisomal disorders (bile acid synthesis disorders)

3/10/15: Unituxin (dinutuximab): To treat pediatric patients with high-risk neuroblastoma

3/6/15: Cresemba (isavuconazonium sulfate): To treat adults with invasive aspergillosis and invasive mucormycosis, rare but serious infections

2/25/15: Avycaz (ceftazidime-avibactam): To treat adults with complicated intra-abdominal infections (cIAI), in combination with metronidazole, and complicated urinary tract infections (cUTI), including kidney infections (pyelonephritis), who have limited or no alternative treatment options

2/23/15: Farydak (panobinostat): To treat patients with multiple myeloma

2/13/15: Lenvima (lenvatinib): To treat patients with progressive, differentiated thyroid cancer (DTC) whose disease progressed despite receiving radioactive iodine therapy (radioactive iodine refractory disease)

2/3/15: Ibrance (palbociclib): To treat advanced (metastatic) breast cancer

1/23/15: Natpara (parathyroid hormone): To control hypocalcemia (low blood calcium levels) in patients with hypoparathyroidism

1/21/15: Cosentyx (secukinumab): To treat adults with moderate-to-severe plaque psoriasis

1/8/15: Savaysa (edoxaban): To reduce the risk of stroke and dangerous blood clots (systemic embolism) in patients with atrial fibrillation that is not caused by a heart valve problem (atrial fibrillation) (venous thromboembolism)

12/22/14: Opdivo (nivolumab): To treat patients with unresectable (cannot be removed by surgery) or metastatic (advanced) melanoma who no longer respond to other drugs

12/19/14: Rapivab (peramivir): To treat influenza infection in adults

12/19/14: Zerbaxa (ceftolozane/tazobactam): To treat adults with complicated intra-abdominal infections (cIAI) and complicated urinary tract infections (cUTI)

12/19/14: Ombitasvir, paritaprevir, and ritonavir tablets co-packaged with dasabuvir tablets: To treat patients with chronic hepatitis C virus (HCV) genotype 1 infection, including those with a type of advanced liver disease called cirrhosis

12/19/14: Lynparza (olaparib): To treat advanced ovarian cancer

12/17/14: Xtoro (finafloxacin otic suspension): To treat acute otitis externa, commonly known as swimmer's ear

12/3/14: Blincyto (blinatumomab): To treat patients with Philadelphia chromosome-negative precursor B-cell acute lymphoblastic leukemia (B-cell ALL)

10/15/14: Esbriet (pirfenidone): For the treatment of idiopathic pulmonary fibrosis (IPF)

10/15/14: Ofev (nintedanib): For the treatment of idiopathic pulmonary fibrosis (IPF)

10/10/14: Lumason (sulfur hexafluoride lipid microsphere): For patients whose ultrasound image of the heart (echocardiograms) are hard to see with ultrasound waves

10/10/14: Akynzeo (netupitant and palonosetron): To treat nausea and vomiting in patients undergoing cancer chemotherapy

10/10/14: Harvoni (ledipasvir/sofosbuvir): To treat chronic hepatitis C virus (HCV) genotype 1 infection

9/18/14: Trulicity (dulaglutide): To treat adults with type 2 diabetes

9/16/14: Movantik (naloxegol): To treat opioid-induced constipation in adults with chronic non-cancer pain

9/4/14: Keytruda (pembrolizumab): For treatment of patients with advanced or unresectable melanoma who are no longer responding to other drugs

8/19/14: Cerdelga (eliglustat): For the long-term treatment of adult patients with the type 1 form of Gaucher disease

8/15/14: Plegridy (peginterferon beta-1a): For the treatment of patients with relapsing forms of multiple sclerosis

8/13/14: Belsomra (suvorexant): To treat difficulty in falling and staying asleep (insomnia)

8/6/14: Orbactiv (oritavancin): To treat adults with skin infections

8/1/14: Jardiance (empagliflozin): To improve gylcemic control in adults with type 2 diabetes

7/31/14: Striverdi Respimat (olodaterol): To treat chronic obstructive pulmonary disease

7/23/14: Zydelig (idelalisib): To treat patients with trhee types of blood cancers

7/7/14: Kerydin (tavaborole): For the topical treatment of onychomycosis of the toenails

7/3/14: Beleodaq (belinostat): To treat patients with peripheral T-cell lymphoma (PTCL)

6/20/14: Sivextro (tablet or injection) (tedizolid phosphate): To treat adults with skin infections

6/6/14: Jublia (efinaconazole): Treat mild to moderate onychomycosis (fungal infection)

5/23/14: Dalvance (dalbavancin): To treat adults with skin infections

5/20/14: Entyvio (vedolizumab): To treat adult patients with moderate to severe ulcerative colitis and adult patients with moderate to severe Crohn's disease (ulcerative colitis)

5/8/14: Zontivity (vorapaxar): To reduce the risk of heart attacks and stroke in high-risk patients

4/29/14: Zykadia (ceritinib): To treat patients with a certain type of late-stage (metastatic) non-small cell lung cancer (NSCLC)

4/23/14: Sylvant (siltuximab): To treat patients with multicentric Castleman's disease (MCD), a rare disorder similar to lymphoma (cancer of the lymph nodes)

4/21/14: Cyramza (ramucirumab): To treat patients with advanced stomach cancer or gastroesophageal junction adenocarcinoma

4/15/14: Tanzeum (albiglutide): To improve glycemic control, along with diet and exercise, in adults with type 2 diabetes

3/21/14: Otezla (apremilast): To treat adults with active psoriatic arthritis (PsA)

3/19/14: Impavido (miltefosine): To treat a tropical disease called leishmaniasis

3/19/14: Neuraceq (florbetaben F 18 injection): For positron emission tomography (PET) imaging of the brain

2/24/14: Myalept (metreleptin for injection): To treat the complications of leptin deficiency

2/18/14: Northera (droxidopa): To treat neurogenic orthostatic hypotension (NOH)

2/14/14: Vimizim (elosulfase alfa): Treatment for Mucopolysaccharidosis Type IVA (Morquio A syndrome)

1/31/14: Hetlioz (tasimelteon): To treat non-24-hour sleep-wake disorder ("non-24") in totally blind individuals. Non-24 is a chronic circadian rhythm (body clock) disorder in the blind that causes problems with the timing of sleep

1/8/14: Farxiga (dapaglifozin): To improve glycemic control, along with diet and exercise, in adults with type 2 diabetes

12/18/13: Anoro Ellipta (umeclidinium and vilanterol inhalation powder): For the once-daily, long-term maintenance treatment of airflow obstruction in patients with chronic obstructive pulmonary disease (COPD)

12/6/13: Sovaldi (sofosbuvir): To treat chronic hepatitis C virus (HCV) infection

11/22/13: Olysio (simeprevir): To treat chronic hepatitis C virus infection

11/14/13: Luzu (luliconozole): For the topical treatment of interdigital tinea pedis, tinea cruris, and tinea corporis caused by the organisms *Trichophyton rubrum* and *Epidermophyton floccosum*, in patients 18 years of age and older

11/13/13: Imbruvica (ibrutinib): To treat patients with mantle cell lymphoma (MCL), a rare and aggressive type of blood cancer

11/8/13: Aptiom (eslicarbazepine acetate): As an add-on medication to treat seizures associated with epilepsy

11/1/13: Gazyva (obinutuzumab): For use in combination with chlorambucil to treat patients with previously untreated chronic lymphocytic leukemia (CLL)

10/25/13: Vizamyl (flutemetamol F 18 injection): A radioactive diagnostic drug for use with positron emission tomography (PET) imaging of the brain in adults being evaluated for Alzheimer's disease (AD) and dementia

10/18/13: Opsumit (macitentan): To treat adults with pulmonary arterial hypertension (PAH), a chronic, progressive, and debilitating disease that can lead to death or the need for lung transplantation

10/8/13: Adempas (riociguat): To treat adults with two forms of pulmonary hypertension

10/3/13: Duavee (conjugated estrogens/bazedoxifene): To treat moderate-to-severe hot flashes (vasomotor symptoms) associated with menopause and to prevent osteoporosis after menopause

9/30/13: Brintellix (vortioxetine): To treat adults with major depressive disorder

8/12/13: Tivicay (dolutegravir): To treat HIV-1 infection

7/12/13: Gilotrif (afatinib): For patients with late stage (metastatic) non-small cell lung cancer (NSCLC) whose tumors express specific types of epidermal growth factor receptor (EGFR) gene mutations, as detected by an FDA-approved test

5/29/13: Mekinist (trametinib): To treat patients whose tumors express the BRAF V600E or V600K gene mutations

5/29/13: Tafinlar (dabrafenib): To treat patients with melanoma whose tumors express the BRAF V600E gene mutation

5/15/13: Xofigo (radium Ra 223 dichloride): To treat men with symptomatic late-stage (metastatic) castration-resistant prostate cancer that has spread to bones but not to other organs

5/10/13: Breo Ellipta (fluticasone furoate and vilanterol inhalation powder): For the long-term, once-daily, maintenance treatment of airflow obstruction in patients with chronic obstructive pulmonary disease (COPD), including chronic bronchitis and/or emphysema

3/29/13: Invokana (canagliflozin): Used with diet and exercise, to improve glycemic control in adults with type 2 diabetes

3/27/13: Tecfidera (dimethyl fumarate): To treat adults with relapsing forms of multiple sclerosis (MS)

3/20/13: Dotarem (gadoterate meglumine): For use in magnetic resonance imaging (MRI) of the brain, spine and associated tissues of patients ages two years and older

3/13/13: Lymphoseek (technetium Tc 99m tilmanocept): A radioactive diagnostic imaging agent that helps doctors locate lymph nodes in patients with breast cancer or melanoma who are undergoing surgery to remove tumor-draining lymph nodes

2/26/13: Osphena (ospemifene): To treat women experiencing moderate to severe dyspareunia (pain during sexual intercourse), a symptom of vulvar and vaginal atrophy due to menopause

2/22/13: Kadcyla (ado-trastuzumab emtansine): For patients with HER2-positive, late-stage (metastatic) breast cancer

2/8/13: Pomalyst (pomalidomide): To treat patients with multiple myeloma whose disease progressed after being treated with other cancer drugs

1/29/13: Kynamro (mipomersen sodium): To treat patients with a rare type of high cholesterol called homozygous familial hypercholesterolemia (HoFH)

1/25/13: Nesina (alogliptin): To improve blood sugar control in adults with type 2 diabetes

12/31/12: Fulyzaq (crofelemer): To treat HIV/AIDS patients whose diarrhea is not caused by an infection from a virus, bacteria, or parasite

12/28/12: Sirturo (bedaquiline): As part of combination therapy to treat adults with multi-drug resistant pulmonary tuberculosis (TB) when other alternatives are not available

12/28/12: Eliquis (apixaban): To reduce the risk of stroke and dangerous blood clots (systemic embolism) in patients with atrial fibrillation that is not caused by a heart valve problem

12/21/12: Juxtapid (lomitapide): To reduce low-density lipoprotein (LDL) cholesterol, total cholesterol, apolipoprotein B, and non-high-density lipoprotein (non-HDL) cholesterol in patients with homozygous familial hypercholesterolemia (HoFH)

12/21/12: Gattex (teduglutide): To treat adults with short bowel syndrome (SBS) who need additional nutrition from intravenous feeding (parenteral nutrition)

12/14/12: Signifor (pasereotide): To treat Cushing's disease patients who cannot be helped through surgery

12/14/12: raxibacumab (raxibacumab): To treat inhalational anthrax, a form of the infectious disease caused by breathing in the spores of the bacterium *Bacillus anthracis*

12/14/12: Iclusig (ponatinib): To treat adults with chronic myeloid leukemia (CML) and Philadelphia chromosome positive acute lymphoblastic leukemia (Ph+ ALL), two rare blood and bone marrow diseases

11/29/12: Cometriq (cabozantinib): To treat medullary thyroid cancer that has spread to other parts of the body (metastasized)

11/6/12: Xeljanz (tofacitinib): To treat adults with moderately to severely active rheumatoid arthritis (RA) who have had an inadequate response to, or who are intolerant of, methotrexate

10/26/12: Synribo (omacetaxine mepesuccinate): To treat adults with chronic myelogenous leukemia (CML), a blood and bone marrow disease

10/22/12: Fycompa (perampanel): To treat partial onset seizures in patients with epilepsy ages 12 years and older

10/17/12: Jetrea (ocriplasmin): To treat an eye condition called symptomatic vitreomacular adhesion (VMA)

9/27/12: Stivarga (regorafenib): To treat patients with colorectal cancer that has progressed after treatment and spread to other parts of the body (metastatic)

9/12/12: Choline C 11 Injection: A positron emission tomography (PET) imaging agent used to help detect recurrent prostate cancer

9/12/12: Aubagio (teriflunomide): For the treatment of adults with relapsing forms of multiple sclerosis (MS)

9/4/12: Bosulif (bosutinib): To treat chronic myelogenous leukemia (CML), a blood and bone marrow disease that usually affects older adults

8/31/12: Xtandi (enzalutamide): To treat men with late-stage (metastatic) castration-resistant prostate cancer that has spread or recurred, even with medical or surgical therapy to minimize testosterone

8/30/12: Linzess (linaclotide): To treat chronic idiopathic constipation and to treat irritable bowel syndrome with constipation (IBS-C) in adults

8/29/12: Neutroval (tbo-filgrastim): To reduce the time certain patients receiving cancer chemotherapy experience severe neutropenia, a decrease in infection-fighting white blood cells called neutrophils

8/27/12: Stribild (elvitegravir, cobicistat, emtricitabine, tenofovir disoproxil fumarate): A once-a-day combination pill to treat HIV-1 infection in adults who have never been treated for HIV infection

8/3/12: Zaltrap (ziv-aflibercept): For use in combination with a FOLFIRI (folinic acid, fluorouracil, and irinotecan) chemotherapy regimen to treat adults with colorectal cancer

7/23/12: Tudorza Pressair (aclidinium bromide): For the long-term maintenance treatment of bronchospasm associated with chronic obstructive pulmonary disease (COPD), including chronic bronchitis and emphysema

7/20/12: Kyprolis (carfilzomib): To treat patients with multiple myeloma who have received at least two prior therapies, including treatment with Velcade (bortezomib) and an immunomodulatory

7/16/12: Prepopik (sodium picosulfate, magnesium oxide, and citric acid): To help cleanse the colon in adults preparing for colonoscopy

6/28/12: Myrbetriq (mirabegron): To treat adults with overactive bladder

6/27/12: Belviq (lorcaserin hydrochloride): For chronic weight management

6/8/12: Perjeta (pertuzumab): To treat patients with HER2-positive late-stage (metastatic) breast cancer

5/1/12: Elelyso (taliglucerase alfa): For long-term enzyme replacement therapy to treat a form of Gaucher disease, a rare genetic disorder

4/27/12: Stendra (avanafil): To treat erectile dysfunction

4/6/12: Amyvid (Florbetapir F 18): Used as a radioactive diagnostic agent for positron emission tomography (PET) imaging of the brain to estimate β-amyloid neuritic plaque density in adult patients with cognitive impairment who are being evaluated for Alzheimer's Disease (AD) and other causes of cognitive decline

3/27/12: Omontys (peginesatide): To treat anemia, a condition in which the body does not have enough healthy red blood cells, in adult dialysis patients who have chronic kidney disease (CKD)

3/6/12: Surfaxin (lucinactant): For the prevention of respiratory distress syndrome (RDS), a breathing disorder that affects premature infants

2/10/12: Zioptan (tafluprost): For reducing elevated intraocular pressure in patients with open-angle glaucoma or ocular hypertension

1/31/12: Kalydeco (ivacaftor): For the treatment of a rare form of cystic fibrosis (CF) in patients ages six years and older who have the specific G551D mutation in the Cystic Fibrosis Transmembrane Regulator (CFTR) gene

1/30/12: Erivedge (vismodegib): To treat adult patients with basal cell carcinoma, the most common type of skin cancer

1/27/12: Inlyta (axitinib): To treat patients with advanced kidney cancer (renal cell carcinoma) who have not responded to another drug for this type of cancer

1/23/12: Picato (ingenol mebutate): For the topical treatment of actinic keratosis

1/17/12: Voraxaze (glucarpidase): To treat patients with toxic levels of methotrexate in their blood due to kidney failure

11/18/11: Erwinaze (asparaginase *Erwinia chrysanthemi*): To treat patients with acute lymphoblastic leukemia (ALL), who have developed an allergy (hypersensitivity) to *E. coli*–derived asparaginase and pegapargase chemotherapy drugs used to treat ALL

11/18/11: Eylea (aflibercept): To treat patients with wet (neovascular) age-related macular degeneration (AMD), a leading cause of vision loss and blindness in Americans ages 60 and older

11/16/11: Jakafi (ruxolitinib): To treat patients with the bone marrow disease myelofibrosis

10/24/11: Onfi (clobazam): For use as an adjunctive (add-on) treatment for seizures associated with Lennox-Gastaut syndrome in adults and children two years of age and older

10/14/11: Ferriprox (deferiprone): To treat patients with iron overload due to blood transfusions in patients with thalassemia, a genetic blood disorder that causes anemia, who had an inadequate response to prior chelation therapy

8/26/11: Xalkori (crizotinib): To treat certain patients with late-stage (locally advanced or metastatic), non-small cell lung cancers (NSCLC) who express the abnormal anaplastic lymphoma kinase (ALK) gene

8/25/11: Firazyr (icatibant): For the treatment of acute attacks of a rare condition called hereditary angioedema (HAE) in people ages 18 years and older

8/19/11: Adcetris (brentuximab vedotin): For the treatment of Hodgkin's lymphoma and ALCL (systemic anaplastic large cell lymphoma)

8/17/11: Zelboraf (vemurafenib): To treat patients with late-stage (metastatic) or unresectable (cannot be removed by surgery) melanoma, the most dangerous type of skin cancer

7/20/11: Brilinta (ticagrelor): To reduce cardiovascular death and heart attack in patients with acute coronary syndromes (ACS)

7/01/11: Arcapta Neohaler (indacaterol inhalation powder): For the long term, once-daily maintenance bronchodilator treatment of airflow obstruction in people with chronic obstructive pulmonary disease (COPD) including chronic bronchitis and/or emphysema

7/01/11: Xarelto (rivaroxaban): To reduce the risk of blood clots, deep vein thrombosis (DVT), and pulmonary embolism (PE) following knee or hip replacement surgery

6/15/11: Nulojix (belatacept): To prevent acute rejection in adult patients who have had a kidney transplant

6/10/11: Potiga (ezogabine): For use as an add-on medication to treat seizures associated with epilepsy in adults

5/27/11: Dificid (fidaxomicin): For the treatment of *Clostridium difficile*–associated diarrhea (CDAD)

5/23/11: Incivek (telaprevir): To treat certain adults with chronic hepatitis C infection

5/20/11: Edurant (rilpivirine): For the treatment of HIV-1 infection in adults who have never taken HIV therapy

5/13/11: Victrelis (boceprevir): To treat certain adults with chronic hepatitis C

5/02/11: Tradjenta (linagliptin): An adjunct to diet and exercise to improve glycemic control in adults with type 2 diabetes mellitus

4/28/11: Zytiga (abiraterone acetate): In combination with prednisone (a steroid) to treat patients with late-stage (metastatic) castration-resistant prostate cancer who have received prior docetaxel (chemotherapy)

4/06/11: Caprelsa (vandetanib): To treat adult patients with late-stage (metastatic) medullary thyroid cancer who are ineligible for surgery and who have disease that is growing or causing symptoms

4/06/11: Horizant (gabapentin enacarbil): A once-daily treatment for moderate-to-severe restless legs syndrome (RLS)

3/25/11: Yervoy (ipilimumab): To treat patients with late-stage (metastatic) melanoma, the most dangerous type of skin cancer

3/14/11: Gadavist (gadobutrol): For use in patients undergoing magnetic resonance imaging (MRI) of the central nervous system

3/9/11: Benlysta (belimumab): To treat patients with active, autoantibody-positive lupus (systemic lupus erythematosus) who are receiving standard therapy, including corticosteroids, antimalarials, immunosuppressives, and nonsteroidal anti-inflammatory drugs

2/28/11: Daliresp (roflumilast): To decrease the frequency of flare-ups (exacerbations) or worsening of symptoms from severe chronic obstructive pulmonary disease (COPD)

2/25/11: Edarbi (azilsartan medoxomil): To treat high blood pressure (hypertension) in adults

1/21/11: Viibryd (vilazodone hydrochloride): To treat major depressive disorder in adults

1/18/11: Natroba (spinosad): For the treatment of head lice infestation in patients ages four years and older

1/14 /11: Datscan (ioflupane i-123): An imaging drug used to assist in the evaluation of adult patients with suspected Parkinsonian syndromes (PS)

ADDITIONAL READING

Abdelnabi R, Jacobs S, Delang L, Neyts J. Antiviral drug discovery against arthritogenic alphaviruses: tools and molecular targets. *Biochem Pharmacol.* 2020;174:113777.

Abduelkarem AR, Anbar HS, Zaraei SO, Alfar AA, Al-Zoubi OS, Abdelkarem EG, El-Gamal MI. Diarylamides in anticancer drug discovery: a review of pre-clinical and clinical investigations. *Eur J Med Chem.* 2020;188:112029.

Ain QU, Batool M, Choi S. TLR4-targeting therapeutics: structural basis and computer-aided drug discovery approaches. *Molecules.* 2020;25(3):627.

Alsafadi HN, Uhl FE, Pineda RH, Bailey KE, Rojas M, Wagner DE, Königshoff M. Applications and approaches for three-dimensional precision-cut lung slices. disease modeling and drug discovery. *Am J Respir Cell Mol Biol.* 2020;62(6):681–691.

Altamura F, Rajesh R, Catta-Preta CMC, Moretti NS, Cestari I. The current drug discovery landscape for trypanosomiasis and leishmaniasis: challenges and strategies to identify drug targets. *Drug Dev Res.* 2020. doi:10.1002/ddr.21664. Epub ahead of print. PMID: .

Arora R, CAB International. *Medicinal Plant Biotechnology.* Cambridge, MA: CABI; 2010.

Asai A, Konno M, Ozaki M, Otsuka C, Vecchione A, Arai T, Kitagawa T, Ofusa K,Yabumoto M, Hirotsu T, Taniguchi M, Eguchi H, Doki Y, Ishii H. COVID-19 drug discovery using intensive approaches. *Int J Mol Sci.* 2020;21(8):2839.

Atun RA, Sheridan DJ. *Innovation in the Biomedicine Industry.* London, NJ: World Scientific Pub.; 2007.

Ayuso M, Buyssens L, Stroe M, Valenzuela A, Allegaert K, Smits A, Annaert P,Mulder A, Carpentier S, Van Ginneken C, Van Cruchten S. The neonatal and juvenile pig in pediatric drug discovery and development. *Pharmaceutics.* 2020;13(1):E44.

Bai J, Wang C. Organoids and microphysiological systems: new tools for ophthalmic drug discovery. *Front Pharmacol.* 2020;11:407.

Bawa R, Szebeni JN, Webster TJ, Audette GF. *Immune Aspects of Biomedicines and Nanomedicines.* Singapore: Pan Stanford Publishing; 2018.

Bayoumi A, Grønbæk H, George J, Eslam M. The epigenetic drug discovery landscape for metabolic-associated fatty liver disease. *Trends Genet.* 2020;36(6):429–441.

Beck A. *Glycosylation Engineering of Biomedicines: Methods and Protocols.* New York: Humana Press; 2013.

Beckman MF, Morton DS, Bahrani Mougeot F, Mougeot JC. Allogenic stem cell transplant-associated acute graft versus host disease: a computational drug discovery text mining approach using oral and gut microbiome signatures. *Supportive Care in Cancer: Official Journal of the Multinational Association of Supportive Care in Cancer.* 2021;29(4):1765–1779. doi:10.1007/s00520-020-05821-2. PMID:

Behera BK. *Biomedicines: Challenges and Opportunities.* 1st ed. Boca Raton: CRC Press; 2021.

Bender A, Cortés-Ciriano I. Artificial intelligence in drug discovery: whatis realistic, what are illusions? Part: ways to make an impact, and why we arenot there yet. *Drug Discov Today.* 2020;S1359-6446(20): 30527–4.

Benns HJ, Wincott CJ, Tate EW, Child MA. Activity- and reactivity-based proteomics: recent technological advances and applications in drug discovery. *Curr Opin Chem Biol.* 2020;60:20–29.

Bhattacharya A, Corbeil A, do Monte-Neto RL, Fernandez-Prada C. Of drugs and trypanosomatids: new tools and knowledge to reduce bottlenecks in drug discovery. *Genes (Basel).* 2020;11(7):722.

Bian Y, Jun JJ, Cuyler J, Xie XQ. Covalent allosteric modulation: an emerging strategy for GPCRs drug discovery. *Eur J Med Chem.* 2020;206:112690. doi:10.1016/j.ejmech.2020.112690. Epub 2020 Aug 9. PMID: .

Bianco G, Goodsell DS, Forli S. Selective and effective: current progress in computational structure-based drug discovery of targeted covalent inhibitors. *Trends Pharmacol Sci.* 2020;41(12):1038–1049.

Biernacki K, Daśko M, Ciupak O, Kubiński K, Rachon J, Demkowicz S. Novel1,2,4-oxadiazole derivatives in drug discovery. *Pharmaceuticals (Basel).* 2020;13(6):111.

Bordon KCF, Cologna CT, Fornari-Baldo EC, Pinheiro-Júnior EL, Cerni FA,Amorim FG, Anjolette FAP, Cordeiro FA, Wiezel GA, Cardoso IA, Ferreira IG, deOliveira IS, Boldrini-França J, Pucca MB, Baldo MA, Arantes EC. From animal poisons and venoms to medicines: achievements, challenges and perspectives in drug discovery. *Front Pharmacol.* 2020;11:1132.

Borsari C, Trader DJ, Tait A, Costi MP. Designing chimeric molecules for drug discovery by leveraging chemical biology. *J Med Chem.* 2020;63(5):1908–1928.

Brooks G. *Biotechnology in Healthcare: An Introduction to Biomedicines.* London: Medicine Press; 1998.

Brummer T, McInnes C. RAF kinase dimerization: implications for drug discovery and clinical outcomes. *Oncogene.* 2020;39(21):4155–4169.

Burke M, Walmsley S. *Biomedicines: A New Era of Discovery in the Biotechnology Revolution?* Richmond: PJB Publications; 2001.

Buskes MJ, Blanco MJ. Impact of cross-coupling reactions in drug discovery and development. *Molecules.* 2020;25(15):3493.

Cai C, Wang S, Xu Y, Zhang W, Tang K, Ouyang Q, Lai L, Pei J. Transfer learning for drug discovery. *J Med Chem.* 2020;63(16):8683–8694.

Caruso G, Musso N, Grasso M, Costantino A, Lazzarino G, Tascedda F,Gulisano M, Lunte SM, Caraci F. Microfluidics as a novel tool for biological and toxicological assays in drug discovery processes: focus on microchip electrophoresis. *Micromachines (Basel).* 2020;11(6):593.

Cassar S, Adatto I, Freeman JL, Gamse JT, Iturria I, Lawrence C, Muriana A,Peterson RT, Van Cruchten S, Zon LI. Use of Zebrafish In Drug Discovery Toxicology. *Chem Res Toxicol.* 2020;33(1):95–118.

Castilho LdR. *Animal Cell Technology: From Biomedicines to Gene Therapy.* New York: Taylor & Francis; 2008.

Cavagnaro JA. *Preclinical Safety Evaluation of Biomedicines: A Science-Based Approach to Facilitating Clinical Trials.* Hoboken, NJ: Wiley; 2008.

Cavasotto CN, Di Filippo JI. Artificial intelligence in the early stages of drug discovery. *Arch Biochem Biophys.* 2021;698:108730. doi:10.1016/j.abb.2020.108730. Epub 2020 Dec 19. PMID: .

Chandrasekaran SN, Ceulemans H, Boyd JD, Carpenter AE. Image-based profiling for drug discovery: due for a machine-learning upgrade? *Nat Rev Drug Discov.* 2021;20:145–159. doi:10.1038/s41573-020-00117-w.

Chaudhari R, Fong LW, Tan Z, Huang B, Zhang S. An up-to-date overview of computational polypharmacology in modern drug discovery. *Expert Opin Drug Discov.* 2020;15(9):1025–1044.

CHEBI: Reference chemical structures, nomenclature and ontological classification. [https://www.ebi.ac.uk/chebi/] 2020.

Chellapandi P, Saranya S. Genomics insights of SARS-CoV-2 (COVID-19) into target-based drug discovery [published online ahead of print, 2020 Jul 31]. *Med Chem Res.* 2020;1–15. doi:10.1007/s00044-020-02610-8.

ChEMBL database in 2017, Gaulton et al., *Nucleic Acids Res.* 2017, http://bit.ly/2AhBcxV; portal for target browser: http://bit.ly/2zVIUNy; blog about drug targets: http://bit.ly/2hGgGvN. The graphic below shows the target browser and selection screen from ChEMBL_20. The current version is ChEMBL_23.

CHEMBL: An open data resource of binding, functional and ADMET bioactivity data. [https://www.ebi.ac.uk/chembl/] 2020.

Chen B, Garmire L, Calvisi DF, Chua MS, Kelley RK, Chen X. Harnessing big 'omics' data and AI for drug discovery in hepatocellular carcinoma. *Nat Rev Gastroenterol Hepatol.* 2020;17(4):238–251.

Chen Y, Kirchmair J. Cheminformatics in natural product-based drug discovery. *Mol Inform.* 2020;39(12):e2000171.

Chen Z, Zhang N, Chu HY, Yu Y, Zhang ZK, Zhang G, Zhang BT. Connective tissue growth factor: from molecular understandings to drug discovery. *Front Cell Dev Biol.* 2020 Oct 29;8:593269. doi:10.3389/fcell.2020.593269. PMID: ; PMCID: PMC7658337.

Cieślik P, Wierońska JM. Regulation of glutamatergic activity via bidirectional activation of two select receptors as a novel approach inantipsychotic drug discovery. *Int J Mol Sci.* 2020;21(22):8811.

Congreve M, de Graaf C, Swain NA, Tate CG. Impact of GPCR structures on drug discovery. *Cell.* 2020;181(1):81–91.

Conrado DJ, Duvvuri S, Geerts H, Burton J, Biesdorf C, Ahamadi M, Macha S,Hather G, Francisco Morales J, Podichetty J, Nicholas T, Stephenson D, Trame M,Romero K, Corrigan B; Drug development tools in the Alzheimer disease continuum (DDT-AD) working group. Challenges in Alzheimer's disease drug discovery and development: the role of modeling, simulation, and open data. *Clin Pharmacol Ther.* 2020;107(4):796–805.

Costa AF, Campos D, Reis CA, Gomes C. Targeting glycosylation: a new road for cancer drug discovery. *Trends Cancer.* 2020;6(9):757–766.

Cota-Coronado A, Durnall JC, Díaz NF, Thompson LH, Díaz-Martínez NE. Unprecedented potential for neural drug discovery based on self-organizing hipsc platforms. *Molecules.* 2020;25(5):1150.

Crick F, Knablein Jr. *Modern Biomedicines: Design, Development and Optimization.* Chichester: Wiley-VCH; 2005.

Crooke ST, Liang XH, Crooke RM, Baker BF, Geary RS. Antisense drug discovery and development technology considered in a pharmacological context. *Biochem Pharmacol.* 2020:114196.

Cruwys S, Hein P, Humphries B, Black D. Drug discovery and development in idiopathic pulmonary fibrosis: challenges and opportunities. *Drug Discov Today.* 2020;25(12):2277–2283.

Cui Y, Zhao H, Wu S, Li X. Human female reproductive system organoids: applications in developmental biology, disease modelling, and drug discovery. *Stem Cell Rev Rep.* 2020;16(6):1173–1184.

Dalton SE, Campos S. Covalent small molecules as enabling platforms for drug discovery. *Chembiochem.* 2020;21(8):1080–1100.

Damale MG, Pathan SK, Shinde DB, Patil RH, Arote RB, Sangshetti JN. Insights of tankyrases: a novel target for drug discovery. *Eur J Med Chem.* 2020;207:112712. doi:10.1016/j.ejmech.2020.112712. Epub 2020 Aug 17. PMID: .

Das TK. *Biophysical Methods for Biotherapeutics: Discovery and Development Applications.* Hoboken, NJ: Wiley; 2014.

David L, Thakkar A, Mercado R, Engkvist O. Molecular representations in AI-driven drug discovery: a review and practical guide. *J Cheminform.* 2020;12(1):56.

Davis RL. Mechanism of action and target identification: a matter of timing in drug discovery. *iScience.* 2020;23(9):101487.

De Masi C, Spitalieri P, Murdocca M, Novelli G, Sangiuolo F. Application of CRISPR/Cas9 to human-induced pluripotent stem cells: from gene editing to drug discovery. *Hum Genomics.* 2020;14(1):25.

De Simone A, Naldi M, Tedesco D, Bartolini M, Davani L, Andrisano V. Advanced analytical methodologies in Alzheimer's disease drug discovery. *J PharmBiomed Anal.* 2020;1:112899.

de Souza Neto LR, Moreira-Filho JT, Neves BJ, Maidana RLBR, Guimarães ACR,Furnham N, Andrade CH, Silva FP Jr. *In silico* strategies to support fragment-to-lead optimization in drug discovery. *Front Chem.* 2020;8:93. Published 2020 Feb 18. doi:10.3389/fchem.2020.00093.

Dehyab AS, Bakar MFA, AlOmar MK, Sabran SF. A review of medicinal plant of Middle East and North Africa (MENA) region as source in tuberculosis drug discovery. *Saudi J Biol Sci.* 2020;27(9):2457–2478.

Deng L, Meng T, Chen L, Wei W, Wang P. The role of ubiquitination in tumorigenesis and targeted drug discovery. *Signal Transduct Target Ther.* 2020;5(1):11.

Deng X, Tavallaie MS, Sun R, Wang J, Cai Q, Shen J, Lei S, Fu L, Jiang F. Drug discovery approaches targeting the incretin pathway. *Bioorg Chem.* 2020;99:103810. doi:10.1016/j.bioorg.2020.103810. Epub 2020 Apr 2. PMID: .

Dhuri K, Bechtold C, Quijano E, Pham H, Gupta A, Vikram A, Bahal R. Antisense oligonucleotides: an emerging area in drug discovery and development. *J Clin Med.* 2020;9(6):2004.

Diethelm-Varela B. Using NMR spectroscopy in the fragment-based drug discovery of small-molecule anticancer targeted therapies. *ChemMedChem.* 2021;16(5):725–742. doi:10.1002/cmdc.202000756. Epub 2020 Dec 16. PMID: .

Drug discovery effectiveness from the standpoint of therapeutic mechanisms and indications, Shih et al., *Nature Revs. Drug Disc.* 2017; http://go.nature.com/2AgsDnf

Dutton RL, Scharer JM. *Advanced Technologies in Biomedicine Processing.* 1st ed. Ames, IA: Blackwell Pub.; 2007.

Ekins S, Mottin M, Ramos PRPS, Sousa BKP, Neves BJ, Foil DH, Zorn KM, BragaRC, Coffee M, Southan C, Puhl AC, Andrade CH. Déjà vu: stimulating open drug discovery for SARS-CoV-2. *Drug Discov Today.* 2020;25(5):928–941.

Elbadawi M, Gaisford S, Basit AW. Advanced machine-learning techniques indrug discovery. *Drug Discov Today.* 2020;S1359-6446(20):30521–3.

Elsheikha HM, Siddiqui R, Khan NA. Drug discovery againstAcanthamoeba infections: present knowledge and unmet needs. *Pathogens.* 2020;9(5):405.

ENZYME PORTAL: integrated enzyme data from EMBL-EBI resources. [https://www.ebi.ac.uk/enzymeportal/]

Ermogenous C, Green C, Jackson T, Ferguson M, Lord JM. Treating age-related multimorbidity: the drug discovery challenge. *Drug Discov Today.* 2020;25(8):1403–1415.

Fader KA, Zhang J, Menetski JP, Thadhani RI, Antman EM, Friedman GS,Ramaiah SK, Vaidya VS. A biomarker-centric approach to drug discovery and development: lessons learned from the coronavirus disease 2019 pandemic. *J Pharmacol Exp Ther.* 2021;376(1):12–20.

Falcicchio M, Ward JA, Macip S, Doveston RG. Regulation of p53 by the 14-3-3 protein interaction network: new opportunities for drug discovery in cancer. *Cell Death Discov.* 2020;6(1):126.

Fernandes RS, Freire MCLC, Bueno RV, Godoy AS, Gil LHVG, Oliva G. Reporter replicons for antiviral drug discovery against positive single-stranded RNA viruses. *Viruses.* 2020;12(6):598.

Finan et al., The druggable genome and support for target identification and validation in drug development. *Science Trans Med.* 2017. http://bit.ly/2hQ5Ua3 (available in manuscript form on bioRxiv, http://bit.ly/2zlZFlY)

Fontana F, Raimondi M, Marzagalli M, Sommariva M, Gagliano N, Limonta P. Three-dimensional cell cultures as an in vitro tool for prostate cancer modeling and drug discovery. *Int J Mol Sci.* 2020;21(18):6806.

Fryszkowska A, Devine PN. Biocatalysis in drug discovery and development. *Curr Opin Chem Biol.* 2020 Apr;55:151–160. doi:10.1016/j.cbpa.2020.01.012. Epub 2020 Mar 10. PMID: .

Gao K, Oerlemans R, Groves MR. Theory and applications of differential scanning fluorimetry in early-stage drug discovery. *Biophys Rev.* 2020;12(1):85–104.

Geigert J. *The Challenge of CMC Regulatory Compliance for Biomedicines.* 3rd ed. Cham: Springer; 2019.

Gopal P, Dick T. Targeted protein degradation in antibacterial drug discovery? *Prog Biophys Mol Biol.* 2020 May;152:10–14. doi:10.1016/j.pbiomolbio.2019.11.005. Epub 2019 Nov 16. PMID: ; PMCID: PMC7145722.

Greene CS, Krishnan A, Wong AK, Ricciotti E, Zelaya RA, Himmelstein DS, Zhang R, Hartmann BM, Zaslavsky E, Sealfon SC, Chasman DI, FitzGerald GA, Dolinski K, Grosser T, Troyanskaya OG. Understanding multicellular function and disease with human tissue-specific networks. *Nature Genetics.* 2015;47(6):569–576. doi:10.1038/ng.3259w. Epub 2015 Apr 27. PMID: ; PMCID: PMC4828725.

Grigalunas M, Burhop A, Christoforow A, Waldmann H. Pseudo-natural products and natural product-inspired methods in chemical biology and drug discovery. *Curr Opin Chem Biol.* 2020 Jun;56:111–118. doi:10.1016/j.cbpa.2019.10.005. Epub 2020 May 1. PMID: .

Grindley JN, Ogden JE. *Understanding Biomedicines: Manufacturing and Regulatory Issues.* Denver, CO: Interpharm Press; 2000.

Grüber G. Introduction: novel insights into TB research and drug discovery. *Prog Biophys Mol Biol.* 2020;152:2–5.

Grygorenko OO, Volochnyuk DM, Ryabukhin SV, Judd DB. The symbiotic relationship between drug discovery and organic chemistry. *Chemistry.* 2020;26(6):1196–1237.

Gupta MN, Alam A, Hasnain SE. Protein promiscuity in drug discovery, drug-repurposing and antibiotic resistance. *Biochimie.* 2020;175:50–57.

Ha J, Park H, Park J, Park SB. Recent advances in identifying proteintargets in drug discovery. *Cell Chem Biol.* 2020;S2451-9456(20):30476–1.

Hampel H, Vergallo A, Caraci F, Cuello AC, Lemercier P, Vellas B, GiudiciKV, Baldacci F, Hänisch B, Haberkamp M, Broich K, Nisticò R, Emanuele E, LlaveroF, Zugaza JL, Lucía A, Giacobini E, Lista S; Alzheimer Precision MedicineInitiative. Future avenues for Alzheimer's disease detection and therapy: liquidbiopsy, intracellular signaling modulation, systems pharmacology drug discovery. *Neuropharmacology.* 2020;185:108081.

Hatzipantelis CJ, Langiu M, Vandekolk TH, Pierce TL, Nithianantharajah J,Stewart GD, Langmead CJ. Translation-focused approaches to GPCR drug discovery for cognitive impairments associated with schizophrenia. *ACS Pharmacol TranslSci.* 2020;3(6):1042–1062.

Hazafa A, Ur-Rahman K, Haq IU, Jahan N, Mumtaz M, Farman M, Naeem H, AbbasF, Naeem M, Sadiqa S, Bano S. The broad-spectrum antiviral recommendations fordrug discovery against COVID-19. *Drug Metab Rev.* 2020;52(3):408–424.

Hefferon KL. *Biomedicines in Plants: Toward the Next Century of Medicine.* Boca Raton, FL: CRC Press/ Taylor & Francis; 2010.

Herholt A, Galinski S, Geyer PE, Rossner MJ, Wehr MC. Multiparametric assays for accelerating early drug discovery. *Trends Pharmacol Sci.* 2020;41(5):318–335.

Herzig V, Cristofori-Armstrong B, Israel MR, Nixon SA, Vetter I, King GF. Animal toxins – Nature's evolutionary-refined toolkit for basic research and drug discovery. *Biochem Pharmacol.* 2020;181:114096.

Hill RG, Rang HP. *Medicine Discovery and Development: Technology in Transition.* 2nd ed. Edinburgh: Churchill Livingstone/Elsevier; 2013.

Ho RJY, Gibaldi M. *Biotechnology and Biomedicines: Transforming Proteins and Genes into Medicines.* 2nd ed. Hoboken, NJ: Wiley-Blackwell; 2013.

Hothersall JD, Jones AY, Dafforn TR, Perrior T, Chapman KL. Releasing thet echnical 'shackles' on GPCR drug discovery: opportunities enabled by detergent-free polymer lipid particle (PoLiPa) purification. *Drug Discov Today.* 2020;S1359-6446(20):30337–8.

Houde DJ, Berkowitz SA. *Biophysical Characterization of Proteins in Developing Biomedicines.* Waltham, MA: Elsevier; 2015.

How many drug targets are there?, Overington et al., *Nature Revs. Drug Disc.* 2006, http://go.nature.com /2hMX2Sv; (available on researchgate.net, http://bit.ly/2AVheWd)

Hu J. Toward unzipping the ZIP metal transporters: structure, evolution, and implications on drug discovery against cancer. *FEBS J.* 2020. doi:10.1111/febs.15658

Hu Z, Li H, Wang X, Ullah K, Xu G. Proteomic approaches for the profiling of ubiquitylation events and their applications in drug discovery. *J Proteomics.* 2021;231:103996.

Huang J, Wang D, Huang LH, Huang H. Roles of reconstituted high-density lipoprotein nanoparticles in cardiovascular disease: a new paradigm for drug discovery. *Int J Mol Sci.* 2020;21(3):739.

Huang X, editor. Alzheimer's disease: drug discovery [Internet]. *Brisbane(AU): Exon Publications.* 2020. PMID: 33400453.

Huxsoll JF. *Quality Assurance for Biomedicines.* Chichester: Wiley; 1994.

Ibhazehiebo K, Rho JM, Kurrasch DM. Metabolism-based drug discovery in zebrafish: an emerging strategy to uncover new anti-seizure therapies. *Neuropharmacology.* 2020;1:107988.

Irurzun-Arana I, Rackauckas C, McDonald TO, Trocóniz IF. beyond deterministic models in drug discovery and development. *Trends Pharmacol Sci.* 2020;41(11):882–895.

Jacobson KA. Tribute to Prof. Geoffrey Burnstock: transition of purinergic signaling to drug discovery. *Purinergic Signal.* 2020;17(1):3–8.

Jaffe EK. Wrangling shape-shifting morpheeins to tackle disease and approach drug discovery. *Front Mol Biosci.* 2020;7:582966.

Jakopin Ž. 2-aminothiazoles in drug discovery: privileged structures or toxicophores? *Chem Biol Interact.* 2020;330:109244.

Jameel F, Hershenson S. *Formulation and Process Development Strategies for Manufacturing Biomedicines.* Oxford: Wiley; 2010.

Jing X, Jin K. A gold mine for drug discovery: strategies to develop cyclic peptides into therapies. *Med Res Rev.* 2020;40(2):753–810.

Johnson MR, Kaminski RM. A systems-level framework for anti-epilepsy drug discovery. *Neuropharmacology.* 2020;170:107868.

Jørgensen L, Nielsen HM. *Delivery Technologies for Biomedicines: Peptides, Proteins, Nucleic Acids and Vaccines.* Hoboken, NJ: Wiley; 2009.

Jugran AK, Rawat S, Devkota HP, Bhatt ID, Rawal RS. Diabetes and plant-derived natural products: from ethnopharmacological approaches to thei rpotential for modern drug discovery and development. *Phytother Res.* 2020;35(1):223–245.

Kaemmerer E, Loessner D, Avery VM. Addressing the tumour microenvironment in early drug discovery: a strategy to overcome drug resistance and identify novel targets for cancer therapy. *Drug Discov Today.* 2020;S1359-6446(20):30514–6.

Katoch S, Patial V. Zebrafish: an emerging model system to study liver diseases and related drug discovery. *J Appl Toxicol.* 2021;41(1):33–51.

Keeley A, Petri L, Ábrányi-Balogh P, Keserű GM. Covalent fragment libraries in drug discovery. *Drug Discov Today.* 2020;25(6):983–996.

Khan S, Soni S, Veerapu NS. HCV replicon systems: workhorses of drug discovery and resistance. *Front Cell Infect Microbiol.* 2020;10:325.

Khare P, Sahu U, Pandey SC, Samant M. Current approaches for target-specific drug discovery using natural compounds against SARS-CoV-2 infection. *Virus Res.* 2020;290:198169.

Knäblein Jr. *Modern Biomedicines: Recent Success Stories.* Weinheim: Wiley-Blackwell; 2013.

Komives C, Zhou W. *Bioprocessing Technology for Production of Biomedicines and Bioproducts.* 1st edi. Hoboken, NJ: John Wiley & Sons, Inc.; 2019.

Krause SO. *Validation of Analytical Methods for Biomedicines: A Guide to Risk-Based Validation and Implementation Strategies.* Bethesda, MD: PDA; 2007.

Krishnan A, Zhang R, Yao V, Theesfeld CL, Wong AK, Tadych A, Volfovsky N, Packer A, Lash A, Troyanskaya OG. Genome-wide prediction and functional characterization of the genetic basis of autism spectrum disorder. *Nature Neuroscience.* 2016;19(11):1454–1462.

Lakshmi PK, Kumar S, Pawar S, Kuriakose BB, Sudheesh MS, Pawar RS. Targeting metabolic syndrome with phytochemicals: focus on the role of molecular chaperones and hormesis in drug discovery. *Pharmacol Res.* 2020;1:104925.

Lang Y, Chen K, Li Z, Li H. The nucleocapsid protein of zoonotic betacoronaviruses is an attractive target for antiviral drug discovery. *LifeSci.* 2020;282:118754.

Lautié E, Russo O, Ducrot P, Boutin JA. Unraveling plant natural chemical diversity for drug discovery purposes. *Front Pharmacol.* 2020;397. doi:10.3389/fphar.2020.00397

Law JW, Law LN, Letchumanan V, Tan LT, Wong SH, Chan KG, Ab Mutalib NS, LeeLH. Anticancer drug discovery from microbial sources: the unique mangrove streptomycetes. *Molecules.* 2020;25 (22):5365.

Lee C-J. *Clinical Trials of Medicines and Biomedicines.* Boca Raton, FL: Taylor & Francis; 2006.

Lee J, Bayarsaikhan D, Bayarsaikhan G, Kim JS, Schwarzbach E, Lee B. Recent advances in genome editing of stem cells for drug discovery and therapeuticapplication. *Pharmacol Ther.* 2020 107501.

Lee J, Noh S, Lim S, Kim B. Plant extracts for type 2 diabetes: from traditional medicine to modern drug discovery. *Antioxidants (Basel).* 2021;10(1):E81.

Lenci E, Trabocchi A. Peptidomimetic toolbox for drug discovery. *Chem SocRev.* 2020;49(11):3262–3277.

Li J, Ge Y, Huang JX, Strømgaard K, Zhang X, Xiong XF. Heterotrimeric G proteins as therapeutic targets in drug discovery. *J Med Chem.* 2020;63(10):5013–5030.

Li J, Hua Y, Miyagawa S, Zhang J, Li L, Liu L, Sawa Y. hiPSC-derived cardiac tissue for disease modeling and drug discovery. *Int J Mol Sci.* 2020;21(23):8893.

Li Q. Application of fragment-based drug discovery to versatile targets. *Front Mol Biosci.* 2020;7:180.

Li Q, Kang C. A practical perspective on the roles of solution nmr spectroscopy in drug discovery. *Molecules.* 2020;25(13):2974.

Li Q, Kang C. Mechanisms of action for small molecules revealed by structural biology in drug discovery. *Int J Mol Sci.* 2020;21(15):5262.

Liang D, Yu Y, Ma Z. Novel strategies targeting bromodomain-containing protein 4 (BRD4) for cancer drug discovery. *Eur J Med Chem.* 2020;200:112426.

Lin S, Schorpp K, Rothenaigner I, Hadian K. Image-based high-content screening in drug discovery. *Drug Discov Today.* 2020;25(8):1348–1361.

Liu H, Liu K, Dong Z. Targeting CDK12 for cancer therapy: function, mechanism, and drug discovery. *Cancer Res.* 2020;81(1):18–26.

Liu ZQ. Bridging free radical chemistry with drug discovery: a promising way for finding novel drugs efficiently. *Eur J Med Chem.* 2020;1:112020.

Lu C, Di L. In vitro and in vivo methods to assess pharmacokinetic drug-drug interactions in drug discovery and development. *Biopharm Drug Dispos.* 2020;41(1–2):3–31.

Macalino SJY, Billones JB, Organo VG, Carrillo MCO. *In silico*strategies in tuberculosis drug discovery. *Molecules.* 2020;25(3):665.

Macdonald SJF, Hatley RJD. Sprinkling the pixie dust: reflections oni nnovation and innovators in medicinal chemistry and drug discovery. *Drug Discov Today.* 2020;25(3):599–609.

Madden SK, Itzhaki LS. Structural and mechanistic insights into the Keap1-Nrf2 system as a route to drug discovery. *Biochim Biophys Acta ProteinsProteom.* 2020;1868(7):140405.

Maghembe R, Damian D, Makaranga A, Nyandoro SS, Lyantagaye SL, Kusari S, Hatti-Kaul R. Omics for bioprospecting and drug discovery from bacteria and microalgae. *Antibiotics (Basel).* 2020;9(5):229.

Mansoldo FRP, Carta F, Angeli A, Cardoso VDS, Supuran CT, Vermelho AB. Chagas disease: perspectives on the past and present and challenges in drug discovery. *Molecules.* 2020;25(22):5483.

Massink A, Amelia T, Karamychev A, IJzerman AP. Allosteric modulation of G protein-coupled receptors by amiloride and its derivatives. Perspectives for drug discovery? *Med Res Rev.* 2020;40(2):683–708.

Maveyraud L, Mourey L. Protein X-ray crystallography and drug discovery. *Molecules.* 2020;25(5):1030.

Meier K, Bühlmann S, Arús-Pous J, Reymond JL. The generated databases (GDBs) as a source of 3D-shaped building blocks for use in medicinal chemistry and drug discovery. *Chimia (Aarau).* 2020;74(4):241–246.

Mendel HC, Kaas Q, Muttenthaler M. Neuropeptide signalling systems – An underexplored target for venom drug discovery. *Biochem Pharmacol.* 2020;181:114129.

METABOLIGHTS: a cross-species repository and reference database for metabolomics. [https://www.ebi.ac.uk/metabolights/]

Miyawaki I. Application of zebrafish to safety evaluation in drug discovery. *J Toxicol Pathol.* 2020;33(4):197–210.

Mohammad Nezhady MA, Rivera JC, Chemtob S. Location bias as emerging paradigm in GPCR biology and drug discovery. *iScience.* 2020;23(10):101643.

Moustaqil M, Gambin Y, Sierecki E. Biophysical techniques for target validation and drug discovery in transcription-targeted therapy. *Int J Mol Sci.* 2020;21(7):2301.

Mullane K, Williams M. Alzheimer's disease beyond amyloid: can the repetitive failures of amyloid-targeted therapeutics inform future approaches to dementia drug discovery? *Biochem Pharmacol.* 2020;177:113945.

Mun J, Choi G, Lim B. A guide for bioinformaticians: omics-based drug discovery for precision oncology. *Drug Discov Today.* 2020:S1359-6446(20):30335–4.

Munir A, Vedithi SC, Chaplin AK, Blundell TL. Genomics, computational biology and drug discovery for mycobacterial infections: fighting the emergence of resistance. *Front Genet.* 2020;11:965.

Naito M, Komatsu H. [Intermolecular interaction-based ubiquitin-proteasome system-targeting drug discovery]. *Nihon Yakurigaku Zasshi.* 2021;156(1):9–12. Japanese.

Nembo EN, Hescheler J, Nguemo F. Stem cells in natural product and medicinal plant drug discovery-An overview of new screening approaches. *Biomed Pharmacother.* 2020;131:110730.

Niazi S. *Biosimilarity: The FDA Perspective.* Boca Raton, FL: CRC Press; 2018; ISBN 9781498750394.

Niazi S. *Biosimilars and Interchangeable Biologicals: Strategic Elements.* Boca Raton, FL: CRC Press; 2015; ISBN 9781482298918.

Niazi S. *Biosimilars and Interchangeable Biologics: Tactical Elements.* Boca Raton, FL: CRC Press; 2015; ISBN 9781482298918.

Niazi S. *Disposable Bioprocessing Systems.* Boca Raton, FL: CRC Press; 2012; ISBN-13: 9781439866702.

Niazi S. *Filing Patents Online.* Boca Raton, FL: CRC Press; 2003; ISBN-13: 9780849316241.

Niazi S. *Fundamentals of Modern Bioprocessing, Sarfaraz K. Niazi and Justin L. Brown*, Boca Raton, FL: CRC Press; 2015; ISBN 9781466585737.

Niazi S. *Handbook of Bioequivalence Testing.* New York: Informa Healthcare; 2007 and 2014.

Niazi S. *Handbook of Biogeneric Therapeutic Proteins: Manufacturing, Regulatory, Testing and Patent Issues.* Boca Raton, FL: CRC Press; 2005; ISBN-13: 9780971474611.

Niazi S. *Handbook of Medicine Manufacturing Formulations*, Volume 6, 2nd ed: *Sterile Products.* New York: Informa Healthcare; 2004, 2009, 2020.

Niazi S. *Handbook of Medicine Manufacturing Formulations*, Volume 1, 2nd ed: *Compressed Solids.* New York: Informa Healthcare; 2009; ISBN-13: 9781420081169.

Niazi S. *Handbook of Medicine Manufacturing Formulations*, Volume 2, 2nd ed: *Uncompressed Solids.* New York: Informa Healthcare; 2004, 2009, 2020.

Niazi S. *Handbook of Medicine Manufacturing Formulations*, Volume 3, 2nd ed: *Liquid Products*. New York: Informa Healthcare; 2004, 2009, 2020.

Niazi S. *Handbook of Medicine Manufacturing Formulations*, Volume 4, 2nd ed: *Semisolid Products*. New York: Informa Healthcare; 2004, 2009, 2020.

Niazi S. *Handbook of Medicine Manufacturing Formulations*, Volume 5, 2nd ed: *Over the Counter Products*, New York: Informa Healthcare; 2004, 2009, 2020.

Niazi S. *Handbook of Preformulation: Chemical, Biological and Botanical Medicines*. New York: Informa Healthcare, 2006 and 2019.

Niazi S. Pharmacokinetic and pharmacodynamic modeling in early medicine development, in Charles G. Smith and James T. O'Donnell (eds.), *The Process of New Medicine Discovery and Development* (2nd ed.). New York: CRC Press, 2004 and 2020.

Niazi S. *Textbook of Biopharmaceutics and Clinical Pharmacokinetics*. New York: J Wiley & Sons; 1979; ISBN-13: 9789381075043.

Noble M, Lin QT, Sirko C, Houpt JA, Novello MJ, Stathopulos PB. Structural mechanisms of store-operated and mitochondrial calcium regulation: initiation points for drug discovery. *Int J Mol Sci*. 2020;21(10):3642.

Olotu F, Agoni C, Soremekun O, Soliman MES. An update on the pharmacological usage of curcumin: has it failed in the drug discovery pipeline? *Cell Biochem Biophys*. 2020;78(3):267–289.

Öztürk H, Özgür A, Schwaller P, Laino T, Ozkirimli E. Exploring chemical space using natural language processing methodologies for drug discovery. *Drug discov Today*. 2020;25(4):689–705.

Pálfy G, Menyhárd DK, Perczel A. Dynamically encoded reactivity of Ras enzymes: opening new frontiers for drug discovery. *Cancer Metastasis Rev*. 2020;39(4):1075–1089.

Park J, Langmead CJ, Riddy DM. New advances in targeting the resolution of inflammation: implications for specialized pro-resolving mediator GPCR drug discovery. *ACS Pharmacol Transl Sci*. 2020;3(1):88–106.

Partridge FA, Forman R, Bataille CJR, Wynne GM, Nick M, Russell AJ, Else KJ,Sattelle DB. Anthelmintic drug discovery: target identification, screening methods and the role of open science. *Beilstein J Org Chem*. 2020;16:1203–1224.

Partridge L, Fuentealba M, Kennedy BK. The quest to slow ageing through drug discovery. *Nat Rev Drug Discov*. 2020;19(8):513–532.

Patel H, Kukol A. Integrating molecular modelling methods to advance influenza A virus drug discovery. *Drug Discov Today*. 2020;S1359-6446(20):30480–3.

Patel L, Shukla T, Huang X, Ussery DW, Wang S. Machine learning methods in drug discovery. *Molecules*. 2020;25(22):5277.

Paul D, Sanap G, Shenoy S, Kalyane D, Kalia K, Tekade RK. Artificial intelligence in drug discovery and development. *Drug Discov Today*. 2020;S1359-6446(20):30425–6.

PDBECHEM: provides comprehensive search over the dictionary of chemical components referred to in PDB entries and maintained by the wwPDB [http://www.pdbe.org/chem]d

Pillaiyar T, Meenakshisundaram S, Manickam M, Sankaranarayanan M. A medicinal chemistry perspective of drug repositioning: recent advances and challenges in drug discovery. *Eur J Med Chem*. 2020;195:112275. doi:10.1016/j.ejmech.2020.112275.

Porterfield V. Neural progenitor cell derivation methodologies for drug discovery applications. *Assay Drug Dev Technol*. 2020;18(2):89–95.

Prazeres DMF. *Plasmid Biomedicines: Basics, Applications, and Manufacturing*. Oxford: Wiley-Blackwell; 2011.

Pulya S, Amin SA, Adhikari N, Biswas S, Jha T, Ghosh B. HDAC6 as privileged target in drug discovery: a perspective. *Pharmacol Res*. 2021;163:105274. doi:10.1016/j.phrs.2020.105274.

Qin HL, Zhang ZW, Lekkala R, Alsulami H, Rakesh KP. Chalcone hybrids as privileged scaffolds in antimalarial drug discovery: a key review. *Eur J MedChem*. 2020;193:112215.

Rampacci E, Stefanetti V, Passamonti F, Henao-Tamayo M. Preclinical models of nontuberculous mycobacteria infection for early drug discovery and vaccine research. *Pathogens*. 2020;9(8):641.

Ramzy GM, Koessler T, Ducrey E, McKee T, Ris F, Buchs N, Rubbia-Brandt L,Dietrich PY, Nowak-Sliwinska P. Patient-derived in vitro models for drug discovery in colorectal carcinoma. *Cancers (Basel)*. 2020;12(6):1423.

Rask-Andersen et al., The druggable genome: evaluation of drug targets in clinical trials suggests major shifts in molecular class and indication. *Ann. Rev. Pharmacol. Toxicol*. 2014, http://bit.ly/2zYLSP9

Rathore AS, Mhatre R. *Quality by Design for Biomedicines: Principles and Case Studies*. Oxford: Wiley; 2009.

Rathore AS, Sofer GK. *Process Validation in Manufacturing of Biomedicines: Guidelines, Current Practices, and Industrial Case Studies*. Boca Raton, FL: Taylor & Francis; 2005.

Rathore AS, Sofer GK. *Process Validation in Manufacturing of Biomedicines*. 3rd ed. Boca Raton, FL: Taylor & Francis/CRC Press; 2012.

Rathore AS. *Process Validation in Manufacturing of Biomedicines*. 3rd ed. Hoboken, NJ: CRC Press; 2012.

Raut D, Bhatt LK. Evolving targets for anti-epileptic drug discovery. *Eur J Pharmacol*. 2020;887:173582. doi:10.1016/j.ejphar.2020.173582

Razinkov VI, Kleemann GR. *High-Throughput Formulation Development of Biomedicines: Practical Guide to Methods and Applications*. Amsterdam: Elsevier/Woodhead Publishing; 2017.

Rehbinder E. *Pharming: Promises and Risks of Biomedicines Derived from Genetically Modified Plants and Animals*. Berlin: Springer; 2009.

Reid ECT. *A Tool-Kit for In-Process Determination and Control of Structural and Conformational Authenticity of Complex Biomedicines* [Thesis (Ph.D.)], University of London; 2007.

RHEA: A curated database of enzyme-catalyzed reactions. [https://www.rhea-db.org/]

Riches A, Hart CJS, Trenholme KR, Skinner-Adams TS. Anti-*Giardia* drug discovery: current status and gut feelings. *J Med Chem*. 2020;63(22):13330–13354.

Rickwood S, Southworth A. *New Technologies in Biomedicines*. London: Financial Times Medicines & Healthcare Publishing; 1995.

Rojanasakul Y, Wu-Pong S. *Biomedicine Medicine Design and Development*. 2nd ed. Totowa, NJ: Humana Press; 2008.

Rosales Mendoza S. *Algae-Based Biomedicines*. Switzerland: Springer; 2016.

Rosenbaum MI, Clemmensen LS, Bredt DS, Bettler B, Strømgaard K. Targeting receptor complexes: a new dimension in drug discovery. *Nat Rev Drug Discov*. 2020;19(12):884–901.

Rosner M, Reithofer M, Fink D, Hengstschläger M. Human embryo models and drug discovery. *Int J Mol Sci*. 2021;22(2):E637.

Rossi GM, Regolisti G, Peyronel F, Fiaccadori E. Recent insights into sodium and potassium handling by the aldosterone-sensitive distal nephron: implications on pathophysiology and drug discovery. *J Nephrol*. 2020;33(3):447–466.

Rusnati M, D'Ursi P, Pedemonte N, Urbinati C, Ford RC, Cichero E, Uggeri M,Orro A, Fossa P. Recent strategic advances in CFTR drug discovery: an overview. *Int J Mol Sci*. 2020;21(7):2407.

Russ and Lampel. The druggable genome: an update. *Drug Disc Today*. 2015, http://bit.ly/2jGwdzY

Salick MR, Lubeck E, Riesselman A, Kaykas A. The future of cerebral organoids in drug discovery. *Semin Cell Dev Biol*. 2020;S1084–9521(19):30302–7.

Sandset T. *Ending AIDS in the Age of Biomedicines: The Individual, the State and the Politics of Prevention*. 1st ed. New York: Routledge; 2020.

Santos R, et al. A comprehensive map of molecular drug targets. *Nature Revs Drug Disc*. 2017, http://go.nature.com/2AePzmX (available on semanticscholar.net, http://bit.ly/2jJm5Xn)

Schaduangrat N, Lampa S, Simeon S, Gleeson MP, Spjuth O, Nantasenamat C. Towards reproducible computational drug discovery. *J Cheminform*. 2020;12(1):9.

Schmidt SR. *Fusion Protein Technologies for Biomedicines: Applications and Challenges*. Hoboken, NJ: Wiley; 2013.

Schwarz J, Rosenthal K, Snajdrova R, Kittelmann M, Lütz S. The development of biocatalysis as a tool for drug discovery. *Chimia (Aarau)*. 2020;74(5):368–377.

Segarra C. *Development of an Integrated Platform for the Production of Recombinant Biomedicines* [Thesis (Ph.D.)], University of Sheffield; 2013.

Seimiya H. Crossroads of telomere biology and anticancer drug discovery. *Cancer Sci*. 2020;111(9):3089–3099.

Sepúlveda-Crespo D, Reguera RM, Rojo-Vázquez F, Balaña-Fouce R, Martínez-Valladares M. Drug discovery technologies: *Caenorhabditis elegans* as a model for anthelmintic therapeutics. *Med Res Rev*. 2020;40(5):1715–1753.

Seshadri S, Hoeppner DJ, Tajinda K. Calcium imaging in drug discovery for psychiatric disorders. *Front Psychiatry*. 2020;11:713. doi:10.3389/fpsyt.2020.00713

Sessions Z, Sánchez-Cruz N, Prieto-Martínez FD, Alves VM, Santos HP Jr,Muratov E, Tropsha A, Medina-Franco JL. Recent progress on cheminformatics approaches to epigenetic drug discovery. *Drug Discov Today*. 2020;25(12):2268–2276.

Shankaraiah N, Sakla AP, Laxmikeshav K, Tokala R. Reliability of click chemistry on drug discovery: a personal account. *Chem Rec*. 2020;20(4):253–272.

Sharma A, Sances S, Workman MJ, Svendsen CN. Multi-lineage human iPSC-derived platforms for disease modeling and drug discovery. *Cell Stem Cell*. 2020;26(3):309–329.

Sheik Amamuddy O, Veldman W, Manyumwa C, Khairallah A, Agajanian S, OluyemiO, Verkhivker G, Tastan Bishop O. Integrated computational approaches and tools for allosteric drug discovery. *Int J Mol Sci*. 2020;21(3):847.

Shibeshi MA, Kifle ZD, Atnafie SA. Antimalarial drug resistance and novelt argets for antimalarial drug discovery. *Infect Drug Resist*. 2020;13:4047–4060. doi:10.2147/IDR.S279433

Shou WZ. Current status and future directions of high-throughput ADME screening in drug discovery. *J Pharm Anal*. 2020;10(3):201–208.

Shyr ZA, Gorshkov K, Chen CZ, Zheng W. Drug discovery strategies for SARS-CoV-2. *J Pharmacol Exp Ther*. 2020;375(1):127–138.

SignaLink 2. A signaling pathway resource with multi-layered regulatory networks, Fazekas et al., *BMC Syst Biol*. 2013, http://bit.ly/2hNkXBe; portal: http://signalink.org

Soeda Y, Takashima A. New insights into drug discovery targeting tau protein. *Front Mol Neurosci*. 2020;13:590896. doi:10.3389/fnmol.2020.590896

Song M, Hwang GT. DNA-encoded library screening as core platform technology in drug discovery: its synthetic method development and applications in DEL synthesis. *J Med Chem*. 2020;63(13): 6578–6599.

Srinivasan B. Explicit treatment of non-michaelis-menten and atypical kinetics in early drug discovery. *ChemMedChem*. 2020;16(6).

Steinke I, Ghanei N, Govindarajulu M, Yoo S, Zhong J, Amin RH. Drug discovery and development of novel therapeutics for inhibiting TMAO in models of atherosclerosis and diabetes. *Front Physiol*. 2020;11:567899. doi:10.3389/fphys.2020.567899

Su H, Zhou F, Huang Z, Ma X, Natarajan K, Zhang M, Huang Y, Su H. Molecular insights into small-molecule drug discovery for SARS-CoV-2. *Angew Chem Int EdEngl*. 2020;60(18):9789–9802.

Sun DJ, Zhu LJ, Zhao YQ, Zhen YQ, Zhang L, Lin CC, Chen LX. Diarylheptanoid: a privileged structure in drug discovery. *Fitoterapia*. 2020;142:104490. doi:10.1016/j.fitote.2020.104490

SURECHEMBL: A publicly available large-scale searchable resource containing compounds extracted from the full text, images and attachments of patent documents. [https://www.surechembl.org/search/]

Swinney DC, Lee JA. Recent advances in phenotypic drug discovery. *F1000Res*. 2020;F1000:944.

Takahashi M. *Proceedings of the 2015 International Conference on Medicine and Biomedicines: 2015 International Conference on Medicine and Biomedicines*, China, 15–16 August 2015.

Tavakoli-Keshe R. *Quantifying the Impact of the Physical Environment during Processing and Storage of Biomedicines* [Thesis (Ph.D.)], University College London (University of London); 2014.

Taylor DG. The political economics of cancer drug discovery and pricing. *Drug Discov Today*. 2020;25(12):2149–2160.

Thomaz-Soccol V, Pandey A, Resende RR. *Current Developments in Biotechnology and Vioengineering. Human and Animal Health Applications*. Amsterdam: Elsevier; 2017.

Thompson DC, Bentzien J. Crowdsourcing and open innovation in drug discovery: recent contributions and future directions. *Drug Discov Today*. 2020;25(12):2284–2293.

Tian JY, Chi CL, Bian G, Guo FJ, Wang XQ, Yu B. A novel GPCR target in correlation with androgen deprivation therapy for prostate cancer drug discovery. *Basic Clin Pharmacol Toxicol*. 2021;28(2):195–203. doi:10.1111/bcpt.13499

Tibon NS, Ng CH, Cheong SL. Current progress in antimalarial pharmacotherapy and multi-target drug discovery. *Eur J Med Chem*. 2020;188:111983. doi:10.1016/j.ejmech.2019.111983

Tovey MG. *Detection and Quantification of Antibodies to Biomedicines: Practical and Applied Considerations*. Hoboken, NJ: Wiley; 2011.

Tran N, Pham B, Le L. Bioactive compounds in anti-diabetic plants: from herbal medicine to modern drug discovery. *Biology (Basel)*. 2020;9(9):252.

Troelsen NS, Clausen MH. Library design strategies to accelerate fragment-based drug discovery. *Chemistry.* 2020;26(50):11391–11403.

Trusler O, Goodwin J, Laslett AL. BRCA1 and BRCA2 associated breast cancer and the roles of current modelling systems in drug discovery. *Biochim BiophysActa Rev Cancer.* 2020;1875(1):188459.

UNICHEM: Rapid lookup of small molecule structures across chemically-aware resources. [https://www.ebi.ac.uk/unichem/]

Urra FA, Araya-Maturana R. Putting the brakes on tumorigenesis with snakevenom toxins: new molecular insights for cancer drug discovery. *Semin CancerBiol.* 2020;S1044–579X(20):30102-4.

Van Drie JH, Tong L. Cryo-EM as a powerful tool for drug discovery. *BioorgMed Chem Lett.* 2020;30(22):127524.

Vatansever S, Schlessinger A, Wacker D, Kaniskan HÜ, Jin J, Zhou MM, ZhangB. Artificial intelligence and machine learning-aided drug discovery in central nervous system diseases: state-of-the-arts and future directions. *Med Res Rev.* 2021;41(3):1427–1473. doi:10.1002/med.21764

Vázquez J, López M, Gibert E, Herrero E, Luque FJ. Merging ligand-based and structure-based methods in drug discovery: an overview of combined virtual screening approaches. *Molecules.* 2020;25(20):4723.

Veeravalli V, Cheruvu HS, Srivastava P, Vamsi Madgula LM. Three-dimensional aspects of formulation excipients in drug discovery: a critical assessment on orphan excipients, matrix effects and drug interactions. *J Pharm Anal.* 2020;10(6):522–531.

Völkner C, Liedtke M, Hermann A, Frech MJ. pluripotent stem cells for disease modeling and drug discovery in niemann-pick type C1. *Int J Mol Sci.* 2021;22(2):E710.

Waddington JL, Zhen X, O'Tuathaigh CMP. Developmental genes and regulatory proteins, domains of cognitive impairment in schizophrenia spectrum psychosis and implications for antipsychotic drug discovery: the example of dysbindin-1 isoforms and beyond. *Front Pharmacol.* 2020;10:1638. doi:10.3389/fphar.2019.01638

Walker PA, Ryder S, Lavado A, Dilworth C, Riley RJ. The evolution of strategies to minimise the risk of human drug-induced liver injury (DILI) indrug discovery and development. *Arch Toxicol.* 2020;94(8):2559–2585.

Walsh G, Murphy B. *Biomedicines, an Industrial Perspective.* Boston, MA: Kluwer Academic; 1999.

Walsh G. *Medicine Biotechnology: Concepts and Applications.* Hoboken, NJ: John Wiley & Sons; 2007.

Walsh G. *Post-translational Modification of Protein Biomedicines.* Weinheim: Wiley-VCH; 2009.

Wang M, Li H, Liu W, Cao H, Hu X, Gao X, Xu F, Li Z, Hua H, Li D. Dammarane-type leads panaxadiol and protopanaxadiol for drug discovery: biological activity and structural modification. *Eur J Med Chem.* 2020;1:112087.

Wang X, McFarland A, Madsen JJ, Aalo E, Ye L. The potential of ^{19}F NMR application in GPCR biased drug discovery. *Trends PharmacolSci.* 2021;42(1):19–30.

Wang Y, Yu Z, Xiao W, Lu S, Zhang J. Allosteric binding sites at the receptor-lipid bilayer interface: novel targets for GPCR drug discovery. *Drug Discov Today.* 2020;S1359-6446(20):30519–5.

Weert Mvd, Møller EH. *Immunogenicity of Biomedicines.* New York: Springer; 2008.

Wei S, Ma X, Zhao Y. Mechanism of hydrophobic bile acid-induced hepatocytel injury and drug discovery. *Front Pharmacol.* 2020;11:1084. doi:10.3389/fphar.2020.01084

Willems H, De Cesco S, Svensson F. Computational chemistry on a budget: supporting drug discovery with limited resources. *J Med Chem.* 2020;63(18):10158–10169.

Wittrup KD, Verdine GL. *Protein Engineering for Therapeutics. Part* B. 1st ed. San Diego, CA: Academic; 2012.

Wu F, Zhou Y, Li L, Shen X, Chen G, Wang X, Liang X, Tan M, Huang Z. Computational approaches in preclinical studies on drug discovery and development. *Front Chem.* 2020;8:726. doi:10.3389/fchem.2020.00726

Xiao J, Glasgow E, Agarwal S. Zebrafish xenografts for drug discovery and personalized medicine. *Trends Cancer.* 2020;6(7):569–579.

Yang D, Zhou Q, Labroska V, Qin S, Darbalaei S, Wu Y, Yuliantie E, Xie L,Tao H, Cheng J, Liu Q, Zhao S, Shui W, Jiang Y, Wang MW. G protein-coupledr eceptors: structure- and function-based drug discovery. *Signal Transduct TargetTher.* 2021;6(1):7.

Yang H. *Emerging Nonclinical Biostatistics in Biomedicine Development and Manufacturing.* New York: CRC Press; 2017.

Yang N, Dong YQ, Jia GX, Fan SM, Li SZ, Yang SS, Li YB. ASBT(SLC10A2): a promising target for treatment of diseases and drug discovery. *Biomed Pharmacother.* 2020;132:110835.

Yang W, Bhattachar SN, Patel PJ, Landis M, Patel D, Reid DL, Duvnjak RomicM. Modulating target engagement of small molecules via drug delivery: approaches and applications in drug discovery and development. *Drug Discov Today*. 2020;26:713–726.

Yang Y, Zhou Q, Gao A, Chen L, Li L. Endoplasmic reticulum stress and focused drug discovery in cardiovascular disease. *Clin Chim Acta*. 2020 May;504:125–137. doi:10.1016/j.cca.2020.01.031. Epub 2020 Feb 1. PMID: .

Yu Q, Jiang Y, Sun Y. Anticancer drug discovery by targeting cullinneddylation. *Acta Pharm Sin B*. 2020;10(5):746–765.

Yu Q, Xiong X, Sun Y. [Targeting cullin-RING E3 ligases for anti-cancer therapy: efforts on drug discovery]. *Zhejiang Da Xue Xue Bao Yi Xue Ban*. 2020;49(1):1–19.

Zanandrea R, Bonan CD, Campos MM. Zebrafish as a model for inflammation and drug discovery. *Drug Discov Today*. 2020;25(12):2201–2211.

Zeng S, Huang W, Zheng X, Liyan Cheng, Zhang Z, Wang J, Shen Z. Proteolysis targeting chimera (PROTAC) in drug discovery paradigm: recent progress and future challenges. *Eur J Med Chem*. 2021 Jan 15;210:112981. doi:10.1016/j.ejmech.2020.112981. Epub 2020 Oct 31. PMID: .

Zhang L, Song J, Kong L, Yuan T, Li W, Zhang W, Hou B, Lu Y, Du G. The strategies and techniques of drug discovery from natural products. *Pharmacol Ther*. 2020;107686.

Zhang Y, Xie X, Hu J, Afreen KS, Zhang CL, Zhuge Q, Yang J. Prospects of directly reprogrammed adult human neurons for neurodegenerative disease modeling and drug discovery: iN vs. iPSCs models. *Front Neurosci*. 2020;14:546484. doi:10.3389/fnins.2020.546484. PMID: ; PMCID: PMC7710799.

Zhang ZD, Milman S, Lin JR, Wierbowski S, Yu H, Barzilai N, Gorbunova V,Ladiges WC, Niedernhofer LJ, Suh Y, Robbins PD, Vijg J. Genetics of extreme human longevity to guide drug discovery for healthy ageing. *Nat Metab*. 2020;2(8):663–672.

Zhao L, Ciallella HL, Aleksunes LM, Zhu H. Advancing computer-aided drug discovery (CADD) by big data and data-driven machine learning modeling. *Drug Discov Today*. 2020;25(9):1624–1638.

Zhavoronkov A, Vanhaelen Q, Oprea TI. Will artificial intelligence for drug discovery impact clinical pharmacology? *Clin Pharmacol Ther*. 2020;107(4):780–785.

Zhou J, Theesfeld CL, Yao K, Chen KM, Wong AK, and Troyanskaya OG. Deep learning sequence-based ab initio prediction of variant effects on expression and disease risk. *Nature Genetics*. 2018;50(8):1171–1179. doi:10.1038/s41588-018-0160-6. Epub 2018 Jul 16. PMID: ; PMCID: PMC6094955.

Zhou J, Troyanskaya OG. Predicting the effects of noncoding variants with deep learning-based sequence model. *Nature Methods*. 2015;12(10):931–934. doi:10.1038/nmeth.3547. Epub 2015 Aug 24. PMID: ; PMCID: PMC4768299.

Zhu L, Chen X, Abola EE, Jing L, Liu W. Serial crystallography for structure-based drug discovery. *Trends Pharmacol Sci*. 2020;41(11):830–839.

Zhu L, Zhang Y, Guo Z, Wang M. Cardiovascular biology of prostanoids and drug discovery. *Arterioscler Thromb Vasc Biol*. 2020;40(6):1454–1463.

Zhu W, Chen CZ, Gorshkov K, Xu M, Lo DC, Zheng W. RNA-dependent RNA polymerase as a target for COVID-19 drug discovery. *SLAS Discov*. 2020;25(10):1141–1151.

Zhu Y, Li J, Pang Z. Recent insights for the emerging COVID-19: drug discovery, therapeutic options and vaccine development. *Asian J Pharm Sci*. 2021;16(1):4–23. doi:10.1016/j.ajps.2020.06.001. Epub 2020 Jul 4. PMID: ; PMCID: PMC7335243.

3

Artificial Intelligence

3.1 Background

In the 1950s, artificial intelligence (AI) pioneers predicted that machines would sense, reason, and think like humans—a proof of concept known as universal AI. I disagree with the vocabulary; there is nothing artificial about intelligence. Instead, humans acquire the same intelligence, except it is held within a machine—a better tag would have been MI (machine intelligence), but we can leave that aside.

Rapid growth in computing power and memory storage, an unprecedented wealth of data, and the development of advanced algorithms have resulted in significant breakthroughs in AI applications such as computer vision, voice recognition, natural language understanding, and digital pathology data analysis. Similarly, AI has revolutionized drugs by uncovering previously unknown patterns and evidence in biomedical data.

Intelligence is defined as the ability to acquire and use knowledge and skill. In contrast, intellect is defined as the faculty of objective reasoning and understanding, particularly in abstract or intellectual issues. For example, a programmed factory robot is flexible, accurate, and consistent but not intelligent; a computer algorithm can be intelligent but not intellectual, at least for now.

Mathematicians and philosophers in early history first studied mechanical or "formal" reasoning. For example, Alan Turing argued that a machine might reproduce any conceivable act of logical deduction by shuffling symbols as simple as "0" and "1" based on his knowledge of mathematical logic. The Church–Turing thesis is the idea that digital computers can imitate any formal reasoning process.

Artificial intelligence (AI) is commonly understood as the intelligence shown by machines, compared to the natural intelligence shown by humans, as suggested by John McCarthy in 1956 at a workshop at Dartmouth College because he wanted to escape the influence of "cybernetics" coined by Norbert Wiener—a sort of rivalry. However, the term AI did not catch up until the early 1980s when computers began simulating human experts' knowledge and analytical skills, as demonstrated by AlphaGo that successfully defeated a professional Go player in 2015.

Artificial intelligence (AI) encompasses (Figure 3.1):

- Machine learning: A system can automatically learn and improve from experience without being explicitly programmed. Computers with learning abilities improve their perception using a Bayesian approach leading manipulations of statistics, psychology, neuroscience, economics, and control theory. Humanized machines (HMs) simulate human behavior based on billions of human expressions, such as the Generative Pre-trained Transformer 3 (GPT-3), an autoregressive language model that uses deep learning to produce human-like text (Figure 3.2).
- Neural networks: A set of algorithms that recognize underlying links in a batch of data using a mechanism that mimics the way neurons in the human brain work (Figure 3.3).
- Deep learning: Machine learning without human supervision combines more complex neural structures that can detect objects, recognize speech, translate languages, and make decisions. It uses large multi-layer (artificial) neural networks that compute with continuous (actual number) representations, a little like the hierarchically organized neurons in human brains (Figure 3.3). The artificial neurons in a fully connected feedforward neural network (FNN) are connected layer by layer from input features to output destinations. Each connection has a

DOI: 10.1201/9781003146933-3

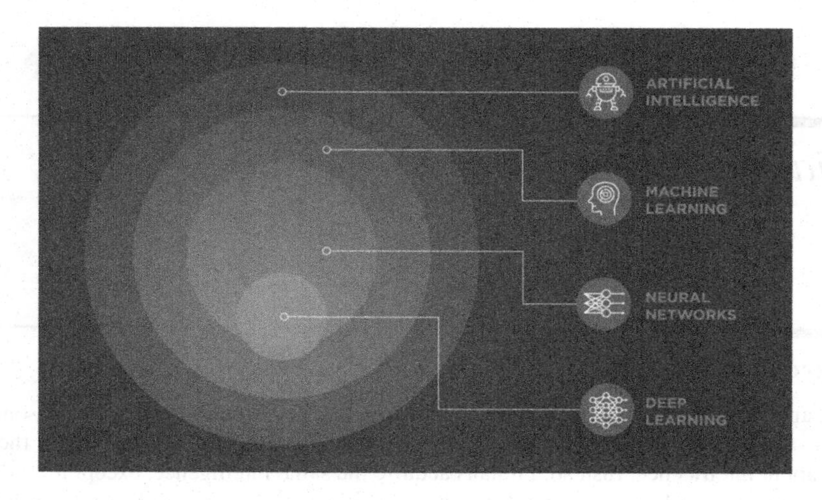

FIGURE 3.1 Domains of artificial intelligence.

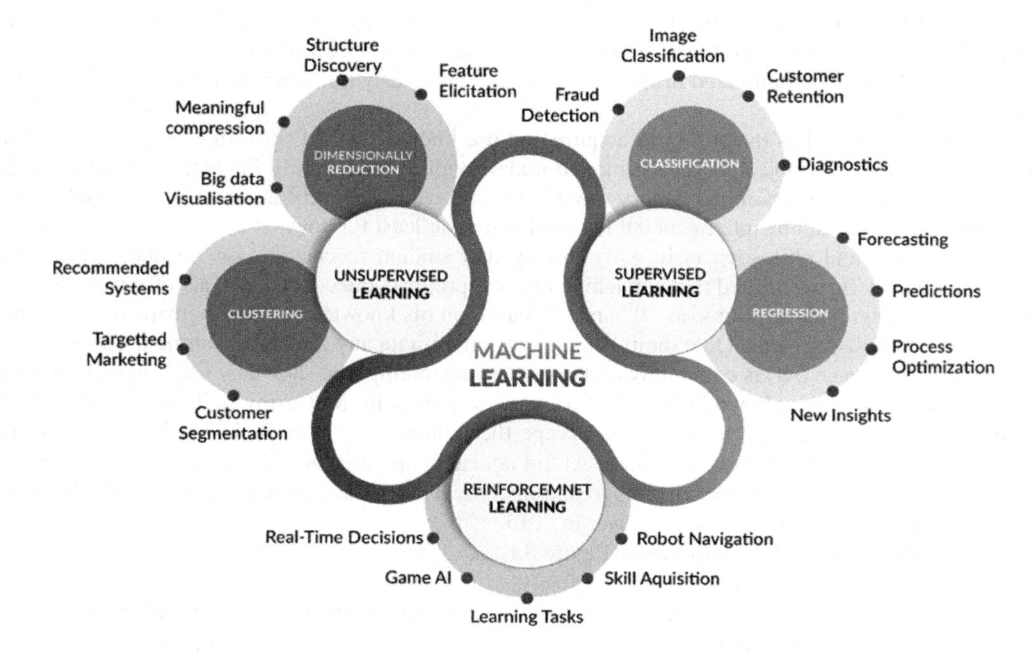

FIGURE 3.2 Elements of machine learning.

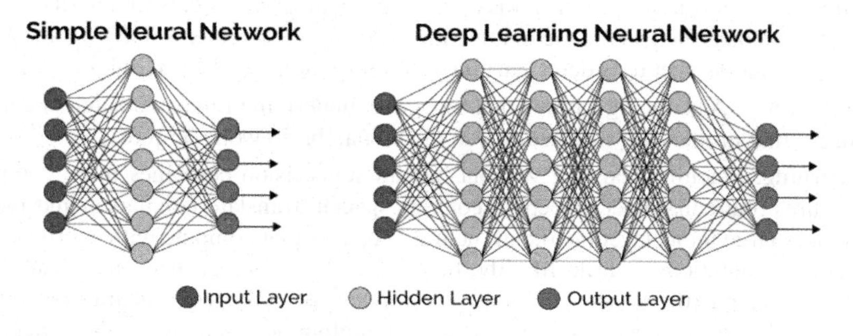

FIGURE 3.3 Comparison of simple neural networks and more varied networks is leading to deep learning.

weight optimized by backpropagating on training samples to minimize the output targets' prediction loss. For data samples expressed as vectors, FNNs are commonly utilized. For example, FNN can classify drugs into pharmaceutical therapeutic classes based on the drugs' transcriptome profile vectors. FNN outperforms other machine learning approaches such as logistic regression.

To better understand what AI is and what it is not, the analysis is presented in Table 3.1; note that certain qualifiers will change the application's definition.

AI and machine learning were put to the test in 2020 to manage the COVID-19 pandemic by creating several vaccines in the shortest time. The AI drug discovery transforms the initial screening process to the predicted success rate based on multiple biological factors. For example, it is now possible to project future mutations of viruses and, based on these projections, design antibodies and vaccines to respond to future pandemics more efficiently. In addition, precision drug or next-generation sequencing techniques will help discover drugs and tailor drugs for individual patients, an era of treatment that is fast emerging.

The machines will construct novel molecules and predict their properties virtually or create molecules to provide specific physicochemical and binding properties. DeepMind (https://deepmind.com/about) has cracked a serious scientific problem that has stumped researchers for half a century; its AlphaFold using the AI can now predict how proteins fold into 3D shapes, making it possible to discover the mechanisms that drive some diseases and pave the way for designer drugs. As a result, the testing of new drugs will become more efficient. I will identify the right candidate for the trial based on history and disease conditions, infection rates, demographics, and ethnicity to represent the most impacted population.

The next decade will bring in quantum computing to give the high throughput screening a big boost. Quantum computing is based on qbits instead of bits that are either 0 or 1; in quantum computing, we cool down the processes almost at the absolute temperature when there remains no resistance to the movement of electrons. The quantum behavior is called superposition when an electron can be both 0 and 1 simultaneously and also communicate with other electrons, which is labeled entanglement. The net result of superpositioning and entanglement is that the information is processed several million times faster which will allow the modeling of drug-receptor binding given the millions of permutations and combinations possible. Quantum computing will forever change how we will discover new drugs.

3.2 Bioinformatics

The application of mathematics, statistics, and computational, quantitative data processing is known as bioinformatics. Bioinformatics is the science of organizing, managing, and analyzing large sets of data. In high throughput screening (HTS) labs, bioinformatics is critical in properly storing and analyzing all aspects of compound heredity through screening results. Incorporating computer science and biology, bioinformatics allows scientists to store and access large amounts of data. In addition, bioinformatics allows data mining, a computational process of discovering patterns in large data sets. For example, pharmaceutical companies have implemented programs to allow for rational and systematic screening of drug-like compounds against biological targets. Using data, scientists can determine which biological targets should be studied and what drug-like compounds would most likely affect this target. This process requires efficient technology and an organized data source and it will become increasingly more important as new screening techniques gather more data.

Under the Human Genome Project (www.genome.gov/human-genome-project), we now have a comprehensive identification of genes that can help identify new drug discovery targets to create therapies for various neglected/orphan diseases and inherited disorders.

Proteomics is the study of the protein products that come from specific genes and their function and interactions. Proteomics is essential in drug discovery as it is most often an abnormality associated with a protein that contributes to the disease process. Thus, if we know the gene that controls the suspect protein, drug-like compounds can probe its biology to understand the particular protein's function and interactions.

All three of these fields combine science and technology to organize data better and predict reactivity between drug-like compounds and biological targets.

TABLE 3.1

Example of the Definition of AI Applications

Applications	Yes	No	Maybe
A spreadsheet that calculates sums and other pre-defined functions on given data		The user-specified formula determines the outcome. No AI is needed	
Plotting of molecular properties from thousands of structures and creating regression analysis	Plotting alone is not AI unless the output also evaluates hidden correlations		
Predicting the stock market by fitting a curve to past data about stock prices	Although a simple curve is not AI, there are plenty to choose from. They will gain from machine learning/AI even if there is a lot of data to confine them	?	?
A GPS navigation system for finding the fastest route	The signal processing and geometry used to determine the coordinates isn't AI but providing good suggestions for navigation (shortest/fastest routes) is AI, especially if variables such as traffic conditions are taken into account		?
Spotify, for example, is a music recommendation system that provides music based on the users' listening habits	The system learns from the users' (not only yours alone) listening behavior		
Big data storage systems that can store large volumes of data (such as photographs or video) and stream it to multiple users simultaneously are known as big data storage solutions		Storing and retrieving specific items from a data collection is neither adaptive nor autonomous	
In photo editing software like Photoshop, settings like brightness and contrast are available		Adjustments such as color balance, contrast, and so on are neither adaptive nor autonomous, but application developers may use some AI to tune the filters automatically	?
Style transfer filters in Prisma applications (https://prisma-ai.com) take a photo and transform it into different art styles (impressionist, cubist, etc.)	Such methods typically learn image statistics (read: what small patches of the image in a particular style look like up close) and transform the input photo so that its statistics match the style, so the system is adaptive		

With recent advances in computational tools, it is now possible to analyze and mine large sets of biological data about patients, with the goals of creating robust, quantitative computer models of normal human physiology, of the natural history of certain diseases, and of the course of a disease as affected by standard treatments.

The concept of model-based product development can also be applied to drug, device, and biological product safety. It should be possible to exploit a variety of existing toxicology and adverse events data to facilitate more accurate predictions of product safety and more rapid post-market identification of safety issues that could not be identified during product development. Using data to improve knowledge about key aspects of product development, such as exposure-response relationships and long-term performance of devices, and supporting innovative trial designs, a model-based development program could reduce uncertainty about dose selection and device design and other key safety and efficacy issues.

3.3 Artificial Intelligence

The AI and machine learning advances have already been in practical use for some time in many industries, including smart cars, natural language processing (NLP), image recognition, smart online search and recommendations, fraud detection, financial trading, weather forecasting, personal and data security, and chatbots, to name a few. However, the biodrug industry is just beginning to adopt the new computational technologies, though quite rapidly.

The potential of AI-based tools is now being investigated at all stages of medical discovery and development, from research data mining to assisting in target identification and validation to assist in the development of novel lead compounds and drug candidates and predict their properties risks. And finally, AI-based software can now assist in planning chemical synthesis to obtain compounds of interest. AI is also applied to planning preclinical and clinical trials and analyzing biomedical and clinical data.

AI is used in various research domains besides target-based drug development, such as phenotypic drug discovery systems, which analyze data from high-content screening approaches. While AI-driven firms primarily focus on small molecule drug discovery, there is also interest in using this technology to identify and develop biologics. The term "machine intelligence" or "machine learning" is more applicable for the subset of AI techniques used in medical research. These can be supervised by human supervision in their inner workings, as in classifiers and statistical learning methods, or unsupervised in their inner workings, as in artificial neural networks. Also important are language and semantic processing and probabilistic methods for uncertain (or fuzzy) reasoning. Understanding how these diverse tasks might be merged into the broader field of "AI" is a difficult undertaking that all parties involved should take on (Figure 3.4).

3.4 Deep Learning Architecture

Deep learning is a machine learning area that refers to a hierarchical approach to data exploration that employs layers of linear and nonlinear transformations. Artificial neural networks are the most extensively used deep learning model. An artificial neuron is the fundamental building component, transforming the weighted sum of input feature variables nonlinearly.

The artificial neurons in a fully connected feedforward neural network (FNN) are connected layer by layer from input features to output destinations. Each connection has a weight optimized by backpropagating on training samples to minimize the output targets' prediction loss. For data samples expressed as vectors, FNNs are commonly utilized. However, when photos are used as the input, and each pixel

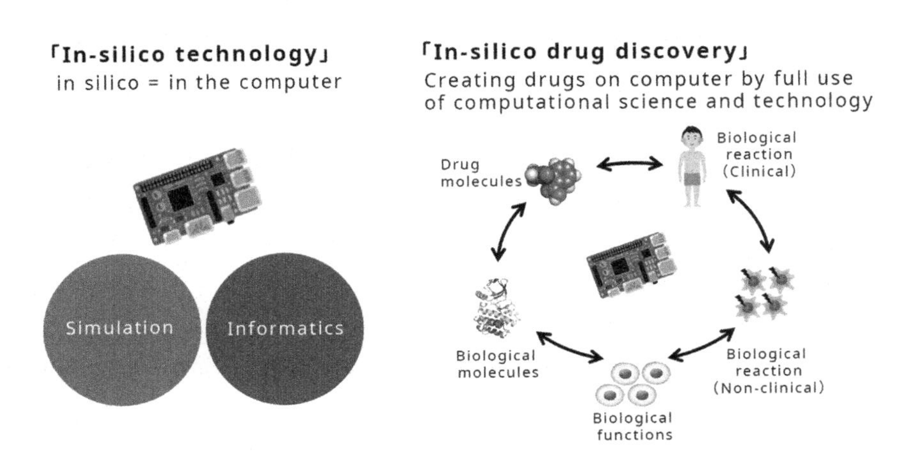

FIGURE 3.4 Digital technology impacting the trends in drug discovery. Source: www. ds-pharma.com/rd/drug_discovery/drug_discovery_research.html.

represents a feature variable, FNNs become impractical due to the enormous number of weights. However, for image processing, a convolutional neural network (CNN panel) is extremely useful. Rather than fully linking neurons in consecutive layers, CNN employs filters (small matrices of weights) that perform a convolution operation on local patches of the pictures, reducing the weights significantly. Chemical pictures are analyzed using CNN to provide knowledge into therapeutic drug actions. AtomNet (www.atomwise.com), for example, uses the structural information collected by CNN to predict the binding affinities of tiny compounds to proteins.

Biological sequences are another sort of data that has been extensively studied for drug repurposing. However, neither FNN nor CNN take into account the data's sequential nature. RNNs (recurrent neural networks) are created specifically for sequences. A recurrent cell, which appears at each timestamp or sequence location and keeps previous information while learning new information in a sequence, is the main building block. The compounds are represented as sequences using simplified molecular input line entry system codes, and RNN models are utilized to generate focused molecule libraries for drug development. To predict drug–target interactions, a hybrid approach involves combining graph neural networks and RNNs. The pre-trained deep learning–based drug–target interaction model, Molecule Transformer-Drug Target Interaction (MT-DTI), was used to identify commercially available drugs that could act on viral proteins of COVID-19. MT-DTI is a self-attention-based deep learning model designed for predicting an affinity score between a drug and a protein.

3.4.1 Graph Representation Learning

The development of medical knowledge graphs, including linkages between different types of medical entities (e.g., diseases, drugs, and proteins) and the prediction of new associations between current licensed drugs and disorders, is a classic technique to repurpose drugs (e.g., done for COVID-19). Based on graph embedding, methods have gained attention for link prediction in graphs representing nodes and edges as low-dimensional feature vectors. We can easily compare the feature vectors of drugs and diseases and identify effective drugs for a given ailment using feature vectors. However, scalability is an issue for the graph embedding method. The size of real-world (knowledge) graphs is usually quite huge. In a medical knowledge graph, the number of entities could be in the millions. Machine learning systems like TensorFlow (www.tensorflow.org) and PyTorch (https://pytorch.org) are primarily geared for regular structures, not large-scale graphs. As a result, various systems have been built specifically designed for learning representations from large-scale graphs. For example, GraphVite (https://graphvite.io), a high-performance system capable of processing tens or hundreds of millions of nodes, looks promising for future drug repurposing. The knowledge graph of BenevolentAI (www.benevolent.com) is a massive store of organized medical data containing multiple machine-learned links derived from scholarly literature.

For example, to treat COVID-19, a graph neural network with 81 probable repurposing candidates was discovered. Understanding the inhibition of AP2-associated protein kinase 1, BenevolentAI has projected that baricitinib, used in rheumatoid arthritis, may treat COVID-19 (encoded by AAK1; Figure 3.5). More than 24 million PubMed publications are used to create a comprehensive COVID-19 knowledge graph (labeled as CoV-KGE: https://pubs.acs.org/doi/pdf/10.1021/acs.jproteome.0c00316?ref=vi-chemistry_coronavirus_research), which includes 15 million edges across 39 types of interactions connecting drugs, illnesses, proteins, genes, pathways, and gene and protein expressions.

3.5 Repurposing

Biological sequences are another sort of data that has been extensively studied for drug repurposing. By combining genetic, transcriptomic, proteomic, and phenomic profiles from individuals, AI techniques help speed up precision drugs.

Visible neural networks, for example, embed the AI model's underlying workings with natural systems in biological sciences; for example, visible machine learning algorithms could lead to model architectures of data heterogeneity and translate patient data to effective therapies. Biological systems are sequences, protein complexes, cells, tissues, organs, and organisms, all complex and hierarchical.

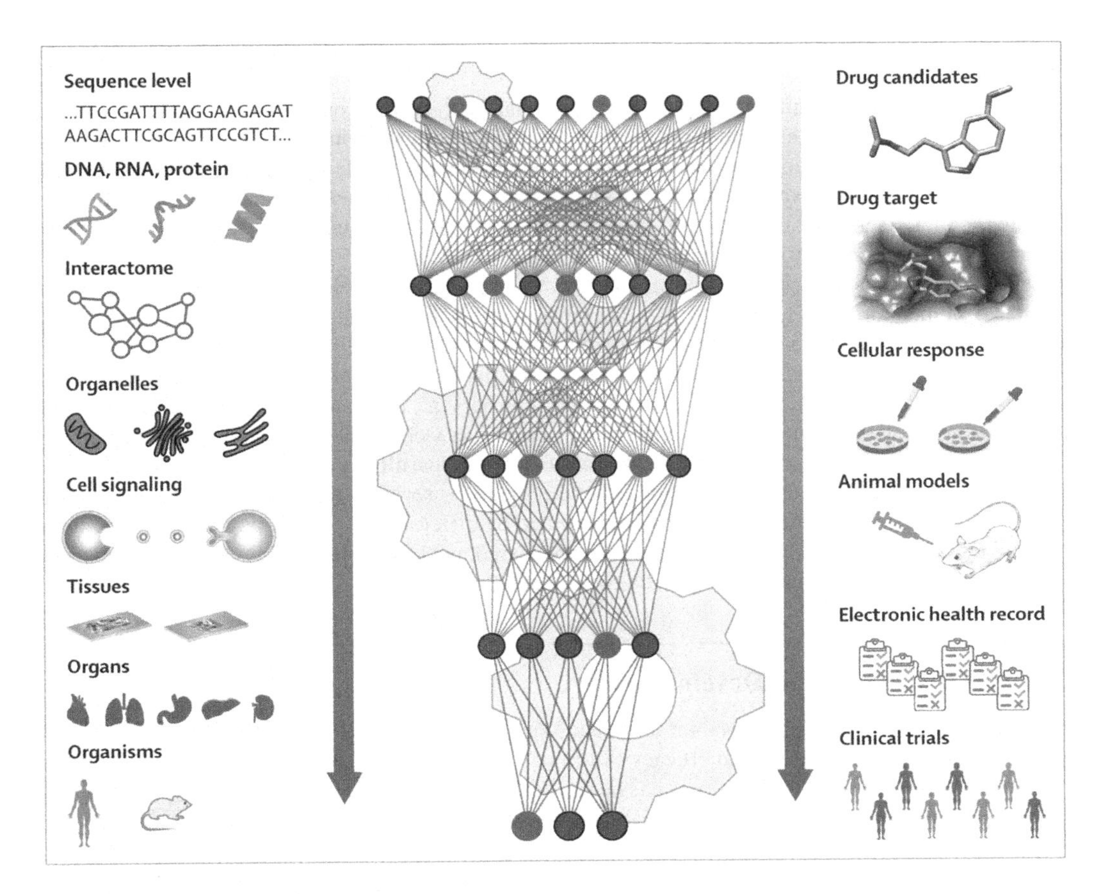

FIGURE 3.5 AI for drug repurposing in an integrative context. By combining biological knowledge with AI techniques, drug repurposing can be considerably accelerated (e.g., human interactome, organelles, tissues, and organs). Computer programs and algorithms are represented by the cogs. Deep neural network neurons are represented by red and black circles. This neuron is colored red because it transports crucial information from the biological processes. People with different shades of green and blue represent different subgroups that may have different reactions to the treatment. The downward arrows demonstrate how AI algorithms can generate more powerful models by combining multi-level biological systems and drug development pipelines. The biological systems are shown on the left, and the drug development pipeline is shown on the right. Source: www.thelancet.com/journals/landig/article/PIIS2589-7500(20)30192-8/fulltext.

Drug discovery involves a multi-level interaction between chemical substances and biological systems that is difficult to master. As a result, adding drug-related items like chemical compounds and disorders to the biologically inspired visual neural network model could help construct a more successful and interpretable drug discovery model. The design of the corresponding computational modules can be guided by biomedical knowledge of how distinct entities interact with one another, unlike existing deep learning methods, which model the entire system with a complex model all at once, our divide-and-conquer scheme models the many components of the complex design and how they interact with one another plainly and transparently. As with other deep learning models, the model parameters can be optimized from start to finish.

3.6 Data and Model Harmonization

Data harmonization is the process of standardizing and integrating information from disparate sources to form a unified database. Data harmonization is a crucial step for guaranteeing that the developed machine-learning-based models are widely applicable in different scenarios. Establishing a high-quality data model (which is a prerequisite for organizing and standardizing the data) is the foundation for the harmonization process.

Model harmonization, which specifies a single standard for storing computational models, is also a crucial feature to improve the generalizability and utility of computational drug repurposing tools, in addition to data harmonization. One such endeavor to build interoperable model transferring standards is the open neural network exchange (ONNX). ONNX defines implemented models as an extensible acyclic graph model. Each node in the graph represents a call to one of the built-in operators, which accepts standard data types as inputs and outputs.

Concerns about data security and privacy have been raised as health-related data (particularly patient data) has become more widely available. Demographics and DNA sequencing data, for example, have a higher likelihood of identifying patients. The data life cycles are evaluated with a lot of detail. Questions such as what type of data will be gathered, whether the data are required and who should secure the data, how the data will be used, kept, and transferred. The person's rights whose data are being collected are carefully considered. Furthermore, increasing public knowledge on regulations and transparency is critical for proper data gathering and utilization. Federated learning, which trains algorithms across decentralized edge devices (e.g., individual mobile phones) or servers storing multiple local samples, could be a viable route toward this aim (e.g., data owned by different samples). There are no common or centralized data samples. Only the trained models are shared, potentially improving patient data security and drug–disease outcome validation in drug repurposing.

3.7 Drug Discovery and Development

The application of AI drug discovery for less than a quarter of a century has yielded many new drugs, repurposed drugs, testing safety and efficacy of drugs, and automated manufacturing of complex products. The difficult drug discovery process has benefited from AI, and we now have AI in various parts of the drug research and development process. Over the next few years, AI's role will expand exponentially as the future applications of AI become more evident (Figure 3.6).

The goals of applying AI in drug discovery and medicinal chemistry involve identifying drug targets, identifying lead compounds, optimizing their designs against multiple property profiles of interest, and identifying synthetic routes to realize the composition of matter. De novo molecular design can combine

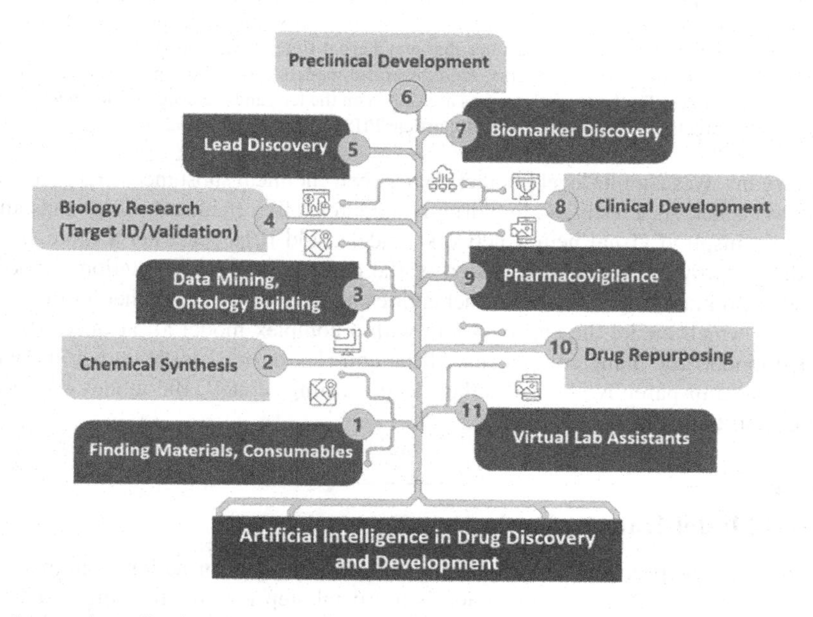

FIGURE 3.6 Systematic application of AI in drug discovery.

optimization parameters such as predictive models and molecular similarity with molecule generation and search to simulate scenario–make–test cycles. These in silico design loops then provide a list of candidate solutions that identify chemical structures predicted to be optimal for the profile defined. However, significant challenges remain concerning the synthetic tractability of these candidates.

Since the 1960s, medicinal chemistry has applied AI in various forms and varying degrees of success to the design compounds. Supervised learning, where labeled training datasets are used to train models, is extensively applied. An example is the quantitative structure–activity relationship (QSAR) approach, which is widely used to predict properties, such as logP, solubility, and bioactivity, for a given chemical structure. Conversely, unsupervised learning, which does not rely on labels, is also popular in medicinal chemistry. Examples such as hierarchical clustering, algorithms, and principal components analysis are used extensively to analyze and break down large molecular libraries into smaller collections of similar compounds.

An approach to molecular design can apply analogs of evolution to optimize chemical structures against a defined set of objectives. A structure with the desired profile emerges, known as multiparameter optimization. The multi-objective automated replacement of fragments algorithm proceeds by initializing a population of candidate structures, which are iteratively evaluated, sampled, and scored to optimize against the structure profile of interest. The multi-objective automated replacement of fragments algorithm uses a database of derived building blocks from synthetic organic chemistry, called synthetic disconnection rules. The bonding patterns and frequency of occurrence of each are retained. Replacement substructures are selected using a new algorithm called the rapid alignment of topological structures to simultaneously balance the exploration of the replacements while minimizing the disruption of the information in the candidate structures. As an example, this approach has optimized the potency of a CDK2 inhibitor while also improving its cell permeability.

The challenges in the automated design of synthetic tractability compounds are resolved using models based on synthetic rules, which combine building blocks using standard synthetic couplings. However, these approaches tend to limit the exploration of the relevant chemical space. An alternative way to generate new chemical structures is the AI-based generative models for molecules. The models are trained on large datasets of molecular structures from exemplified medicinal chemistry space, for example, ChEMBL (www.ebi.ac.uk/chembl/). These generative models learn a distribution over the molecules in the dataset. From this distribution, these approaches permit the sampling of novel molecules from the chemistry space learned to be more "drug-like." I created Figure 3.7 using the ChEMBL to describe thousands of compounds' characteristics to understand property regression. The graphs listed do not count as AI, but if the machine learning improved the prediction of properties based on one other attribute, this would count as an AI application.

From the origins of the atomistic theory, chemists have endeavored to predict compounds' properties without requiring synthesizing these compounds. Alexander Crum Brown stated in 1869 that the physiological response of a compound is merely a function of its chemical constitution. However, defining that function remains challenging. QSAR remains an active area of research leading to advances in the routine of particular physicochemical property predictions, notably exemplified by ClogP, to calculate the octanol/water partition coefficient (https://daylight.com/dayhtml/doc/clogp/index.html).

Since the formal advent of QSAR over 50 years ago, the numbers of modeling techniques, representations of molecules, and volume of data and compute resources available have increased significantly. The advances in all of these fields mean that techniques such as deep learning that previously were not appropriate or available to these datasets can now be utilized. As a result, we now have access to massive volumes of chemical structure data and quantitative endpoints, which we may utilize to construct prediction models. However, there remains a limited quantity of these data, and even when access is available, the quality is highly variable. Here, the expectation is that more modern ML methods will be able to tackle these noisy data.

Computer-aided synthesis planning (CASP) assists in providing alternative routes to prioritize compounds that can be readily synthesized, working backward from the target using transformation rules. Meanwhile, heuristics, which is now known as retrosynthetic analysis, turned out to be tremendously helpful for humans, but less so for machines.

The manual analysis of large datasets to identify potential new drug candidates is particularly time-consuming. Machine learning and deep learning algorithms used in AI can substantially speed up this

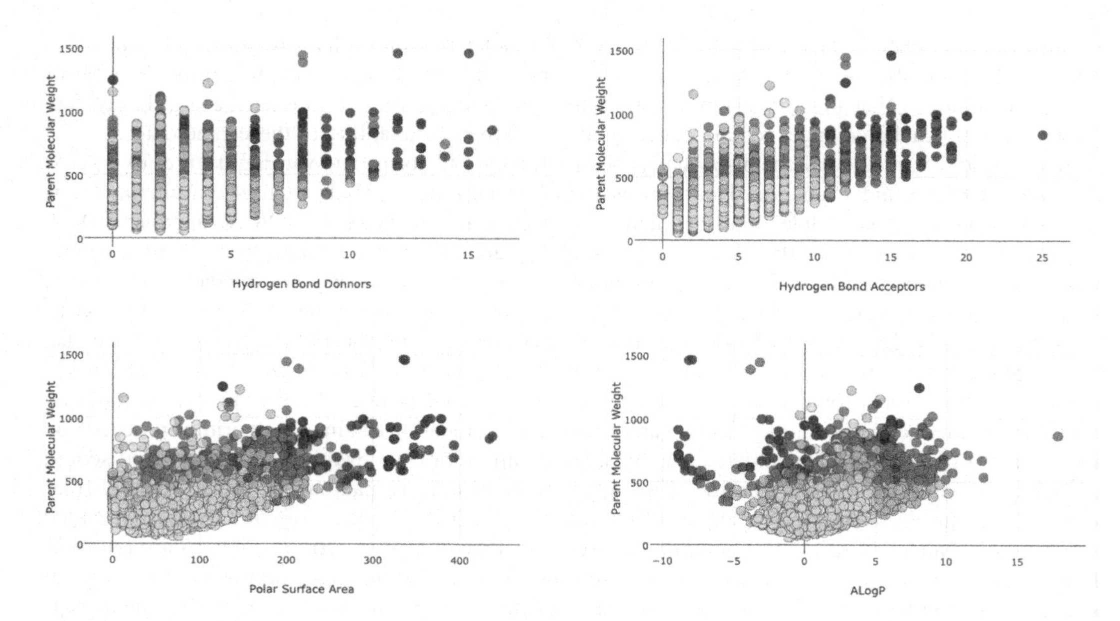

FIGURE 3.7 Graphic representation of 6,717 compounds and their properties relating to molecular weight. Darker shading means higher violations of RO5. ChEMBL is a database of bioactive compounds with drug-like characteristics that have been carefully selected. It combines chemical, bioactivity, and genetic data to turn genomic data into useful novel drugs. ChEMBL has 6,810 small molecules, 57 proteins, and 33 unknown compounds (as of early 2021). The above figure includes only those compounds for which the property variables are known. In silico drug discovery is a virtual screening of many chemical structures to find hits that are more closely aligned with the target in terms of interaction energy and other derived parameters, based on available structural information about target proteins. Source: www.ebi.ac. uk/chembl/.

process. AI and machine learning also allow for an extensive review of the scientific literature to discover new disease insights using the IBM Watson for Drug Discovery (www.ibm.com/watson), a cloud-based platform to assist with the discovery of novel cancer drug targets that IBM recently discontinued. More recently, the AI-based literature search and drafting is the near era, including the GPT3 (https://openai.com/blog/openai-api/).

The FDA sees excellent potential in using AI and machine learning in healthcare and is keen to see its use expanding across the sector. In 2017, the FDA issued a "Digital Health Innovation Action Plan" outlining its approach to implementing effective digital health technologies. The agency has expanded upon this program to support the use of AI and machine learning in drug development, including the introduction of Information Exchange and Data Transformation (INFORMED), a science and health technology incubator that will use Big Data and advanced analytics to provide scientific insights and improve health outcomes (https://pubmed.ncbi.nlm.nih.gov/29622786/).

While AI and machine learning do not currently have a significant role in the drug review process, the FDA researches potential advanced predictive and analytical machine learning initiatives that could create a more streamlined process. The FDA is also working to establish and de-risk AI use in the design of clinical trials as a tool for drug development, particularly where there is a high unmet need for product innovation.

3.7.1 Stepwise Approach

AI applications in drug development include:

- Stage 1: Identifying targets for intervention. Biologists identify a disease's likely mechanism and recommend a biological "target"—usually a protein implicated in a cascade of processes behind the disease—in a frequently utilized target-based method to drug discovery. Inhibiting or otherwise affecting such a protein can usually have a significant impact on pathogenesis, and therefore the disease can be repressed and healed. After the target has been proposed, hundreds of thousands or even millions of tiny molecules are screened against it to find "hits," or compounds with a high affinity for the target protein. Furthermore, the hits are subjected to a slew of additional testing and chemical alterations, with just a small percentage of small molecules making it to clinical trials. Understanding the disease's biological origins (pathways) and resistance mechanisms is the first stage in finding a treatment. Then you must find appropriate targets (usually proteins) to treat the condition. The growing availability of high-throughput tools like shRNA screening and deep sequencing has considerably enhanced the quantity of data accessible for identifying suitable target pathways. (Screening with RNAi is a powerful method for perturbing gene activity in cultured cells to enable gene function, pathway analysis, and target identification. shRNA is utilized for stable gene knockdown and two formats are commonly used for shRNA screening: arrayed libraries and pooled libraries.) On the other hand, traditional methods still struggle to integrate the large number and variety of data sources—and then uncover the appropriate patterns. Machine learning algorithms can quickly examine data and even learn to recognize good target proteins on their own.

- Stage 2: Finding therapeutic candidates entails screening a huge number of possible compounds—frequently hundreds or even millions—for their effect on the target (affinity), as well as any off-target negative effects (toxicity). Natural, synthetic, or bioengineered substances are all possibilities. Based on structural fingerprints and molecular descriptors, machine learning algorithms learn to predict the appropriateness of a molecule.
- Stage 3: Accelerating clinical trials. Machine learning helps speed up the design of clinical trials by automatically selecting acceptable candidates and ensuring that groups of trial participants are distributed correctly. In addition, algorithms can aid in the detection of patterns that distinguish good candidates from bad. They can also act as an early warning system for clinical trials that aren't yielding solid findings, allowing researchers to intervene sooner and potentially save the drug's development.
- Stage 4: Identifying biomarkers for disease diagnosis. Biomarkers are chemicals found in bodily fluids (usually human blood) that enable 100% certainty in determining whether a patient has an illness, making disease diagnosis safe and inexpensive.

Because of their expressly pre-programmed character and pre-determined models utilized for computations, traditional in silico approaches are still limited and not accurate enough to replace real-world experimental screens and trials. This is where new drug research startups and machine learning algorithms come into play.

Automation refers to technological advancements that have the potential to revolutionize the drug development process. Automation can improve laboratory efficiency, lower overall attrition, and lower costs along the drug discovery value chain. New technologies like microfluidics, robotics, and artificial intelligence, when combined with automated data analysis, can assist and speed up the drug research and approval process, allowing patients to receive therapies sooner. Automation enhances data accuracy, precision, repeatability, and traceability, in addition to lowering costs and shortening timescales, allowing researchers to use high-quality data in hypothesis-driven research.

Robotics improves a process's overall efficiency by developing efficient ways of accomplishing preset tasks with precision, consistency, and data capture quality, which is difficult to achieve manually. In addition, the homogeneity of the assay contributes to data accuracy. The obvious benefit of automation and automated liquid handling is that highly calibrated liquid handling instruments handle critical processes in dispensing tiny quantities.

3.7.2 Application Types

Modern biology is becoming increasingly data-rich, such as the massive amount of genetic data that has resulted in thousands of genomic databases. However, in order to produce statistically accurate models that can make predictions, these enormous datasets necessitate the use of competent analytical procedures. To gather these enormous datasets and use them for early target identification and validation, artificial intelligence (AI) can be used.

The machine needs algorithms to evaluate existing data and uncover trends in attributes to forecast drug discovery outcomes. ML can be employed at several phases of drug development. Validation of biological targets, finding of drug candidate compounds, and identification of illness biomarkers are all areas where machine learning can be used. ML can be employed at several phases of drug development. Validation of biological targets, finding of drug candidate compounds, and identification of illness biomarkers are all areas where machine learning can be used.

Since most AI-driven organizations employ a combination of methodologies and rely on interdisciplinary data sources for their modeling work, the primary uses of AI include:

- Preclinical candidates screening: A virtual compound library of several billion compounds can be screened using AI, and preclinical candidates can be identified in a fraction of the time it takes with traditional approaches. Linking genes to diseases:
  - Finding proteins that can be used as therapeutic targets for certain disorders.
  - Examining the feasibility of repurposing each known drug against every potential target for each known disease in detail.
  - Using fast chemoinformatics, rapidly screening millions of potential or current drug-like molecules as possible drugs, weeding out those with poor ADMET (absorption, distribution, metabolism, excretion, and toxicity) and solubility, and selecting those that may be active (possibly by fast docking or pharmacophore searches).
  - Possible adverse effects are predicted.
  - Linking treatment efficacy to human genetic variation at both a group and individual level.
  - Improving the process of getting a drug from concept to patients.
- Drug target identification and validation: Finding a druggable biological target—a target is druggable if its activity (behavior or function) may be altered by a therapy, whether it's a small molecule drug or a biologic. Proteins and nucleic acids, for example, are biological targets. What constitutes a "good" target?
  - Characteristics of a potential pharmacological target.
  - The target has been proven to play a function in disease pathogenesis and is disease-modifying.
  - The expression of the target is not spread uniformly throughout the body.
  - The 3D structure of the target can be used to determine druggability.
  - Because the target is easily "assayable," high-throughput screening is possible.
  - The target has a good toxicity profile, and phenotypic data can forecast probable side effects.
  - The intended target's intellectual property (IP) situation is good. (This is important for pharmaceutical businesses.)
- Target-based and phenotypic drug discovery: By applying AI-driven image analysis technology, phenomic AI can broadly approach drug discovery through high-throughput phenotypic screening. A phenotypic screen doesn't rely on a known drug target but instead aims to identify molecules that alter a cell's phenotype. Automated drug discovery employing data collection and analysis to map the hundreds of genes can resolve the treatment issues for Alzheimer's, Parkinson's, and ALS.
- Biomedical, clinical and patient data: Using biomedical and clinical data to draw unintuitive insights about drug candidates or attempting to model the whole biological systems to identify novel pathways, targets, and biomarkers.
- Drug repurposing: This brings a lot of value since much data is already known about the drug in question.

- Biomarkers: Biomarkers are useful medical diagnostic tools, but they can also be used in drug discovery and development. Predictive biomarkers, for example, are used to detect likely responders to a targeted molecular therapy before human testing.
- Research literature, publications, and patents: One of the most developed application cases for AI-based algorithms is reading, grouping, and understanding enormous amounts of textual data. AI enables knowledge aggregation since the number of research articles in the field is rapidly increasing, making it difficult for academics to keep up with the latest developments.
- Manufacturing process improvement: This applies to quality control, shortening design time, reducing materials waste, improving production reuse, performing predictive maintenance, and more. The AI machine learning algorithms ensure that activities are completed accurately while also analyzing the process to identify places where it might be simplified. As a result, there is less waste, production is faster, and Critical Quality Attributes are met more consistently (CQAs). The benefits of using MES include compliance with guaranteed legal regulations, minimized risks, increased transparency, shortened production cycles, optimized resource utilization, controlled and monitored production steps, and optimized up to batch release.
- Genome research: The genome is a sort of "instruction" for the organism to say which proteins and other molecules should be produced. Linking the genome with large-scale data regarding the output of particular genes at specific times, in specific places, in response to specific environmental stressors leads to a deeper knowledge of the genome. This is referred to as "multi-omic" analysis. The term "omic" refers to the several "layers" of the biological system. Such a multidimensional approach is promising for understanding diseases' mechanisms, especially such complex ones as cancer and diabetes. Research on biology systems generates enormous data, which needs to be stored, processed, and analyzed. If the three billion molecular coding units that make up a person's DNA are typed line by line into an Excel spreadsheet, the result would be a 7,900-mile-long table. More than 30,000 different proteins have been found in the human proteome so far. In addition, the body contains around 40,000 tiny compounds known as metabolites. Data mapping generates trillions of data points from a variety of studies, associations, and combinations of elements and situations. Big data analysis and machine learning algorithms make it possible to identify previously undiscovered data patterns, as well as previously unknown linkages and associations. For example, large-scale modeling of gene expression data using an automated protocol can predict differential gene expression as a function of the compound structure. Unlike the traditional in silico design paradigm, which examines a specific target-based response, the newly established technique allows for virtual screening and lead optimization for desired multitarget gene expression profiles.
- High-throughput screening: After scientists have proposed an excellent biological target, it is time to look for molecules that may selectively interact with the target, generating the desired action—a "hit" molecule. To find hit compounds, a range of screening paradigms are available. A common high-throughput screening (HTS) method, for example, includes screening millions of chemical compounds against a therapeutic target. This is a kind of "trial and error" method to find a needle in the haystack. This screening paradigm involves using complex robotic automation, it is costly, and the success rate is relatively low. What's nice about it is that it doesn't require any prior knowledge of the chemical compounds that are likely to have activity at the target protein. As a result, HTS appears to be an experimental supply of research ideas, as well as beneficial "negative" results to consider using automated technology; high-throughput screening (HTS) evaluates the activity of a large number of chemicals against a specified biological target quickly. The real benefit of adopting high-throughput screening in lead discovery is that it allows you to consistently and rapidly evaluate tens of thousands to hundreds of thousands of agents (small compounds or functional genomics techniques). HTS can be thought of as a quick scan of biological processes that allows candidates with insufficient or no effect to be quickly ruled out of the drug discovery pipeline. HTS labs employ various assay formats, and the automation of assays plays a central role in the process. These assays aim to reduce a

large number of agents to a small number that produces promising findings in the test. Liquid handling equipment, robots, plate readers as detectors, and specific instrumentation control and data processing software are used to automate the process. For example, with the automation's precision, all of the plates in the assay will be run under very similar conditions. We can ensure assay homogeneity throughout the screen by using plate-based controls. Furthermore, automation enables researchers to test a greater number of hypotheses and create complicated workflows and screening scenarios that would be difficult or impossible to accomplish manually.

- CADD: Other ways include fragment screening and physiological screening, a more specialized focused screening approach. Instead of targeting one specific pharmacological target, this is a tissue-based strategy that looks for a more aligned response with the final targeted in vivo effect. Computational scientists advanced computer-aided drug discovery (CADD) approaches using pharmacophores and molecular modeling to conduct so-called "virtual" screens of compound libraries to reduce the costs of the above complex laboratory screens while increasing their efficiency and predictability. We can now use in silico approach to screen millions of compounds against a known 3D structure of a target protein (structure-based technique); if the structure is unknown, drug candidates can be identified based on knowledge of other molecules known to have an action against the target of interest.

The drug discovery paradigm's classic notion of "one gene, one drug, one disease" may have led to the poor success rate in drug development. Without prior knowledge of the complete drug target information (i.e., the molecular "promiscuity" of drugs), developing promising strategies for efficacious treatment of multiple complex diseases is difficult due to unintended therapeutic effects or multiple drug–target interactions leading to off-target toxicities and suboptimal effectiveness. To improve efficacy while limiting negative effects in clinical trials, molecular targets for known drugs must be identified. However, while experimentally determining drug–target interactions is costly and time-consuming, computational techniques provide innovative testable hypotheses for the systematic and impartial identification of known drugs' molecular targets.

Recent advances in omics technologies and pharmacology approaches have generated considerable knowledge from chemical, phenotypic, genomic, and cellular networks. It is feasible to infer whether two drugs share a target using a network that incorporates these parameters. The drug–target network is a bipartite graph made up of FDA-approved drugs and proteins linked by drug–target/protein binary relationships that have been empirically validated. Target identification for known drugs has been made using network-based techniques, which helps to reduce adverse effects and speed up drug repurposing. On the other hand, traditional network topology-based algorithms are based on a single homogeneous drug–target network and perform poorly on pharmaceuticals in known drug–target networks with low connectedness (degree). Heterogeneous data sources provide diverse information and a multi-view viewpoint for predicting novel drug–target indications (DTIs). Incorporating heterogeneous data improves DTI prediction accuracy and provides fresh insights into drug repurposing.

3.7.3 An Example of AI Application

Translational science has struggled for decades to turn research discoveries into novel, effective drugs, and technologies that can be delivered quickly. This problem has prompted basic and translational scientists to collaborate to achieve this critical goal. De novo drug discovery has been a stumbling block for generations of scientists. A drug repurposing technique, in which drug has already been studied and approved by the US FDA, can theoretically overcome de novo drug discovery constraints. The amount of authorized or clinically unsuccessful drugs, on the other hand, is immense, underscoring the difficulties in deciding which drug would be highly beneficial for the ailment at hand.

Drug repurposing is a viable strategy because of the potential for shorter development timetables and lower total costs. In addition, artificial intelligence (AI) can accelerate drug repurposing or repositioning, particularly in precision drugs, such as those required to treat COVID-19 and similar pandemics.

These advantages are evident in the COVID-19 global pandemic caused by the severe acute respiratory syndrome coronavirus 2 (SARS-CoV-2) when finding new drugs is nearly impossible (see Figure 4.5

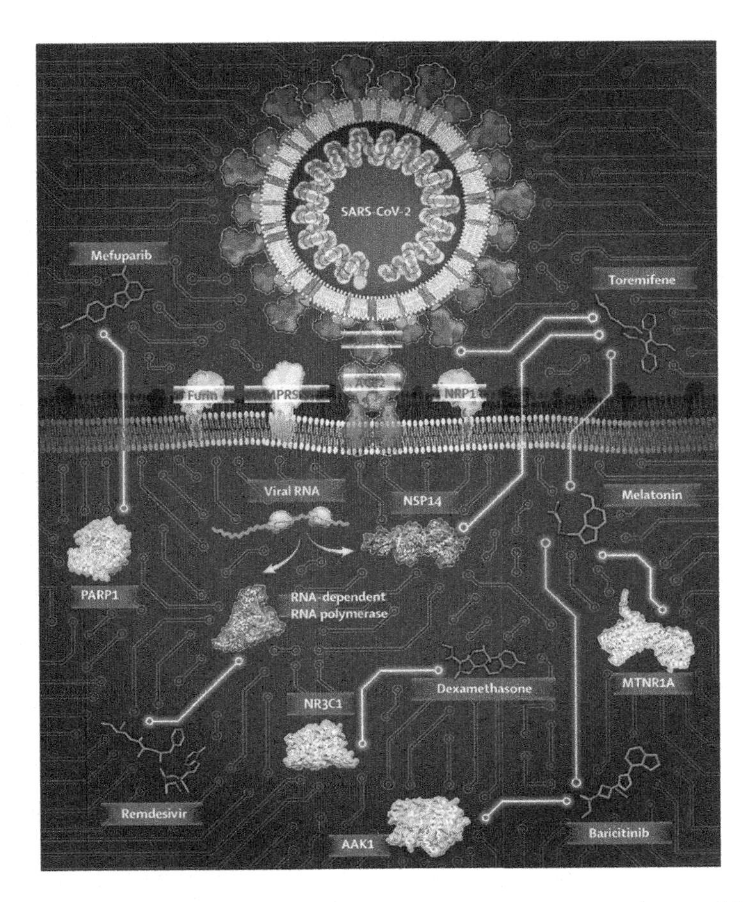

FIGURE 3.8 Overview of AI-assisted drug repurposing for COVID-19. Drug repurposing, a quick and cost-effective technique to find novel therapy choices for developing diseases, can be done with AI algorithms. AI = artificial intelligence. PARP1 = poly-ADP-ribose polymerase 1. NR3C1 = nuclear receptor subfamily 3 group C member 1. AAK1 = AP2-associated protein kinase 1. MTNR1A = melatonin receptor 1A. TMPRSS2 = transmembrane serine protease 2. ACE2 = angiotensin I converting enzyme 2. NRP1 = neuropilin 1. NSP14 =non-structural protein 14. Forty-one repurposed drug candidates (including dexamethasone and melatonin) are identified for COVID-19 treatment. Sources: reproduced with permission from the Cleveland Clinic Center for Medical Art and Photography; www. thelancet.com/journals/landig/article/PIIS2589-7500(20)30192-8/fulltext.

in Chapter 4). Thus, the pandemic is an excellent opportunity for introducing advanced AI algorithms combined with network drugs for drug repurposing (Figure 3.8).

3.8 AI Tools

Multimodal PaML (Predictive Analysis and Machine Learning) Tools hold AI applications' future since AI is fundamentally composed of machine learning (ML) models and divided into three segments: multimodal, notebook-based, and automation-focused. The majority of multimodal PaML vendor products can assist data scientists in completing their tasks. These solutions may be used to obtain data, create a data transformation pipeline, apply transformations, view results, select from a variety of analytical approaches, and deploy models. However, the importance and scope of PaML have expanded to become strategic versus tactical. The essential building blocks of AI, which will become a vital force in the digital future, are machine learning models. To achieve their AI goals, businesses must now choose a multimodal PaML solution (see Figure 3.9).

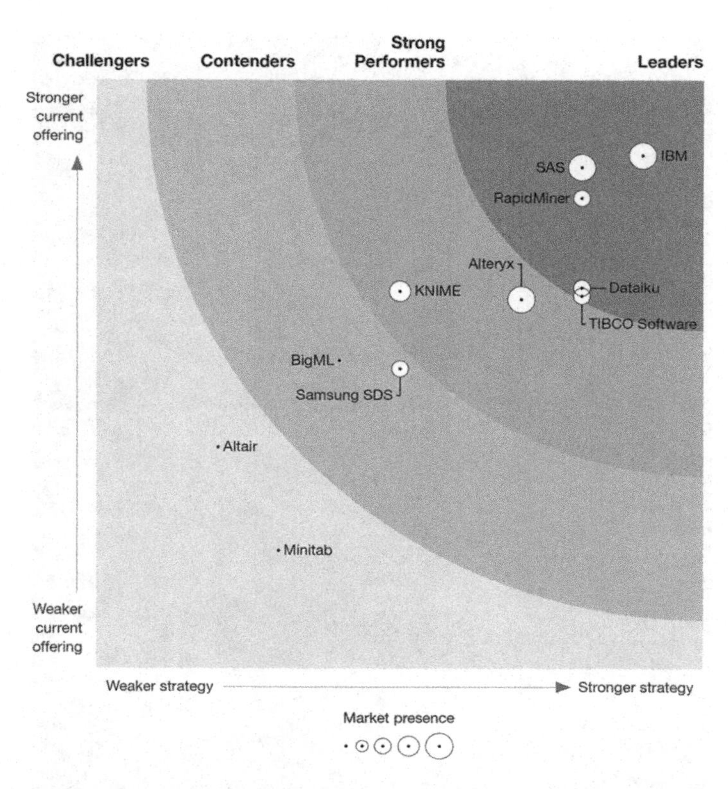

FIGURE 3.9 Comparison of PaML tools available as of end 2020. Source: www.lorenzoni. de/de/archiv/electronics/artikel/parasoft-leading-position-in-forrester-wave-report-2018.html.

Automated machine learning (autoML) helps run repetitive tasks in the model development lifecycle, such as feature engineering, training, and evaluation. Some multimodal PaML providers, such as Datarobot (www.datarobot.com) and H2O (www.h2oai.com), offer autoML capabilities that compete with automation-focused PaML vendors.

Model operations (Modelops) are used to scale up machine learning. However, organizations' ability to implement more business-worthy AI use cases faster is hampered by installing machine learning models in production, frenzied handoffs, manual monitoring, and weak governance. Traditionally, multimodal PaML suppliers have concentrated their product development on analytical tools and machine learning methodologies. That's still crucial, but now that AI is becoming more ubiquitous, businesses want machine learning to be done more quickly. Cross-functional AI teams can use PaML products' Modelops features to deploy, monitor, retrain, and regulate AI models in production systems.

- IBM offers a microservices platform that may run on-premises, in the private cloud, and across various public clouds, with services ranging from data management to PaML to business intelligence. IBM Cloud Pak for Data is a service that makes PaML lifecycle features available to your users when and where they need them. Watson Studio is a fundamental component of Cloud Pak for Data. This PaML solution blends simple, SPSS-inspired workflows with open-source machine learning libraries and notebook-based interfaces. Fairness monitoring, bias prevention, autoML, and federated learning are all examples of IBM research innovations. IBM provides an attractive, scalable, increasingly integrated, and harmonized platform that spans the entire PaML lifecycle and can be deployed anywhere on any cloud. Users will have to handle some technical previews and rapidly growing features, but they will avoid having to piece together a mishmash of commercial and open-source software elsewhere (www. ibm.com/Watson).

- Viya is a totally re-engineered platform that underpins all of SaS's offerings, including SaS visual analytics, SaS visual data mining, machine learning, and SaS Model Manager. With aPis, Viya cloud makes SaS products possible, unifies user interfaces, and provides interoperability, integration, and extension. SaaS allows companies to innovate more quickly, provide cloud solutions, and interface with third-party services and open-source software. SaS has a lot of advantages, including extremely well-integrated autoML and other guided analytics features. Open-source programming languages, such as Python and R, are increasingly supported by SaS, allowing data science teams to take advantage of the SaS engine. With SaS Model Manager, it is now possible to operationalize models that were not created in SaS, bringing it closer to becoming a comprehensive PaML platform (www.sas.com/enus/home.html).
- RapidMiner is a data science tool that combines ease of use and rigor. It includes one of the most extensive visual interfaces for developing data and ML pipelines and some of the most productivity-enhancing technologies for automated data preparation (Turbo Prep) and model creation (Auto Model) in the multimodal industry. Python (www.python.org) is also supported by RapidMiner (www.rapidminer.com).
- PaML is available from Dataiku for various positions inside an organization, ranging from business analysts to data scientists. It also provides persona-specific training and enablement programs to assist businesses in equipping many users with data science skills (www.dataiku.com).
- TIBco Data Science takes on challenging, high-impact use cases. Unlike most vendor machine learning solutions, TiBCo focuses on AI applications rather than ML models. TiBCo Data Science not only facilitates the building of machine learning models throughout their full lifecycle, but it also seamlessly connects with the company's other platform solutions to provide insights and AI apps. TiBCo Data Science interfaces with TiBCo Spotfire to provide insights. The ML model-building lifecycle for AI solutions integrates smoothly with the rest of TiBCo's application portfolio, such as TiBCo Streaming. Customers use TiBCo Data Science to construct a variety of AI apps, ranging from customer engagement to silicon fabrication, as well as a variety of Internet of Things (IoT) apps. TiBCo's most robust features include data exploration, data preparation, security, and modeling tools. More automation features come to its autoML tools designed to augment analysts and data scientists (with seamless integration in both Spotfire and TiBCo Data Science) by outputting reusable pipelines and Python code (www. tibco.com).
- The KNIME Analytics Platform comprises over 4,000 analytical, statistical, data transformation, and machine learning methods that are free to download. For individual users, that's a lot of value. Small, medium, and large subscriptions to the KNIME Server, which provides data science teams with extra features for collaboration, automation, deployment, and management, are available to support the company's open-source community stewardship. KNIME excels at visual modeling tools, a wide range of analytical approaches, automation, and application development. Users can now package and parameterize elements of pipelines into reusable, shareable "components" and then tag parts of model development pipelines to generate rapid production pipelines, which improves collaboration and deployment time. Noncoding data science teams are the ideal fit for the KNIME Analytics Platform (www.knime.com).
- In addition to its Brightics AI (www.brightics.ai) platform, Samsung offers a full PaML platform that aids in the development and deployment of ML and AI apps, including data prep, a visual environment for building data and ML pipelines, autoML capabilities for guided analytics, and hyperparameter optimization, as well as capabilities for deploying your models. Brightics AI is the technology that Samsung SDS utilizes to deliver digital transformation projects ranging from demand forecasts to chemotherapy treatment suggestions, so it should come as no surprise. Samsung's greatest strengths are the ease and speed with which customers can

construct simple machine learning programs, from data input to simple analytics apps—and it has a few tricks up its sleeve, particularly for deep learning applications (e.g., pre-trained models and features for accelerating data labeling). Citizen data scientists and citizen developers can be created fast by business users (www.sra.samsung.com/artificial-intelligence/).

- With a few clicks on bigml.com, you can get an immediate, stylish ML. BigML's complex yet straightforward graphical user interface allows professional and aspiring data scientists to train and deploy machine models. Because of the free-to-low entry-point cost, more than 120,000 users have signed up for the website. BigML's concentration on individual users and small teams has shifted in recent years to suit the needs of major companies, including on-premise deployments. BigML's main advantages are its overall simplicity and support for unsupervised learning techniques (such as clustering, anomaly detection, topic modeling, and association finding) as well as autoML capabilities (www.bigml.com).
- Altair Knowledge Studio is suitable for users of all skill levels, from subject matter experts with no formal data science experience to seasoned data scientists working to improve an existing model's performance. Knowledge Studio supports a wide range of machine learning approaches, but it stands out by offering a highly effective yet user-friendly visual interface for constructing, browsing, and altering decision and strategy trees. Data discovery, visual modeling interfaces, governance, and Modelops are all strengths of Altair Knowledge Studio. To be more competitive, Altair should invest in automation features, integrate open-source technologies more firmly, and become truly cloud-native (www.altairdata.com).
- Minitab makes authoritative machine learning technologies available to the rest of the Minitab community. SPM is most recognized for its implementation of specific algorithms such as CarT, MarS, random forests, and Treenet. These and additional techniques are available in most other vendor solutions. However, Minitab's methods are implemented and fine-tuned by its creators (www. minitab.com).
- Deep learning is a machine learning area that refers to a hierarchical approach to data exploration that employs layers of linear and nonlinear transformations. Artificial neural networks are the most extensively used deep learning model. An artificial neuron is the basic building block, which modifies the weighted sum of input feature variables nonlinearly. The creation of promising and affordable ways to treat human diseases is complex without a prior understanding of the complete drug target information. DeepDTnet (https://github.com/ChengF-Lab/deepDTnet) is a deep learning system for identifying new targets and repurposing drugs in a heterogeneous drug–gene–disease network that embeds 15 types of chemical, genomic, phenotypic, and cellular network profiles. In a recent test, the model was trained on 732 FDA-approved small molecule drugs, and deepDTnet outperformed previously reported state-of-the-art approaches in discovering novel molecular targets for existing treatments. For example, topotecan (an authorized topoisomerase inhibitor) predicted by deepDTnet was verified as a novel, direct inhibitor (IC50 0.43 [M]) of the human retinoic-acid-receptor-related orphan receptor-gamma t (ROR-gt) and potentially effective in multiple sclerosis. In Figures 3.10 and 3.11, deepDTnet embeds 15 types of chemical, genomic, phenotypic, and cellular networks to develop physiologically and pharmacologically relevant characteristics for both drugs and targets by learning low-dimensional yet useful vector representations.

3.9 Conclusion

Artificial intelligence is a comprehensive process of using machines to understand big data, make conclusions about the networked dependencies, make projections through machine learning based on decision-making abilities. The discovery of future drugs will depend heavily on how the developers adopt AI as the primary tool of the invention. With the exponential growth of the machine capability, it will be possible to expedite target identification, target development, and evaluation of target safety and efficacy.

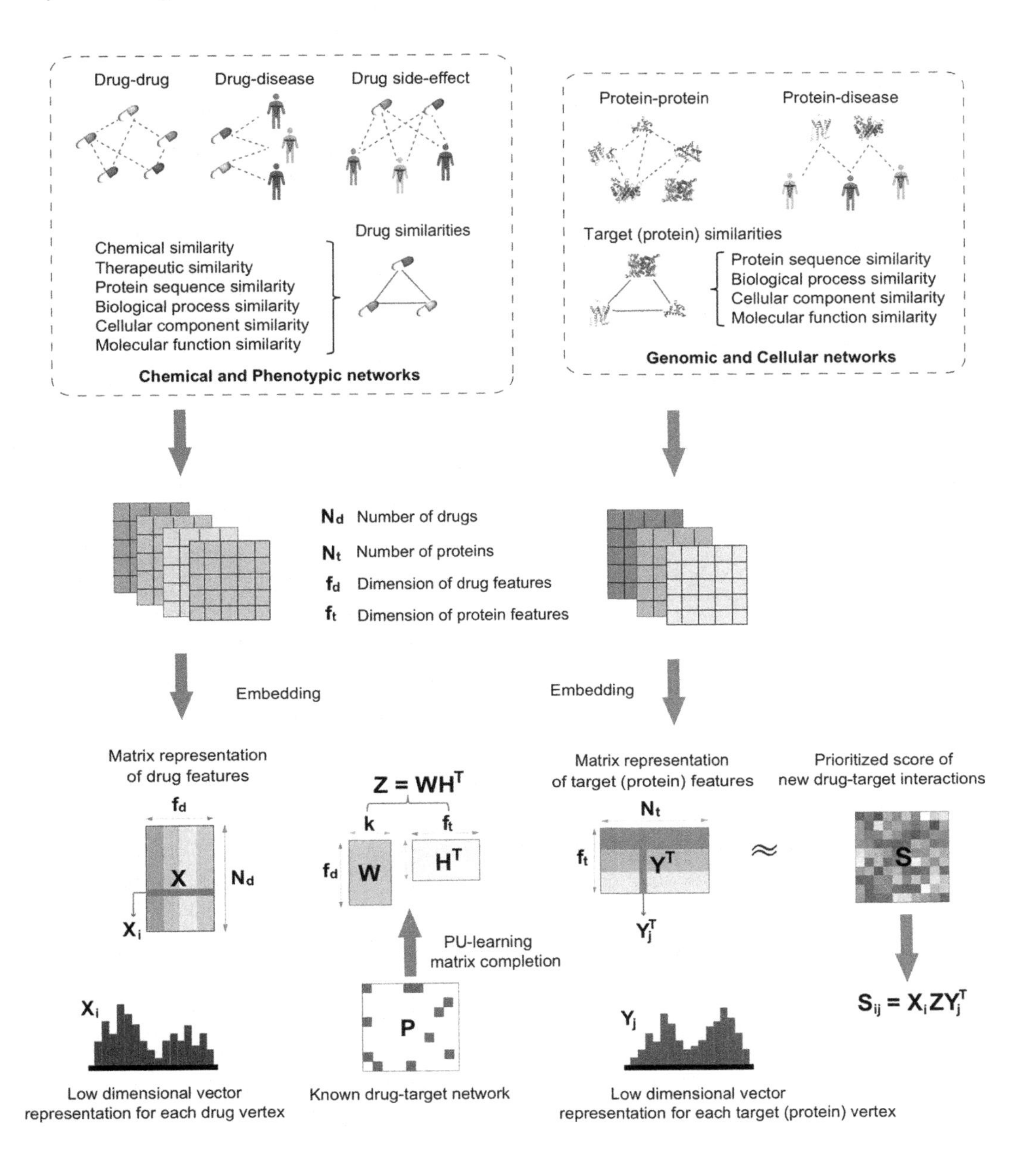

FIGURE 3.10 A diagram illustrating the workflow of deepDTnet. DeepDTnet uses PU-matrix completion to find the best projection from drug space onto target (protein) space. The projected feature vectors of drugs are geometrically close to feature vectors of known interacting targets. Finally, deepDTnet generates new drug targets based on their geometric proximity to the drug's projected feature vector in the projected space.

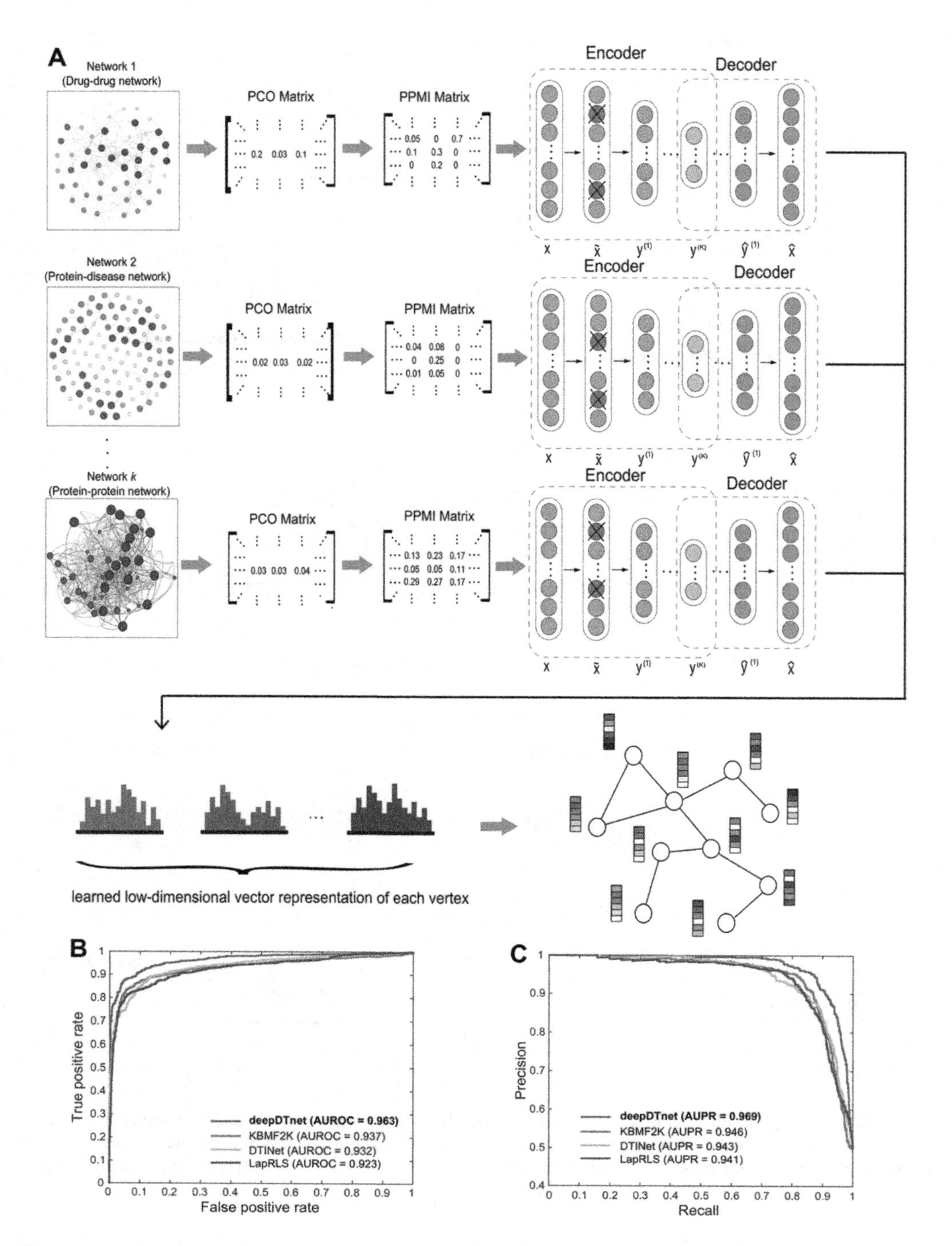

FIGURE 3.11 A workflow illustrating the network embedding and performance of deepDTnet. (A) The deep neural networks model for graph representations (DNGR) consists of three major steps: (i) a random surfing model to capture the structural graph information and generate a probabilistic co-occurrence (PCO) matrix; (ii) calculation of the shifted positive pointwise mutual information (PPMI) matrix based on the probabilistic co-occurrence matrix; and (iii) a stacked denoising autoencoder to generate compressed, low-dimensional vectors from the original high-dimensional vertex vectors. The learned low-dimensional feature vectors encode the relational properties, association information, and topological context of each node in the heterogeneous drug–gene-disease network. (B and C) Performance of deepDTnet was assessed by both (B) the area under the receiver operating characteristic curve (AUROC) and (C) the area under the precision-recall curve (AUPR) of deepDTnet against the top k predicted list during cross-validation.

ADDITIONAL READING

Ahuja AS, Reddy VP, Marques O. Artificial intelligence and COVID-19: a multidisciplinary approach. *Integr Med Res.* 2020;9(3):100434.

Álvarez-Machancoses Ó, Fernández-Martínez JL. Using artificial intelligence methods to speed up drug discovery. *Expert Opin Drug Discov.* 2019;14(8):769–777.

Bajorath J, Kearnes S, Walters WP, Georg GI, Wang S. The future is now: artificial intelligence in drug discovery. *J Med Chem.* 2019;62(11):5249.

Bajorath J, Kearnes S, Walters WP, Meanwell NA, Georg GI, Wang S. Artificial intelligence in drug discovery: into the great wide open. *J Med Chem.* 2020;63(16):8651–8652.

Basu K, Sinha R, Ong A, Basu T. Artificial intelligence: how is it changing medical sciences and its future? *Indian J Dermatol.* 2020;65(5):365–370.

Bhhatarai B, Walters WP, Hop CECA, Lanza G, Ekins S. Opportunities and challenges using artificial intelligence in ADME/Tox. *Nat Mater.* 2019;18(5):418–422.

Díaz Ó, Dalton JAR, Giraldo J. Artificial intelligence: a novel approach for drug discovery. *Trends Pharmacol Sci.* 2019;40(8):550–551.

Dlamini Z, Francies FZ, Hull R, Marima R. Artificial intelligence (AI) and big data in cancer and precision oncology. *Comput Struct Biotechnol J.* 2020;18:2300–2311.

Dovey D. For the first time ever, a drug developed by AI will be tested in human trials. 2020. Retrieved 4 April 2020, from https://www.forbes.com/sites/danadovey/2020/02/11/first-time-ever-artificial-intelligence-develops-drug-candidate/#6b2dc7b260de

Fernández A. Artificial intelligence teaches drugs to target proteins by tackling the induced folding problem. *Mol Pharm.* 2020;17(8):2761–2767.

Fleming N. How artificial intelligence is changing drug discovery. *Nature.* 2018;557(7707):S55–S57.

Fujiwara T, Kamada M, Okuno Y. [Artificial intelligence in drug discovery]. *Gan To Kagaku Ryoho.* 2018;45(4):593–596.

Gasteiger J. Chemistry in times of artificial intelligence. *Chemphyschem.* 2020 doi:10.1002/cphc.202000518.

Griffen EJ, Dossetter AG, Leach AG, Montague S. Can we accelerate medicinal chemistry by augmenting the chemist with Big Data and artificial intelligence? *Drug Discov Today.* 2018;23(7):1373–1384.

Hassanzadeh P, Atyabi F, Dinarvand R. The significance of artificial intelligence in drug delivery system design. *Adv Drug Deliv Rev.* 2019;151–152:169–190.

Hessler G, Baringhaus KH. Artificial intelligence in drug design. *Molecules.* 2018 Oct;23(10):2520.

Ho D. Artificial intelligence in cancer therapy. *Science.* 2020;367(6481):982–983.

Jing Y, Bian Y, Hu Z, Wang L, Xie XQ. Correction to: deep learning for drug design: an artificial intelligence paradigm for drug discovery in the Big Data era. *AAPS J.* 2018;20(4):79.

Jing Y, Bian Y, Hu Z, Wang L, Xie XQ. Deep learning for drug design: an artificial intelligence paradigm for drug discovery in the Big Data era. *AAPS J.* 2018;20(3):58.

Kabra R, Singh S. Evolutionary artificial intelligence based peptide discoveries for effective Covid-19 therapeutics. *Biochim Biophys Acta Mol Basis Dis.* 2020;1867(1):165978.

Keshavarzi Arshadi A, Salem M, Collins J, Yuan JS, Chakrabarti D. DeepMalaria: artificial intelligence driven discovery of potent antiplasmodials. *Front Pharmacol.* 2019;10:1526.

Li JY, Chen HY, Dai WJ, Lv QJ, Chen CY. Artificial intelligence approach to investigate the longevity drug. *J Phys Chem Lett.* 2019;10(17):4947–4961.

Liu B, He H, Luo H, Zhang T, Jiang J. Artificial intelligence and big data facilitated targeted drug discovery. *Stroke Vasc Neurol.* 2019;4(4):206–213.

Mak KK, Pichika MR. Artificial intelligence in drug development: present status and future prospects. *Drug Discov Today.* 2019;24(3):773–780.

Mamoshina P, Ojomoko L, Yanovich Y, et al. Converging blockchain and next-generation artificial intelligence technologies to decentralize and accelerate biomedical research and healthcare. *Oncotarget.* 2018;9(5):5665–5690.

Méndez-Lucio O, Baillif B, Clevert DA, Rouquié D, Wichard J. De novo generation of hit-like molecules from gene expression signatures using artificial intelligence. *Nat Commun.* 2020;11(1):10.

Merk D, Friedrich L, Grisoni F, Schneider G. De novo design of bioactive small molecules by artificial intelligence. *Mol Inform.* 2018 Jan;37(1–2):1700153.

Mitchell JB. Artificial intelligence in pharmaceutical research and development. *Future Med Chem.* 2018;10(13):1529–1531.

Mohanty S, Harun Ai, Rashid M, Mridul M, Mohanty C, Swayamsiddha S. Application of artificial intelligence in COVID-19 drug repurposing. *Diabetes Metab Syndr.* 2020;14(5):1027–1031.

Nogrady B. Artificial intelligence shakes up drug discovery. 2019. Retrieved 4 April 2020, from https://www.the-scientist.com/bio-business/artificial-intelligence-shakes-up-drug-discovery-65787

Noorbakhsh-Sabet N, Zand R, Zhang Y, Abedi V. Artificial intelligence transforms the future of health care. *Am J Med.* 2019;132(7):795–801.

Oliveira AL. Biotechnology, Big Data and artificial intelligence. *Biotechnol J.* 2019;14(8):e1800613.

OneThree Biotech. Redesigning drug discovery with biology-driven AI. 2020. Retrieved 7 April 2020, from https://onethree.bio/

Paul D, Sanap G, Shenoy S, Kalyane D, Kalia K, Tekade RK. Artificial intelligence in drug discovery and development. *Drug Discov Today.* 2021 Jan;26(1):80–93.

Rogers MA, Aikawa E. Cardiovascular calcification: artificial intelligence and big data accelerate mechanistic discovery. *Nat Rev Cardiol.* 2019;16(5):261–274.

Rohall SL, Auch L, Gable J, et al. An artificial intelligence approach to proactively inspire drug discovery with recommendations. *J Med Chem.* 2020;63(16):8824–8834.

Romeo-Guitart D, Forés J, Herrando-Grabulosa M, et al. Neuroprotective drug for nerve trauma revealed using artificial intelligence. *Sci Rep.* 2018;8(1):1879.

Saikin SK, Kreisbeck C, Sheberla D, Becker JS. Closed-loop discovery platform integration is needed for artificial intelligence to make an impact in drug discovery. *Expert Opin Drug Discov.* 2019;14(1):1–4.

Sato K, Ikegaya Y. [Challenges to improve the prediction accuracy of the non-clinical tests for human CNS adverse effects: potentials of artificial intelligence and human ESC/iPSC-derived Neurons]. *Yakugaku Zasshi.* 2018;138(6):807.

Schneider P, Walters WP, Plowright AT, et al. Rethinking drug design in the artificial intelligence era. *Nat Rev Drug Discov.* 2020;19(5):353–364.

Sellwood MA, Ahmed M, Segler MH, Brown N. Artificial intelligence in drug discovery. *Future Med Chem.* 2018;10(17):2025–2028.

Serebrov M. FDA looks to AI to streamline drug development and approval process. 2019. Retrieved 4 April 2020, from https://www.bioworld.com/articles/429315-fda-looks-to-ai-to-streamline-drug-development-and-approval-process

Sharma S, Sharma D. Intelligently applying artificial intelligence in chemoinformatics. *Curr Top Med Chem.* 2018;18(20):1804–1826.

Sirois S, Tsoukas CM, Chou KC, Wei D, Boucher C, Hatzakis GE. Selection of molecular descriptors with artificial intelligence for the understanding of HIV-1 protease peptidomimetic inhibitors-activity. *Med Chem.* 2005;1(2):173–84.

Tanaka H. [Artificial intelligence-based drug discovery and drug repositioning]. *Brain Nerve.* 2019;71(9):981–989.

Tayarani NMH. Applications of artificial intelligence in battling against Covid-19: a literature review. *Chaos Solitons Fractals.* 2021 Jan;142:110338.

Yang X, Wang Y, Byrne R, Schneider G, Yang S. Concepts of artificial intelligence for computer-assisted drug discovery. *Chem Rev.* 2019;119(18):10520–10594.

Yassine HM, Shah Z. How could artificial intelligence aid in the fight against coronavirus? *Expert Rev Anti Infect Ther.* 2020;18(6):493–497.

Zhavoronkov A. Artificial intelligence for drug discovery, biomarker development, and generation of novel chemistry. *Mol Pharm.* 2018;15(10):4311–4313.

Zhavoronkov A. Medicinal chemists versus machines challenge: what will it take to adopt and advance artificial intelligence for drug discovery? *J Chem Inf Model.* 2020;60(6):2657–2659.

Zhavoronkov A, Mamoshina P, Vanhaelen Q, Scheibye-Knudsen M, Moskalev A, Aliper A. Artificial intelligence for aging and longevity research: recent advances and perspectives. *Ageing Res Rev.* 2019;49:49–66.

Zhavoronkov A, Vanhaelen Q, Oprea TI. Will artificial intelligence for drug discovery impact clinical pharmacology? *Clin Pharmacol Ther.* 2020;107(4):780–785.

Zhong F, Xing J, Li X, et al. Artificial intelligence in drug design. *Sci China Life Sci.* 2018;61(10):1191–1204.

Zhu H. Big data and artificial intelligence modeling for drug discovery. *Annu Rev Pharmacol Toxicol.* 2020;60:573–589.

4

Drug Discovery Trends

4.1 Background

The drug discovery process is long, complicated, and expensive. Pharmaceutical companies can spend over $1 billion and 12 years developing a new drug (Figure 4.1) despite significant developments in implementing new technologies such as artificial intelligence, machine learning, genomics, proteomics, and HTS as advancements in bioinformatics and in silico modeling. The classical approaches to drug discovery need updating. New technologies like microfluidics, organ on the chip, and higher computing powers will make a significant change in the process of drug discovery in the near and far future.

Optimization of drug discovery now focuses on comprehensive approaches starting with questions like:

- What makes, and how can we identify, a good target?
- How can we identify the chemical compound which would become the drug?
- How can we optimize that drug?
- How can we test it works in models of disease?
- How can we demonstrate that it would be safe to dose in humans?

Multiple scientific areas including chemistry, biology, pharmacokinetics, pharmacodynamics, animal modeling, and in silico approaches are now merged to deliver clinical candidates, providing a highly structured pathway that is now universally followed (Figure 4.2).

However, there remain many logistic, technical, and regulatory hindrances that need resolutions in order to expedite drug discovery (Table 4.1).

4.2 High-Throughput Screening (HTS)

Over the last three decades, target-based drug discovery has resulted in a significant increase in the number of chemotypes and pharmacophores available to medicinal chemists. New techniques such as high-throughput screening (HTS), fragment-based screening (FBS), crystallography in combination with molecular modeling, and combinatorial and parallel chemistry have resulted in a wide range of chemical lead structures that go far beyond the known natural products and ligands that have previously served as chemical starting points for drug discovery. Furthermore, this wealth of chemotypes can now be used as a source for tool compounds to study uncharted biological territory and discover new drug targets, as well as phenotypic screening using systems-based approaches to identify target-agnostic drug candidates.

One of the most successful approaches incorporated across multiple scientific research fields is high-throughput screening (HTS). CRISPR, for example, is a relatively new genome-editing technique that allows for direct changes to the immediate eukaryotic genome. To enable parallel screening of multiple samples or clones, an HTS strategy is used for its high sensitivity in detection. The HTS technology

DOI: 10.1201/9781003146933-4

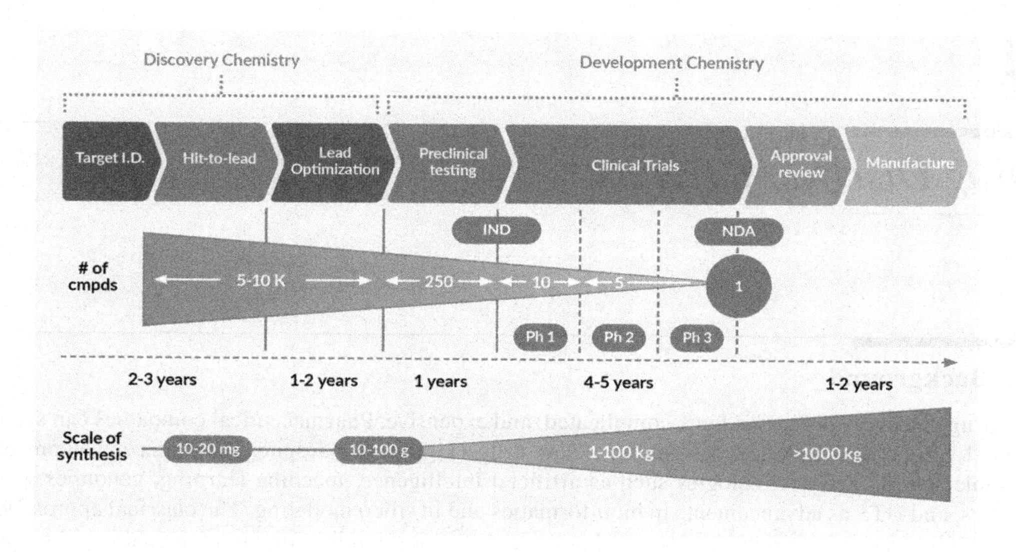

FIGURE 4.1 Timeline of drug development.

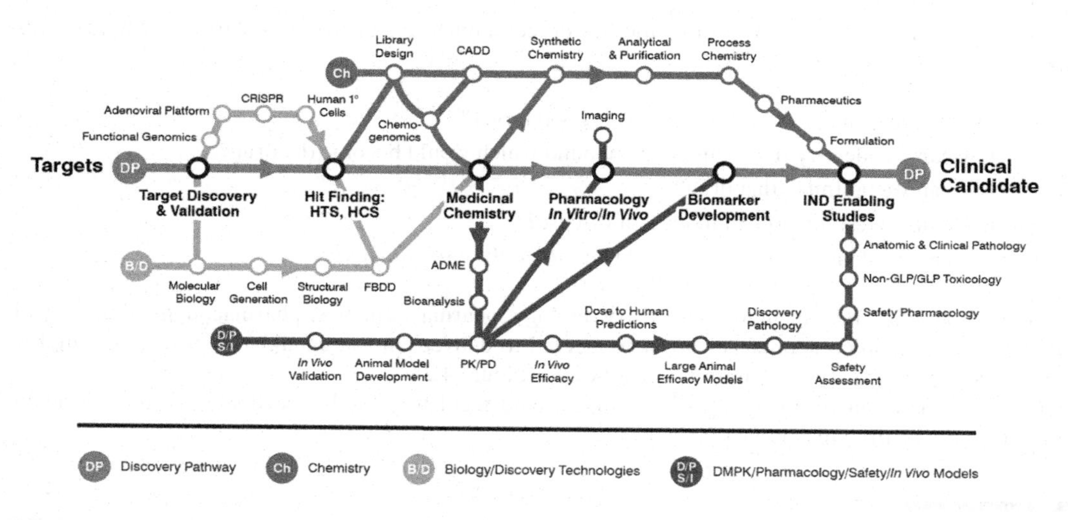

FIGURE 4.2 Modern, multifaceted approach to drug discovery.

typically provides much more accurate data and activity estimates than previously used detection assays (Figure 4.3).

Increasing in its complexity, HTS can also be applied with label-free detection methods such as MS. These techniques are becoming more common as they are highly sensitive and useful in ligand detection. Without using MS, false positives and negatives can be created because of molecular labels that can change or alter the binding between targeted proteins and ligands. To avoid this, MS differentiates ligands based on masses and can be screened. The HTS method allows the addition of separation steps to assess more than one compound at a time.

A final frontier that is being investigated with the help of HTS is to implement primary human cells to produce induced neurons (iNs) for research to replace the use of primary mouse neurons and takes us one step further towards humanized models for neurologic disorder's HTS.

The target-based HTS involves understanding the biological process involved in the disease targeted as derived from animal disease models and clinical patient observations. For example, with this understanding, a specific enzyme or receptor can be targeted to control the process.

TABLE 4.1

Factors Hindering Drug Discovery

Availability of API	Formulation Issues	Insufficient Capacity	Unexpected TK
Single most common reason for delay Quantity and quality of API Clinical formulation Contingency	Also very common Higher doses than previous studies Appropriate vehicles for test species Check solubility at appropriate concentrations Suspensions more appropriate?	Repeat dose tox is rate-limiting CROs have finite capacity; select CRO early Know strategy Avoid last-minute changes	May invalidate studies Include additional dose groups Animals—API, money, and time wasted Conduct lead optimization with TK
Unanticipated Toxicity	**Analytical Method Development**	**Species Selection**	**Late Reports**
Can result in significant delay Can result in unnecessary use of Tl Conduct appropriately designed lead optimization	Bioanalysis and formulation analysis methods required Formulation analysis a GLP requirement Fully validated (in each matrix) Start as early as possible	Fundamental basis of all non-clinical programs Traditional 'rat and dog' approach no longer acceptable Species selection impacts on API Biologicals—relevant species	Can delay regulatory submission Avoid by careful CRO selection Track record of quality reports delivered on time Experience in FIM programs Communication is key

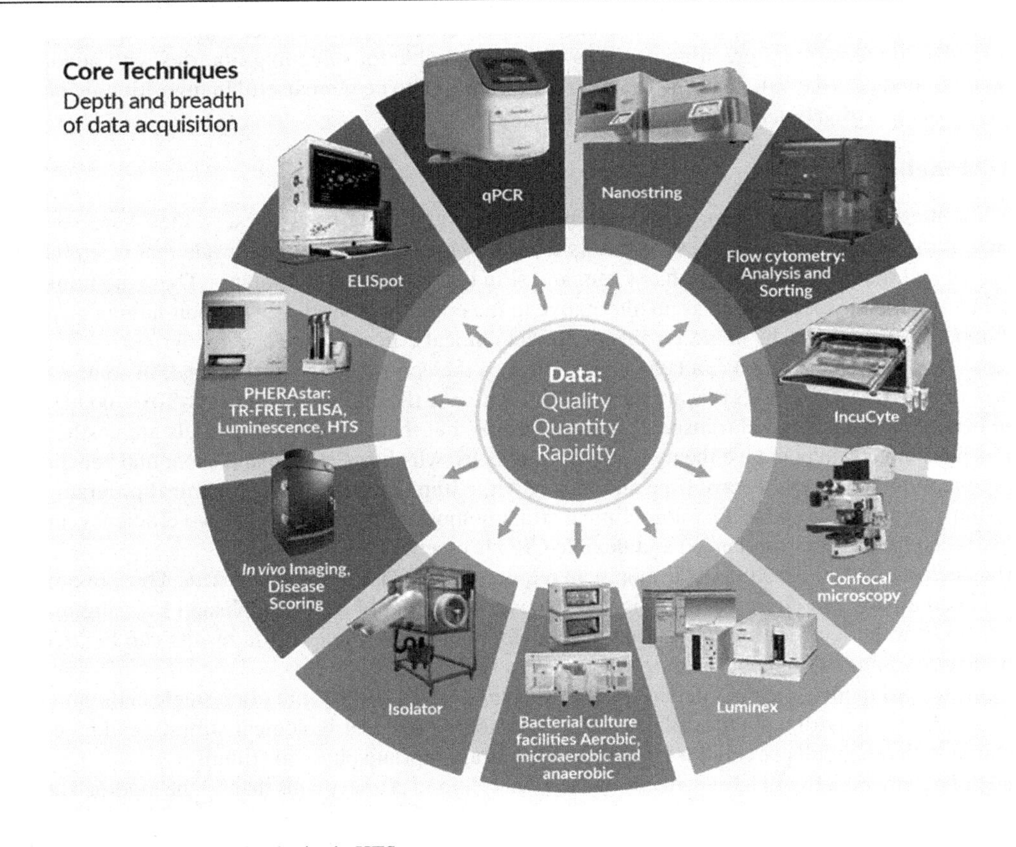

FIGURE 4.3 Evolving technologies in HTS.

4.2.1 Phenotypic Screening

Phenotypic screening is valuable when little is known about the disease process. Phenotypic HTS involves introducing compounds into a cell-based system and measuring the response. Unlike the targeted approach, there is no identified biological component for the drug interaction. Instead, a selection is based on a desired elicited response (e.g., cancer cell apoptosis, protein trafficking, receptor translocation). Thus, a process or pathway is tested instead of a specific targeted enzyme or receptor. Hence, any component along the process pathway that produces the sought results can result in potential therapeutic leads. After a compound is found to have the desired result, the process can be isolated to determine which step the compound affects and, thus, which biological target is the major contributor to the disease.

The most straightforward phenotypic screens employ cell lines and monitor a single parameter such as cell death or particular protein production. However, high-content screening, which monitors changes in the expression of multiple proteins simultaneously, is also widespread.

Phenotypic screening is best exemplified in whole animal-based techniques, where a drug is examined for possible therapeutic effect across various animal models representing multiple disease states. Model organisms are used in phenotypic screening in animal-based systems to determine the effects of a test substance in entirely constructed biological systems. Fruit flies (*Drosophila melanogaster*), zebrafish (*Danio rerio*), and mice (*Mus musculus*) are examples of creatures utilized for high-content screening. In some cases, the term phenotypic screening refers to unexpected findings in clinical trials, especially when novel and unexpected therapeutic effects of a therapeutic candidate are discovered.

Researchers can investigate test agents or changes in targets of interest in the context of fully integrated, assembled biological systems using model organisms, revealing information that would otherwise be unavailable in cellular systems. For example, cell-based systems are frequently unable to accurately represent human disease processes involving many distinct cell types across many different organ systems. This level of complexity can only be replicated in model organisms. The efficiency of drug discovery by phenotypic screening in organisms, including surprising discoveries in the clinic, supports this theory.

Animal-based phenotypic screening methods aren't as suitable for screening libraries with hundreds of tiny compounds. As a result, these methods have been proven to be more useful in repositioning previously authorized medications or late-stage drug candidates.

4.2.2 Modeling

When it comes to animal models, mini pigs are increasingly being used because they have several advantages, including omnivore digestion that is similar to humans', an estrogen cycle that is similar to humans' sexual maturity by six months of age, and skin that is similar to humans'. Thus, the mini pig is a viable non-rodent species used as an alternative to the commonly used dog and non-human primate (NHP) models. In addition, he might be able to predict clinical efficacy more accurately.

Disease models (typical mice) can help assess safety in the context of the disease and, in some cases, can show toxicological responses that are more representative of the response in patients. Toxicology studies can benefit from humanized transgenic animal models, but these humanized models are costly. The use of various models may reduce the use of NHPs and dogs, which has ethical and economic benefits.

There are numerous ways to save time and money while implementing the non-clinical program, but quality must always come first. The non-clinical strategy must be defined to improve efficiency, and a good partnership with an experienced and flexible CRO is essential.

Early studies and later preclinical development require the availability of safety data. Thus, improved safety-related attrition in clinical studies is a key focus, which could be accomplished by using model systems closer to humans and producing more reliable, translatable data. These results can be used to identify toxicity flags throughout the discovery process reliably.

The current cell models are insufficient to provide accurate data. Models are often single cells cultured in a simple 2D setup with a glass or plastic substrate, lacking relevant biological stimuli, and no communication with other cells or cellular models, as well as appropriate physical stimuli.

Next-generation models will have better access to stem cells and primary cells that can be modified using CRISPR technology. In addition, to simulate in vivo activity, multiple cell types can be cultured together; newer models could include 3D spheroids without supports, matrix gels, or even patient-derived organoids.

Validation and use of humanized isolated organ-on-a-chip models (OOC) and connected on-chip models that better mimic a typical biological environment for use in efficacy and safety determination will be required to exploit more complex cell models.

A critical step is developing isolated models and multiple organ models using the latest technology and identifying promising models that can be used. Industrial experience can provide the expertise to characterize the model, elucidate how good it is, how robust it is, and identify limitations.

4.2.3 Screening Using Fragments (FBS)

Fragment-based screening is a type of HTS based on the idea that smaller molecules (usually under 250 Da) are better suited to sampling the chemical space because it is much less complex for small molecules than for larger ones. As a result, hits are more common, but they may only bind weakly to the biological target, necessitating their growth or combination to produce a high-affinity lead. FBS can be used to map a target's binding site in great detail, providing chemists and molecular modelers with useful ideas for developing new chemotypes and, perhaps more importantly, optimizing lead structures. As a result, lead discovery is no longer viewed as a one-time activity at the start of a drug discovery project but rather as a continuous activity in tandem with compound optimization. In addition, cross-fertilization is possible between lead generation and lead optimization. The former can be done in iterative cycles, with previous cycles and lead optimization efforts feeding into the next.

Compound collections for high-throughput screening are typically made up of chemically diverse molecules and chemotypes from previous projects and contain up to two million substances. The compounds are screened in biological test systems, and hits are further optimized to drug candidates after being validated by independent biochemical or biophysical methods. The fragment library is a carefully curated collection of 1,300 fragments that follow the rule of three and include both 2D and 3D fragments that can run in parallel. These elements work together to ensure that all of the hits from the screen are high-quality compounds with a good chemical starting point.

4.2.4 Ligandomics

In contrast to traditional methods of discovering one ligand at a time, ligandomics is a new technology that uses molecular probes to map disease-specific cellular ligands systematically. High efficacy, minimal side effects, wide therapeutic indices, and low safety-related attrition rates are advantages of biologics targeting these ligands with disease selectivity. As a result, ligandomics represents a paradigm shift in addressing the biologics development bottleneck of target discovery.

The curation and analysis of known drug–target databases have allowed them to be classified into protein families. These are four main target classes of privileged "druggable" families—rhodopsin-like GPCR ligands, ion channels, nuclear receptors, and protein kinases (Figure 4.4). Approximately 53% of historical drug targets and 70% of approved drugs modulate one of these four targets, so investing in screening technologies, in compound libraries, and expertise around the system biology and signaling of these proteins support the drug discovery process, alongside the use of informatics to gather data on the desired target (Figure 4.5).

The use of databases such as the ChEMBL (www.ebi.ac.uk/chembl/) shows known drug targets such as GPCR ligands that yield a good return on investment; almost 18% of compounds published in lead optimization studies are GPCR ligands 30% of approved the market are GPCR drugs. So while the identification of a novel drug target is more exciting, it is also the riskier path to take.

X-ray crystallography provides a high-resolution crystal structure of an exemplar protein-ligand complex, the CN group fitted into the narrow pocket in the kinase, forming a hydrogen bond to lysine.

4.2.5 Gene-Based Testing

Genetics reveals gene-disease links in many ways. For example, Alzheimer's disease appears as plaque formation, but genes determine these plaques' activity—no one had thought of it; it happened in serendipitous discovery. Thus, genetics makes excellent contributions to the drug industry. For example,

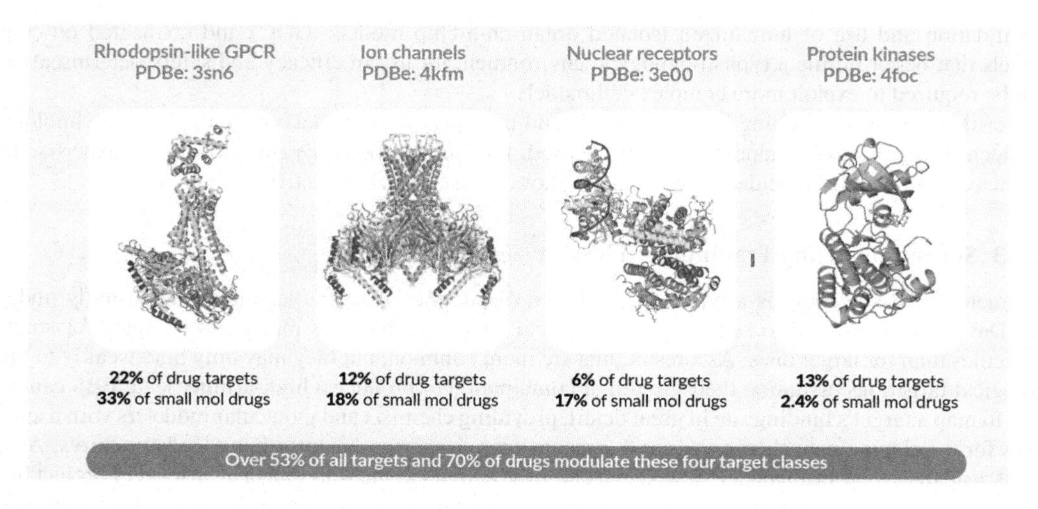

FIGURE 4.4 Privileged historical target families.

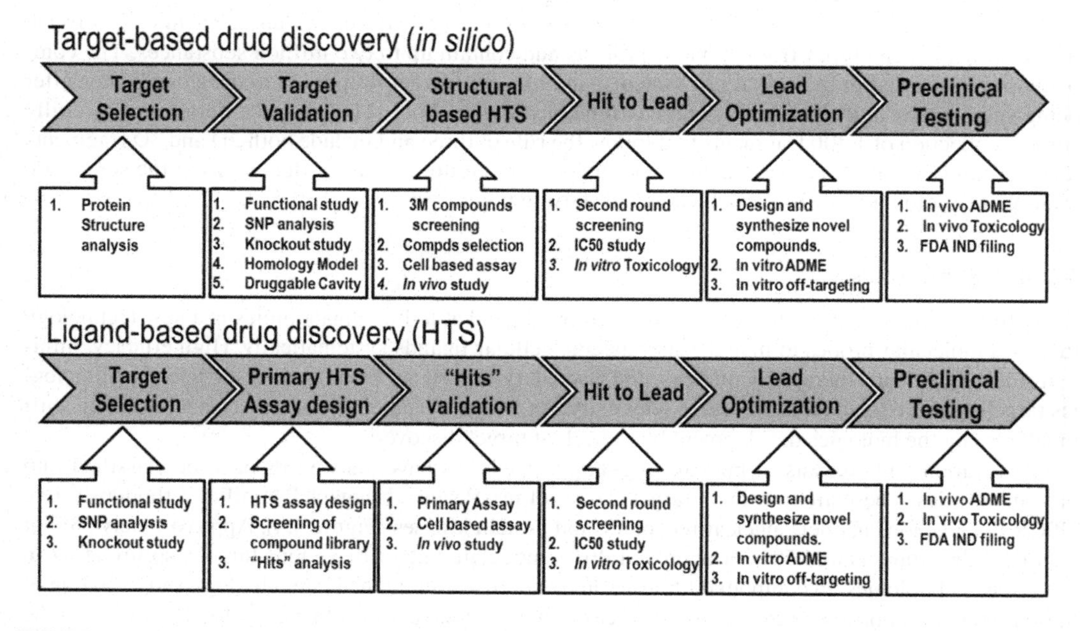

FIGURE 4.5 Two types of approaches to drug discovery. Source: www.drugdiscoverycenter.org/drug-discovery/.

disease-associated genes constitute a promising source of targets. Furthermore, the pathogenesis revealed by genetics is extremely valuable. For example, suppose a disease arises from a gain of function (GOF) mutation of a target gene. In that case, the complementary drugs must be antagonists or inhibitors. In contrast, for a disease induced by loss of function (LOF) mutation of a gene, the targeted drugs must be agonists.

Traditional Mendelian genetics and recently developed genome- and phenome-wide association studies have identified thousands of disease-associated genes (GWAS and PheWAS, respectively). On the other hand, almost every study linked diseases to changes in a single genetic locus. Because a combination of pathogenic factors causes most diseases, most of the links discovered between diseases and single genetic variations aren't strong enough to be therapeutically useful. Only 5% of the drug–disease associations derived from PheWAS (https://phewascatalog.org), for example, are backed up by clinical evidence. Thus, to find potential drugs using medical genetic information, we should look for multiple genes associated with specific diseases rather than a single pathogenic factor.

Genetic linkage to disease and model translatability are critical features associated with reduced clinical efficacy are widely explored, leading to building an integrated target discovery translatable model and genetic target validation to identify, prioritize and validate novel drug targets. A good example is the use of genomic data and CRISPR gene editing to identify and validate new drug targets. In addition, the development of a CRISPR-Cas9 DOX system has further increased the relevance of screening and precision and minimizes off-target effects using an insulator, doxycycline.

Several systems genetics methods have been developed to enrich and screen the driver genes underlying complex traits in the post-GWAS (genome-wide association studies) era. A gene-based association method called PrediXcan directly tests the molecular mechanisms through which genetic variation affects phenotype. NetWAS, a network-guided GWAS analysis method that integrates tissue-specific networks and nominally significant *p*-values in GWAS, identifies biologically critical disease–gene associations.

Antisense oligonucleotides are nucleic acid pieces that stop protein formation by either degrading mRNA, affecting the translational machinery, or rerouting a bound protein for degradation. The effect of removing that protein can then be studied to validate the target. Ribozymes are RNA molecules that can act as enzymes and can be used to target the mRNA that synthesizes the protein being studied. Small-interfering RNA or si-RNA is a cost-effective method that uses RNA to target the gene involved in the disease process. Targeting this gene allows for protein knockout or knockdown and, thus, target validation. These methods allow for studying specific proteins in the disease process by removing them or inhibiting their function.

Conversely, many disease processes function by downregulation of a particular gene or protein expression. Hence, upregulation or turning on gene expression increases protein function, which may be the desired outcome, and targets can be validated accordingly, that is, by looking at disease phenotype upon modulation and upregulation of the concordant transcription and translation processes. Regardless of the method, if the protein is found to be important for the disease process, the target can be said to be validated. Thus, once the target is validated, an assay can be developed and be considered for HTS.

4.2.6 Target Identification

Because existing compound collections were built in small molecule designs targeting known biological targets, new biological targets necessitate new designs and new ideas rather than reusing chemistry. Before, the automation of drug discovery utilizing HTS was a big challenge; now, we can screen up to one million samples in a day due to the availability of bulk reagent dispensers, compound transfer devices, and plate readers.

The drug discovery starts with determining the cause of the disease and suggests a potential biological target. A target can be any biological entity from RNA to a protein to a gene that is "druggable" or accessible to binding with a drug-like compound.

Drug interactions with a biological target change the shape or conformation of some facet of the target when bound to a small molecule and alter its ability to function. This conformational change ideally triggers a desired biological response involved in the particular disease process explored. A target is usually identified before testing to discover drug-like compounds that alter a disease process. A target-based approach focuses on a specific aspect of a target protein's function and substrate interactions. It is typically applied when scientists have a thorough understanding of a disease process.

A target may also be identified after a cell-based disease model is tested with drug-like compounds. This case is called a phenotypic cell-based screen since drug selection is based on a desired biological response without knowing the exact interaction or target responsible. Once the desired outcome against disease is discovered, we can reverse engineer and test the individual cellular processes versus the hits to deduce the biological component most responsible for the disease. Often target-based biochemical approaches are implemented when there is a greater understanding of the disease, but phenotypic screening is important in diseases that are not yet completely understood. In both cases, target identification is critically important to grasp which drug-like compounds to use when testing for reactivity and understanding the disease process. However, for the most high-priority diseases, both target-based screening and phenotypic-based HTS are often used in parallel with each other to help drive the drug discovery process faster, allowing for rapid analysis of both outcomes providing a synergistic drug discovery portfolio.

A successful drug target needs to demonstrate two fundamental properties:

- It has to have a site capable of binding drug-like molecules, i.e., a druggable site.
- It has to have a causal link to a disease process.

Historical drug targets have both of these properties by definition, and analysis of their features can help guide and derisk future drug discovery.

Whereas knowledge of target druggability is essential, so is the efficacy component. Mendelian randomization can provide evidence of the causal relationship between the target and disease and provide a way of anticipating the likely success (Figure 4.6). However, the real benefit of pre-validating these targets' success is that it can be done before large-scale, expensive phase II trials.

When considering drug targets for analysis, triage, and so forth, the use of online resources can support these decisions. Examples include Open Target, a collaborative project between several industry partners, the EMBL-EBI, and the Sanger Institute, who publish a richly curated and integrated data collection. Illuminating the Druggable Genome (IDG) is a global project whose aim is to identify and provide information on more minor well-studied proteins within commonly drug-targeted protein families. Finally, the CanSAR platform at the Institute of Cancer Research provides data on somatic diseases (see Tables 4.2 and 4.3).

4.2.6.1 Hit Identification

Drug discovery scientists must confirm activity in an assay to validate a "hit" as a statistically significant reaction. Many reactions will give false positives for reasons such as organic impurities, reader

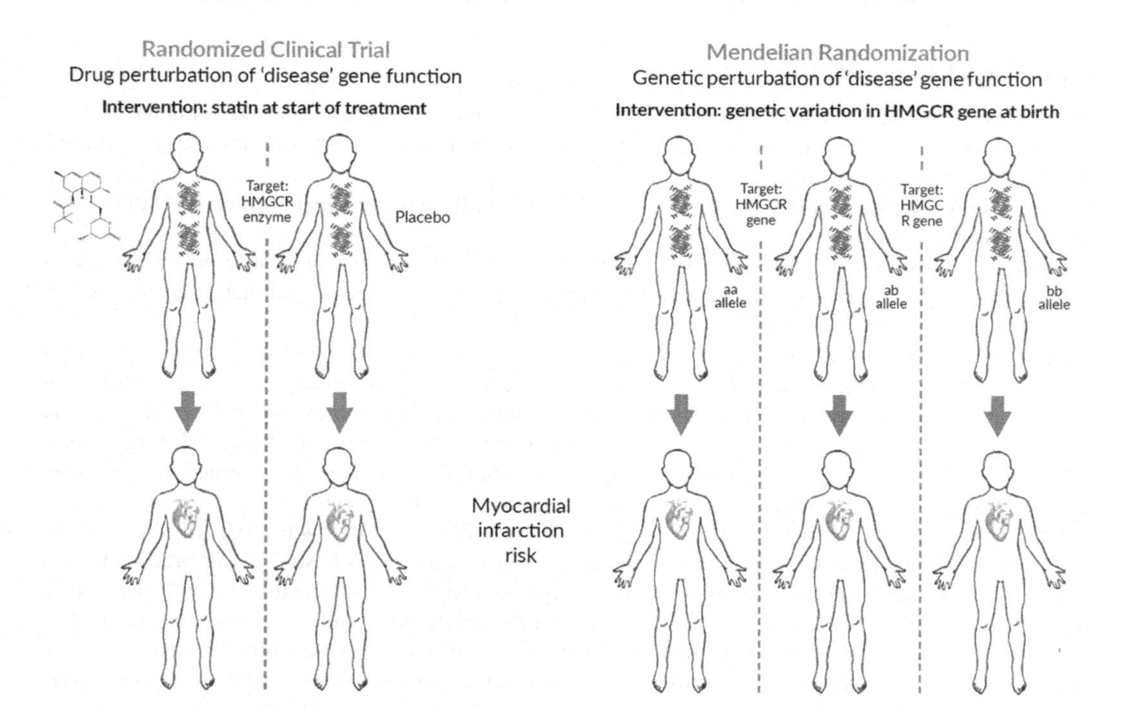

FIGURE 4.6 Mendelian randomization in target validation.

TABLE 4.2

Online Resources on Drug Discovery Initiatives

ATOM	A data-driven modeling pipeline capable of rapidly building and optimizing ML models for bioassay activity and molecular property predictions. This modeling pipeline is essential for developing predictive models for public and private pharmaceutical assay datasets. While ML-based techniques to predict drug properties from structures are regularly used in computational drug design, there remains a need for an automated modular pipeline for everyday modeling tasks. Some critical features for such a software package are to enable reproducibility, incorporate new models, support a variety of chemical representations, allow for hyperparameter optimization, and validate predictive performance. (https://atomscience.org)
BindingDB	A searchable database of experimentally measured binding affinities, focusing chiefly on the interactions of proteins considered to be drug targets with small, drug-like molecules. BindingDB contains 1,419,347 binding data, for 7,000 protein targets and 635,301 small molecules. (www.bindingdb.org/bind/index.jsp)
BioGRID	The Biological General Repository for Interaction Datasets is an open-access database on protein, genetic and chemical interactions for humans and all major model organism species and humans. To facilitate network-based approaches for drug discovery, BioGRID now incorporates 27,501 chemical-protein interactions for human drug targets.
BioPath	BioPath is a biochemical pathway database that provides access to metabolic transformations and cellular regulations derived from the Roche Applied Science "Biochemical Pathways" wall chart. In the current version 3, BioPath also provides access to biological transformations reported in the primary literature. The BioPath database is available in Symyx MOL/RDF format for integration into existing retrieval systems or, optionally, fully integrated into the web-based retrieval system BioPath.Explore. (www.mn-am.com/databases/biopath)
canSAR	Cancer research and drug discovery knowledgebase contain chemical and pharmacological data for over one million bioactive, small molecule drugs and compounds corresponding to approximately eight million pharmacological bioactivities and over ten million calculated chemical properties intended to enable target selection and validation in drug discovery.
CARLSBAD	A confederated database of more than one million bioactivity values for over 400,000 compounds associated with 3,500 protein targets. A one-click user query can determine potential leads for a target, associated off-targets, and druggable targets in associated disease pathways.
ChEMBL	A large-scale database of bioactive drug-like small molecules contains 2D structures, calculated properties (e.g., logP, Molecular Weight, *Lipinski* Parameters, etc.), and abstracted bioactivities (e.g., binding constants, pharmacology, and ADMET information). Target data can be searched via keyword, protein sequence search (BLAST), or navigating the target classification hierarchy. These include primary chemistry resources (ChEMBL and ChEBI) and other resources. The main focus is not small molecules but may contain some small-molecule information (e.g., Gene Expression Atlas, PDBe). The historical definition of drug targets includes catalytic sites, substrate binding sites, or epigenetic modification sites. Current understanding that protein-protein interactions are druggable, along with the emerging realization that "nodes" in signaling pathways and biological networks themselves can be manipulated with small molecules in non-traditional ways, has opened up new targeting options. So far, we have identified about 2,400 mechanisms for 1,400 indications and the combination of those two yields about 15,000 mechanism or indication pairs that can be regarded as another version count of the drug–disease targeting set.
CSNAP	Chemical Similarity Network Analysis Pull-down is a computational approach for compound target identification. Query and reference compounds are populated on the network connectivity map, and a graph-based neighbor counting method is applied to rank the consensus targets. The CSNAP approach facilitates high-throughput target discovery and off-target prediction.
DataWarrior	An open-access software, whereas Spotfire appears to be most widely used in the industry. (www.openmolecules.org/datawarrior/index.html)

(*Continued*)

TABLE 4.2 (CONTINUED)

Online Resources on Drug Discovery Initiatives

DeepSEA	A deep learning-based algorithmic framework for predicting the chromatin effects of sequence alterations with single nucleotide sensitivity. DeepSEA can accurately predict the epigenetic state of a sequence, including transcription factors binding, DNase I sensitivities, and histone marks in multiple cell types, and further utilize this capability to predict the chromatin effects of sequence variants and prioritize regulatory variants.
DEL	DNA-encoded chemical libraries (DEL) is a technology for the synthesis and screening on an unprecedented scale of collections of small molecule compounds (www.apexbt.com). DEL is used in medicinal chemistry to bridge the fields of combinatorial chemistry and molecular biology. DEL technology aims to accelerate the drug discovery process and, in particular, early-phase discovery activities such as target validation and hit identification. DEL technology involves the conjugation of chemical compounds or building blocks to short DNA fragments that serve as identification bar codes and, in some cases, also direct and control the chemical synthesis. The technique enables the mass creation and interrogation of libraries via affinity selection, typically on an immobilized protein target. A homogeneous method for screening DNA-encoded libraries has recently been developed, which uses water-in-oil emulsion technology to isolate, count, and identify individual ligand-target complexes in a single-tube approach. In contrast to conventional screening procedures such as high-throughput screening, biochemical assays are not required for binder identification, in principle allowing the isolation of binders to a wide range of proteins historically challenging to tackle with conventional screening technologies. In addition to the general discovery of target-specific molecular compounds, the availability of binders to pharmacologically essential but so-far "undruggable" target proteins opens new possibilities to develop novel drugs for diseases that could not be treated so far. In eliminating the requirement to initially assess the activity of hits, it is hoped and expected that many of the high-affinity binders identified will be shown to be active in independent analysis of selected hits, therefore offering an efficient method to identify high-quality hits and pharmaceutical leads. An alternative approach to access new medicine-like chemical space for hit exploration is using DNA-encoded library technology (DELT). Owing to the "split-and-pool" nature of DELT synthesis, it becomes possible to make huge numbers of compounds in a cost and time-efficient manner (millions to billions of compounds).
DGIdb 3.0	The drug–gene interaction database consolidates, organizes, and presents drug–gene relationships and gene druggability information from papers, databases, and web resources. It encapsulates multiple gene categories (e.g., kinases, G-protein coupled receptors) expected to be good drug targets.
DINIES	Drug–target interaction network inference engine built on supervised analysis enables predicting potential interactions between drug molecules and target proteins, based on drug data and omics-scale protein data.
DIP	The DIP database catalogs experimentally determined interactions between proteins. It combines information from a variety of sources to create a single, consistent set of protein–protein interactions. The data stored within the DIP database are curated manually by expert curators and automatically using computational approaches that utilize the knowledge about the protein–protein interaction networks extracted from the most reliable, core subset of the DIP data. (https://dip.doe-mbi.ucla.edu/dip/Main.cgi)
DisGeNET	A platform is integrating information on human disease-associated genes and variants. It can be used for investigation of the molecular underpinnings of specific human diseases, analysis of the properties of disease genes, generation of hypothesis on drug therapeutic action and drug adverse effects, validation of computationally predicted disease genes, and retrieval of druggable targets and biological pathways for a disease of interest.
DrugBank 3.0	A combination of detailed drug data with comprehensive drug target information, including searchable details on the nomenclature, ontology, chemistry, structure, function, action, pharmacology, pharmacokinetics, metabolism, and pharmaceutical properties. Content covers 10,510 drug entries, 871 approved biotech (protein/peptide) drugs, 105 nutraceuticals, and over 5,028 experimental drugs.

(*Continued*)

TABLE 4.2 (CONTINUED)

Online Resources on Drug Discovery Initiatives

DrugCentral	Online drug compendium integrating structure, bioactivity, regulatory, pharmacologic actions, and indications for active pharmaceutical ingredients. At the molecular level, DrugCentral bridges drug–target interactions with pharmacological action and indications to provide the mechanistic understanding and relate protein targets to human disease and symptoms.
DTO	Drug Target Ontology offers searchable database access to classify and integrate drug discovery data based on formalized and standardized classifications and annotations of druggable protein targets. DTO integrates phylogenecity, function, target development level, disease association, tissue expression, chemical ligand, substrate characteristics, and target-family specific features.
ECOdrug	A research platform tool is connecting drugs and conservation of their targets across species. It harmonizes ortholog predictions from multiple sources via a simple user interface underpinning critical applications for a wide range of pharmacology studies, ecotoxicology, and comparative evolutionary biology.
EnamineStore	337 million molecules searchable (by similarity) at EnamineStore. (https://enaminestore.com/search)
ExPecto	Makes highly accurate cell-type-specific predictions of gene expression solely from DNA sequence. With ExPecto, the tissue-specific impact of gene transcriptional dysregulation can be systematically probed 'in silico,' at a scale not yet possible experimentally. ExPecto leverages deep learning-based sequence models trained on chromatin profiling data and integrated with spatial transformation and regularized linear models.
GDB-17	GDB-17 (https://gdb.unibe.ch/downloads/) is a database of virtual molecules containing 166.4 billion molecules and FDB-17 of ten million fragment-like molecules with up to 17 heavy atoms. (www.ncbi.nlm.nih.gov/pubmed/283750)
Github	A web application for interactive exploration of the target, biological process, and disease trends. https://rguha.shinyapps.io/MovingTargets/ is based on Github and provides publications detail on targets and diseases. (https://github.com/BZdrazil/Moving_Targets)
HitGen	Contain 400 billion molecules, X-chem provides 200 million compounds for screening. (www.hitgen.com)
HitPick	A web server that facilitates the analysis of chemical screenings by identifying hits and predicting their molecular targets, focusing on analysis and interpretation of chemical phenotypic screens. The target prediction functionality can also be used in a stand-alone fashion.
Human Metabolome Database	The Human Metabolome Database (HMDB) is a freely available electronic database containing detailed information about small molecule metabolites found in the human body. It is intended to be used for metabolomics, clinical chemistry, biomarker discovery, and general education. The database is designed to contain or link three kinds of data: 1) chemical data, 2) clinical data, and 3) molecular biology/biochemistry data. The database contains 114,260 metabolite entries, including both water-soluble and lipid-soluble metabolites as well as metabolites that would be regarded as either abundant (> 1 uM) or relatively rare (< 1 nM). Additionally, 5,702 protein sequences are linked to these metabolite entries. Each MetaboCard entry contains 130 data fields, with 2/3 of the information being devoted to chemical/clinical data and the other 1/3 devoted to enzymatic or biochemical data. Many data fields are hyperlinked to other databases (KEGG, PubChem, MetaCyc, ChEBI, PDB, UniProt, and GenBank) and various structure and pathway viewing applets. The HMDB database supports extensive text, sequence, chemical structure, and relational query searches. Four additional databases, DrugBank, T3DB, SMPDB, and FooDB are also part of the databases' HMDB suite. DrugBank contains equivalent information on ~2,280 drug and drug metabolites, T3DB contains information on ~3,670 common toxins and environmental pollutants, SMPDB contains pathway diagrams for ~25,000 human metabolic and disease pathways, while FooDB contains equivalent information on ~28,000 food components and food additives. (https://hmdb.ca)

(Continued)

TABLE 4.2 (CONTINUED)

Online Resources on Drug Discovery Initiatives

HumanBase	HumanBase is a "one-stop shop" for biological researchers interested in data-driven predictions of gene expression, function, regulation, and interactions in humans, particularly in the context of specific cell types/tissues and human disease. This resource is not merely a public database of primary genomics data or biological literature. The data-driven integrative analyses (i.e., algorithms that "learn" from sizeable genomic data collections) presented in HumanBase are compelling because they separate signal from noise in extensive biological data collections to reach beyond "existing biological knowledge" represented in the biological literature to identify novel associations that are not biased toward well-studied areas of biomedical research. Carefully designed algorithms can drive the development of experimentally testable hypotheses. Thus, HumanBase is a resource for biomedical researchers to incorporate into their research workflows, which they can interpret their experimental results and generate hypotheses for experimental follow-up. HumanBase is actively developed by the genomics group at the Flatiron Institute. (https://hb.flatironinstitute.org)
iDrug-Target	A package of web services for predicting drug-target interactions between drug compounds and target proteins in cellular networking via a benchmark dataset optimization approach. It contains four predictors: iDrug-GPCR, iDrug-Chl, iDrug-Ezy, and iDrug-NR, specialized for GPCRs (G protein-coupled receptors), ion channels, enzymes, and NR (nuclear receptors), respectively.
idTarget	A web server that can predict possible binding targets of a small chemical molecule via a divide-and-conquer docking approach. It is also intended to reproduce known off-targets of drugs or drug-like compounds. Unlike previous approaches that screen against a specific class of targets or a limited number of targets, idTarget addresses nearly all protein structures deposited in the Protein Data Bank (PDB).
IsoStar	IsoStar is a web application that provides thousands of interactive 3D scatterplots that show the probability of occurrence and spatial characteristics of interactions between pairs of chemical functional groups. Accessed using just a few intuitive buttons clicks these scatterplots facilitate the rapid exploration and assessment of intermolecular interactions without the need to construct complex search queries or carry out detailed data analyses. (www.ccdc.cam.ac.uk/solutions/csd-core/components/isostar/)
IUPHAR/BPS	An interactive guide to pharmacology is aggregating drug target information from Ensembl, UniProt, PubChem, ChEMBL, and DrugBank, as well as curated citations from PubMed. Coverage includes the key properties and selective ligands and tool compounds available for each target family. Queries can then be expanded into each target's pharmacological, physiological, structural, genetic, and pathophysiological properties.
KiggLigand	KEGG LIGAND is a composite database name for COMPOUND, GLYCAN, REACTION, RCLASS, and ENZYME databases, whose entries are identified by C, G, R, RC, and EC numbers, respectively. (www.genome.jp/dbget/ligand.html)
MANTRA	Mode of Action by NeTwoRk Analysis is a computational tool for evaluating the target mode of action (MoA) of novel drug structures and identifying known and approved candidates for "drug repositioning." Structural queries are automatically integrated into a network of compounds where the topology reveals similarities and differences in MoA compared to reference compounds in the known pharmacopeia.
MarkTB	Reliable biomarkers can shorten the time needed to develop improved TB cures and diagnostics that can save millions of lives.
NetWas	GWAS re-prioritization (NetWAS): tissue-specific networks provide a new means to generate hypotheses related to the molecular basis of human disease. In NetWAS, the statistical associations from a standard GWAS guide the analysis of functional networks. NetWAS, in conjunction with tissue-specific networks, effectively reprioritizes statistical associations from GWAS to identify disease-associated genes. This reprioritization method is driven by GWAS discovery and does not depend on prior disease knowledge.
Neuvolution	Nuevolution, now part of Amgen, has assembled a collection of 40 trillion compounds. (www.nuevolution.com)

(Continued)

TABLE 4.2 (CONTINUED)

Online Resources on Drug Discovery Initiatives

OMIM	OMIM is a comprehensive, authoritative compendium of human genes and genetic phenotypes that is freely available and updated daily. (www.ncbi.nlm.nih.gov/omim)
Open Targets	A platform for therapeutic target identification and validation provides either a target-centric workflow to identify diseases that may be associated with a specific target or a disease-centric workflow to identify targets related to a specific disease. Coverage includes genetic associations, somatic mutations, know drugs, gene expression, affected pathways, literature mining, and animal models.
PASS	Prediction of Activity Spectra for Substances is an online tool for evaluating an organic drug-like molecule's general biological potential. PASS provides simultaneous forecasts of many biological activity types, including molecular and cellular targets, with readouts modeled after the Anatomical Therapeutic Chemical classification system (ATC). In this context, see also SuperPred.
PharmMapper	A web server for potential drug target identification with a target database of over 53,000 receptor-based pharmacophore models created with ~23,000 protein poses predicted to qualify as druggable binding sites. The expanded target data repository in Version 7 now covers 450 indications and 4,800 molecular functions.
Pharos	A multimodal web interface and target search portal at the front end of the underlying databases illuminated the Druggable Genome initiative. It also integrates with the DrugCentral and DTO resources (also cited in this compendium). Pharos now serves as an entry point to targets in the entire human proteome. Its design is intended to shed light on the dark corners, thereby expanding what is considered druggable.
PhID	A network pharmacology portal of targets, diseases, genes, side-effects, pathways, and drugs is designed to provide visualization of complex relationships and precisely predict drug-target interactions. The underlying databases cover approximately 330,000 chemical structures, including the known pharmacopeia, 24,000 targets, 8,500 diseases, 43,000 genes; 4,500 side effects; and 867 pathways.
PPB	The Polypharmacology Browser is a multi-fingerprint target prediction tool using ChEMBL bioactivity data. It allows users to find out if a newly identified bioactive molecule, or any compound, is closely related to molecules with documented bioactivity and, therefore, is likely to interact with the corresponding biological target.
PrediXcan	A gene-based association method called PrediXcan directly tests the molecular mechanisms through which genetic variation affects phenotype. PrediXcan is a computational algorithm developed to exploit GTEx data, including eQTLs identification and their relationship to complex traits. PrediXcan evaluates the aggregate effects of cis-regulatory variants (within 1 MB upstream or downstream of genes of interest) on gene expression via an elastic net regression method. Consequently, PrediXcan may identify loci with modest to weak effect sizes that do not achieve significance in variant-based association studies. In theory, PrediXcan has a significantly reduced multiple testing burden as compared to single-variant-single-trait association tests. For example, given one trait and a genotypic dataset of ten million SNPs, there are at most about 20,000 tests for PrediXcan (~20,000 genes), but ten million tests for single-variant-single-trait association study. Putative eQTLs and their effect sizes on gene expression level in each GTEx tissue type are available online in PredictDB. (http://predictdb.org/)
PROMISCUOUS	A database and visualization tool for network-based drug-repositioning designed to deliver complex relations among drugs, their respective targets, and side-effects of the drugs. The web portal has been designed with a novel interface that offers a natural way of exploring the network: database entities (drugs, targets, and side effects) are represented as nodes in a network with edges representing the relations between them. Coverage of the 25,000 drugs plus drug-like molecules collection includes annotations on drug-protein and protein-protein relationships. (http://bioinformatics.charite.de/promiscuous2/)

(*Continued*)

TABLE 4.2 (CONTINUED)

Online Resources on Drug Discovery Initiatives

PROSITE	The ProRule section of PROSITE comprises manually created rules that can automatically generate annotation in the UniProtKB/Swiss-Prot format based on PROSITE motifs. In most cases, rules are based on PROSITE profiles as they are more specific than patterns, but occasionally rules make use of patterns. In these cases, the rules will not work independently but will be called by another rule, triggered by a profile. In addition to these rules corresponding to a unique PROSITE motif, rules are triggered by a specific combination of PROSITE motifs called metamotifs. Metamotifs allow the definition of arrangements of domains separated by spacers of variable size and the anchoring to the N- and C-termini and excluding a PROSITE motif. ProRule uses the UniRule format common to all types of rules created to annotate UniProtKB/Swiss-Prot, including the HAMAP rules. Each rule contains information used to provide template-based annotation associated with the domain or family detected by the PROSITE motif. ProRule is used to create UniProtKB/Swiss-Prot lines with basic and complex annotation derived from the domain and biologically critical amino acids: domain name and boundaries, EC number, function, keywords, associated PROSITE patterns, PTMs, active sites, disulfide bonds, etc. ProRule contains notably the position of structurally and functionally critical amino acid(s), as well as the condition(s) they must fulfill to play their biological role(s). Part of these supplementary data is used by ScanProsite that not only provides the protein sequence matched by a profile but also information about the relevance of biologically meaningful residues, like active sites, binding sites, post-translational modification sites, or disulfide bonds, to help function determination. (https://prosite.expasy.org)
REAL	Readily Available (REAL) chemical space by Enamine has ~650 million molecules searchable via REAL Space Navigator software. (www.biopharmatrend.com/post/56-navigating-real-chemical-space-in-a-pursuit-of-novel-medicines/#comments)
RTECS	RTECS is a compendium of data extracted from the open scientific literature. The data are recorded in the RTECS staff's format and arranged in alphabetical order by prime chemical name. Six types of toxicity data are included in the file: 1) primary irritation; 2) mutagenic effects; 3) reproductive effects; 4) tumorigenic effects; 5) acute toxicity; and 6) other multiple dose toxicity. Specific numeric toxicity values such as LD50, LC50, TDLo, TCLo are noted, species studied, and administration route. For each citation, the bibliographic source is listed, enabling the user to access the actual studies cited. (www.cdc.gov/niosh/rtecs/default.html)
SEA	The Similarity Ensemble Approach categorizes proteins by comparing the set-wise chemical similarity among their ligands. It can be used to search large compound databases rapidly and to build cross-target similarity maps. A collection of ~65,000 ligands annotated for drug targets are incorporated into the query algorithms. According to ligand chemistry, these related targets reveal unexpected relationships that may be assayed using the ligands themselves.
SIDER2	SIDER contains information on marketed medicines and their recorded adverse drug reactions. The information is extracted from public documents and package inserts. The available information includes side effect frequency, drug and side effect classifications as well as links to further knowledge, for example, drug–target relations. (http://sideeffects.embl.de)
SLAP	Semantic Link Association Prediction uncovers "missing links" from a wide range of databases, including compound–gene, drug–drug, protein–protein, and drug–side effects, to create a complex network of compound–target interactions for which there is no experimental data but which are statistically probable.
SPiDER	Computer-assisted drug design identifies the macromolecular targets of chemical entities using self-organizing maps, consensus scoring, and statistical analysis to successfully identify targets for both known drugs and computer-generated molecular scaffolds.
SuperDRUG2	Knowledge-based of approved and marketed drugs covering 4,587 active pharmaceutical ingredients, including small molecules and biological products. The database is intended as a one-stop resource providing data on chemical structures, regulatory details, indications, drug targets, side effects, physicochemical properties, pharmacokinetics, and drug–drug interactions.

(*Continued*)

TABLE 4.2 (CONTINUED)
Online Resources on Drug Discovery Initiatives

SuperPred	A prediction web server for ATC codes and target prediction of compounds. Predicting ATC codes or targets of small molecules, and thus gaining information about the compounds, assists in the drug development process for new compounds. The web server's ATC prediction and target prediction are based on an internal pipeline consisting of a 2D fragment and 3D similarity search results. In this context, also see PASS.
SuperTarget	A web-based, searchable data warehouse is integrating drug-related information associated with medical indications, adverse drug effects, drug metabolism, pathways, and Gene Ontology (GO) terms for target proteins. The current database version contains more than 6,000 target proteins, annotated with more than 330,000 relationships to 196,000 compounds (including approved drugs).
SwissTargetPrediction	A web server for target prediction of small bioactive molecules using drawn structures or SMILES notation for input. By analyzing a combination of 2D and 3D similarity measures, the underlying software compares the query molecule to a library of 280,000 compounds active on more than 2,000 targets in five different organisms. Mapping predictions by homology within and between different species is enabled for close paralogs and orthologs.
TargetMine	An integrative data analysis platform for gene set analysis and knowledge discovery in a data warehouse framework. The current version has been optimized for target prioritization in response to queries while also surveying the broader biological and chemical data space relevant to drug discovery and development. Search functions permit users to identify chemicals and drugs that interact with a given set of genes/proteins and integrate them into gene-disease associations and regulatory networks.
T3DB	SOON TO BE NAMED AS Toxic Exposome Database is a unique bioinformatics resource that combines detailed toxin data with comprehensive toxin target information. The database currently houses 3,678 toxins described by 41,602 synonyms, including pollutants, pesticides, drugs, and food toxins, linked to 2,073 corresponding toxin target records. Altogether there are 42,374 toxins, toxin target associations. Each toxin record (ToxCard) contains over 90 data fields and holds information such as chemical properties and descriptors, toxicity values, molecular and cellular interactions, and medical information. This information has been extracted from over 18,143 sources, including other databases, government documents, books, and scientific literature. (www.t3db.ca)
TargetNet	A web service for predicting potential drug-target interaction profiling via multi-target SAR models. Naïve Bayes models, together with various molecular fingerprints, are employed to construct prediction models against 623 human proteins with highly validated druggable features.
TransPortal	The FDA Transporter Database is a repository of information on transporters necessary in the drug discovery process as a part of the US Food and Drug Administration-led Critical Path Initiative. Information includes transporter expression, localization, substrates, inhibitors, and drug–drug interactions.
TTD	Therapeutic Target Database is a resource for facilitating bench-to-clinic research of targeted therapeutics. Current coverage for searches based on similarities to the input query includes related information on 3,100 target and 34,000 drugs and drug-like compounds, consisting in part of 2,500 approved drugs and 18,900 investigational agents.
UniChem	Awhile the simple, large-scale non-redundant database of pointers between chemical structures and EMBL-EBI chemistry resources. Its purpose is to optimize the efficiency with which structure-based hyperlinks may be built and maintained between chemistry-based resources and is particularly suitable for creating such links "on the fly" (using REST web services). Primarily, this service has been designed to maintain cross-references between EBI chemistry resources.
UniPort	The mission of UniProt is to provide the scientific community with a comprehensive, high-quality, and freely accessible resource of protein sequence and functional information. (www.uniprot.org)

(Continued)

TABLE 4.2 (CONTINUED)

Online Resources on Drug Discovery Initiatives

WITHDRAWN	A resource for withdrawn and discontinued drugs to be used as heuristic templates for future predictions. The searchable database comprises 578 withdrawn or discontinued drugs, their structures, important physicochemical properties, protein targets, and relevant signaling pathways. A unique feature of the database calls out the drugs withdrawn due to adverse reactions and toxic effects so that that similarity searches can uncover possible liabilities in query molecules. (https://academic.oup.com/nar/article/44/D1/D1080/25026)

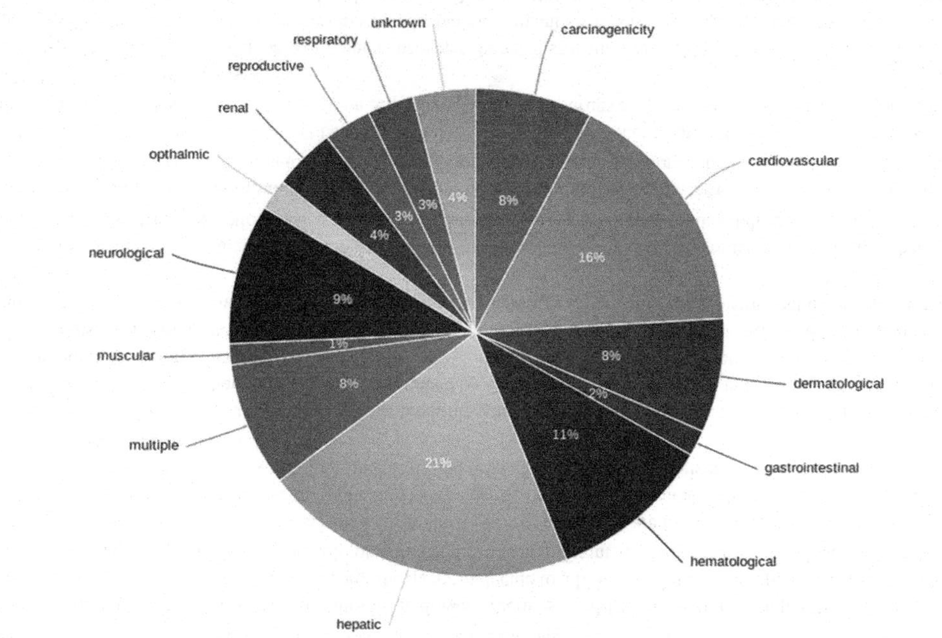

ZINK	A free database of commercially available compounds for virtual screening, containing 750 million molecules, including 230 million in 3D formats ready for docking. (http://zinc15.docking.org/)

TABLE 4.3
ChEMBL Targets for Targets

Target	No in ChEMBL
Adhesion	18
Auxilliary transport protein	26
Enzyme	3,983
Epigenetic regulator	155
Ion channel	441
Membrane receptor	948
Other cytosolic protein	98
Other membrane protein	15
Other nuclear protein	11
Secreted protein	87
Structural protein	32
Surface antigen	29
Transcription factor	195
Transporter	260
Unclassified protein	1,312
TOTAL	7,610

interference, and nonspecific binding. The hit can be identified using a fluorescence output or transient output, such as kinetic-based observations using image readers in the Molecular Devices FLIPR Tetra. When a hit is identified, a confirmation screen is done. This confirmation screen establishes the reproducibility of the hit by repeating the test with the same compound.

The Z-factor is commonly used to determine the quality of high-throughput assay screens. A Z coefficient of 1 is ideal, and any value above 0.5 shows a high-quality assay. As shown in Equation 4.1, the Z-factor uses the means (μ) and standard deviations (σ) of both the positive and negative values. The Z coefficient reflects the variation of data as well as the signal strength. It is dimensionless and allows a uniform means for comparing the quality of HTS assays. The Z' prime factor, on the other hand, is used to find the quality of the assay development and its optimization. Using the same equation as Equation 4.1, the Z' equation replaces the mean and standard deviation with those measured from the control. Thus, Z' helps HTS scientists determine the quality of a particular assay for an individual experiment. Therefore, the Z-factor is an indicator of the overall quality of an HTS assay.

The equation for Z-factor used in HTS

$$\text{Z-factor} = 1 - \frac{3(\text{Standard deviation of sample} + \text{Standard deviation of control})}{|\text{Mean of sample} - \text{mean of control}|}$$

The identified hit should be a high-quality compound translatable to an optimization program and delivered into the drug candidate requiring integration of chemistry, protein science, and assay biology. To identify a suitable quality compound and good quality hits, one can utilize the LeadBuilder virtual screening platform (www.domainex.co.uk/services/leadbuilder-virtual-screening). Using the information on the target protein or the ligand of interest utilizes structural information or homology models and screens up to 1,000 compounds. The interrogation of different virtual libraries and the NICE library consisting of commercially available compounds enables rapid hit expansion (see Table 4.4).

Critical to good quality protein production is intensive quality control of the protein for purity, activity, compound binding. Another approach is to perform testing using orthogonal methods such as multiple-step chromatography. One can also use microscale thermophoresis, a solution-based system to assess the protein that requires small protein samples, typically 5–15 nM concentration in about 5 ml. It has the advantage of focusing on suitable protein. It also uses multiple labeling strategies, directed by the structural information gathered about the target, enabling proteins' delivery in their near-physiological states.

TABLE 4.4
Compound Libraries

Compound Type	Compound Collection	Number of Compounds	Ideal Application	Description
Academic/government	MLSMR	350,478	Identification of novel modulators of drug target	The Molecular Libraries Small Molecule Repository (MLSMR) is a chemically diverse collection of small molecules used for probe discovery as part of the now-retired Molecular Libraries Probe Production Centers Network (MLPCN).
Academic/government	NExT Diversity Libraries	84,000+	Identification of novel modulators of drug target	The NExT Diversity Libraries contain chemical scaffolds across ten commercial suppliers and compounds that are selected to fall within the boundaries of drug-like chemical space (e.g., Lipinski's rule of five, high QED scores).
Commercial	Assorted collections	1,000+	Assay validation, identification of control compounds	Commercially available chemical libraries are available to help validate HTS-amenable assays and identify potential small molecule controls. These libraries contain several privileged scaffolds and are often biased toward known bioactivity and polypharmacology.
NCATS exclusive	Genesis	100,000+	Identification of novel modulators of drug target	NCATS has assembled the Genesis collection to provide a novel modern chemical library that emphasizes high-quality chemical starting points, sp3-enriched chemotypes, and core scaffolds that enable immediate purchase and derivatization via medicinal chemistry.
NCATS exclusive	Sytravon	44,000	Identification of novel modulators of drug target	The Sytravon library is a retired pharma screening collection that contains a diversity of novel small molecules, emphasizing medicinal chemistry-tractable scaffolds.
NCATS exclusive	NPACT	11,000+	Characterization of target/pathway biology	The NCATS Pharmacologically Active Chemical Toolbox (NPACT) is a library of annotated compounds that inform on novel phenotypes, biological pathways, and cellular processes. More than 7,000 mechanisms and phenotypes are identified in the literature and worldwide patents that cover biological interactions within mammals, microbial, plant, and other model systems.
NCATS exclusive	NPC	2,400	Drug repurposing	The NCATS Pharmaceutical Collection (NPC) is a library of all compounds that have been approved for use by the Food and Drug Administration, along with several approved molecules from related agencies in foreign countries.

To see how long a compound must be bound to a target before it can affect an electrospun scaffold material onto which cells are seeded. The magnetic scaffold allows an adherent monolayer of cells to move from well to well, i.e., from wells containing the tracer to wells containing the compound. The plates can then be directly inserted into the plate reader. The resulting graph shows the time versus BRET (bioluminescence resonance energy transfer) ratio, with different compounds competing at different rates for the receptor.

PROTAC (proteolysis targeted chimeras) induces protein degradation at the proteasome using a ubiquitin-proteasome system. A small chimeric molecule is used in the technology; one end selectively binds to the protein target of interest. The other end attaches to an E3 ligase and is held together by a linker. The protein is ubiquitinated by the E3 ligase, which marks it for degradation. The PROTAC molecules dissociate and can be reused once the degradation process has begun. This system has the advantage of degrading rather than inhibiting the target protein, making it an excellent technique for studying undruggable proteins.

4.2.6.2 Hit to Lead

A drug-like compound is classified as a lead when it is deemed selective for a particular pathway or protein and does not have adverse cytotoxic properties. Selectivity is essential as many compounds will work on a specific protein and affect many other proteins in a cell. This means that the drug is not selective and may bring about side effects if it progressed to in vivo testing. Also, this counter screen often determines whether or not the compound is toxic to cells. Therefore, the cytotoxicity of a drug-like compound is imperative to understand whether or not a drug will be toxic to the cell and potentially the patient. The next step is to determine how different concentrations of the compound affect biological activity. This is known as dose-response titration or concentration-response curve and is recorded on a semilog graph, which gives a sigmoidal curve. A broad hillslope means that a slight increase in dosage has little effect on the drug's activity.

A steep hillslope means that a slight increase in dosage significantly affects the drug's activity. The drug potency is established by the EC50, which is the concentration at which the drug elicits 50% of its maximum response. A potent drug is a small dosage needed to elicit 50% of its maximal response. The maximum is the point at which increasing the drug dose no longer produces any different response. A higher maximum response is important in determining a compound's effectiveness or efficacy. A more effective compound will elicit a higher percent response at a particular dosage. The potency, efficacy, and safety of a drug can be observed using multiple assays and their respective dose-response curves. This information is necessary to advance from a hit to a lead.

4.2.6.3 Target Validation and Efficacy

Target validation is required to increase confidence in the biological hypothesis. The hypothesis's strength grows as the system's complexity grows, from cell lines to primary cells to complex cell systems and animal disease models before efficacy is tested in human clinical trials.

The biological hypothesis must be tested as part of the target validation process to improve clinical attrition. It's crucial to determine whether a lack of efficacy is caused by the compound failing to engage with the intended target or by the compound engaging with the target. The goal isn't to change the disease pathway.

When compared to isolated protein or protein domain approaches, cellular target engagement models the complexity of the cell environment. When compared to targets on the cell surface, achieving this for intracellular targets can be more difficult, as three broad categories can be exemplified.

- CETSA is reliant on the structural confirmation of its target being stabilized by small-molecule binding. When a heat pulse is applied to the target protein, the ligand-bound form unfolds at a higher temperature than the unbound form, resulting in a shift in the melt curve. A variety of detection methods can be used to read out this difference caused by ligand-induced stabilization, ranging from the Western blot and antibody-based detection to mass spectrometry-based proteomics. It's worth noting that CETSA can produce false-negative results for compounds that genuinely bind the target but don't cause thermal stabilization; however, it's a versatile method with minimal reagent requirements.

- BRET is a cell-based assay that uses a fluorescent tracer ligand and a luciferase enzyme tag. While BRET is similar to fluorescence resonance energy transfer (FRET), it has a better signal because there is no widefield illumination with the luciferase tag producing the donor emission. Instead, compound binding is detected by a shift in the tracer and a drop in the BRET signal, allowing real-time monitoring of the compound's binding. In addition, it's one of the few techniques that can measure intracellular residence times, which could open up new avenues for improving drug efficacy and safety profiles.
- FRET is the third category.

Validating proximal markers downstream of the target is frequently used to demonstrate modulation of the disease-relevant pathway. Therefore, these markers should ideally be specific to the desired ligand–target interaction and well validated.

Target engagement should show that the ligand reaches its target, that the ligand–target interaction and mechanism are confirmed, and that proximal markers that can report disease pathway modulation are identified and measured. This idea of target engagement is carried over. Various detection methods can be used to read out this difference caused by ligand-induced stabilization, ranging from mass spectrometry–based proteomics to western blot and antibody-based detection. CETSA can produce false-negative results for compounds that bind the target but don't cause thermal stabilization; however, it's a versatile method with few reagent requirements. From early discovery in vitro cascades to the use of proof of mechanism biomarkers to inform clinical trial outcomes

4.2.6.4 Cell-Based Models

Beyond just comparing phenotypic and target-based approaches, there is a clear trend toward more complex cellular assays, like going from immortal cell lines to primary cells, patient cells, co-cultures, and 3D cultures. In HTS, roughly 50–60% of the assays are cell-based assays. The experimental setup is also becoming more sophisticated, with changes in subcellular compartments, single-cell analysis, and even cell imaging being observed in addition to univariate readouts.

Before developing an assay, it is critical to consider the type of model required and whether it can adequately reflect the disease's complexity. A clear understanding of the actionable data required and how to characterize the relevant biology in the model and, as a result, which model approach is best for the study, should be established. It's sometimes enough to have a simple model that faithfully reproduces a critical functional requirement. However, at times, a more complex model may be required. The most crucial factor is that the model accurately reflects the essential biology.

The use of primary cell models has both benefits and drawbacks, as well as some opportunities. First, primary cells have the advantage of being native cells, which allows for a better understanding of the physiological, morphological, and molecular processes that occur naturally in human cells, and thus provide the most in vivo–like cellular biology possible.

The disadvantages of using primary cells include the difficulty of maintaining cellular phenotypes in culture, the need for regular access, the scale/numbers required for higher throughput screening models, and thus the need to frequently source cells from individual donors interindividual variation within the assay. While interindividual variation can be a disadvantage in some situations (e.g., screening), it can also be advantageous in others. In the end, it more accurately reflects the variation that may be observed in the clinic.

The increasing ability to perform/access high volume isolations for specific cell types, such as PBMCs, which can be cryopreserved for future studies and provide consistency across multiple assays, are critical opportunities with primary cells. Also, the ongoing development of more sophisticated multicellular culture platforms can offer a relevant function for a long time.

In most cases, primary cell-based assays are used in the tertiary screening or candidate selection stages. In addition, however, bioequivalence data can be generated using appropriately validated primary cell-based assays to support marketing authorization applications. Finally, the preclinical development cascade must consider the model and positioning of the assay and relevant clinical translation of biomarkers carried through to clinical development.

Primary cell assays can help explain the pharmacology and show differences between primary cells and other cell lines. The use of primary cellular models can support the validation of the target and therapeutic efficacy and demonstrate the potential for any safety issues. It's equally important to appropriately model both the novel drug's efficacy and disposition/safety characteristics (Figure 4.7).

The model's clinical translation is critical to its success. It is possible to model native biology at native receptors in simple or complex systems. The format, complexity, different cell types, the required throughput, and the source materials must all be considered for it to succeed. The model must then be characterized as fit for purpose and capable of generating the required data.

4.2.6.5 *In Vivo Testing*

Several steps are required for testing a molecule before in vivo, as shown in the drug discovery cascade in Figure 4.7. First, large numbers of compounds are used in the initial in vitro high-throughput screening to identify "hits." On the other hand, using in vivo pharmacology, the number of target compounds tested is limited to those with the desired in vitro profile and properties.

Several preclinical murine models serve as surrogates for patients, including syngeneic models, human cell line–derived models, genetically modified models, patient-derived explant models, and humanized mouse models. The model selection is influenced by the target, the in vitro cell line data, and the tested hypothesis.

The main elements that are important to assure the success of in vivo study are:

- Design of the experiment: a suitable tool molecule for testing (confidence in potency, selectivity, PK).
    - Understand PK—dosing, and timing (acute and chronic dosing).
    - At the start of the in vivo cascades, the PKPD relationship isn't always known.

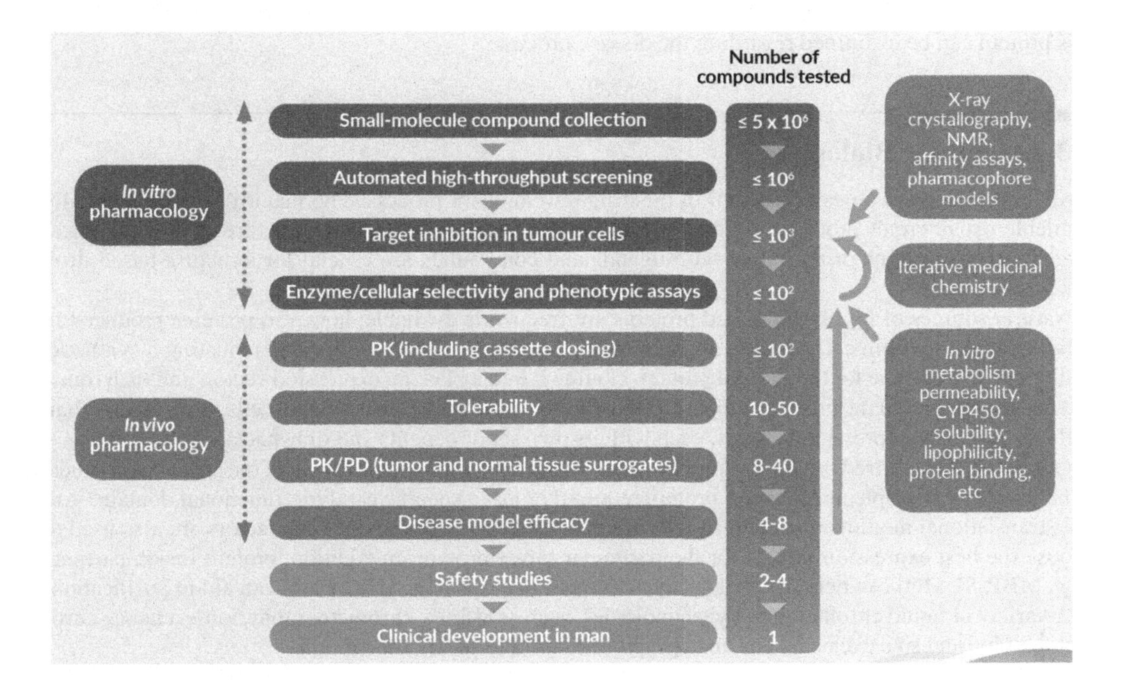

FIGURE 4.7 Success rate of target compounds through various testing models.

   - Use the appropriate formulation.
   - Vehicles and positive controls are examples of appropriate controls.
   - Treatment options include monotherapy and combination therapy.
   - PK, tumor biomarker assessment, and other tissue biomarker samples should all be taken.
- Model selection—based on the mode of action of the molecule.
   - The model needs to be well-defined—immunophenotype, gene expression, mutational analysis.
   - Cell line-derived or patient-derived xenograft models expressing the target of interest are used in targeted therapy.
   - Immune therapy necessitates models with a functioning immune system, such as syngeneic or humanized models.
   - Recognize your preferred model.
   - Recognize the significance.
- Understand how to interpret and apply data.

Selecting the right in vivo model to answer the scientific question, better understanding PK, PD, potential biomarkers, and establishing PK/PD and efficacy relationships are vital to validating your target and increasing the probability of success of your project.

Target validation is also made in vivo using transgenic animals. By knocking out a gene, for example, a biological target can be confirmed. Not only does the gene knockout method validate a target, but it also gives insight into how a drug should affect a disease. For example, if a protein is overexpressed, knocking out the genes associated with it may stop the disease process. This draws attention to compounds that can stop or modulate the activity of a particular protein. This can also be done using antibodies, dominant-negative controls, antisense oligonucleotides, ribozymes, and small-interfering RNAs.

Antibodies are desirable as they can be specific to an antigen or a protein being studied. To validate an antibody's response, profiling protein expression patterns using western blotting to determine whether or not the antibody is bound to the desired antigen is required. Dominant-negative controls work by finding a mutant that will block the function of a specific protein. By blocking function, the effect of inhibiting this protein can be examined regarding the disease process.

4.3 Structural Biology

Structural biology is an essential tool in the drug development process. The majority of commercially available drugs target proteins. As a result, the high-resolution molecular structure of the biological target and interactions of the target with ligands and compounds are crucial for structure-based drug design.

Natural sources of highly expressed proteins are frequently available; however, proteins produced in small quantities within cells must be recombinantly produced. This usually entails creating a synthetic, codon-optimized gene for the desired protein, cloning it into a plasmid expression vector, and then transfecting the recombinant protein into cultured cells. *E. coli*, baculovirus/insect cells, and mammalian cells are common expression systems, each with its own set of benefits and drawbacks.

Obtaining the required protein frequently necessitates meticulous engineering of the protein constructs to be used. For example, is the entire protein required or just a specific catalytic/functional domain? Are post-translational modifications required for function/stability? And so on. Such factors are also used to choose the best expression system for the particular target protein. In addition, protein fusion partners (e.g., MBP, SUMO) can help with solubility, while affinity tags (e.g., His6, Flag) can aid in purification.

A variety of liquid chromatography technologies, such as affinity chromatography, ion-exchange chromatography, and size exclusion chromatography, are used to purify the protein.

It's critical to keep track of and assess the quality of the protein being produced, which can be done in various ways. SDS-PAGE gels indicate purity and approximate molecular size, 280 nm absorbance estimates protein concentration, and analytical size exclusion chromatography determines the molecular size or complex in a protein solution. Mass spectrometry provides a precise molecular mass that can be used to confirm the purified protein's identity. If one is available, a functional assay can be used to see if the purified protein still has the expected activity.

Protein structure is important because it provides information about protein function and allows for the rational chemical design of drug molecules. X-ray crystallography is a common method for determining the atomic structure of proteins. This is based on proteins' ability to form crystals that can diffract x-rays. However, because there is currently no way to predict which conditions will produce suitable crystals in advance, an empirical process is needed. Therefore, many different combinations of precipitants, buffers, and salts are incubated with the protein of interest to determine which conditions will produce suitable crystals. Such crystallization screening is frequently carried out by robotic systems in 96-well plates using vapor diffusion methodologies.

After successfully obtaining crystals, data are collected by exposing them to intense x-ray beams, often done at specialized x-ray synchrotron facilities. Diffraction data are typically made up of many x-ray diffraction patterns taken as the crystal rotates in the x-ray beam.

Knowledge of the position and intensity of each diffracted spot or reflection in such images is generally not sufficient to reconstruct the protein's electron density within a crystal. Information on the relative phase angle of each reflection is also required, and this can be determined using a variety of methods. Molecular replacement relies on the availability of similar/homologous protein structures. Sequence ID of > 30% is used as an initial model. Multiple anomalous dispersion (MAD) methods, in which native methionine residues are replaced with selenomethionine during protein expression, can be used if no homologous structures are available. The required phase information is then calculated using the small differences in diffraction intensities that result (Figure 4.8).

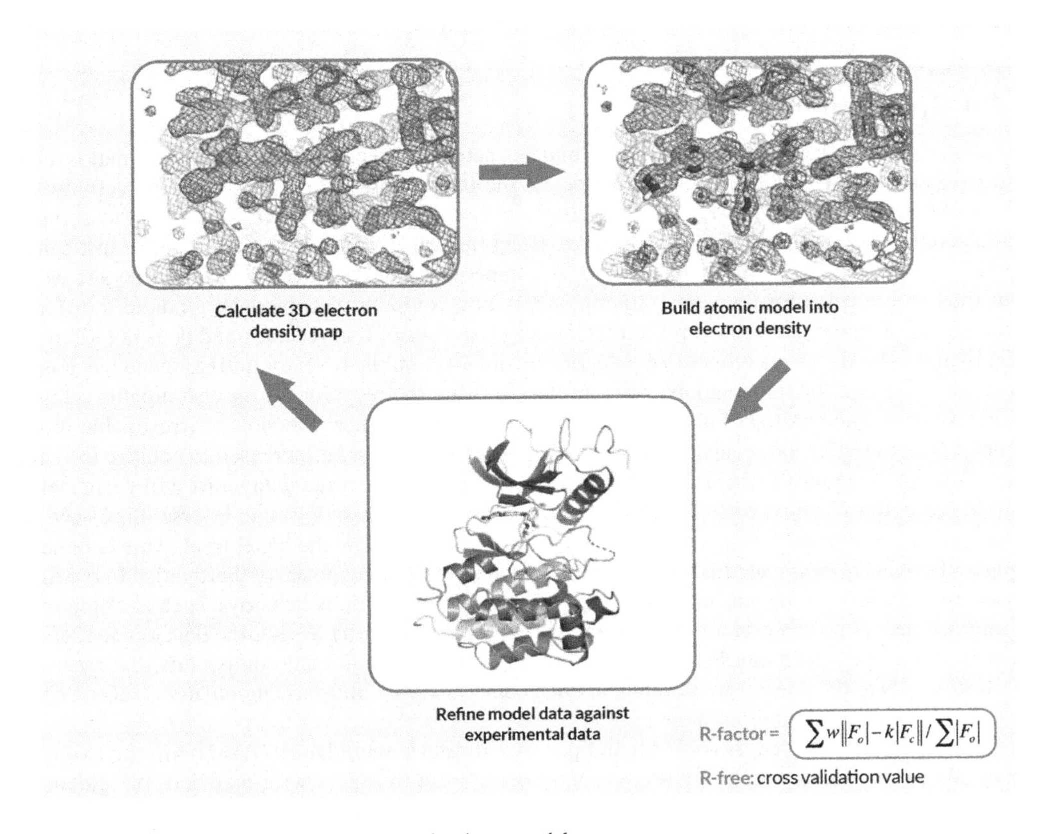
Calculate 3D electron density map
Build atomic model into electron density
Refine model data against experimental data
R-factor = $\sum w \| F_o | - k | F_c \| / \sum | F_o |$
R-free: cross validation value

FIGURE 4.8 Protein crystallography: electron density to model.

Once initial estimates of the phases have been obtained, electron density maps of the protein within the crystal can be calculated and visualized using computer graphics. This enables creating a protein model, which can then be refined against experimental data to improve the model and provide even better phases until convergence.

The experimental data should explain protein structures determined by x-ray crystallography, such as having low Rfactor and Rfree values. The resolution, completeness, redundancy, signal-to-noise ratio, and merging statistics of the experimental data should all be monitored. Finally, protein models must be stereochemically correct. A simple way to determine this is to check Ramachandran plots to see if the amino acid backbone phi/psi angles are within expected limits.

Cryo-electron microscopy (CryoEM) is a powerful structural biology technique that can be used to investigate a wide range of macromolecular complexes and questions in drug development. We can now routinely resolve structures for a wide range of macromolecular complexes to resolutions of around three angstroms thanks to recent advances in software and hardware in CryoEM. CryoEM can be used to determine the structure of potential targets, to examine the location of a small molecule directly, or to examine antibody or non-antibody protein binding. CryoEM can often generate high-quality structural information even when heterogeneity (both compositional and conformational heterogeneity). Single-particle CryoEM can typically determine the structure of proteins and macromolecular complexes ranging in size from 100 Kda to thousands of Kda. Large macromolecular complexes with many subunits and complexes with disordered regions can benefit from cryoEM. X-ray crystallography and other structure-determining techniques may not be suitable.

Protein complexes can also benefit from cryoEM. Because cryoEM requires lower volumes and concentrations of material, it is difficult to generate sufficient volumes or concentrations for other structural techniques such as x-ray crystallography. CryoEM paves the way for structure-based drug design approaches to be applied to previously unsolvable targets, as well as analysis of membrane proteins and other difficult-to-work-with complexes (www.nature.com/articles/d41586-020-00341-9).

4.4 Hit Optimization

An agonist, or activator, is a compound that stimulates activity higher than the basal or normal level by activating receptors. An antagonist, or inhibitor, on the other hand, takes this stimulated activity and lowers it. An antagonist does not lower the activity below the basal level since its role is to compete with the agonist. An antagonist by itself does not affect the activity of a reaction. An antagonist can be competitive, noncompetitive, or uncompetitive. A competitive antagonist binds to the same site as the ligand; thus, it competes for the same binding site. A non-competitive antagonist binds to a different location on the receptor. This changes the function or properties of that receptor and does not allow the natural ligand to bind. An uncompetitive antagonist cannot act on the receptor until a ligand has bound. Thus, a natural ligand or some agonist must already activate the receptor for an uncompetitive ligand to inhibit activity. The binding of an agonist or antagonist can be either reversible or irreversible. When an agonist and reversible antagonist compete, the agonist's dose must be increased to achieve the same activity. Adding an agonist to an irreversible antagonist will not affect the antagonist will permanently bind to the receptor. If an irreversible agonist binds, no amount of antagonist can reverse this effect. An inverse agonist, an inhibitor, is a compound that lowers activity below the basal level. This is done by binding to the same receptor sites as the agonist but eliciting an effect opposite to the agonist. In research, agonists, antagonists, and inverse agonists can study specific interactions in assays, such as compound/drug interactions between a protein and a ligand. However, in particular assays, the development of and work with a specific ligand can be complex. In these situations, additional compounds that react and bind allosterically to the protein are developed. Such compounds are allosteric modulators and can either inhibit or enhance ligand binding to the protein.

Negative allosteric modulators (NAMs) and positive allosteric modulators (PAMs) are the two most common allosteric modulators. They are currently being used in assays with metabotropic glutamate receptors and muscarinic acetylcholine receptors and have potential utility for treating cognitive disorders, schizophrenia, Alzheimer's disease, and addiction (Figure 4.9).

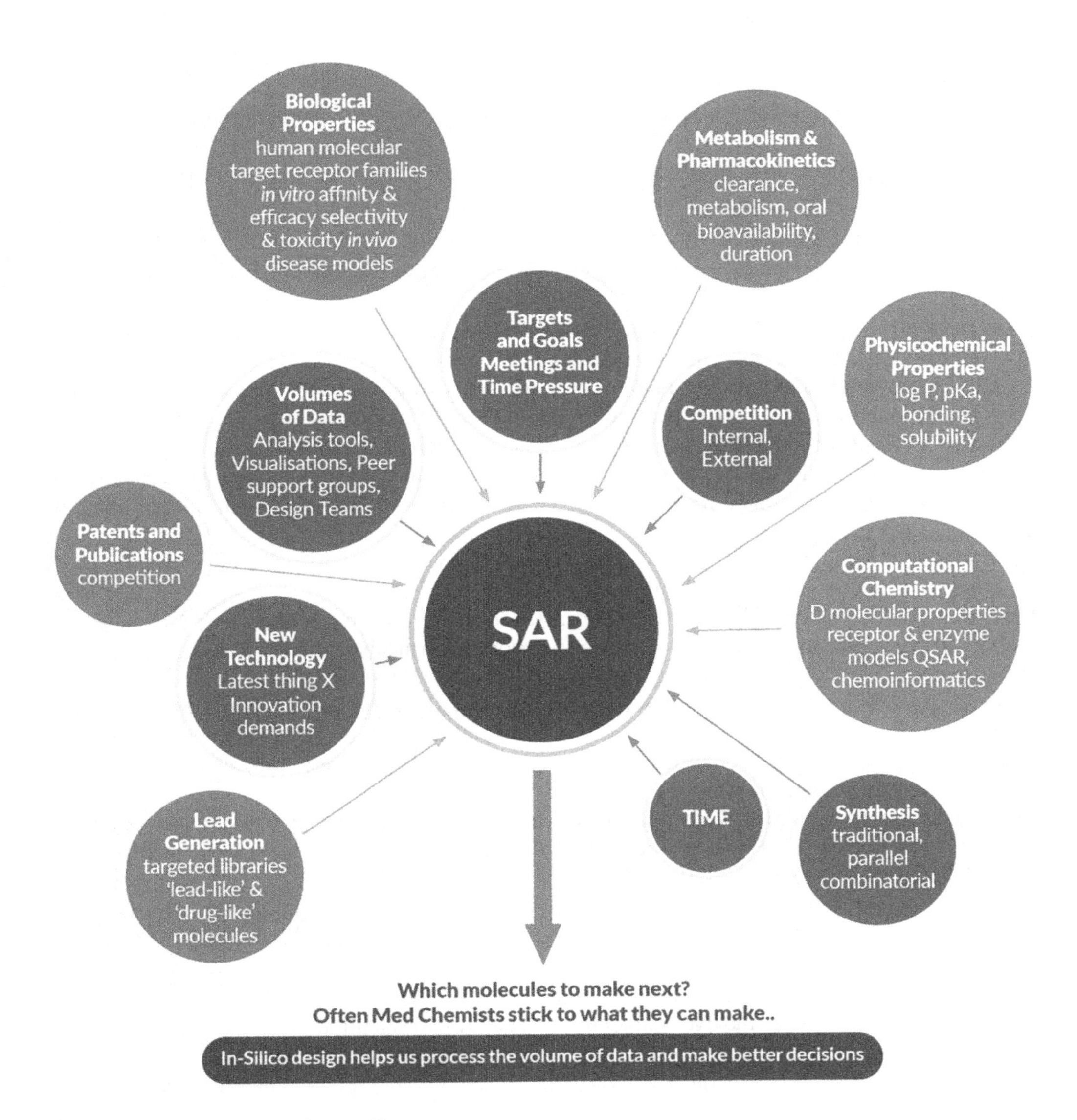

FIGURE 4.9 Medicinal Chemist's Toolbox.

Single-molecule structures, conformational and torsional analysis, protein/ligand structures, docking and scoring, and force field/scoring can all be used in 3D design/structure-based drug design. In addition, free energy perturbation, quantum mechanics, and molecular dynamics can all be used in 3D design.

Compound development requires structural modifications, size, and lipophilicity. Calculated lipophilicity can be used to estimate a molecule's lipophilicity (ClogP). On the LogD/P scale, this should be between 1–3; too polar or too lipophilic can cause problems with the compound.

Literature references are essential for a thorough understanding of the subject. A library of references is available from MedChemica at www.medchemica.com/bucket-list/.

4.4.1 PK–PD Relationship

Improved physicochemical data on prospective new active entities (NAEs) helps in the development with improvements in pre-formulation science for a better projection of the downstream processes, including hit-to-lead (HTL), lead optimization (LO), and in vitro absorption, distribution, metabolism, elimination, and toxicology (ADMET) studies.

The common four mistakes made and how to identify and resolve the key issues include:

- What good does it do to optimize in vitro clearance?
- The significance of the concentration of unbound drugs.
- The key to a drug's development ability is its bioavailability.
- DMPK is not an afterthought in an integrated drug discovery program; it is an integral part.

For a variety of reasons, intrinsic clearance is not always regarded as a method worth optimizing. As a result of the poor correlation between Clint and in vivo clearance, the assay is not always used. Basic science can be used to improve a plot's correlations. The well-stirred model can be used, which corrects for unbound Clint as well as plasma protein binding. If any outliers with significant under or over-prediction are discovered, they can be investigated further. A standard hepatocyte assay can be used to measure compound loss due to metabolism. Total Clint in vivo, on the other hand, should take into account the various elimination parameters, such as hepatic metabolism, hepatic uptake, and renal clearance.

For drugs like statins, a standard hepatic uptake assay and an assay that measures loss from the media alone can be much more predictive of elimination.

According to the free drug hypothesis, efficacy is determined solely by the free drug (unbound) concentration at a receptor. In the absence of active transport, a permeable compound will have the same unbound concentration on both sides of a cellular membrane at a steady state. Under these circumstances, the free compound concentration at the receptor of the target tissue should be equal to the unbound concentration in blood. The amount of drug bound non-specifically to plasma must be measured to determine the free drug concentration. It is impossible to optimize plasma protein binding. All that is required is for it to be known.

PPB measurements are critical for translating in vitro to in vivo data for the IVIVE, and they should be compared across species. PPB should be measured in the same animals that are used for PK/efficacy and tox. Differences in data can be significant.

When a compound is delivered orally, bioavailability measurements are used to determine the extent and rate of absorption and the fraction that enters the systemic circulation. Bioavailability is influenced by metabolism and absorption, so you want to create an easily absorbed compound and have low hepatic clearance. The goal of formulation strategies is to increase the amount of material that is absorbed. The amount of drug metabolized by the liver cannot be controlled by formulations. Hepatic clearance must be measured because it is an intrinsic property of the drug, allowing compounds with a high inherent clearance rate, which results in an inadequate drug exposure level, to be eliminated before a candidate drug is chosen. When a compound is delivered orally, bioavailability measurements are used to determine the extent and rate of absorption and the fraction that enters the systemic circulation. Bioavailability is influenced by metabolism and absorption, so you want to create an easily absorbed compound and have low hepatic clearance. The goal of formulation strategies is to increase the amount of material that is absorbed. The amount of drug metabolized by the liver cannot be controlled by formulations. Hepatic clearance must be measured because it is an intrinsic property of the drug, allowing compounds with a high inherent clearance rate, which results in an inadequate drug exposure level, to be eliminated before a candidate drug is chosen.

Drug metabolism and pharmacokinetics (DMPK) are multifaceted processes that should be identified and addressed early on in the drug development process. Structure, bioavailability, human PK and dose prediction, and drug–drug interaction risk should be considered during the evaluation. The influence of DMPK should be extended through phase Iia clinical trials with a robust dataset.

There are numerous imaging modalities in preclinical and clinical use. Each modality has distinct ranges, spatial resolution, penetration depth, and distinct advantages and disadvantages, such as the requirement for sophisticated technology or bolus contrast.

Examples of imaging techniques that can be used include:

- Fluorescence near-infrared imaging device for longitudinal Cy-7 biodistribution. Cy-7 imaging allows deep biological penetration within the body and images the whole-body distribution with good signal-to-noise. In addition, there are many ways to label a molecule with a dye enabling it to be tracked.
- 89Zr PET can also look at whole-body distribution and off-target toxicity, and nonspecific binding. 89Zr PET is an ideal tracer due to its half-life, allowing repeated images to assess the compound's distribution longitudinally. This technique can also be used to assess tumor penetration longitudinally.
- Three imaging techniques can be used to assess distribution and penetration across the blood–brain barrier (BBB), including PET, near-infrared imaging, and bioluminescence probes which offer a non-invasive method, and mass spectrometry imaging, which has the potential to define drug distribution while the small brain structures with a non-labeled approach.
- Non-invasive mass spectrometry imaging has broad potential in the drug distribution space. Two main mass spectrometry imaging techniques used include desorption electrospray ionization (DESI) and matrix-assisted laser desorption ionization (MALDI).

Understanding the pharmacokinetic–pharmacodynamic (PK–PD) relationship in preclinical models is crucial to predicting an efficacious dose regime in man. Preclinical PK–PD analysis investigates the dose–response relationship of exposure and biological effect. PK analysis in the plasma or target tissue is used to determine a drug's post-dosing exposure levels. A PD marker's measurement reveals how the drug affects the biological target.

PK modeling can be useful in early-stage drug discovery. For example, suppose the plasma exposure is known from a single 10 mg/kg dose in a mouse. In that case, modeling could help define a hypothesis for the pharmacology stage by predicting what would happen to trough concentrations with a twice-daily 30 mg/kg dose.

The simplest PK–PD models are direct PK–PD models, in which the plasma concentration is directly related to the effect at all time points. When there is a delayed response in vivo, indirect PK–PD occurs, and the maximum effect occurs later. The underlying PK and EC50 are the same in both plots. The direct PK–PD needs to be taken twice a day. Furthermore, an oral compartment can be added to the model, adding to its complexity. A PD effect (effect versus concentration) can be added to this, and a direct PK–PD relationship, i.e., the integrated relationship between plasma exposure time (PK) and development versus dosing for a > 70% effect, can be observed. An indirect PK–PD, on the other hand, achieves a > 80% effect from once-daily dosing. For one drug concentration, a hysteresis loop indicates two different response levels.

The simplest PK–PD models are direct PK–PD models, in which the plasma concentration is directly related to the effect at all time points. When there is a delayed response in vivo, indirect PK–PD occurs, and the maximum effect occurs later. The underlying PK and EC50 are the same in both plots. The direct PK–PD needs to be taken twice a day.

Preclinical pharmacokinetic–pharmacodynamic (PK–PD) analysis can aid in the drug discovery process by examining the dose–response relationships between exposure and biological effect in the plasma and the target tissue. Benefits include the prediction of time course and pharmacological effects of drug doses (single or multiple doses), as well as an understanding of target modulation and the dosing schedules required to achieve statistically significant efficacy while minimizing toxicity (Figure 4.10).

PK analysis can be used to determine a drug's exposure levels in plasma and target tissue after dosing. PD analysis looks at how a drug works at the site of action and can help answer questions like, "Does it modulate the target?"

Analyzing a variety of doses, as well as looking at effectiveness over time, is essential. Furthermore, it may be possible to link the PK–PD parameters to any negative effects observed.

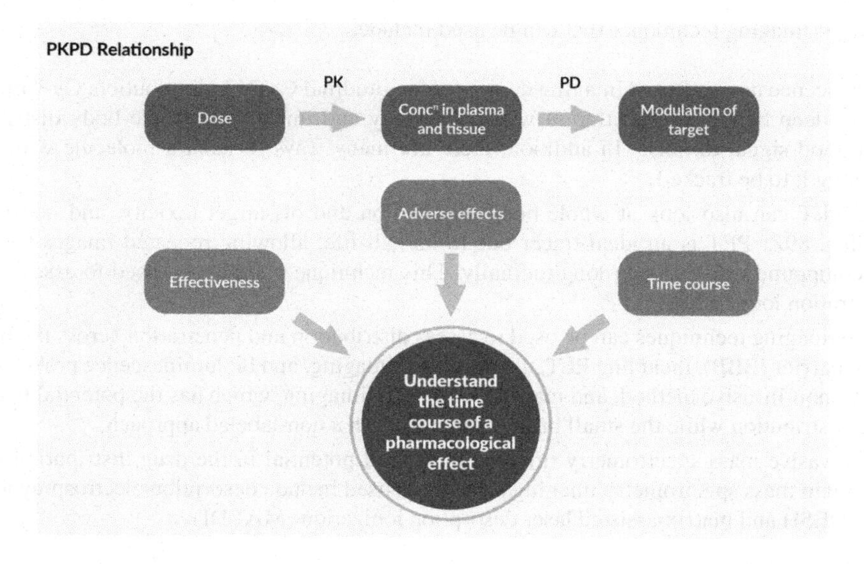

FIGURE 4.10 PK–PD relationship to understand the course of response.

A successful PK–PD study should include:

- A range of doses, for example, three.
- A set of time intervals, such as 5–6 around Tmax.
- A washout phase used to see if there are any direct or indirect effects on the target.
- Measured plasma and target tissue levels.
- Several samples from different animals.

Previously obtained PK data from naïve and diseased animals, in vitro data, and modeling data are used to design a PK–PD study with a 14-day optimized dosing schedule.

4.5 Chemistry and Formulation

Specific skills are required of the chemist to successfully navigate the earlier and later stages of the drug discovery process, and the two disciplines have apparent differences (Figure 4.11).

- Discovery/medicinal chemists.
    - Design, synthesize and purify small libraries of compounds.
    - Use screening cascades to establish structure-activity or property relationship.
    - Understand target biology to ensure desired therapeutic effects are achieved and DMPK liabilities are considered.
    - Uses computational modeling to generate new ideas for synthesis.
- Development chemists.
    - Focus specifically on the synthesis of a small number of compounds nominated as candidates at the end of a lead optimization campaign.
    - Design robust, highly efficient, and cost-effective routes to the candidate compounds.
    - Require mechanistic understanding of each stage in this synthetic scheme.
    - Can identify impurities formed during the reaction and design them out of the process.

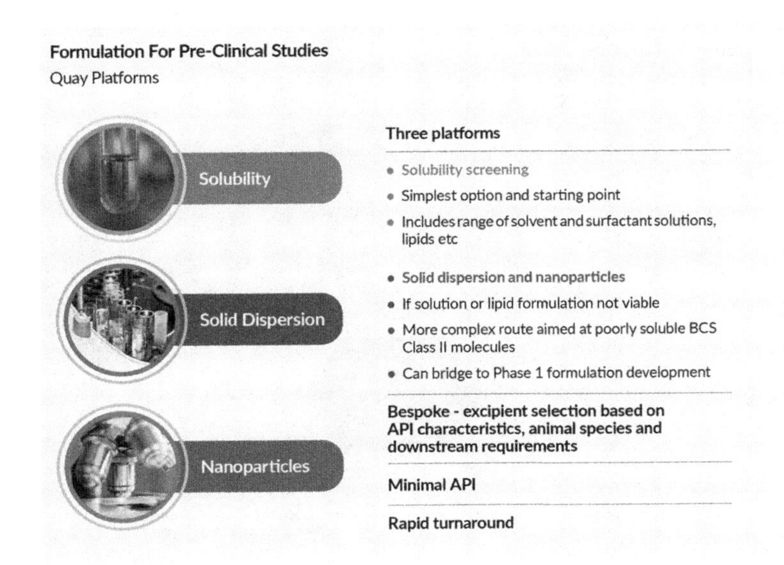

Formulation For Pre-Clinical Studies
Quay Platforms
Solubility
Solid Dispersion
Nanoparticles
Three platforms
Solubility screening
Simplest option and starting point
Includes range of solvent and surfactant solutions, lipids etc
Solid dispersion and nanoparticles
If solution or lipid formulation not viable
More complex route aimed at poorly soluble BCS Class II molecules
Can bridge to Phase 1 formulation development
Bespoke - excipient selection based on API characteristics, animal species and downstream requirements
Minimal API
Rapid turnaround

FIGURE 4.11 Basic approaches to formulation designs.

- Understand the regulatory framework and chemical engineering process to better facilitate the transfer to the pilot plants and beyond.

The goal is to maximize dose and absorption, typically accomplished by using a liquid dose and insoluble in water molecules with limited available API. Excipients should be carefully considered due to the possibility of adverse effects that vary by animal species. Chemical structure, solubility data, logP, pKa, melting point, Caco-2 data, amount of API available, maximum target dose required in animal species, and intended preclinical species are valuable data to aid in this process.

Before formulation, data on the API's physicochemical properties, particle size, distribution, shape or density, flow properties, polymorphic form, and stability are required. In addition, the following are considered biological characteristics: permeability, Caco-2 cell data, any potential efflux mechanisms, and existing pharmacokinetic data.

Preclinical data can aid in the definition of the developability classification system (DCS) and target dose from the target product profile. Molecules are classified into four classes: class 1, which exhibits high solubility and permeability; class 2, which exhibits low solubility or permeability; and class 3, which exhibits low solubility or permeability. And due to their low solubility and permeability, class 4 molecules are difficult to formulate. The majority of compounds are classified as class 2 (Figure 4.12).

4.5.1 Lipinski's Rule of Five (RO5)

Lipinski's rule of five, alternatively referred to as Pfizer's rule of five or simply the rule of five (RO5), is a rule of thumb used to determine whether a chemical compound with a particular pharmacological or biological activity possesses chemical and physical properties consistent with its being an orally active drug in humans. Christopher A. Lipinski proposed the rule in 1997 based on the observation that most drugs administered orally are relatively small and moderately lipophilic molecules. The rule defines a drug's molecular properties critical for its pharmacokinetics in the human body, including absorption, distribution, metabolism, and excretion ("ADME"). The rule, however, does not indicate whether a compound is pharmacologically active. Thus, during drug discovery, the rule is critical to remember when a pharmacologically active lead structure is optimized step-wise to increase the compound's activity and selectivity while maintaining drug-like physicochemical properties consistent with Lipinski's rule.

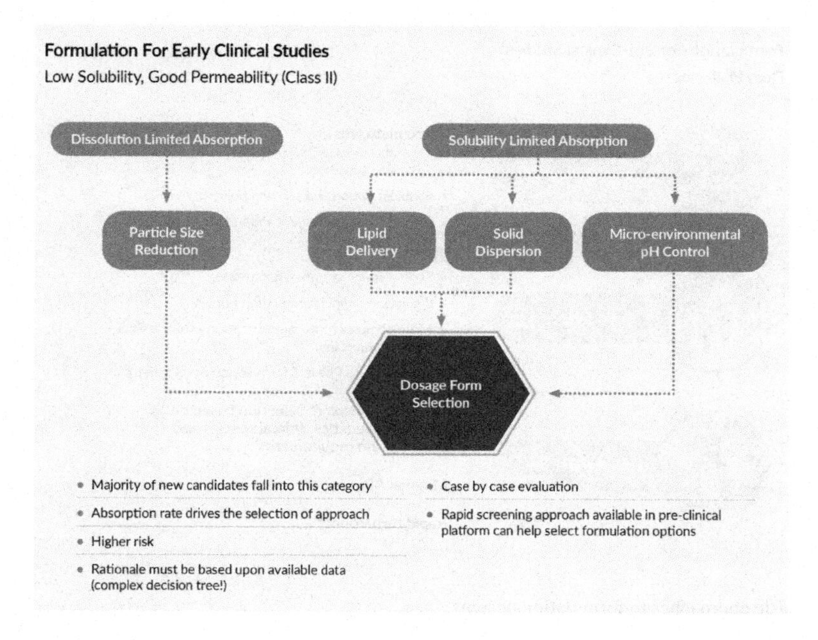
Formulation For Early Clinical Studies
Low Solubility, Good Permeability (Class II)
Dissolution Limited Absorption
Solubility Limited Absorption
Particle Size Reduction
Lipid Delivery
Solid Dispersion
Micro-environmental pH Control
Dosage Form Selection
Majority of new candidates fall into this category
Absorption rate drives the selection of approach
Higher risk
Rationale must be based upon available data (complex decision tree!)
Case by case evaluation
Rapid screening approach available in pre-clinical platform can help select formulation options

FIGURE 4.12 Formulation for early clinical studies (low solubility, good permeability [Class II]).

Candidate drugs that adhere to the RO5 have a lower attrition rate during clinical trials and a higher probability of reaching the market.

- No more than five hydrogen bond donors (the total number of nitrogen–hydrogen and oxygen–hydrogen bonds).
- No more than ten hydrogen bond acceptors (all nitrogen or oxygen atoms).
- A molecular mass of fewer than 500 daltons.
- An octanol–water partition coefficient (log P) that does not exceed 5.

Not that all of the numbers are multiples of five, which is how the rule got its name. As with many other rules of thumb, such as Baldwin's rules for ring closure, there are many exceptions.

To improve the predictions of drug-likeness, the rules have spawned many extensions, for example, the Ghose filter:

- Additionally, Veber's Rule Coefficient of partition log P in the range of 0.4 to + 5.6.
- Molar refractivity ranges between 40 and 130.
- The molecular weight ranges between 180 and 480.
- Between 20 and 70 atoms (includes H-bond donors [e.g., Ohs and NHs and H-bond acceptors {e.g., Ns and Os}]) question a 500 molecular weight cutoff.
- It is predicted that compounds with ten or fewer rotatable bonds and a polar surface area of less than 1,402 have a high oral bioavailability.

During drug discovery, lipophilicity and molecular weight are frequently increased to increase the affinity and selectivity of the drug candidate. Hence it is often challenging to maintain drug-likeness (i.e., RO5 compliance) during the hit and lead optimization. As a result, it has been proposed that members of screening libraries from which hits are discovered be biased toward lower molecular weight and lipophilicity to make it easier for medicinal chemists to deliver optimized drug development candidates that are also drug-like. Thus, to define lead-like compounds, the rule of five has been extended to three (RO3).

A rule of three compliant compound is defined as one that has:

- Octanol-water partition coefficient log P not greater than 3.
- Molecular mass less than 300 daltons.
- Not more than three hydrogen bond donors.
- Not more than three hydrogen bond acceptors.
- Not more than three rotatable bonds.

4.6 Safety Testing

In vitro drug activity aims to determine the potential side effects of a compound before it reaches living organisms. The compound is screened against a wide range of targets from receptors to ion channels to enzymes in an artificial environment outside of a living organism. This identifies any other reactions that may occur when the drug candidate is introduced into an animal than humans. One required assay screen for possible interaction with the hERG channel is a voltage-gated potassium channel. Interactions with this channel are unwanted as these interactions can lead to heart arrhythmias. Some side effects or adverse drug reactions (ADRs) are mild such as a rash, but others, like heart arrhythmias, can be life-threatening and illustrate the importance of in vitro drug safety testing. This screening can also be done earlier in the drug discovery testing to eliminate potentially harmful drugs before additional time and money are spent. An in vitro study is very important before in vivo study is taken as it is a faster way to test for safety and catch problems before animal testing begins. It also uses fewer compounds than in vivo studies, again saving time and money. In vitro studies strive to emulate in vivo processes essential when understanding side effects during clinical trials.

Safety risks can occur as a result of target-mediated risk, off-target activity, pharmacodynamic effects on major body systems such as the cardiovascular, central nervous, and respiratory systems, as well as gross behavioral and pathological changes in animals. Therefore, the optimal time to optimize novel compound safety characteristics is during the early discovery phase, incorporating chemistry, biology, and DMPK. Three critical areas must be considered: safety risks associated with the drug target itself, chemical space risks, and patient safety.

Safety concerns regarding the primary target continue to be a significant cause of drug project failure. On average, up to 25% of discovery projects and 50% of early clinical phase studies are halted due to concerns about the primary target's safety. Understanding the target in normal physiology may allow for predicting potential toxicities, differentiation of on- and off-target toxicity, and influence dosing schedules, route of administration, or combination opportunities. It may also influence selection criteria and play a role in determining whether to pursue the drug lead.

Numerous in silico approaches can be used to investigate chemical-related toxicity or risks associated with liabilities other than the target that could constrain an effective dose range. Key liabilities can be evaluated through in vitro safety screenings, secondary pharmacology screenings, or genotoxicity testing of the primary compound, for example.

Integrating additional measurements can help maximize the value of toxicology studies. For example, genotoxicology endpoints can be added to pivotal repeat dose rodent toxicity studies using flow cytometry analysis of micronuclei, reducing animal usage and cost. In addition, non-invasive telemetry and Irwin style observations and combining a male fertility element in sub-chronic or chronic rodent toxicity studies can all be used to include safety pharmacology in repeat-dose toxicity studies.

The critical endpoint of toxicity studies, histopathology, can be rate-limiting in and of itself. Time will be saved by transferring all tissues from all animals to slides and making the slides available for evaluation when needed. The development of clinically relevant biomarkers in tandem with non-clinical studies allows for a direct comparison of non-clinical and clinical data, informing clinical trial design and dose level selection. By reducing or eliminating satellite animals for toxicokinetic samples, microsampling allows for more efficient science with fewer animals.

The current cell models are frequently insufficient and too simple to provide these data. Models are often single cells, cultured in a simple 2D setup, used with a glass or plastic substrate, lacking in relevant biological stimuli, no communication with other cells or cellular models, and relevant physical stimuli are absent; cells are immortalized and have aberrant cellular metabolism; models are often single cells, cultured in a simple 2D setup, used with a glass or plastic substrate, lacking in relevant biological stimuli, and no communication with other cells or cellular models, and relevant physical stimuli are absent.

More biologically relevant models are primary cells that can be modified using CRISPR. To mimic in vivo situations, multiple cell types should be cultured together. For example, 3D spheroids with unsupported structures, matrix gels, or even patient-derived organoids are more recent models.

Validation and use of humanized isolated OOC models and connected on-chip models, which better mimic a typical biological environment for use in efficacy and safety determination, will be required to exploit more complex cell models.

Neurotoxicity is also a significant issue, and the blood–brain barrier (BBB) provides an opportunity to develop a model that can provide more accurate and predictive results. In vitro BBB models are currently used in transwell plates with Caco-2 or MDCK-MDR1 cell lines and in vivo rodent models for compound permeability and neurotoxicity. They do, however, have limited physiological significance.

After preliminary in vitro testing, a compound can advance to in vivo testing. Because of their cost-effectiveness, rats are often the first line of in vivo testing. These animals also require low dosages of the compound. These experiments illustrate how quickly the drug is cleared from the system, safe dosages, and the compound's breakdown. All of this is important to understand the pharmacokinetics of the potential drug candidate. However, even with animal testing, some side effects may not be found due to the human body's complexity. In vivo testing allows for further understanding of how a drug functions with the broad and diverse range of targets in an organism, but animal testing will never fully understand interactions in the human body. Thus, many drugs that advance to clinical testing may not succeed in human trials.

4.6.1 Animal Models

The FDA's Animal Model Qualification Program (AMQP) is voluntary (i.e., not required for product approval or licensure under the Animal Rule). CDER and CBER jointly support the AMQP. The qualification process is limited to animal models used in the Animal Rule for product approval. A qualified model may be used to evaluate the efficacy of multiple investigational drugs for the same targeted disease or condition in development programs. These animal models are regarded as product-independent (i.e., not linked to a specific drug). A model developed for use in a single investigational drug development program is not eligible for qualification. The Animal Rule states that the FDA may rely on animal studies to provide substantial evidence of a drug's effectiveness only if all four of the following criteria are met.

- There is a reasonably well-understood pathophysiological mechanism for the substance's toxicity and how the product can prevent or significantly reduce it.
- Unless the effect is demonstrated in a single animal species that is a sufficiently well-characterized animal model for predicting human response, the effect must be shown in multiple animal species expected to react similarly to humans.
- An animal study aims to achieve the desired benefit in humans, which is usually increased survival or the avoidance of significant morbidity.
- Data or information on the product's kinetics and pharmacodynamics and other relevant data or information in animals and humans aid in selecting an effective dose in humans.

The FDA has recognized that when a specific animal species is exposed to a specific challenge agent via a specific route, a disease process or condition is produced that is significantly similar to the human disease or condition of interest. The FDA will decide based on the adequacy of data from human disease or condition studies and data from animal model natural history studies. Once an animal model is qualified, the FDA does not have to reevaluate this conclusion each time this model is used within the bounds of its stated context of use. Due to the increased economies of time, animals, and resources associated with using an animal model for efficacy testing in development programs, multiple drug development programs for the same targeted disease or condition are qualified.

Animal models are assessed and qualified for a specific context of use (COU), a comprehensive and precise statement describing the qualified animal model's appropriate use and application in drug development and regulatory review. It also specifies the details necessary to replicate the model. These details include:

- Characterization of the animals to be used.
- Characterization and preparation of the challenge agent.
- Procedural information for the challenge agent exposure.
- Identification of the primary and secondary endpoints.
- Triggers for intervention.
- When the model is replicated, the ranges of key disease or condition parameter values will be used as quality control and quality assurance measures.

The submission of additional data may support the expansion of the COU of a qualified animal model. Expansion of a COU may include but are not limited to additional clinical indications, use of a different challenge agent, or different routes of exposure.

Before using a qualified animal model in an efficacy study of an investigational drug, sponsors should demonstrate that the animal model is a suitable test system for their drug concerning the drug's mechanism of action, related host factors, and the ability to select a dose and regimen in humans. Similarly, because animal models are qualified without regard to a specific drug, using one does not guarantee that it will be accepted as a single animal species that represents a sufficiently well-characterized animal model for predicting the response in humans, as the Animal Rule's second criterion states. The FDA may not accept evidence of efficacy from a single animal model (even if it is qualified) for an investigational drug unless it determines sufficient evidence that the results generated in this model accurately predict the response to the drug in humans. The review division will decide whether or not to allow approval of a drug based on using an animal model in a single species on a case-by-case basis.

Qualification does not imply that data obtained from adequate and well-controlled efficacy studies using a qualified animal model are sufficient to approve products under the Animal Rule without review or without supporting data. The qualification also does not imply that the model will be acceptable under the second criterion of the Animal Rule.

Because qualification is a regulatory conclusion, FDA recommends that model-defining natural history studies submitted to support the qualification of an animal model follow good laboratory practice (GLP) for nonclinical laboratory studies to the extent practicable. This will make study conduct easier and ensure data quality and integrity. Submitters will be expected to submit a plan to ensure data integrity for studies not performed following GLP regulations. The model-defining natural history studies submitted for qualification, regardless of the data quality and integrity assurance plan used, will be subject to inspection by FDA to verify the quality and integrity of the data.

4.6.2 Replacing Animal Testing

Animal models were the only way to get in vivo data that could predict human pharmacokinetic responses in the early stages of drug development. Experiments on animals, on the other hand, are time-consuming, costly, and divisive. In addition, animal models, for example, are frequently subjected to mechanical or chemical techniques that mimic human injuries. Concerns about the validity of such animal models have also been raised due to a lack of cross-species extrapolation.

Moreover, animal models offer limited control of individual variables, and it can be cumbersome to harvest specific information.

As a result, simulating human physiological responses in an in vitro model must be made more affordable. In addition, biological experiments must include cellular level control; biomimetic microfluidic systems could replace animal testing. Finally, many fields, including toxicology and pharmaceuticals, and cosmetics that rely on animal testing and clinical trials, could benefit from developing MEMS-based biochips that reproduce complex organ-level pathological responses.

Perfusion in vitro systems based on physiological principles have recently been developed to provide a cell culture environment similar to that found in vivo. New testing platforms based on multi-compartmental perfused systems have sparked a lot of interest in pharmacology and toxicology. Its goal is to create a cell culture environment that is as close to in vivo as possible to more accurately reproduce in vivo mechanisms or ADME processes involving absorption, distribution, metabolism, and elimination. In vitro, perfused systems combined with kinetic modeling are promising tools for studying the various processes involved in xenobiotic toxicokinetics in vitro.

Microfabricated cell culture systems are being developed to create models that as closely as possible replicate aspects of the human body and provide examples of their potential use in drug development, such as identifying synergistic drug interactions and simulating multi-organ metabolic interactions. Multi-compartment microfluidic-based devices, particularly those representing the mass transfer of compounds in compartmental models of the mammalian body using physical representations of physiologically based pharmacokinetic (PBPK) models, may help to improve the drug development process.

Based on the initial drug dose, mathematical pharmacokinetic (PK) models aim to estimate concentration-time profiles within each organ. In such mathematical models, the body is treated as a single compartment in which drug distribution reaches a rapid equilibrium after administration. When all of the parameters are known, mathematical models can be highly accurate. Time-dependent pharmacological effects of a drug can be predicted using models that combine PK or PBPK models with PD models. With PBPK, we can almost predict the PK of any chemical in humans from the first principles. These models can be simple, like statistical dose-response models, or sophisticated, like systems biology models, depending on the goal and data available. For those models, all we need are good parameter values for the molecule in question.

PBPK models could be used in conjunction with microfluidic cell culture systems such as micro-cell culture analogs (CCAs). These scaled-down CCAs devices, also known as body-on-a-chip devices, can simulate multi-tissue interactions with realistic tissue-to-tissue size ratios and near-physiological fluid flow conditions. These systems' data can be used to test and refine mechanistic hypotheses. Microfabricating devices also enable us to customize them and scale the compartments of the organs correctly about one another.

Cross-species extrapolation is made more accessible by the device's ability to work with animal and human cells. When combined with PBPK models, the devices can estimate effective concentrations that can be used in animal model studies or predict human response. PBPK models, for example, can aid in the development of multicompartment devices by guiding device design decisions about chamber placement and fluidic channel connections, resulting in more successful clinical trials.

4.7 Synthetic Biology

Synthetic biology has now progressed to a stage where we can readily synthesize genes of any size and even commercially manufacture DNA using PCRs and other in vitro methods; I see significant progress in this field to make synthetic biology a cost-competitive modality to plasmid DNA production. Having a synthetic platform will reduce the risk of contamination and lower the cost of DNA and mRNA vaccines and many novel antibodies.

The availability of three-dimensional structures and ever more sophisticated computer modeling programs also enable the in silico discovery of chemical starting points. Today, in many cases, a target's x-ray crystal structure is available early during a drug discovery project. Even the structures of membrane receptors can now be solved. With this structural information, it is often possible to combine the different lead-finding approaches into a broader, integrated lead-finding strategy. The structural information gained from each individual hit thereby adds to an overall understanding of how best to fill the binding pocket of a target and can be used to design new chemotypes based on a holistic experience of the contributions of many diverse molecular substructures.

The vast majority of new compounds discovered in the last 75 years are the result of synthetic chemistry. Cardiology has been transformed by β-blockers and calcium channel blockers. Agonists in respiratory therapy and H2 antagonists in the treatment of gastrointestinal ulcer disease are just a few examples of how synthetic chemists' work has transformed clinical treatment strategies. The established model of identifying a functional transmitter in a physiological system, then identifying the receptor with which the transmitter interacts, and finally modifying the agonist structure to identify a specific antagonist has proven to be effective in the drug discovery process. Technological advancements will continue to uncover novel receptors and physiological system targets. As a result, the synthetic chemist will undoubtedly continue to make significant contributions to drug discovery, despite the information age's influence. With the availability of software to assist in determining the structure of receptors, potential receptor blockers have become critical tools in the discovery process. Additionally, computer-assisted drug synthesis has tremendous potential. The revolution is comparable to the one that occurred in the animation industry as a result of computers.

The path forward is to apply computers to the steps beyond modeling systems in order to identify chemical structures and then develop synthetic approaches. Synthetic antagonists with the highest possible potency can be developed from a variety of chemical options. The development of more selective and potent agents will increase the yield of these approaches.

The information age applications to synthetic modeling will improve with improvements in screening techniques. A new, promising compound is processed through hundreds of models, looking for possible pharmacologic activity. Newer testing models based on a Bayesian theory will improve the screening. Combining screening with gene expression targeting will further increase the potential for success. Although we are transitioning from synthetic chemistry to the age of biotechnology and gene manipulation, synthetic discovery will remain with us for all time to come because it is the chemical–biological interaction that creates a pharmacologic response and that will not change.

4.8 Libraries

Typically, libraries are targeted at specific classes of enzymes, such as kinases, serine proteases, or bromodomains. Additionally, they can consist of molecules directed toward specific areas of the body, such as the central nervous system. Additionally, libraries can be designed to act via specific mechanisms, such as by including reactive moieties capable of covalently modifying the target—a strategy that has been successfully used with kinases and serine proteases. Analogs of transition states have also garnered recent attention.

A targeted library aims to include as many bioactive compounds as possible from the entire library in as small a subset as possible. One can enrich bioactivity collections by utilizing informatics-based approaches such as conventional similarity searches or machine learning models built on bioactivity databases. These approaches should be used with caution; one highly efficient way for a machine-learning algorithm to maximize the number of bioactive molecules in the selected subset is to choose unselective or frequently hitting molecules that do not represent useful starting points for drug discovery. Prefiltering for frequent hitters based on prior behavior in screens where possible and using substructural filters is critical. While physicochemical properties are typically used to describe CNS-directed libraries, physicochemical "whole molecule" descriptors have been found to be useful in target class-directed libraries as well. These descriptors are less reliant on explicit substructural features as demonstrated in the training set.

Targeted libraries must strike a balance between increasing the probability of discovering hits, allowing for serendipity to uncover novel chemotypes, and minimizing the number of promiscuous molecules. The application of structure-based and physicochemical property–based approaches has the potential to compensate for the inherent chemotype bias in fingerprinting methods. Increasing the sophistication of pre-selection filtering through the use of machine learning approaches to identify undesirable molecules is also likely to gain prominence.

Today, large and diverse compound libraries, combined with great advances in cell and organoid culture technologies, make phenotypic screening an exciting approach for target and drug discovery.

Genetic disease genes are viewed as a potentially lucrative source of drug targets. Because the majority of diseases are caused by multiple pathogenic factors, it is reasonable to assume that chemical agents targeting multiple disease genes will have the desired effect. This assertion is backed up by a thorough examination of the relationships between agent activity and target genetic characteristics. The therapeutic potential of agents increases steadily as the number of targeted disease genes increases and can be enhanced further by strengthening the genetic link between targets and diseases.

Data libraries and drug and disease modeling approaches have the potential of unlocking knowledge about patterns that cannot be seen today—patterns in product efficacy and failures, in product-related safety signals, and in relationships between animal and human test results. The findings from in silico testing (computer simulation, rather than laboratory or animal testing) could reduce the risk and cost of human testing by helping product sponsors make more informed decisions on how to proceed with product testing and when to remove a product from further development.

Table 4.2 lists the Online Resources on Drug Discovery Initiatives. Table 4.4 lists the Compound Libraries.

4.8.1 DNA Libraries

High-throughput screening has enabled the identification of potent hit molecules for a wide variety of structural and functionally diverse protein targets, but at a high cost due to the screening and maintenance of large compound collections. The discovery of affinity binders based on biomolecules (e.g., proteins, peptides, antibodies, RNA, and DNA aptamers) is uncomplicated, and streamlined affinity-selection protocols enable the discovery of such binders for most proteins quickly and at a lower cost. Encoding compounds with appended DNA sequences that define the library compounds' structural information are collections of small molecules each modified with oligonucleotide tags enabling their identification—the concept of using nucleic acids to encode chemical libraries in the form of DNA-encoded one-bead-one-compound libraries. The development of high-throughput DNA sequencing technologies has made it possible to decipher millions of sequences read simultaneously.

Recent years have seen tremendous progress toward the goal of developing DNA-encoded chemical libraries as an enabling technology for drug discovery. Numerous critical issues have been successfully addressed. As evidenced by the increasing number of hits discovered by screening DNA-encoded chemical libraries, the technology is now routinely used in drug discovery efforts. These libraries have the potential to disrupt the conventional medicinal chemistry workflow, and it will be exciting to see what new applications emerge in the coming years.

Using DNA-encoded library technology is another way to gain access to new drug-like chemical space for hit exploration (DELT). Due to the "split and pool" nature of DELT synthesis, it is possible to produce large quantities of compounds in a cost-effective and timely manner (millions to billions of compounds). The "split and pool" method enables the construction of libraries with up to 1,010 compounds, in comparison to the size of a shared HTS library, which is limited to several million compounds due to the prohibitively high cost of synthesizing and managing larger collections.

DELs are carried out in single test tubes by incubating the target protein with a library. The target proteins can be covalently linked to a solid support, most frequently magnetic beads. Only high-affinity ligands remain bound to a target following thorough washing. Following DNA sequencing and decoding the structure of active compounds, the latter should be resynthesized in order to perform the affinity binding assay again. Numerous selection strategies are compatible with DELs, including phenotypic screening.

DEL is an excellent method for synthesizing and screening small molecules, macrocyclic compounds, and peptides. Scientists are exploiting the chemical properties of DNA, particularly the complementarity principle, to develop novel strategies for library design.

One of the more sophisticated methods of library construction is to determine the sequence of chemical reactions using DNA code. Prior to synthesis, templates are created that contain regions complementary to the barcodes of BBs. When barcodes are coupled to the template, the relative sterility of the building blocks enables a chemical reaction to occur. This technique is advantageous when building libraries of macrocycles and peptides.

The benefit of dual-pharmacopeia libraries consists of the flexibility of two chemical moieties in reaching adjoining uncomplicated binding sites. Two sublibraries are made up of dual-pharmacopeia libraries. They form two compounds when combined. They form heteroduplexes. The most popular method is ESAC (encoded self-assembly chemicals).

DEL-compatible chemistry is limited to DNA-compatible reactions. DNA is a water-soluble molecule that should therefore translate traditional organic responses into the appropriate conditions. At first, the chemical toolbox had just a few reactions, but its number has increased, leveraging different approaches for synthesis.

DNA-encoded libraries are now a standard method for identifying protein binders. The increasing use of DNA-encoded libraries has resulted in an exponential increase in the number of screening hits identified using these libraries. Numerous hits exhibit novel chemotypes and novel binding modes, including first-in-class compounds and allosteric regulators. Additionally, screening protocols have become more sophisticated in recent years. Parallel screening experiments with DNA-encoded libraries complement simple hit discovery efforts by providing valuable information about protein binding and target selectivity.

DNA offers unique properties as a readable barcode for chemical libraries. Nucleic acids store information at high density and conveniently amplify and read this information by PCR and DNA sequencing. The extensive toolbox of enzymes for processing nucleic acids greatly facilitates library assembly, and the polyanionic backbone imparts excellent solubility to conjugates of small molecules. The utility of nucleic acids to encode combinatorial compound libraries is well precedented by display technologies used to discover biomolecules. These methods use simple affinity-selection protocols combined with sequencing the linked genome (or another coding nucleic acid) to find target binders. Phage display is a prototypical example of such a technology. In phage display, bacteriophages are engineered to express polypeptides on the filamentous protein coat based on sequences engineered into the phage's genome. Panning phages over immobilized targets are followed by amplifying the retained viruses in host organisms to provide binder-enriched libraries. Iterative screening cycles are repeated until the high-affinity phages can be identified by sequencing a representative number of genomes. Related technologies include ribosome display, mRNA display, and SELEX. However, the dependence of these technologies on processes for transferring the genetic information into phenotypic proteins (i.e., transcription and translation) limits the value of such methods for medicinal chemistry.

The prospect of discovering low-molecular-weight protein binders with the efficacy, throughput, and economics of phage display motivated the development of several methods to assemble compound libraries with conjugated DNA barcodes. A key challenge in the conception of DNA-encoded libraries (DECL) as a drug discovery technology is linking library molecules to readable barcodes. In contrast to biological display technologies, the synthetic nature of molecules in DNA-encoded libraries prevents the use of biological transcription and translation machinery for library synthesis. DECL synthesis methods can be divided into three categories. One approach referred to as DNA-recorded synthesis achieves library assembly by iterative cycles of compound synthesis and encoding steps. A second approach termed DNA-directed synthesis relies on mechanisms that convert DNA sequences into molecular structures. The third approach harnesses hybridization to self-assemble sub-libraries of DNA fragment conjugates into DNA-encoded libraries.

A fundamental advantage of DNA-directed relative to DNA-recorded library synthesis is the conceptual possibility to iterate screening-amplification cycles because of the option to convert amplified sequences into molecular structures. Such a translation step is incompatible with DNA recorded library synthesis and, in the case of self-assembled libraries, depends on the library design. Initially, it was assumed that series of affinity-selection cycles would be required for effective hit discovery in large libraries. However, tremendous advances in DNA sequencing technologies made it possible to achieve sufficient sequencing depth that a single affinity screening cycle (which may include several panning steps) is enough for hit identification obviating the need for information transfer from DNA to molecules.

The most widely used approach for the preparation of DNA-encoded libraries is a split-and-pool synthesis scheme involving cycles of DNA elongation and chemical reaction steps. In these approaches, individual sequences with a chemical handle are modified in separate reaction vessels with a panel of chemical building blocks. Additional cycles of pooling, chemical modification, and encoding of the incoming molecular entities will provide the desired combinatorial library with appended DNA barcodes. Several methods are available for extending the coding oligonucleotides during library preparation, including a) parallel solid-phase synthesis of oligonucleotides and compounds, b) enzymatic or chemical DNA ligation, and c) polymerase extension.

Enzymatic ligation is the prevalent method to introduce DNA codes during the preparation of DNA-recorded libraries. One approach is the enzymatic ligation of single-stranded DNA codes. In single-strand ligation, a splint oligonucleotide juxtaposes the incoming coding sequence and the DNA-compound conjugate and serves as a template for enzymatic strand joining by DNA ligase. Ligation requires pairs of adjoining 5'-phosphate and 3'-hydroxy termini. Removal of the template is possible by enzymatic or chemical digestion or by chromatography.

Similarly, one can encode libraries by ligation of double-stranded DNA. Short overhang sequences ("sticky-ends") allow sequences to align for enzymatic ligation. An advantage of this approach, in addition to preventing the need for a template sequence, is that double-stranded DNA protects nucleobases from potentially damaging reagents during compound synthesis. Ligation-based encoding has also been applied to one-bead-one-compound libraries.

Chemical ligation is an alternative for the synthesis of DNA-encoded chemical libraries. This approach harnesses the well-established rate-enhancing effect of hybridizing two nucleic acids with adjoining reactive termini on a common strand to ligate them without the need for an enzyme.

Another method to encode chemical structures is to extend two partially hybridized DNA sequences by enzymatic replication. The incoming coding strand and the oligonucleotide linked to the synthetic compound have conserved non-coding sequences that form a short duplex. The coding sequences remain single-stranded; a polymerase (e.g., Klenow fragment) bidirectionally extends the duplex establishing a fully double-stranded DNA.

Ligating self-assembled library members generates a single readable sequence containing all information for affinity selection and hit discovery. There are two principal strategies for the preparation of DNA-encoded libraries by DNA-directed synthesis, relying either on DNA-templated chemical reactions or on the hybridization-based routing of intermediates. In both cases, the original DNAs contain coding sequences to instruct the synthesis of the compounds.

Diverse chemical reactions compatible with DNA-templated synthesis have been reported. In principle, it is possible to add the various reactive conjugates simultaneously and use hybridization to guide parallel reactions in a single batch; however, library synthesis generally involved performing the individual reactions separately to allow for better synthesis control and facile purification of the products.

Libraries of coding DNA strands are divided into separate compartments by hybridization to defined capture tags for modification with diverse synthons. Elution of the conjugates, pooling, and hybridization-based redistribution into reaction compartments will be repeated for translating the coding sequences into chemical structures. Considerable refinement of technical protocols allows highly parallelized synthesis with large fragment sets using mesofluidic devices.

4.9 Microphysiometry

Microphysiometry is the in vitro measure of life or living-life functions and activities (such as organs, tissues, or cells) with the small-scale physical and chemical phenomena involved. The main parameters evaluated in microphysiometry include pH and oxygen dissolved, glucose, and lactic acid concentrations, which emphasize the first two. The quantitative output parameters of extracellular acidification rates (EAR), oxygen consumption rates (OUR), and glucose consumption rates or lactate releases characterize the metabolic situation are used in the quantitative measurement of these parameters combined with a fluidic system for cell culture maintenance and a defined application of drugs or toxins. The dynamic monitoring of the cells or tissues for several days or even longer is possible because of the sensor-based measurements' label-free nature. A dynamic cell metabolic response analysis can identify acute (e.g., one hour after treatment), early (e.g., 24 hours), and delayed chronic responses on a longer time scale (e.g., at 96 hours).

4.9.1 Microfluidics

Microfluidics have a major interest in drug discovery and development. The advantage of system miniaturization is clearly the microfluidism. Microfluidics help to miniaturize assays and increase the experimental flow by modulating the movement of small amounts of fluids. The use of microfluid technology, like 3D cell cultivation systems, organ-on-a-chip, and laboratory-on-a-chip technology, and gout techniques has grown rapidly over recent years. The volume of the microfluidic device is low and several features on one chip can be integrated. The inner size of the chip ranges from micrometers to millimeters, enabling even the picoliters to handle samples and reagents. In combination with multichannel and dispatch designs, microfluidic chips allow a high-performance process to be achieved which increases your screen speed. Microfluidics reduce reagent use and cost through their miniaturized devices, apart from quick check-ups and analyses.

Organ-on-a-chip is a promising technology that uses microfluidics. A biomimetic organ physiological system constructed on a microfluidic chip is called an organ-on-a-chip. Due to their capacity to carefully mimic in vivo microenvironments' dynamic interactions, organ-on-a-chip systems and body-on-a-chip systems are very promising for high-performance development assays that might prove useful in drug screening and toxicity studies.

Microfluidics, complex organoid cultures, and nano detection of phenotypic and genomic outputs turn many metaphors into reality. The fundamental idea began with an arrangement of cells into collaborative 3D cultures, tissues-like organoids, cell phenotypes that share interconnections in order to imitate the exchange of ions and metabolites found in true organs. An example of such an early incarnation might be that the liver-to-chip functions as hepatitis of other cells that are representative of the functional unit. The obvious next step in the evolution towards a "body-on-a-chip" would then array emulations of, for example, liver, gut, and pancreas on the same chip and so forth, culminating in a modern incarnation of the homunculus. Not only has the concept been embraced by regulatory and funding agencies, but pharmaceutical companies and academia are increasingly utilizing it as a platform for drug discovery. On-chip systems represent over two dozen organ systems.

The read-outs of on-chip study also accommodate advanced imaging and cell viability tests, ELISA, intracellular detection of proteins, RT-PCR, BrdU, and actin stain.

Living human cell-lined microchips have the potential to revolutionize drug development, disease modeling, and personalized medicine. These microchips, called "organs-on-chips," offer a potential alternative to traditional animal testing. Ultimately, connecting the systems altogether is a way to have the whole "body-on-a-chip" system ideal for drug discovery and drug candidate testing and validation. Regulatory and funding agencies embraced the concept, but it is now increasingly adopted as a drug research platform by pharma and academia. Over two dozen organ systems are represented in on-chip systems.

4.9.2 Organs-on-a-Chip (OOC)

A laboratory on a chip is a device that includes one or more laboratory functions on one single chip dealing with particle handling in hollow, microfluidic channels. For over a decade it has been developed. The advantages in the handling of particulates at such a small scale include lower consumption of fluid volumes (lower reagent costs, less waste), increased device portability, improved control of the process (due to faster thermo-chemical reactions), and lower production costs. Furthermore, the microfluidic flow is completely laminar (i.e., no turbulence). There is therefore virtually no mixing in a hollow channel between neighboring streams. This rare property was exploited in order to investigate more complicated cell behaviors, such as chemotactic stimulus cell motility, stem cell differentiation, axon guidance, biochemical subcell propagation, and embryonic development during cell biological convergence.

4.9.3 Brain-on-a-Chip

Brain-on-a-chip systems are designed to create an interface between microfluidics and neuroscience by 1) enhancing culture viability; 2) supporting high-performance screening; 3) enabling in vitro/ex vivo modeled physiologies and diseases; and 4) improving microfluid devices' accuracy and tunability. Brain-on-a-chip devices cover a multitude of complexities with respect to the methodology of cell culture. Devices have been developed with platforms that vary in organotypic brain sections from traditional 2D cell cultivation to 3D tissue.

4.9.4 Lung-on-a-Chip

Lungs-on-a-chip have been designed to increase the physiology of existing alveolar-capillary in vitro interface models. A multifunctional microdevice such that a system contains two closely applied micro-channels, a thin (10 μm) flexible porous membrane made from PDMS, comprising, in large part, three microfluidic channels, can reproduce the fundamental structural, functional, and mechanical properties of the human capillary interface (i.e., the fundamental functional unit of the life lung). On either side of the membrane, the cultivated cells are human alveolar epithelial cells on one side of the membrane and human pulmonary endothelial microvascular cells.

4.9.5 Heart-on-a-Chip

Past efforts to replicate heart tissue environments have been challenging as contractility and electro-physiological responses have been imitated. The accuracy of in vitro experiments would be significantly increased by this feature.

In vitro tests of cardiomyocytes, which generate electrical impulses that control the heart rate, have already been contributed by microfluidics. In order to electrochemically and optically monitor the metabolism of cardiomyocytes, for instance, researchers have built a series of PDMS microchambers that are in line with sensors and electrode stimulation tools. Another laboratory on a chip similarly combined an extracellular potential from a single adult moray cardiomyocyte with a planar microelectrode microfluidic network in PDMS.

4.9.6 Kidney-on-a-Chip

Microfluid devices that have the potential to accelerate research including the artificial substitution of lost kidney function have already been simulated with renal cells and nephrons. In dialysis patients, this means they now need to go to the clinic up to three times a week. Instead of increasing patient health (by increasing the rate of treatment), a transportable and accessible way of treatment would make the entire process more efficient and tolerable. The research into artificial kidneys seeks to ensure that innovative disciplines such as microfluidics, miniaturization, and nanotechnology can be transported, wearable, and possibly implanted.

4.9.7 Nephron-on-a-Chip

The nephron consists of a glomerulus and a tubular component and is the functional unit of the kidney. A bio-artificial device that replicates the glomerulus function, the proximal tubing, and the Henle loop has two microfabricated layers separated by a membrane. Each part consists of two layers. The only inlet for the blood sample in the microfluidic device is designed. In the glomerular section of the nephron, the membrane permits certain blood particles, which include the endothelial, basement membrane, and epithelial podocytes, through its wall of capillary cells. Fluid is called a filtrate or primary urine which is filtered out of the capillary blood into the Bowman's space. As part of the urine formation of the tubules, some substances are added to the filtrate and returned to the blood. The proximal tubule is the first segment of these tubules. This is where nutritionally significant substances are almost completely absorbed. This section is simply the straight channels of the device, but the above-mentioned membrane and the layer of renal proximal tubular cells have to cross the blood particles that go to the filtrate. The second section of the tubules is the Henle loop, where water and ions are absorbed from the urine. The looping canals of the device attempt to simulate the Henle loop's counteracting mechanism. Similarly, the Henle loop requires a variety of cell types because each cell type has different characteristics and properties for transport. These include lower limb cells, thin upward limb cells, thick upward limb cells, the cells in which the cortical duct is collected, and the cells in which the medullary duct is collected.

4.9.8 Vessel-on-a-Chip

Cardiovascular diseases are often caused by changes in the structure and function of small blood vessels. A microfluidic platform simulating the biological response of an artery could not only enable organ-based screens to occur more frequently throughout a drug development trial but also yield a comprehensive understanding of the underlying mechanisms behind pathologic changes in small arteries and develop better treatment strategies. Conventional methods used to examine intrinsic properties of isolated resistance vessels (arterioles and small arteries with diameters varying between 30 µm and 300 µm) include the pressure myography technique. However, such methods currently require manually skilled personnel and are not scalable. An artery-on-a-chip could overcome several of these limitations by accommodating an artery onto a platform that would be scalable, inexpensive, and possibly automated in its manufacturing.

The artery-on-a-chip is designed for reversible implantation of the sample. The device contains a microchannel network, an artery loading area, and a separate artery inspection area. There is a microchannel used for loading the artery segment. When the loading well is sealed, it is also used as a perfusion channel to replicate the process of nutritional delivery of arterial blood to a capillary bed in the biological tissue. Another pair of microchannels serves to fix the two ends of the arterial segment. Finally, the last couple of microchannels are used to provide superfusion flow rates to maintain the organ's physiological and metabolic activity by delivering a constant sustaining medium over the abluminal wall. A thermoelectric heater and a thermoresistor are connected to the chip and maintain physiological temperatures at the artery inspection area.

Vessel-on-chips are used to study many disease processes such as viral hemorrhagic syndrome, which involves virus-induced vascular integrity loss.

4.9.9 Skin-on-a-Chip

Human skin is the first line of defense against many pathogens and can be subject to various diseases and issues, such as cancers and inflammation. As such, skin-on-a-chip applications include testing of topical pharmaceuticals and cosmetics, studying the pathology of skin diseases and inflammation, and "creating noninvasive automated cellular assays" to test for the presence of antigens or antibodies that could denote the presence of a pathogen. Despite the wide variety of potential applications, relatively little research has gone into developing a skin-on-a-chip compared to many other organ-on-a-chips, such as lungs and kidneys. Issues such as detachment of the collagen scaffolding from microchannels, incomplete cellular differentiation, and the predominant use of poly(dimethylsiloxane) (PDMS) for device fabrication have been shown to leach chemicals into biological samples. They cannot be mass-produced stymie standardization of a platform. One additional difficulty is the variability of cell-culture scaffolding or the base substance in which to culture cells, that is used in skin-on-a-chip devices. In the human body, this substance is known as the extracellular matrix.

4.9.10 Human-on-a-Chip

Researchers are building a multifunctional 3D cell culturing system that shares micro-environments where 3D cell aggregates are grown to imitate several organs in the organism. The researchers are involved in this process. Today most models of an organ-on-a-chip only cultivate one cell type, which makes it impossible to ascertain the systemic impact of a drug on the human body, although it may be a valid model with which to study organ whole functions.

The development and inclusion of lung cellulars, drug liver, and fat cells were particularly followed by an integrated cell culture analogy (µCCA). The cells are linked together as a blood substitute in a 2D liquid system, and therefore a nutrient supply system is efficiently provided while at the same time waste is removed from the cells.

4.10 Clinical Trials

Within the context of medical product development, clinical trials are tools for evaluating the performance of investigational medical products in people. Clinical testing is the most expensive aspect of medical product development, often requiring the enrollment of large numbers of people and the collection of massive amounts of data. Stakeholders point to the costs of clinical trials as a barrier to innovation.

- Advancing innovative trial designs: The majority of clinical trials currently conducted during product development, particularly for pharmaceuticals, are empirical (i.e., designed to assess whether patients improve or have adverse reactions, not designed to explore the underlying physiologic mechanisms of product performance). This is due to a dearth of knowledge and evaluative tools for exploring pharmacologic mechanisms (either of benefit or risk). Another major drawback of empirical trials is their limited ability to address more than a few questions within a single trial. Consequently, after a long and expensive development program, numerous questions about product performance frequently remain unanswered. The situation is better for some medical devices, where there are reliable metrics to evaluate specific aspects of device performance (e.g., physical, electrical, mechanical, imaging). However, for other devices (e.g., certain drug–device combination products), problems similar to those of pharmaceuticals also occur. As tools to elucidate the causal mechanisms underlying product safety and efficacy become available, new trial designs and clinical development programs will need to evolve to use the knowledge gained. Such unique designs are often referred to as learning trials. Learning trials have a different underlying conceptual framework and require a statistical approach different from empirical trials. One type of learning trial in use today is the dose- or concentration-controlled trial, which uses biomarkers or other intermediate measures as endpoints to explore dose- or concentration-response relationships. In the future, we hope that such trials can employ multiple biomarker assays, such as advanced imaging techniques and genomic- and proteomics-based tests, to reduce uncertainties around product performance quickly. Knowledge gained from learning trials can be incorporated into quantitative computer models of disease and product performance to refine their precision and lead to more efficient confirmatory trials. More conceptual work needs to be done in advancing the design and analysis of these trials. In the Opportunities List, several projects are delineated—appropriate use of enrichment designs within a development program and methods for using prior knowledge—intended to stimulate innovation in trial design in the areas discussed above. Additionally, the list identifies several serious challenges in existing trial design and analysis that require resolution to improve clinical development innovation. Challenges include developing reliable methods for noninferiority designs, treatment of missing data, and use of multiple endpoints.
- Improving the measurement of patient responses: Today, most clinical trials investigating product effectiveness compare the overall response of the treated population to the untreated population (i.e., the control population). These trials do not seek to understand which individuals respond to an intervention or why they respond. Again, this is primarily due to a lack of tools to perform such evaluations. However, as a new generation of biomarkers emerges—capable of distinguishing among individuals with different variations of a disease or rapidly signaling status changes in organ systems or disease processes—trial designs will need to evolve to effectively use this information. Trials that define and measure variations in individual response and seek correlation with biomarker status are the necessary first steps toward personalized medicine.
- Disease- or indication-specific trial designs: As new designs and analytical principles of innovative trials are implemented, effort must also be invested in developing trials and outcome measures tailored to specific diseases. Because each disease has a particular time course, a constellation of symptoms, a need for monitoring, and a set of therapeutic alternatives, disease-specific trial designs that incorporate appropriate safety monitoring and standardized

disease-specific efficacy measures are highly desirable. Standardized designs and metrics will 1) reduce the need to reinvent the wheel for each new trial, 2) assist clinical investigators and study personnel (who often conduct multiple trials in a given disease), 3) help reduce variation and error, and 4) facilitate cross-study analyses. The list opportunities only scratch the surface of the work needed to advance disease-specific trial designs.

- Measuring patient preferences: During the development of disease-specific outcome measures, substantial attention must be given to patient values and preferences (e.g., assigning weight to the value of relief of various symptoms in composite endpoints). Much more effort needs to be expended in eliciting patient points of view about the burden of disease and the relief of symptoms. Improved linkage of outcome measures to established patient benefit will help identify the overall benefit of therapies with more precision and enhance product development.
- Streamlining and automating clinical trials: Finally, standardizing and automating clinical trial procedures, conduct, and data processing to the greatest extent possible could dramatically improve clinical development efficiency. Efforts are underway in many areas, including standardizing terminology and developing data standards. Yet many opportunities remain in this area.

4.10.1 Biomarkers

The key to greater success will be to understand the key clinical issues and provide testable and scientific evidence for the transition from preclinical to clinical.

A biomarker strategy is developed to answer a range of key clinical questions and help develop a robust clinical study. For example,

- What disease is the drug going to treat?
- In that disease, who are the targeted patients?
- How often, e.g., daily, weekly, etc. will the dose be used?
- How does the drug work in comparison with current treatments? A drug similar to an established standard of care will not succeed.
- Will the combination therapy with the treatment standard improve treatment results further?
- Can an acquired resistance after long-term therapy develop?

Understanding these key questions allows them to be tested in a preclinical setting to help mitigate some risks.

At the beginning of the drug discovery pipeline at the target selection phase, biomarkers should be introduced. The mechanism of action with the objective and all the markers involved must be understood. The tests and techniques shown below can be determined by means of various multianalytes to identify certain key markers which can be controlled once the compound is reached by a robust biomarker identification test (Table 4.5).

Important considerations to build into a clinical trial design include:

- In the treated patient, pharmacodynamic markers, i.e., the hitting compound. In turn, this allows for the determination of the dosing schedule, mechanism, and dose range evidence.
- Does the morphology change due to target modulation, e.g., proliferation markers or cell death markers?
- Concept evidence, i.e., what are the clinical effects?
- Predictive biomarkers—can an effect on the target be predicted?
- Selecting patients—which patients will be responding to the most common biomarker to measure?
- Biomarkers for safety are key to your biomarker strategy.
    - Are there resistance markers?
    - How do you compare this with the current care standard?

TABLE 4.5
FDA-Approved Markers

Qualified Biomarker(s)	Abbreviated Biomarker Description	Abbreviated COU	Qualification Decision
Albumin, β2-microglobulin, clusterin, cystatin C, KIM-1, total protein, and trefoil factor-3	Urinary nephrotoxicity biomarkers as assessed by immunoassays	Safety biomarker to be used with traditional indicators to indicate renal injury in rat	Qualified, 4/14/2008
Clusterin, renal papillary antigen (RPA-1)	Urinary nephrotoxicity biomarkers as assessed by immunoassays	Safety biomarker to be used with traditional indicators to indicate renal injury in rat	Qualified, 9/22/2010 Not qualified: alpha-s-glutathione transferase
Cardiac troponins T (cTnT) and I (cTnI)	Serum/plasma cardiotoxicity biomarkers as assessed by immunoassay	Safety biomarker to indicate cardiotoxicity in rats, dogs, or monkeys when testing known cardiotoxic drugs and may be used to help estimate a non-toxic human dose	Qualified, 2/23/2012
Galactomannan	Serum/broncho-alveolar lavage fluid biomarker as assessed by immunoassay	Diagnostic biomarker used with other clinical and host factors to identify patients with invasive *Aspergillosis*	Qualified, 11/14/2015
Fibrinogen	Plasma biomarker as assessed by immunoassay	Prognostic biomarker used with other characteristics to enrich for COPD exacerbations	Qualified, 9/14/2016
Total kidney volume (TKV)	TKV as assessed by MRI, CT, and US	Prognostic biomarker with patient age and baseline glomerular filtration rate for autosomal dominant polycystic kidney disease	Qualified, 9/15/2016
Clusterin (CLU), cystatin-C (CysC), kidney injury molecule-1 (KIM-1), N-acetyl-beta-D-glucosaminidase (NAG), neutrophil gelatinase-associated lipocalin (NGAL), and osteopontin (OPN)	Urinary nephrotoxicity biomarker panel as assessed by immunoassays	Safety biomarker panel to aid in the detection of kidney tubular injury in phase I trials in healthy volunteers	7/25/2018
Plasmodium 18S rRNA/rDNA	*Plasmodium falciparum* 18S rRNA/rDNA (copies/ml) measured in blood samples by a nucleic acid amplification test	Monitoring biomarker informs initiation of treatment with anti-malarial drug following controlled human malaria infection (CHMI) with *P. falciparum* sporozoites in healthy subjects in clinical studies for vaccine and drug development	Qualified, 10/12/2018

Source: www.fda.gov/drugs/biomarker-qualification-program/list-qualified-biomarkers.

Changes in biomarkers following treatment reflect the clinical response to the product. Techniques as disparate as imaging, serum or genetic assays, or psychological tests can yield useful product development biomarkers. Biomarkers can reduce uncertainty by providing quantitative predictions about performance. The existence of predictive efficacy biomarkers, in particular, can revolutionize product development in a disease area.

There is a clear consensus that new biomarkers and animal models—qualified for a wide range of product testing purposes—are urgently needed to unlock innovation in product development and treatment and could be developed with concerted scientific effort.

The use of mini pigs, which has many advantages, including equal omnivorous digestion to humans, an estrogen cycle like humans, sexual maturity at the age of six months, and skin similar to human beings, is increasing specifically in animals. The mini pig offers a viable, non-rodent species as an alternative to the commonly used NHP models, which can provide an improved clinical efficacy forecast.

In carrying out a safety evaluation in the context of the disease, (usually mice) models can be of value and, in some situations, may have toxicological responses that are more representative of patient reaction. The toxicology studies may include humanized transgenic animal models for better reading, but humanized models are expensive. The use of various models could lead to a concurrent decrease in the ethical and economic advantages of NHPs and dogs.

Biomarkers (incorporated into relevant diagnostics) used to select high-risk populations for clinical trials will also, once the product is on the market, help physicians target treatment to the patients who are likely to benefit most. Such tools will help bring individualized medicine into the physician's office to help shape the future's medical practice. Right now, the work necessary to prove that a given biomarker is sufficiently correlated with the clinical response is rarely undertaken.

Many of the biomarkers used in medical product development today have been in use for many years, even decades. These longstanding biomarkers are empirically derived; they often lack predictive and explanatory power. New biomarker development has stalled. Many potential new biomarkers have been proposed, but the essential work needed to evaluate their utility—known as biomarker qualification—has not been carried out. The opportunities to qualify new biomarkers that are particularly promising include:

- Genomic, proteomic, and metabolomic technologies: The new -omic technologies (genomics, proteomics, and metabolomics) hold great promise as a source of powerful biomarkers. Some in vitro diagnostic tests that detect specific genetic variations that affect an individual's response to treatment are ready for use. For example, recently FDA approved several genomic tests for drug-metabolizing enzymes. These assays can identify patients who are at high risk for serious toxicity from cancer therapies because the recommended doses are too high for them. Pharmacogenetic tests for drug metabolism status are only the first in a new generation of diagnostics that could transform product development.
- Safety biomarkers: The development of more predictive safety biomarkers for use in animal toxicology studies would improve the effectiveness of safety screening before introducing products into humans, enable better selection of initial human doses, and help target toxicity monitoring in early trials. Clinical trial safety could be improved, as could overall development efficiency. New safety biomarkers are also crucial to improving the safety of products used in clinical practice. Biomarkers are urgently needed to monitor for early signs of toxicity and signal severe toxicity potential. Such biomarkers could significantly improve the development and use of products that patients will take overtime periods far longer than the length of clinical trials, such as implanted devices and drugs that treat chronic conditions. Also, the development of markers and diagnostics to identify individuals at high risk for serious drug side effects—such as cardiac arrhythmias—could dramatically improve medical product safety while simplifying product development.
- Personalized medicine: Biomarkers are crucial for individualizing, or personalizing, medical treatment. For example, markers can create more precise classifications of disease to target or stratify therapy. Similarly, for a therapy directed at a molecular target (e.g., many cancer treatments under development), markers of that target may provide reliable predictions of who

will respond—and thus who should receive that therapy. Markers of drug metabolism can individualize drug dosage, preventing, for example, predictable underdosing (and resultant lack of efficacy) in more rapid metabolizers and severe side effects from overdosing in slow metabolizers. For example, we now know that genetic variants in metabolizing enzymes play a significant role in the large variability among patients in warfarin dosing. Harnessing this knowledge to develop rigorous dosing protocols based on a patient's unique genetic profile should reduce safety problems associated with warfarin therapy initiation. Biomarkers are also useful for predicting dose-response characteristics and for monitoring response during treatment.

- Surrogate endpoints: There is great interest in qualifying additional surrogate endpoints. A surrogate endpoint is a biomarker used to predict clinical benefit (direct measurement of how a patient feels, functions, or survives). Often, changes in such biomarkers can be detected earlier or more readily than the corresponding clinical endpoint (an outcome being used to measure drug effect). In disorders where the clinical endpoint is hard to assess (e.g., joint deterioration in rheumatoid arthritis) or takes a long time to occur (e.g., certain preventive therapies), the use of a qualified surrogate endpoint can markedly accelerate the development process for treatment breakthroughs. There is a great deal of confidence, nevertheless, that changes in the marker reliably predict the wanted clinical endpoints before a biomarker is accepted as a surrogate endpoint. There must also be a comprehensive and thoughtful discussion of possible risks (e.g., trials using a surrogate endpoint for effectiveness can be shorter and will not evaluate longer-term risks). One opportunity in the list involves more clearly laying out a path for qualifying a biomarker as a surrogate endpoint.
- New imaging techniques: New imaging techniques hold vast potential for use as biomarkers for various purposes in product development—measuring treatment efficacy, patient stratification, and improved diagnosis. Although preliminary data are promising, the predictive capacity of most new imaging techniques has not been rigorously evaluated. Their application in product development is complicated further by the lack of standardizing imaging methods and evaluation techniques. Research to qualify imaging techniques for particular uses in product development would enable developers to measure the effects of candidate products earlier and more accurately. Also, data gained from the standardization and qualification processes could provide the evidence base for clinical use.
- Improving predictions of human responses from disease models: Animal models of disease are additional important tools in selecting and refining candidate medical products. Frequently, candidate products need to succeed in animal models before moving into testing in humans. Current animal models have not been predictive of success in humans for some diseases, leading to a succession of failed clinical development programs in that indication (e.g., neuroprotection).

4.10.1.1 BEST

The biomarker, endpoints, and other tools are defined by BEST and BNB as defining characteristics measured as indicators of normal biological processes, pathogenic processes, or exposure or intervention responses, including therapeutic interventions (www.ncbi.nlm.nih.gov/books/NBK326791/?report=reader). Types of biomarkers are molecular, histological, x-ray, or physiological characteristics. A biomarker does not evaluate the way a person feels, works, or survives. BEST defines seven categories of biomarkers: sensitivity/risk, diagnosis, surveillance, prognosis, prediction, drugs/response, and safety. A full description of the biomarker includes the name of the biomarker, the source/matrix, the measurable property(s), and the analytic method for the biomarker. A biomarker may be a single feature or a multiple feature panel. Qualified biomarkers can provide valuable information, which in regulatory decision-making during drug development could reduce uncertainty.

When a biomarker is qualified, it means that the biomarker has undergone a formal regulatory process to ensure we have a specific interpretation and application within the indicated context of an application for medical product development and regulatory review (COU). It should be noted that a biomarker is qualified rather than a biomarker method.

The qualification process is collaborative, where the Biomarker Qualification Program works with the requestor(s) in guiding biomarker development. Multiple interested parties often work together in working groups or consortia to develop a biomarker for qualification. This approach enables shared resources and reduces the burden on employees. This may in turn encourage stakeholders, despite the limited resources, to join the DDT development effort.

Immune system modulation unravels treatment from infectious diseases to autoimmunity and immunology across various therapeutic areas. Many strong techniques for measuring immune function biomarkers are available. For a particular study, the experimental solution must be selected on the basis of an understanding of the target immune component and its logistics. In order to confirm the target commitment (or proof of mechanism) from preclinical to clinical phases, immune biomarkers can be integrated into the drug discovery process. An optimum strategy calls for informed choices as to the immune parameter, how to measure it, and the amount of validation needed. In the end, biomarkers with PD can have a positive effect.

In the context of PD biomarkers, a "window of impact," after modulation by the test compound of interest, is established between the biomarker level. Various test platforms can be used to identify biomarkers of the immune system. In order, for example, to identify a protein product, such as an antigen-specific antibody, like titers or cytokines/chemokines produced in response to an antigen, ELISA or multiplex platforms (e.g., Luminex) can be utilized. qPCR or nanostring can be used in the biological sample to study or evaluate modulation by sample treatment or stimulation of the molecular "message" for a specific biomarker (mRNA or DNA). Nanostring technology is a strong technique that can simultaneously measure, profile, and select a smaller biomarker panel, expressing up to 800 genes by higher-throughput methods. In vaccination studies, ELISpot can be used at the cellular level to confirm the success of antigen-specific T cell frequency increase. Flow cytometry is simultaneously a potent technique, which can simultaneously quantify in a biologic sample the frequency of multiple sub-sets of immune cells. The technique chosen to identify, validate and quantify biomarkers is best suited to the needs of the study.

For successfully identifying biomarkers, sample logistics considerations are also essential—how are samples to be taken, how are they to be saved, how are they to be shipped? For a pre-clinical trial to be translated successfully into a clinical trial, this is especially important. A clinical test is typically preceded by a validation phase, which imitates conditions under which the test samples are exposed—such as freezing exposure or attachment—to stabilize the markers before the test. Finally, the tests require fit-for-use validation, including confirmation of parameters such as the performance of the default curve and intra- and inter-test accuracy, allowing for batch analysis of the samples.

4.11 Exploratory IND

Plans describing the progress of new drugs, reconstituted or refined, commercialized drugs into human and clinical evidence of conceptual studies using the traditional or traditional early drug development, the IND approach, as previously outlined in these guidelines. This section describes a new approach in order to accelerate the development of new drugs and imaging molecules for people who use phase 0 (exploratory IND). The IND exploratory research strategy was first published as draft guidance in April 2005. Following numerous feedback from the public and private sectors, the final guidance was published in January 2006.

Phase 0 is a description of clinical studies which occur very soon in the development stage of phase I. Phase 0 studies limit human drug exposure (up to seven days) and have no therapeutic purpose. The phase 0 studies are seen as an essential tool for speeding up new drugs in the clinic by the FDA and the National Cancer Institute (NCI). Data requirements for an exploratory IND are somewhat flexible. These conditions are determined by research goals (e.g., receptor occupancy, pharmacokinetics, human biomarker validation), the approach of clinical testing, and expected risks.

Exploratory IND studies give the sponsor a chance to evaluate up to five chemical entities or formulas simultaneously (optimized chemical lead candidates). The exploratory IND is close, and subsequent drug development takes place along the traditional IND pathway, when an optimized chemical lead candidate or formulation is chosen. This approach enables the human pharmacokinetics and the target interaction of chemical lead candidates to be characterized if appropriate. Exploratory IND goals generally include:

- The previously defined plans in these guidelines describe the development in human and clinical evidence of concept trials using the conventional or earlier IND approach of new drug and recycled or re-proposed drug products. This section of the guidelines outlines an approach to accelerating new drug development and imaging molecules for people who use phase 0 (exploratory IND). First, a draft guideline was published as part of the IND strategy for exploratory research in April 2005. Following numerous feedback from the private and public sectors, the final guidance was published in January 2006.
- Phase 0 describes the clinical trials which occur in the phase I development phase very early. Phase 0 tests limit human drug exposure (up to seven days) and do not have a therapeutic purpose. The FDA and the National Cancer Institute (NCI) regard phase 0 studies as essential tools to speed up the development of new drugs in the clinic. Data requirements for a scanning IND are flexible. These requirements depend on research objectives (e.g., receptor occupancy, pharmacy kinetics, validation of human biomarkers), clinical testing approach, and expected risks.
- Exploratory IND studies give the sponsor an opportunity to evaluate up to five chemical entities or formulations at once. When the candidate for an optimized chemical lead or formula is chosen, the explorative IND is closed, which is the traditional pathway for the development of drugs.

Exploratory IND studies are broadly referred to as microdosing studies and clinical trials to show a pharmacological effect. Prior to implementation, exploratory IND or phase 0 strategies shall be discussed with the appropriate regulatory agency. The following studies are described.

The pharmacokinetics of chemical lead candidates or the imaging of specific drug targets are intended for microdosing studies. No pharmacological effect is to be achieved through microdosing studies. In order to generate a pharmacological effect in humans or a dose of less than 100 μg/subject, doses are reduced to less than 1/100th of the dose expected (by preclinical data). The preclinical security requirements for microdosing studies that permit exploratory INDs are significantly lower than the conventional IND approach. In the United States, a single dose of the toxicity study using the clinical route is necessary. Fourteen days from the single dose of animals are observed. Endstages are collected for routine toxicology. The objective of these studies is to identify or demonstrate a high degree of safety for the minimally toxic dose (e.g., 100x). There is no need for genotoxicity studies. Contrary to the FDA, before starting microdosing trials, the EMEA needs to undergo toxicology studies using two routes of administration—intravenous and clinical. Studies of genotoxicity (bacterial micronucleus and mutation) must be carried out. In the workshops on exploratory INDs, the allowances for up to five micro-supplements administered to each subject participating in the IND exploratory study were discussed or proposed, subject to a dose not exceeding 1:100 of a dose NOAEL or 1:100 of a pharmacologically active dose, or to a total dose of less than 100 mcg. In this case, at least six pharmacokinetic terminal half-lives would be separated by doses for washing. Fourteen days of repeat toxicity studies covering the predicted therapeutic dose range, however below the MTD, were also proposed in micro-dosing studies to support the extension of dosing.

In May 2004, the PhRMA suggested exploratory IND clinical studies to produce a pharmacological effect, based on a retrospective analysis of 106 drugs supporting the accelerated paradigm of preclinical safety assessments. Up to five compounds can be studied in phase 0 studies to produce a pharmacological effect. The compounds should have a common pharmaceutical goal but do not have a structural relationship. The clinic can receive up to seven repeat doses for healthy volunteers or for minimum-ill patients. The objective is not to define MTD but to achieve a pharmacological response. In comparison to microdosing studies, preclinical safety requirements are higher. A full clinical and histopathological assessment is necessary and is carried out in 14 days of repeated toxicology studies in rodents (e.g., rats). In addition, as described in ICH S7a a complete safety pharmacology battery is required. In other words, before phase 0, unpredictable pharmacological consequences are characterized for cardiovascular, respiratory, and central nervous systems. In addition, studies of genotoxicity involving bacterial mutation and micronucleus tests are conducted. A repeat dose study in non-rodent species (typically the dog) is carried out at the rat NOAEL in addition to the 14-day rodent toxicology study. The duration of the non-rodent dose repeat study corresponds to the dose duration planned for the phase 0 test. The chemical lead applicant will not proceed with phase 0 if toxicity is observed in the non-rodent species of the rat NOAEL.

For phase 0, the starting dose is usually defined as 1/50 of NOAEL rat, based on a squared base of one meter. Dose increases in these studies are ended when 1) the pathological effect or the target modulation is observed; 2) the human systemic exposure reflectable in the AUC reaches one-half of the AUC observed in rats or dogs in 14-day repeat toxicology studies, whichever is less. Dose increases are concluded when the pharmacological effect or objective modulation is observed.

Early-stage clinical research involving potentially promising drugs for life-threatening diseases with terminally ill patients without therapeutic options can be conducted under limited conditions (e.g., up to three days dosage) with a facilitated IND strategy. As with the above phase 0 strategy, this approach has to be defined before implementation in partnership with the FDA.

The reduced preclinical safety requirements are measured against phase 0 studies in terms of objectives, duration, and extent. Phase 0 is good if the initial clinical knowledge is not toxic when the primary determinant of selecting pharmacokinetic drugs in a group of chemical lead candidates is the pharmacodynamic end-stage method (for example blood or tumor tissue), or when the main interest of pharmacodynamic end-stage drugs is the bioanalytic method for quantifying microdose concentrations (e.g., receptor occupancy studies employing PET scanning).

The exploratory IND approach has its limitations. Doses used in phase 0 studies may not be predictive of human doses (up to the maximum tolerated dose). Phase 0 patient studies raise ethical problems as compared with the conventional phase I, since the exploratory IND guidance could not permit escalation to a pharmacologically active dose range. Phase 0 is designed to kill drugs early on which the PK or PK/PD are likely to fail. If phase 0 leads to a decision on the "go." In subsequent clinical studies, however, a conventional IND is required, adding time and cost. The characterization of the tissue distribution (e.g., occupancy after PET studies) after the micro-supplement is perhaps one of the most compelling arguments for the use of an exploratory IND strategy.

4.12 Repurposing

Reusing or repositioning drugs is a technique used to treat new and challenging diseases with existing medications. The reuse of drugs has turned into a promising approach as development schedules and overall costs have been lowered. In the Big Data era, AI and network drugs offer state-of-the-art applications for information science to define diseases as well as drug and therapeutical products, and to identify goals with the lowest error. In this review, we present guidelines on how to use AI to accelerate drug repurposing and repositioning, which are not only excellent but necessary for AI approaches. Therapeutic development can be accelerated quickly, strongly, and innovatively by developing AI and network drugs technology.

Drug repurposing (including clinically defective) is a strategy to identify new indications for approved or investigative medications not approved (including clinically failed ones) (panel). Because the safety of such drugs has already been tested for other applications in clinical trials, repurposing of known drugs can bring drugs to patients much faster and less expensive than developing new drugs. For decades the idea of screening the libraries of drugs with various tests could uncover new applications and observations have been promoted by academic bodies and science funding agencies that have led to drugs designed to find applications for one disease in another.

The drug repurposing strategy is a powerful solution for emerging diseases, yet, without foreknowledge of the complete drug-target network, the development of promising and affordable approaches for the effective treatment of complex diseases is challenging. As drug targets are not isolated from the complex protein system comprising the molecular machinery of cell association they should be examined in an integrative context, each interaction between drug and target (panel). Therapeutic interventions must take account and have little to do functionally with genetic and genomic events, and the disturbance of disease system properties (termed network medicine panel). Observations and advances in network medicine further indicate that the disease, which is essential to drug discovery and development, is driven by cellular systems and the human interactome (panel). Observations and advances in network medicine further indicate that the disease, which is essential to drug discovery and development, is driven by cellular systems and the human interactome (panel).

Translational science has been confronted for decades by the challenge of translating research findings into new, efficient, and quickly delivering drugs. The basic and translational sciences have encouraged this challenge to collaborate in this key objective. Generations of researchers have struggled to make progress in the discovery of drugs. A drug repurposing strategy in which the US FDA has already tested and approved a drug can overcome barriers to the discovery of de novo drugs in principle. The volume of approved or clinically failed medicinal products is however huge, highlighting the difficulties of selecting the drug that would be extremely effective in this disease.

Despite their enthusiasm for repurposing drugs, there are still challenges. Cellular or animal tests may not reflect the virus infection host environment in people. In the original indications repurposed drugs could also be optimized for a specific target, dose, or tissue.

Progress in pharmacogenetics and pharmacogenomics has shown a significant improvement in the treatment of the disease if treatments are guided by the genomic profiles of individuals. In some diseases, including cancer, this hypothesis has achieved initial success. Genetic, epigenetic, and environmental factors influence drug responsiveness.

4.13 Orphan Drugs

Cancer drug development programs are often much more complex than drugs used in many other indications. This complexity often leads to extended timelines for development and approval. In comparison with other more common indications, patient populations in oncology are also often much smaller. These factors (e.g., limited patent life and smaller populations of patients) complicate marketing strategies often and ultimately make access to crucial new therapies for patients more challenging.

In order to manage and speed up the marketing of drugs used in rare diseases such as numerous cancers, the orphan drug law was signed in 1983. This law provides incentives for sponsors and researchers to develop new treatments for conditions and diseases with fewer than 200,000 cases per year to allow more realistic marketing.

Orphan-designated drugs have many incentives:

- The sponsor of a designated orphan medication product has seven years' exclusive marketing rights, once the FDA has received a market authorization.
- A tax credit for qualified expenses for clinical research in the development of a designated orphan product.
- Eligibility to apply for orphan drug subsidies.
- A sponsor can request the designation of orphan drugs for:
- An earlier drug not authorized.
- A new indication for a medication on the market.
- A drug that is already orphan—if the sponsor can provide valid proof that his drug is clínically superior to the first drug.

A sponsor, an investigator, or a person may request an orphan drug designation or apply at any stage of development (e.g., phases 1–3) before establishing an active clinical program. If the designation of orphan drugs is granted, the proposed indication must be supported through clinical studies. Until the FDA approves a marketing application, a drug will not be accorded orphan drug status and marketing exclusivity. The first sponsor is granted to obtain FDA authorization and not forcibly the sponsor originally submitting an application for orphan drug designation. Orphan drug status is granted.

An orphan drug designation is not formally requested. However, it does identify the components to include in the regulations (e.g., 21 CRF 316). An orphan application for designation is typically a five-to-ten-page literature document, with references appended in support of the less than 200,000 cases per year prevalence statements. The orphan drug designation request generally includes:

- The particular rare disease or condition to be appointed for an orphan drug sponsor contact, as well as the name or source of the sponsor.
- Description and medically feasible reason of the rare disease or condition of any sub-set approach.
- Description of the drug and the scientific rationale for the rare disease or disease use.
- Summary of the drug's status and marketing history.
- Documents (for treatment for disease or condition) showing that less than 200,000 people in the United States are affected by the drug (prevalence).
- Documentation (for the prevention of disease [or a vaccine or drug]) that the drug in the United States is affecting fewer than 200,000 individuals annually (incidence).

4.14 Conclusion

Drug discovery technologies are evolving fast and truly demonstrate how a nonlinear model is built. The transition from anecdotal trial and error continues to be practiced. Still, it is quickly replaced by an "automated" trial and error, the HTS that provides many possibilities. Still, the success rate from hits to clinical remains very low, reminding us of the human body's complexity, the theories surrounding diseases, and receptor interactions. What appears to be significant progress today may turn out to be a steady evolution in the future. We have, however, moved so far that a variety of diseases can be avoided, including autoimmune disorders, cancer management, and slow cell aging. The technologies of organ-on-a-chip and microfluidics have changed how we design a drug discovery project; unfortunately, the cost of entering the game has also risen exponentially. Still, smaller innovative companies and academia continue to contribute to new drug discovery faster than big pharma.

ADDITIONAL READING

Astashkina A, Mann B, Grainger DW. A critical evaluation of in vitro cell culture models for high-throughput drug screening and toxicity. *Pharmacol Ther.* 2012;134(1):82–106.

Beutner GL, et al. TCFH-NMI: direct access to N-acyl imidazoliums for challenging amide bond formations. *Org Lett.* 2018;20(14):4218–4222.

Brown DG, Boström J. Analysis of past and present synthetic methodologies on medicinal chemistry: where have all the new reactions gone? *J Med Chem.* 2016;59(10):4443–4445.

Brown DG, Boström J. Where do recent small molecule clinical development candidates come from? *J Med Chem.* 2018;61:9442–9468.

Chi CW, Ahmed AR, Dereli-Korkut Z, Wang S. Microfluidic cell chips for high-throughput drug screening. *Bioanalysis.* 2016;8(9):921–937.

Dickey CA, Eriksen J, Kamal A, et al. Development of a high throughput drug screening assay for the detection of changes in tau levels – proof of concept with HSP90 inhibitors. *Curr Alzheimer Res.* 2005;2(2):231–238.

Engel JC, Ang KK, Chen S, Arkin MR, McKerrow JH, Doyle PS. Image-based high-throughput drug screening targeting the intracellular stage of *Trypanosoma cruzi*, the agent of Chagas' disease. *Antimicrob Agents Chemother.* 2010;54(8):3326–3334.

Eren RO, Kopelyanskiy D, Moreau D, et al. Development of a semi-automated image-based high-throughput drug screening system. *Front Biosci (Elite Ed).* 2018;10:242–253.

Fan Y, Nguyen DT, Akay Y, Xu F, Akay M. Engineering a brain cancer chip for high-throughput drug screening. *Sci Rep.* 2016;6:25062.

Guo WM, Loh XJ, Tan EY, Loo JS, Ho VH. Development of a magnetic 3D spheroid platform with potential application for high-throughput drug screening. *Mol Pharm.* 2014;11(7):2182–2189.

Gupta R, Netherton M, Byrd TF, Rohde KH. Reporter-based assays for high-throughput drug screening against. *Front Microbiol.* 2017;8:2204.

Hong B, Xue P, Wu Y, Bao J, Chuah YJ, Kang Y. A concentration gradient generator on a paper-based microfluidic chip coupled with cell culture microarray for high-throughput drug screening. *Biomed Microdevices.* 2016;18(1):21.

Ishaq O, Negri J, Bray MA, Pacureanu A, Peterson RT, Wählby C. AUTOMATED QUANTIFICATION OF ZEBRAFISH TAIL DEFORMATION FOR HIGH-THROUGHPUT DRUG SCREENING. *Proc IEEE Int Symp Biomed Imaging.* 2013:902–905.

Kainkaryam RM, Woolf PJ. poolHiTS: a shifted transversal design based pooling strategy for high-throughput drug screening. *BMC Bioinformatics.* 2008;9:256.

Kainkaryam RM, Woolf PJ. Pooling in high-throughput drug screening. *Curr Opin Drug Discov Devel.* 2009;12(3):339–350.

Krutzik PO, Nolan GP. Fluorescent cell barcoding in flow cytometry allows high-throughput drug screening and signaling profiling. *Nat Methods.* 2006;3(5):361–368.

Lievens S, Caligiuri M, Kley N, Tavernier J. The use of mammalian two-hybrid technologies for high-throughput drug screening. *Methods.* 2012;58(4):335–342.

Ohlson S, Duong-Thi MD, Bergström M, et al. Toward high-throughput drug screening on a chip-based parallel affinity separation platform. *J Sep Sci.* 2010;33(17–18):2575–2581.

Roughley SD, Jordan AM. The medicinal chemist's toolbox: an analysis of reactions used in the pursuit of drug candidates. *J Med Chem.* 2011;54(10):3451–3479.

Stilwell GE, Saraswati S, Littleton JT, Chouinard SW. Development of a Drosophila seizure model for in vivo high-throughput drug screening. *Eur J Neurosci.* 2006;24(8):2211–2222.

Zhang L, He M, Zhang Y, Nilubol N, Shen M, Kebebew E. Quantitative high-throughput drug screening identifies novel classes of drugs with anticancer activity in thyroid cancer cells: opportunities for repurposing. *J Clin Endocrinol Metab.* 2012;97(3):E319–28.

Zhou M, Li W, Li J, et al. Phase-separated condensate-aided enrichment of biomolecular interactions for high-throughput drug screening in test tubes. *J Biol Chem.* 2020;295(33):11420–11434.

5

Drug Development Assays

5.1 Background

5.1.1 Assay Optimization

The process of HTS begins with standard 96-, 384-, or 1,536-well microtiter plates. Each well holds a particular compound and every assay is tested against a protein (biochemical assay) or a whole cell (cell-based assay). Before the assay ever reaches the robotics system, the assay and all its components must be prepared and optimized by the HTS scientists. The scientist or compound manager prepares the drug-like compounds in the chosen microtiter plate. Before the biological targets and drug-like compounds are tested, the lab biologists prepare solutions for this assay plate. These solutions consist of many variables that may be an enzyme, cofactors, a substrate, a mix of nutrients, and buffers needed for cell survival. Assay optimization is critically important to ensure that the developed assay works at a miniaturized level. Lower density test plates are used as a head-to-head comparison point to understand changes that affect the outcome. The appropriate positive and negative controls are always included on each test plate at an N of 24 per plate. An example of a positive control is using the IC100 concentration of a known pharmacologic inhibitor, while the negative control might be vehicle only. There are hundreds of methods to use as a readout to determine the biological effect on an assay. Listing and explaining all of them would require an additional chapter, but you can think about all of them in the sense that they typically exploit the physical properties of light energy. An alternative to that is to use radioactive isotopes to determine a rise or fall in assay signal. Many times tests are done using fluorescence and luminescence tags to determine which assay is the most conducive to the survival of the biological target and its activity. Here, HTS scientists want to maximize the Z'-factor, which assesses the statistical reliability of the assay's performance for HTS. A Z'-factor close to 1 is ideal, and any value above 0.5 is considered a high-quality HTS assay. Once the assay is optimized, it can be prepared to enter the robotics system to measure reactivity between the drug-like compound and biological target. Using absorbance, fluorescence, luminescence, time-resolved fluorescence resonance energy transfer (TR-FRET), Flou-Pol, Ca++ detection, bioluminescence (BRET), high-content analysis, etc., HTS scientists can determine if there is an activity between the biological target and drug-like compound. If activity is found, then the drug-like compound and biological target are said to be active.

Drug efficacy can be measured in HTS using absorbance, luminescence, and fluorescence. These three techniques are used to determine the optimal conditions assay and measure the extent to which interaction occurred between the compound and its biological target. Absorbance is the extent to which a sample absorbs light at a given wavelength. Luminescence occurs when excited electrons in a molecule fall to the ground state, and energy is emitted in light. The electrons' excitation can occur after the molecule absorbs energy in light or during a chemical reaction. Among the different types of luminescence, we find bioluminescence. It is located in some living organisms (e.g., fireflies) and occurs when light is emitted after an organism's biochemical reaction. Fluorescence is another form of luminescence that allows some atoms and molecules to absorb light at a shorter wavelength, which excites an electron to a higher state. When this electron returns to its ground state, it releases energy, in light, at a longer wavelength. Absorbance, luminescence, and fluorescence measurements can be used to determine whether or not an interaction occurred between a drug-like compound and its biological target.

DOI: 10.1201/9781003146933-5

The Fluorescent Imaging Plate Reader (FLIPR) measures kinetic changes such as ion influxes simultaneously for each well. This allows for a quick reading of all wells, up to 1,536 simultaneously, and the reading occurs in real-time, limiting the variable of time. This is also important as it can accurately measure processes such as calcium flux, which occur quickly. Ion fluxes are measured via fluorescent tagging. These dyes are introduced to the assay to measure intracellular ion changes, such as calcium fluxes, a vital signaling method within cells. These dyes are fluorescent ligands, which attach to calcium. The signal emits light at a higher wavelength when calcium is bound. Thus, the wavelength at which light is absorbed can tell the HTS scientists the calcium location in the assay giving information about the cell's activity.

TR-FRET is used as a tag in many assays to determine activity. TR-FRET is based on the transfer of energy between two entities. Each part is labeled with a fluorescent marker. When the donor is excited, it releases energy, which is picked up by the acceptor. This means that the donor and acceptor have to be close in proximity. This acceptor then emits an alternate yet specific fluorescence at a given wavelength. Thus, the interaction of proximal proteins can be measured. In practice, this assay occurs in the presence of buffers, proteins, lysate, or other components. Each of these also emits some fluorescence, but since the decay is in the nanosecond domain and the signal fluorophore is in the microsecond time domain, the signals can be separated by time, in other words, time-resolved (TR), as shown below. Thus, TR-FRET can be used to eliminate this quick measurement of fluorescence to measure the target molecules alone. Amplified Luminescent Proximity Homogeneous Assay (AlphaScreen) is a bead-based assay used to study biomolecular interactions in a microtiter plate format. There is both a donor bead and an acceptor bead in each assay. When a molecule is bound to the bead, an energy transfer occurs from one bead to another, which produces a luminescent/fluorescent signal. When the donor bead is hit with a light at 680 nm, a photosensitizer in the donor bead converts oxygen to an excited state of 0 2•. In this excited state, the oxygen can diffuse 200 nm in solution. If an acceptor bead lies within this distance, it will accept that energy. The acceptor bead will then produce light at 520–620 nm. If there is no acceptor in that distance, the oxygen will simply lose that energy, and it will fall back down to the ground state without eliciting a response. Similar to TR-FRET, this is a method for measuring whether or not an interaction took place. This technique's advantage is the removal of autofluorescent biologics and compounds that could create the discovery of false hits.

Fluorescence polarization (PP) is a testing method that allows the analysis of activity with drug-like compounds and biological targets. This method stems from the theory that the degree of a fluorophore's polarization is inversely related to molecular rotation. Thus, it measures the difference between perpendicular light intensity and parallel to the light used to excite the fluorophore. PP is not used for measuring the concentration of fluorophore or the intensity of light but rather the difference between the planes of light. It can be used in various interactions such as protein-protein, protein-DNA, protein-ligand interactions, and G protein-coupled receptors, nuclear receptors, and enzymes. FP is a favorable method as few, inexpensive reagents are necessary. This is in keeping with the low volume desired in HTS. It also does not destroy samples, so more than one reading can be conducted on one plate. With its wide range of applications and accurate results, FP is popular in HTS to analyze activity between drug-like compounds and biological targets.

Analytical techniques using MS, LC-MS, and nuclear magnetic resonance (NMR) are also practical in determining assay results. Each method has analytical figures of sensitivity, speed of analysis, selectivity, and cost-effectiveness that are desirable. LC-MS, in particular, is a method used in the Lead Identification Lab at Scripps Florida. In the quality control process, LC is utilized for purity detection. Then MS spectra analysis is used for compound identification, entered into a searchable database as results.

5.2 Assay Development and Validation

The developer must validate a biological assay system and methodology by proceeding through a series of steps along the HTS and SAR pathway. The overall objective of any assay validation procedure is to demonstrate that the assay is acceptable for its intended purpose. As mentioned above, the purpose

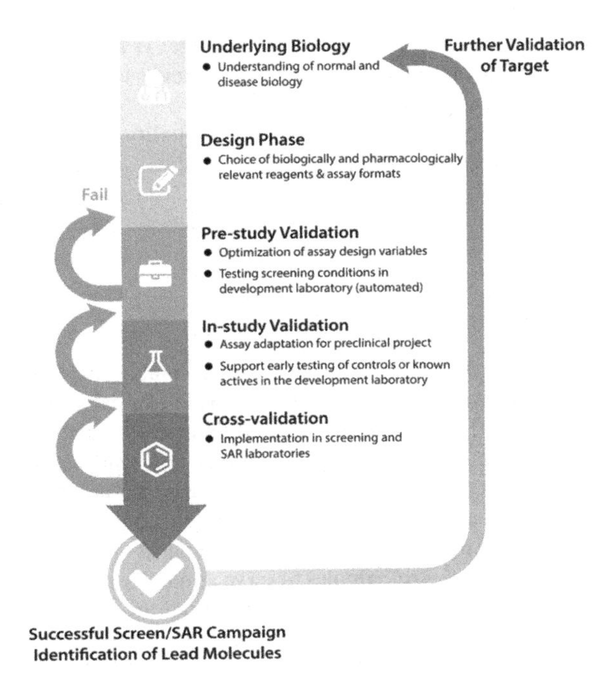

FIGURE 5.1 The assay development and validation cycle. The cycle begins in the design phase, which is followed by multiple validation steps that are executed at different stages throughout the assay life cycle, including pre-study (pre-screen) validation, in-study (in-screen) validation, and cross-validation (assay transfer validation). Failure to validate the assay in any of these steps requires either addressing the deficiency or developing a new assay that meets the validation requirements.

is to determine the biological and/or pharmacological activities of new chemical entities on pathways involved in normal and disease processes. An assay's acceptability begins with its design, construction, and execution in automated or semi-automated procedures, which can significantly affect its performance and robustness.

The assay development and validation cycle is a process with multiple validation steps (Figure 5.1). Successful completion of assay validation increases the likelihood of success in drug discovery or chemical probe development programs. During the design phase, assay conditions and procedures are selected to minimize the impact of potential sources of invalidity on the measurement of an analyte or biological endpoint in targeted sample matrices or test solutions. False-positive and false-negative hit rates are related to the selectivity and sensitivity of an assay. Additionally, technology-related artifacts, such as interference with the reporter system, also contribute to invalid results. Many other variables, including assay automation, pipetting, reagent stability, quantities of available reagents, and data analysis models, impact an assay's overall validity.

There are three fundamental areas in assay development, and validation: a) pre-study (pre-screen) validation, b) in-study (in-screen) validation, and c) cross-validation or assay transfer validation. These stages encompass the systematic scientific steps within the assay development and validation cycle. Rigorous validation is critical considering that assays are expected to perform robustly over several years during preclinical development.

5.2.1 Pre-Study Validation

There are several choices of assay format and design available. For many well-characterized target classes, there are several assays and commercially available kits. At this stage, the choice of an assay format is made. Important factors include selecting reagents with appropriate biological relevance (e.g., cell type, enzyme-substrate combination, a form of enzyme/protein target, readout labels, etc.), specificity, and stability. The choice of detection is also made at this stage. If fluorescent labels are chosen, the wavelength is selected to ensure low interference by test compound's compatibility with microtiter plate plastics and appropriate filter plate readers' availability.

Validation of assay performance proceeds smoothly if high-quality reagents and procedures are chosen. Assessment of assay performance requires appropriate statistical analysis of confirmatory data using appropriate reagents, assay conditions, and control compounds. The assessment is made from planned experiments, and the analytical results must satisfy predefined acceptance criteria. If control compounds or reagents are available, the assay sensitivity and pharmacology are quickly evaluated.

5.2.2 In-Study Validation

In-study validation is needed to verify that an assay remains acceptable during its routine use. For assays to be conducted in automated (larger compound screening, HTS) or even semi-automated (a series of compounds during SAR) modes, the assay must be adapted to microtiter plate volumes that are standard in preclinical screening laboratories. Therefore, plate acceptance testing is required where the assay is run in several microtiter plates (at least 96-well plates). From this data, statistical measures of assay performance, such as Z-factors, are calculated. Some assays might require additional experiments to validate the automation and scale-up that might not have been addressed in earlier stages. The plates should contain appropriate maximum and minimum control samples to serve as quality controls for each run and indicate the assay performance. If positive and negative control compounds are available, they are used to establish maximum and minimum (or basal) signals as appropriate. This will allow the developer to identify procedural errors and evaluate the assay's ability over time. Examining a randomly selected subset of test compounds at multiple concentrations monitors parallelism of the test and standard curve samples.

5.2.3 Cross-Validation

Cross-validation is required if an assay is transferred from the individual developer's team to a high-throughput screening center or other laboratories collaborating on the project. More broadly, this procedure is used at any stage to verify that an acceptable level of agreement exists in analytical results before and after procedural changes to an assay (reagents, instrumentation, personnel, lab location, etc.) and between results from two or more assays or laboratories. Typically, each laboratory performs the assay with a subset of compounds using the same well-documented protocols. The agreement in results is compared to predefined criteria that specify the assay's allowable performance during transfer. Note that the modification of assays to miniaturized 384-and 1,536-well microtiter plate formats, which minimize costly reagent use, and increase throughput, is not trivial. These formats should be rigorously validated before changing the assay operation from a 96-well format to higher density plates. The assumption that a reduction in volume will not affect the results is not valid. Note that this might happen inadvertently if assay methods are transferred to collaborators and remote labs.

5.2.4 Critical Path

Whether intended for a chemical probe or drug discovery efforts, the entire compound development program encompasses a series of assays, which have been subjected to the process described above. These assays are set in place to answer key questions along the development path to identify compounds with desired properties. For example, assays acting as "counter-screens" can identify direct interference with the detection technology. Orthogonal assays serve to provide additional evidence for targeted activity. Selectivity assays can provide information on the general specificity of a compound or compound series. Biophysical assays are used to confirm the direct binding of a compound to the target. Cell-based assays are implemented to measure the efficacy of a compound in disease-relevant cell types with specific biomarkers. In vivo assays can serve as models of the disease, while proof-of-concept clinical assays serve as a measure of efficacy in humans. Placing the right assays at the appropriate points will define the success of a program, and the chosen configuration of these assays is referred to as the "critical path."

5.3 Receptor Binding Assays in HTS

Receptor binding assay formats for HTS and lead optimization applications are critical considerations requiring appropriate selection of detection technologies, instrumentation, assay reagents, reaction conditions, and basic concepts in receptor binding analysis as applied to assay development. Circumstances that address high-affinity binders and Hill slope variations are also described as most useful for data analysis and troubleshooting. A discussion on scintillation proximity (SPA), filtration binding, and fluorescence polarization (FP) assays for receptor binding analysis is also included with detailed accounts on assay development using these technologies.

There are two typical assay formats used to analyze receptor-ligand interactions in screening applications, filtration, and scintillation proximity assay (SPA). Both formats utilize a radiolabeled ligand and a receptor source (membranes, soluble/purified). Receptor binding assays using non-radioactive formats (fluorescence polarization, time-resolved fluorescence, etc.), which are continually being investigated for feasibility, would have similar assay development schemes to those presented in this document.

Selection of the detection method to be used (SPA, filtration, non-radioactive) is the first step to receptor binding assay development. In some cases, the investigation into more than one format may be required to meet the following desired receptor binding criteria:

- Low nonspecific binding (NSB): 80% specific binding at the Kd concentration of the radioligand.
- Less than 10% of the added radioligand should be bound (zone A).
- Steady-state obtained and stability of signal maintained.
- For competition assays, the radioligand concentration should be at or below the dose-response in the absence of an added receptor.
- Reproducible.
- Appropriate signal window (i.e., Z-factor > 0.4, SD window > 2 SD units).

While developing receptor binding assays, some experiments are performed iteratively to achieve full optimization. Also, preliminary experiments are required to assess the system.

In many instances, a multi-variable experimental design is set up to investigate the impact of several parameters simultaneously or to determine the optimum level of a factor. It is recommended that full assay optimization be performed in collaboration with an individual trained in experimental design (Figure 5.2).

Quality reagents are one of the most important factors involved in assay development. Validated reagents of sufficient quantity are critical for successful screen efforts over a long period. The primary reagents required for a radioactive receptor binding assay, which are discussed on the following pages, are receptors (membranes or purified) and radioligands.

5.3.1 Scintillation Proximity Assays (SPA)

SPA assays do not require a separation of free and bound radioligand, and therefore are amenable to screening applications. A diagram for a standard receptor binding SPA is shown in Figure 5.3.

The advantages of the SPA assay include:

- Non-separation method.
- No scintillation cocktail required.
- Reduced liquid radioactive waste.
- Reduced handling steps (add, incubate, read).
- Multiple bead types (WGA, PEI-coated, etc.).

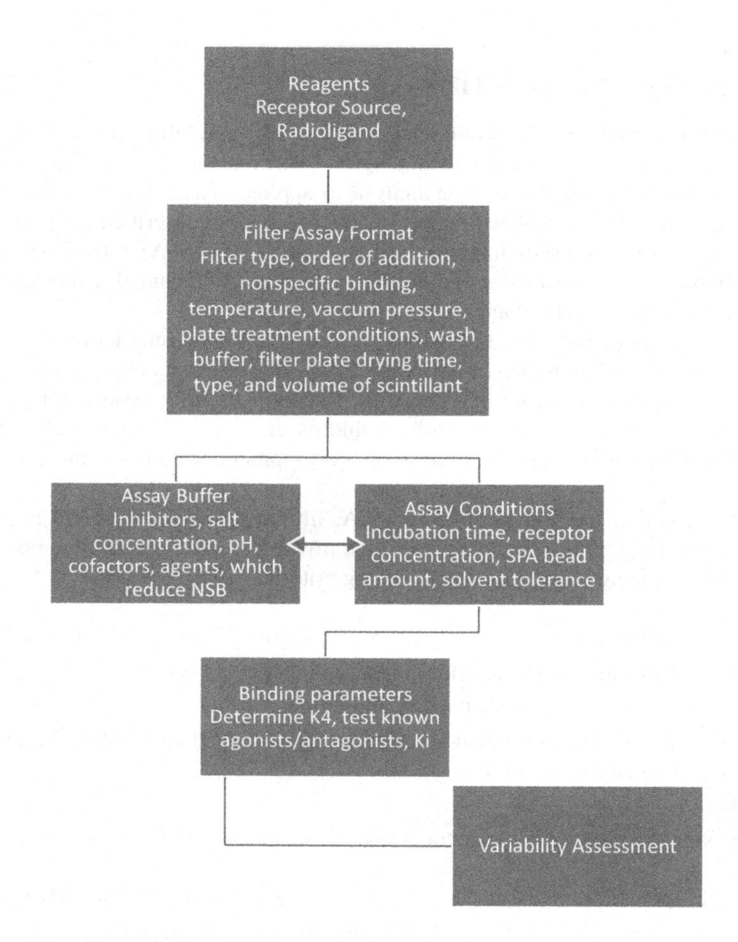

FIGURE 5.2 Flowchart of steps to assay development for filter format.

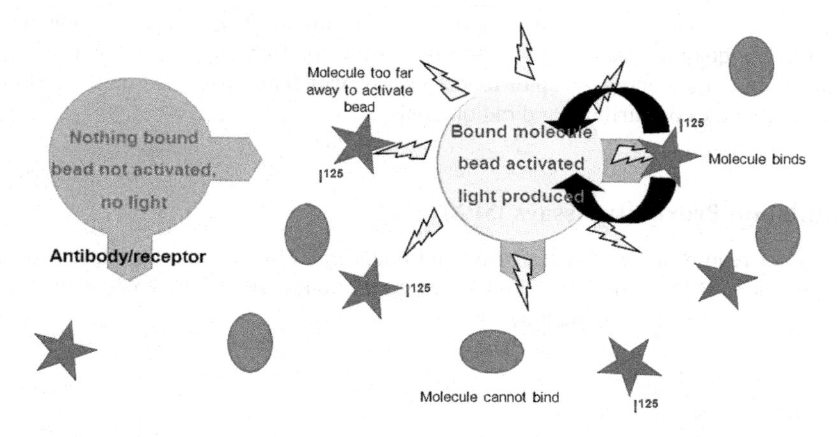

FIGURE 5.3 HTS radioligand binding assay for multiple radioligands such as I125, 3H, and 33P.

The disadvantages include:

- More expensive—requires license.
- Lower counting efficiency.
- Primarily for 3H and 125I (33P, 35S possible).
- Non-proximity effects.
- Quenching by colored compounds.
- Difficult to perform kinetic experiments.
- Bead settling effects.

General steps for a SPA assay:

1. Add and incubate test compound radioligand, receptor, and SPA beads in a plate (in some cases, the SPA beads are added at a later time point).
2. Count plates in the microplate scintillation counter. The appropriate settling time needs to be determined experimentally.

The main components of a SPA receptor binding assay format include bead type, plate type, the order of addition, non-specific binding (NSB)/non-proximity effects, and temperature. The SPA bead surface-coupling molecule selected for use in a receptor binding assay must be able to capture the receptor of interest with minimal interaction to the radioligand itself. Two types of SPA beads are available: plastic SPA beads, made of polyvinyl toluene (PVT), act as a solid solvent for diphenylanthracine (DPA) scintillant incorporated into the bead A Glass SPA bead, or Yttrium silicate (YSi), uses cerium ions within a crystal lattice scintillation process. YSi is a more efficient scintillator than PVT, but YSi SPA beads require continuous mixing even during dispensing.

Typical experiments to investigate the nonspecific binding of radioligand to SPA beads include varying the amount of radioligand (above and below the predicated Kd value) and the number of SPA beads (0.1 mg to 1 mg) in the absence of added membrane protein. This experiment's results can identify the proper type of SPA beads to use in future experiments and the baseline background due to non-proximity effects. Additives are useful in decreasing high levels of nonspecific binding of radioligand to the SPA beads.

5.3.2 Filtration Assays

Filter assays differ from SPA because the separation of free radioligand and radioligand bound to the receptor is required for measurement. However, many of the assay development and optimization steps are the same.

Advantages:

- Less color quenching.
- A traditional, trusted method.
- Higher efficiency than SPA.
- Easier kinetic experiments (association/dissociation).

Disadvantages:

- Separation method (dissociation of ligand).
- Generated large volumes of liquid waste.
- Variable vacuum across the plate.
- Nonspecific binding to filters.

- Accumulation of radioactivity on unit.
- Requires more handling steps.

General steps for a filtration assay:

- Add and incubate test compound radioligand and receptor in a plate (this is a separate plate or, if validated, the filtration plate directly).
- Apply vacuum to "trap" receptor, bound radioligand onto the filter, and remove the unbound radioligand. Wash several times with an appropriate buffer to minimize nonspecific binding.
- Allow filters to dry. Add liquid scintillation cocktail or other scintillant (i.e., solid Meltilex).
- Count filters in a microplate scintillation counter. Some time between adding the scintillant and counting is required.

Depending on the radioligand, receptor, and other assay factors, it is necessary to perform experiments with more than one type of filter to determine the best system under investigation.

The speed of separation is important, particularly for lower affinity interactions (< 1 nM), and is influenced by the filter plate type. Dissociation of bound radioligand from a receptor interaction with an affinity of 1 nM can occur under 2 min. Lower affinity interactions can dissociate even more quickly when the separation process disrupts the equilibrium (Figure 5.4).

5.4 In Vitro Biochemical Assays

When developing enzyme assays for HTS, the target enzyme's integrity is critical to the quality of the HTS, and the actives, or "hits," identified through the screens. The incorrect identity or lack of enzymatic purity of the enzyme preparation will significantly affect a screen's results. Of significance are the consequences of impure and misidentified enzyme preparations, potential steps taken to avoid measurement of the wrong activity, and methods to validate the enzymatic purity of enzyme preparation.

5.4.1 Definitions

- Enzyme identity: Enzyme identity determination confirms that the protein preparation in, fact, contains the enzyme of interest. Enzyme identity is confirmed by demonstrating that

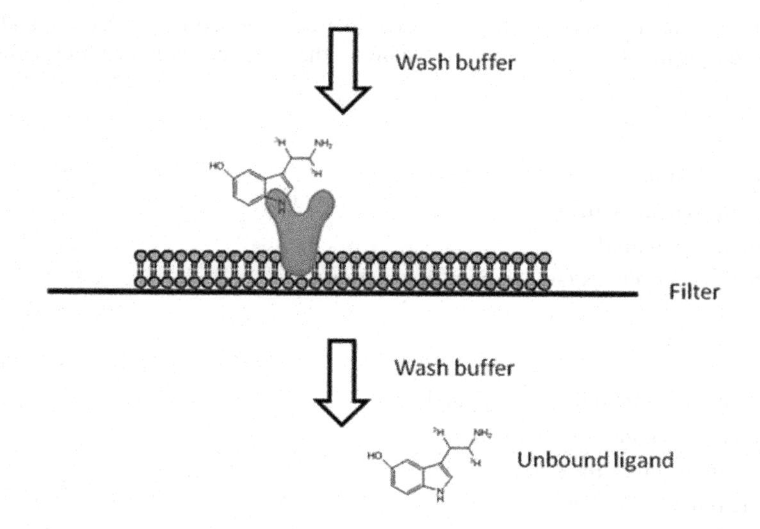

FIGURE 5.4 Diagram for a standard filtration assay.

the experimentally determined primary amino acid sequence matches the predicted primary amino acid sequence.

- Mass purity: Mass purity refers to the protein percentage in a preparation that is the target enzyme or protein. For instance, 90 μg of the enzyme in a solution containing 100 μg of protein is considered 90% pure.
- Enzymatic purity or activity purity: Enzymatic purity or activity purity refers to the fraction of activity observed in an assay that comes from a single enzyme. Typically, suppose 100% (or nearly so) of the observed activity in an enzyme assay is derived from a single enzyme. In that case, the enzyme preparation is considered enzymatically pure, even if it lacks mass purity. If two or more activities are detected in an enzyme assay, the enzyme preparation is enzymatically impure. Note that enzymatic purity is not the same as specific activity, enzymatic activity (in defined units) per unit mass of protein (typically mg of protein).
- Interrelationships between identity, mass, and enzymatic purity: High mass purity and high specific activity are highly desirable in an enzyme used for screening because it decreases the probability of measuring contaminating enzyme activities. However, high mass purity or high specific activity alone does not guarantee enzymatic purity. On the other hand, enzymatically pure preparations may have poor mass purity. It is also possible to have an enzymatically pure preparation with all the activity coming from the wrong enzyme! For enzyme assays, enzymatic purity must be established before the screening (unless intentionally screening with mixed enzymes). Arguably, enzyme identity and enzymatic purity are the most critical factors. It is possible to have a valid enzyme assay with poor (or no) mass purity if it is demonstrated that 100% of the observed activity comes from the target enzyme.
- Consequences of using enzymatically impure enzyme preparations: The consequences of using enzymatically impure enzyme preparations for a screen are multiple and far-reaching. First, if the lot of enzymes used for assay development is enzymatically impure with the chosen substrate and format, the assay conditions could be optimized wrong enzyme activity. The contaminating activity may not be revealed until after the screen, when abnormally shaped IC50 curves are obtained. Inhibitors obtained from such a screen will likely be a mixture of target and/or non-target inhibitors. Depending on the fraction of the signal contributed by the contaminating activity, the most potent inhibitors are non-selective and inhibit both/all enzyme activities present. In other words, the screen may produce hits that are biased towards non-selective inhibitors. These compounds interfere with the assay format (like colored compounds), "nuisance" hits such as aggregators/reactive compounds, or a combination of these undesirable results. Thus, many or most target selective compounds may not appear as hits. Furthermore, compounds in the screening database would be annotated with false and misleading data.

5.4.2 Signs of Enzymatic Contamination

- Inhibitor IC50 values $\geq$ 10-fold different compared to literature or gold standard assay.
- Inhibitor IC50 slopes are shallow (Hill slope < 1).
- Unable to reach complete inhibition of activity at high concentrations of inhibitor.
- Biphasic IC50 curves.
- IC50 curves that plateau at significantly less than 100% enzyme activity at low inhibitor concentrations.
- Km values do not match the expected value.
- Abnormally shaped Km plot.
- Unexpected substrate specificities.
- Lack of reproducible activity and/or IC50 values between two different assay formats with the same enzyme preparation.

- Different enzyme sources (e.g., from different vendors) or different batches of the enzyme (produced in the same lab) produce different IC50 values or Hill slopes.
- Post-screen: a high percentage of screen hits display Hill slopes that are very broad or do not reach complete inhibition.

5.4.3 Solutions for Enzymatic Contamination

- Purify enzyme further (add more steps to eliminate contaminating enzymes) or evaluate enzyme preparations from external or commercial suppliers.
- Use a substrate that is a more specific target enzyme.
- Optimize/change buffer conditions to eliminate other activities' detection (e.g., change pH or NaCl concentration).
- Change assay format to one that is a more specific target of interest.
- Use multiple inhibitors for IC50 experiments, instead of just one, in case the problem lies with the reference inhibitor compound.
- Use inhibitors of contaminating activity in the assay buffer: The use of protease and phosphatase inhibitor cocktails is necessary to inhibit contaminating activities. EDTA can sometimes be used to eliminate Mg^{2+}-dependent contaminating activities, assuming the target enzyme does not require a divalent metal ion like Mg^{2+} or Mn^{2+}. Control experiments should be undertaken to ensure any inhibitors do not interfere with the target protein activity.

5.4.4 Batch Testing

Each new batch of enzymes should be subject to some level of enzymatic purity testing since there may be contaminating enzymes present in each new preparation due to variability in expression and purification. Thus, both large- and small-scale purifications of enzymes need to be validated, even when the purification protocol remains the same. Batch-to-batch variability and scale-up of enzyme purifications for screening could result in subtle changes that result in, for example, differences in the percentage of target protein proteolysis or host enzyme impurities. At a minimum, new batch testing might include performing SDS-PAGE analysis for mass purity and identity along with using the most selective reference inhibitor and confirming that the IC50 value and Hill slope obtained using the new batch of enzyme matches the original batch. Ideally, there should only be one or two lots of enzymes—one small one for assay development and one large bulk lot for screening/follow-up. Multiple smaller batches are pooled before assay development/validation. In theory, but not necessarily in practice, the screening lot should get the most rigorous validation (before screening).

5.4.4.1 Identity and Mass Purity

Confirming enzyme identity is important because it prevents screening with the wrong enzyme. This problem occasionally arises, particularly when the target is expressed in a heterologous host. Thus, the determination of protein identity and mass purity is essential before any assay development and HTS. In reality, no protein is purified to absolute homogeneity. After purification, the target protein may contain contaminants derived either from the target protein itself or from host proteins. The remaining contaminants in a protein preparation may or may not interfere with the assay format under consideration.

5.4.4.2 Methods for Confirming Identity and Mass Purity

Proteins used for HTS are expressed as a recombinant form in a heterologous host. This form of expression may result in denatured, aggregated, or proteolyzed forms of the target protein. Several methods are used to assess sample purity with the choice depending on sample availability, required accuracy, and sensitivity. A simple wavelength scan also allows an assessment of non-proteinaceous contamination such as DNA/RNA.

5.4.4.3 Protein Stain of SDS-PAGE

A typical first assessment for sample purity is the use of sodium dodecyl sulfate-polyacrylamide gel electrophoresis (SDS-PAGE) with either Coomassie Blue staining or the more sensitive silver staining. These techniques are easy, rapid, and inexpensive. Gradient SDS gels (e.g., 4–20%) allow the detection of a wide range of molecular weights and are very useful for assessing sample purity. Overloading the gel with 25–50 µg of protein allows more sensitive detection of contaminating proteins. Densitometry of the stained gel allows some estimation of purity.

5.4.4.4 Western Blot with the Specific Antibody

Western blotting with antibodies specific to the target protein allows confirmation of identity and a determination of the target protein's intactness.

5.4.4.5 Analytical Gel Filtration

Analytical gel filtration is used to assess some contaminants' presence under native conditions and the presence and amount of target protein aggregates. A symmetrical peak eluting at the predicted molecular weight is indicative of a pure single species with no aggregation or degradation. Additional peaks eluting before the protein of interest be aggregates, and peaks eluting after may be degradation products. To confirm, fractions are collected and analyzed by western blotting and mass spectrometry to assess if the additional peaks are derived from the protein of interest.

5.4.4.6 Reversed-Phase HPLC

Reversed-phase HPLC (RP-HPLC) using a stationary phase, such as C4 or C8, is another rapid method for assessing target purity and contaminants in the protein sample. UV detection at 280 nm is typically used to monitor proteins, but when RP-HPLC is used in combination with a diode array detector, the simultaneous monitoring of a large number of wavelengths allows for detecting non-proteinaceous material as well.

5.4.4.7 Mass Spectrometry

Mass spectrometry (MS) is the best technique (least ambiguous) for establishing protein identity because it provides an accurate direct measurement of protein mass. Mass accuracy will depend on the size of the protein but is typically around 0.01%. Furthermore, mass spectrometry provides the best approach to measuring the presence of impurities and their mass as well, hence the possibility of identification. Although many labs do not possess the requisite equipment or expertise for mass spectrometry, many mass spectrometry facilities will characterize samples as a fee-based service.

5.4.4.8 Whole Mass for Protein

Matrix-assisted laser desorption ionization (MALDI) time-of-flight (TOF) mass spectrometry is typically used for mass protein measurement because it can analyze proteins over a wide mass range, up to 200 kDa or higher. Proteins should be desalted, e.g., using a C4 ZipTip (Millipore Co.). Samples are deposited onto an α-cyano-4-hydroxycinnamic acid matrix prepared in an aqueous solvent containing 50% acetonitrile and ten mM ammonium citrate. Protein mass is determined using a MALDI TOF mass spectrometer. A comparison of the measured mass with the predicted mass allows confirmation of identity. Masses higher than predicted may indicate protein modifications, either post-translational or experimental, e.g., oxidation. Masses lower may be degradation products. Additional peaks in the spectrum may indicate contaminants' presence, although it should be remembered that ionization efficiencies may differ. For MALDI TOF, depending on the measured molecular size and the instrument used, mass accuracy is typically approximately 10 ppm to 0.01%.

5.4.4.9 Peptide Mass Finger Printing

The identity of a protein is confirmed using peptide mass fingerprinting. In this technique, peptide fragments are generated by in-gel tryptic digestion of a Coomassie Blue–stained protein band excised from a 1-D SDS-PAGE gel. The resulting peptides are analyzed using MALDI TOF/TOF MS, and observed peptide masses compared to the NCBI non-redundant database using a search algorithm such as the MASCOT MS/MS Ions search algorithm (Matrix Science: www.matrixscience.com). The observed masses of all the peptides are compared to the calculated masses of the expected peptides resulting from the target protein's tryptic cleavage.

5.4.4.10 Edman Sequencing

In addition to mass spectrometry, N-terminal Edman sequencing is used to confirm protein identity and assess the homogeneity among primary amino acid sequences in the purified target protein. To identify internal sequences from the target protein, proteins are separated by SDS-PAGE and then transferred to sequencing-grade PVDF membranes. Membranes are stained with Coomassie Blue R-250 for three minutes, then bands excised for tryptic peptide analysis. Peptides are separated by reversed-phase HPLC, and N-terminal Edman sequencing is then performed on the peptides using a protein sequencer.

5.4.4.11 Crude Enzyme Preparations

Enzyme assays are available for less pure proteins, and even cell lysates, and whole serum. For example, an activity-based probe is a highly selective substrate for measuring the protease dipeptidyl aminopeptidase 1 (DPAP1) activity in *Plasmodium falciparum* cell lysates and for Cathepsin C in rat liver extracts is available. Furthermore, the whole serum is used as a source of the enzyme serum paraoxonase/arylesterase 1 (PON1) to develop an enzyme assay for HTS. PON1 is the only enzyme in serum capable of hydrolyzing the chemical paraoxon. In these cases, a highly selective substrate is used such that only the target enzyme can efficiently convert it to the product in the time frame of the reaction. Enzyme assays that use these crude sources of enzyme require extra rigor in validating enzymatic purity and identity. These assays are validated with known selective inhibitors and/or multiple methods outlined below.

5.4.4.12 Commercial Enzymes

Commercial enzymes may be misidentified, have poor mass purity, and display poor enzymatic purity under a particular assay condition. Therefore, even for a commercially obtained enzyme, it is recommended that the identity of the target protein be confirmed to ensure that not only is the correct protein being used but that it is also from the correct species. Carrying out a high throughput screen on the incorrect target or a target from the wrong species is an expensive control experiment. The identity of the target, including primary sequence confirmation, is critical.

5.4.4.13 Co-Purification of Contaminating Enzymes

Host enzymes can co-purify with the recombinant target enzyme. These contaminating host enzymes may have the size and physical-chemical properties (like the isoelectric point) that are indistinguishable from those of the target enzyme, making their presence in a preparation difficult to detect. This can lead to misleading purity determinations. Multiple identity and mass purity determination methods can reveal co-purifying contaminants that may have activity in the assay. Enzymatic purity analysis can also reveal this contaminating activity.

5.4.4.14 Mock Parallel Purification

One method used to aid in establishing the identity of a recombinant enzyme preparation is to use an enzymatically inactive site-directed mutant (a mutant of the target that loses all activity) to make inactive enzyme and then apply the same purification protocol to both the wild-type enzyme, and the mutant. The idea is that, unlike the wild-type enzyme, the mutant-derived enzyme preparation should have no activity in the assay, demonstrating that the activity originates from the recombinant protein, not from contaminating host proteins. An assumption is that the mutation does not alter the overall structure of the enzyme. This is sometimes also done with empty vector constructs instead of mutant enzymes. While this is a useful technique, it is still recommended that all enzyme preparations to be used for screening be tested for identity, mass, and enzymatic purity.

5.4.4.15 Reversal of Enzyme Activity

Contaminating enzymes can reverse the enzyme reaction by converting the product back to substrate or into a different, undetected product. For instance, a contaminating phosphatase in a kinase preparation may dephosphorylate the product and alter the observed enzyme kinetics, depending on the kinase format chosen. Inhibitors of the contaminating activity, e.g., phosphatase inhibitors, are used to prevent this. The presence of phosphatases in kinase assays may be difficult to detect. A common method is to test the kinase activity in the presence and absence of broad activity phosphatase inhibitors, such as sodium orthovanadate. Lack of an effect by these inhibitors suggests that phosphatase activity is not a problem in the assay. Increasing the mass purity of the enzyme preparation can also eliminate such issues.

5.4.5 Detecting Enzyme Impurities

How an assay is designed and configured can influence whether or not contaminating enzyme activity is detected in the assay. In practice, if a contaminating enzyme is present, but not detected in the final assay, then there is no problem. The choice of substrate, enzyme concentration, and assay format can profoundly impact the probability of detecting any enzyme impurities if present.

5.4.5.1 Consequences of Substrate Selectivity

- Selective substrates: The use of a selective substrate is an excellent method of reducing the chances of detecting any contaminating enzymes present in an enzyme preparation. If only the target enzyme generates a detectable signal, any contaminating enzymes present become irrelevant since they do not contribute to the assay window. Extremely selective substrates have been used to detect specific enzyme activity in whole-cell lysates (e.g., luciferin for cell-based luciferase assays) or whole serum (e.g., hydrolysis of paraoxon by PON1 in serum).
- Non-selective substrates: Using less selective substrates, those that are converted to product by many enzymes, increases the probability that contaminating enzymes will cause a problem. Therefore, non-selective substrates require the developer to obtain more data to demonstrate that the correct activity is being measured. For a kinase assay, the presence of a contaminating kinase may impact the assay depending on the substrate's selectivity. For instance, the polymer substrate poly-(Glu, Tyr) is phosphorylated by most tyrosine kinases, so this substrate will also detect contaminating tyrosine kinase activity if present. In contrast, using a natural protein or selective peptide substrate may reduce the chances of detecting contaminating kinase activity. Another example of a non-selective substrate is para-nitrophenol phosphate (pNPP), which is used as a substrate for a wide variety of phosphatases.

5.4.5.2 Substrate Km

Substrate selectivity has the largest impact on whether contaminating enzyme activity is detected in an assay. However, when choosing between equally selective substrates, the substrate with the lowest Km is preferable (with all other considerations being equal). When substrates are used that have a high Km value, higher amounts of the substrate are needed in the reaction to obtain a good assay signal. However, with higher substrate concentration, especially for non-selective substrates, the chances are greater for detecting any contaminating enzyme activity that may be present. The use of substrates at concentrations at or below Km value will select for detection of the enzyme in the preparation with the greatest activity towards the substrate. Furthermore, the substrate concentration should be kept at $\leq$ Km to ensure the sensitive detection of competitive substrate inhibitors, if desired.

5.4.5.3 Enzyme Concentration

The concentration of enzyme used in an assay can determine whether contaminating enzymes, if present, are detected or not. Using high concentrations of the target enzyme, based on the mass purity, increases the risk of detecting contaminating activity, especially for non-selective substrates. Conversely, using a low 1 nM enzyme concentration, for example, means that picomolar levels of contaminating activity would need to be detected to interfere with the assay. Coupled enzyme assays are particularly vulnerable to the detection of impurity activities because high concentrations of the coupling enzymes, which may also be contaminated with interfering activities, are usually added to not be a rate-limiting factor in the assay.

5.4.5.4 Format Selection

Assay formats that are broadly applicable to a large class of enzymes are convenient but increase the odds of detecting any contaminating activity present. For example, adenosine diphosphate detection methods for measuring kinase activity will detect all kinases in preparation and even any ATPases present. Thus, these assay formats should be used with care, and enzymatic purity should be verified by multiple methods. Highly specific formats will reduce the odds of detecting non-target activity. A kinase assay can use a natural substrate protein and an antibody to detect phosphorylation at a specific residue. Formats that allow very sensitive detection of the product allow the use of low concentrations of enzyme, which avoids the detection of very low activity/low concentration contaminating enzymes

5.4.6 Validating Enzymatic Purity

Enzymatic purity is assessed using inhibitor-based studies, substrate-based studies, and/or comparison studies. Inhibitor-based studies are the most commonly used and the single best way to validate enzymatic purity. Combinations of these methods can also be used to enhance confidence in the assay. Enzymatic purity is highly substrate- and format-dependent. The same enzyme preparation is used with one substrate/format and has 100% of the detected activity come from the intended target enzyme. Still, a different substrate or format may reveal multiple enzyme activities that are present in the preparation. Note that high specific activity preparations may be obtained, but there could still be multiple enzymes present that perform the same reaction, and therefore the preparation would lack enzymatic purity. This can occur, if for instance, the contaminating enzyme(s) are the same size as the target or if the contaminating enzymes are present at a small percent by mass but with higher specific activity than the target enzyme.

5.4.6.1 Inhibitor-Based Studies

Inhibitors of enzymatic activity are critical tools and are the only practical tool to validate the enzymatic purity of enzyme preparations. Once an enzymatic assay has been established under kinetically valid conditions and optimized, inhibitors described in the literature enzyme are used to validate that only one enzyme activity is being measured. Inhibitors are usually small organic molecules but can also be small peptides or analogs of the natural substrate. In general, two types of inhibitors are used for this purpose—relatively selective inhibitors and non-selective inhibitors. Selective inhibitors are preferable in verifying activity purity, but non-selective or modestly selective inhibitors are also useful when there is no practical alternative. Inhibition by selective inhibitors increases the confidence that the correct activity is being measured. However, non-selective inhibitors within a given enzyme class will frequently have a reported IC50 value, and critical data is ascertained concerning activity purity. For example, staurosporine is a broad-spectrum kinase inhibitor used when a selective kinase inhibitor is not available. A small panel of non-selective inhibitors with a range of potencies can also be used to compare results to literature and increase confidence in the activity purity of the assay/enzyme preparation. Any known activators of enzyme activity can also be used as evidence of enzymatic identity. Three important values are derived from concentration-response inhibition curves that aid in enzymatic purity validation: IC50 value, Hill slope, and maximal inhibition.

For a complete evaluation of IC50 data as outlined here, maximum and minimum signal controls must be performed along with the inhibitor titration. Maximum controls should consist of enzyme reactions with no inhibitor—just DMSO. Minimum signal controls should be performed using DMSO only (no inhibitor) and leaving the enzyme out of the reaction (adding just buffer instead) to represent 100% enzyme inhibition.

5.4.6.2 IC50 Value

IC50 values for known inhibitors should match or be close to the literature values, with the caveat that different assay conditions (e.g., substrate concentration, total protein, pH, etc.) may alter apparent potencies. Alternatively, inhibitors are tested in a different validated assay format using the same enzyme preparation or a completely different enzyme source, for example, a commercially available enzyme. IC50 values can then be compared between the different formats. IC50 values are generally considered to be in close agreement if they differ by a factor of three or less.

5.4.6.3 Hill slope

The steepness or shallowness of the IC50 curve referred to as the Hill slope, can provide valuable information on whether a single enzyme is being inhibited. Inhibitors bind to a single binding site on the enzyme should yield concentration-response curves with a Hill slope of 1.0, based on the law of mass action. A negative sign in front of the Hill slope value may be ignored—the ± sign on a Hill slope signifies the curve's direction, which changes if the data is plotted using percent activity or percent inhibition. Both selective and non-selective enzyme inhibitors should display a concentration-response curve with a Hill slope of close to 1.0. Thus, after plotting a concentration-response curve for an inhibitor, there are three possible results when analyzing the slope:

- Hill slope = 1.0. This indicates a high probability that a single enzyme is generating the observed signal in the assay. An acceptable slope range under careful, manually performed experimental conditions is 0.8 to 1.2. The observation of this normal Hill slope using multiple inhibitors with a range of potencies greatly enhances confidence in the assay's enzymatic purity. Multiple inhibitors are particularly useful when only non-selective inhibitors are available.
- Hill slope < 1.0. A shallow slope (for example < 0.8) derived from the IC50 curve may indicate more than one enzyme contributing to the assay signal. This occurs when two or more enzymes generate the signal, but they have different but non-resolvable affinities inhibitors. The result is a blended IC50 curve that is broader than expected. If the two affinities are different enough to be resolved in the experiment, a biphasic curve will result. Thus, biphasic curves are also strongly suggestive of multiple activities present. However, in standard 10 points (1:3 dilutions) IC50 curves, a partial biphasic curve may appear as a single curve where the low concentrations of inhibitor produce a plateau significantly less than the expected 100% enzyme activity as determined by controls. This type of curve is due to multiple enzyme activities or an artifact of the experiment caused by misleading controls due to, for example, well position or edge effects. Differentiating these two possibilities requires follow-up experiments.
- Hill slope > 1.0. A steep slope (Hill slope >> 1.0, for example, > 1.5) may indicate that the inhibitor is either forming aggregates in aqueous solution and inhibiting non-specifically, chemically reacting with the enzyme, or chelating a required co-factor. This type of inhibitor

cannot be used in enzymatic purity validation studies. One important exception to this rule is inhibitors with IC50 values lower than half the active enzyme concentration in the assay—these inhibitors are sometimes referred to as tight-binding inhibitors. These inhibitors are sometimes exquisitely specific to the enzyme target, and very potent, but result in steep Hill slopes because they are titrating enzymes. If assay sensitivity allows, it may be possible to lower the enzyme concentration in the reaction below twice the IC50 value (even if only for validation studies) and thus demonstrate a Hill slope of 1.0 with tight-binding inhibitors.

5.4.6.3.1 Understanding Hill Slope

- A normal Hill slope supports evidence for enzymatic purity in the developed assay, while an unexpected Hill slope requires further investigation into the enzymatic purity of the enzyme preparation.
- Incomplete curves may give a less accurate Hill slope—the best data is obtained when a complete top and bottom of the curve are obtained. When partial curves are obtained because high concentrations of an inhibitor cannot be achieved, Hill slope information is obtained by fitting the inhibition data using a three-parameter logistic fit with the 100% inhibition value (max or min) set equal to the average value of the "no enzyme" control. Achieving high compound concentrations in an assay may be limited by compound solubility or DMSO tolerance.
- Imprecise and/or inaccurate pipetting will shift the Hill slope.
- High assay variability or too few data points can lead to unreliable Hill slope determinations.
- Method of dilution is important—the purpose of verifying enzymatic purity, change tips between different concentrations in a serial dilution, since this prevents carry-over of a compound that could result in erroneous concentrations. For HTS hit confirmation and automated follow-up assays, tip changing is often impractical because tips are expensive or because compounds are being diluted using automated equipment with fixed tips.
- For small molecules, use 100% DMSO as a diluent in the initial serial dilution series. These dilutions can then be further diluted into assay buffer for assaying. This minimizes compound precipitation at high concentrations when diluted into aqueous solutions, altering actual compound concentrations.
- An impure compound (a mixture of different inhibitors) may also generate shallow Hill slopes due to different affinities targets.
- Compound solubility problems can result in a shallow or steep slope.
- Graphing software programs capable of fitting inhibition data with a four-parameter logistic fit will return a value Hill slope.
- For a Hill slope of 1.0, there should be an 81-fold inhibitor concentration difference between 10% and 90% inhibition.
- Errant data points will alter the slope—suspected outlier data points should be masked (temporarily removed from the curve). The curve fitting is repeated to see if masking the data point(s) dramatically improves the fit quality.
- Rarely, an enzyme may have more than one binding site, and the Hill slope should be a higher integer (e.g., 2.0, 3.0, or higher).
- It is conceivable that multiple forms of the same enzyme might be present in the assay (for example, due to heterogeneous post-translational modification) and that they may have different affinities for an inhibitor. If the two affinities cannot be resolved, the result will broaden the IC50 curve.
- It is theoretically possible to have two very similar enzymes (i.e., isozymes or isoforms) present in the enzyme preparation with identical affinities for an inhibitor resulting in ideally shaped IC50 curves. Isoform selective inhibitors (sometimes discovered later) may show the contamination.

5.4.6.3.2 Maximal Inhibition

The highest concentrations in a complete IC50 curve should result in close to 100% inhibition of the assay signal based on controls with and without enzyme. Even with a Hill slope = 1.0, lack of complete inhibition is strongly suggestive that more than one enzyme activity is being measured. This can occur if the inhibitor only inhibits one of the enzymes present but does not inhibit the other enzymes contributing to the assay signal.

Such curves can have a "normal" shape, but at the highest concentrations of inhibitor, the curve plateaus (flattens out) at significantly less than 100% inhibition. Partial curves with normal Hill slopes are exempted from this criterion. Partial or incomplete curves show some inhibition at the highest inhibitor concentrations but lack data points displaying complete (100%) inhibition based on controls, i.e., no clear plateau.

Generally, the most accurate Hill slopes for partial curves will be obtained using a three-parameter fit where 100% inhibition is fixed to equal the average value from control wells that represent no enzyme activity (such as by leaving the enzyme out of the reaction). The most common cause of partial curves is simply the compound's low potency to inhibit the target enzyme. Poor compound solubility at higher concentrations could also explain a lack of complete inhibition. Still, in that case, the curve is unlikely to have a normal appearance and a Hill slope of 1.0.

In summary, while inhibitor studies that result in expected IC50 values, display expected Hill slopes, and reach complete inhibition are not infallible proof of enzymatic purity, they provide strong evidence that only one enzyme species is being measured. Conversely, inhibitor studies that result in un-expected IC50 values, have unexpected Hill slopes, and/or fail to achieve complete signal inhibition are not proof of contaminating enzyme activity but are strong warning signs that should not be ignored. These results require further investigation to either rule out enzyme contamination, lay the blame elsewhere, prove enzyme contamination, and require a change of enzyme source before proceeding. It is especially troubling when these warning signs are observed for multiple inhibitors.

5.4.7 Substrate-Based Studies

If no suitable inhibitors are available, or to further confirm enzymatic purity, substrate-based studies are employed. Two approaches are used: substrate Km determinations and substrate selectivity studies.

5.4.7.1 Substrate Km Determination

Substrate Km determinations are usually done during assay development. The Km value should be close to the literature value (less than ten-fold difference), though different assay conditions can alter observed Km values. The Km plot (initial velocity versus substrate concentration) should follow a single-site rectangular hyperbolic curve giving a defined Vmax. Km values $\geq$ 10-fold different from literature values, and/or abnormally shaped curves suggest possible enzyme contamination or an error in enzyme identity. Hyperbolic curves may not be achievable if the Km value is very high, and assay format limitations preclude testing sufficiently high substrate concentrations.

5.4.7.2 Substrate Selectivity Studies

Different substrates with the same enzyme target are tested to demonstrate selectivity. These studies are done by performing Km determinations and comparing kcat/Km values to the literature or expected selectivity. However, it is more easily performed by testing the different substrates at the same concentration, a concentration well below the expected Km value. In this case, the initial velocity will be proportional to kcat/Km, and therefore the measured velocities will allow a relative determination of how good a substrate is a target (Figure 5.5).

If substrate selectivity does not match expectations, it is a sign of contamination or misidentification of the enzyme preparation. Similar substrates that should not result in measurable activity using the target enzyme can also exclude certain enzymes that might be contaminants in the primary assay.

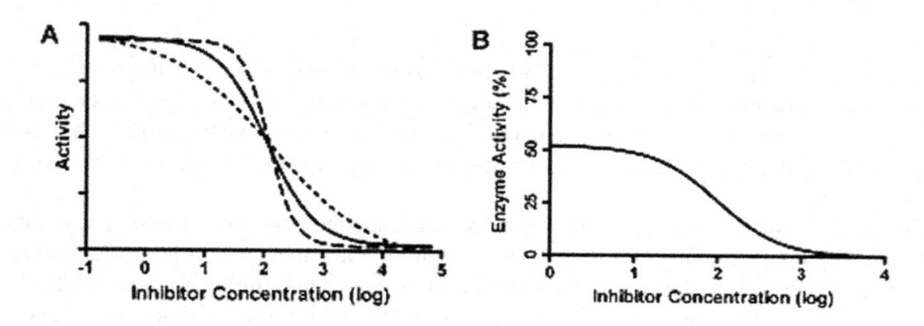

FIGURE 5.5 Left: IC50 curves with a Hill slope of 1.0 (solid line), 2.0 (dashed), 0.5 (dotted) (A); partial biphasic graph (B). Right: complete IC50 curve (solid line) compared to an incomplete maximal inhibition curve (dashed line). Note that both curves have a Hill slope of 1.0.

5.4.7.3 Comparison Studies

For some little-studied enzymes, no or few inhibitors have been identified, and substrate selectivity is unknown. For these targets, inhibitor studies and substrate studies are limited or not possible due to the availability of inhibitors and substrates. In these cases, comparison studies are done to aid in verifying purity. However, the evidence for enzymatic purity generated is not as strong as with the inhibitor and substrate-based studies.

5.4.7.4 Enzyme Source

The enzyme preparation under scrutiny may be compared to other enzyme preparations from different sources, such as a commercially generated enzyme. The basis for this comparison study is that different purification methods (and ideally different source organisms, e.g., mammalian versus insect cells) are unlikely to generate the same contaminating enzymes at the same concentrations. An exception would be enzymes that co-purify due to physical association. Different enzyme sources are compared by performing Km determination studies with each enzyme using the same substrate. The Km values should be within three-fold of each other if the same enzyme activity is being measured. The curve should also follow a single-site rectangular hyperbolic curve giving a defined Vmax (assuming high enough concentrations of the substrate are used). For recombinant enzymes, one can also generate enzyme inactive mutants (at least empty vector control cells) to help establish that a host enzyme is not being measured. It may also be possible for a highly selective substrate to demonstrate that there is no measurable target enzyme activity in host cell lysates, so there is little possibility of detecting host enzyme contaminants in the assay.

5.4.7.5 Format Comparison

In format comparison studies, the same enzyme preparation activities are determined using two different formats. If the same enzyme is measured in both formats (in the same assay buffer and substrate concentration), then such a comparison should yield similar activity in both assays (within ten-fold). Since different formats are used, standards would likely be required to convert assay signal to the product produced. Lack of activity in one format would be a potential warning sign that different enzymes are being measured in the two assays. This is most useful if one format is a highly selective enzyme in question (e.g., a gold-standard assay), and this assay is used to validate a less selective format. For example, for kinases, an assay where a specific antibody is used to detect phosphorylated protein products could be compared to an ADP detection format, which detects all ATPase activity. Similar results would support the purity of the enzyme preparation. Furthermore, format comparison studies are useful if even just one non-selective weak inhibitor is a known target. In this case, an IC50 value comparison is made using different formats to gain confidence in the assay's enzymatic purity.

5.5 Enzymatic Assays for HTS

Enzymes are important to drug targets. Many marketed drugs today function through the inhibition of enzymes mediating disease phenotypes. To design, develop, and validate robust enzymatic assays for HTS applications, it is critical to have a thorough understanding of enzyme biochemistry and the kinetics of enzyme action. The basic concepts of enzyme kinetics, selection of appropriate substrates for assay design, estimation and significance of Km and Vmax, and the intrinsic kinetic parameters of enzyme targets are presented here.

Enzyme inhibitors are an important class of pharmacological agents. Often these molecules are competitive, reversible inhibitors of substrate binding. This section describes the development and validation of assays for the identification of competitive, reversible inhibitors. In some cases, other mechanisms of action may be desirable, which would require a different assay design. A separate approach should be used if seeking a non-competitive mechanism that is beyond the scope of this document and should be discussed with an enzymologist and chemist.

5.5.1 Basic Concept

Enzymes are biological catalysts involved in important pathways that allow chemical reactions to occur at higher rates (velocities) than would be possible without the enzyme. Enzymes are generally globular proteins that have one or more substrate binding sites. The kinetic behavior for many enzymes is explained with a simple model proposed during the 1900s:

$$E + S \underset{k_{-1}}{\overset{k_1}{\rightleftarrows}} ES \xrightarrow{k_2} E + P$$

E is an enzyme, S is a substrate, and P is a product (or products). ES is an enzyme-substrate complex that is formed before the catalytic reaction. Term k1 is the rate constant for enzyme-substrate complex (ES) formation, and k-1 is the dissociation rate of the ES complex. In this model, the overall rate-limiting step in the reaction is the ES complex's breakdown to yield product, which can proceed with rate constant k2. The reverse reaction (E + P → ES) is generally assumed to be negligible.

Assuming rapid equilibrium between reactants (enzyme and substrate) and the enzyme-substrate complex resulted in mathematical descriptions of enzymes' kinetic behavior based on the substrate concentration. The most widely accepted equation, derived independently by Henri and subsequently by Michaelis and Menten, relates the velocity of the reaction to the substrate concentration as shown in the equation below, which is typically referred to as the Michaelis-Menten equation:

$$v = \frac{v_{\max}[S]}{[S] + K_m}$$

where

v = rate if reaction
Vmax = maximal reaction rate
S = substrate concentration
Km = Michaelis-Menten constant

For an enzymatic assay to identify competitive inhibitors, it is essential to run the reaction under initial velocity conditions with substrate concentrations at or below the Km value given substrate. The substrate should either be the natural substrate or a surrogate substrate, like a peptide, that mimics the natural substrate. The optimal pH and buffer component concentrations should be determined before measuring the Km.

5.5.1.1 Initial Velocity

- Initial velocity is the initial linear portion of the enzyme reaction when less than 10% of the substrate has been depleted, or less than 10% of the product has formed. Under these conditions, it is assumed that the substrate concentration does not significantly change, and the reverse reaction does not contribute to the rate.

- Initial velocity depends on enzyme and substrate concentration and is the region of the curve in which the velocity does not change with time. This is not a predetermined time and can vary depending on the reaction conditions.
- What are the consequences of not measuring the initial velocity of an enzyme reaction?
- The reaction is non-linear concerning enzyme concentration.
- There is an unknown concentration of substrate.
- There is a greater possibility of saturation of the detection system.
- The steady-state or rapid equilibrium kinetic treatment is invalid.

Measuring an enzyme reaction rate when 10% or less of the substrate has been depleted is the first requirement for steady-state conditions. At low substrate depletion, i.e., initial velocity conditions, the factors listed below contribute to non-linear progression curves for enzyme reactions that do not have a chance to influence the reaction.

- Product inhibition.
- Saturation of the enzyme with substrate decreases as reaction proceeds due to a decrease in the concentration of substrate (substrate limitation).
- Reverse reaction contributes as the concentration of product increases over time.
- The enzyme may be inactivated due to instability at given pH or temperature.

5.5.2 Reagents and Method Development

It is critical for any enzyme target to ensure that the appropriate enzyme, substrate, necessary co-factors, and control inhibitors are available before beginning assay development. The following requirements should be addressed during the method design phase:

- Identity of the enzyme target, including amino acid sequence, purity, and the amount and source of enzyme available for development, validation, and support of screening/SAR activities. One should also ensure that contaminating enzyme activities have been eliminated. Specific activities should be determined for all enzyme lots.
- Identify the source, and acquire native or surrogate substrates with appropriate sequence, chemical purity, and adequate available supply.
- Identify, and acquire buffer components, co-factors, and other necessary additives for enzyme activity measurements according to published procedures and/or exploratory research.
- Determine the stability of enzyme activity under long-term storage conditions and during on-bench experiments. Establish lot-to-lot consistency for long-term assays.
- Identify and acquire enzyme-inactive mutants purified under identical conditions (if available) to compare with wild-type enzymes.

5.5.2.1 Detection System Linearity

Instrument capacity needs to be determined by detecting the product's signal and plotting it versus product concentration. If a detection system has a limited linear range such as 20%, the system becomes non-linear at concentrations of greater than 10% of the total product generated. This limited linear range compromises measurements since the enzyme reaction condition must be within the instrument capacity's linear portion. The linear range of detection for an instrument is determined using various product concentrations and measuring the signal. Plotting the signal obtained (Y-axis) versus the amount of product (X-axis) yields a curve used to identify the detection instrument's linear portion.

5.5.2.2 Enzyme Reaction Progress Curve

A reaction progress curve is obtained by mixing an enzyme and its substrate and measuring the subsequent product generated over time. The initial velocity region of the enzymatic reaction needs to be determined, and subsequent experiments should be conducted in this linear range, where less than 10% of the substrate has been converted to product. If the reaction is not linear, the enzyme concentration is modified to retain linearity during the experiments. These steps (modifying the enzyme and analyzing the reaction linearity) are conducted in the same experiment.

In this data set, the product is measured at various times for three different concentrations of enzyme and one substrate concentration. The curves 1x and 2x relative levels of enzyme reach a plateau early due to substrate depletion. To extend the time that the enzyme-catalyzed reaction exhibits linear kinetics, the enzyme level is reduced, as shown as a 0.5x curve. These curves are used to define the amount of enzyme used to maintain initial velocity conditions over a given period. These time points should be used for subsequent experiments.

5.5.2.3 Measuring the Initial Velocity of an Enzyme Reaction

- Keep the temperature constant in the reaction by having all reagents equilibrated at the same temperature.
- Design an experiment so pH, ionic strength, and composition of the final buffer are constant. Initially, use a buffer known enzyme of interest by consulting the literature or using the buffer recommended enzyme. This buffer could be further optimized in later stages of development.
- Perform the time course of reaction at three or four enzyme concentrations.
- Measure the signal generated when 10% product is formed to detect 10% loss of substrate.
- Measure the signal at $t = 0$ to correct for the background (leave out enzyme or substrate).

For kinase assays, the background is determined by leaving out the enzyme or the substrate. The condition resulting in the highest background level should be used. EDTA is not recommended for use as the background control during the validation of a kinase assay. Once the assay has been validated, if the background measured with EDTA is the same as both the no enzyme, and no substrate control, then EDTA can be used.

5.5.2.4 Measurement of Km and Vmax

Once the initial velocity conditions have been established, the substrate concentration should be varied to generate a saturation curve determination of Km and Vmax values. Initial velocity conditions must be used. The Michaelis-Menten kinetic model shows that the Km = [S] at Vmax/2. For competitive inhibitors to be identified in a competition experiment that measures IC50 values, a substrate concentration around or below the Km must be used. Using substrate concentrations higher than the Km will identify competitive inhibitors (a common goal of SAR) more difficult.

For kinase assays, the Km for ATP should be determined using saturating concentrations of the substrate undergoing phosphorylation. Subsequent reactions need to be conducted with optimum ATP concentration, around or below the Km value using initial velocity conditions. However, it would be best to determine Km for ATP and the specific substrate simultaneously. This would allow maximum information to be gathered during the experiment and address any potential cooperativity between a substrate and ATP.

A requirement for steady-state conditions to be met means that a large excess of the substrate over enzyme is used in the experiment. Typical ratios of the substrate to the enzyme are greater than 100 but can approach one million.

5.5.2.5 What Does the Km Mean?

- If Km >>> [S], then the velocity is very sensitive to changes in substrate concentrations. If [S] >>> Km, then the velocity is insensitive to changes in substrate concentration. A substrate concentration around or below the Km is ideal for the determination of competitive inhibitor activity.

- Km is constant for a given enzyme and substrate and is used to compare enzymes from different sources.
- If Km seems "unphysiologically" high, then activators may miss the reaction that would normally lower the Kmin vivo or that the enzyme conditions are not optimum.

5.5.2.6 How to Measure Km

- Measure the initial velocity of the reaction at substrate concentrations between 0.2–5.0 Km. If available, use the Km reported in the literature to determine the range of concentration to be used in this experiment. Use eight or more substrate concentrations (Figure 5.6).
- Measuring Km is an iterative process. For the first iteration, use six substrate concentrations covering a wide range of substrate concentrations to get an initial estimate. For subsequent iterations, use eight or more substrate concentrations between 0.2–5.0 Km. Make sure there are multiple points above and below the Km.
- For enzymes with more than one substrate, measure the substrate's Km of interest with the other substrate at saturating concentrations. This is also an iterative process. Once the second Km is measured, it is necessary to check that the first Km was measured under saturating second substrate concentrations.
- Fit the data to a rectangular hyperbola function using non-linear regression analysis. To determine the Km for a substrate, the reaction product is measured at various times for different substrate levels. The product generated (Y-axis) is plotted against the reaction time (X-axis). Each curve represents a different concentration of substrate. If all the curves are linear, this indicates that initial velocity conditions (< 10% of substrate conversion) have been met.

The initial velocity (Vo) for each reaction progress curve is equivalent to the line's slope, which is defined as the change in the product formed divided by the change in time. This is expressed by the equation below and is calculated using linear regression or another standard linear method:

$$\frac{\Delta Y}{\Delta X} = Slope = vo$$

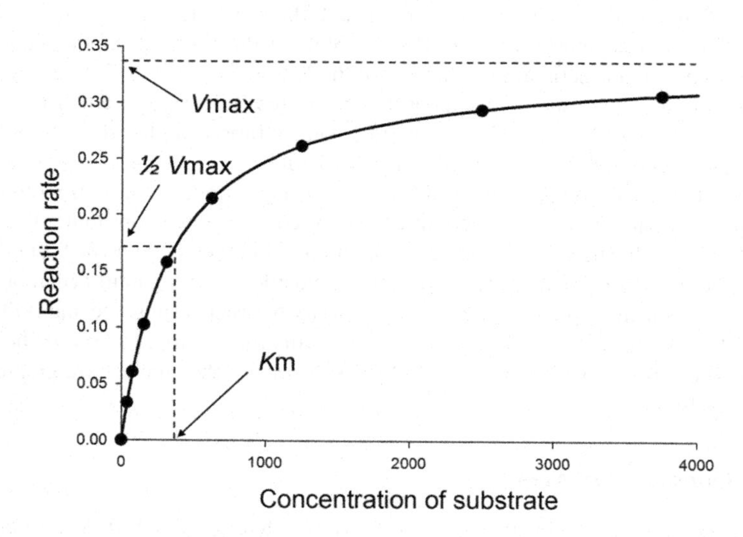

FIGURE 5.6 Initial velocity versus substrate concentration.

The resulting slopes (initial velocity, vo) for each reaction progress curve are plotted on the Y-axis versus the concentration of substrate (X-axis), and nonlinear regression analysis using a rectangular hyperbola model is performed.

The Vmax and Km system is calculated from the nonlinear regression analysis. The meaning of each term is shown in Figure 5.5. The Km is the substrate concentration, which results in an initial reaction velocity that is one-half the maximum velocity determined under saturating substrate concentrations.

Linear transformations, such as a double reciprocal Lineweaver-Burke plot of the initial velocity/substrate concentration data (i.e., 1/vo versus 1/[S]), should not be used for calculating the Km, and Vmax from saturation type experiments such as those described above. These linear transformations tend to distort the error involved with the measurement and were used before programs that can perform nonlinear regression analysis were widely available.

An additional parameter that is useful to describe an enzyme's efficiency is the catalytic constant (or turnover number) that is termed kcat that is determined from saturation data. The catalytic rate constant, kcat, is a first-order rate constant that gives the frequency of decomposition of the E•S complex to products. Note that its units are inverse time. Sometimes kcat is referred to as the turnover number. One can think of kcat as the frequency with which an enzyme, operating at saturation, can convert substrate to the product—how frequently the enzyme turns over.

For kinase reactions where the Km for ATP and substrate need to be determined, it is best if a multidimensional analysis is used to measure both Km's simultaneously. An example is shown in Figure 5.11.

If this method is used, it is important to demonstrate that in extreme conditions (particularly low substrate, high ATP concentrations), the instrument's linearity is maintained. Also, it is important that the linearity of the reaction is maintained at all conditions. Proper background controls must be used. The best condition would be combining the best signal-to-noise ratio while maintaining the substrate and ATP concentration as low as possible. Consult with a biochemist and statistician experienced in these techniques to ensure appropriate data analysis methods are utilized.

5.5.2.7 Determination of IC50 for Inhibitors

Concentration-response plots are used to determine the effects of an inhibitor on an enzymatic reaction. These experiments are performed at constant enzyme and substrate concentrations and are the primary type of analysis performed for structure-activity relationship (SAR) measurements for compounds of interest.

A typical concentration-response plot is shown in Figure 5.7. Fractional activity (Y-axis) is plotted as a function of inhibitor concentration (X-axis). The data are fit using a standard four-parameter logistic, nonlinear regression analysis.

The compound concentration that results in 50% inhibition of maximal activity is termed the IC50 (inhibitor concentration yielding 50% inhibition). It is important to use enough inhibitor concentrations

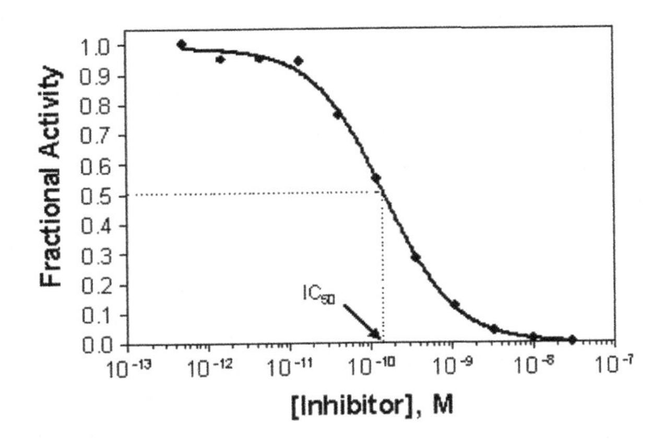

FIGURE 5.7 Concentration-response plot for an enzyme inhibitor.

to provide well-defined top and bottom plateau values. These parameters are critical mathematical models used to fit the data. Other criteria for successful concentration-response curves are listed in the following discussion.

IC50 Determination for SAR:

1. Use a minimum of ten inhibitor concentrations for an accurate IC50 determination. Equally spaced concentration ranges (i.e., three-fold or half-log dilutions) provide the best data sets for analysis.
2. Ideally, half the data points on the IC50 curve are above the IC50 value, and half are below the IC50 value, including a minimum and maximum signal.
3. The lower limit for determining an IC50 is one-half the enzyme concentration (tight-binding inhibitors, 3).
4. Screening strategies for defining an initial SAR include determining the % inhibition at a single concentration, determining the % inhibition at a high and a low concentration of inhibitor, and finally, determining an apparent IC50 using fewer concentrations.

Criteria for reporting IC50s:

1. The maximum % inhibition should be greater than 50%.
2. Top and bottom values should be within 15% of the theory.
3. The 95% confidence limits IC50 should be within a 2–5-fold range.

Since the IC50 value is the most common result reported for enzymatic assays, it is important to understand how experimental conditions affect IC50 determinations. Generally, the substrate concentrations relative to the Km and the amount of product produced have the greatest effect on the measured IC50. Figure 5.12 demonstrates the effect of both substrate concentration and percent conversion on measured IC50 values for a competitive inhibitor.

Chosen assay conditions of pH, temperature, ionic strength, etc. Also, for enzymes that are dimerized, a large dilution into assay buffer may result in inactivation.

Parameters such as substrate Km and control inhibitor IC50's need to be determined in three separate experiments to assess variability. Refer to HTS assay validation to assess the variability of the assay.

5.5.2.8 Optimization Experiments

Published literature information should be used in selecting these factors. For example, a factorial design experiment could be conducted while varying:

- Divalent cations, for example, Ca^{2+}, Mg^{2+}, Mn^{2+}.
- Salts, for example, NaCl, KCl.
- EDTA.
- Reducing agents such as βME, DTT, glutathione.
- Bovine serum albumin.
- Detergents such as Triton, CHAPS.
- DMSO.
- Buffer source, for example, HEPES versus acetate.
- pH.

In addition to assay conditions, enzyme stability may be affected if appropriate measures are not taken during long-term storage. Many enzymes need to be stored at –70° C to maintain activity, but freeze–thaw cycles are not recommended. Other enzymes are stored for long periods of time at –20° C using an additive in the storage buffer such as 50% glycerol.

The presence of carrier proteins in the buffer (bovine serum albumin, ovalbumin, others), and the use of polypropylene plates (or non-binding polystyrene plates) may be essential to retain proper enzyme activity.

5.6 ELISA-Type Assays

5.6.1 Basic Concept

Enzyme-linked immunosorbent assays (ELISAs) follow the basic design shown in Figure 5.1. These formats are used to measure PPI and measure competition between a PPI and a small-molecule inhibitor. One of the proteins is attached to a plate surface to measure a PPI, and the second protein is then allowed to bind to the first protein. The second protein is detected by the binding of an antibody that is linked to an enzyme. When the substrate is added, the enzyme produces a measurable readout quantitatively linked to the amount of the second protein. ELISAs are very sensitive because the readout is amplified by using an enzyme. Further amplification is achieved by using multiple layers, such as secondary antibodies.

ELISA technically means that the detection event uses an antibody and enzyme-based detection; however, this term is commonly used to describe plate-bound detection of a reagent, even if the affinity reagent is not an antibody or if the detection reagent is not an enzyme. One commonly used, the non-enzymatic format, is called dissociation-enhanced lanthanide fluorescent immunoassay (DELFIA, Perkin Elmer). In DELFIA, the detection signal is the time-resolved fluorescence of a lanthanide ion (such as europium). The lanthanide ion is bound to the affinity reagent through a chemical linkage; upon adding a proprietary detergent mixture, the europium fluoresces, providing a highly sensitive measurement of the concentration of bound protein. Three features of lanthanide fluorescence lead to highly sensitive and selective assays: a) a long emission lifetime (milliseconds) allows the measurement to start after the fluorescence of organic material (proteins, test compounds) has decayed, b) the emission occurs at around 600 nm, where few biological materials absorb or emit light, and c) the narrow emission spectrum of lanthanides allow them to be multiplexed.

ELISA-style assays are designed in many ways. The surface-bound protein's attachment can occur by passive adsorption to a plastic plate, by capture with an adsorbed antibody, or by biotinylation and avidin capture.

Detection of the second protein can occur by directly labeling the protein with a signal-generating enzyme by binding an enzyme-labeled antibody by binding an unlabeled primary antibody followed by a labeled secondary antibody, or by biotinylation followed by enzyme-linked avidin. Detection enzymes can include colorimetric, fluorogenic, or luminogenic reactions. The selection criteria for each of these steps are described below.

5.6.2 General Considerations

Consider the affinity of the PPI when designing a plate-based assay. Such assays involve multiple wash steps, which will remove unbound protein. If binding kinetics are rapid, signals will be lower with most weak interactions (ca. > 1 μM). The fewer amplification steps (e.g., direct conjugation of the enzyme to the solution-phase protein), the less the signal is lost to washing. Assay format is, therefore, a compromise between assay complexity and signal amplification.

In principle, either member of the PPI could be immobilized, but several issues should be considered:

- Is there a potential for avidity in the interaction? Avidity occurs when multiple contacts are made simultaneously. A trimeric protein binds to a trimeric ligand or when a trimeric protein binds to a plate with a high density of ligand. This Velcro-like effect results in slowed unbinding kinetics (off-rates), and thus an apparent affinity is tighter than the 1:1 binding affinity. For weak interactions, such avidity allows the PPI to survive washing, but it also complicates quantitative analysis. If one member of the PPI is monomeric, it is generally recommended to use this protein as the solution-phase protein, while a multimeric partner is immobilized on the plate.

- Is one protein more likely to bind to the small molecule? Compounds are more likely to bind to the PPI side that is concave, such as when a bit of secondary structure from the other protein binds into a groove (examples include MDM2/p53, PDZ domains). If the grooved protein is kept in solution, then the ELISA will monitor a solution-phase binding event.
- Is one protein more apt to precipitate or aggregate? If one protein is known to precipitate, it might be more stable as the captured, plate-bound partner.
- Is one PPI partner limiting? Generally, more of the immobilized protein is used, so if one protein is easier to obtain and purify, it should be considered immobilization.
- Another option is if one of the proteins is expressed with a tag such as his or GST or FLAG, a plate coated with antibodies to the tag would serve to immobilize the protein to the plate. A protein is biotinylated, and the streptavidin-coated plate is used.

If there is no compelling reason to use one protein for surface immobilization, then both assay orientations should be evaluated. In the ideal case, the same IC50 values should be obtained from both formats.

5.6.2.1 Assay Design and Development

- Instrumentation: The assays described here are performed with most multimodal plate readers, and the readout is selected based on available instrumentation. Typical readouts are absorbance, fluorescence, luminescence, or time-resolved fluorescence (TRF). Time-resolved fluorescence, used by DELFIA, is the least-standard modality, but most HTS facilities will have TRF-compatible instruments.
- Plates: ELISA-type assays are generally performed in polystyrene microwell plates with high-binding surfaces to adsorb proteins. The color of the plate is selected based on the readout: clear (absorbance), black (fluorescence), and white (luminescence). DELFIA is performed in clear, white, or yellow plates.
- Binding of first protein (protein 1): The first immobilized protein is bound to the plate by passive adsorption or capture. Passive adsorption is simple—the protein is added to a base plate; however, some proteins will denature upon adsorption, and the orientation of proteins on the surface will be random. After the protein is adsorbed, the rest of the well surface is blocked with a nonspecific protein, such as casein (1%), nonfat milk (5%), or bovine serum albumin (1%). Critical steps for passive adsorption include a) selecting a protein concentration to maximize ELISA signal and b) selecting a blocking protein that reduces nonspecific binding of the second protein partner and detection reagents. At any step in the ELISA process, a blocking protein or detergent is used to reduce nonspecific binding. If assay sensitivity is low when the protein is adsorbed, a capture step is added. In this format, an antibody or avidin is adsorbed to the plate first. Generally, the capture protein is plated in a saturating condition. The plate is then blocked with nonspecific proteins, and protein one is added. If an antibody is used for capture, it should not block the PPI and should be available in a sufficient supply scale of the assay. If avidin is used, different versions (e.g., streptavidin and neutravidin) could alter the degree of nonspecific binding. The protein to be captured must be biotinylated, accomplished during expression (via AviTag; Avidity) or chemically (via reaction with amines, acids, or cysteine residues). Biotinylation using AviTag sequences will provide homogeneous labeling near the N- or C-terminal of the protein.
- Binding of the second protein (protein 2): Protein 2 in the PPI can also be added to the ELISA plate in several formats. The protein is unmodified. It is biotinylated (if the first protein was not immobilized by biotin/avidin binding) or labeled directly with the detector (e.g., enzyme or DELFIA probe). As mentioned above, the decision to label or use secondary detection balances the number of washing steps and signal amplification. Directly labeled proteins, such as

horseradish peroxidase (HRP)-protein conjugates, are less soluble and more prone to artifacts; compounds can also interfere with the detection, such as by inhibiting the detection enzyme itself. Therefore, ELISAs usually use a secondary detection step. In either case, protein two should be titrated to achieve a robust but non-saturating signal. Incubation times should allow equilibrium to be reached. After incubation, the unbound protein two should be thoroughly washed from the plate, usually using three phosphate-buffered saline cycles with 0.01% Tween 20 (or another detergent).

- Affinity reagents (e.g., antibodies or streptavidin): When protein 2 is not directly labeled with a detection reagent, one or two binding steps must add the detector. When protein 2 is biotinylated, avidin is conjugated with the detection reagent. When the protein is unmodified, an antibody to protein two is usually used. This primary antibody is labeled with a detection reagent, or a secondary antibody (e.g., rabbit anti-murine IgG) is labeled and bound. The affinity reagents should be titrated to reach a maximal signal-to-background; the binding is saturated, but care should be taken to ensure that the reagent is not binding non-specifically to wells without protein 2. Incubation time is another optimize-able parameter and can vary from one hour to overnight. After incubation, the plate should be thoroughly washed to remove unbound reagents.
- Detection methodology: The final step of the ELISA involves adding a substrate; when the linked enzyme turns over the substrate, a measurable change (e.g., color) occurs. Two commonly used enzymes are horseradish peroxidase (HRP) and alkaline phosphatase (AP); avidin and antibody conjugates of these enzymes are widely available, as are chromogenic and luminogenic substrates. Generally speaking, luminescent substrates are more sensitive, requiring smaller amounts of material and/or less incubation time than chromogenic substrates, and have a more comprehensive dynamic range than chromogenic substrates. On the other hand, chromogenic products tend to be more stable over time. ELISAs are read kinetically (monitoring the color change over time) or at a fixed endpoint. Endpoint readings can include a quenching step, such as adding acid (e.g., an equal volume of 1 M HCl or H3PO4) or base (e.g., 1 M ammonium chloride) to stop enzyme turnover and stabilize the ELISA signal.

DELFIA assays are processed similarly to ELISAs. Some europium-labeled reagents are commercially available, including anti-IgGs, anti-tag antibodies (such as anti-Histag antibodies), and streptavidin, and others are prepared in the lab or by custom synthesis. Detection requires the addition of a commercial "dissociation-enhancement solution."

ELISA and DELFIA have some essential benefits. They are very flexible and sensitive and are inexpensive to run. They are also less likely to have compound interference since the compound is not present in the processing step. They also have significant limitations that have led to their reduced use in HTS. Most ELISAs have multiple incubations and washing steps, which are time-consuming for automated and bench-top assays. Washing can also disrupt weak interactions (e.g., Kd > 1 μM). Finally, it is crucial to demonstrate that potential PPI inhibitors do not interfere with the detection system or act nonspecifically with the proteins and detection reagents. Changing formats and using complementary detection methods (such as those described below) will validate potential inhibitors.

5.6.3 Fluorescence Polarization/Anisotropy

Fluorescence polarization (FP) is a sensitive nonradioactive method study of molecular interactions in solution. This method is used to measure association and dissociation between two molecules if one of the molecules is relatively small and fluorescent. When a fluorescently labeled molecule is excited by polarized light, it emits light with a degree of polarization inversely proportional to the molecular rotation rate. Molecular rotation is mainly dependent on molecular mass, with larger masses showing slower rotation. Thus, when a small, fluorescent biomolecule, such as a small peptide or ligand (typically < 1,500 Da), is free in solution, it will emit depolarized light. When this fluorescent ligand is bound to a more extensive (e.g., > 10,000 Da) molecule, such as a protein, the fluorophore's rotational movement

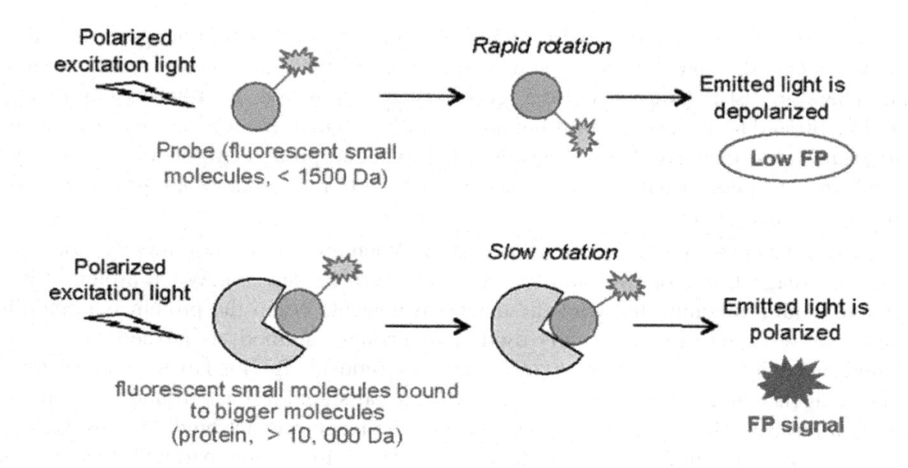

FIGURE 5.8 Diagram of a fluorescence polarization assay. Rapidly rotating small-molecule fluorophore gives a low FP signal (low mP). The association of a relatively large molecule, such as a protein, with the small molecule fluorophore slows down the fluorophore's motion, leading to an increased FP signal.

becomes slower. Thus the emitted light will remain polarized. Therefore, the binding of a fluorescently labeled small molecule or peptide to a protein is monitored by the change in polarization (Figure 5.8).

5.6.3.1 Assay Design

- Selection of FP probe: FP monitors protein–protein interactions if one of the PPI components is negligible. Typically, the ligand/probe's molecular weight is less than 1,500 Da, although up to 5,000 Da is acceptable if the binding partner is very large. For most PPI, FP will be practical only a) if one side of the PPI is minimized to a peptide, b) if there is a synthetic peptide known to bind at the interface (e.g., via phage display), or c) if an organic compound binds at the interface (or to a mutually exclusive binding site). Fortunately, several examples of peptides mimic the epitope of a protein in a PPI, including PDZ domains, IAPs, Bcl2-family proteins, and others.
- Selection of fluorescent dye: Once a probe molecule has been selected, it must be labeled with a fluorescent dye. Dyes are typically available in amine-reactive, cysteine-reactive, and acid-reactive forms and are chemically attached to the probe peptide/molecule using simple chemistry. Typical fluorophores used in FP are fluorescein, rhodamine, and BODIPY dyes. The BODIPY dyes have longer excited-state lifetimes than fluorescein, and rhodamine, making their fluorescence polarization sensitive to binding interactions over a larger molecular weight range (11). Red-shifted dyes are preferable to reduce the number of compounds that will cause interference with the 405 nm (e.g., fluorescein) range.
- Selection of buffer: The buffer must have low fluorescence background. Frequently used buffers have neutral pHs, such as PBS or HEPES.
- Instrumentation for FP measurement with microtiter plate: Many commercially available instruments are capable of measuring the FP signal from solution in 96/384/1,536-well microtiter plate format for high throughput screening (HTS). The fluorescence is measured using polarized excitation and emission filters. Two measurements are performed on every well, and fluorescence polarization is defined and calculated as:

$$Polarization = P = (Ivertical - Ihorizontal) / \left(Ivertical + Ihorizontal\right)$$

Ivertical is the intensity of the emission light parallel to the excitation light plane, and Ihorizontal is the intensity of the emission light perpendicular to the excitation light plane (10). All polarization values are expressed as the milli-polarization units (mP).

All commercial microplate readers have built-in software for mP calculation. Depending on the instrument used, three sets of data are generally reported, including calculated mP values, raw fluorescence intensity counts of vertical (or parallel/S-channel), and horizontal (or perpendicular/P-channel) measurements for each well. mP calculation for different instruments requires the proper use of measured fluorescence intensity of parallel/S-channel and perpendicular/P-channel. As optical parts of fluorometers possess unequal transmission or varying sensitivities for vertically or horizontally polarization light, such instrument artifacts should be corrected for accurate calculation of the molecule's absolute polarization state using fluorescent readers. This correction factor is known as the "G Factor," which is instrument-dependent. G-factor corrects for any bias toward the horizontal (or perpendicular/P-channel) measurement. Most commercially available instruments have an option for correcting the single-point polarization measurement with the G factor. For example, the mP values for FP measurement with Envision Multilabel plate reader are calculated as:

$$mP = 1000 * (SG * P)/(S + G * P)$$

In practice for HTS applications, however, it is unnecessary to measure absolute polarization states; the assay window is important. The assay window is insignificantly changed by G Factor variation.

- Determining the concentrations of fluorescent probes FP binding assay: To select the proper fluorescent probe binding assay concentrations, increasing concentrations of the fluorescent probe is prepared in assay buffer without the binding protein. The fluorescence intensity (FI) in the parallel channel is then measured with defined settings in a plate reader with FP mode. A concentration of the fluorescent probe with at least ten-fold or higher FI signal than that of buffer should only be selected subsequent binding assay. Notice that the FP signal is expressed as a ratio of fluorescence intensities. Thus, the signal is not influenced by changes in intensity brought about by changes in the tracer concentration.
- FP Binding assay development: To determine the binding of the fluorescent probe with the protein of interest, increasing protein concentrations are mixed with a fixed concentration of the probe. The FP signal as expressed in mP is then measured with a plate reader. mP versus (protein) is then plotted to generate a binding isotherm calculation of association parameters such as Kd and maximal binding. For the FP inhibition assay, select a concentration of protein that provides ca. 80% of the maximum change in polarization probe (e.g., 80% bound).
- Data analysis: The dynamic range of the FP assay, i.e., assay window, is defined as mPb – mPf, where mPb is recorded mP value specific binding in the presence of a particular protein concentration, and mPf is the recorded mP value for free tracer from specific binding proteins (12). Typically, the assay window is 3–5-fold (e.g., 50 mP – 150 mP).
- Selectivity: Once the probe and protein concentrations are determined, the interaction's specificity should be assessed. First, an unlabeled version of the probe is titrated into a mixture of the FP-probe and protein. As the concentration of the unlabeled probe competes with the bound fluor-probe, the FP should decrease. The IC50 for this interaction should be similar to the Kd measured above. Similarly, other known inhibitors should yield the expected IC50 values.
- Fluorescence of the bound probe: Often, the fluorescence of the probe changes when it binds to the protein. In this case, anisotropy measurements should be used in place of polarization, since, unlike FP, anisotropy is directly proportional to fluorescence intensity. Anisotropy is calculated with the following expression: r = (Ivertical – Ihorizontal)/(Ivertical + 2 Ihorizontal), where Ivertical is the intensity of the emission light parallel to the excitation light plane, and Ihorizontal is the intensity of the emission light perpendicular to the excitation light plane. FP-based technology has several key advantages for monitoring biomolecular interactions, especially for HTS applications. It is non-radioactive and is in a homogeneous "mix-and-read" format without wash steps, multiple incubations, or separations. FP measurement is directly carried out in solution; no perturbation of the sample is required, making the measurement faster and perhaps more

native-like than immobilization-based methods like ELISA. It is readily adaptable to low volume (30 μl for a 384-well plate or 5 μl for a 1,536-well plate). In addition to measuring PPI, FP assays have been used to study a wide variety of targets, including protein-nucleic acid interactions, kinases, phosphatases, proteases, G-protein-coupled receptors (GPCRs), and nuclear receptors. FP is subject to optical interference from compounds that absorb the fluorescent probe's excitation or emission wavelengths as a fluorescence-based technology. Being a ratiometric technique makes FP somewhat resistant, though enough light must be available to obtain an emission signal. FP is also sensitive to the presence of fluorescence from test compounds. The use of red-shifted probes will minimize background fluorescence interference.

5.6.4 Fluorescent/Förster Resonance Energy Transfer and Time-Resolved (TR) FRET

Fluorescence/Förster Resonance Energy Transfer (FRET) is the phenomenon of non-radiative energy transfer between two fluorophores with specific spectral properties. For FRET to occur, the emission spectrum of one fluorophore, i.e., the "donor," must overlap the excitation spectrum of the second fluorophore, i.e., the "acceptor." When the donor is excited by incident light, energy is transferred to the acceptor via long-range dipole-dipole interactions, resulting in acceptor emission; however, this FRET event will only occur if the donor and acceptor are in sufficient proximity to one another. The equation defines FRET efficiency E:

$$E = \frac{1}{1 + (r / R0)^6}$$

where r is the distance between the fluorophores and Ro is the Förster distance and, which FRET efficiency is 50% specific donor/acceptor pair. Two key factors arise from this equation. First, the amount of energy transfer decays with the sixth power of the distance between the fluorophores. Second, the term Ro depends on the donor emission spectrum's spectral overlap and the acceptor absorbance spectrum; FRET is observed over longer distances when the spectral overlap is large. Fortunately, the proximity limit for several donor/acceptor pairs is approximately 10 nm, which happens to be the distance over which many biomolecular interactions occur. Therefore, FRET is used to monitor biomolecular interactions in a homogeneous mix-and-read assay format by tagging or labeling interacting biomolecules "A" and "B" with the acceptor, and donor fluorophores, respectively. In such a scenario, the ratio of acceptor to donor emission following donor excitation is used to quantify and monitor "AB" binding.

Due to the spectral properties of biological media and traditional FRET donor/acceptor pairs, the FRET signal is significantly contaminated by 1) autofluorescence of biological media and test compounds; 2) a wide acceptor excitation spectrum that allows the acceptor to be directly excited by incident light; and 3) a broad donor emission spectrum that bleeds through into the acceptor emission detection window. These signal contaminants must be corrected for and can significantly diminish the sensitivity of traditional FRET assays.

One elegant solution to the problem of FRET signal contamination is the use of donor fluorophores with exceptionally long emission half-lives (up to 1,500 μs), such as the rare earth metals Europium or Terbium, in a modification of FRET known as Time-Resolved (TR) FRET (also called HTRF). In TR-FRET, Europium or Terbium cryptates (ligands that coordinate the metal ion and provide an "antenna" dye) serve as donors that have a very long luminescence half-life. This long emission decay allows for a time delay (50–150 μs) between donor excitation and acceptor emission recording. During this time delay, both media autofluorescence and acceptor excitation due to incident light will rapidly decay (ns scale) and be extinguished by the time acceptor emission is measured. This essentially eliminates signal contaminants 1 and 2 above. Signal contaminant 3—donor emission bleed-through into acceptor detection—is attenuated by the use of acceptors with red-shifted emission such as allophycocyanin, Alexa 680 (Invitrogen), Cy5, or d2 (Cisbio Bioassays). Another advantage of TR-FRET is that the rare earth metals have a modestly larger proximity limit for FRET (up to 20 nm), allowing the detection of larger biomolecular complexes. TR-FRET assays are well suited for certain HTS applications due to their homogeneous mix-and-read design, high signal-to-background ratios, and enhanced proximity detection range (Figure 5.9).

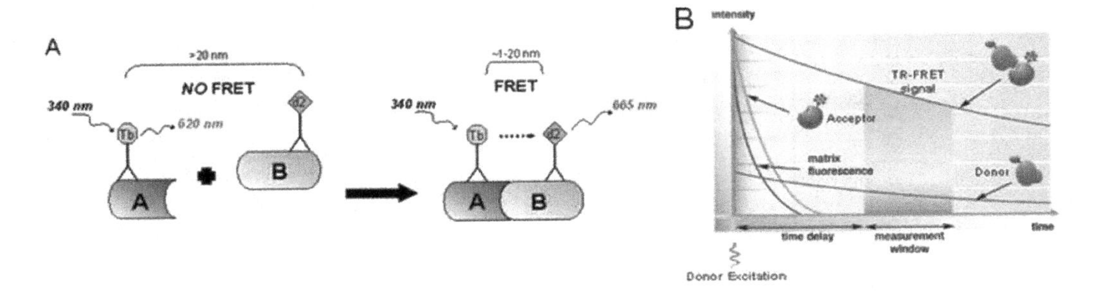

FIGURE 5.9 Principles of TR-FRET. A: schematic of a typical FRET bioassay. Protein 1 is bound to an antibody fused to a donor fluorophore, e.g., Terbium (Tb), and Protein 2 is bound to an antibody fused to an acceptor fluorophore, e.g., d2 or XL665. If A and B interact, the donor and acceptor are brought into sufficient proximity for FRET. In the case of a positive FRET event, acceptor emission is detected upon donor excitation. B: the primary sources of FRET signal contamination (matrix fluorescence, direct excitation of the acceptor) are avoided in TR-FRET by inserting a time delay between donor excitation and detection of acceptor emission ("measurement window").

5.6.5 AlphaScreen Format

AlphaScreen™ is a bead-based format commercialized by PerkinElmer (www.perkinelmer.com) and used to study biomolecular interactions in a microplate format. A newer, more sensitive version of the technology is called AlphaLISA. The acronym ALPHA stands for Amplified Luminescent Proximity Homogeneous Assay. Like FRET, AlphaScreen is a non-radioactive, homogeneous proximity assay. The binding of two molecules captured on the beads leads to an energy transfer from one bead to another, ultimately producing a fluorescent signal. Excitation of the donor bead leads to the formation of singlet oxygen, diffuses to the acceptor, and stimulates emission. Unlike FRET, acceptor emission occurs at higher energy (lower wavelength) than donor excitation.

The AlphaScreen assay beads are latex-based and approximately 250 nm in diameter. Both bead types (donor and acceptor) are coated with a hydrogel that minimizes non-specific binding and self-aggregation and provides reactive aldehyde groups for conjugating biomolecules to the bead surface. The beads are small enough that they do not sediment in biological buffers, and bead suspensions do not clog the tips used commonly in liquid handling devices. The beads are typically used at ug/mL concentration and are very stable, even if heated to 95° C, for example, for PCR or lyophilized.

Donor beads contain a photosensitizer, phthalocyanine, which converts ambient oxygen to an excited form of O2, singlet oxygen, upon illumination at 680 nm. Like other excited molecules, singlet oxygen has a limited lifetime before returning to the ground state. Within its four μsec half-lives, singlet oxygen can diffuse approximately 200 nm in solution. If an acceptor bead is within that distance, energy is transferred from the singlet oxygen to thioxene derivatives within the acceptor bead, resulting in light production. Without the interaction between donor, and acceptor bead, singlet oxygen falls to the ground state, and no signal is produced. AlphaScreen acceptor beads use rubrene as the final fluorophore, emitting light between 520 and 620 nm. AlphaLISA acceptor beads use a Europium chelate as the final fluorophore, emitting light in a narrower peak at 615 nm (Figure 5.10). The AlphaLisa light is less likely to be affected by particles and other substances commonly found in biological samples (for example, plasma and serum), thereby reducing background noise and optimizing precision.

AlphaScreen assays have been developed to quantify enzymes, molecular (protein, peptide, small molecule) interactions, and DNA and RNA hybridizations. Due to the large diffusion distance of singlet oxygen, the binding interactions of even very large proteins and phage particles are quantified by AlphaScreen and AlphaLISA. The high sensitivity and large distance range have led to the increasing use of these technologies in HTS settings.

The hook effect is common when using any sandwich-type assay, including AlphaScreen, ELISA, and some of the FRET-based formats described above. When the PPI components are titrated (e.g., during assay development), both donor and acceptor beads become progressively saturated by their target molecules, and the signal increases with increasing protein concentration. At the "hook" point, either

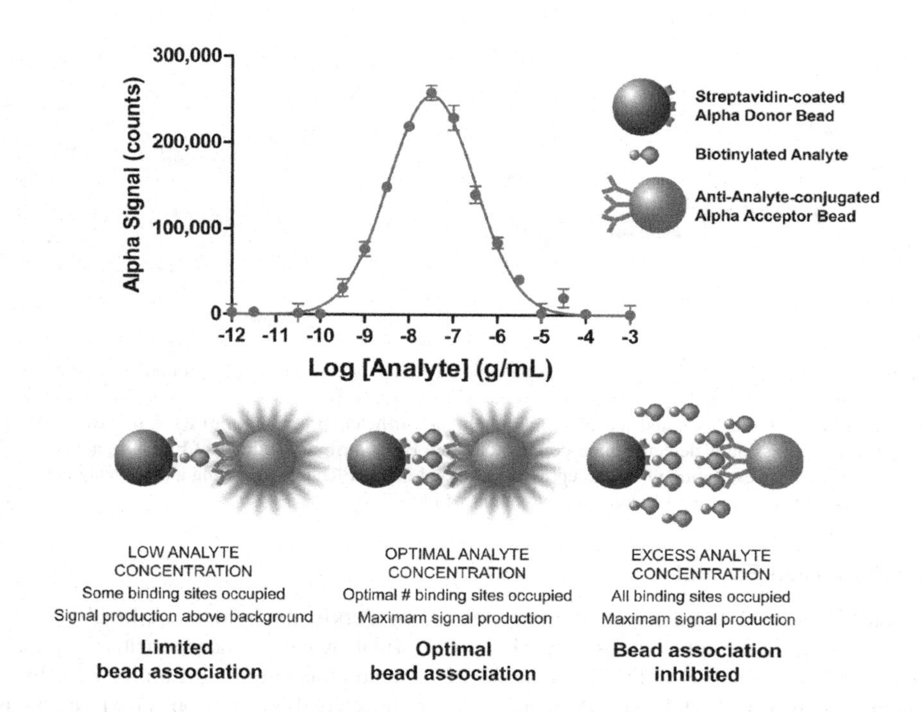

FIGURE 5.10 AlphaScreen and AlphaLisa. Left: binding of biological partners (represented by small ovals A and B) brings donor and acceptor beads (represented by the large blue and yellow circles) into proximity (≤ 200 nm), and thus a fluorescent signal between 520–620 nm is produced in the case of AlphaScreen, and 615 nm in the case of the AlphaLisa. When there is no binding between biological partners, donor and acceptor beads are not nearby. Singlet oxygen decays, and no signals are produced. Right: comparison of emission spectra for AlphaScreen (red) and AlphaLISA (blue).

the donor or the acceptor component is saturated with the target molecule, and a maximum signal is detected. Above the hook point, there is an excess of target molecules donor or the acceptor beads, which inhibits their association, and causes a progressive signal decrease (Figure 5.10). When the PPI affinity is higher (weaker) than the concentrations used in the assay, the hooking effect is masked, resulting in what looks like a traditional saturation curve that reaches a plateau rather than hooking. In this case, two competing equilibria occur: the signal is decreasing because of the hooking effect on the bead, but the protein-protein interaction is still increasing because higher concentrations of protein drive the equilibrium toward the more protein-protein complex. In either event, choose a protein concentration below the hook point (or saturation point) for your assay.

The goal of primary screening is to select a set of compounds that might be active. However, among "actives," many compounds act by mechanisms that will not be optimizable into a qualified drug lead or biological probe. Some of the artifactual mechanisms that lead to activity in a primary assay are specific to the assay format; as described above, compounds could cause autofluorescence or quench the fluorescence signal used to detect the PPI. Thus, it is precious to develop at least one orthogonal assay format, an in vitro assay, and a cell-based assay, plus an independent way to measure binding directly.

Other artifacts are less selective to the assay methodology, though they may be somewhat selective proteins or assay conditions. A well-described and very common example is compound aggregation. Aggregates are quite large (30–200 nM) and can interfere with protein structure in a number of pathological ways. Aggregation can also be very dependent on the assay condition; rather than thinking of compounds as "aggregators," it is more accurate to think of aggregation as a form of molecular interaction, dependent on salt, pH, detergents, carrier proteins, and concentration of the compound. Thus, it is not sufficient to demonstrate that a compound is selective for a particular screen over other screens; to be a bona fide PPI inhibitor, the compound must bind at a different site(s) on one of the proteins the complex. Binding stoichiometry is, therefore, a key metric for selecting useful and optimizable probes/leads.

Several biophysical assays measure the binding of the small molecule to the protein. It is very beneficial to use at least two assays since no assay is infallible, and various types of information are gleaned from each format. Depending on the size of the protein(s), the binding affinity of the molecule, and other details, the following methods are used.

5.6.5.1 Optical Biosensors

Several related technologies measure the binding of a surface-immobilized "ligand" to a soluble "analyte." In general, optical biosensors detect changes in the angle, color, or phase of light reflected off of a solid/liquid interface. Many instruments are sensitive enough to monitor the binding of a small-molecule analyte to a surface-bound protein. These systems can also be used in competition experiments, in which a PPI is monitored in the presence of increasing concentrations of inhibitors. Because the signals are proportional to the analyte change in mass, PPI is usually easier to monitor than protein/small-molecule interactions. The first popular optical biosensor was the surface plasmon resonance (SPR) instrument developed by Biacore (GE Healthcare). The technology is now widely used, and numerous companies market SPR instruments (e.g., Bio-Rad, ICX, and others). Most SPR instruments use microfluidics to introduce the analyte and monitor the binding in real-time. The concentration of the analyte is varied to develop a dose-response. SPR provides a measure of binding stoichiometry, reversibility, and affinity to a protein bound to a surface through kinetic and steady-state experiments. Other technologies include optical gradients (SRU BIND, Corning Epic) and interferometry (Forte Bio Octet Red). The optical gradient systems are plate-based, allowing high throughput but more limited kinetic resolution. In interferometry, the ligand is coated onto fiber optic sensors that are then dipped into the analyte solutions. This technology is developing rapidly and could soon have the throughput, cost/assay, and sensitivity to rival SPR for measuring small-molecule/protein interactions.

5.6.5.2 Nuclear Magnetic Resonance (NMR)

NMR measures nuclei's response in a magnetic field and is very sensitive to the nucleus's chemical environment. Due to the method's flexibility, NMR has many uses in small-molecule characterization and protein structure determination. Small-molecule/protein NMR experiments come in two general formats—ligand-detected and protein-detected. Ligand-detected experiments measure the change in the compound's NMR signals ("resonances") as a function of binding to the protein. Energy is transferred from the solvent and protein to the compounds (saturation transfer difference, WaterLOGSY). The compound's apparent mass is increased due to binding a large protein (translation, diffusion). Ligand-detected measurements are often used qualitatively to assess the presence of binding to the target. Saturation transfer difference is prevalent for moderate-throughput applications because the protein concentration is low (micromolar), and it is particularly effective for compounds in fast exchange (weaker than micromolar). There is no limit on the protein size for ligand-detected experiments. Protein-detected NMR provides a measurement of the effect of the compound on the protein. The most popular moderate-throughput methods are 15N-1H HSQC, and 13C-1H HSQC, and the related 15N-and 13C-TROSY. N-H HSQC measures the amide N-H bond's environment and thus provides a single peak for each amino acid in a protein sequence (except for proline; asparagine and glutamine also have primary NH signals). 13C-1H HSQC uses labeled methyl groups to detect changes to valine, methionine, isoleucine, and leucine. If the NMR spectrum has been assigned, modifications to the resonances in the compound's presence will suggest the binding site. However, even without giving the protein resonances, compounds are binned by binding site, and non-binders or multi-site binders are identified. Protein-detected NMR was reserved for relatively small proteins; however, technical improvements in NMR hardware, pulse sequences, deuteration of the protein, and selective labeling have made many more proteins amenable to these experiments.

5.6.5.3 Isothermal Calorimetry (ITC)

ITC measures the heat generated or absorbed by a binding interaction. For weakly binding PPI inhibitors (in the mid micromolar range), ITC is challenging because protein usage is high, compound solubility is limited, and the heats of binding are small. It is essential to match the protein and compound buffers and control heat-of-dilution as the compound sample is added to the protein (or vice versa). Despite these challenges, ITC is very valuable because, unlike some other methods, ITC is truly label-free, and all components are in solution. By directly measuring the binding energy, ITC provides information on the entropy and enthalpy of the interaction, the binding affinity (by titrating one of the partners), and the binding stoichiometry.

Thermal stabilization-differential scanning calorimetry (DSC) and differential scanning fluorimetry (DSF, thermafluor, protein thermal shift): One way to define protein stability is by the temperature at which the protein unfolds. Unfolding is usually a highly cooperative process and gives a defined melting temperature (Tm) under a given condition of concentration, buffer, etc. When a compound binds to the protein, the complex is more stable than the protein alone, and the protein's Tm increases. To measure the binding affinity of a compound for a protein, one monitors the increase in Tm (ΔTm) as the compound's concentration increases. Tm measurements are generally done with micromolar concentrations of protein and are therefore most sensitive to determining binding affinities in this range. This method also has the advantage that all components are in solution. There are several methods for measuring the change in Tm. Differential scanning calorimetry (DSC) monitors the heat absorbed by the protein as the temperature increases; the energy/degree increases at the Tm.

Differential scanning fluorimetry (DSF) monitors a hydrophobic dye's binding to the protein as the temperature is increased. The dye binds preferentially to hydrophobic portions of a protein exposed when a protein melts; this binding is accompanied by a change in fluorescence as a function of temperature. Typical DSF dyes include SYPRO orange and 1,8-ANS; DSF measurements are read in specialized instruments or real-time PCR machines. The magnitude of DSC and DSF signals, and the ΔTms obtained from small-molecule binding studies, is dependent on both the protein and the assay conditions. Thermodynamic statements are only valid in the cases that thermal denaturation is reversible. Nevertheless, ΔTm measurements can provide a rapid assessment of binding affinity and are increasingly being used in primary screening assays as single-concentration measurements.

5.6.5.4 Sedimentation Analysis (SA; Analytical Ultracentrifugation)

Sedimentation analysis measures the sedimentation of proteins in response to a centrifugal force. The protein concentration is measured along the length of a centrifugation cell using the proteins' absorbance, refractive index, or fluorescence. Two general types of SA experiments are Velocity Sedimentation and Equilibrium Sedimentation. Equilibrium sedimentation gives the first principle measurement of molecular mass and is often used to measure self-association (e.g., dimerization) constants. However, it can also be used to assess the binding of a small molecule to the protein, particularly if the molecule has an absorbance at wavelengths distinct from the protein (e.g., > 300 nm). The compound's aggregation state and the compound's effect on the protein's apparent molecular mass provide a quick readout of aggregation-based artifacts. Direct binding of the compound to protein can also be assessed. Analytical centrifuges are sold by Beckman Coulter, and add-on fluorescence detection is available from Aviv Biomedical.

5.6.5.5 X-Ray Crystallography

X-ray crystallography continues to be the gold standard for characterizing protein/small molecule interactions. The high-resolution (ca. 1.5–3 angstrom) structure fit from x-ray diffraction data provides information on the binding site and the specific contacts between compound and protein. The presence of a single molecule bound to a single binding site suggests—but does not prove—that the compound's inhibition of a PPI arises from binding at that site. Co-structures of compounds and proteins are generally prepared by soaking the compound into a protein crystal or by co-crystallization of the protein and compound together. It is challenging to obtain co-crystal structures in many cases, either because the protein does not crystallize well. The compound induces changes to the protein structure that inhibit crystallization (e.g., binding at a crystal contact, changing the protein conformation), or the compound is not soluble enough.

5.7 In Vitro Toxicity and Drug Efficacy Testing

An increasing need for robust and reliable in vitro models for toxicity and drug efficacy testing is potentiated not only by the urge to make the process of bringing therapeutics from the bench to the bedside faster and more cost-effective but also by increasing regulatory and safety challenges. However, one of the significant concerns of in vitro toxicity/efficacy testing remains its predictive power and translation into in vivo situations. As discussed in the introductory section, 3D cell culture formats such as spheroids present a powerful alternative to traditional 2D cell culture for in vitro studies. The 3D spheroid model helps mimic solid tumors from a physiologically relevant architectural perspective when grown with multiple cell types prevalent in these tumors.

The choice of the 3D model and the endpoint for toxicity/efficacy testing should depend on both the physiological question to be answered and the screen scale. In general, treatment with a toxicant can affect cellular and 3D cell culture morphology, viability, metabolic activity (such as oxygen consumption or metabolic enzyme activation), or tissue-specific function. Here, the spectrum of possible tissue-specific endpoints is continually widening, together with the development of specialized 3D tissue models. In the case of liver microtissues of co-cultured hepatocytes and non-parenchymal cells (NPCs), established approaches include monitoring albumin, urea secretion, bile acid secretion, Kupffer cell-dependent IL-6, and TNFα secretion, to list a few. Contractile responsiveness of the myocardial microtissue model or glucose-stimulated insulin secretion by pancreatic microislets adds yet further options to the growing list of functionality tests. Additionally, cultivated 3D cell culture models are further analyzed using transcriptomic and proteomic methods, allowing RNA and protein expression profiling upon toxicant exposure.

Although very powerful and promising, the use and predictivity of the 3D models have to be carefully validated for each given application, and conditions of cultivation and sample collection need to be standardized and controlled. For screening purposes, 3D cell culture models are treated with many substances (e.g., small molecules, biologicals, siRNA/RNAi). It is good practice to include an appropriate model- or cellular process-specific control compound of known toxic effect, such as chlorpromazine for drug-induced hepatotoxicity, aflatoxin B for apoptotic cell death induction, or trovafloxacin for inflammation-mediated toxicity.

The toxic agents' effect on microtissue morphology, cell viability, and tissue functionality is further investigated, depending on the study goal, endpoint of interest, and compatibility with the screening approach.

The GravityPLUS™ Hanging Drop System is designed to generate organotypic microtissues in the scaffold-free aggregation of cells and enable or prolonged cultivation and multiple compound re-dosing. Microtissues are formed within two to four days from cell suspensions in hanging drops on the GravityPLUS™ Plates and are subsequently harvested into the ultra-low adhesive GravityTRAP™ ULA Plates. The unique design of GravityTRAP™ ULA wells allows for numerous media exchanges without microtissue disturbance and microtissue imaging. This 96-well platform is compatible with liquid handling stations and suitable for HT-screening applications.

Testing toxicity/drug efficacy in 3D cell culture formats presents multiple advantages over conventional 2D cell culture systems. Firstly, cells aggregated into a 3D structure exhibit native tissue-mimicking organization, metabolic characteristics, and specialized functions and retained them for significantly more extended periods, enabling prolonged and repeated exposure. This, in turn, allows for the detection of effects caused by more prolonged exposure of lower compound concentrations, which frequently appear in vivo. For example, more prolonged exposure tends to shift IC50 values towards lower compound concentrations, increasing the assay's sensitivity and better predicting false-negative compounds. Additionally, a comparison between shorter and longer toxic exposures may give an idea about the system's sensitization to a given treatment. Secondly, several commercially available solutions allow for 3D cell culture cultivation in HT-friendly 96- or 384-well format with multiple re-dosing of tested compounds. An appealing concept of multiplexing endpoints to generate simultaneous data-reach readouts is currently under development and shall provide more experimental flexibility on the assay development side.

5.8 In Vivo Assay Validation

There is always a need for the development and statistical validation of in vivo assays residing in discovery projects' flow schemes. This includes a statistical methodology for pre-study, cross-study (lab-to-lab transfers and protocol changes), and in-study (quality control monitoring) validation (Figure 5.11).

- Identifying potential assay formats of in vivo models compatible with single-dose screens (SDSs) and dose-response curves (DRCs) for evaluating structure–activity relationships (SAR).
- Statistical validation of the assay performance parameters (pre-study, in-study, and cross-study validation).
- Optimizing assay protocols with respect to sensitivity, dynamic range, and stability.

A biological assay is defined by a set of methods that produce a detectable signal allowing a biological process to be quantified. In general, the quality of an assay is defined by the robustness and reproducibility of this signal in the absence of any test compounds or the presence of inactive compounds. This robustness will depend on the type of signal measured (biochemical, physiological, behavioral, etc.) and the analytical and automation instrumentation employed. The SDS quality is then defined by this assay system's behavior when screened against a collection of compounds. These two general concepts, assay quality and screen quality, are discussed with specific examples in this manual.

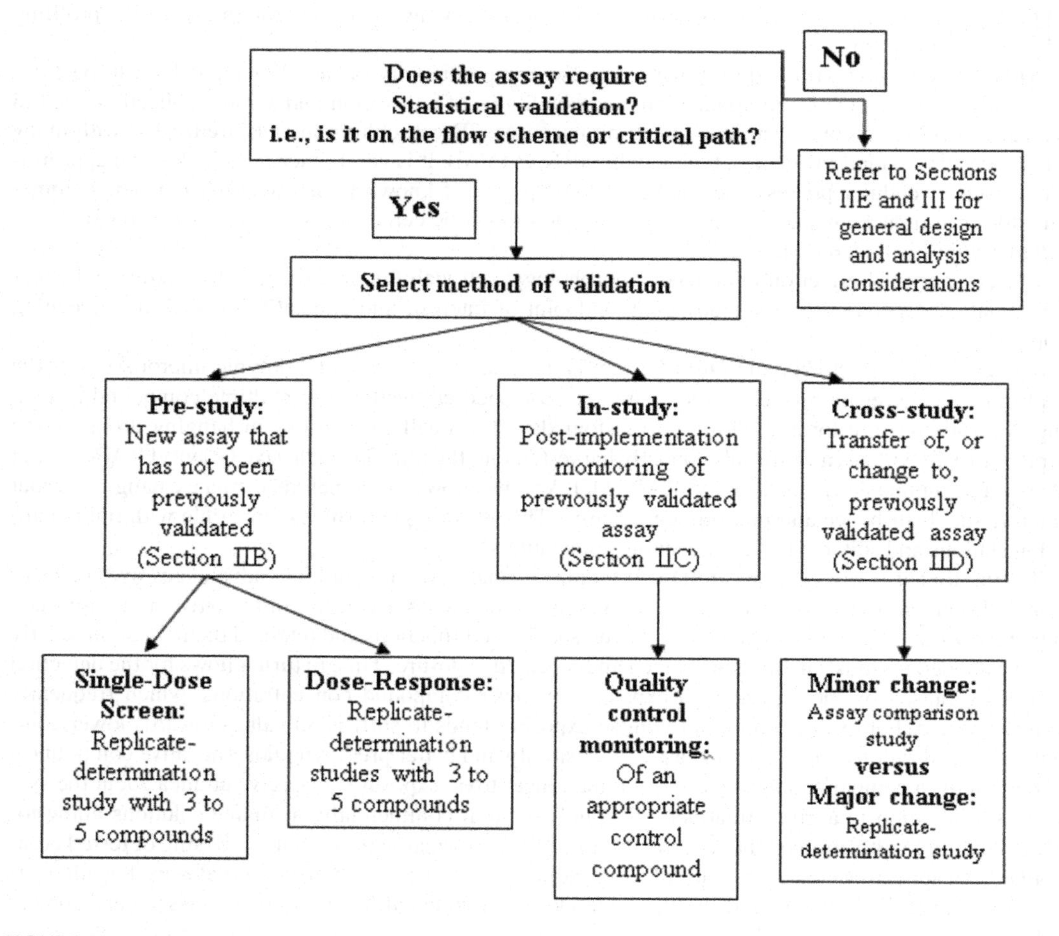

FIGURE 5.11 Flowchart for assay validation.

5.8.1 General Concepts

The overall objective of any method validation procedure is to demonstrate that the method is acceptable for its intended purpose. Usually, the goal is to determine the biological and or pharmacological activity of new chemical entities (NCE). The acceptability of a measurement procedure or bioassay method begins with its design and construction, affecting its performance and robustness.

The validation process originates during the identification and design of a model and method development and continues throughout the assay life cycle (Figure 5.1). During method development, assay conditions and procedures are selected that minimize the impact of potential sources of invalidity (e.g., so-called false positives or false negatives) on the measurement of the analyte or the biological endpoint (e.g., biochemical, physiological, or behavioral changes). There are three fundamental general areas in method development and validation: a) pre-study (identification and design phase) validation, b) in-study (development and production phase) validation, and c) cross-validation or method transfer validation. These stages encompass the systematic scientific steps in the assay development and validation cycle.

5.8.1.1 Pre-Study Validation

This validation occurs before implementing the assay. At this stage, the choice of an assay format is made. Close attention must be paid to factors such as the selection of methods with appropriate specificity and stability. The assay must be designed. The protocol is written to facilitate the statistical analysis (i.e., appropriate design, analysis method, an adequate sample size), and ensure that proper randomization technique is used. This requires the generation and statistical analysis of confirmatory data from planned experiments to document that analytical results satisfy pre-defined acceptance criteria. Within-run statistical measures of assay performance such as the minimum significant difference (MSD) for SDSs and minimum significant ratio (MSR) for DRCs are calculated. If available, the assay sensitivity and pharmacology are evaluated using control compounds.

5.8.1.2 In-Study Validation

These procedures are needed to verify that a method remains acceptable during its routine use. To compare data for compounds tested at different times, the pre-study statistical measures of assay performance (MSD or MSR) are updated to include between-run variability. Each run of the assay should contain appropriate

Maximum and minimum control groups or treatments serve as quality controls of each run and to check overall performance. (Maximum and minimum quality controls differ conceptually from "active" positive or negative controls. This will allow the developer to check for procedural errors and evaluate the method's stability over time. Control charts illustrate procedures, which may be used to evaluate assay performance over time [i.e., control chart monitoring].)

5.8.1.3 Cross-Validation

This portion includes the assay hand-off from the individual developer's team to another laboratory or a screening center. More broadly, this procedure is used at any stage to verify that an acceptable level of agreement exists in analytical results before and after procedural changes in a method and between results from two or more processes or laboratories. Typically, each laboratory assays a subset of compounds, and the agreement in results are compared to predefined criteria that specify the acceptable performance of the assay.

5.8.1.4 Resources

The validation guidelines described here should apply to most in vivo models encountered in drug discovery research. However, situations could arise in which their verbatim application would be impractical given resource constraints, the assay's intended use, or other reasons. In these situations, and in general, the following principles should apply:

- Some form of statistical validation should always be performed and is better than no validation.
- The number of resources, including time, spent on validation should be kept to a reasonably small fraction of the total resources used for testing compounds. What is "reasonable" will have to be determined by the key personnel involved with each project.

These guidelines are intended to be used as "guidelines" and not exact "requirements." The specified assay performance measures serve to quantify how well the assay is performing and should be used to guide the proper interpretation of the data. Determining whether an assay is "fit for its intended purpose" should be based on a combination of these assay performance measures and the team's sound scientific judgment.

5.8.2 Assay Validation Procedures

The statistical validation requirements for an assay vary, depending upon the prior history of the assay. The four main components of the statistical validation are:

- Good study design and data analysis method.
- Proper randomization of animals.
- Appropriate statistical power and sample size.
- Adequate reproducibility across assay runs.

Assays should be designed so that all biologically meaningful effects are statistically significant. In an exploratory study, this "meaningful effect" might correspond to any pharmacologically relevant effect. A project/program team might correspond to the effect that meets the critical success factors (CSFs) defined in the compound development flow scheme. Power and sample size analyses are especially relevant for experiments designed to address critical endpoints in a flow scheme. It is not acceptable to set a CSF equal to the effect size that is statistically significant since that effect size may or may not be biologically relevant. A CSF should be established based upon its biological relevance to the discovery effort. The assay is designed, optimized, and validated so that biologically meaningful effects (e.g., CSFs) are statistically significant. Quantifying the reproducibility of an in vivo flow scheme assay will enable a team to discern whether compounds tested in different assay runs are exhibiting differential activity. This will result in better decisions about SAR directions and compound prioritization.

If the assay is new or has never been previously validated relative to the assay's targeted purpose or mechanism of action, then full validation should be performed. If the assay has been previously validated in a different laboratory and is being transferred to a new laboratory, then a replicate-determination study (pre-study validation) and a formal comparison between the new assay and the existing (old) assay (i.e., cross-study validation; cross validation) should be performed. If an assay is being transferred, it is considered validated if it has previously been assessed by all the methods and moved to a new laboratory without undergoing any substantive changes to the protocol. If the intent is to store the data under the same assay method version (or AMV) in an electronic database as the previous laboratory's AMV, then an assay comparison study (cross validation) should be done as part of the replicate-determination study. Otherwise, only the intra-laboratory part of the replicate-determination study (pre-study validation) is recommended.

If the assay is updated from a previous version run in the same facility, then the requirements vary, depending upon the change's extent. Significant changes require a validation study equivalent to the validation of a new assay. Minor changes require bridging studies that demonstrate the equivalence of the assay before and after the change.

An assay methodology, which has been previously validated for a different target or mechanism of action should be validated in full when used for a new or different target or mechanism as the variability, in particular, and reproducibility may be quite different for different mechanisms even though the methods may be very similar or identical. This concept is analogous to separately validating receptor binding assays for different receptors.

5.8.2.1 Pre-Study Validation

It is important to verify that assay results from multiple determinations or assay runs have acceptable reproducibility with no systematic material trends in the critical endpoints. In this section, we define how to quantify assay variability and determine assay equivalence. We also explain the statistical rationale methods employed in calculating the reproducibility of activity and potency. We strongly recommend consultation with a statistician before designing experiments to estimate variability, and the sources described below. In particular, you should discuss with a statistician alternatives for assays with significant time, resource, or expenditure constraints, and assays, which will be used to test a minimal number of compounds to balance validation requirements with these constraints properly.

Replicate-determination studies with two runs are used to formally evaluate the within-run assay variability (i.e., pre-study validation) or to formally compare a new assay to an existing (old) assay (i.e., cross-study validation). Replicate-determination studies also allow a preliminary assessment of the overall or between-run assay variability, but two runs are not enough to adequately assess overall variability. In-study methods (in-study validation) are used to formally evaluate the overall variability in the assay in routine use. Note that the replicate-determination study is a diagnostic and decision tool used to establish that the assay is ready to go into production by showing that the assay's endpoints are reproducible over a range of efficacies or potencies. It is not intended as a substitute for in-study monitoring or to estimate the overall MSD or MSR.

It may seem counter-intuitive to call the differences between two independent assay runs "within-run." However, the terminology results from the way those terms are defined. Experimental variation is categorized into two distinct components: between-run and within-run sources.

Consider the following examples:

- Between-run variation: If there is variation in the concentrations of the vehicle components between two runs, then the assay results could be affected. However, assuming that the exact vehicle is used with all compounds within the run, each compound will be equally affected. So the difference will only show up when comparing the results of two runs: one run will appear higher on average than the other run. This variation is called between-run variation.
- Within-run variation: If the concentration of one compound in the vehicle varies from the intended concentration (or dose), all animals receiving that compound will be affected. However, animals receiving other compounds will be unaffected. This type of variation is called within-run as the source of variation affects different compounds in the same run differently. Therefore, it is necessary to compare results for one compound on each of two occasions.
- Some sources of variability affect both within-and between-run variation. For example, environmental conditions in an animal room can contribute to both types of variability. Suppose within a run of a particular in vivo assay, the animal room temperature exhibits spatial variation, and animal response is sensitive to temperature. Animals will then respond differently depending upon their location in the room, and these differences are within-run as not all animals are equally affected. In comparison, suppose that the room temperature on average is higher or lower during a particular run of the assay than in previous runs. In this instance, the animals will respond differently on average during this run relative to other runs, and since all animals are affected, this is a between-run variation. Thus, a variable such as animal room temperature is a source of both within-and between-run variation.

The total variation is the sum of both sources of variation. When comparing two compounds across runs, one must consider both the within-run and between-run sources of variation. But when comparing two compounds in the same run, one must only consider the within-run sources since, by definition, the between-run sources affect both compounds equally.

In a replicate-determination study, the between-run sources of variation cause one determination to be on average higher than another resolution. However, it would be doubtful that the difference between the two decisions would be the same for every compound in the study. These individual compound "differences from the average difference" are caused by the within-run sources of variation. The higher the within-run variability, the greater the individual compound variation within assay runs.

The analysis approach used in the replicate-determination study is to estimate and factor out between-run variability and then estimate the magnitude of within-run variability. The between-and within-run sources of variability assessed during assay validation calculations apply to the treatment group means, not animal level data. Animal-to-animal variability is present in vivo experiments, and this variability affects the reproducibility of the resulting treatment group means. Still, as shown subsequently, the animal-to-animal variability is not directly used to calculate the MSD and MSR. It is used to assess whether a data transformation is needed and to assess sample size adequacy.

5.9 Pharmacokinetics and Drug Metabolism

Assessment of the pharmacological properties of small molecule chemical compounds is critical to the initial selection or identification of a chemical lead, during the further lead optimization to elucidate the structure–activity relationships (SAR) and structure–property relationships (SPR), and ultimately to select the compound(s) that will enter investigational new drug (IND)-enabling studies. While extensive discussion of how absorption, distribution, metabolism, and excretion (ADME) of compounds affect their ultimate pharmacokinetics (PK) is beyond the scope of this chapter, herein, we provide guidelines for ADME and PK assessments, benchmarks, and practical "rules of thumb" for selecting compounds with sufficient PK to be viable efficacious drugs.

The in vivo efficacy of an optimized lead will be better served by having good pharmacological properties. The compound administered at a given dose achieves the required concentration for sufficient duration in the target tissue to achieve the desired biological effect while minimizing undesired off-target effects. Improvement in these ADME properties is sought before actual dosing in animals to assess PK. Indeed, for more extensive compound efficacy studies, animals are expensive, and the ethics of sacrificing animals in poorly designed studies uninformed by pharmacological guidance are indefensible.

An exemplary compound(s) emerges from the structure–activity relationship (SAR) systematic elucidation by examining the potency, specificity, and selectivity of analogs around a chemical scaffold. This comprises identifying a chemical lead, where the most potent, specific, and selective compound(s) are chosen.

Assessments of the pharmacological properties of absorption, distribution, metabolism, and excretion (ADME) of a candidate chemical lead(s) are critical to their initial selection and establishes benchmarks against which compounds are synthesized during lead optimization can be evaluated. Further improvements in ADME properties during lead optimization are sought while preserving the potency, and selectivity of the chemical lead(s), though sometimes more efficacious compounds have lower in vitro potencies, better ADME properties.

These activities often reside in an experimental pharmacology group that provides in vitro, in vivo pharmacologic, and physicochemical property analysis of biologically active small molecules supporting small molecule probe/drug discovery projects. Early pharmacological assessment is necessary for a powerful drug or probe discovery process because functional molecules' development and optimization is a multi-parameter process. Simply designing new analogs and developing a SAR for increased potency against the biological target is inadequate development of small molecule probes or drugs suitable for cellular, tissue, or whole animal disease model(s).

The assessment and optimization of structure–pharmacologic/property relationships (SPR) is a further critical step for efficacy evaluation. In addition to assessing compound characteristics such as solubility, protein binding, and serum stability, the data prioritizing different structural classes and rank order them not only based on potency but also potential downstream absorption or metabolism liabilities. An excellent additional overview of pharmacokinetics (PK) can be found on the online version of the Merck Manual (www.merckmanuals.com/professional/clinical-pharmacology/pharmacokinetics/overview-of-pharmacokinetics).

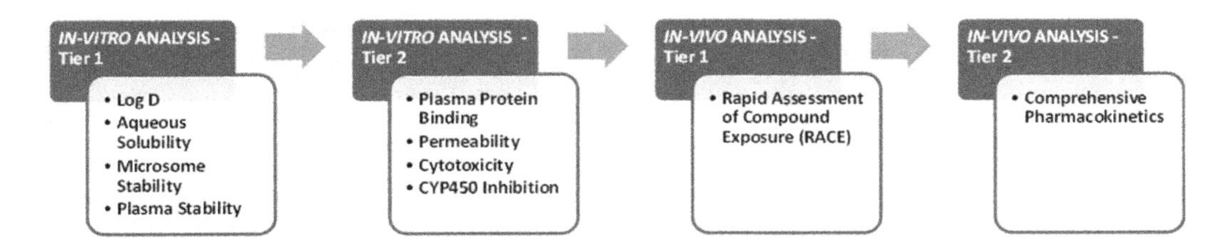

FIGURE 5.12 Flowchart of a two-tier approach for in vitro and in vivo.

Before actual dosing in animals, several relatively rapid and cost-effective in vitro assays can serve as surrogates and indicators of compounds' ADME fate in vivo. Improvements in ADME properties of compounds translate to their improved PK properties. Suppose a compound is rapidly absorbed, well distributed, minimally metabolized, and not rapidly eliminated while not being toxic. In that case, it more likely will rapidly achieve peak levels in the blood, maintain the desired levels (n-fold above the IC50) for a longer duration before falling to low trough levels, and ultimately being cleared by the body (Figure 5.12).

5.9.1 In Vitro Analysis

5.9.1.1 Lipophilicity

Understanding where the drug distributes in the body fat (lipid compartment) or the aqueous compartment (the blood and interstitial fluids) is important to relate lipophilicity to ADME properties since a target binding takes place mostly where the compound is concentrated.

Lipophilicity is an important physicochemical property of a potential drug. It plays a role in solubility, absorption, membrane penetration, plasma protein binding, distribution, CNS penetration, and partitioning into other tissues or organs such as the liver and impacting the routes of clearance. It is important in ligand recognition of the target protein, CYP450 interactions, HERG binding, and PXR mediated enzyme induction.

Lipophilicity is typically measured as the neutral (non-ionized) compound distribution between the non-aqueous (octanol) and aqueous (water) phase, and the result is expressed as a 10-base logarithm of the concentration ratios between these phases (partition coefficient), log P.

Another standard measure for lipophilicity is the distribution coefficient, log D, which considers the compound's ionized and non-ionized forms. Therefore the measurement is done at different pH values. Typically the most interesting is pH 7.4 since most known drugs contain ionizable groups and are likely to be charged at physiological pH.

Assay design:

- Test articles are assayed in triplicate.
- One concentration of test article (typically ten μM).
- n-Octanol is the partition solvent.
- The ratio of the buffer to Octanol is 1:1 (other ratios available).
- Positive control: testosterone (high log D 7.4 value).
- Negative control: tolbutamide (low log D 7.4 value).
- Analysis: LC/MS/MS measurement of the parent compound.
- Report: log D 7.4 value.
- Quantity of test article required: 1.0–2.0 mg.

Summary of assay:

The lipophilicity of compounds is assessed using the golden standard "shake-flask" method. The compound is dissolved in a solution with equal amounts of octanol, and water, shaken for three hours and then measured the amount of compound in each phase. Log D values are calculated by the log ([compound]octanol / [compound]buffer).

5.9.1.2 Solubility

The bioavailability of a compound depends on its aqueous and lipid solubility since the drug molecules pass through both types of membranes. Aqueous solubility is a critical analysis as it reflects the bioavailability of the compound. A compound's ability to dissolve in a solvent to give a homogenous system is an important parameter to achieve the desired drug concentration in systemic circulation aimed (anticipated) pharmacological response. Formulation and administration routes, especially oral dosing, are challenging for poorly soluble drugs, limiting the absorption of the compound from the gastrointestinal tract. Also, poor solubility will affect other AMDE/DMPK analyses if some fraction of the compound precipitates and is unavailable (e.g., in assays for metabolite stability and various CYP identification/inhibition/induction assays). Also, since most known drugs contain ionizable groups, the aqueous solubility is assessed over a range of pH values.

Assay design:

- Test articles are assayed in duplicate.
- One concentration of test article (typically one μM).
- Phosphate-buffered solution (other buffers available).
- Three-stage pH range (5.0, 6.2, 7.4).
- Positive control: diclofenac (high solubility).
- Negative control: dipyridamole (low solubility).
- Background control: DMSO only.
- Analysis: UV spectrophotometry measurement of the parent compound.
- Report: amount of compound dissolved (μM).
- Quantity of test article required: 1.0–2.0 mg.

Summary of assay:

The compound is dissolved in buffer solutions at the indicated pH values. The compound is allowed to reach thermodynamic equilibrium by incubating for 18 hours. Compound UV absorption is compared to a fully saturated solution in 1-propanol.

5.9.1.3 Hepatic Microsome Stability

The mode and duration of an unknown compound's action will be determined by how long the compound stays in the plasma. This is determined by the assay that uses subcellular fractions of the liver, microsomes, to investigate compounds' metabolic fate. Liver microsomes consist mainly of the endoplasmatic reticulum and contain many drug-metabolizing enzymes, including cytochrome P450s (CYPs), flavin monooxygenases, carboxylesterases, and epoxide hydrolase. Liver microsomes are available commercially (for example, Xenotech, LifeTechnologies, and DB Biosciences) as frozen preparations usually prepared in bulk with pooled livers from sacrificed mice, rats, or human cadavers. As a result, the hepatic microsomal metabolic activity can vary significantly from batch to batch. Therefore, in critical studies, it is recommended that planning to obtain the same lot of microsomes be considered in the experimental plans. If lots of microsomes do run out, a few bridging comparisons to establish comparable values for reference compounds' microsomal stability should be made.

Assay design:

- Test articles are assayed in triplicate.
- Human liver microsomes (or other species as needed) (0.5 mg/mL).

- One concentration of test article (typically 10 μM).*
- Two time stages: t = 0 and t = 60 min.*
- Positive control: substrates with known activity.
- Negative control: NADPH deficient.

Analysis: LC/MS/MS measurement of parent compound at specific time stages.

Report: % metabolism of the test article (single time stage); also, intrinsic clearance and half-life (multiple time stages).*

Quantity of test article required: 1.0–2.0 mg.

Summary of assay:

Metabolic stability of compounds is assessed at a single concentration (typically 10 μM) at t = 0 and t = 60 min. The stability of compounds is tested in human (other species available) liver microsomes. Compounds are tested in triplicate with or without NADP wells as a negative control for P450 metabolism. Each assay will include a substrate with known activity (such as the CYP3A4 substrate testosterone) as a positive control.

5.9.1.4 Plasma Stability

In addition to hepatic metabolism, compounds are also subjected to degradation, and modification by enzymes in plasma, particularly hydrolysis and esterases. Thus, the stability of test compounds in plasma is an important parameter, which affects not only the in vivo results but also the bioanalytical assay strategy and design.

Investigation of plasma stability should be performed early in the discovery process to assess potential degradation and protein binding issues.

Assay design:

- Test articles are assayed in triplicate.
- Two concentrations (10 μM and 100 μM or if known, Cmax and 10x Cmax).
- Two time stages: t = 0 and t = 180 min.
- Positive control: procaine (50 μM).
- Negative control: procainamide (50 μM).
- Analysis: LC/MS/MS detection of the remaining test article.
- Report: % parent compound remaining.
- Quantity of test article required: 1.0–2.0 mg.

Summary of assay:

A solution of the test compound in plasma is prepared and incubated for a predetermined period. Aliquots are removed at pre-defined time stages and analyzed by LC/MS/MS. The peak area parent compound is compared to the time zero sample to assess the amount of compound still available.

5.9.1.5 Plasma Protein Binding

The binding of test compounds to plasma proteins is an important factor affecting drug efficacy, metabolism, and pharmacokinetic properties. In many cases, drug efficacy is determined by the free drug concentration (unbound) rather than the total concentration in plasma. If the drug is highly bound to plasma proteins, the amount of drug available to reach the target is reduced. Subsequently, the efficacy of that compound may be significantly reduced. Therefore, information on the free drug fraction is essential for drug development and may correlate with in vivo efficacy.

---

* The number of concentrations/time stages in the assay can be expanded for drug development SAR efforts.

Rapid equilibrium dialysis (RED) is an accurate and reliable method for determining the degree to which a compound binds to plasma proteins. Plasma spiked with test compound is added to the center chamber of a commercial plate-based RED device. Blank, isotonic sodium phosphate buffer is added to the RED device's peripheral chamber, and the plate is incubated at 37° C for four hours. Equilibrium of free compound is achieved by the diffusion of the unbound compound across the dialysis membrane. Several manufacturers provide RED devices (e.g., Thermo Scientific). Aliquots of the buffer and the plasma are taken at pre-determined time stages, and the concentration of free and bound test compound is determined by LC/MS/MS analysis.

Assay design:

- Test articles are assayed in duplicate.
- Test articles are mixed with human plasma (other species available).
- One concentration of test article (10 μM, different concentrations available).
- One time stage (t = 4 hours at 37° C).
- Positive control: propranolol (high binding) and metoprolol (low binding).
- Negative control: no plasma (PBS only).

Analysis: LC/MS/MS detection of the test compound in plasma and the buffer.

Report: % compound bound.

Quantity of test article required: 1.0–2.0 mg.

Summary of assay:

The sample chamber's human or specific interest plasma species are spiked with test compounds at 100x dilution of stock solution (typically 10 mM in DMSO). The chamber is sealed, and the compound is dialyzed against PBS, pH 7.4 at 37° C for four hours. Aliquots from each chamber (plasma and PBS) are collected, and the concentrations of a compound in each sample are determined by LC/MS/MS. Adjustments are made for non-specific binding.

5.9.1.6 Screening Cytotoxicity and Hepatotoxicity Test

Cytotoxicity is a well-established and easily accessible endstage to gather early information about the general and acute toxic potential of a new compound. The in vitro cytotoxicity test with primary hepatocytes is used to identify a test substance's cytotoxic potential. The relative cell viability upon incubation with the test article compared to the solvent control is determined (single-stage).

The ATPlite 1step Luminescence Assay System (PerkinElmer) is a single reagent addition, homogeneous, luminescence ATP detection assay that measures the number of live cells in culture wells.

Assay design:

- Primary hepatocytes (other cells available).
- 12-dose concentration-response curve (CRC) of the test article (100x IC50 or 50 μM maximum concentration).
- Two replicates of CRC.
- One incubation time: 24 hours.
- Positive control: compounds with known toxicity.
- Negative control: compound with known non-toxicity.
- Background control: vehicle only.
- Analysis: luminescence is measured from 550–620 nm.

Report: IC50.

Quantity of test article required: 1.0–2.0 mg.

Summary of assay:

Hepatocyte cells are incubated for 24 hours with known toxic and non-toxic compounds at a range of different concentrations. At the end of the incubation period, the cells are loaded with the ATPlite 1step ATP monitoring reagent and scanned using an automated plate reader with luminescence detection (Tecan Infinite M200 reader) to determine the number of active cells.

5.9.1.7 CYP450 Inhibition Profiling

This assay extends the microsomal stability assay findings to determine if the new compound inhibits a key oxidative metabolic enzyme that would lead to subsequent drug–drug interactions.

Cytochrome P450s (CYPs) are a superfamily of heme-containing enzymes that mediate the inactivation and metabolism of many drugs and endogenous substances. Compounds that inhibit P450s may cause the toxic accumulation of other substrates. CYP inhibition profiling examines the effects of a test compound on the metabolism of other known enzyme substrates of the five primary drugs human metabolizing CYP: 1A2, 2B6, 2C9, 2D6, 3A4. The levels of the CYP isoform marker substrate and metabolites are measured in the presence and absence of a test compound by LC/MS/MS.

Assay design:

- Five CYP isoenzymes: 1A2, 2B6, 2C9, 2D6, 3A4.
- Test articles are run in triplicate.
- One concentration of human liver microsomes (0.5 mg/mL).
- One concentration of test item (10 μM).
- One time stage: 0.5 hours.
- Positive control: CYP marker reaction (Table 5.1).
- Negative control: NADPH deficient reaction control.

Analysis: LC/MS/MS detection (appearance of metabolite).

Report: data are expressed as % inhibition of selected metabolites formation for each CYP450 enzyme (1A2, 2B6, 2C9, 2D6, 3A4).

(See FDA guideline for CYP substrates: www.fda.gov/Drugs/DevelopmentApprovalProcess/DevelopmentResources/DrugInteractionsLabeling/ucm093664.htm.)

Quantity of test article required: 1.0–2.0 mg.

Summary of assay:

In an assay similar to the metabolic stability assay, liver microsomes are used to determine the CYP450 inhibition profile of test compounds by measuring the % metabolism of a known substrate. Microsomes (an NADPH regenerating system) are dispensed into a 96-well plate containing a substrate and test compound (10 μM), and the reaction is allowed to proceed for 0.5 hours at 37° C with shaking. The reaction is quenched by the addition of MeOH, centrifuged, and the amount of product is measured by LC/MS/MS. Each plate will contain a known inhibitor of each CYP450 profiled as a positive control and NADP–/– negative controls (Table 5.1).

TABLE 5.1

Inhibition Profiling Five Primary Drug–Human Metabolizing Cytochrome P450s

CYP Enzyme	Substrate	Metabolite	Known Inhibitor
1A2	Phenacetin	Acetaminophen	Furafylline
2B6	Bupropion	Hydroxybupropion	Ticlopidine
2C9	Diclofenac	4-hydroxydiclofenac	Tienilic acid
2D6	Dextromethorphan	Dextrorphan	Paroxetine
3A4	Testosterone	6β-hydroxytestosterone	Azamulin

5.9.1.8 Permeability

The pharmacologic question addressed is: "How well is my drug absorbed in the gastrointestinal tract?"

Evaluating compound permeability through a cell monolayer is a good indication of intestinal permeability and oral bioavailability. The parallel artificial membrane permeability assay (PAMPA) provides a high throughput, non-cell-based method for predicting passive, transcellular intestinal absorption, the process by which the majority of small-molecule drugs enter circulation. An artificial membrane immobilized on a filter is placed between a donor and acceptor compartment in the PAMPA method. The compound is introduced in the donor compartment. Following the permeation period, the amount of compound in the donor and acceptor compartments are quantified using scanning UV spectrophotometry.

The gastrointestinal tract (GT) has a pH range from pH 1–8. The pH of the blood is constant at pH 7.4; therefore, it is possible for a pH gradient to exist between the GT and the plasma that can affect ionizable molecules' transport. To mimic this pH gradient in vitro, alternative assays with pH 7.4 acceptor compartment and pH values 5.0, 6.2, and 7.4 in the donor compartment are used.

PAMPA is a well-established and predictive assay that models the absorption of drugs in the gut. However, PAMPA is an artificial system that may provide inaccurate and potentially misleading results. Despite these limitations, PAMPA can be a useful tool to prioritize lead compounds in the early development stages. The colon carcinoma (Caco-2) cell permeability assay is the industry standard for in vitro prediction of drugs' intestinal absorption, but it also has limitations. Caco-2 cells require extensive culturing (> 20 days) and often fail to form the cohesive monolayer necessary for the uniform transport of compounds across the cell layer. The assay requires a significant amount of compound to perform the assay (typically ~20 mg). Together, the limitations of time and compound consumption decrease the value of the results obtained by Caco-2 at the early stages of drug discovery. One variant of PAMPA is the blood–brain barrier (BBB) PAMPA in where the artificial monolayer contains brain-specific membrane components, such as sphingolipids.

Assay design:

- Test articles are run in triplicate.
- One concentration (25 μM).
- One time stage (18 hours).
- One pH (7.4) or three-stage pH range (5.0, 6.2, 7.4) for acceptor compartment.
- Single polar membrane lipid (phosphatidylcholine in dodecane).
- Multiscreen PVDF membrane (0.45 μm).
- Positive control: verapamil (high permeability).
- Negative control: theophylline (low permeability).

Analysis: the concentration of the compound remaining in the donor well, diffused through the membrane and into the acceptor well, and reference compounds are measured by UV spectrophotometry.

Report: bin the results as high, medium, or low predicted absorption, and report direct permeability units (10–6 cm/s).

Quantity of test article required: 5.0–7.0 mg.

Summary of assay:

A lipid bilayer is established on a membrane filter, and a test compound solution is added to the top of the membrane-lipid interface. The ability of compounds to passively diffuse through the lipid-treated membrane indicates the overall compound permeability. This approach is helpful in compound profiling and supporting the relative rank ordering of compounds.

Analysis: LC/MS/MS detection of the test compound(s) in individual plasma samples.

Report: time course of plasma drug concentration versus time, PK parameters (for example, AUC, t1/2, oral bioavailability), and metabolite identification.

Quantity of test article required: 10–100 mg.

5.10 Conclusion

New drug discovery is highly dependent on efficient, accurate, and reproducible assays of biological activity; future science will allow newer technologies for studying drug–receptor interactions enabling newer drugs that are more specific to a mode of action. While drug discovery teams are often divided into particular focuses of work, a solid understanding of how the assays are used and can be used more creatively is key to successful drug discovery. It is for this reason that I have added this chapter to the book and included some reflections on how future drug activity assays will be developed.

ADDITIONAL READING

Aitken L, Baillie G, Pannifer A, et al. In vitro assay development, and HTS of small-molecule human ABAD/17β-HSD10 inhibitors as therapeutics in Alzheimer's disease. *SLAS Discov.* 2017;22(6): 676–685.

Alvarado C, Stahl E, Koessel K, et al. Development of a fragment-based screening assay focal adhesion targeting domain using SPR, and NMR. *Molecules.* 2019;24(18):3352.

Baniecki ML, Wirth DF, Clardy J. High-throughput *Plasmodium falciparum* growth assay for malaria drug discovery. *Antimicrob Agents Chemother.* 2007;51(2):716–723.

Binder C, Lafayette A, Archibeque I, et al. Optimization, and utilization of the SureFire phospho-STAT5 assay for a cell-based screening campaign. *Assay Drug Dev Technol.* 2008;6(1):27–37.

Butkiewicz M, Wang Y, Bryant SH, Lowe EW, Weaver DC, Meiler J. High-throughput screening assay datasets from the pubchem database. *Chem Inform.* 2017;3(1):1.

Caballero I, Lafuente MJ, Gamo FJ, Cid C. A high-throughput fluorescence-based assay for Plasmodium dihydroorotate dehydrogenase inhibitor screening. *Anal Biochem.* 2016;506:13–21.

Cai SX, Drewe J, Kasibhatla S. A chemical genetics approach discovery of apoptosis inducers: from phenotypic cell based HTS assay, and structure-activity relationship studies, to identification of potential anticancer agents, and molecular targets. *Curr Med Chem.* 2006;13(22):2627–2644.

Chan B, Cottrell JR, Li B, et al. Development of a high-throughput AlphaScreen assay for modulators of synapsin I phosphorylation in primary neurons. *J Biomol Screen.* 2014;19(2):205–214.

Chen Y, Fu Z, Li D, Yue Y, Liu X. Optimizations of a novel fluorescence polarization-based high-throughput screening assay for β-catenin/LEF1 interaction inhibitors. *Anal Biochem.* 2021;612:113966.

Cho EJ, Devkota AK, Stancu G, Edupunganti R, Powis G, Dalby KN. A fluorescence-based high-throughput assay identification of anticancer reagents targeting fructose-1,6-bisphosphate aldolase. *SLAS Discov.* 2018;23(1):1–10.

Cho EJ, Devkota AK, Stancu G, et al. A robust, and cost-effective luminescent-based high-throughput assay for fructose-1,6-bisphosphate aldolase A. *SLAS Discov.* 2020;25(9):1038–1046.

Chopra P, Nanda K, Chatterjee M, Bajpai M, Dastidar SG, Ray A. An improved zinc cocktail-mediated fluorescence polarization-based kinase assay for high-throughput screening of kinase inhibitors. *Anal Biochem.* 2008;380(1):143–145.

Chung TD, Sergienko E, Millán JL. Assay format as a critical success factor for identification of novel inhibitor chemotypes of tissue-nonspecific alkaline phosphatase from high-throughput screening. *Molecules.* 2010;15(5):3010–3037.

Coussens NP, Sittampalam GS, Guha R, et al. Assay guidance manual: quantitative biology, and pharmacology in preclinical drug discovery. *Clin Transl Sci.* 2018;11(5):461–470.

Decker AM, Mathews KM, Blough BE, Gilmour BP. Validation of a high-throughput calcium mobilization assay human trace amine-associated receptor 1. *SLAS Discov.* 2021;26(1):140–150.

Drake KM, Watson VG, Kisielewski A, Glynn R, Napper AD. A sensitive luminescent assay histone methyltransferase NSD1, and other SAM-dependent enzymes. *Assay Drug Dev Technol.* 2014;12(5):258–271.

Du Y, Fu RW, Lou B, et al. A time-resolved fluorescence resonance energy transfer assay for high-throughput screening of 14–3-3 protein-protein interaction inhibitors. *Assay Drug Dev Technol.* 2013;11(6):367–381.

Du Y, Nikolovska-Coleska Z, Qui M, et al. A dual-readout F2 assay that combines fluorescence resonance energy transfer, and fluorescence polarization for monitoring bimolecular interactions. *Assay Drug Dev Technol.* 2011;9(4):382–393.

Forbes L, Ebsworth-Mojica K, DiDone L, et al. A high throughput screening assay for anti-mycobacterial small molecules based on adenylate kinase release as a reporter of cell lysis. *PLoS One.* 2015;10(6):e0129234.

Harbert C, Marshall J, Soh S, Steger K. Development of a HTRF kinase assay for determination of Syk activity. *Curr Chem Genomics.* 2008;1:20–26.

Haubrich BA, Ramesha C, Swinney DC. Development of a bioluminescent high-throughput screening assay for nicotinamide mononucleotide adenylyltransferase (NMNAT). *SLAS Discov.* 2020;25(1):33–42.

Hendricson A, Umlauf S, Choi JY, et al. High-throughput screening for phosphatidylserine decarboxylase inhibitors using a distyrylbenzene-bis-aldehyde (DSB-3)-based fluorescence assay. *J Biol Chem.* 2019;294(32):12146–12156.

Ho YH, Chen L, Huang R. Development of a continuous fluorescence-based assay for. *Int J Mol Sci.* 2021 Jan 8;22(2):594.

Honarnejad S, van Boeckel S, van den Hurk H, van Helden S. Hit discovery for public target programs in the european lead factory: experiences, and output from assay development, and ultra-high-throughput screening. *SLAS Discov.* 2021;26(2):192–204.

Horiuchi KY, Eason MM, Ferry JJ, et al. Assay development for histone methyltransferases. *Assay Drug Dev Technol.* 2013;11(4):227–236.

Imamura RM, Kumagai K, Nakano H, Okabe T, Nagano T, Kojima H. Inexpensive high-throughput screening of kinase inhibitors using one-step enzyme-coupled fluorescence assay for ADP detection. *SLAS Discov.* 2019;24(3):284–294.

Istrate MA, Spicer TP, Wang Y, et al. Development of an HTS-compatible assay for discovery of RORα modulators using AlphaScreen® technology. *J Biomol Screen.* 2011;16(2):183–191.

Jia Y, Quinn CM, Kwak S, Talanian RV. Current in vitro kinase assay technologies: the quest for a universal format. *Curr Drug Discov Technol.* 2008;5(1):59–69.

Johansson T, Norris T, Peilot-Sjögren H. Yellow fluorescent protein-based assay to measure GABA(A) channel activation, and allosteric modulation in CHO-K1 cells. *PLoS One.* 2013;8(3):e59429.

Johnston PA, Foster CA, Shun TY, et al. Development, and implementation of a 384-well homogeneous fluorescence intensity high-throughput screening assay to identify mitogen-activated protein kinase phosphatase-1 dual-specificity protein phosphatase inhibitors. *Assay Drug Dev Technol.* 2007;5(3):319–332.

Kim TG, Lee JH, Lee MY, et al. Development of a high-throughput assay for inhibitors of the polo-box domain of polo-like kinase 1 based on time-resolved fluorescence energy transfer. *Biol Pharm Bull.* 2017;40(9):1454–1462.

Kimos M, Burton M, Urbain D, et al. Development of an HTRF assay detection, and characterization of inhibitors of catechol-*O*-methyltransferase. *J Biomol Screen.* 2016;21(5):490–495.

Kumar M, Lowery RG. A high-throughput method for measuring drug residence time using the transcreener ADP assay. *SLAS Discov.* 2017;22(7):915–922.

Lariosa-Willingham KD, Rosler ES, Tung JS, Dugas JC, Collins TL, Leonoudakis D. Development of a high throughput drug screening assay to identify compounds that protect oligodendrocyte viability, and differentiation under inflammatory conditions. *BMC Res Notes.* 2016;9(1):444.

Law CJ, Ashcroft HA, Zheng W, Sexton JZ. Assay development, and multivariate scoring for high-content discovery of chemoprotectants of endoplasmic-reticulum-stress-mediated amylin-induced cytotoxicity in pancreatic beta cells. *Assay Drug Dev Technol.* 2014;12(7):375–384.

Li H, Totoritis RD, Lor LA, et al. Evaluation of an antibody-free ADP detection assay: ADP-Glo. *Assay Drug Dev Technol.* 2009;7(6):598–605.

Li JQ, Deng CL, Gu D, et al. Development of a replicon cell line-based high throughput antiviral assay for screening inhibitors of Zika virus. *Antiviral Res.* 2018;150:148–154.

Li Q, Chen C, Kapadia A, et al. 3D models of epithelial-mesenchymal transition in breast cancer metastasis: high-throughput screening assay development, validation, and pilot screen. *J Biomol Screen.* 2011;16(2):141–154.

Li Q, Maddox C, Rasmussen L, Hobrath JV, White LE. Assay development, and high-throughput antiviral drug screening against Bluetongue virus. *Antiviral Res.* 2009;83(3):267–273.

Lim KT, Zahari Z, Amanah A, Zainuddin Z, Adenan MI. Development of resazurin-based assay in 384-well format for high throughput whole cell screening of Trypanosoma brucei rhodesiense strain STIB 900 identification of potential anti-trypanosomal agents. *Exp Parasitol.* 2016;162:49–56.

Liu B, Tang L, Zhang X, et al. A cell-based high throughput screening assay discovery of cGAS-STING pathway agonists. *Antiviral Res.* 2017;147:37–46.

Liu H, Gao ZB, Yao Z, et al. Discovering potassium channel blockers from synthetic compound database by using structure-based virtual screening in conjunction with electrophysiological assay. *J Med Chem.* 2007;50(1):83–93.

Lorenz DA, Vander Roest S, Larsen MJ, Garner AL. Development and implementation of an HTS-compatible assay discovery of selective small-molecule ligands for pre-microRNAs. *SLAS Discov.* 2018;23(1):47–54.

Lucantoni L, Duffy S, Adjalley SH, Fidock DA, Avery VM. Identification of MMV malaria box inhibitors of plasmodium falciparum early-stage gametocytes using a luciferase-based high-throughput assay. *Antimicrob Agents Chemother.* 2013;57(12):6050–6062.

Luthra P, Anantpadma M, De S, et al. High-throughput screening assay to identify small molecule inhibitors of marburg virus VP40 protein. *ACS Infect Dis.* 2020;6(10):2783–2799.

Massai F, Saleeb M, Doruk T, Elofsson M, Forsberg Å. Development, optimization, and validation of a high throughput screening assay for identification of Tat, and Type II secretion inhibitors of. *Front Cell Infect Microbiol.* 2019;9:250.

Massé N, Davidson A, Ferron F, et al. Dengue virus replicons: production of an interserotypic chimera, and cell lines from different species, and establishment of a cell-based fluorescent assay to screen inhibitors, validated by the evaluation of ribavirin's activity. *Antiviral Res.* 2010;86(3):296–305.

McElroy SP, Jones PS, Barrault DV. The SULSA assay development fund: accelerating translation of new biology from academia to pharma. *Drug Discov Today.* 2017;22(2):199–203.

McMahon JB, Beutler JA, O'Keefe BR, Goodrum CB, Myers MA, Boyd MR. Development of a cyanovirin-N-HIV-1 gp120 binding assay for high throughput screening of natural product extracts by time-resolved fluorescence. *J Biomol Screen.* 2000;5(3):169–176.

McWhirter C, Tonge M, Plant H, Hardern I, Nissink W, Durant ST. Development of a high-throughput fluorescence polarization DNA cleavage assay identification of FEN1 inhibitors. *J Biomol Screen.* 2013;18(5):567–575.

Meleza C, Thomasson B, Ramachandran C, O'Neill JW, Michelsen K, Lo MC. Development of a scintillation proximity binding assay for high-throughput screening of hematopoietic prostaglandin D2 synthase. *Anal Biochem.* 2016;511:17–23.

Mezna M, Wong AC, Ainger M, Scott RW, Hammonds T, Olson MF. Development of a high-throughput screening method for LIM kinase 1 using a luciferase-based assay of ATP consumption. *J Biomol Screen.* 2012;17(4):460–468.

Miguel-Blanco C, Lelièvre J, Delves MJ, et al. Imaging-based high-throughput screening assay to identify new molecules with transmission-blocking potential against Plasmodium falciparum female gamete formation. *Antimicrob Agents Chemother.* 2015;59(6):3298–3305.

Minuesa G, Antczak C, Shum D, et al. A 1536-well fluorescence polarization assay to screen for modulators of the MUSASHI family of RNA-binding proteins. *Comb Chem High Throughput Screen.* 2014;17(7):596–609.

Miraglia S, Swartzman EE, Mellentin-Michelotti J, et al. Homogeneous cell-, and bead-based assays for high throughput screening using fluorometric microvolume assay technology. *J Biomol Screen.* 1999;4(4):193–204.

Mitachi K, Siricilla S, Yang D, et al. Fluorescence-based assay for polyprenyl phosphate-GlcNAc-1-phosphate transferase (WecA), and identification of novel antimycobacterial WecA inhibitors. *Anal Biochem.* 2016;512:78–90.

Moynié L, Hope AG, Finzel K, et al. A substrate mimic allows high-throughput assay of the FabA protein, and consequently the identification of a novel inhibitor of *Pseudomonas aeruginosa* FabA. *J Mol Biol.* 2016;428(1):108–120.

Mukherjee A, Syeb K, Concannon J, Callegari K, Soto C, Glicksman MA. Development of a fluorescent quenching based high throughput assay to screen for calcineurin inhibitors. *PLoS One.* 2015;10(7):e0131297.

Multipurpose HTS coagulation analysis: assay development, and assessment of coagulopathic snake venoms. *Toxins (Basel).* 2017;9(12):382.

Ngo M, Wechter N, Tsai E, et al. A high-throughput assay for DNA replication inhibitors based upon multivariate analysis of yeast growth kinetics. *SLAS Discov.* 2019;24(6):669–681.

Nilam M, Gribbon P, Reinshagen J, et al. A label-free continuous fluorescence-based assay for monitoring ornithine decarboxylase activity with a synthetic putrescine receptor. *SLAS Discov.* 2017;22(7):906–914.

Pais E, Cambridge JS, Johnson CS, Meiselman HJ, Fisher TC, Alexy T. A novel high-throughput screening assay for sickle cell disease drug discovery. *J Biomol Screen.* 2009;14(4):330–336.

Park JY, Arnaout MA, Gupta V. A simple, no-wash cell adhesion-based high-throughput assay discovery of small-molecule regulators of the integrin CD11b/CD18. *J Biomol Screen.* 2007;12(3):406–417.

Peng J, Gong L, Si K, Bai X, Du G. Fluorescence resonance energy transfer assay for high-throughput screening of ADAMTS1 inhibitors. *Molecules.* 2011;16(12):10709–10721.

Pytel D, Seyb K, Liu M, et al. Enzymatic characterization of ER stress-dependent kinase, PERK, and development of a high-throughput assay for identification of PERK inhibitors. *J Biomol Screen.* 2014;19(7):1024–1034.

Qing M, Liu W, Yuan Z, Gu F, Shi PY. A high-throughput assay using dengue-1 virus-like particles for drug discovery. *Antiviral Res.* 2010;86(2):163–171.

Rectenwald JM, Hardy PB, Norris-Drouin JL, et al. A general TR-FRET assay platform for high-throughput screening, and characterizing inhibitors of methyl-lysine reader proteins. *SLAS Discov.* 2019;24(6):693–700.

Ribeiro CJA, Kankanala J, Shi K, et al. New fluorescence-based high-throughput screening assay for small molecule inhibitors of tyrosyl-DNA phosphodiesterase 2 (TDP2). *Eur J Pharm Sci.* 2018;118:67–79.

Risse E, Nicoll AJ, Taylor WA, et al. Identification of a compound that disrupts binding of amyloid-β to the prion protein using a novel fluorescence-based assay. *J Biol Chem.* 2015;290(27):17020–17028.

Rosenberg LH, Lafitte M, Grant W, Chen W, Cleveland JL, Duckett DR. Development of an HTS-compatible assay discovery of Ulk1 inhibitors. *J Biomol Screen.* 2015;20(7):913–920.

Sborgi L, Ude J, Dick MS, et al. Assay for high-throughput screening of inhibitors of the ASC-PYD inflammasome core filament. *Cell Stress.* 2018;2(4):82–90.

Segers K, Klaassen H, Economou A, Chaltin P, Anné J. Development of a high-throughput screening assay discovery of small-molecule SecA inhibitors. *Anal Biochem.* 2011;413(2):90–96.

Smith KP, Kirby JE. Validation of a high-throughput screening assay for identification of adjunctive, and directly acting antimicrobials targeting carbapenem-resistant enterobacteriaceae. *Assay Drug Dev Technol.* 2016;14(3):194–206.

Song Y, Li L, Chen Y, et al. Discovery of potent DOT1L inhibitors by AlphaLISA based high throughput screening assay. *Bioorg Med Chem.* 2018;26(8):1751–1758.

Soriano A, Radice AD, Herbitter AH, et al. Escherichia coli acetyl-coenzyme A carboxylase: characterization, and development of a high-throughput assay. *Anal Biochem.* 2006;349(2):268–276.

Sotoud H, Gribbon P, Ellinger B, et al. Development of a colorimetric, and a fluorescence phosphatase-inhibitor assay suitable for drug discovery approaches. *J Biomol Screen.* 2013;18(8):899–909.

Stowell AI, James DI, Waddell ID, et al. A high-throughput screening-compatible homogeneous time-resolved fluorescence assay measuring the glycohydrolase activity of human poly(ADP-ribose) glycohydrolase. *Anal Biochem.* 2016;503:58–64.

Sturchler E, Chen W, Spicer T, Hodder P, McDonald P, Duckett D. Development of an HTS-compatible assay discovery of ASK1 signalosome inhibitors using alphascreen technology. *Assay Drug Dev Technol.* 2014;12(4):229–237.

Tang Y, Luo J, Fleming CR, et al. Development of a sensitive, and HTS-compatible reporter gene assay for functional analysis of human adenosine A2a receptors in CHO-K1 cells. *Assay Drug Dev Technol.* 2004;2(3):281–289.

Thomas-Fowlkes B, Cifelli S, Souza S, et al. Cell-based in vitro assay automation: balancing technology, and data reproducibility/predictability. *SLAS Technol.* 2020;25(3):276–285.

Thorne N, Auld DS, Inglese J. Apparent activity in high-throughput screening: origins of compound-dependent assay interference. *Curr Opin Chem Biol.* 2010;14(3):315–324.

Tiong-Yip CL, Plant H, Sharpe P, et al. Development of a high-throughput replicon assay identification of respiratory syncytial virus inhibitors. *Antiviral Res.* 2014;101:75–81.

Turek-Etienne TC, Kober TP, Stafford JM, Bryant RW. Development of a fluorescence polarization AKT serine/threonine kinase assay using an immobilized metal ion affinity-based technology. *Assay Drug Dev Technol.* 2003;1(4):545–553.

Vasilyev DV, Shan QJ, Lee YT, et al. A novel high-throughput screening assay for HCN channel blocker using membrane potential-sensitive dye, and FLIPR. *J Biomol Screen.* 2009;14(9):1119–1128.

Veloria JR, Devkota AK, Cho EJ, Dalby KN. Optimization of a luminescence-based high-throughput screening assay for detecting apyrase activity. *SLAS Discov.* 2017;22(1):94–101.

Vempati UD, Przydzial MJ, Chung C, et al. Formalization, annotation, and analysis of diverse drug, and probe screening assay datasets using the BioAssay Ontology (BAO). *PLoS One.* 2012;7(11):e49198.

Walhart T, Isaacson-Wechsler E, Ang KH, Arkin M, Tugizov S, Palefsky JM. A cell-based. *SLAS Discov.* 2020;25(1):79–86.

Wang J, Fang P, Chase P, et al. Development of an HTS-compatible assay for discovery of melanoma-related microphthalmia transcription factor disruptors using alphascreen technology. *SLAS Discov.* 2017;22(1):58–66.

Watson VG, Drake KM, Peng Y, Napper AD. Development of a high-throughput screening-compatible assay discovery of inhibitors of the AF4-AF9 interaction using AlphaScreen technology. *Assay Drug Dev Technol.* 2013;11(4):253–268.

Wu G, Irvine J, Luft C, Pressley D, Hodge CN, Janzen B. Assay development, and high-throughput screening of caspases in microfluidic format. *Comb Chem High Throughput Screen.* 2003;6(4):303–312.

Zhang HZ, Kasibhatla S, Wang Y, et al. Discovery, characterization, and SAR of gambogic acid as a potent apoptosis inducer by a HTS assay. *Bioorg Med Chem.* 2004;12(2):309–317.

Zhang RY, Qin Y, Lv XQ, et al. A fluorometric assay for high-throughput screening targeting nicotinamide phosphoribosyltransferase. *Anal Biochem.* 2011;412(1):18–25.

Zhou W, Madrid P, Fluitt A, Stahl A, Xie XS. Development, and validation of a high-throughput screening assay for human long-chain fatty acid transport proteins 4, and 5. *J Biomol Screen.* 2010;15(5):488–497.

Zhu MR, Du DH, Hu JC, et al. Development of a high-throughput fluorescence polarization assay discovery of EZH2-EED interaction inhibitors. *Acta Pharmacol Sin.* 2018;39(2):302–310.

Zielinski T, Reichman M, Donover PS, Lowery RG. Development, and validation of a universal high-throughput UDP-glycosyltransferase assay with a time-resolved FRET signal. *Assay Drug Dev Technol.* 2016;14(4):240–251.

6

Nanomedicine

6.1 Background

The term "nano" signifies one billionth of a meter (1 nm = 10^{-9} M) (Figures 6.1 and 6.2). The thickness of plasma membranes varies between 5 and 10 nm; human red blood cells are roughly 1,000 times wider than a plasma membrane. As the particle size (solid or liquid) gets smaller, many things change, from its surface properties to its ability to enter body cells, including crossing the formidable blood–brain barrier.

The natural scene of biological phenomena is used to develop precise prevention, diagnosis, and treatment solutions in nanomedicine, applying nanotechnology in medicine. The integration of nanomaterials with biology has provided many diagnostic devices, contrast agents, analytical tools, physical therapy applications, and drug delivery vehicles (Figure 6.1).

Some applications of nanotechnology include:

- Gold nanoparticles as samples to detect specific nucleic acid sequences, cancer treatments, and other conditions.
- Better imaging and nanotechnology diagnostic tools pave the way for earlier diagnosis, more individualized treatment options, and better success rates in therapy.
- Atherosclerosis or a higher plaque in nanopharmaceuticals that imitate "good" cholesterol in the body, called HDL (high-density lipoprotein), helps shrink plates.
- The development of new technologies for gene sequencing for single-molecule detection could be permitted by solid-state nanopores.
- Nanoparticles encapsulated in cancer cells provide direct medication, reducing healthy tissue exposure.
- Knob and neural tissue engineering where novel materials are designed to imitate human bone's crystal mineral structure or used for restore purposes.
- Instead of organ transplantation, growing complex tissues.
- Graphene nanoribbons can be used to repair backbone damage as the neuron well grows on the conductive surface of graphene.
- Improvement without needles of vaccines and their delivery.
- Universal vaccine ground covering multiple strains for an annual influenza vaccine.
- Biosensors for nanoelectronics.
- Biological machinery molecular nanotechnology.

Nanomaterials have a size like most bio-molecules and structures; therefore, in vivo and in vitro biomedical research and useful applications can be made with nanomaterials. Furthermore, by interacting with biological molecules or structures, nanomaterials are given additional functionalities.

The National Nanotechnology Initiative (www.nano.gov) is a United States federal government program for the science, engineering, and technology research and development for nanoscale projects.

DOI: 10.1201/9781003146933-6

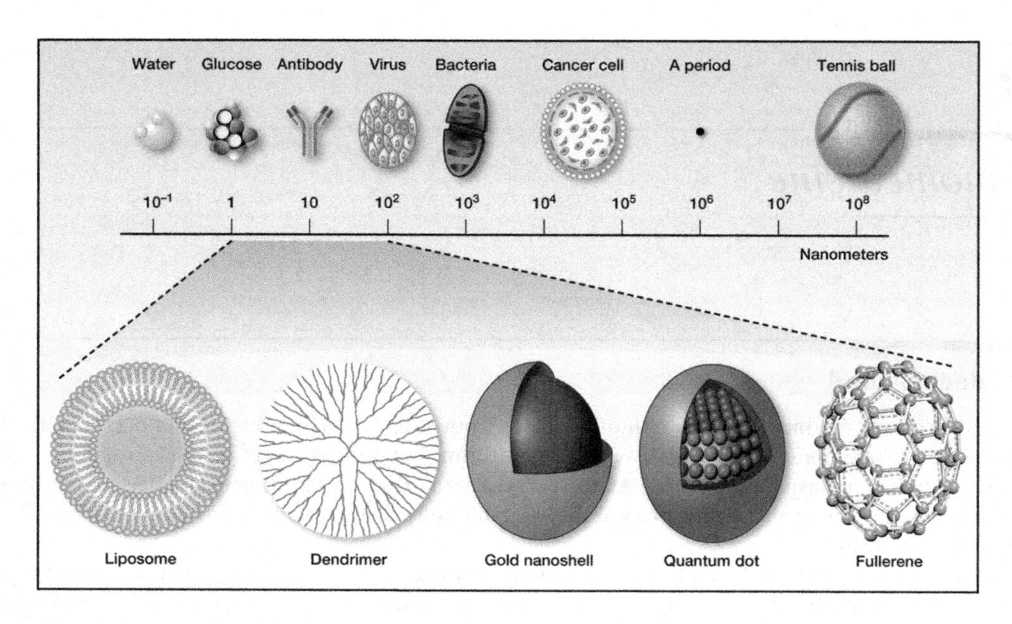

FIGURE 6.1 Nanomedicine elements. Source: https://clincancerres.aacrjournals.org/content/18/12/3229.

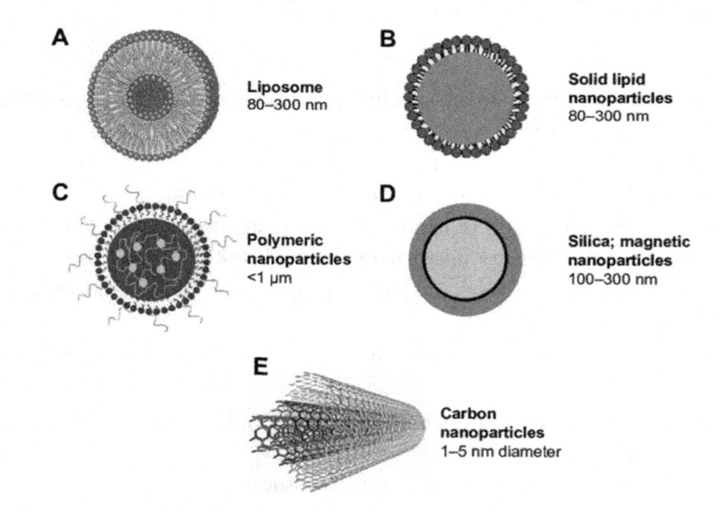

FIGURE 6.2 Types of nanoparticles used in nanomedicine. Source: Voltan, A, Quindós, G, Medina-Alarcón, K, Almeida, A, Mendes Giannini, MJ, Chorilli, M. Fungal diseases: Could nanostructured drug delivery systems be a novel paradigm for therapy? *International Journal of Nanomedicine*. 2016;11:3715–3730. 10.2147/IJN.S93105.

The NNI serves as the central point of communication, cooperation, and collaboration for all Federal agencies engaged in nanotechnology research, bringing together the expertise needed to advance this broad and complex field. The goals of the initiative include:

- Promoting an R&D program for world-class nanotechnologies.
- Promoting the commercial and public transfer of new technologies into products.
- Developing and sustaining educational resources, skilled staff, nanotechnology-advancing infrastructures and tools, and encouraging responsible nanotechnology development.

New commercial applications for the pharmaceutical industry are anticipated by the National Nanotechnology Initiative, covering advanced drug delivery systems, new therapies, and in vivo imaging.

A part of the Cancer Nanotechnology Alliance at the Federal Research and Development Center (NCI) is the Nanotechnology Characterization Lab (NCL) (managed by SAIC Frederick, Inc.). It is a resource for preclinical development of drug delivery based on nanomaterials and imaging agents with proven biological effectiveness outside the proof of development stage. The facility has been set up to speed up the clinical translation of promising formulations derived from nanotechnology. This NCI-funded resource, available to academic investigators, industry collaborators, and government laboratories, was established by NCI in collaboration with the FDA and the National Institute of Standards and Technology. Once a project is approved through a simple submission and material transfer agreement process, a large-scale batch is obtained from the collaborator for testing at NCL facilities. The laboratory conducts preclinical assessment through an established assay cascade that includes thorough physicochemical assessment, relevant in vitro studies to investigate biocompatibility, and in vivo absorption, distribution, metabolism, excretion, toxicity, efficacy, and imaging studies rodent models as appropriate. In addition to the preclinical assessment, NCL actively engages in standard protocol development and reference material standards development through collaborations. The NCL also plays an active role in educational and knowledge-sharing efforts to advance the nanomedicine field. For further information, visit http://ncl.cancer.gov.

6.2 Delivery Routes

Nanotechnology provides novel opportunities for delivering drugs to specific cells or targeted delivery using nanoparticles with a substantially lower dose and side effects. Drug supply concentrates on maximizing bioavailability by molecular targeting nanotechnology devices in particular locations in the body and over time. The nanoscale is advantageous for medical technology because smaller devices are less invasive and implantable within the body, and their biochemical response times are considerably shorter. These devices are quicker and more sensitive than typical medicinal products. A) Efficient encapsulation of drugs, b) successful drug delivery in the target region of a person, and c) successful release of medicines are the keys to the efficacy of nanomedicine supply (Figure 6.3).

Drug delivery systems, lipid- or polymer-based nanoparticles help alter the drug's pharmacokinetics and biodistribution to avoid the body's disposition mechanisms and prolong exposure to the body. The nanomedicines get drugs through cell membranes and into the cell cytoplasm rapidly and efficiently. Nanomedicines can activate interactions in body cells when introduced in the body and activated on a particular signal. Nanoparticles can demonstrate hydrophilic and hydrophobic properties improving their distribution across many biological barriers and reaching difficult target receptors in the body.

They can be made of natural or artificial polymers, lipids, dendrimers, and micelles and are of a size from 10–1,000 nm (or 1 μm). Various delivery methods are available, including the peroral, intranasal, intravenous, and intracranial transport of these drugs to the body. Most studies have shown an increase in intravenous delivery for nanoparticles. In addition, there are various modes of operation or activation of the carriers of nanoparticles, along with delivery and transport methods. These means include the dissolution or absorption of a drug throughout the nanoparticle, the encapsulation of a drug in the particle, or the attachment of a drug on the surface of that particle.

Different routes, including topical, periocular, suprachoroidal, and intravitreal, are available to administer nanoparticles. However, intravitreal nanoparticle injection often results in the clouding of the glass because of the light scattering properties of polymeric particulate matter. In addition, the possible loss of bio-activity, low protein stability, and extensive nanoencapsulation methods complicate the provision of nano-formulations of proteins due to interactions with the nanoparticle matrix. So far, fewer delivery systems for protein drugs with nanoparticles have been reported and are in the early stage of development.

Redox-activated nanocarriers are also considered effective supply systems for medicines and genes, often sensitive to glutathione as a cell redox regulator.

A long residence in the nasal cavity is ensured through the nasal administration of protein drugs using nano parts with mucoadhesive nanoparticles such as chitosan for the nasal delivery of insulin. When covered with a polymer matrix of 10–1,000 nm, the nanoparticles improve the physical-chemical stability of the gastrointestinal tract. Nanoparticles < 100 nm, but not for nanoparticles > 500 nm, are well-absorbed throughout the intestinal mucosa.

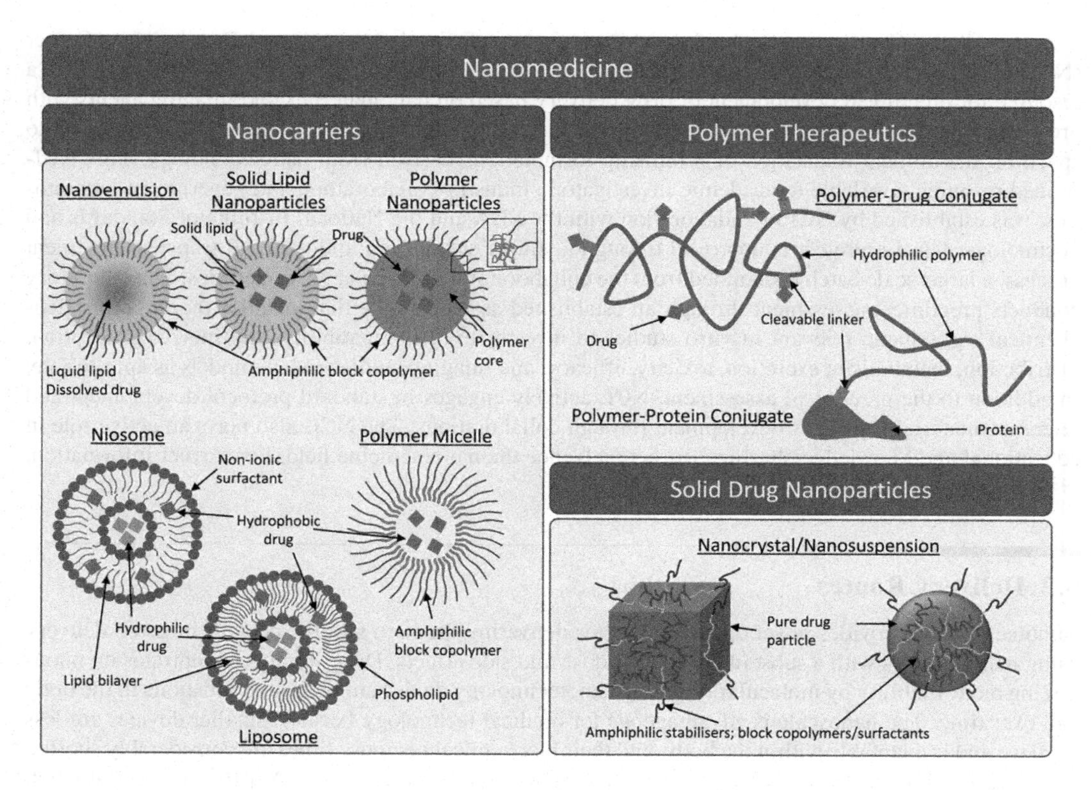

FIGURE 6.3 Types of nanomedicine routes. Source: https://onlinelibrary.wiley.com/doi/full/10.1002/jin2.61.

Nanoparticles and mucoadhesive nanoparticles have a more extended residence in the nasal cavity for the nasal use of protein medicines. For example, the nasal delivery of insulin was extensively studied with chitosan nanoparticles.

The human corneal epithelia has several layers of epithelial cells linked by close interconnections, severely limiting the ocular penetration of drugs, particularly many types of hydrophilic molecules. In addition, topical medicines are often used in the fore-eye segment by clearance mechanisms, including blinking the eyes, tear film, tear turnover, drying of solutions, and tearing. Nanoparticles possess lipid-fluidizing functions that modify extracellular lipids of the stratum corneum and play an essential role in the skin's permeability.

For ocular protein delivery, the nanocarriers of lipid-based lipids such as liposomes, nanoparticles of solid lipid, and nanostructured lipid carriers were examined. Several repeated intravitreal injections may increase the risk of ocular complications, including vitreous hemorrhage, endophthalmitis, retinal detachment, and cataracts. Therefore, they should help reduce the risk of such ocular complications based on the sustained release of drugs. However, intravitreal nanoparticle injection often results in the clouding of the glass, as the light dissemination properties of polymeric particles lead to the loss of bioactivity, which has limited these applications. Nevertheless, ocular drug delivery is successful with polymeric nanoparticles, including a thermo-gelling system based upon polymer.

Because of its chemical stability, biodegradability, biocompatibility, immunogenicity lack, and low toxicity, self-assembling nanovesicles consisting of nonionic surfactants, which are compatible with liposomes, are also preferred for the topical delivery of ocular drugs. The lipophilic and hydrophilic drugs can also encapsulate and provide structural flexibility. Disks are a modified form of large niosomes produced by Solulan C24 (12–16 mm) (nonionic surfactant). Their large dimensions can prevent their drainage into the systems pond. Therefore, they are suitable for the ocular route. In addition, discomforts are disc-like and can fit into the sinus of the eyes better. Early-stage development of niosomes and discomfort continues, and their potential as an ocular protein delivery system should be further explored.

The stratum cornea efficiently enters nanocarriers scattered through lipophilic vehicles since it is a hydrophobic stratum. Nanoemulsion is a nano-carrier system containing two immiscible phases of fluid that have low-viscosity isotropic dispersion.

Ocular drug delivery is successful with polymeric nanoparticles, including a thermo-gelling system based upon polymer.

The method for the transportation of medication molecules through the blood–brain barrier (BBB) using nanoparticles is nanoparticles for delivering drugs into the brain. These medications cross BBB and supply the brain with pharmaceuticals to treat neurological disturbances for therapy. Parkinson's disease, Alzheimer's disease, schizophrenia, depression, and brain tumors are examples of neurological disorders. Unfortunately, one of the difficulties in finding cures for CNS disorders is that no genuinely effective supply of BBB drugs is available. A few examples of molecules that cannot pass the BBB alone are antibiotics, antineoplastic, and several CNS-active drugs, especially neuropeptides. But some medicines can now cross the BBB with the aid of nanoparticles and are even less toxic and less harmful to the body.

The BBB is not the only physiological barrier to drug supply to the brain; other biological factors influence the movement of drugs across the body and target specific areas. These factors include alteration of the blood flow, edema, increased intracranial pressure, metabolism, altered gene expression, and protein synthesis. Nanoparticles in the CNS can overcome many of these barriers.

In 1995, the first successful drug delivery across the whole BBB was the embodiment of an intravenous injection of hexapeptide dalargin (an anti-nociceptive peptide).

Many polymers are natural, biocompatible, and biodegradable and prevent CNS contamination for nanoparticles supply systems. Various existing methods for delivering drugs to the brain include liposomes, medicines, and carriers.

Their possible accumulation in the body is one issue with the use of nanoparticles. Polymer nanoparticles could develop in the body, causing unwanted effects by more prolonged and frequent injections often required to treat chronic conditions such as Alzheimer's disease.

6.3 Liposomes

Liposomes consist of bilayer vesicles, laminae made of biocompatible, biodegradable lipids, for example, sphingomyelin, phosphatidylcholine, and glycerophospholipids. These are the composition. Lipid-nanoparticles also often contain cholesterol, a type of lipid. Cholesterol can improve the stability of a liposome by preventing the leakage of a bilayer as the hydroxyl group can interact with its polar heads.

Liposomes can protect the drug from degradation, target sites for action, and reduce toxicity and adverse effects. In addition, lipid nanoparticles can be manufactured by high-pressure homogenization, a current method used to produce parenteral emulsions.

For rectal administration, nano-sized liposomes are also used. As an additional nanocarrier, solid lipid nanoparticles are applicable for rectal drug delivery. Modified nanoliposomes containing hepatitis B surface antigen can be used for mucosal immunization, composed of 1,2-dipalmitoyl-sn-glycerol-3-phosp hocholine bilayer engulfing a solid fat core (mainly glyceryl tripalmitate) and use monophosphoryl lipid A as an adjuvant. These hybrid liposomes show greater stability and significant humoral and cellular immune responses in rats after intracolonic administration.

Because nanoemulsion is a thermodynamically unstable system, physical instability such as creaming and flocculation during long-term storage is their major drawback. However, optimizing the particle size and surfactant composition can produce a metastable state in the system. Thus, equal to its thermodynamic instability, transcutaneous nanodispersion immunization has demonstrated some potential as a transdermal antigen delivery vehicle, although nanoemulsions are less popular for transdermal delivery.

Liposomes can also be worked out by attaching different ligands to the surface to improve brain delivery.

Free diffusion, a type of facilitated diffusion or endocytosis lipid-mediated, is a liposome transport mechanism throughout the BBB. Many receptors of lipoprotein bind lipoproteins into complexes that transport the liposome nano supply system throughout the BBB. Apolipoprotein E is a protein that makes lipid and cholesterol transportation easier. ApoE components link to nanoparticles and then bind to the LDLR in the BBB, enabling the transport of these complex components.

A liposome cationic can also be used for delivery in the brain as a lipid nanoparticle. These are positively charged lipid molecules. The nanovesicle boundary of a drug as a cationic liposome that contains hydrophilic groups around the hydrophobe chain is strengthened by bola amphiphiles. Bola amphiphile nanovesicles can cross the BBB and allow the pharmaceutical to enter the target area in a controlled manner. Lipoplexes can also be formed by cationic liposomes and transfection solutions for DNA. Cationic liposomes cross the BBB through adsorption and endocytosis and then internalize the endothelial cell endosomes. Physical changes in the cells could be achieved by transfecting endothelial cells through lipoplexes. These physical changes may enhance how some nanoparticle carriers traverse the BBB.

Solid-lipid nanoparticles have many advantages, such as physical stability, targetability, and controlled release, as they are composed of physiologic lipids, easy to scale up, and non-toxicity. It also improves the corneal uptake of drugs and enhances the eye bioavailability of hydrophilic and lipophilic drugs.

The solid lipid nanoparticle is shown in Figure 6.2 (SLN). The inside of the particle is solid, so there is only one phospholipid layer. Therefore, the SLN surface can be bound to molecules like antibodies, targeting peptides and medical molecules.

The liquid lipid oil employed in the emulsion process can be replaced by a solidified lipid by SLNs. The drug molecules in solid lipid nanoparticles are dissolved in the solid hydrophobic core of the particle and called drug payload and are surrounded by an aqueous solution. Many SLNs come from triglycerides, wax, and fatty acids. The production can be carried out with high pressure or micro-emulsification homogenization. In addition, it is possible to increase the BBB permeability by the functionalization of nanoparticles on the surface with polyethylene glycol (PEG). However, several colloidal carriers such as liposomes, polymer nanoparticles, and emulsions have reduced the stableness, shelf-life, and encapsulation efficacy. Solid lipid nanoparticles are developed to overcome these deficiencies and have, apart from a targeted supply of drugs, excellent drug release, and physical stability.

Oil-in-water emulsions using common biocompatible oils such as triglycerides and fatty acids combined with water and surface coating surfactants are also used for nanoparticles supply systems. In particular, omega-3 fatty acid-rich oils contain essential factors which help penetrate the BBB's tight intersections.

6.4 Dendrimers

Dendrimers are nano-sized polymeric carriers that can entrap and conjugate high molecular weight molecules. They are radially symmetric molecules with well-defined, homogeneous, and monodisperse structures consisting of treelike branches. Some commonly used dendrimers are poly amido amines, polyamines, polyamides (polypeptides), poly (aryl ethers), polyesters, and carbohydrates; poly amidoamine are the most common and commercially available. Their molecular weight and surface charge play a crucial role in determining tissue accumulation profiles and drug release rates from the polymer. The absorption is maximal in the cationic dendrimers due to their ability to interact with lipid bilayers, and it is decreased with the uncharged or anionic dendrimers. Additionally, the multiple functional groups on their surface make it possible to target any location in the body, reinforcing ligand-receptor binding, ameliorating the targeting of attached components, and accelerating dendrimer stimuli-responsive functions.

6.5 Polymers

Natural biodegradable polymers nanoparticles can target specific organ and body tissue, carry gene therapy DNA, and provide larger molecules like proteins, peptides, and genes. The drugs are first dissolved or encapsulated, or attached to a polymer nanoparticle matrix to produce these polymers. There are then three different structures: nanoparticles, nanocapsules (in which the drug is encapsulated, and the polymer matrix surrounds it), and nanospheres.

Polybutyl cyanoacrylate (PBCA), poly(isohexyl cyanoacrylate) (PISCA), polylactic acid (PLA), or polylactide co-glycolide are common polymer materials that are used in pharmaceutical deliveries (PLGA). PBCA is degraded in the alkyl chain via the enzyme cleavage of its ester bond to produce water-soluble by-products. The most rapid biodegradable material is also PBCA, with studies showing an 80% decrease following 24 hours of intravenous therapy injection. The PIHCA rate of degradation is slower, which reduces toxicity further in turn.

The production of nanoparticle delivery systems is also using human serum albumin (HSA) and chitosan. Nanoparticles with albumin may overcome many constraints for stroke therapy. Albumin nanoparticles, for example, can improve the permeabilities of BBB, increase solubility and increase circulatory half-life. In addition, brain cancer patients naturally increase albumin uptake in the brain by overexpressing albumin binding proteins such as SPARC and gp60. This is the relation by which albumin nanoparticles co-encapsulate a type of cell-penetrating protein used for anti-glioma therapy, paclitaxel, fenretinide, modified with the low weight molecle protamine (LMWP). Once injected into the patient's body, nanoparticles of the albumin can more easily cross the BBB, tie to the proteins, penetrate glioma cells and release all drugs.

Natural and synthetic polymers are polylactic acid, poly-co-glycolic acid, chitosan, gelatin, polymethyl methacrylate, and poly alkyl-cyanoacrylate been used in nanoparticles. Chitosan is a copolymer consisting of glucosamine and N-acetyl glucosamine derived from chitin deacetylation. Much of the chitosan properties, including biocompatibility, mucoadhesion, and low toxicity, make it an adequate protein supplier. By opening the narrow junction, Chitosan also improves cellular uptake. Chitosan is commonly used to manufacture and deliver polymeric nanoparticles, PLGa, PLA, and methacrylic acid copolymers. In addition, these polymeric nanoparticles frequently undergo surface modifications to provide additional assets such as site-specificity or extended circulation periods.

Chitosan can overcome the limitation of internal administration in the brain with its adsorptive and mucoadhesive properties. In addition, cationic chitosan nanoparticles have been shown to interact with a negative brain endothelium.

Chitosan nanoparticles have prolonged their time of contact between insulin and the nasal mucosal membrane, improving the bioavailability of insulin. The intranasal administration of nanoparticles of chitosan-N-acetyl-L-cysteine and PEG-g-chitosan nanoparticles also improves insulin bioavailability. Intranasal vaccination focuses on the nasal-associated lymphoid, and chitosan, PLGA, and polymer nanoparticles are useful in antigen uptake. The residence of antigen and enhanced IgA and IgG production increase trimethane chitosan nanoparticles. Phytosanitary nanoparticles also increase the brain's absorption by nasal administration of the nerve growth factor.

Alginate is a natural anionic polymer commonly used as a carrier of medicinal products. It can easily be gel-formulated via electrostatic interaction with cationic materials through its anionic surface charge. Alginate beads, however, have high porosity, leading to drug leakage. Chitosan or dextran sulfate are often employed together with alginate to overcome this problem.

The receptor-mediated endocytosis through brain capillaries is the mechanism for the transport of polymer-based nanoparticles across the BBB. Transcytosis then occurs in the endothelial cell tightly and in the brain to transport the nanoparticles. Nanoparticles covered by surfactant products such as polysorbate 80 or poloxamer 188 increase the brain absorption of the medicine. It also uses specific receptors situated on the luminous surface of the BBB's endothelial cells. To make a formational change, ligands that are coated on the surface of the article are attached to specific receptors. Transcytosis may start once bound to these receptors, involving the formation of vesicles from the plasma membrane, which after internalization, pinch out of the nanoparticulate system.

The scavenger receptor class B type I (SR-BI), the LDL receptor (LRP1), the transferrin receptor, and the insulin receptor are also receptors for nanoparticle delivery systems. Thus, as long as an endothelial surface of the BBB is equipped with a receptor, the ligand may be attached to the surfaces of the nanoparticles so that it can bind and undergo endocytosis.

Adsorption-mediated transcytosis is another method, which involves electrostatic interactions in mediating the crossing of the BBB nanoparticles. This mechanism is of interest to cationic nanoparticles (including the cationic fibers) because they help bind endothelial cells in the brain with their positive charges. In addition, a cell-penetrating peptide, TAT-peptides, can further improve drug transport within the brain to functionalize the surface of cationic nanoparticles.

The covering with various surfactants of these polymeric nanoparticles may help BBB get through and into the brain. The functionality of the polyethylene glycol (PEG) surface of nanoparticles may induce the "stealth impact," which allows drug-laden nanoparticles to circulate across the body for extended periods. Due in part to the hydrophilic and flexible properties of PEG chains, the stealth effect facilitates the location of the drug at the target tissue and organ sites.

Based on biocompatibility and ease of surface alteration and copolymerization, polymeric nanoparticles are widely used as pulmonary suppliers. Chitosan, alginate, and gelatin are the most used natural polymer carriers. Similarly, the most used synthetic nanocarriers to deliver pulmonary drugs are poloxamer, poly(lactic-co-glycolic) acid, and polyethylene glycol.

The polymeric micelles consist of amphiphile copolymers with hydrophilic chains forming a shell and hydrophobic chains, which are nano-carriers with sized ranges from 10 to 100 nm. They can be assembled in aqueous media to form an organized supramolecular structure at levels above their critical mice. Polymeric ocular micelles are produced using a variety of polymers, including poloxamer 407, poloxamer 188, methoxy-poly(e-caprolactone), poly(butylene oxide)-poly(butylene oxygen), polyhydroxyethylaspartamide and isopropylacrylamide (Figure 6.4).

The most advanced non-viral gene delivery system is lipid nanoparticles (LNPs). Lipid nanoparticles deliver nuclear acids safely and effectively, overcoming a significant barrier to the development and use of genetic medicines. The application of genetics is diverse, for instance, for the editing of genes, rapid vaccine development, immuno-oncology, and treatment, usually impaired by the inefficiency of nucleic acid delivery. Lipid nanoparticles offer many advantages over previous lipid-based nucleic acid delivery systems, including:

- High enclosure and powerful transfection efficiency.
- Enhanced tissue penetration for therapeutic use.
- Cytotoxicity and immunosuppression.
- Outstanding nuclear acid supply candidates.

The Pfizer-BioNTech COVID-19 vaccine contains the following ingredients: mRNA, lipids ([4-hydrox ybutyl]azanediyl)bis(hexane-6,1-diyl)bis(2-hexyldecanoate), 2 ([polyethylene glycol]-2000)-N,N-ditetradecylacetamide, 1,2-Distearoyl-sn-glycero-3- phosphocholine, and cholesterol), potassium chloride, monobasic potassium phosphate, sodium chloride, dibasic sodium phosphate dihydrate, and sucrose.

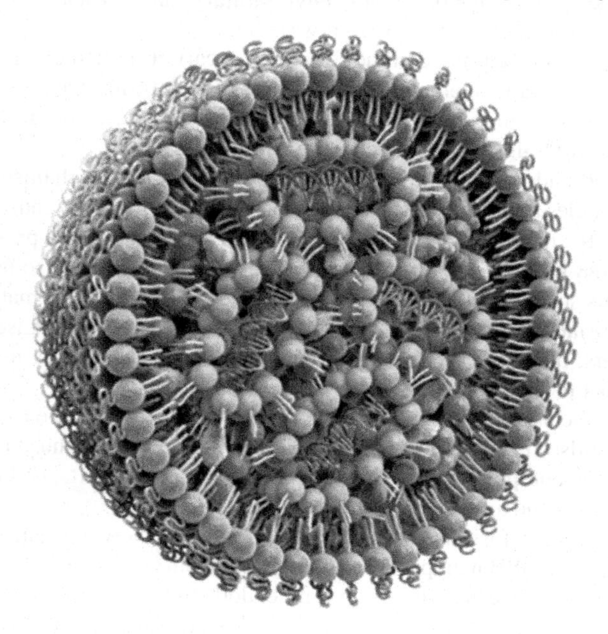

FIGURE 6.4 Lipid nanoparticle for mRNA vaccine.

The Moderna COVID-19 vaccine contains the following ingredients: messenger ribonucleic acid (mRNA), lipids (SM-102, polyethylene glycol [PEG] 2000 dimyristoyl glycerol [DMG], cholesterol, and 1,2-distearoyl-sn-glycero-3-phosphocholine [DSPC]), tromethamine, tromethamine hydrochloride, acetic acid, sodium acetate, and sucrose.

6.6 Metal Particles

Due to the biocompatibility of nanoparticles, gold, silver, and platinum are commonly used in nanoparticles. Due to their large volume range, these metal nanoparticles have geometric and chemical tuning properties and endogenous antimicrobial properties. In addition, the silver cations released from silver nanoparticles can be fixed to the negative cell membrane of the bacterium and enhance membrane permeability to allow foreign chemicals into the intracellular fluid.

Reducing reactions are used to synthesize metal nanoparticles chemically. For example, the presence of ionic compounds results in drug-conjugated silver nanoparticles by reducing silver nitrate to sodium borohydride. The medication is attached to the silver surface and is used to stabilize nanoparticles.

Metal nanoparticles usually cross the BBB via transcytosis. The delivery of nanoparticles to the central nervous system can be increased through the introduction of peptide conjugates. For example, recent research has improved the efficiency of delivering the gold nanoparticles by combining a peptide that connects the brain endothelial cells with the transferrin receptors.

Gold nanoparticles (AuNPs) are also a potential tool for cancer therapy and CT imaging to influence tumor vascular permeability. AuNPs absorb radiation and release short-scale low-energy photoelectrons, which increase the local radiation dose during external radiation therapy by the beam (RT).

The risk of neurotoxicity and cytotoxicity is associated with metal nanoparticles. These heavy metals produce reactivated oxygen, causing oxidative stress and damaging the mitochondria and reticule of the cells. This leads to additional problems in cell toxicity, such as DNA damage and cellular disturbance. Silver nanoparticles, in particular, are more toxic than others, for example, gold or iron. As discovered by an analysis of the distribution of silver nanoparticles in rats, silver nanoparticles can circulate across the body and accumulate quickly in various organs. After the injection of nanoparticles, subcutaneous traces of silver are collected in the lungs, spleen, kidney, liver, and brain of the rats. Silver nanoparticles also produce more reactive oxygen species than other metals, leading to a larger overall toxicity problem.

Magnetic field delivery does not depend heavily on the brain's biochemistry. The use of a magnetic field gradient pulls nanoparticles across the BBB in this case. It is only through the direction of the slope that nanoparticles are drawn into and removed from the brain. The nanoparticles have a non-zero magnet moment and a diameter of below 50 nm for the work approach. The requirements are met by both magnetic and non-magnetic nanoparticles (MEN). But the non-zero magnetoelectric (ME) effects are only displayed in MENs. Because of the ME effect, MENs can access nanoscale local electric fields directly, allowing two-way communication with a single-neuron network.

The nanotechnological platform for super magnetic iron oXides (SPIUN) can target, control release, and visualize the metal nature of nanotechnology. Magnetism may target SPIONs to the tissue of concern or trigger the release of drugs, and the SPIONs can be imaged via MRI.

6.7 Quantum Dots

Quantum dots (QDs) are semiconductor particles a few nanometers in size with optical and electronic characteristics that vary from larger particles due to quantum mechanics. In nanotechnology, they are a central subject. When UV light is applied to the quantum dots, a source dot electron may excite a higher energy state. This process corresponds to a transition of the electron from the valence band to the conducting band with the semiconducting quantum dot. Then, the aroused electron can fall back to the valence band, releasing its energy through light emissions. This light emission is illustrated in the right figure (photoluminescence). The color depends on the difference in energy between the driving band and the valence band.

Nano-scale semiconductor materials contain either electrons or electron holes in the language of materials science tightly. Quantum dots are sometimes referred to as artificial atoms that emphasize their unique characteristics and bound electronic states, such as atoms or molecules that occur naturally. The electronic wave functions in quantum points are similar to those in real atoms. Combining a few such quantum points and hybridizing even at room temperature, an artificial molecule can be made.

Quantum points have intermediate characteristics between large semiconductors and discrete atoms or molecules. As a function of both size and form, the optoelectronic properties change. Larger 5–6 nm diameter QDs with orange or red colors emit longer wavelengths. Smaller (2–3 nm) QDs emit shorter wavelengths, which yield blue and green colors. However, depending on the exact composition of the QD, the colors are different.

Applications of potentially single-electron transistors, solar cells, lasers, single-photon sources, second-harmonic generations, quantum computing, research into cell biology, and medical imagery include potentially quantum dots. In addition, thanks to its small size, certain QDs are suspended into solution and can be printed with inkjet and spin-coated.

6.8 Fullerenes

A complement is a carbon allotrope whose molecule contains carbon-atoms connected by a single and a two-bond mesh with a fused ring of five to seven atoms and forming a closed and partially closed mesh. The molecule can be hollow, elliptical, tube, or any other form and dimension. The graphite, a flat mesh of regular hexagonal rings, can be regarded as an extreme family member (isolated graphite atomic layers).

The empirical formula CN, often written CN where n is the number of carbon atoms, informally denotes fullerenes with a closed mesh topology. There may, however, be more than one isomer for some values of n.

Fullerenes were forecast for some time, but they were only detected in natural and outer space after their accidental synthesis in 1985. Fullerene discovery has significantly expanded the number of known carbon allotropes previously confined to graphite, diamond, and amorphous carbon such as soot and charcoal. They were intensively researched for both their chemicals and their technical applications, particularly in materials science, electronics, and nanotechnology (Figure 6.5.)

Carbon nanotubes belong to the fullerene family of carbon allotropes with cylindrical shapes and exhibit unique physicochemical properties with easy surface modification. They also possess superior mechanical properties, high thermal conductivities, and, more importantly, the ability to penetrate cell membranes, making them suitable as nanocarriers for targeted or controlled drug delivery, biosensing, and bioimaging.

6.9 Theranostics

Nanoparticles are attractive candidates for better therapeutic applications for various diseases due to their controlled release properties, cell and tissue-targeting ability, and selectiveness. The surface of nanoparticles can easily be modified with ligands to make them useful for active targeting and consequently improve their targeting efficiencies. Imaging agents can be introduced with the drug carriers to make treatment much less troublesome and prognosis bright. Nano theranostics can be a general approach in which diagnosis and therapy are interwoven to solve clinical issues and improve treatment outcomes. In most cases, theranostic nanomedicines' interesting results in the literature are available only for in vitro studies. In vivo applications at the preclinical and clinical levels, there are more challenges to face. It appears that advanced nano theranostics becomes an approach of the future generation.

Theranostics is a combination of therapy and diagnosis. Theranostics is the term for combining one radioactive medicine for the identification (diagnosis) and the second radioactive medicine for the treatment of the primary tumor and all metastatic tumors. Nano theranostics integrates theranostic nanomaterials with diagnostic and therapy integration, enabling diagnosis, therapy, and monitoring progress and

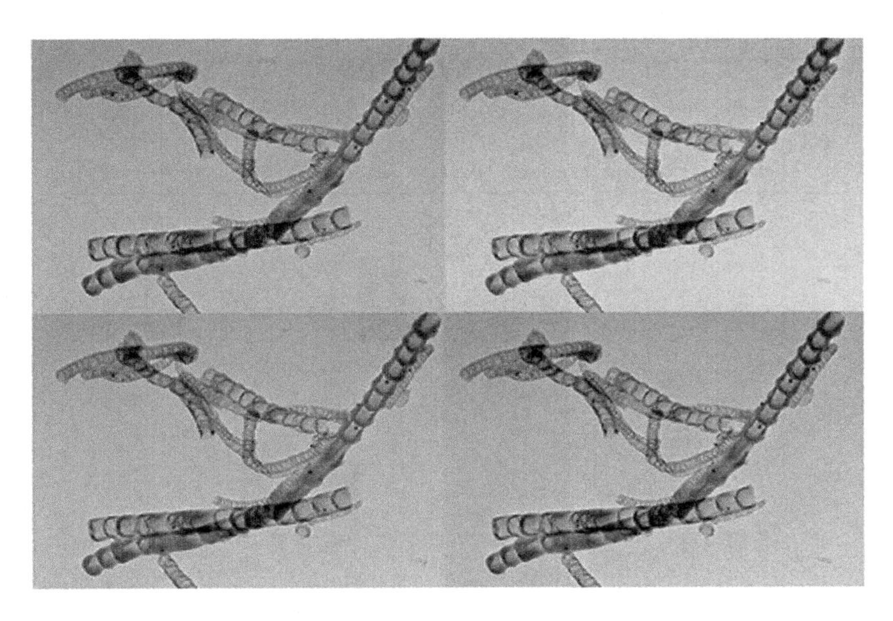

FIGURE 6.5 The bamboo-like structure of nitrogen-doped carbon nanotubes for the treatment of cancer. Source: courtesy of Wake Forest and the National Cancer Institute.

effectiveness in treatment in real-time. Diagnostic and medical agents are adsorbed, conjugated, trapped, and enclosed in nanomaterials in theranostic nanocarriers of 10–1,000 nm for simultaneous cells and molecules diagnostics and treatment (Figure 6.6.)

Hydrophobic drugs, proteins, peptides, and genetic materials are among the therapeutic agents in theranostic nanomedicine. In addition to therapeutic agents, commonly used diagnostics in theranostic includes fluorescent dyes, quantum dots, iron oxides super-paramagnétic (SPIOs), and iodine radionuclides. This strategy can provide better theranostics effects and reduce adverse effects by delivering diagnostic and therapeutic agents continuously in targeted tissues. Even for fatal conditions, such as cancer, inflammatory bowel (IBD), cardiovascular conditions (CBD), diabetes, ocular diseases, and AIDS, nano theranostics can be promising to improve the prognosis while increasing patients' tolerance for treatment and saving resources.

Theranostic nanomedicine is multifunctional and can use ligands and biomarkers to diagnose and treat diseased cells. Applications include the imaging guidance on drug delivery, molecular sensing, and tissue engineering of polymer nanoparticles responsive to external pH stimuli. Theranostics can also promote a wide range of different treatments, including photothermal treatment (PTT), photodynamic treatment (PDT), and immunotherapy, using nanotechnology.

To develop theranostic agents, imaging materials are conjugated to delivery carriers loaded with drugs, and a variety of imaging methods were used to visualize the agent. The most widely employed noninvasive imaging methods include magnetic resonance imaging (MRI), computed tomography (CT), positron emission tomography (PET), and optical imaging to monitor biodistribution, drug release kinetics, and therapeutic efficacy of theranostic nanomaterials. The design of nano theranostics materials is shown in Figure 6.3.

Theranostics enables the visualization and monitoring of diseased tissue, delivery kinetics, and the efficacy of the anticancer treatment while allowing controlled and rational tuning of the therapeutic strategy. For example, most anticancer medications, such as doxorubicin (DOX) and paclitaxel (PTX), are toxic to normal cells. Targeted delivery of cancer treatment may reduce this problem; in this regard, nanomedicine offers hope. With NIR fluorescent probes incorporated into nano-drug carriers, nanoparticles can be tracked in vivo in real-time.

Theranostic applications mean different combinations of the combined therapy and imaging methods. Several non-invasive imaging methods are used to monitor biodistribution, pharmacokinetics, and

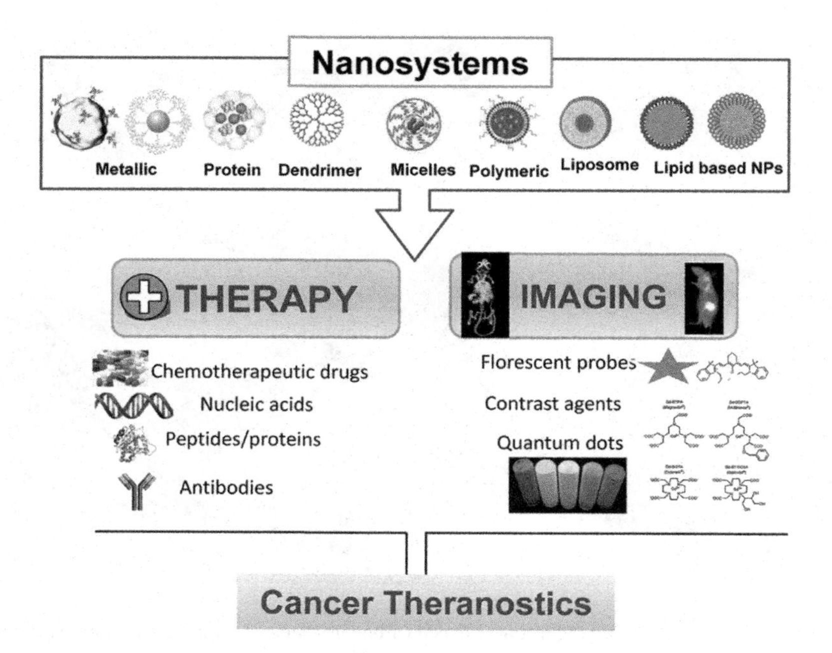

FIGURE 6.6 Basic concept of theranostic applications using nanosystems. Source: www.frontiersin.org/articles/10.3389/fphar.2019.01264/full.

therapeutic efficacy of theranostic nanoparticles (for example, optical, magnetic resonance [MR], CT, PET, and ultrasound [US] imaging techniques).

6.10 Diagnostics

MRI is an efficient, non-invasive imagery method used to acquire cross-section tomographic images of tissues by magnetic fields and radio waves. MRI benefits from high spatial resolution, deep penetration, and nonionizing radiation compared with other image techniques.

Computer tomography (CT) is one of the most commonly used computerized x-ray images for the production of intersectional tomographic 3D images of tissues of interest. In functional imagery, contrasting agents allow the structure to be highlighted despite a lack of contrast.

Nanoparticles containing iodine are used to imagine the tumor in dual-mode for x-ray CT and US.

PET is a technique that generates 3D functional body images. PET is ideal for tracking and quantifying physiological processes in vivo with advantages like higher sensitivity, non-invasiveness, and quantitative real-time imaging. PET uses radiotracers (like fluorine-18) that are biologically active in producing a positron and an electron, which decay and cause widespread destruction. PET can be used to track radiolabeled nano molecules potentially used to diagnose cancer or other indications. For example, 18F-labeled PEGylated liposomes are used to their biodistribution under the PET imaging format.

The imaging techniques routinely used for cardiovascular disease diagnosis are electrocardiography (ECG), chest X-ray, echocardiography, cardiac catheterization, and blood tests. In addition, nanoparticle imaging techniques cover advanced optical and luminescence imaging and spectroscopy, ultrasound, X-ray imaging, MRI, and nuclear imaging with radioactive tracers, most of which depend on targeting agents or contrast agents introduced into the body to mark the disease site.

Magnetically sensitive nanoparticles are an essential tool in the diagnostic application of detecting disease as early as possible. For example, FDA has approved gadolinium (Gd) as a TI relaxation paramagnetic MRI contrast agent. In addition, dextran-coated iron oxide nanoparticles loaded with NIR fluorophores and phototoxic nanoparticles specifically target macrophages and are activated by light to induce apoptosis in the targeted macrophages.

6.11 Specific Diseases

6.11.1 IBD

IBD represents a promising frontier in drug targeting since it is characterized by segmental inflammation of the bowel. IBD is made up of ulcerative colitis and Crohn's disease. Mucosal lesions are seen in the rectum and extend a certain distance up the colon in ulcerative colitis (and rarely to the terminal ileum). The inflammation of Crohn's disease usually occurs only in short segments of the whole bowel. Thus, most of the bowels in IBD are healthy and should not be exposed to any medication to reduce or prevent systemic adverse effects. Maintaining an effective drug concentration in inflamed mucosa is the major challenge when reducing IBD reoccurrences. In modifying the pharmacokinetics and the effectiveness of existing medicines in intestinal inflammatory cells, nanotechnology offers advantages. The Brownian movement of the luminous nanoparticles increases their mucoadhesive properties. Since luminal streaming does not affect nanoparticles, adherence, and insertion into the intestinal mucosa are improved. This improves. The intestinal epithelial monolayer disrupts the integrity of the intestinal cell under inflammatory conditions and loses its barrier function. The gaps or trout in the epithelial membrane significantly improve the introduction to the mucosa of the nanoparticles. In addition, the small size could facilitate endocytosis and transcytosis, which were responsible respectively for the uptake of particles less than 100 nm and 500 nm in diameter.

Nano molecules to deliver existing or experimental IBD drugs to inflamed intestinal tissue include prednisolone, budesonide, curcumin (CC), and TNFa siRNA. Prednisolone is one of the two most commonly used oral glucocorticoids for IBD, working through broad anti-inflammatory actions. It can be used for mild, moderate, or severe IBD, depending on the route of administration.

6.11.2 Diabetes

Diabetes mellitus or diabetes is caused by low insulin secretion by pancreatic islet cells, leading to hyperglycemia. The loss of insulin-produced beta cells in the pancreas of islets of Langerhans in type 1 (insulin-dependent) diabetes mellitus, which leads to insulin deficiency. In contrast, type 2 (non-insulin-dependent) diabetes is caused by insulin resistance or reduced insulin secretion. Glycemic control can be achieved through diet, physical activity, insulin therapy, and oral medications. Applications of nanoparticles for the treatment of type 1 diabetes through effective insulin delivery are possible. The major obstacles in developing oral insulin formulations are either enzymatic barriers or physical barriers. Insulin is degraded by gastric pH and intestinal enzymes, and the intestinal epithelial cell membranes serve as a formidable absorption barrier itself. Together, this results in $< 1\%$ bioavailability of total oral insulin intake. One solution is to use nanocarriers as the best-suited vehicle for the oral delivery of insulin (Figure 6.7).

Chitosan-based nanoparticles enhance paracellular transport across the intestinal epithelium and prolong small intestinal residence time, both of which augment absorption. In addition, the intestinal residence time is increased because chitosan can adhere to the mucosal surface.

6.11.3 Cancer

History has led to the weakening and systemic toxicities, poor bioavailability, and unfavorable pharmacokinetics in treating cancer patients with chemotherapeutic agents. The systems of drug delivery based on nanotechnology can focus specifically on cancer cells, prevent rapid clearance, and be administered without toxic solvents while preventing their healthy neighbors. Nanomaterials open up new forms of cancer therapy, such as photodynamic and hyperthermic treatments, in addition to established therapeutic modes of action. Nanoparticle carriers can also tackle multiple drug delivery issues that have not in the past been successfully resolved. They include overcoming formulation problems, multidrug resistance, and pervasive cellular barriers that may limit device readiness to targets such as the blood–brain barrier. Thus, nanoscale devices are promising for the diagnosis and treatment of new methods of cancer.

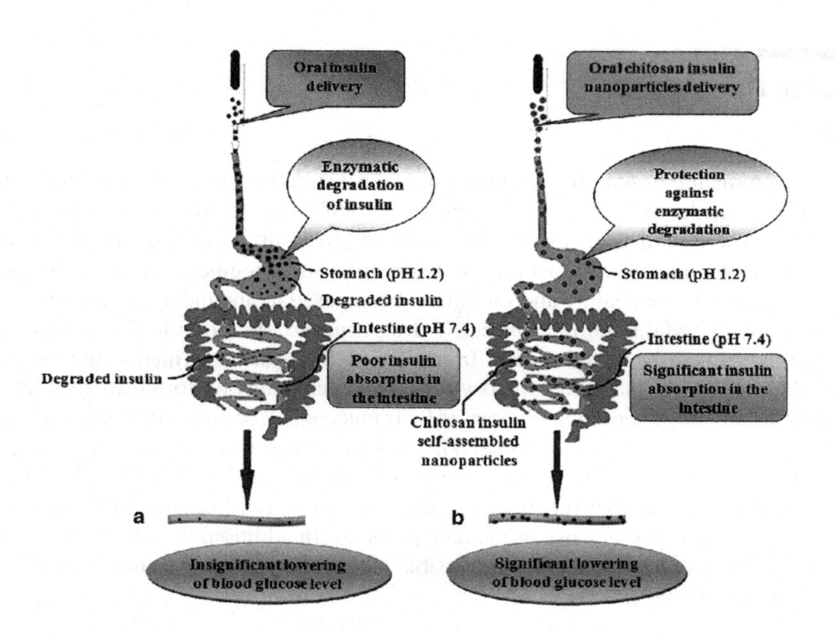

FIGURE 6.7 Novel delivery systems for insulin. Source: www.semanticscholar.org/paper/Nanoparticle-Insulin-Drug-Delivery-—-Applications-Elçioğlu-Sezer/7009a7a9e4e6d6f730a8fb44be3f181c897582c9.

New nanomaterial multifunctional structures can be transmitted directly to a tumor site and selectively eradicate cancer cells. A proper nano-construction design enables better pharmaceutical efficiency at lower doses than small-molecule medication treatment, a broader therapy scope, and reduced adverse events. Nanomaterials open up entire new cancer therapy methods, such as photodynamics and hyperthermic, in addition to established therapeutic modes of action. Furthermore, nanoparticle carriers may also deal with several problems related to drug delivery, which have not been effectively resolved in the past, including overcoming the phenomenon of multidrug resistance and penetrating cellular barriers that could limit device access to intended goals such as the blood–brain barrier. The only members of this related new class of agents approved in the United States are polyethylene glycol (PEG)ylated-liposomal doxorubicin liposomal cytarabine, and paclitaxel albumin-bound particles.

Many anti-cancer medicinal products could significantly improve the therapeutic effects of cancer and the result of anti-cancer therapies if 1) tumor (cancer cell) or preferably cell organelle–specific drug delivery occurs and 2) toxic drugs are reduced. Solubility and bioavailability issues could also be overcome in poorly soluble drug candidates. Several nanocarriers have been utilized to prepare new dosage formulations with high bioavailability and drug delivery to tumors (such as liposomes, polymer micelles, and polymeric nanoparticles). The biocompatibility of these nanocarriers is affected by zeta potential, size, cationic surface charging, and solution (Figure 6.3). This affects the cytotoxicity (surface reactivity), clearance (renal or bile) process (RES), and enhanced permeability/retention (EPR) effect of the mononuclear phagocyte (MPS) system (RES) (Figure 6.8).

The multifunctional nanomedicines combine different biological properties (e.g., increased blood circulation, tumor buildup capacity via EPR, and sensitivity to stimulates) and contain a combination of several labels and markers of diagnosis. Also emerging are target nanosystems that can focus specifically on cell or intracellular surfaces and, as such, contribute to increased drug accumulation in the tumor—almost all nanomedicines for cancer use certain aspects of the targeting. The majority rely exclusively on "passive" targeting, known as EPR, which allows nanoparticles to be extravasate from the circulation through abnormal tumor vasculature fenestration. "Active" targeted nanomedicine provides an additional targeting mechanism of nanoparticles that bind recipient-mediated nanoparticles on the surface of tumor cells or blood vessels.

A successful active nanomedicine requires a delicate ligand and surface-expenditure balance, which minimizes immunological recognition and clearance to ensure sufficient nanoparticle circulation time is

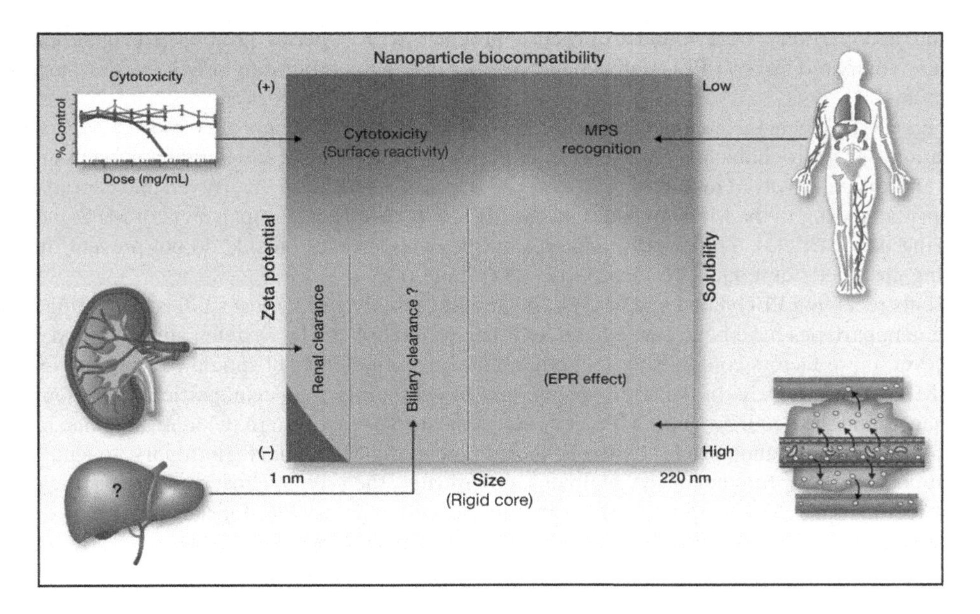

FIGURE 6.8 Nanoparticle biocompatibility trends. The zeta potential, size, and solubility affect the cytotoxicity (surface reactivity), clearance process (renal or biliary), MPS/RES recognition, and EPR effect.

available to reach the target cells while attaining appropriate surface receptor binding affinity expressed in tumor cells or blood vessels. In addition, the presence of multiple ligands targeting by nanoparticles produces a binding affinity more strongly than that of the ligand alone, which improves the interaction between the ligand-receptor and the nanoparticle.

A paradox of targeted delivery is that the most administered dose ends in normal tissues throughout the body even with effective targeting resulting in pronounced non-targeted off-target toxicity. The dramatic decrease of the overall administered dose, thus significantly decreasing the toxicity to normal tißues and still supplying more drug to the tumor than after "traditional" administrations, could be achieved if target efficiency is so increased that less than 3% of the injected dose reaches the tumor site. As such, many anti-cancer medicines can only be found in the tumor with high cytotoxicity. A new type of nanocarrier able to control drug release is an example of on-request drug delivery using mesoporous silicon nanoparticles functionalized with the pH-sensitive nano valve, only opened in intracellular acidified endosomal compartments.

The pharmacokinetic disposition of the nanoparticles depends on the carrier and not on the parent drug until they are released. An inactive drug is a drug that remains encapsulated in or linked to nanoparticles or a conjugate or polymer, thus releasing it from the carrier to be active. It depends on the formulation of the carrier and the mechanism of release to determine if the medication must be released outside the cell into or within the extracellular tumor (ECF) fluid. After the release of the medicine from the carrier, the pharmaceutical disposition will be the same as after non-carrier administration of the medicine. Unencapsulated medicine and the encapsulated drug could be used to explain the complex pharmacokinetics, separation, and quantification of each of these species. A combination of cancer medicines is used in many formulations. In this case, the efficiency and release profiles of encapsulation, conjugation, and drug discharge can differ depending on the hydrophobicity and hydrophilicity of the drug and the formula.

By taking the drug into account the pharmacokinetic characteristics of the carrier, nanoparticles may alter both the tissue distribution and the clearance rate of a drug. The physicochemical characteristics of the nanoparticles include dimensions, surface load, form, nature, and density of coating (for example), composition, stability, membranes of lipid (for liposomal particles), steric stabilization, deformability, dose, and route of administration, depend on the physicochemical characteristics. The tumor, liver, and spleen are the primary sites for the accumulation of nanoparticles compared to non-nanoparticles.

PEGylated nanoparticles were found to produce products with superior prolonged plasma exposure and tumor compared to non-PEGylated nanoparticles when incorporating PEG on the surface of nanoparticles.

The RES carrier clears the nanoparticles, also called the MPS. The carriers are removed. MPS absorption of cationic or hydrophobic nanoparticles leads to quick blood removal and buildup of the tissues, like the liver and spleen, involved in the MPS. The use by the MPS can lead to the irreversible degradation of the encapsulated drug in the MPS. In addition, the MPS may cause acute impairment of MPS and toxicity by using nanoparticles. The negative charges on the nanoparticles outside do not prevent the MPS from being absorbed but reduce the absorption rate (Figure 6.9.)

In patients receiving PEGylated and non-PEGylated liposomal agents, most studies evaluating factors affecting nanoparticles have been carried out, and therefore these carrier systems are described. In theory, however, these factors could also affect other nanocarrier systems but should be assessed in future studies. MPS dendritic cells in the liver, spleen, and blood mainly clear nanoparticles via monocytes, macrophages, and the dendritic cells. MPS cells also appear to be involved in the lung and bone marrow. The tumor can deliver nanoparticles by the EPR and potentially MPS effects in tumors. In age, gender, body composition, liver tumors, doses, regimens, other drugs, the type of cancer, and prior therapy, the factors affecting the pharmacokinetics (PK) and pharmacodynamics (PD) for nanoparticular drugs in patients and animal patterns. PBMC, mononuclear cell peripheral blood.

A scalable, reproducible production process is a critical element for the successful development and marketing of any pharmaceutical product. Nanotechnology-based products are also additional cancer challenges and typical considerations and challenges with scale-up and commercial production. Among the critical aspects of the manufacturing of cancer, nanomedicines are sterility, size, and polydispersion (mainly administered intravenously), encapsulation efficiency, removal of free drugs, and drug release.

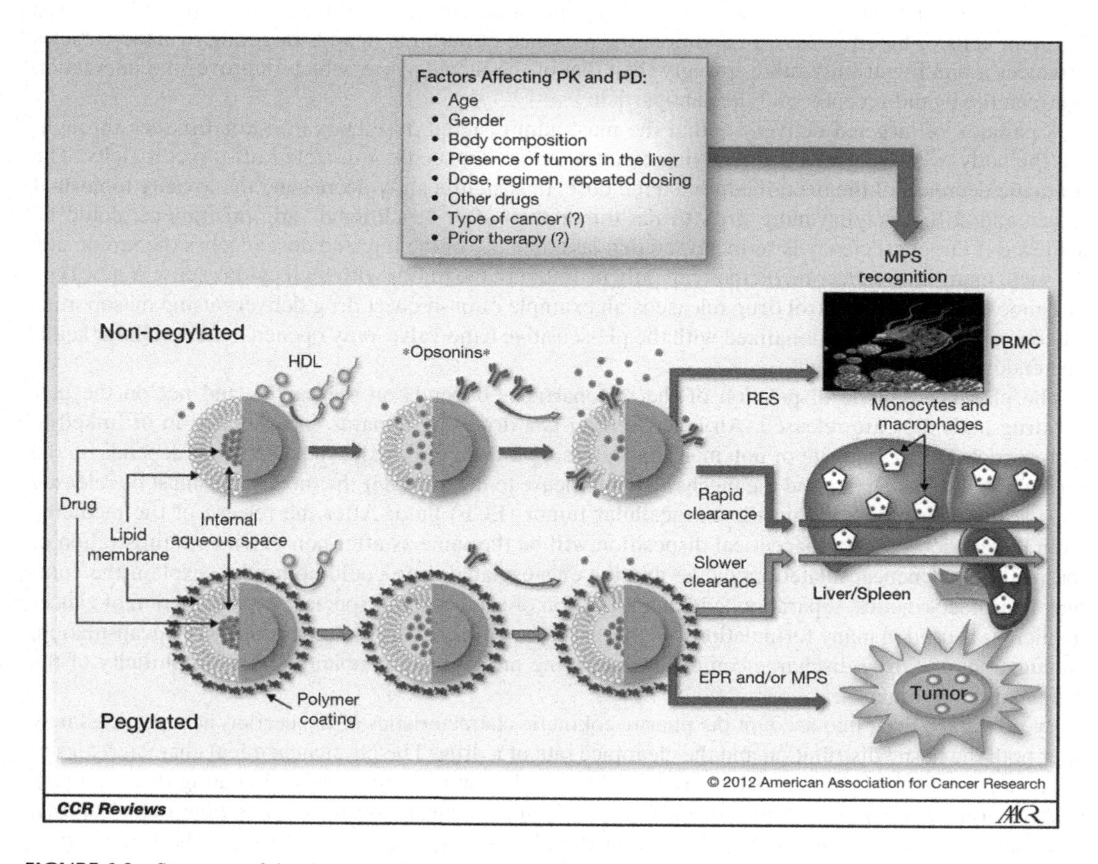

FIGURE 6.9 Summary of the clearance of nanoparticle agents via the MPS.

In addition, the quantity and adequate surface exposure of the targeting ligand must be addressed for active cancer nanomedicines which use receptor-mediated binding of nanoparticles to tumors.

6.12 Regulatory

For injectable products, sterility is the main quality parameter. However, sterility can be very difficult as terminal thermal sterilization may affect the size and polydispersion of nanoparticles and negatively impact trafficking and biodistribution. Furthermore, sterile filtration may not work if the size of nanoparticles is well more than 100 nm and polydispersion is wide. This leaves few options, including the use of very costly, sterile, and aseptic raw materials or radiation that cannot be withstood by many nanoparticle products.

It is often difficult to remove the nonencapsulated medication from nanoparticles, yet free or nonencapsulated medicinal contamination is a risk to its effectiveness and safety. Also, suppose that the production process cannot control nanoparticles' drug release rate. If a drug explosion is released quickly or heavily from the carrier, its performance will be unreliable and potentially unsafe. Finally, the well-controlled process requires actively targeted nanomedicines, providing consistent ligand exposure on the surfaces of nanoparticles, to benefit fully from an effective nanoparticular bond to produce increased tumor-drug concentrations and cellular trafficking.

Considering the novel characteristics and often multipart nature of nanoparticle therapeutics, there are three elements in the rational characterization strategy: physicochemical characterization, in vitro tests, and in vivo studies. Reproducible synthesis and characterization tests to achieve consistency batch-to-batch, predictive of in vivo fate, are required in physicochemical characterization.

Besides these parameters, the stability of the formulations should be measured with appropriate methods for predicting biological effects as a function of time, storage, temperature, pH and light (photostability), diluents, vehicles, freezing, and centrifuges. The multifunctional nanomaterials intended for drug delivery or imaging are more challenging for these characterization methods. In multiple-step synthetic methodology, some of these challenges can be addressed during synthesis, purging, and characterization steps to ensure uniformity from multiple lot components and have controls. For example, the characterization of a multi-component system is significantly more complicated for self-assembly methodologies in the case of liposomes or emulsions. Therefore, it is crucial for success in translation to optimize the method itself with adequate controls. For targeted systems of the delivery of drugs, for example, those with actively targeted ligands binding to over-expressed tumor receptors, it would be essential to carry out a bioassay predictor of in vivo behavior as part of the analysis techniques.

The main goal of in vitro characterization is to clarify biological interactions and mechanisms of toxicity and not to check biocompatibility strictly. These in vitro studies could help identify areas that need attention while conducting animal studies in vivo. At the same time, many in vitro studies can be performed in primary and transformed tissue culture cells to assess features such as the uptake of nanoparticles, subcellular tracking, intracellular drug delivery, cytotoxic killing, reactive oxygen generation, and proinflammatory effects in the blood or blood cell. Several in vitro tests could explain possible problems during the in vivo evaluation phase. While not all in vitro tests predict the in vivo outcome, several relevant in vitro tests can characterize the potential issues with the wording of the nanoparticles. Since most animal rodent models are non-human immunotoxicity forecasts, the use of human blood, though an in vitro environment, could point to potential problems during the clinical stage of development. Sterility and endotoxin contamination is also essential in vitro analyses. The most clinically relevant animal model should be carried out in preclinical pharmacology and animal toxicity studies, as described earlier.

ADDITIONAL READING

Abazari M, Ghaffari A, Rashidzadeh H, Momeni Badeleh S, Maleki Y. Current status and future outlook of nano-based systems for burn wound management. *J Biomed Mater Res B Appl Biomater.* 2020;108(5):1934–1952.

Abed Z, Beik J, Laurent S, et al. Iron oxide-gold core-shell nano-theranostic for magnetically targeted photothermal therapy under magnetic resonance imaging guidance. *J Cancer Res Clin Oncol.* 2019;145(5):1213–1219.

Abou-ElNaga A, Mutawa G, El-Sherbiny IM, et al. Novel nano-therapeutic approach actively targets human ovarian cancer stem cells after xenograft into nude mice. *Int J Mol Sci.* 2017;18(4)

Adrienn K, Peter S, Romana Z. Medical application possibilities of nano- and microfibrous systems. *Acta Pharm Hung.* 2016;86(2):53–59.

Ahmad J, Gautam A, Komath S, Bano M, Garg A, Jain K. Topical nano-emulgel for skin disorders: formulation approach and characterization. *Recent Pat Antiinfect Drug Discov.* 2019;14(1):36–48.

Ahmad MZ, Ahmad J, Haque A, Alasmary MY, Abdel-Wahab BA, Akhter S. Emerging advances in synthetic cancer nano-vaccines: opportunities and challenges. *Expert Rev Vaccines.* 2020;19(11):1053–1071.

Al Ameri J, Alsuraifi A, Curtis A, Hoskins C. Effect of poly(allylamine) molecular weight on drug loading and release abilities of nano-aggregates for potential in cancer nanomedicine. *J Pharm Sci.* 2020;109(10):3125–3133.

Al-Asmari AK, Ullah Z, Al Balowi A, Islam M. In vitro determination of the efficacy of scorpion venoms as anti-cancer agents against colorectal cancer cells: a nano-liposomal delivery approach. *Int J Nanomedicine.* 2017;12:559–574.

Ali I. Nano anti-cancer drugs: pros and cons and future perspectives. *Curr Cancer Drug Targets.* 2011;11(2):131–4.

Ali I. Nano drugs: novel agents for cancer chemo-therapy. *Curr Cancer Drug Targets.* 2011;11(2):130.

Ali I, Rahis-Uddin, Salim K, Rather MA, Wani WA, Haque A. Advances in nano drugs for cancer chemotherapy. *Curr Cancer Drug Targets.* 2011;11(2):135–146.

Ali R, Jain GK, Iqbal Z, et al. Development and clinical trial of nano-atropine sulfate dry powder inhaler as a novel organophosphorous poisoning antidote. *Nanomedicine.* 2009;5(1):55–63.

Allen C. Why I'm holding onto hope for nano in oncology. *Mol Pharm.* 2016;13(8):2603–2604.

Alphandéry E. Nano-therapies for glioblastoma treatment. *Cancers (Basel).* 2020a;19;12(1):242.

Alphandéry E. Natural metallic nanoparticles for application in nano-oncology. *Int J Mol Sci.* 2020b;21(12).

Ambalavanan R, John AD, Selvaraj AD. Nano-encapsulated. *IET Nanobiotechnol.* 2020;14(9):803–808.

Andreu I, Natividad E, Solozábal L, Roubeau O. Nano-objects for addressing the control of nanoparticle arrangement and performance in magnetic hyperthermia. *ACS Nano.* 2015;9(2):1408–19.

Andrew MacKay J, Almutairi A, Hennink W, Hoffman AS. NanoDDS 2013: the 11th international nano drug delivery symposium. *J Control Release.* 2014;191:1–3.

Andrews LE, Chan MH, Liu RS. Nano-lipospheres as acoustically active ultrasound contrast agents: evolving tumor imaging and therapy technique. *Nanotechnology.* 2019;30(18):182001.

Ansari MA, Badrealam KF, Alam A, et al. Recent nano-based therapeutic intervention of bioactive sesquiterpenes: prospects in cancer therapeutics. *Curr Pharm Des.* 2020;26(11):1138–1144.

Anton N, Atzenhoffer M, Daubeuf F, et al. Do iodinated nano-emulsions designed for preclinical vascular imaging alter the vascular reactivity in rat aorta? *Int J Pharm.* 2013;454(1):143–148.

Antonietti M. Small is beautiful: challenges and perspectives of nano/meso/microscience. *Small.* 2016;12(16):2107–2114.

Anwar MM, Abd El-Karim SS, Mahmoud AH, Amr AEE, Al-Omar MA. A comparative study of the anticancer activity and PARP-1 inhibiting effect of benzofuran-pyrazole scaffold and its nano-sized particles in human breast cancer cells. *Molecules.* 2019;24(13):2413.

Aoki I. Nano-theranostics and nitroxyl radical-labeled antitumor agents for magnetic resonance imaging. *Yakugaku Zasshi.* 2016;136(8):1087–1091.

Ardekani SM, Dehghani A, Ye P, Nguyen KA, Gomes VG. Conjugated carbon quantum dots: potent nano-antibiotic for intracellular pathogens. *J Colloid Interface Sci.* 2019;552:378–387.

Arnardottir HH, Dalli J, Colas RA, Shinohara M, Serhan CN. Aging delays resolution of acute inflammation in mice: reprogramming the host response with novel nano-proresolving medicines. *J Immunol.* 2014;193(8):4235–4244.

Asemani D, Haemmerich D. A unified mathematical model for nano-liposomal drug delivery to solid tumors. *IEEE Trans Nanobioscience.* 2018;17(1):3–11.

Ashokan A, Somasundaram VH, Gowd GS, et al. Biomineral nano-theranostic agent for magnetic resonance image guided, augmented radiofrequency ablation of liver tumor. *Sci Rep.* 11 2017;7(1):14481.

Assali M, Shakaa A, Abu-Hejleh S, et al. A cross-sectional study of the availability and pharmacist's knowledge of nano-pharmaceutical drugs in Palestinian hospitals. *BMC Health Serv Res.* 2018;18(1):250.

Augustine R, Kalva N, Kim HA, Zhang Y, Kim I. pH-responsive polypeptide-based smart nano-carriers for theranostic applications. *Molecules.* 2019;24(16):2961.

Avadhani KS, Manikkath J, Tiwari M, et al. Skin delivery of epigallocatechin-3-gallate (EGCG) and hyaluronic acid loaded nano-transfersomes for antioxidant and anti-aging effects in UV radiation induced skin damage. *Drug Deliv.* 2017;24(1):61–74.

Azeem A, English A, Kumar P, et al. The influence of anisotropic nano- to micro-topography on in vitro and in vivo osteogenesis. *Nanomedicine (Lond).* 2015;10(5):693–711.

Bahadori F, Topçu G, Eroğlu MS, Onyüksel H. A new lipid-based nano formulation of vinorelbine. *AAPS Pharm Sci Tech.* 2014;15(5):1138–1148.

Bahmani B, Bacon D, Anvari B. Erythrocyte-derived photo-theranostic agents: hybrid nano-vesicles containing indocyanine green for near infrared imaging and therapeutic applications. *Sci Rep.* 2013;3:2180.

Bahreyni A, Yazdian-Robati R, Hashemitabar S, et al. A new chemotherapy agent-free theranostic system composed of graphene oxide nano-complex and aptamers for treatment of cancer cells. *Int J Pharm.* 2017;526(1–2):391–399.

Balabathula P, Whaley SG, Janagam DR, et al. Lyophilized iron oxide nanoparticles encapsulated in amphotericin B: a novel targeted nano drug delivery system for the treatment of systemic fungal infections. *Pharmaceutics.* 2020;10;12(3):247.

Barenholz Y, Peer D. Liposomes and other assemblies as drugs and nano-drugs: from basic and translational research to the clinics. *J Control Release.* 2012;160(2):115–116.

Bartkowski M, Giordani S. Supramolecular chemistry of carbon nano-onions. *Nanoscale.* 2020;12(17): 9352–9358.

Battaglia L, Gallarate M. New formulative strategies for lipid nano and microparticles preparation. *Recent Pat Drug Deliv Formul.* 2011;5(3):176–177.

Beeran AE, Fernandez FB, Nazeer SS, et al. Multifunctional nano manganese ferrite ferrofluid for efficient theranostic application. *Colloids Surf B Biointerfaces.* 2015;136:1089–1097.

Belardi JA, Albertal M. Nano version of the XIENCE stent: good things may come in small packages. *Catheter Cardiovasc Interv.* 2012;80(4):554–555.

Benckiser G. Nanotechnology and patents in agriculture, food technology, nutrition and medicine - advantages and risks: worldwide patented nano- and absorber particles in food nutrition and agriculture. *Recent Pat Food Nutr Agric.* 2012;4(3):171–175.

Bencsik A, Lestaevel P, Guseva Canu I. Nano- and neurotoxicology: an emerging discipline. *Prog Neurobiol.* 2018;160:45–63.

Bennett MG, Naranja RJ. Getting nano tattoos right – a checklist of legal and ethical hurdles for an emerging nanomedical technology. *Nanomedicine.* 2013;9(6):729–731.

Bhardwaj V, Kaushik A, Khatib ZM, Nair M, McGoron AJ. Recalcitrant issues and new frontiers in nanopharmacology. *Front Pharmacol.* 2019;10:1369.

Bhargava A, Mishra DK, Jain SK, Srivastava RK, Lohiya NK, Mishra PK. Comparative assessment of lipid based nano-carrier systems for dendritic cell based targeting of tumor re-initiating cells in gynecological cancers. *Mol Immunol.* 11 2016;79:98–112.

BioStar 2006 2nd international congress on regenerative biology and ICBN 2006 2nd international congress on bio-nano-interface, October 9–11, 2006, Stuttgart, Germany. Abstracts. *Tissue Eng.* 2007;13(4):865–925.

Björnmalm M, Thurecht KJ, Michael M, Scott AM, Caruso F. Bridging bio-nano science and cancer nanomedicine. *ACS Nano.* 2017;11(10):9594–9613.

Bollhorst T, Rezwan K, Maas M. Colloidal capsules: nano- and microcapsules with colloidal particle shells. *Chem Soc Rev.* 2017;46(8):2091–2126.

Bosetti R, Jones SL. Cost-effectiveness of nanomedicine: estimating the real size of nano-costs. *Nanomedicine (Lond).* 2019;14(11):1367–1370.

Brouwer DH, Spaan S, Roff M, et al. Occupational dermal exposure to nanoparticles and nano-enabled products: part 2, exploration of exposure processes and methods of assessment. *Int J Hyg Environ Health.* 2016;219(6):503–512.

Bunkar N, Shandilya R, Bhargava A, et al. Nano-engineered flavonoids for cancer protection. *Front Biosci (Landmark Ed).* 2019;24:1097–1157.

Burgess MT, Porter TM. Acoustic cavitation-mediated delivery of small interfering ribonucleic acids with phase-shift nano-emulsions. *Ultrasound Med Biol.* 2015;41(8):2191–2201.

Burris KP, Wu TC, Vasudev M, Stroscio MA, Millwood RJ, Stewart CN. Mega-nano detection of foodborne pathogens and transgenes using molecular beacon and semiconductor quantum dot technologies. *IEEE Trans Nanobioscience.* 2013;12(3):233–238.

Cai K, Wang AZ, Yin L, Cheng J. Bio-nano interface: the impact of biological environment on nanomaterials and their delivery properties. *J Control Release.* 2017;263:211–222.

Cai P, Leow WR, Wang X, Wu YL, Chen X. Programmable nano-bio interfaces for functional biointegrated devices. *Adv Mater.* 2017;29(26). doi: 10.1002/adma.201605529.

Cai P, Zhang X, Wang M, Wu YL, Chen X. Combinatorial nano-bio interfaces. *ACS Nano.* 2018;12(6):5078–5084.

Canal F, Sanchis J, Vicent MJ. Polymer--drug conjugates as nano-sized medicines. *Curr Opin Biotechnol.* 2011;22(6):894–900.

Cannon LA, Simon DI, Kereiakes D, et al. The XIENCE nano everolimus eluting coronary stent system for the treatment of small coronary arteries: the SPIRIT small vessel trial. *Catheter Cardiovasc Interv.* 2012;80(4):546–553.

Canton I, Ustbas B, Armes SP. Galactosylated block copolymers: a versatile nano-based tool for effective intracellular drug delivery? *Ther Deliv.* 2014;5(2):105–107.

Carrara S. Nano-bio-technology and sensing chips: new systems for detection in personalized therapies and cell biology. *Sensors (Basel).* 2010;10(1):526–543.

Cassano D, Pocoví-Martínez S, Voliani V. Ultrasmall-in-nano approach: enabling the translation of metal nanomaterials to clinics. *Bioconjug Chem.* 2018;29(1):4–16.

Chauhan SS, Shetty AB, Hatami E, Chowdhury P, Yallapu MM. Pectin-tannic acid nano-complexes promote the delivery and bioactivity of drugs in pancreatic cancer cells. *Pharmaceutics.* 2020;22;12(3):285.

Cheah HY, Kiew LV, Lee HB, et al. Preclinical safety assessments of nano-sized constructs on cardiovascular system toxicity: a case for telemetry. *J Appl Toxicol.* 2017;37(11):1268–1285.

Chen J, Chen Q, Liang C, et al. Albumin-templated biomineralizing growth of composite nanoparticles as smart nano-theranostics for enhanced radiotherapy of tumors. *Nanoscale.* 2017;9(39):14826–14835.

Chen J, Gao C, Zhang Y, et al. Inorganic nano-targeted drugs delivery system and its application of platinum-based anticancer drugs. *J Nanosci Nanotechnol.* 2017;17(1):1–17.

Chen P, Huang NT, Chung MT, Cornell TT, Kurabayashi K. Label-free cytokine micro- and nano-bio-sensing towards personalized medicine of systemic inflammatory disorders. *Adv Drug Deliv Rev.* 2015;95:90–103.

Chen Q, Chen J, Liang C, et al. Drug-induced co-assembly of albumin/catalase as smart nano-theranostics for deep intra-tumoral penetration, hypoxia relieve, and synergistic combination therapy. *J Control Release.* 2017;263:79–89.

Chen Q, Guan G, Deng F, et al. Anisotropic active ligandations in siRNA-Loaded hybrid nanodiscs lead to distinct carcinostatic outcomes by regulating nano-bio interactions. *Biomaterials.* 2020;251: 120008.

Chen Q, Wang X, Wang C, Feng L, Li Y, Liu Z. Drug-induced self-assembly of modified albumins as nano-theranostics for tumor-targeted combination therapy. *ACS Nano.* 2015;9(5):5223–5233.

Chen W, Guo M, Wang S. Anti prostate cancer using PEGylated bombesin containing, cabazitaxel loading nano-sized drug delivery system. *Drug Dev Ind Pharm.* 2016;42(12):1968–1976.

Chen W, Liu X, Xiao Y, et al. Nano regulation of cisplatin chemotherapeutic behaviors by biomineralization controls. *Small.* 2014;10(18):3644–3649.

Chen X, Chen Y, Jiang J, et al. Nano-pulse stimulation (NPS) ablate tumors and inhibit lung metastasis on both canine spontaneous osteosarcoma and murine transplanted hepatocellular carcinoma with high metastatic potential. *Oncotarget.* 2017;8(27):44032–44039.

Chen Z, Deng S, Yuan DC, et al. Novel nano-microspheres containing chitosan, hyaluronic acid, and chondroitin sulfate deliver growth and differentiation factor-5 plasmid for osteoarthritis gene therapy. *J Zhejiang Univ Sci B.* 2018;19(12):910–923.

Chien CS, Wang CY, Yang YP, et al. Using cationic polyurethane-short branch PEI as microRNA-driven nano-delivery system for stem cell differentiation. *J Chin Med Assoc.* 2020;83(4):367–370.

Chintamaneni PK, Krishnamurthy PT, Rao PV, Pindiprolu SS. Surface modified nano-lipid drug conjugates of positive allosteric modulators of M1 muscarinic acetylcholine receptor for the treatment of Alzheimer's disease. *Med Hypotheses.* 2017;101:17–22.

Chng EL, Zhao G, Pumera M. Towards biocompatible nano/microscale machines: self-propelled catalytic nanomotors not exhibiting acute toxicity. *Nanoscale.* 2014;6(4):2119–2124.

Cho Y, Borgens RB. Polymer and nano-technology applications for repair and reconstruction of the central nervous system. *Exp Neurol.* 2012;233(1):126–144.

Choi B, Lee SH. Nano/micro-assisted regenerative medicine. *Int J Mol Sci.* 2018;19(8):2187.

Chowdhury EH, Akaike T. Bio-functional inorganic materials: an attractive branch of gene-based nano-medicine delivery for 21st century. *Curr Gene Ther.* 2005;5(6):669–676.

Chowdhury EH, Akaike T. High performance DNA nano-carriers of carbonate apatite: multiple factors in regulation of particle synthesis and transfection efficiency. *Int J Nanomedicine.* 2007;2(1):101–106.

Chugh H, Sood D, Chandra I, Tomar V, Dhawan G, Chandra R. Role of gold and silver nanoparticles in cancer nano-medicine. *Artif Cells Nanomed Biotechnol.* 2018;46(supl):1210–1220.

Cicciù M, Fiorillo L, Herford AS, et al. Bioactive titanium surfaces: interactions of eukaryotic and prokaryotic cells of nano devices applied to dental practice. *Biomedicines.* 2019;2;7(1):12.

Colletti M, Paolo VD, Galardi A, et al. Nano-delivery in pediatric tumors: looking back, moving forward. *Anticancer Agents Med Chem.* 2017;17(10):1328–1343.

Corrie SR, Thurecht KJ. Nano-bio interactions: guiding the development of nanoparticle therapeutics, diagnostics, and imaging agents. *Pharm Res.* 2016;33(10):2311–2313.

Costa RR, Alatorre-Meda M, Mano JF. Drug nano-reservoirs synthesized using layer-by-layer technologies. *Biotechnol Adv.* 2015;33(6 Pt 3):1310–1326.

Cui J, Hibbs B, Gunawan ST, et al. Immobilized particle imaging for quantification of nano- and microparticles. *Langmuir.* 2016;32(14):3532–3540.

Cui X, Bao L, Wang X, Chen C. The nano-intestine interaction: understanding the location-oriented effects of engineered nanomaterials in the intestine. *Small.* 2020;16(21):e1907665.

Curnis F, Fiocchi M, Sacchi A, Gori A, Gasparri A, Corti A. NGR-tagged nano-gold: a new CD13-selective carrier for cytokine delivery to tumors. *Nano Res.* 2016;9(5):1393–1408.

Curtin CM, Cunniffe GM, Lyons FG, et al. Innovative collagen nano-hydroxyapatite scaffolds offer a highly efficient non-viral gene delivery platform for stem cell-mediated bone formation. *Adv Mater.* 2012;24(6):749–754.

Da Silva CG, Rueda F, Löwik CW, Ossendorp F, Cruz LJ. Combinatorial prospects of nano-targeted chemoimmunotherapy. *Biomaterials.* 2016;83:308–320.

Dai L, Si C. Recent advances on cellulose-based nano-drug delivery systems: design of prodrugs and nanoparticles. *Curr Med Chem.* 2019;26(14):2410–2429.

Darwiche K, Zarogoulidis P, Krauss L, et al. "One-stop shop" spectral imaging for rapid on-site diagnosis of lung cancer: a future concept in nano-oncology. *Int J Nanomedicine.* 2013;8:4533–4542.

Datta NR, Krishnan S, Speiser DE, et al. Magnetic nanoparticle-induced hyperthermia with appropriate payloads: Paul Ehrlich's "magic (nano)bullet" for cancer theranostics? *Cancer Treat Rev.* 2016;50:217–227.

De La Iglesia D, Chiesa S, Kern J, et al. Nanoinformatics: new challenges for biomedical informatics at the nano level. *Stud Health Technol Inform.* 2009;150:987–991.

de Oliveira Carvalho H, Gonçalves DES, Picanço KRT, et al. Actions of *Cannabis sativa* L. fixed oil and nano-emulsion on venom-induced inflammation of *Bothrops moojeni* snake in rats. *Inflammopharmacology.* 2020.

Delaney M. Nano comes to HIV. *Proj Inf Perspect.* 2008;(45 Suppl):7–8.

Delpiano GR, Casula MF, Piludu M, et al. Assembly of multicomponent nano-bioconjugates composed of mesoporous silica nanoparticles, proteins, and gold nanoparticles. *ACS Omega.* 2019;4(6):11044–11052.

Deng T, Wang J, Li Y, et al. Quantum dots-based multifunctional nano-prodrug fabricated by ingenious self-assembly strategies for tumor theranostic. *ACS Appl Mater Interfaces.* 2018;10(33):27657–27668.

Denning D, Bennett S, Mullen T, et al. Maturation of adenovirus primes the protein nano-shell for successful endosomal escape. *Nanoscale.* 2019;11(9):4015–4024.

Desantis V, Saltarella I, Lamanuzzi A, et al. MicroRNAs-based nano-strategies as new therapeutic approach in multiple myeloma to overcome disease progression and drug resistance. *Int J Mol Sci.* 2020;27;21(9):3084.

Dey P, Zhu S, Thurecht KJ, Fredericks PM, Blakey I. Self assembly of plasmonic core-satellite nano-assemblies mediated by hyperbranched polymer linkers. *J Mater Chem B.* 2014;2(19):2827–2837.

Di DR, He ZZ, Sun ZQ, Liu J. A new nano-cryosurgical modality for tumor treatment using biodegradable MgO nanoparticles. *Nanomedicine.* 2012;8(8):1233–1241.

Di Martino P, Censi R, Gigliobianco MR, et al. Nano-medicine improving the bioavailability of small molecules for the prevention of neurodegenerative diseases. *Curr Pharm Des.* 2017;23(13):1897–1908.

Doyle S. Promise of nano revolution hasn't materialized. *CMAJ.* 2012;184(2):E133–E134.

Du J, El-Sherbiny IM, Smyth HD. Swellable ciprofloxacin-loaded nano-in-micro hydrogel particles for local lung drug delivery. *AAPS PharmSciTech.* 2014;15(6):1535–1544.

du Toit LC, Pillay V, Choonara YE. Nano-microbicides: challenges in drug delivery, patient ethics and intellectual property in the war against HIV/AIDS. *Adv Drug Deliv Rev.* 2010;62(4–5):532–546.

Dua K, de Jesus Andreoli Pinto T, Chellappan DK, Gupta G, Bebawy M, Hansbro PM. Advancements in nano drug delivery systems: a challenge for biofilms in respiratory diseases. *Panminerva Med.* 03 2018;60(1):35–36.

Duro-Castano A, Movellan J, Vicent MJ. Smart branched polymer drug conjugates as nano-sized drug delivery systems. *Biomater Sci.* 2015;3(10):1321–1334.

Eftekhari A, Dizaj SM, Chodari L, et al. The promising future of nano-antioxidant therapy against environmental pollutants induced-toxicities. *Biomed Pharmacother.* 2018;103:1018–1027.

El-Hammadi MM, Arias JL. Nano-sized platforms for vaginal drug delivery. *Curr Pharm Des.* 2015;21(12):1633–1644.

Elbayoumi TA. Nano drug-delivery systems in cancer therapy: gains, pitfalls and considerations in DMPK and PD. *Ther Deliv.* 2010;1(2):215–219.

Ellis-Behnke R. Nano neurology and the four P's of central nervous system regeneration: preserve, permit, promote, plasticity. *Med Clin North Am.* 2007;91(5):937–962.

Ellis-Behnke RG, Liang YX, Tay DK, et al. Nano hemostat solution: immediate hemostasis at the nanoscale. *Nanomedicine.* 2006;2(4):207–215.

Ellis-Behnke RG, Liang YX, You SW, et al. Nano neuro knitting: peptide nanofiber scaffold for brain repair and axon regeneration with functional return of vision. *Proc Natl Acad Sci U S A.* 2006;103(13):5054–5059.

Fadeel B. Nano på gott och ont: möjligheter och risker med nanoteknologi [Nano for better or worse: opportunities and risks with nanotechnology]. *Lakartidningen.* 2017;114:201.

Fanciullino R, Ciccolini J, Milano G. Challenges, expectations and limits for nanoparticles-based therapeutics in cancer: a focus on nano-albumin-bound drugs. *Crit Rev Oncol Hematol.* 2013;88(3):504–513.

Farjadian F, Moghoofei M, Mirkiani S, et al. Bacterial components as naturally inspired nano-carriers for drug/gene delivery and immunization: set the bugs to work? *Biotechnol Adv.* 2018;36(4):968–985.

Feng L, Yang X, Shi X, et al. Polyethylene glycol and polyethylenimine dual-functionalized nano-graphene oxide for photothermally enhanced gene delivery. *Small.* 2013;9(11):1989–1997.

Fernandes C, Soni U, Patravale V. Nano-interventions for neurodegenerative disorders. *Pharmacol Res.* 2010;62(2):166–178.

Finlay WH, Moussa W. Medical and pharmaceutical nanoengineering conference/International conference on MEMS, nano and smart systems. *Expert Opin Drug Deliv.* 2004;1(1):177–180.

Fiorillo M, Verre AF, Iliut M, et al. Graphene oxide selectively targets cancer stem cells, across multiple tumor types: implications for non-toxic cancer treatment, via "differentiation-based nano-therapy". *Oncotarget.* 2015;6(6):3553–3562.

Fischer S. At the interface of disciplines: Jeffrey Karp pulls from nature and nano to transform medicine. *IEEE Pulse.* 2014;5(2):30–33.

Fischer S. Regulating nanomedicine: new nano tools offer great promise for the future--if regulators can solve the difficulties that hold development back. *IEEE Pulse.* 2014;5(2):21–24.

Foong TR, Chan KL, Hu X. Structure and properties of nano-confined poly(3-hexylthiophene) in nano-array/polymer hybrid ordered-bulk heterojunction solar cells. *Nanoscale.* 2012;4(2):478–485.

Forsberg E. Nanomaterial måste EU-regleras bättre – Risk att bristen på lagstiftning stör teknikutvecklingen och skapar misstro för nanotekniken hos allmänheten [Nano materials need stricter EU regulation]. *Lakartidningen.* 2017;114.

Francia V, Montizaan D, Salvati A. Interactions at the cell membrane and pathways of internalization of nano-sized materials for nanomedicine. *Beilstein J Nanotechnol.* 2020;11:338–353.

Francia V, Reker-Smit C, Boel G, Salvati A. Limits and challenges in using transport inhibitors to characterize how nano-sized drug carriers enter cells. *Nanomedicine (Lond).* 2019;14(12):1533–1549.

Fu H, Huang Y, Lu H, et al. A theranostic saponin nano-assembly based on FRET of an aggregation-induced emission photosensitizer and photon up-conversion nanoparticles. *J Mater Chem B.* 2019;7(35):5286–5290.

Fu X, Li YS, Zhao J, et al. Will arsenic trioxide benefit treatment of solid tumor by nano- encapsulation? *Mini Rev Med Chem.* 2020;20(3):239–251.

Gaber M, Elhasany KA, Sabra S, et al. Co-administration of tretinoin enhances the anti-cancer efficacy of etoposide via tumor-targeted green nano-micelles. *Colloids Surf B Biointerfaces.* 2020;192:110997.

Gadoue SM, Toomeh D. Radio-sensitization efficacy of gold nanoparticles in inhalational nanomedicine and the adverse effect of nano-detachment due to coating inactivation. *Phys Med.* 2019;60:7–13.

Gajbhiye KR, Chaudhari BP, Pokharkar VB, Pawar A, Gajbhiye V. Stimuli-responsive biodegradable polyurethane nano-constructs as a potential triggered drug delivery vehicle for cancer therapy. *Int J Pharm.* 2020;588:119781.

Gan S, Zhong L, Han D, Niu L, Chi Q. Probing bio-nano interactions between blood proteins and monolayer-stabilized graphene sheets. *Small.* 2015;11(43):5814–5825.

García JL, Lozano R, Misiewicz-Krzeminska I, et al. A novel capillary nano-immunoassay for assessing androgen receptor splice variant 7 in plasma. Correlation with CD133 antigen expression in circulating tumor cells. A pilot study in prostate cancer patients. *Clin Transl Oncol.* 2017;19(11):1350–1357.

Garcia-Guerra A, Dunwell TL, Trigueros S. Nano-scale gene delivery systems: current technology, obstacles, and future directions. *Curr Med Chem.* 2018;25(21):2448–2464.

Gaurav C, Saurav B, Goutam R, Goyal AK. Nano-systems for advanced therapeutics and diagnosis of atherosclerosis. *Curr Pharm Des.* 2015;21(30):4498–4508.

George A, Shah PA, Shrivastav PS. Natural biodegradable polymers based nano-formulations for drug delivery: a review. *Int J Pharm.* 2019;561:244–264.

Ghavami S, Lahouti F. Abnormality detection in correlated gaussian molecular nano-networks: design and analysis. *IEEE Trans Nanobioscience.* 2017;16(3):189–202.

Gholami YH, Josephson L, Akam EA, et al. A chelate-free nano-platform for incorporation of diagnostic and therapeutic isotopes. *Int J Nanomedicine.* 2020;15:31–47.

Ghoneum A, Sharma S, Gimzewski J. Nano-hole induction by nanodiamond and nanoplatinum liquid, DPV576, reverses multidrug resistance in human myeloid leukemia (HL60/AR). *Int J Nanomedicine.* 2013;8:2567–2573.

Ghosh S, Chatterjee S, Roy A, et al. Resonant oscillation language of a futuristic nano-machine-module: eliminating cancer cells & Alzheimer aβ plaques. *Curr Top Med Chem.* 2015;15(6):534–541.

Ghosh S, Ucer KB, D'Agostino R, et al. Non-covalent assembly of meso-tetra-4-pyridyl porphine with single-stranded DNA to form nano-sized complexes with hydrophobicity-dependent DNA release and anti-tumor activity. *Nanomedicine.* 2014;10(2):451–461.

Giordani S, Camisasca A, Maffeis V. Carbon nano-onions: a valuable class of carbon nanomaterials in biomedicine. *Curr Med Chem.* 2019;26(38):6915–6929.

Gioria S, Caputo F, Mehn D. Nano-enabled medicinal products: time for an international advanced community? *Nanomedicine (Lond).* 07 2019;14(14):1787–1790.

Giubilato E, Cazzagon V, Amorim MJB, et al. Risk management framework for nano-biomaterials used in medical devices and advanced therapy medicinal products. *Materials (Basel).* 2020;13(20):4532.

Greish K, Nehoff H, Bahman F, Pritchard T, Taurin S. Raloxifene nano-micelles effect on triple-negative breast cancer is mediated through estrogen receptor-β and epidermal growth factor receptor. *J Drug Target.* 09 2019;27(8):903–916.

Grieneisen ML. The proliferation of nano journals. *Nat Nanotechnol.* 2010;5(12):825.

Guevara ML, Persano F, Persano S. Nano-immunotherapy: overcoming tumour immune evasion. *Semin Cancer Biol.* 2021;69:238–248.

Gujrati V, Prakash J, Malekzadeh-Najafabadi J, et al. Bioengineered bacterial vesicles as biological nano-heaters for optoacoustic imaging. *Nat Commun.* 2019;10(1):1114.

Gulati K, Aw MS, Findlay D, Losic D. Local drug delivery to the bone by drug-releasing implants: perspectives of nano-engineered titania nanotube arrays. *Ther Deliv.* 2012;3(7):857–873.

Gulzar A, Xu J, Yang D, et al. Nano-graphene oxide-UCNP-Ce6 covalently constructed nanocomposites for NIR-mediated bioimaging and PTT/PDT combinatorial therapy. *Dalton Trans.* 2018;47(11): 3931–3939.

Guo H, Jornet JM, Gan Q, Sun Z. Cooperative Raman spectroscopy for real-time in vivo nano-biosensing. *IEEE Trans Nanobioscience.* 2017;16(7):571–584.

Guo J, Zeng H, Chen Y. Emerging nano drug delivery systems targeting cancer-associated fibroblasts for improved antitumor effect and tumor drug penetration. *Mol Pharm.* 04 2020;17(4):1028–1048.

Haj-Ahmad R, Rasekh M, Nazari K, et al. EHDA spraying: a multi-material nano-engineering route. *Curr Pharm Des.* 2015;21(22):3239–3247.

Hameed S, Zhang M, Bhattarai P, Mustafa G, Dai Z. Enhancing cancer therapeutic efficacy through ultrasound-mediated micro-to-nano conversion. *Wiley Interdiscip Rev Nanomed Nanobiotechnol.* 2020;12(3):e1604.

Hammond PT. A growing place for nano in medicine. *ACS Nano.* 2014;8(8):7551–7552.

Hampton T. Healing power found in "nano knitting". *JAMA.* 2007;297(1):31.

Han HS, Choi KY, Lee H, et al. Gold-nanoclustered hyaluronan nano-assemblies for photothermally maneuvered photodynamic tumor ablation. *ACS Nano.* 2016;10(12):10858–10868.

Harashima H. Multifunctional envelope type nano device for non-viral gene delivery: concept and application for nanomedicine. *Nucleic Acids Symp Ser (Oxf).* 2008;52:87.

Harilall SL, Choonara YE, Modi G, et al. Design and pharmaceutical evaluation of a nano-enabled cross-linked multipolymeric scaffold for prolonged intracranial release of Zidovudine. *J Pharm Pharm Sci.* 2013;16(3):470–485.

Hayashi Y, Hatakeyama H, Kajimoto K, Hyodo M, Akita H, Harashima H. Multifunctional envelope-type nano device: evolution from nonselective to active targeting system. *Bioconjug Chem.* 2015;26(7):1266–1276.

He X, Luo Q, Zhang J, et al. Gadolinium-doped carbon dots as nano-theranostic agents for MR/FL diagnosis and gene delivery. *Nanoscale.* 2019;11(27):12973–12982.

Heng D, Lee SH, Ng WK, Tan RB. The nano spray dryer B-90. *Expert Opin Drug Deliv.* 2011;8(7):965–72.

Henrich-Noack P, Nikitovic D, Neagu M, et al. The blood-brain barrier and beyond: nano-based neuropharmacology and the role of extracellular matrix. *Nanomedicine.* 2019;17:359–379.

Ho LWC, Liu Y, Han R, Bai Q, Choi CHJ. Nano-cell interactions of non-cationic bionanomaterials. *Acc Chem Res.* 2019;52(6):1519–1530.

Hoang NH, Sim T, Lim C, et al. A nano-sized blending system comprising identical triblock copolymers with different hydrophobicity for fabrication of an anticancer drug nanovehicle with high stability and solubilizing capacity. *Int J Nanomedicine.* 2019;14:3629–3644.

Hodgins NO, Wang JT, Al-Jamal KT. Nano-technology based carriers for nitrogen-containing bisphosphonates delivery as sensitisers of γδ T cells for anticancer immunotherapy. *Adv Drug Deliv Rev.* 2017;114:143–160.

Hong SI, Rhim JW. Antimicrobial activity of organically modified nano-clays. *J Nanosci Nanotechnol.* 2008;8(11):5818–5824.

Hosnedlova B, Kepinska M, Skalickova S, et al. Nano-selenium and its nanomedicine applications: a critical review. *Int J Nanomedicine.* 2018;13:2107–2128.

Huang C, Liang J, Ma M, et al. Evaluating the treatment efficacy of nano-drug in a lung cancer model using advanced functional magnetic resonance imaging. *Front Oncol.* 2020;10:563932.

Huang Y, Chen Y, Zhou S, et al. Dual-mechanism based CTLs infiltration enhancement initiated by Nano-sapper potentiates immunotherapy against immune-excluded tumors. *Nat Commun.* 2020;11(1):622.

Huynh E, Rajora MA, Zheng G. Multimodal micro, nano, and size conversion ultrasound agents for imaging and therapy. *Wiley Interdiscip Rev Nanomed Nanobiotechnol.* 2016;8(6):796–813.

Huynh E. From nano to micro and back. *Nat Nanotechnol.* 2015;10(4):380.

Hwang SR, Kim K. Nano-enabled delivery systems across the blood-brain barrier. *Arch Pharm Res.* 2014;37(1):24–30.

Ibrahim S, Tagami T, Kishi T, Ozeki T. Curcumin marinosomes as promising nano-drug delivery system for lung cancer. *Int J Pharm.* 2018;540(1–2):40–49.

In't Veld RH, Da Silva CG, Kaijzel EL, Chan AB, Cruz LJ. The potential of nano-vehicle mediated therapy in vasculitis and multiple sclerosis. *Curr Pharm Des.* 2017;23(13):1985–1992.

Indrakumar J, Korrapati PS. Steering efficacy of nano molybdenum towards cancer: mechanism of action. *Biol Trace Elem Res.* 2020;194(1):121–134.

Ishijima A, Minamihata K, Yamaguchi S, et al. Selective intracellular vaporisation of antibody-conjugated phase-change nano-droplets in vitro. *Sci Rep.* 2017;7:44077.

Jabeen N, Maqbool Q, Sajjad S, et al. Biosynthesis and characterisation of nano-silica as potential system for carrying streptomycin at nano-scale drug delivery. *IET Nanobiotechnol.* 2017;11(5):557–561.

Jacobs K. Nano- and microfluidics. Preface. *J Phys Condens Matter.* 2011;23(18):180301.

Jain A, Kesharwani P, Garg NK, et al. Nano-constructed carriers loaded with antioxidant: boon for cardiovascular system. *Curr Pharm Des.* 2015;21(30):4456–4464.

Jebali A, Nayeri EK, Roohana S, et al. Nano-carbohydrates: synthesis and application in genetics, biotechnology, and medicine. *Adv Colloid Interface Sci.* 2017;240:1–14.

Jeevanandam J, Danquah MK, Debnath S, Meka VS, Chan YS. Opportunities for nano-formulations in type 2 diabetes mellitus treatments. *Curr Pharm Biotechnol.* 2015;16(10):853–870.

Jia J, Limongi T, Liu Y, Su G, Zhou H. Editorial: nano-bio interactions: ecotoxicology and cytotoxicity of nanomaterials. *Front Bioeng Biotechnol.* 2020;8:918.

Jiang H, Du Y, Chen L, et al. Multimodal theranostics augmented by transmembrane polymer-sealed nano-enzymatic porous MoS. *Int J Pharm.* 2020;586:119606.

Jiang W, Li Q, Zhu Z, et al. Cancer chemoradiotherapy duo: nano-enabled targeting of DNA lesion formation and DNA damage response. *ACS Appl Mater Interfaces.* 2018;10(42):35734–35744.

Jin SE, Bae JW, Hong S. Multiscale observation of biological interactions of nanocarriers: from nano to macro. *Microsc Res Tech.* 2010;73(9):813–823.

Jones RA, Gnanam AJ, Arambula JF, et al. Lanthanide nano-drums: a new class of molecular nanoparticles for potential biomedical applications. *Faraday Discuss.* 2014;175:241–255.

Kajimoto K, Sato Y, Nakamura T, Yamada Y, Harashima H. Multifunctional envelope-type nano device for controlled intracellular trafficking and selective targeting in vivo. *J Control Release.* 2014;190: 593–606.

Kalishwaralal K, Barathmanikanth S, Pandian SR, Deepak V, Gurunathan S. Silver nano - a trove for retinal therapies. *J Control Release.* 2010;145(2):76–90.

Kalluru P, Vankayala R, Chiang CS, Hwang KC. Nano-graphene oxide-mediated In vivo fluorescence imaging and bimodal photodynamic and photothermal destruction of tumors. *Biomaterials.* 2016;95:1–10.

Kamaleddin MA. Nano-ophthalmology: applications and considerations. *Nanomedicine.* 2017;13(4):1459–1472.

Karagkiozaki V, Logothetidis S, Lousinian S, Giannoglou G. Impact of surface electric properties of carbon-based thin films on platelets activation for nano-medical and nano-sensing applications. *Int J Nanomedicine.* 2008;3(4):461–469.

Karimi Z, Karimi L, Shokrollahi H. Nano-magnetic particles used in biomedicine: core and coating materials. *Mater Sci Eng C Mater Biol Appl.* 2013;33(5):2465–2475.

Kaur J, Tikoo K. Ets1 identified as a novel molecular target of RNA aptamer selected against metastatic cells for targeted delivery of nano-formulation. *Oncogene.* 2015;34(41):5216–5228.

Kaushik A, Jayant RD, Nair M. Advancements in nano-enabled therapeutics for neuroHIV management. *Int J Nanomedicine.* 2016;11:4317–4325.

Kaushik A, Nikkhah-Moshaie R, Sinha R, et al. Investigation of ac-magnetic field stimulated nanoelectroporation of magneto-electric nano-drug-carrier inside CNS cells. *Sci Rep.* 2017;7:45663.

Kecman S, Škrbić R, Badnjevic Cengic A, et al. Potentials of human bile acids and their salts in pharmaceutical nano delivery and formulations adjuvants. *Technol Health Care.* 2020;28(3):325–335.

Kerry RG, Malik S, Redda YT, Sahoo S, Patra JK, Majhi S. Nano-based approach to combat emerging viral (NIPAH virus) infection. *Nanomedicine.* 2019;18:196–220.

Khan F, Ali A, Iqbal A, Musharraf SG. Profiling of hydroxyurea-treated β-thalassemia/ serum proteome through nano-LC-ESI-MS/ MS in combination with microsol-isoelectric focusing. *Biomed Chromatogr.* 2020;34(3):e4753.

Khorsandi K, Fekrazad S, Vahdatinia F, Farmany A, Fekrazad R. Nano antiviral photodynamic therapy: a probable biophysicochemical management modality in SARS-CoV-2. *Expert Opin Drug Deliv.* 2021 Feb;18(2):265–272.

Kim B, Yalaz C, Pan D. Synthesis and characterization of membrane stable bis(arylimino)isoindole dyes and their potential application in nano-biotechnology. *Tetrahedron Lett.* 2012;53(32):4134–4137.

Kim JW, Kim DH. Introduction to the special section on the 8th international conference on nano/molecular medicine and engineering (IEEE-NANOMED 2014). *IEEE Trans Nanobioscience.* 2015;14(8):809–810.

Kingham E, Oreffo RO. Embryonic and induced pluripotent stem cells: understanding, creating, and exploiting the nano-niche for regenerative medicine. *ACS Nano.* 2013;7(3):1867–1881.

Kogure K, Akita H, Yamada Y, Harashima H. Multifunctional envelope-type nano device (MEND) as a non-viral gene delivery system. *Adv Drug Deliv Rev.* 2008;60(4–5):559–571.

Kokkinos J, Ignacio RMC, Sharbeen G, et al. Targeting the undruggable in pancreatic cancer using nano-based gene silencing drugs. *Biomaterials.* 2020;240:119742.

Korde JM, Kandasubramanian B. Microbiologically extracted poly(hydroxyalkanoates) and its amalgams as therapeutic nano-carriers in anti-tumor therapies. *Mater Sci Eng C Mater Biol Appl.* 2020;111:110799.

Kose N, Çaylak R, Pekşen C, et al. Silver ion doped ceramic nano-powder coated nails prevent infection in open fractures: in vivo study. *Injury.* 2016;47(2):320–324.

Krasnoslobodtsev AV, Torres MP, Kaur S, et al. Nano-immunoassay with improved performance for detection of cancer biomarkers. *Nanomedicine.* 2015;11(1):167–173.

Kumar P, Choonara YE, Khan RA, Pillay V. The chemo-biological outreach of nano-biomaterials: implications for tissue engineering and regenerative medicine. *Curr Pharm Des.* 2017;23(24):3538–3549.

Kydd J, Jadia R, Rai P. Co-administered polymeric nano-antidotes for improved photo-triggered response in glioblastoma. *Pharmaceutics.* 2018 Dec;10(4):226.

Lakkireddy HR, Bazile DV. Nano-carriers for drug routeing – towards a new era. *J Drug Target.* 2019;27(5–6):525–541.

Lammers T, Storm G. Setting standards to promote progress in bio-nano science. *Nat Nanotechnol.* 2019;14(7):626.

Laube N, Grabowy U, Bernsmann F. [Nano-coatings: principle, range of applications, threats]. *Dtsch Med Wochenschr.* 2013;138(33):1665–1669.

Layek B, Sadhukha T, Panyam J, Prabha S. Nano-engineered mesenchymal stem cells increase therapeutic efficacy of anticancer drug through true active tumor targeting. *Mol Cancer Ther.* 2018;17(6): 1196–1206.

Lee N, Choi SH, Hyeon T. Nano-sized CT contrast agents. *Adv Mater.* 2013;25(19):2641–2660.

Lee S, Kim J, Bark CW, et al. Spotlight on nano-theranostics in South Korea: applications in diagnostics and treatment of diseases. *Int J Nanomedicine.* 2015;10:3–8.

Lee SH, Heng D, Ng WK, Chan HK, Tan RB. Nano spray drying: a novel method for preparing protein nanoparticles for protein therapy. *Int J Pharm.* 2011;403(1–2):192–200.

Lettieri S, d'Amora M, Camisasca A, Diaspro A, Giordani S. Carbon nano-onions as fluorescent on/off modulated nanoprobes for diagnostics. *Beilstein J Nanotechnol.* 2017;8:1878–1888.

Li G, Kang W, Jin M, et al. Synergism of wt-p53 and synthetic material in local nano-TAE gene therapy of hepatoma: comparison of four systems and the possible mechanism. *BMC Cancer.* 2019;19(1):1126.

Li H, Gan S, Feng ST, et al. Nano-sized ultrasound contrast agents for cancer therapy and theranostics. *Curr Pharm Des.* 2017;23(35):5403–5412.

Li J, Lyv Z, Li Y, et al. A theranostic prodrug delivery system based on Pt(IV) conjugated nano-graphene oxide with synergistic effect to enhance the therapeutic efficacy of Pt drug. *Biomaterials.* 2015;51:12–21.

Li L, Chao T, Brant J, O'Malley B, Tsourkas A, Li D. Advances in nano-based inner ear delivery systems for the treatment of sensorineural hearing loss. *Adv Drug Deliv Rev.* 2017;108:2–12.

Li R, Gao R, Wang Y, et al. Gastrin releasing peptide receptor targeted nano-graphene oxide for near-infrared fluorescence imaging of oral squamous cell carcinoma. *Sci Rep.* 07 2020;10(1):11434.

Li W, Zhao M, Ke C, et al. Nano polymeric carrier fabrication technologies for advanced antitumor therapy. *Biomed Res Int.* 2013;2013:305089.

Li Z, Hu Y, Chang M, et al. Highly porous PEGylated Bi2S3 nano-urchins as a versatile platform for in vivo triple-modal imaging, photothermal therapy and drug delivery. *Nanoscale.* 2016;8(35):16005–16016.

Lim C, Moon J, Sim T, et al. A nano-complex system to overcome antagonistic photo-chemo combination cancer therapy. *J Control Release.* 2019;295:164–173.

Lin FC, Hsu CH, Lin YY. Nano-therapeutic cancer immunotherapy using hyperthermia-induced heat shock proteins: insights from mathematical modeling. *Int J Nanomedicine.* 2018;13:3529–3539.

Lin L, Xiong L, Wen Y, et al. Active targeting of nano-photosensitizer delivery systems for photodynamic therapy of cancer stem cells. *J Biomed Nanotechnol.* 2015;11(4):531–554.

Liu J, Huang Y, Kumar A, et al. pH-sensitive nano-systems for drug delivery in cancer therapy. *Biotechnol Adv.* 2014;32(4):693–710.

Liu L, Guo W, Liang XJ. Move to nano-arthrology: targeted stimuli-responsive nanomedicines combat adaptive treatment tolerance (ATT) of rheumatoid arthritis. *Biotechnol J.* 2019;14(1):e1800024.

Liu L, Li H, Zhang M, Lv X. Effects of targeted nano-delivery systems combined with hTERT-siRNA and Bmi-1-siRNA on MCF-7 cells. *Int J Clin Exp Pathol.* 2015;8(6):6674–6682.

Liu W, Mao Y, Zhang X, et al. RGDV-modified gemcitabine: a nano-medicine capable of prolonging half-life, overcoming resistance and eliminating bone marrow toxicity of gemcitabine. *Int J Nanomedicine.* 2019;14:7263–7279.

Liu X, Jiang J, Meng H. Transcytosis – An effective targeting strategy that is complementary to "EPR effect" for pancreatic cancer nano drug delivery. *Theranostics.* 2019;9(26):8018–8025.

Liu Y, Lou C, Yang H, Shi M, Miyoshi H. Silica nanoparticles as promising drug/gene delivery carriers and fluorescent nano-probes: recent advances. *Curr Cancer Drug Targets.* 2011;11(2):156–163.

Liu Y, Wang J, Xiong Q, Hornburg D, Tao W, Farokhzad OC. Nano-bio interactions in cancer: from therapeutics delivery to early detection. *Acc Chem Res.* 2021;54(2):291–301.

Liu Z, Liu J, Wang R, Du Y, Ren J, Qu X. An efficient nano-based theranostic system for multi-modal imaging-guided photothermal sterilization in gastrointestinal tract. *Biomaterials.* 2015;56:206–218.

Ljubimova JY, Sun T, Mashouf L, et al. Covalent nano delivery systems for selective imaging and treatment of brain tumors. *Adv Drug Deliv Rev.* 2017;113:177–200.

Lu CH, Willner I. Stimuli-responsive DNA-functionalized nano-/microcontainers for switchable and controlled release. *Angew Chem Int Ed Engl.* 2015;54(42):12212–12235.

Lu S, Tu D, Hu P, et al. Multifunctional nano-bioprobes based on rattle-structured upconverting luminescent nanoparticles. *Angew Chem Int Ed Engl.* 2015;54(27):7915–7919.

Lukyanenko V, Salnikov V. Gold nanoparticle as a marker for precise localization of nano-objects within intracellular sub-domains. *Methods Mol Biol.* 2013;991:33–39.

Lukyanenko V. Delivery of nano-objects to functional sub-domains of healthy and failing cardiac myocytes. *Nanomedicine (Lond).* 2007;2(6):831–846.

Lukyanenko V. Permeabilization of cell membrane for delivery of nano-objects to cellular sub-domains. *Methods Mol Biol.* 2013;991:57–63.

Luo L, Iqbal MZ, Liu C, et al. Engineered nano-immunopotentiators efficiently promote cancer immunotherapy for inhibiting and preventing lung metastasis of melanoma. *Biomaterials.* 2019;223:119464.

Lymberis A. Converging micro-nano-bio technologies towards integrated biomedical systems: state of the art and future perspectives under the EU-information & communication technologies program. *Annu Int Conf IEEE Eng Med Biol Soc.* 2008;2008:6–8.

Lymberis A. Micro-nano-biosystems: an overview of European research. *Minim Invasive Ther Allied Technol.* 2010;19(3):136–143.

Lymberis A. The era of micro and nano systems in the biomedical area: bridging the research and innovation gap. *Annu Int Conf IEEE Eng Med Biol Soc.* 2011;2011:1548–1551.

Lynch I, Feitshans IL, Kendall M. 'Bio-nano interactions: new tools, insights and impacts': summary of the Royal Society discussion meeting. *Philos Trans R Soc Lond B Biol Sci.* 2015;370(1661):20140162.

Mahmoodi Chalbatani G, Dana H, Gharagouzloo E, et al. Small interfering RNAs (siRNAs) in cancer therapy: a nano-based approach. *Int J Nanomedicine.* 2019;14:3111–3128.

Mahmoudi M. Debugging nano-bio interfaces: systematic strategies to accelerate clinical translation of nanotechnologies. *Trends Biotechnol.* 08 2018;36(8):755–769.

Mansur HS, Mansur AAP, Curti E, De Almeida MV. Functionalized-chitosan/quantum dot nano-hybrids for nanomedicine applications: towards biolabeling and biosorbing phosphate metabolites. *J Mater Chem B.* 2013;1(12):1696–1711.

Marassi V, Casolari S, Roda B, et al. Hollow-fiber flow field-flow fractionation and multi-angle light scattering investigation of the size, shape and metal-release of silver nanoparticles in aqueous medium for nano-risk assessment. *J Pharm Biomed Anal.* 2015;106:92–99.

Marchesan S, Prato M. Nanomaterials for (Nano)medicine. *ACS Med Chem Lett.* 2013;4(2):147–149.

Marchetti M, Wuite G, Roos WH. Atomic force microscopy observation and characterization of single virions and virus-like particles by nano-indentation. *Curr Opin Virol.* 2016;18:82–88.

Martin-Sanchez F, Maojo V. Biomedical informatics and the convergence of Nano-Bio-Info-Cogno (NBIC) technologies. *Yearb Med Inform.* 2009:134–142.

Marycz K, Smieszek A, Targonska S, Walsh SA, Szustakiewicz K, Wiglusz RJ. Three dimensional (3D) printed polylactic acid with nano-hydroxyapatite doped with europium(III) ions (nHAp/PLLA@Eu. *Mater Sci Eng C Mater Biol Appl.* 2020;110:110634.

Mazibuko Z, Choonara YE, Kumar P, et al. A review of the potential role of nano-enabled drug delivery technologies in amyotrophic lateral sclerosis: lessons learned from other neurodegenerative disorders. *J Pharm Sci.* 2015;104(4):1213–1229.

Medina-Ramírez IE, Díaz de León Olmos MA, Muñoz Ortega MH, Zapien JA, Betancourt I, Santoyo-Elvira N. Development and assessment of nano-technologies for cancer treatment: cytotoxicity and hyperthermia laboratory studies. *Cancer Invest.* 2020;38(1):61–84.

Mehta P, Justo L, Walsh S, et al. New platforms for multi-functional ocular lenses: engineering double-sided functionalized nano-coatings. *J Drug Target.* 2015;23(4):305–310.

Mei KC, Ghazaryan A, Teoh EZ, et al. Protein-corona-by-design in 2D: a reliable platform to decode bio-nano interactions for the next-generation quality-by-design nanomedicines. *Adv Mater.* 2018: e1802732.

Mei L, Zhang X, Yin W, et al. Translocation, biotransformation-related degradation, and toxicity assessment of polyvinylpyrrolidone-modified 2H-phase nano-MoS. *Nanoscale.* 2019;11(11):4767–4780.

Meng E, Sheybani R. Micro- and nano-fabricated implantable drug-delivery systems: current state and future perspectives. *Ther Deliv.* 2014;5(11):1167–1170.

Meng H, Nel AE. Use of nano engineered approaches to overcome the stromal barrier in pancreatic cancer. *Adv Drug Deliv Rev.* 2018;130:50–57.

Meng H, Zou Y, Zhong P, et al. A smart nano-prodrug platform with reactive drug loading, superb stability, and fast responsive drug release for targeted cancer therapy. *Macromol Biosci.* 2017;17(10).

Merchant Z, Buckton G, Taylor KM, et al. A new era of pulmonary delivery of nano-antimicrobial therapeutics to treat chronic pulmonary infections. *Curr Pharm Des.* 2016;22(17):2577–2598.

Mfouo Tynga I, Abrahamse H. Nano-mediated photodynamic therapy for cancer: enhancement of cancer specificity and therapeutic effects. *Nanomaterials (Basel).* 2018 Nov 8;8(11):923.

Mier W, Babich J, Haberkorn U. Is nano too big? *Eur J Nucl Med Mol Imaging.* 2014;41(1):4–6.

Mikelez-Alonso I, Aires A, Cortajarena AL. Cancer nano-immunotherapy from the injection to the target: the role of protein corona. *Int J Mol Sci.* 2020 Jan;21(2):519.

Minakshi P, Ghosh M, Brar B, et al. Nano-antimicrobials: a new paradigm for combating mycobacterial resistance. *Curr Pharm Des.* 2019;25(13):1554–1579.

Minakshi P, Kumar R, Ghosh M, Brar B, Barnela M, Lakhani P. Application of polymeric nano-materials in management of inflammatory bowel disease. *Curr Top Med Chem.* 2020;20(11):982–1008.

Mirzaie V, Ansari M, Nematollahi-Mahani SN, et al. Nano-graphene oxide-supported APTES-spermine, as gene delivery system, for transfection of pEGFP-p53 into breast cancer cell lines. *Drug Des Devel Ther.* 2020;14:3087–3097.

Misra SK, Kim B, Kolmodin NJ, Pan D. A dual strategy for sensing metals with a nano 'pincer' scavenger for in vitro diagnostics and detection of liver diseases from blood samples. *Colloids Surf B Biointerfaces.* 2015;126:444–4451.

Mitragotri S, Lammers T, Bae YH, et al. Drug delivery research for the future: expanding the nano horizons and beyond. *J Control Release.* 01 2017;246:183–184.

Moawad HM, Jain H. Development of nano-macroporous soda-lime phosphofluorosilicate bioactive glass and glass-ceramics. *J Mater Sci Mater Med.* 2009;20(7):1409–1418.

Moghimi SM, Chirico G, Zaichenko A. A special issue on nano- and micro-technologies for biological targeting, tracking, imaging and sensing. *J Biomed Nanotechnol.* 2009;5(6):611–613.

Mohamed S, Parayath NN, Taurin S, Greish K. Polymeric nano-micelles: versatile platform for targeted delivery in cancer. *Ther Deliv.* 2014;5(10):1101–1121.

Mohammadzadeh P, Cohan RA, Ghoreishi SM, Bitarafan-Rajabi A, Ardestani MS. AS1411 aptamer-anionic linear globular dendrimer G2-iohexol selective nano-theranostaics. *Sci Rep.* 2017;7(1):11832.

Mohammed MI, Makky AM, Teaima MH, Abdellatif MM, Hamzawy MA, Khalil MA. Transdermal delivery of vancomycin hydrochloride using combination of nano-ethosomes and iontophoresis: in vitro and in vivo study. *Drug Deliv.* 2016;23(5):1558–1564.

Molinaro R, Corbo C, Livingston M, et al. Inflammation and cancer: in medio stat nano. *Curr Med Chem.* 2018;25(34):4208–4223.

Moradi Kashkooli F, Soltani M, Souri M. Controlled anti-cancer drug release through advanced nano-drug delivery systems: static and dynamic targeting strategies. *J Control Release.* 2020;327:316–349.

Mousa SA, Bharali DJ. Nanotechnology-based detection and targeted therapy in cancer: nano-bio paradigms and applications. *Cancers (Basel).* 2011;3(3):2888–2903.

Moyano DF, Rotello VM. Nano meets biology: structure and function at the nanoparticle interface. *Langmuir.* 2011;27(17):10376–10385.

Mrówczyński R. Polydopamine-based multifunctional (nano)materials for cancer therapy. *ACS Appl Mater Interfaces.* 2018;10(9):7541–7561.

Mrsny RJ. Lessons from nature: "pathogen-mimetic" systems for mucosal nano-medicines. *Adv Drug Deliv Rev.* 2009;61(2):172–192.

Myerson JW, Anselmo AC, Liu Y, Mitragotri S, Eckmann DM, Muzykantov VR. Non-affinity factors modulating vascular targeting of nano- and microcarriers. *Adv Drug Deliv Rev.* 2016;99(Pt A):97–112.

Nadimi AE, Ebrahimipour SY, Afshar EG, et al. Nano-scale drug delivery systems for antiarrhythmic agents. *Eur J Med Chem.* 2018;157:1153–1163.

Nag S, Bagchi D, Chattopadhyay D, Bhattacharyya M, Pal SK. Protein assembled nano-vehicle entrapping photosensitizer molecules for efficient lung carcinoma therapy. *Int J Pharm.* 2020;580:119192.

Nagano F, Selimovic D, Noda M, et al. Improved bond performance of a dental adhesive system using nanotechnology. *Biomed Mater Eng.* 2009;19(2–3):249–257.

Nakayama M, Okano T. [Drug delivery systems using nano-sized drug carriers]. *Gan To Kagaku Ryoho.* 2005;32(7):935–940.

Naz A, Cui Y, Collins CJ, Thompson DH, Irudayaraj J. PLGA-PEG nano-delivery system for epigenetic therapy. *Biomed Pharmacother.* 2017;90:586–597.

Nguyen MH, Yu H, Kiew TY, Hadinoto K. Cost-effective alternative to nano-encapsulation: amorphous curcumin-chitosan nanoparticle complex exhibiting high payload and supersaturation generation. *Eur J Pharm Biopharm.* 2015;96:1–10.

Niaz T, Hafeez Z, Imran M. Prospectives of antihypertensive nano-ceuticals as alternative therapeutics. *Curr Drug Targets.* 2017;18(11):1269–1280.

Pandit A, Zeugolis DI. Twenty-five years of nano-bio-materials: have we revolutionized healthcare? *Nanomedicine (Lond).* 2016;11(9):985–987.

Pang Y, Liu J, Li X, et al. Nano Let7b sensitization of eliminating esophageal cancer stemlike cells is dependent on blockade of Wnt activation of symmetric division. *Int J Oncol.* 2017;51(4):1077–1088.

Parekh G, Shi Y, Zheng J, Zhang X, Leporatti S. Nano-carriers for targeted delivery and biomedical imaging enhancement. *Ther Deliv.* 2018;9(6):451–468.

Pascal J, Ashley CE, Wang Z, et al. Mechanistic modeling identifies drug-uptake history as predictor of tumor drug resistance and nano-carrier-mediated response. *ACS Nano.* 2013;7(12):11174–11182.

Patra JK, Das G, Fraceto LF, et al. Nano based drug delivery systems: recent developments and future prospects. *J Nanobiotechnology.* 2018;16(1):71.

Peng R, Yang D, Qiu X, Qin Y, Zhou M. Preparation of self-dispersed lignin-based drug-loaded material and its application in avermectin nano-formulation. *Int J Biol Macromol.* 2020;151:421–427.

Peteiro-Cartelle J, Rodríguez-Pedreira M, Zhang F, Gil PR, del Mercato LL, Parak WJ. One example on how colloidal nano- and microparticles could contribute to medicine. *Nanomedicine (Lond).* 2009;4(8):967–979.

Placente D, Ruso JM, Baldini M, et al. Self-fluorescent antibiotic MoO. *Nanoscale.* 2019;11(37):17277–17292.

Pompa PP, Vecchio G, Galeone A, et al. Physical assessment of toxicology at nanoscale: nano dose-metrics and toxicity factor. *Nanoscale.* 2011;3(7):2889–2897.

Prasad R, Aiyer S, Chauhan DS, Srivastava R, Selvaraj K. Bioresponsive carbon nano-gated multifunctional mesoporous silica for cancer theranostics. *Nanoscale.* 2016;8(8):4537–46.

Proceedings of the NanoDDS 2013. The 11th international nano drug delivery symposium, October 25–27, 2014, San Diego, CA. *J Control Release.* 2014;191:1–130.

Qamar Z, Qizilbash FF, Iqubal MK, et al. Nano-based drug delivery system: recent strategies for the treatment of ocular disease and future perspective. *Recent Pat Drug Deliv Formul.* 2019;13(4):246–254.

Qin M, Zhang J, Li M, et al. Proteomic analysis of intracellular protein corona of nanoparticles elucidates nano-trafficking network and nano-bio interactions. *Theranostics.* 2020;10(3):1213–1229.

Qin X, Liu J, Zhang Q, Chen W, Zhong X, He J. Synthesis of yellow-fluorescent carbon nano-dots by microplasma for imaging and photocatalytic inactivation of cancer cells. *Nanoscale Res Lett.* 2021;16(1):14.

Qu Y, Wang P, Man Y, Li Y, Zuo Y, Li J. Preliminary biocompatible evaluation of nano-hydroxyapatite/polyamide 66 composite porous membrane. *Int J Nanomedicine.* 2010;5:429–435.

Rady Raz N, Akbarzadeh TMR. Swarm-fuzzy rule-based targeted nano delivery using bioinspired nanomachines. *IEEE Trans Nanobioscience.* 2019;18(3):404–414.

Rahman M, Ahmad MZ, Ahmad J, et al. Role of graphene nano-composites in cancer therapy: theranostic applications, metabolic fate and toxicity issues. *Curr Drug Metab.* 2015;16(5):397–409.

Rahoui N, Jiang B, Hegazy M, et al. Gold modified polydopamine coated mesoporous silica nano-structures for synergetic chemo-photothermal effect. *Colloids Surf B Biointerfaces.* 2018;171:176–185.

Rai S, Singh N, Bhattacharya S. Concepts on smart nano-based drug delivery system. *Recent Pat Nanotechnol.* 2021. doi:10.2174/1872210515666210120113738

Ramachandra Kurup Sasikala A, Unnithan AR, Thomas RG, et al. Hexa-functional tumour-seeking nano voyagers and annihilators for synergistic cancer theranostic applications. *Nanoscale.* 2018;10(41):19568–19578.

Ramachandran R, Junnuthula VR, Gowd GS, et al. Theranostic 3-dimensional nano brain-implant for prolonged and localized treatment of recurrent glioma. *Sci Rep.* 2017;7:43271.

Raphael AP, Sisney JP, Liu DC, Prow TW. Enhanced delivery of nano- and submicron particles using elongated microparticles. *Curr Drug Deliv.* 2015;12(1):78–85.

Raza K, Singh B, Lohan S, et al. Nano-lipoidal carriers of tretinoin with enhanced percutaneous absorption, photostability, biocompatibility and anti-psoriatic activity. *Int J Pharm.* 2013;456(1):65–72.

Rehman FU, Zhao C, Jiang H, Wang X. Biomedical applications of nano-titania in theranostics and photodynamic therapy. *Biomater Sci.* 2016;4(1):40–54.

Ribeiro IRS, da Silva RF, Silveira CP, Galdino FE, Cardoso MB. Nano-targeting lessons from the SARS-CoV-2. *Nano Today.* 2021;36:101012.

Roberts RA, Shen T, Allen IC, Hasan W, DeSimone JM, Ting JP. Analysis of the murine immune response to pulmonary delivery of precisely fabricated nano- and microscale particles. *PLoS One.* 2013;8(4):e62115.

Rodrigues HF, Capistrano G, Bakuzis AF. Magnetic nanoparticle hyperthermia: a review on preclinical studies, low-field nano-heaters, noninvasive thermometry and computer simulations for treatment planning. *Int J Hyperthermia.* 2020;37(3):76–99.

Roma-Rodrigues C, Rivas-García L, Baptista PV, Fernandes AR. Gene therapy in cancer treatment: why go nano? *Pharmaceutics.* 2020 Mar;12(3):233.

Rozhkova EA, Ulasov IV, Kim DH, et al. Multifunctional nano-bio materials within cellular machinery. *Int J Nanosci.* 2011;10(4):899.

Sadikot RT. The potential role of nano- and micro-technology in the management of critical illnesses. *Adv Drug Deliv Rev.* 2014;77:27–31.

Salapa J, Bushman A, Lowe K, Irudayaraj J. Nano drug delivery systems in upper gastrointestinal cancer therapy. *Nano Converg.* 2020;7(1):38.

Sallustio F, Gesualdo L, Pisignano D. The heterogeneity of renal stem cells and their interaction with bio- and nano-materials. *Adv Exp Med Biol.* 2019;1123:195–216.

Sandhir R, Yadav A, Sunkaria A, Singhal N. Nano-antioxidants: an emerging strategy for intervention against neurodegenerative conditions. *Neurochem Int.* 2015;89:209–226.

Saravanan M, Asmalash T, Gebrekidan A, et al. Nano-medicine as a newly emerging approach to combat human immunodeficiency virus (HIV). *Pharm Nanotechnol.* 2018;6(1):17–27.

Sartori S, Chiono V, Tonda-Turo C, Mattu C, Gianluca C. Biomimetic polyurethanes in nano and regenerative medicine. *J Mater Chem B.* 2014;2(32):5128–5144.

Satalkar P, Elger BS, Shaw D. Naming it 'nano': expert views on 'nano' terminology in informed consent forms of first-in-human nanomedicine trials. *Nanomedicine (Lond).* 2016;11(8):933–940.

Satalkar P, Elger BS, Shaw DM. Defining nano, nanotechnology and nanomedicine: why should it matter? *Sci Eng Ethics.* 2016;22(5):1255–1276.

Sato Y, Nakamura T, Yamada Y, Harashima H. Development of a multifunctional envelope-type nano device and its application to nanomedicine. *J Control Release.* 2016;244(Pt B):194–204.

Sato Y, Nakamura T, Yamada Y, Harashima H. The nanomedicine rush: new strategies for unmet medical needs based on innovative nano DDS. *J Control Release.* 2020;330:305–316.

Saxl T, Khan F, Matthews DR, et al. Fluorescence lifetime spectroscopy and imaging of nano-engineered glucose sensor microcapsules based on glucose/galactose-binding protein. *Biosens Bioelectron.* 2009;24(11):3229–3234.

Schostek S, Schurr MO. Micro-nano-biosystems – technology brought to life. *Minim Invasive Ther Allied Technol.* 2010;19(3):126.

Selvaraj G, Kaliamurthi S, Wei DQ. Emerging trends on nanoparticles and nano-materials in biomedical applications -II. *Curr Pharm Des.* 2019;25(24):2607–2608.

Sengupta S, Kumar S, Das T, Goswami L, Ray S, Bandyopadhyay A. A polyester with hyperbranched architecture as potential nano-grade antibiotics: an in-vitro study. *Mater Sci Eng C Mater Biol Appl.* 2019;99:1246–1256.

Serda RE, Godin B, Blanco E, Chiappini C, Ferrari M. Multi-stage delivery nano-particle systems for therapeutic applications. *Biochim Biophys Acta.* 2011;1810(3):317–329.

Serpooshan V, Sivanesan S, Huang X, et al. [Pyr1]-Apelin-13 delivery via nano-liposomal encapsulation attenuates pressure overload-induced cardiac dysfunction. *Biomaterials.* 2015;37:289–298.

Šetrajčić-Tomić AJ, Popović JK, Vojnović M, Džambas LD, Šetrajčić JP. Review of core-multishell nano-structured models for nano-biomedical and nano-biopharmaceutical application. *Biomed Mater Eng.* 2018;29(4):451–471.

Setyawati MI, Sevencan C, Bay BH, et al. Nano-TiO. *Small.* 2018;14(30):e1800922.

Shamsi M, Mohammadi A, Manshadi MKD, Sanati-Nezhad A. Mathematical and computational modeling of nano-engineered drug delivery systems. *J Control Release.* 2019;307:150–165.

Sharma R, Kaur A, Sharma AK, Dilbaghi N. Nano-based anti-tubercular drug delivery and therapeutic interventions in tuberculosis. *Curr Drug Targets.* 2017;18(1):72–86.

Sheng Z, Song L, Zheng J, et al. Protein-assisted fabrication of nano-reduced graphene oxide for combined in vivo photoacoustic imaging and photothermal therapy. *Biomaterials.* 2013;34(21):5236–5243.

Shi X, Zhan Q, Yan X, Zhou J, Zhou L, Wei S. Oxyhemoglobin nano-recruiter preparation and its application in biomimetic red blood cells to relieve tumor hypoxia and enhance photodynamic therapy activity. *J Mater Chem B.* 2020;8(3):534–545.

Si Y, Chen M, Wu L. Syntheses and biomedical applications of hollow micro-/nano-spheres with large-through-holes. *Chem Soc Rev.* 2016;45(3):690–714.

Siemer S, Westmeier D, Vallet C, et al. Resistance to nano-based antifungals is mediated by biomolecule coronas. *ACS Appl Mater Interfaces.* 2019;11(1):104–114.

Siemer S, Wünsch D, Khamis A, et al. Nano meets micro-translational nanotechnology in medicine: nano-based applications for early tumor detection and therapy. *Nanomaterials (Basel).* 2020 Mar;10(2):233.

Silva VL, Al-Jamal WT. Exploiting the cancer niche: tumor-associated macrophages and hypoxia as promising synergistic targets for nano-based therapy. *J Control Release.* 2017;253:82–96.

Sim T, Lim C, Hoang NH, et al. Synergistic photodynamic therapeutic effect of indole-3-acetic acid using a pH sensitive nano-carrier based on poly(aspartic acid-graft-imidazole)-poly(ethylene glycol). *J Mater Chem B.* 2017;5(43):8498–8505.

Simon L, Marcotte N, Devoisselle JM, Begu S, Lapinte V. Recent advances and prospects in nano drug delivery systems using lipopolyoxazolines. *Int J Pharm.* 2020;585:119536.

Simpson JD, Smith SA, Thurecht KJ, Such G. Engineered polymeric materials for biological applications: overcoming challenges of the bio-nano interface. *Polymers (Basel).* 2019 Sep 2;11(9):1441.

Singh H, Jindal S, Singh M, Sharma G, Kaur IP. Nano-formulation of rifampicin with enhanced bioavailability: development, characterization and in-vivo safety. *Int J Pharm.* 2015;485(1–2):138–151.

Singh MK, Kuncha M, Nayak VL, et al. An innovative in situ method of creating hybrid dendrimer nano-assembly: an efficient next generation dendritic platform for drug delivery. *Nanomedicine.* 2019;21:102043.

Sneider A, VanDyke D, Paliwal S, Rai P. Remotely triggered nano-theranostics for cancer applications. *Nanotheranostics.* 2017;1(1):1–22.

Sofias AM, Dunne M, Storm G, Allen C. The battle of "nano" paclitaxel. *Adv Drug Deliv Rev.* 2017;122:20–30.

Sokolova V, Loza K, Knuschke T, et al. A systematic electron microscopic study on the uptake of barium sulphate nano-, submicro-, microparticles by bone marrow-derived phagocytosing cells. *Acta Biomater.* 2018;80:352–363.

Song Y, Wang XF, Wang YG, Dong F, Lv PJ. [A preliminary study for the effect of nano hydroxyapatite on human adipose-derived mesenchymal stem cells mixture 3D bio-printing]. *Beijing Da Xue Xue Bao Yi Xue Ban.* 2016;48(5):894–899.

Starsich FH, Sotiriou GA, Wurnig MC, et al. Silica-coated nonstoichiometric nano Zn-ferrites for magnetic resonance imaging and hyperthermia treatment. *Adv Healthc Mater.* 2016;5(20):2698–2706.

Sufi SA, Pajaniradje S, Mukherjee V, Rajagopalan R. Redox nano-architectures: perspectives and implications in diagnosis and treatment of human diseases. *Antioxid Redox Signal.* 2019;30(5):762–785.

Sujatha G, Sinha A, Singh S. Cells behaviour in presence of nano-scaffolds. *J Biomed Nanotechnol.* 2011;7(1):43–44.

Sundarabharathi L, Parangusan H, Ponnamma D, Al-Maadeed MAA, Chinnaswamy M. In-vitro biocompatibility, bioactivity and photoluminescence properties of Eu. *J Biomed Mater Res B Appl Biomater.* 2018;106(6):2191–2201.

Szuplewska A, Rozmysłowska-Wojciechowska A, Poźniak S, et al. Multilayered stable 2D nano-sheets of Ti. *J Nanobiotechnology.* 2019;17(1):114.

Tan A, Rajadas J, Seifalian AM. Exosomes as nano-theranostic delivery platforms for gene therapy. *Adv Drug Deliv Rev.* 2013;65(3):357–367.

Tan S. A baby step for nano. *Sci Transl Med.* 2012;4(130):130fs8.

Taneja G, Sud A, Pendse N, Panigrahi B, Kumar A, Sharma AK. Nano-medicine and vascular endothelial dysfunction: options and delivery strategies. *Cardiovasc Toxicol.* 2019;19(1):1–12.

Tasciotti E. Mission: nano. *Nat Nanotechnol.* 2014;9(12):1064.

Thammawongsa N, Mitatha S, Yupapin PP. Optical spins and nano-antenna array for magnetic therapy. *IEEE Trans Nanobioscience.* 2013;12(3):228–232.

Thanekar AM, Sankaranarayanan SA, Rengan AK. Role of nano-sensitizers in radiation therapy of metastatic tumors. *Cancer Treat Res Commun.* 2021;26:100303.

Thang DC, Wang Z, Lu X, Xing B. Precise cell behaviors manipulation through light-responsive nano-regulators: recent advance and perspective. *Theranostics.* 2019;9(11):3308–3340.

Thomas DG, Gaheen S, Harper SL, et al. ISA-TAB-Nano: a specification for sharing nanomaterial research data in spreadsheet-based format. *BMC Biotechnol.* 2013;13:2.

Thomas L. Nano neuro knitting repairs injured brain. *Lancet Neurol.* 2006;5(5):386.

Thorat ND, Bauer J, Tofail SAM, Gascón Pérez V, Bohara RA, Yadav HM. Silica nano supra-assembly for the targeted delivery of therapeutic cargo to overcome chemoresistance in cancer. *Colloids Surf B Biointerfaces.* 2020;185:110571.

Tian X, Chong Y, Ge C. Understanding the nano-bio interactions and the corresponding biological responses. *Front Chem.* 2020;8:446.

Timin AS, Litvak MM, Gorin DA, Atochina-Vasserman EN, Atochin DN, Sukhorukov GB. Cell-based drug delivery and use of nano-and microcarriers for cell functionalization. *Adv Healthc Mater.* 2018 Feb;7(3).

Tran CTM, Tran PHL, Tran TTD. pH-independent dissolution enhancement for multiple poorly water-soluble drugs by nano-sized solid dispersions based on hydrophobic-hydrophilic conjugates. *Drug Dev Ind Pharm.* 2019;45(3):514–519.

Tran TT, Tran PH, Nguyen KT, Tran VT. Nano-precipitation: preparation and application in the field of pharmacy. *Curr Pharm Des.* 2016;22(20):2997–3006.

Truffi M, Mazzucchelli S, Bonizzi A, et al. Nano-strategies to target breast cancer-associated fibroblasts: rearranging the tumor microenvironment to achieve antitumor efficacy. *Int J Mol Sci.* 2019 Mar 13;20(6):1263.

Trusel M, Baldrighi M, Marotta R, et al. Internalization of carbon nano-onions by hippocampal cells preserves neuronal circuit function and recognition memory. *ACS Appl Mater Interfaces.* 2018;10(20):16952–16963.

Ungaro F, d'Angelo I, Miro A, La Rotonda MI, Quaglia F. Engineered PLGA nano- and micro-carriers for pulmonary delivery: challenges and promises. *J Pharm Pharmacol.* 2012;64(9):1217–1235.

Unzueta U, Saccardo P, Domingo-Espín J, et al. Sheltering DNA in self-organizing, protein-only nano-shells as artificial viruses for gene delivery. *Nanomedicine.* 2014;10(3):535–541.

Valentini F, Carbone M, Palleschi G. Carbon nanostructured materials for applications in nano-medicine, cultural heritage, and electrochemical biosensors. *Anal Bioanal Chem.* 2013;405(2–3):451–465.

Vang KB, Safina I, Darrigues E, et al. Modifying dendritic cell activation with plasmonic nano vectors. *Sci Rep.* 2017;7(1):5513.

Verderio P, Avvakumova S, Alessio G, et al. Delivering colloidal nanoparticles to mammalian cells: a nano-bio interface perspective. *Adv Healthc Mater.* 2014;3(7):957–976.

Viti L, Hu J, Coquillat D, Politano A, Knap W, Vitiello MS. Efficient Terahertz detection in black-phosphorus nano-transistors with selective and controllable plasma-wave, bolometric and thermoelectric response. *Sci Rep.* 2016;6:20474.

Vong LB, Nagasaki Y. Nitric oxide nano-delivery systems for cancer therapeutics: advances and challenges. *Antioxidants (Basel).* 2020 Sep;9(9):791.

Vordos N, Giannakopoulos S, Gkika DA, et al. Kidney stone nano-structure – Is there an opportunity for nanomedicine development? *Biochim Biophys Acta Gen Subj.* 2017;1861(6):1521–1529.

Voruganti S, Qin JJ, Sarkar S, et al. Oral nano-delivery of anticancer ginsenoside 25-OCH3-PPD, a natural inhibitor of the MDM2 oncogene: nanoparticle preparation, characterization, in vitro and in vivo anti-prostate cancer activity, and mechanisms of action. *Oncotarget.* 2015;6(25):21379–21394.

Vukomanović M, Žunič V, Kunej Š, et al. Nano-engineering the antimicrobial spectrum of lantibiotics: activity of nisin against gram negative bacteria. *Sci Rep.* 2017;7(1):4324.

Wang C, Hsu CH, Li Z, et al. Effective heating of magnetic nanoparticle aggregates for in vivo nano-theranostic hyperthermia. *Int J Nanomedicine.* 2017;12:6273–6287.

Wang D, Zhang N, Jing X, Zhang Y, Xu Y, Meng L. A tumor-microenvironment fully responsive nano-platform for MRI-guided photodynamic and photothermal synergistic therapy. *J Mater Chem B.* 2020;8(36):8271–8281.

Wang J, Gao W. Nano/microscale motors: biomedical opportunities and challenges. *ACS Nano.* 2012;6(7):5745–5751.

Wang J, Liu G. Imaging nano-bio interactions in the kidney: toward a better understanding of nanoparticle clearance. *Angew Chem Int Ed Engl.* 2018;57(12):3008–3010.

Wang K, Guo C, Zou S, et al. Synthesis, characterization and in vitro/in vivo evaluation of novel reduction-sensitive hybrid nano-echinus-like nanomedicine. *Artif Cells Nanomed Biotechnol.* 2018;46(sup2):659–667.

Wang M, Gustafsson OJR, Siddiqui G, et al. Human plasma proteome association and cytotoxicity of nano-graphene oxide grafted with stealth polyethylene glycol and poly(2-ethyl-2-oxazoline). *Nanoscale.* 2018;10(23):10863–10875.

Wang R, Deng J, He D, et al. Corrigendum to "PEGylated hollow gold nanoparticles for combined X-ray radiation and photothermal therapy in vitro and enhanced CT imaging" [Nanomedicine: nanotechnology, biology, and medicine 16 (2019) 195–205 NANO 1919]. *Nanomedicine.* 2020;35:102313. doi:10.1016/j.nano.2020.102313

Wang W, Zhou S, Guo L, Zhi W, Li X, Weng J. Investigation of endocytosis and cytotoxicity of poly-d, l-lactide-poly(ethylene glycol) micro/nano-particles in osteoblast cells. *Int J Nanomedicine.* 2010;5:557–566.

Wang X, Ma B, Xue J, Wu J, Chang J, Wu C. Defective black nano-titania thermogels for cutaneous tumor-induced therapy and healing. *Nano Lett.* 2019;19(3):2138–2147.

Wang Y, Cai R, Chen C. The nano-bio interactions of nanomedicines: understanding the biochemical driving forces and redox reactions. *Acc Chem Res.* 2019;52(6):1507–1518.

Wang Y, Huang HY, Yang L, Zhang Z, Ji H. Cetuximab-modified mesoporous silica nano-medicine specifically targets EGFR-mutant lung cancer and overcomes drug resistance. *Sci Rep.* 2016;6:25468.

Wang Y, Wang F, Liu Y, et al. Glutathione detonated and pH responsive nano-clusters of Au nanorods with a high dose of DOX for treatment of multidrug resistant cancer. *Acta Biomater.* 2018;75:334–345.

Watal G, Watal A, Rai PK, Rai DK, Sharma G, Sharma B. Biomedical applications of nano-antioxidant. *Methods Mol Biol.* 2013;1028:147–151.

Watanabe M, Kagawa S, Kuwada K, et al. Integrated fluorescent cytology with nano-biologics in peritoneally disseminated gastric cancer. *Cancer Sci.* 2018;109(10):3263–3271.

Watson CY, DeLoid GM, Pal A, Demokritou P. Buoyant nanoparticles: implications for nano-biointeractions in cellular studies. *Small.* 2016;12(23):3172–3180.

Webster TJ, Lee S, An SS. Today's diverse nano-theranostic applications and tomorrow's promises. *Int J Nanomedicine.* 2015;10(Spec Iss):1–2.

Weiss PS. What can nano do? *ACS Nano.* 2013;7(11):9507–9508.

Wijaya A, Maruf A, Wu W, Wang G. Recent advances in micro- and nano-bubbles for atherosclerosis applications. *Biomater Sci.* 2020;8(18):4920–4939.

Witika BA, Makoni PA, Mweetwa LL, et al. Nano-biomimetic drug delivery vehicles: potential approaches for COVID-19 treatment. *Molecules.* 2020;25(24):5592.

Wolfram J, Yang Y, Shen J, et al. The nano-plasma interface: implications of the protein corona. *Colloids Surf B Biointerfaces.* 2014;124:17–24.

Woodruff MA, Lange C, Chen F, Fratzl P, Hutmacher DW. Nano- to macroscale remodeling of functional tissue-engineered bone. *Adv Healthc Mater.* 2013;2(4):546–551.

Wu L, Li Y, Gu N. Nano-sensing and nano-therapy targeting central players in iron homeostasis. *Wiley Interdiscip Rev Nanomed Nanobiotechnol.* 2020:e1667.

Wu M, Liao L, Jiang L, et al. Liver-targeted Nano-MitoPBN normalizes glucose metabolism by improving mitochondrial redox balance. *Biomaterials.* 2019;222:119457.

Wu Y, Shih EK, Ramanathan A, Vasudevan S, Weil T. Nano-sized albumin-copolymer micelles for efficient doxorubicin delivery. *Biointerphases.* 2012;7(1–4):5.

Wu ZL, Zhao J, Xu R. Recent advances in oral nano-antibiotics for bacterial infection therapy. *Int J Nanomedicine.* 2020;15:9587–9610.

Xiong Y, Ren C, Zhang B, et al. Analyzing the behavior of a porous nano-hydroxyapatite/polyamide 66 (n-HA/PA66) composite for healing of bone defects. *Int J Nanomedicine.* 2014;9:485–494.

Xiong Y, Wang Y, Tiruthani K. Tumor immune microenvironment and nano-immunotherapeutics in colorectal cancer. *Nanomedicine.* 2019;21:102034.

Xu C, Pu F, Ren J, Qu X. A DNA/metal cluster-based nano-lantern as an intelligent theranostic device. *Chem Commun (Camb).* 2020;56(39):5295–5298.

Xu M, Li J, Iwai H, et al. Formation of nano-bio-complex as nanomaterials dispersed in a biological solution for understanding nanobiological interactions. *Sci Rep.* 2012;2:406.

Xu X, Bayazitoglu Y, Meade A. Evaluation of theranostic perspective of gold-silica nanoshell for cancer nanomedicine: a numerical parametric study. *Lasers Med Sci.* 2019;34(2):377–388.

Yan S, Zhao W, Wang B, Zhang L. A novel technology for localization of parathyroid adenoma: ultrasound-guided fine needle aspiration combined with rapid parathyroid hormone detection and nano-carbon technology. *Surg Innov.* 2018;25(4):357–363.

Yang B, Dong X, Lei Q, Zhuo R, Feng J, Zhang X. Host-guest interaction-based self-engineering of nano-sized vesicles for co-delivery of genes and anticancer drugs. *ACS Appl Mater Interfaces.* 2015;7(39):22084–22094.

Yang G, Xu L, Chao Y, et al. Hollow MnO. *Nat Commun.* 2017;8(1):

Yang K, Feng L, Shi X, Liu Z. Nano-graphene in biomedicine: theranostic applications. *Chem Soc Rev.* 2013;42(2):530–547.

Yang X, Liu G, Shi Y, Huang W, Shao J, Dong X. Nano-black phosphorus for combined cancer phototherapy: recent advances and prospects. *Nanotechnology.* 2018;29(22):222001.

Yao J, Hsu CH, Li Z, et al. Magnetic resonance nano-theranostics for glioblastoma multiforme. *Curr Pharm Des.* 2015;21(36):5256–5266.

Yao S, Li L, Su XT, et al. Development and evaluation of novel tumor-targeting paclitaxel-loaded nano-carriers for ovarian cancer treatment: in vitro and in vivo. *J Exp Clin Cancer Res.* 2018;37(1):29.

Yeh YC, Huang TH, Yang SC, Chen CC, Fang JY. Nano-based drug delivery or targeting to eradicate bacteria for infection mitigation: a review of recent advances. *Front Chem.* 2020;8:286.

Yumita N, Iwase Y, Umemura SI, Chen FS, Momose Y. Sonodynamically-induced anticancer effects of polyethylene glycol-modified carbon nano tubes. *Anticancer Res* 2020;40(5):2549–2557.

Zabihi E, Babaei A, Shahrampour D, Arab-Bafrani Z, Mirshahidi KS, Majidi HJ. Facile and rapid in-situ synthesis of chitosan-ZnO nano-hybrids applicable in medical purposes; a novel combination of biomineralization, ultrasound, and bio-safe morphology-conducting agent. *Int J Biol Macromol.* 2019;131:107–116.

Zaidi S, Misba L, Khan AU. Nano-therapeutics: a revolution in infection control in post antibiotic era. *Nanomedicine.* 2017;13(7):2281–2301.

Zarogouldis P, Karamanos NK, Porpodis K, et al. Vectors for inhaled gene therapy in lung cancer. Application for nano oncology and safety of bio nanotechnology. *Int J Mol Sci.* 2012;13(9):10828–10862.

Zhang J, Chen Z, Kankala RK, Wang SB, Chen AZ. Self-propelling micro-/nano-motors: mechanisms, applications, and challenges in drug delivery. *Int J Pharm.* 2021;596:120275.

Zhang J, Li S, Li X. Polymeric nano-assemblies as emerging delivery carriers for therapeutic applications: a review of recent patents. *Recent Pat Nanotechnol.* 2009;3(3):225–31.

Zhang J, Mai J, Li F, et al. Investigation of parameters that determine Nano-DC vaccine transport. *Biomed Microdevices.* 2019;21(2):39.

Zhang L, Su H, Wang H, et al. Tumor chemo-radiotherapy with rod-shaped and spherical gold nano probes: shape and active targeting both matter. *Theranostics.* 2019;9(7):1893–1908.

Zhang L, Wang D, Yang K, et al. Mitochondria-targeted artificial "Nano-RBCs" for amplified synergistic cancer phototherapy by a single nir irradiation. *Adv Sci (Weinh).* 2018;5(8):1800049.

Zhang Q, Du Y, Jing L, et al. Infra red dye and endostar loaded poly lactic acid nano particles as a novel theranostic nanomedicine for breast cancer. *J Biomed Nanotechnol.* 2016;12(3):491–502.

Zhang S, Ma X, Sha D, Qian J, Yuan Y, Liu C. A novel strategy for tumor therapy: targeted, PAA-functionalized nano-hydroxyapatite nanomedicine. *J Mater Chem B.* 2020;8(41):9589–9600.

Zhang T, Zhu G, Lu B, Peng Q. Oral nano-delivery systems for colon targeting therapy. *Pharm Nanotechnol.* 2017;5(2):83–94.

Zhang TX, Zhu GY, Lu BY, Zhang CL, Peng Q. Concentration-dependent protein adsorption at the nano-bio interfaces of polymeric nanoparticles and serum proteins. *Nanomedicine (Lond).* 2017;12(22):2757–2769.

Zhang XY, Zhang PY. Mitochondria targeting nano agents in cancer therapeutics. *Oncol Lett.* 2016;12(6):4887–4890.

Zhang Y, Fu H, Liu DE, An J, Gao H. Construction of biocompatible bovine serum albumin nanoparticles composed of nano graphene oxide and AIEgen for dual-mode phototherapy bacteriostatic and bacterial tracking. *J Nanobiotechnology.* 2019;17(1):104.

Zhang Y, Yu C, Huang G, Wang C, Wen L. Nano rare-earth oxides induced size-dependent vacuolization: an independent pathway from autophagy. *Int J Nanomedicine.* 2010;5:601–609.

Zhang YJ, Li BA, Li ZY, Xia N, Yu HY, Zhang YZ. Synthesis and characterization of Tamoxifen citrate modified reduced graphene oxide nano sheets for breast cancer therapy. *J Photochem Photobiol B.* 2018;180:68–71.

Zheng D, Wan C, Yang H, et al. Her2-targeted multifunctional nano-theranostic platform mediates tumor microenvironment remodeling and immune activation for breast cancer treatment. *Int J Nanomedicine.* 2020;15:10007–10028.

Zheng DW, Chen JL, Zhu JY, et al. Highly integrated nano-platform for breaking the barrier between chemotherapy and immunotherapy. *Nano Lett.* 07 2016;16(7):4341–4347.

Zhou H, Mu Q, Gao N, et al. A nano-combinatorial library strategy for the discovery of nanotubes with reduced protein-binding, cytotoxicity, and immune response. *Nano Lett.* 2008;8(3):859–865.

Zhu D, Zhang WG, Nie XD, Ding SW, Zhang DT, Yang L. Rational design of ultra-small photoluminescent copper nano-dots loaded PLGA micro-vessels for targeted co-delivery of natural piperine molecules for the treatment for epilepsy. *J Photochem Photobiol B.* 2020;205:111805.

Zhu G, Xu Z, Yan LT. Entropy at bio-nano interfaces. *Nano Lett.* 2020;20(8):5616–5624.

Zhu Y, Wen LM, Li R, Dong W, Jia SY, Qi MC. Recent advances of nano-drug delivery system in oral squamous cell carcinoma treatment. *Eur Rev Med Pharmacol Sci.* 2019;23(21):9445–9453.

Zhu Z, Zhang Q, Lay Yap P, Ni Y, Losic D. Magnetic reduced graphene oxide as a nano-vehicle for loading and delivery of curcumin. *Spectrochim Acta A Mol Biomol Spectrosc.* 2021;252:119471.

Zullino S, Argenziano M, Stura I, Guiot C, Cavalli R. From micro- to nano-multifunctional theranostic platform: effective ultrasound imaging is not just a matter of scale. *Mol Imaging.* 2018;17:1536012118778216.

7

Antimicrobials

7.1 Background

Louis Pasteur once said, "it's in man's power to eradicate infection from the earth" (Pasteur as cited in Roser et al. 2014). Two infectious diseases, smallpox and rinderpest, have been eradicated by this power. We are also closer to eradicating the diseases polio and Guinea worm. But can all infections in the world be eradicated? To achieve a feasible disease eradication as an option, specific criteria must be met:

- It must be a disorder of infection. (We are unable to eliminate non-infectious conditions, for example, heart disease or cancer.)
- There must be ways of preventing or treating infection.
- It must be transmissible to other humans or animals.

Other aspects of the disease considered include:

- How many disease pathogens are there?
- Do one or more hosts have the disease-causing pathogen?
- Does the disease have any recognizable symptoms?
- Is it possible to remove the disease regionally?
- With financial and political support, is the perceived disease burden high?

The more pathogens cause the disease, the harder it will be to eradicate. However, if a limited number of pathogens cause an infection, they may be eradicated using the same tools and approaches. For example, two types of variola virus have caused smallpox, and the same vaccine has been used to prevent them. Contrast this with a condition that requires different treatments, like pneumonia, which has multiple pathogens, from bacteria to viruses.

Multi-host diseases are difficult to eradicate as they often mean that the disease needs to be eradicated. There is only one host—humans—for pathogenic diseases, such as poliomyelitis, measles, mumps, rubella, diphtheria, and whooping cough. In general, individual-host pathogens are an exception, not a rule. In particular, the Guinea worm disease eradication target for 2020 had to be postponed because we were aware of Guinea worm transmission rates between dog populations, which could lead to the development of new human infections.

In the first place, some diseases cannot be detected easily. Currently, approximately 1.7 billion people are suffering from latent TB infection. Because latent tuberculosis has no symptoms, it is impossible to recognize each person with latent tuberculosis if every person in the world is tested. The stigma surrounding the condition can even limit our treatment capacity if symptoms can be visible or detectable for other diseases. For example, hepatitis C is a disease that meets most of the criteria for eradication. However, given the high prevalence of the disease among drug users, a stigma is attached to an infected person, making it hard to identify all the cases (Roser et al. 2014).

DOI: 10.1201/9781003146933-7

7.2 Eradicable Diseases

The eradication of diseases usually occurs step by step. Proof-of-concept of eradication in one region is a positive indicator of possible eradication at a broader level. Once the reduction of the disease has been achieved, greater support can be gathered for the feasibility of removal elsewhere. The following sections list diseases that are likely to be eradicated by our existing technology, perhaps faster if future technologies such as nucleic acid vaccines are considered (Roser et al. 2014).

7.2.1 Polio

Poliomyelitis, also known as polio, is a disease caused by the poliovirus. In 1953 and 1961, Jonas Salk and Albert Sabin invented two polio vaccines, eradicating the disease in both the United States and Canada in 1979 and rapidly leading to a significant reduction in Western Europe. A needle injection is needed for Salk's vaccine while Sabin's vaccine is oral and may be swallowed. The latter feature enabled its distribution across the developing world, as its administration needed less trained healthcare staff.

In 1988, the Global Polio Eradication Initiative was created to support the eradication of polio on a large scale. Since then, a dramatic reduction in the number of cases of paralytic polio has led to it being endemic in three countries only: Pakistan, Afghanistan, and Nigeria, as of 2018. However, polio also shows that positive trends could reverse. For example, Nigeria's cases increased from 202 in 2002 to 1,143 in 2006 due to rumors of covert infertility and the propagation of HIV in the local communities resulting in an 11-month boycott of the vaccination. This example shows that efforts to eradicate must be successful at international, national, and community levels (Roser et al. 2014).

7.2.2 Guinea Worm Disease (Dracunculiasis)

Dracunculus medinensis is the worm that causes Guinea worm disease. There is no vaccine available to protect against the disease. It can, however, be successfully eradicated by identifying and treating all current cases of the disease. In 2018, there were 28 cases of Guinea worm reported, in Angola (one case), Chad (17 cases), and South Sudan (ten cases). Guinea worm is on the verge of extinction (Roser et al. 2014).

7.2.3 Lymphatic Filariasis

Lymphocytic filariasis is caused by roundworms. It is a disease that is not fatal, but it is extremely debilitating. It causes lymph node swelling, which can cause painful swelling of the arms, legs, and other body parts. In 2017, 62 million people were infected with lymphatic filariasis. The majority of cases are found in sub-Saharan Africa, South Asia, and Indonesia.

Preventive chemotherapy can effectively stop the transmission of the roundworms that cause lymphatic filariasis, spread by mosquitoes. WHO and its partners have been working on mass drug administration campaigns (MDAs) to prevent disease transmission. Rather than targeting infected individuals, MDAs target groups of people living in endemic areas. Since the year 2000, MDA campaigns have provided 7.7 billion preventive chemotherapy treatments (Roser et al. 2014).

7.2.4 Measles, Mumps, and Rubella

Vaccination against measles, mumps, and rubella is available for children. Humans are the only known hosts of these viruses, making them a good target for eradication. One of the major roadblocks to eradicating these diseases is the public misperception of the disease's seriousness, which leads to low vaccination rates. In developing countries, insufficient information on disease prevalence and a lack of resources are also significant factors.

In 2017, the World Health Organization recorded more than 741,000 cases of these three diseases when taken together. However, because not all cases are reported to the WHO, this figure is likely to be underestimated.

Despite the availability of a safe and effective vaccine, measles remains a highly contagious killer of young children worldwide. Measles claimed the lives of 110,000 people in 2017, the majority of whom were children under five. There has been a global increase in one-year-old vaccination coverage and the concurrent decline in reported cases of measles, from nearly 1,000 cases per million people to 28 cases per million. This equates to a 33-fold decrease.

Mumps is spread through direct human contact or airborne droplets. It causes painful swelling of the parotid glands, which are located on the side of the face beneath the ears, and fever, headaches, and muscle aches. In teenagers and adults, it can lead to sterility.

Rubella is usually mild in children, but it can cause complications in up to 90% of pregnant women, with approximately 20% of those cases resulting in fetal death (Roser et al. 2014).

7.2.5 Cysticercosis

The pork tapeworm (*Taenia solium*) causes cysticercosis, a parasitic tissue infection of tissues (including brain and muscle tissue). These infections are a major cause of adult-onset seizures in low-income countries.

Cysticercosis was added to the list of eradicable diseases by the International Task Force for Disease Eradication in 1993. However, millions of people around the world are still affected by the disease. Neurocysticercosis affected 2.56–8.30 million people in 2015, according to the WHO. Tapeworms, which can affect the nervous system and cause severe epileptic seizures, cause the disease.

The tapeworm transmission cycle between humans and pigs must be broken to eradicate cysticercosis in humans. This can be accomplished effectively through sanitary measures, as well as proper pork inspection and cooking. In addition, vaccines against the tapeworm are now available for use in pigs, and the oxfendazole drug can be used to treat animals with the tapeworm (Roser et al. 2014).

7.2.6 Yaws

Yaws is a chronic skin infection characterized by papillomas (noncancerous lumps) and ulcers. It is caused by the bacterium *Treponema pallidum subspecies pertenue*, which belongs to the same group of bacteria that causes venereal syphilis.

Yaws primarily affects children aged under 15 years who live in poor communities in warm, humid, and tropical forested areas of Africa, Asia, Latin America, and the Pacific islands. The majority of affected populations live in rural areas, far from health services. Poverty, low socio-economic conditions, and poor personal hygiene facilitate the spread of yaws.

Although there are over 80,000 cases of yaws each year, experts believe the disease can be controlled and ultimately eradicated for several reasons. First, it only occurs in humans, not animals, making control much easier. It is also easy to treat with readily available drugs and has already been eliminated in some countries, including India. Although there are some remaining pockets of yaws infection, they are usually in remote places, meaning further spread is less likely with proper surveillance and control measures (Medical College Directory 2021).

7.2.7 Trachoma

Trachoma is a bacterial infection caused by *Chlamydia trachomatis*. The disease causes blindness by affecting the eyes. Sanitary measures, such as access to clean water and facial cleanliness, can help to prevent trachoma. In addition, antibiotics in large doses can successfully stop disease transmission, and surgery can reverse disease-related blindness.

7.2.8 Onchocerciasis

Onchocerciasis, also known as river blindness, is a parasitic worm-caused eye infection. The disease causes blindness, skin damage, and epilepsy in some people. According to the Global Burden of Disease study, there were 20.9 million cases of river blindness in 2017; 1.2 million cases resulted in blindness, 14.7 million cases resulted in skin lesions, and five million cases were asymptomatic.

7.2.9 Malaria

Malaria deaths are estimated by the Institute of Health Metrics and Evaluation (IHME) from 1990 onwards. Over this period, we can see a clear rise–peak–fall trend, with deaths rising from around 670,000 in 1990 to around 930,000 in 2004, then falling (at varying rates) to around 620,000 in 2017.

7.3 Vaccines

The types of vaccines include:

- Live-attenuated vaccines.
- Inactivated vaccines.
- Subunit, recombinant, polysaccharide, and conjugate vaccines.
- Toxoid vaccines.

7.3.1 Live-Attenuated Vaccines

Live vaccines use a weakened (or attenuated) version of the disease-causing germ. These vaccines elicit a strong and long-lasting immune response because they are similar to the natural infection they help prevent. Most live vaccines can provide lifetime protection against a germ and the disease it causes with just one or two doses. Live vaccines protect against measles, mumps, rubella (MMR combined vaccine), rotavirus, smallpox, chickenpox, and yellow fever.

7.3.2 Inactivated Vaccines

Inactivated vaccines use a dead version of the disease-causing germ. As a result, inactivated vaccines rarely provide the same level of immunity (protection) as live vaccines. As a result, you may need several doses over time (booster shots) to maintain disease immunity.

7.3.3 Subunit, Recombinant, Polysaccharide, and Conjugate Vaccines

Because these vaccines only use specific germ pieces, they produce a strong immune response targeted to the germ's most important parts. They can also be used on almost anyone who requires them, including those with compromised immune systems and long-term health issues. One drawback of these vaccines is that you may need booster shots in the future to remain disease-free.

Hib (*Hemophilus influenzae* type b) disease, hepatitis B, HPV (human papillomavirus), whooping cough (part of the DTaP combined vaccine), pneumococcal disease, meningococcal disease, and shingles are all protected by subunit, recombinant, polysaccharide, and conjugate vaccines.

7.3.4 Toxoid Vaccines

Toxoid vaccines use a toxin (harmful product) made by the germ that causes a disease. They create immunity to the parts of the germ that cause a disease instead of the germ itself. That means the immune response is targeted to the toxin instead of the whole germ. Like some other types of vaccines, you may need booster shots to get ongoing protection against diseases. Toxoid vaccines are used to protect against diphtheria and tetanus (Office of Infectious Disease and HIV/AIDS Policy 2021).

7.3.5 Nucleic Acid Vaccines

DNA vaccines are simple to make and inexpensive, and they provide effective long-term immunity. In addition, because recombinant vector vaccines (platform-based vaccines) mimic natural infection, they're particularly effective at teaching the immune system to fight germs. Chapter 8 provides details on nucleic acid vaccines.

Nucleic acid vaccines are used against COVID-19, as the first such vaccine approved in 2020.

7.4 Antibiotics

Antibiotics have been used to treat infections for millennia, even though people didn't realize bacteria were to blame until the last century. Some of the world's earliest civilizations used various molds and plant extracts to treat infections—the ancient Egyptians used moldy bread to treat infected wounds. Despite this, infections that we now consider simple to treat—such as pneumonia and diarrhea caused by bacteria—were the leading causes of death in the developed world until the twentieth century.

Scientists didn't start observing antibacterial chemicals in action until the late nineteenth century. According to Paul Ehrlich, a German physician, certain chemical dyes colored some bacterial cells but not others. He concluded that, based on this principle, it should be possible to create substances that can selectively kill bacteria while causing no harm to other cells. In 1909, he discovered that arsphenamine, a chemical, was an effective syphilis treatment. Although Ehrlich referred to his discovery as "chemotherapy" —the use of a chemical to treat a disease—it became the first modern antibiotic. Selman Waksman, a Ukrainian-American inventor and microbiologist who discovered over 20 antibiotics during his lifetime, coined the term "antibiotics" over 30 years later.

Alexander Fleming's work was a little haphazard, and he discovered penicillin by accident. In 1928, he returned from a vacation in Suffolk and discovered that a fungus, *Penicillium notatum*, had infected a culture plate of *Staphylococcus* bacteria that he had left uncovered. Wherever the fungus grew on the plate, it created bacteria-free zones. So Fleming isolated the mold and expanded it in pure culture. He discovered that *P. notatum* was highly effective even at low concentrations, preventing *Staphylococcus* growth even after being diluted 800 times, and was less toxic than the disinfectants in use at the time.

Antibiotics are extremely effective, but there is growing concern about the rise of antibiotic-resistant bacteria, which cause about a million deaths worldwide each year and are expected to reach up to ten million by 2050. Bacteria evolve and develop resistance to the antibiotics that have been used successfully in the past, rendering them useless.

The efforts to discover new antibiotics have changed significantly after a long period of silence; the new stimuli created by governments and private organizations over the last several years are the main drivers of the revived interest. The GAIN (Generating Antibiotic Incentives Now) Act of 2012 (www.congress.gov/bill/112th-congress/house-bill/) is one example in the United States, and a newer qualified infectious disease product (QIDP) designation for antibiotics and antifungals (www.fda.gov/media/111091/download) gives new candidates priority review and five years of market exclusivity if approved. The Antibiotic Development to Advance Patient Treatment (ADAPT) Act, which was approved by the House in July 2015 and allowed the FDA to approve antibacterial medicines to treat serious or life-threatening infections based on small clinical trials, could provide additional support (www.congress.gov/bill/114th-congress/house-bill/).

7.4.1 Antibiotic Discovery

Antibiotic-resistant bacteria, also known as superbugs, are causing increasing concern. They cause about 700,000 deaths each year worldwide, and according to a study conducted by the United Kingdom government, this number could rise to ten million by 2050. Bacteria evolve and develop resistance to antibiotics, which have been used successfully in the past but have since become obsolete.

Antibiotic discovery has historically been critical in outpacing resistance. Success has been linked to systematic procedures—platforms that catalyzed the antibiotic golden age, such as the Waksman platform, followed by semi-synthesis platforms and fully synthetic antibiotics. Aminoglycosides, amphenicols, ansamycins, beta-lactams, lipopeptides, diaminopyrimidines, fosfomycin, imidazoles, macrolides, oxazolidinones, streptogramins, polymyxins, sulphonamides, glycopeptides, quinolones, and tetracyclines are just a few of the antibiotic classes. The target-based platform emerged during the genomics era, and it was widely regarded as a failure due to difficulties in translating drugs to the clinic. As a result, cell-based platforms have been reinstated and remain critical in the fight against infectious diseases. There is an increasingly large set of information available on microbial metabolism in the post-genomic era, even though the antibiotic pipeline is still lacking, particularly in terms of new classes and novel mechanisms of action. The translation of this knowledge into new platforms will hopefully lead to discovering new and better therapeutics, which will help us reclaim the battle against infectious diseases.

7.4.1.1 Semi-Synthetic

Antibacterial semi-synthesis is the alteration of pre-existing scaffolds, or molecular backbones, obtained through a fermentation process. The Waksman platform has historically been the source of most scaffolds. As a result of selective pressures, such as the actinomycete-bacteria "fight," they have evolved to be exceptionally well suited to reach and bind to their target. This, however, does not account for therapeutic efficacy or safety, which can often be improved using semi-synthesis, as well as chemical stability and the reduction of undesirable side effects, among other features that are important in marketing antibiotics, such as patenting derivatives, which increases the profitability of antibiotic development programs, which is critical for this generally unappealing drug. Semi-synthesis began in 1946 with the catalytic hydrogenation of streptomycin, resulting in dihydrostreptomycin, which had greater chemical stability and antimicrobial activity. Unfortunately, even though streptomycin and its novel derivative were quickly adopted into clinical practice, their prescription was eventually reevaluated due to concerns about ototoxicity.

Penicillin G is synthesized, hydrolyzed into 6-APA, purified, and then chemically altered, for example, at the acyl side chain to produce various semi-synthetic penicillins. The semi-synthesis of cephalosporins, which has reduced the incidence of both side effects and resistance while also providing an additional site for chemical modification, is another beta-lactam example similar to penicillins. In 1948, cephalosporin C was discovered as a metabolite of *Cephalosporium acremonium*. The precursor to a variety of semi-synthetic cephalosporins, 7-aminocephalosporanic acid (7-ACA), was obtained from its hydrolysis under acidic conditions by 1959 (Table 7.1).

Another important example of semi-synthesis is chlortetracycline's catalytic hydrogenolysis (discovered in 1948), which resulted in the semi-synthesis of tetracycline by 1953. It was later discovered, however, to be a natural product. Semi-synthetic cephalosporins are primarily derivatives of 7-ACA, which are made by adding different molecular groups to the two adjustable sites, C7 and C3', respectively. Serial structural modifications make semi-synthetic tetracyclines and macrolides. Each iteration necessitates the chemical manipulation of the previous semi-synthetic derivative, preserving its benefits.

Nonetheless, over a series of semi-synthetic generations, the number of chemical changes grows proportionally and becomes increasingly difficult. As a result, only about ten semi-synthetic tetracyclines have been commercialized in the last 60 years, compared to more than 50 commercialized beta-lactam derivatives. Figure 7.1 depicts the evolution of semi-synthetic cephalosporins, their introduction timeline, and the benefits and drawbacks of the subsequent generations currently on the market.

7.4.1.2 Synthetic

Recent advances in fully synthetic routes have reignited interest in tetracycline derivative synthesis, which is critical since semi-synthesis is one of the most essential strategies for antibiotic discovery and is especially important in keeping up with the evolution of resistance mechanisms.

Fully synthetic antibiotics enable production at a scale suitable for clinical use while introducing novel molecules. Chloramphenicol, for example, was the first fully synthetic antibiotic to reach the clinic in 1949, with a scaffold derived from a natural product. Semi-synthesis, or the chemical manipulation of a scaffold, applies to a fully synthetic antibiotic like chloramphenicol, which is unsurprising. In 1952, the nitro group was replaced with methanesulfonyl, resulting in thiamphenicol, which overcomes the most concerning toxicity issues while also having a greater antimicrobial effect, improving its clinical application. The natural product azomycin, discovered in 1953, had little clinical application but established

TABLE 7.1

Beta-Lactam Subclasses Highlighting Their Diversity with Examples of Marketed Antibiotics

Subclasses	Examples of Marketed Antibiotics
Penicillins	Penicillin G, penicillin V, ampicillin, amoxicillin, bacampicillin, cloxacillin, floxacillin, mezlocillin, nafcillin, oxacillin, methicillin,[a] dicloxacillin,[a] carbenicillin,[b] idanyl,[b] piperacillin,[b] ticarcillin[b]
Cephalosporins	Cefalothin,[c] cephradinea,[c] cefadroxyl,[c] cefazolin,[c] cephalexin,[c] cefuroxine,[d] cefaclor,[d] cefotetam,[d] cefmetazole,[d] cefonicd,[d] cefixime,[e] ceftibuten,[e] cefizoxime,[e] ceftriaxone,[e] cefamandol,[e] cefoperazone,[e] cefotaxime,[e] proxetil,[e] cefprozil,[e] ceftazidime,[e] cefuroxime, axetil,[e] cefpodexime,[e] cefepime,[f] ceftobiprole[g]
Other minor subclasses	Flomoref,[h] latamoxef,[h] cefoxitin,[i] loracarbef,[j] imipenem,[j] meropenem,[j] panipenem,[j] azreonam,[k] carumonam[k]

Notes

[a] Penicillinase-resistant penicillin.
[b] Anti-pseudomonal penicillin.
[c] First-generation cephalosporin
[d] Second-generation cephalosporin.
[e] Third-generation cephalosporin.
[f] Fourth-generation cephalosporin.
[g] Fifth-generation cephalosporin.
[h] Oxycepham.
[i] Cefam.
[j] Carbapenem.
[k] Monobactam.

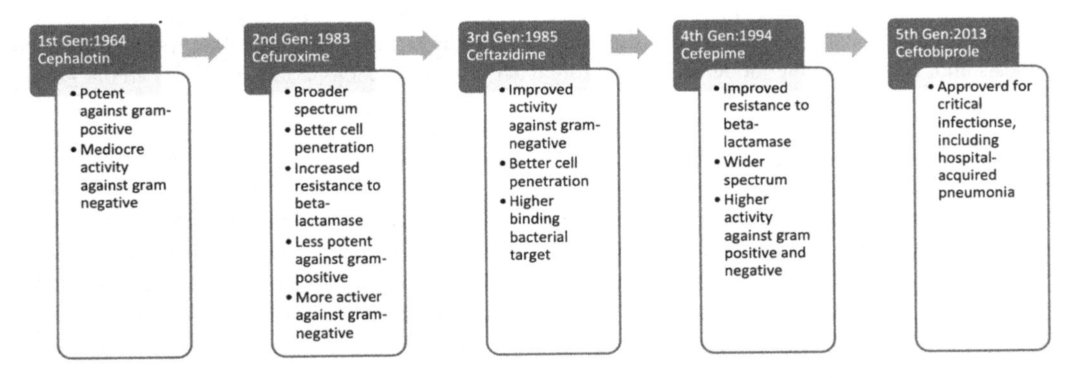

FIGURE 7.1 Evolution of cephalosporin characteristics over semi-synthetic generations. Because each generation is adding different molecular groups to 7-ACA, characteristics are not necessarily inherited by succeeding generations. For instance, second-generation cephalosporins had reduced potency against Gram-positive pathogens, despite their otherwise improved properties.

the nitroimidazole class. Metronidazole, which is currently produced using a fully synthetic protocol and is effective against the trichomoniasis parasite, was discovered in 1962 during a search for optimized derivatives. Surprisingly, its activity against anaerobic bacteria was discovered by chance, and it is still used for that purpose. Similar to metronidazole, the natural product fosfomycin had a practical clinical application only after Merck developed a racemic synthesis protocol, and it is still prescribed today. While there are apparent benefits to chemically synthesizing natural products, fully synthetic antibiotics have also resulted in novel scaffolds. Trimethoprim, a diaminopyrimidine derivative, was introduced in 1962 after synthetic analogs of pyrimidine and purine bases inhibited bacterial growth.

The majority of fully synthetic antibiotics discussed have limited use in uncomplicated infections or cost-effective alternatives in developing countries. Despite the limited activity of acid in 1962, the quinolone class, which was discovered as a by-product of the synthesis of the antimalarial compound chloroquine, was an essential scaffold in the synthesis of nalidixic. Chemical modification was used to create three more generations, the fluoroquinolones. Quinolones, after macrolides and beta-lactams, are the third most commonly prescribed antibiotic to outpatients. Their antimicrobial effect is due to the formation of a DNA gyrase-quinolone-DNA complex in Gram-positive and Gram-negative pathogens, which inhibits replication and causes cellular death. Another important antibiotic class, macrolides, is made by semi-synthesis from erythromycin, ranging from simple modifications (e.g., four steps to derive azithromycin) to more complex ones (e.g., 16 steps for the drug candidate solithromycin). The recent publication of a fully synthetic protocol that produced over 300 macrolides gives this antibiotic class new hope. It depicts the significance of the fully synthetic platform to this day, not only in facilitating synthesis but also in increasing the variety of antibiotics available.

Fully synthetic beta-lactams are of particular importance because they allowed more complex antibiotics to be synthesized, eventually leading to many subclasses. The carbapenem and monobactam subclasses are two notable examples. Carbapenems have a similar core structure to penicillins. Still, they differ at the C2–C3 double bond and replace C1 sulfur with carbon, resulting in increased potency, activity spectrum, and resistance to beta-lactamase action. Since their discovery in 1985, ten carbapenem derivatives have been commercialized or are in clinical trials. Carbapenems are the first-line treatment for multidrug-resistant infections because they have the broadest activity spectrum among beta-lactams, including resistant pathogens.

Monobactams, on the other hand, have higher beta-lactamase stability and are a promising way forward. With the introduction of aztreonam to the clinic in 1984, these monocyclic beta-lactams are now being developed for the siderophore moiety. The bacterial iron uptake machinery is used in this Trojan horse strategy to facilitate entry into Gram-negative bacteria.

The oxazolidinone class is divided into two groups, each with a different mode of action. In 1952, the natural product cycloserine, which is now produced synthetically, was introduced as the first act on cell wall biosynthesis. Cycloserine is still used as a second-line treatment for tuberculosis, particularly in multidrug-resistant strains. The other oxazolidinones group was discovered in 1984 to target protein synthesis and, despite having moderate antimicrobial activity, had toxicity concerns. The DuPont group synthesized various derivatives from these, leading to the discovery of linezolid, which was approved in 2000 as the first novel antibiotic class since the discovery of nalidixic acid, a nearly 50-year gap. Although no major resistance to linezolid has been reported, its limited efficacy against Gram-positive bacteria and toxicity during prolonged treatments limit its therapeutic use as a last resort against multidrug-resistant pathogens in complicated cases. Given their low resistance profile, there has been a lot of interest in developing new oxazolidinones over the last decade. As a result, a few companies have been working on new analogs. Thus, semi-synthesis, along with complete chemical routes, has catalyzed the dawn of the medicinal chemistry era, which has yielded the vast majority of clinically relevant antibiotics, characterized by increasing potency and decreasing side effects with subsequent iterations, giving mankind the upper hand on infectious diseases.

7.4.1.3 Genomic Approaches

The need for a new strategy coincides with the genomics era, which has shaped new high-tech platforms and redefined the scientific paradigm governing antibiotic discovery. The total number of sequenced microbial genomes increased from three to over 200 during the genomics era (1995–2004) and over 30,000 during the post-genomics era (2004–2014). The first platform to emerge in this context was comparative genomics, which identified novel targets essential for pathogen survival from repositories of sequenced and annotated genomes. Comparing genome sequences of pathogenic and non-pathogenic strains revealed that these targets could encode pathogenicity mechanisms. Furthermore, comparing these genomes to those of the host eliminates targets that are not unique to the pathogen, resulting in fewer drug–host interactions and therapeutic side effects (Figure 7.2). The target is then cloned, overexpressed, and used in a high-throughput screening (HTS) assay to search chemical libraries for binding agents.

New MOAs were expected to emerge because bacteria have a manageable number of exclusive and conserved proteins, so some companies launched pioneering target-based screening programs. Although

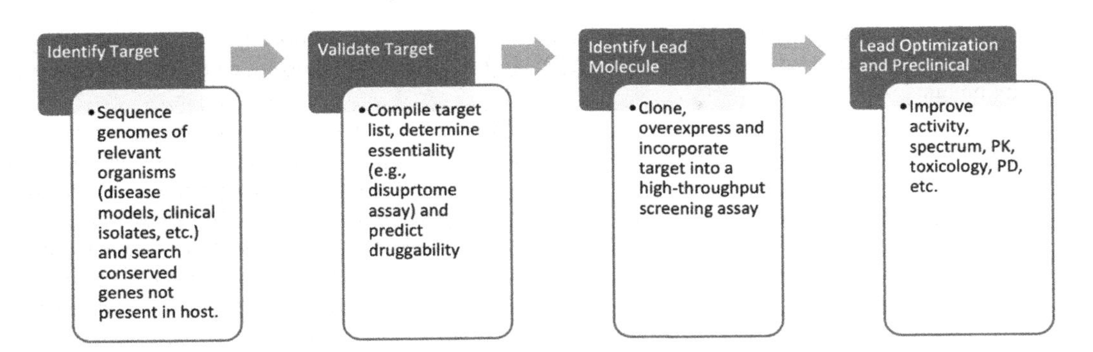

FIGURE 7.2 Schematic representation of the target-based antibiotic discovery platform: potential targets are identified from the genome sequence of pathogens and the host. The products of genes exclusive and essential for bacteria are incorporated into high-throughput screening assays, which identify drug candidates suitable for lead optimization and preclinical development. The latter falls outside the scope of antibiotic discovery. Thus, it is not discussed.

target-based screening is effective for identifying potent inhibitors of specific targets, their inability to reach their target in vivo is hampered by the low permeability of bacterial membranes or the action of efflux pumps. The bacterial cell wall is a very effective barrier against most small-molecule drugs in a physiological context. Furthermore, said targets might have functional redundancy. The target-based screening approach failed because not all targets could be easily cloned, purified, and incorporated into in vitro screening assays, in addition to the difficulties mentioned above.

In some cases, the assay's oversimplified environment excludes cofactors and isn't sensitive enough to detect off-target effects. Merck discovered, for example, that Gram-positive pathogens with low guanine-cytosine have increased resistance to fatty acid biosynthesis targets when grown on media similar to the human host, which a target-based assay cannot account for. In addition, single point mutations conferring resistance are also common in single-gene targets. As a result, they are more likely to choose resistant mutants.

Despite massive bacterial genome sequencing and bioinformatics tools to analyze the sequences, many genes remain uncharacterized in biological function. Furthermore, genetic diversity complicates target-based screening at the model organism level. For example, GlaxoSmithKline researchers discovered an unrelated copy of a gene conferring resistance in 20% of clinical isolates. Thus, antibiotic discovery is still a challenging task that cannot be accomplished solely through target-based genomics. Many people consider the comparative genomics platform to be a failure because no new drugs have been discovered.

Nonetheless, it sparked a quest to learn more about bacterial physiology, which has had undeniable benefits in the development of antimicrobial chemotherapy. Target-based screening evolved from a reductionist approach, such as analyzing a single gene/protein (target) outside of its biological context, to a more holistic phenotypic and pathway-based analysis. Following platforms arose from reviving whole-cell screening, which was the foundation of the Waksman platform, and has the inherent advantage that leads compounds can interact anywhere along the pathway, on multiple network constituents, or even on different metabolisms replicating in vivo conditions. New MOAs were expected to emerge because bacteria have a manageable number of exclusive and conserved proteins, so some companies launched pioneering target-based screening programs. Although target-based screening is effective for identifying potent inhibitors of specific targets, their inability to reach their target in vivo is hampered by the low permeability of bacterial membranes or the action of efflux pumps. The bacterial cell wall is a very effective barrier against most small-molecule drugs in a physiological context. Furthermore, said targets might have functional redundancy. The target-based screening approach failed because not all targets could be easily cloned, purified, and incorporated into in vitro screening assays, in addition to the difficulties mentioned above.

In some cases, the assay's oversimplified environment excludes cofactors and isn't sensitive enough to detect off-target effects. Merck discovered, for example, that Gram-positive pathogens with low guanine-cytosine have increased resistance to fatty acid biosynthesis targets when grown on media similar to the human host, which a target-based assay cannot account for. In addition, single point mutations conferring resistance are also common in single-gene targets. As a result, they are more likely to choose resistant mutants.

Despite massive bacterial genome sequencing and bioinformatics tools to analyze the sequences, many genes remain uncharacterized in biological function. Furthermore, genetic diversity complicates target-based screening at the model organism level. For example, GlaxoSmithKline researchers discovered an unrelated copy of a gene conferring resistance in 20% of clinical isolates. Thus, antibiotic discovery is still a challenging task that cannot be accomplished solely through target-based genomics. Many people consider the comparative genomics platform to be a failure because no new drugs have been discovered.

Nonetheless, it sparked a quest to learn more about bacterial physiology, which has had undeniable benefits in developing antimicrobial chemotherapy. Target-based screening evolved from a reductionist approach, such as analyzing a single gene/protein (target) outside of its biological context, to a more holistic phenotypic and pathway-based analysis. Following platforms arose from reviving whole-cell screening, which was the foundation of the Waksman platform, and has the inherent advantage that leads compounds can interact anywhere along the pathway, on multiple network constituents, or even on different metabolisms replicating in vivo conditions.

7.4.2 Reverse Genomics: Revival of Cell-Based Screening

The case of anti-tuberculosis drug discovery is an excellent example of this shift in strategy: researchers returned to cell-based screening after abandoning target-based ADPs, with tremendous success in discovering novel, more diverse lead molecules for further optimization. However, in general, cell-based screening produces more variability and complex data than target-based screening, which is more difficult to relate to biologic phenomena due to its binary hit/no-hit nature.

After a positive hit, such as a drug interaction with a microorganism that changes its phenotype, counter-screening with human cells allows for cytotoxic evaluation of drug candidates with antimicrobial activity in cell-based assays. Cell-based ADPs first look for antimicrobial activity before moving on to characterizing MOA. They've also coined the term "reversed genomics. This isn't necessarily a drawback, as the FDA doesn't require identifying the molecular target to start clinical trials or get marketing approval (see Figure 7.3).

Cell-based assays, also known as phenotypic screening, involve screening large libraries in a systems-based mindset to evaluate the complex network of responses that antibiotics elicit. The term target-agnostic may be used if the screening probes phenotypic changes independent of the target hypothesis. Furthermore, cell-based screening can take a chemocentric approach, focusing on compounds and their derivatives that have been shown to have a biological effect. Thus, the development of cell-based screening methods is critical. In their simplest form, these focus on determining the minimum inhibitory concentration (MIC) to quantify antimicrobial activity. Because they complement other ADPs, MIC assays are still useful. However, genetic manipulation and the use of a label, either in a fluorescent or radioactive molecule or a reporter gene, are required as alternatives to MIC-type assays. This is a limiting factor because genetic manipulation, on the one hand, necessitates a priori knowledge. On the other hand, the

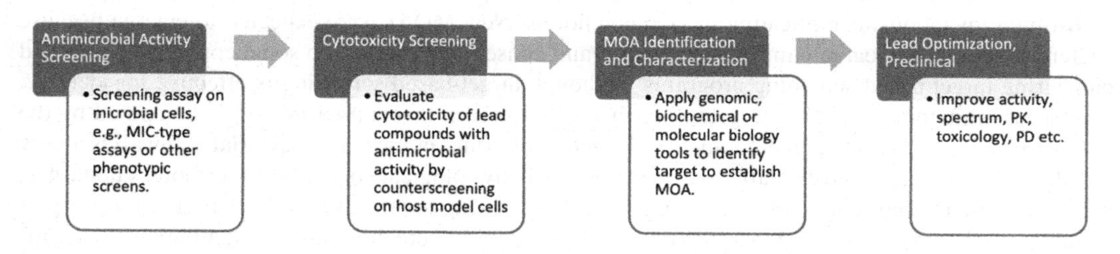

FIGURE 7.3 Schematic representation of the cell-based antibiotic discovery platform: drug candidates are identified from cell-based screening assays, a counter-screen excludes cytotoxic compounds, and subsequently, genomics tools are applied to identify MOA. Although MOA is not a requisite, it may facilitate lead optimization and preclinical development. For instance, structural information on the target can enable a rational modification of the drug candidate.

use of a reporter gene to indicate gene transcription may not always be consistent with changes in enzymatic activity, limiting the sensitivity of these assays.

Furthermore, because these signal transduction events can take a long time to become detectable, assay capacity and throughput are limited. Aside from the impact of the reporter gene, some of these labeled assays are limited in terms of miniaturization. Despite these drawbacks, cell-based screening continues to make significant contributions to antibiotic discovery.

Antibiotic therapy has traditionally relied on the discovery of chemically optimized or manufactured natural scaffolds. As a result, continuing to develop screening strategies that probe nature's repositories, particularly using cell-based assays, remains a rational decision. The primary antibiotic scaffolds currently in use are derived from natural products except for fluoroquinolones, sulphonamides, and trimethoprim. New cell-based ADPs should be able to identify antimicrobial-active molecules without the need for a label. Furthermore, because isolated projects have low success rates, these assays would be ideal for gaining insight into MOA while screening large libraries.

7.4.3 Post-Genomics

7.4.3.1 Transcriptomics, Proteomics, and Lipidomics

Biological research is becoming more specialized as it becomes more focused and localized; however, a system-wide understanding of biological constituents and their interactions is becoming more important. It is now possible to extract, handle, and interpret data from a much wider range of sources, including transcripts (transcriptomics), proteins (proteomics), and other molecules such as lipids (lipidomics), among others. The impact of these omics technologies on antibiotic discovery is undeniable, particularly in understanding antibiotic mode of action, identifying novel targets, and providing information on bacterial metabolism and physiology. Given the importance of screening in the ADPs discussed thus far, future platforms should be built on this foundation. Transcriptomics, proteomics, and lipidomics, on the other hand, have not yet reached the throughput capacity of cell-based screening assays and thus are not the core technology of any ADP. Furthermore, these technologies provide information about the biomolecules they study rather than the overall dynamics of bacterial metabolism, making them complementary, if not essential, tools in the antibiotic discovery process. Because a post-genomics ADP has yet to be developed, this section focuses on the technological foundations and contributions of post-genomics techniques to antibiotic discovery.

Northern blotting and microarrays were the first hybridization-based transcriptomics technologies. By the mid-1990s, microarrays had become the standard until next-generation sequencing expanded to transcriptomics, which is better at dealing with high genetic variation and non-specific hybridizations and being label-free, unbiased, and having a higher upper hand limit of detection. In terms of predicting differentially expressed genes, RNA-seq outperforms microarrays (90% versus 76%). Both technologies, however, estimated the MOA of anti-cancer drugs similarly. In addition, non-coding RNA, which plays a regulatory role in microbial antibiotic responses, can be studied using RNA-seq. As a result, it could be a viable alternative for discovering new antimicrobial targets and developing novel combinatorial therapies. Although next-generation sequencing, unbiased transcriptomics, and non-coding RNA technologies have all been used in drug discovery, few studies have looked at how they can be used to find antibiotics. Whole-genome expression profiling elucidates molecular and cellular responses to antibiotic stresses, which is especially useful for determining MOA, which is still a major gap in antibiotic discovery.

Genome expression technologies go beyond transcripts to include biological events at the protein level. Not only do these occur without any changes to the transcriptome, but the instability of bacterial RNA poses both conceptual and technological challenges, emphasizing the importance of combining transcriptomics and proteomics. Early proteomics research relied on 2D gel-based assays or difference gel electrophoresis, both of which require high-purity protein samples due to their sensitivity to low-abundance proteins, co-migration proteins, and different modifications on the same protein. Furthermore, because gel-based techniques are time-consuming, difficult to automate, and thus difficult to use in large-scale studies, the evolution of MS combined with chromatographic separation offers an alternative.

Proteomics has aided in discovering novel antimicrobial targets, the understanding of resistance mechanisms to therapeutic antibiotics, and the elucidation of MOA, despite its inability to characterize MOA fully. Notably, the application of transcriptomics and proteomics technologies sheds new light on the functions of various genes, resulting in updated annotations and a better understanding of bacterial metabolism and physiology. Although these technologies are not at the core of any ADP, they complement other ADPs by revealing information that helps pave the way forward. Because proteins interact with various biomolecules, such as nucleic acids and lipids, specialized techniques to investigate these interactions have been developed.

Furthermore, the field of phosphoproteomics has emerged from the realm of proteomics. Although thought to be unique to eukaryotes, this type of post-translational modification affects bacterial homeostasis, virulence, and signal transduction. Because the machinery used by bacteria to cause diseases, such as tyrosine kinases and phosphatases, is structurally different from the hosts and thus can be targeted exclusively, virulence mechanisms are fascinating. There are more descriptions of phosphoproteomics for drug discovery, but they are not related to infectious diseases.

Due to a technological gap filling with very selective and sensitive lipidome characterization studies using MS and combining variously targeted and non-targeted approaches, understanding the physiological role of lipids, especially at the molecular level, has been severely limited. Various chromatographic methods, such as hydrophilic interaction liquid chromatography or gas chromatography, are routinely used in conjunction with MS to achieve the required lipid separation. Lipids play a role in various biological processes, including signaling, trafficking, and even metabolite functions, in addition to their structural function. The characterization of the pathogenic microbe's cell wall, which reveals its regulation and role in pathogenesis, is an example of lipidomics application in infectious diseases. This has revealed essential enzymes involved in fatty acid synthesis, such as FabI, FabH, FabF, and acetyl-CoA carboxylase, which are conserved across many clinically relevant pathogens. The inhibitors of these enzymes promise future targets, particularly for mycobacterial infections that use fatty acids as a carbon source.

7.4.3.2 Metabolomics to Meta-Omics

Transcriptomics and proteomics data on gene expression face challenges. For example, due to conceptual and technological limitations associated with bacterial RNA instability, increases in RNA levels may not consistently result in changes in protein levels, and differences in protein levels are often poor metabolic activity estimators. As a result, there has been a surge in interest in small-molecule metabolites. Metabolomics uses complex analytical methods like NMR and chromatographic techniques associated with MS and advanced data analysis algorithms to provide a more in-depth view of the biological reality governing microbial metabolism. Because bacterial antibiotic responses are rapid and involve multiple pathways, metabolomics is well suited to elucidating the MOA. Additionally, metabolic networks can be built that combine catalytic activity (i.e., enzymes) with its coding and expression (i.e., genes and their transcriptional and translational control).

Natural product discovery, which has played a key role in antibiotic discovery and chemotherapy, ranging from oncological to immunologic treatments, has been bolstered by metagenomics and meta-omics in general. For example, approximately half of all FDA-approved therapeutics are natural products or their derivatives. However, according to metagenomic studies, only 10% of natural products have been identified, so the suggestion that only 1% of the total natural product repository has been investigated is not surprising. As a result, there is renewed optimism in the search for new drugs derived from natural sources. In this regard, sampling new natural product sources such as plants and marine organisms and endophytes and epiphytes is expected to reveal an even broader range of metabolic pathways with therapeutic potential. Furthermore, investigating microorganisms that are not culturable in traditional laboratory conditions or pathways that are not activated in typical laboratory conditions necessitates the development of appropriate protocols. Given the meta-omics discovery of nature's "untapped" repositories, these could very well be the next "gold mine" after the actinomycete-fueled Waksman platform, justifying such efforts.

The iChip (www.popsci.com/ichip-new-way-find-antibiotics-and-other-key-drugs/) is an interesting device that allows for high-throughput cultivation of microbial species in their natural habitat, with a growth recovery of 50% versus 1% for traditional recovery methods, allowing access to otherwise "uncultivable" microorganisms. Thousands of isolates can be extracted using the iChip. Teixobactin, a peptidoglycan synthesis inhibitor, was discovered in a new *Betaproteobacteria* species, which is thought to belong to a new genus related to *Aquabacterium*. Teixobactin is most effective against Gram-positive pathogens, including drug-resistant strains. Its bactericidal activity is even higher than vancomycin (a last-resort antibiotic), and it shows no signs of resistance. Metagenomics allows for a new approach. Rather than growing these "uncultivable" microbes, sequences of interest can be identified from metagenomes, which can then be cloned and expressed in laboratory-friendly microbes. This avoids in situ cultivations, as with the iChip, and the time-consuming task of deciphering the conditions required for growth or activation of previously unknown pathways, and could lead to the discovery of novel antibiotics.

Meta-omics has also enabled antibiotic interaction with the human microbiome, allowing for more antibiotic discovery opportunities. Gene clusters with antibiotic potential were discovered in human-associated metagenomic studies. These commensal bacteria, for example, inhibit the presence of *Staphylococcus aureus* strains in *Staphylococcus lugdunensis* nasal colonization, preventing opportunistic infections. This effect was linked to *S. lugdunensis*' production of lugdunin, a novel class antibiotic (macrocyclic thiazolidine peptides) with bactericidal activity against key pathogens and a low risk of resistance development. Lactocillin, a novel thiopeptide antibiotic, was also discovered in the vaginal microbiota and demonstrated significant antimicrobial activity against common pathogens. On a different note, complete microbiome transplantation has been used to treat recurrent *Clostridium difficile* infections, which is a brute-force approach compared to pinpointing the key molecular agent responsible for regulating commensal flora and pathogenic agents. These findings suggest that meta-omics technologies have enabled novel therapeutics such as introducing healthy microbiota, targeted manipulation of commensal microbial populations, and even purified molecular agents of commensal bacteria.

As can be seen, post-genomics technologies have aided in the development of new antibiotic research opportunities, though these have not been the focus of any ADP. The case of teixobactin, for example, was heavily reliant on meta-genomics revelations and the technologies required to build a device like the iChip. However, cell-based assays in a reverse genomics platform revealed which of the molecules recovered with the iChip has antimicrobial activity and insights into their MOA. Because phenotypic screening has a higher success rate in identifying first-in-class molecules, it's a good place to start for ADPs. The disadvantage is that the mechanistic information obtained is limited, whereas omics technologies provide faster insight into the MOA, including the molecular target and regulation. Target-based screening can optimize lead molecules into best-in-class medicines once the required mechanical information is obtained. Even though most new antibiotics in late clinical development belong to established classes, the paradigm of combining target- and cell-based screening offers renewed hope for the future. Returning to compounds that were abandoned in the early stages of development could provide new opportunities.

Infectious diseases, which were once thought to be a solved health problem, have resurfaced as a topic that requires immediate attention. Since the Waksman platform's success, semi-synthesis, and fully synthetic ADPs, antibiotic discovery has come a long way. As previously stated, the development of systematic procedures—platforms—was critical in discovering the major antibiotic classes currently in use. Cell-based ADPs were revived during the genomics era due to the limitations of target-based screening. While some may find the genomics era platforms unsatisfactory, the value of the lessons learned should not be overlooked. Due to significant technological advancements, researchers now have unprecedented access to biological events and have repositioned antibiotic research in a systems biology context. In the field of antibiotic discovery, paradoxically, the more we know, the less we can discover. Omics technologies have proven invaluable as auxiliary tools for antibiotic discovery, despite not being at the core of any ADPs.

Importantly, cell-based screening necessitates MOA characterization, which requires the use of omics technologies. Despite the fact that they provide additional information on biological events, their low throughput capacity and complementarity in terms of resourcing multiple omics at the same time limit their use in ADPs aiming to screen large libraries, such as the reservoir of untapped natural products, which is likely the next antibiotic "gold mine." Between phenotypic screening (high-throughput) and omics-centered assays, there is a gap (high-information). Antimicrobial activity can be supplemented with mechanistic and molecular information without the time-consuming and extensive use of various omics assays. We have yet to fully exploit the potential of various omics technologies due to their novelty, but it appears that these technologies will mature to fill this gap. Alternatively, novel high-throughput technologies could be developed, even if molecular sensitivity is sacrificed to some extent. In any case, the ever-increasing demand for antibiotics fuels the never-ending research at the forefront of antibiotic discovery. This is likely to increase our understanding of the biological events that underpin infectious diseases and, hopefully, lead to better therapeutics that can turn the tide in the war on infectious diseases.

7.5 Phage Therapy

Although not technically "phage therapy," the use of phages as delivery mechanisms for traditional antibiotics is another possible therapeutic application. In addition, in preliminary in vitro experiments for tissue culture cells, the use of phages to deliver antitumor agents has also been described.

The use of bacteriophages to treat bacterial infections is known as phage therapy. When bacteria develop resistance to antibiotics, this could be used instead. With the increased use of antibiotics, superbugs resistant to multiple types of drugs are becoming a concern. Because phages are so specific, they can target these dangerous microbes without harming human cells.

Bacteriophage treatment could be a viable alternative to antibiotics in the treatment of bacterial infections. Although bacteria can develop phage resistance, it is possible that phage resistance is more accessible to overcome than antibiotic resistance. This is because viruses, like bacteria, can evolve resistance and overcome it.

The therapeutic use of bacteriophages to treat pathogenic bacterial infections is known as phage therapy, viral phage therapy, or phagotherapy. Bacteriophages also referred to as phages, are a type of virus. Phages attach to bacterial cells and inject the cell's viral genome. The viral genome successfully replaces the bacterial genome, putting an end to the bacterial infection. Because the infecting bacterial cell is unable to reproduce, it instead produces more phages. The bacteria strains against which phages are effective are particular. Reduced side effects and the risk of the bacteria developing resistance are two advantages. The difficulty of finding an effective phage for a specific infection is one of the disadvantages. Because they can easily be separated from the environment, virulent phages can be isolated much faster than other compounds and natural products. Furthermore, standardized manufacturing processes would significantly speed up delivering phages from the lab to the clinic.

Antibiotics and phages are frequently compared; however, phages are more effective than antibiotics. Antibiotics typically cannot penetrate a biofilm that is covered by a polysaccharide layer. Antibiotics are not as specific as bacteriophages. They are usually safe for the host organism and other beneficial bacteria, such as the gut microbiota, which reduces opportunistic infections. Their therapeutic index is high. That is, even at higher-than-therapeutic doses, phage therapy is expected to have few side effects. Because phages replicate in vivo (in living cells), a lower effective dose can be used.

This uniqueness is also a drawback: a phage will only kill a bacterium if it matches the strain. As a result, phage mixtures (or "cocktails") are frequently used to improve success rates. Alternatively, recovering patients' samples may contain appropriate phages that can be grown to cure other patients infected with the same strain.

In Russia and Georgia, phages are currently being used therapeutically to treat bacterial infections that do not respond to conventional antibiotics. In addition, the FDA approved the first US clinical trial for intravenous phage therapy in 2019 to assess the safety, tolerability, and efficacy of AB-SA01, an experimental bacteriophage combination, in treating people with ventricular assist devices (VADs) infected with resistant *Staphylococcus aureus*.

Human medicine and dentistry, veterinary science, and agriculture could all benefit from phage therapy. If the phage therapy treatment's target host is not an animal, the term "biocontrol" (as in phage-mediated bacterial biocontrol) is usually used instead of "phage therapy."

In 1915, the Englishman Frederick Twort and the French-Canadian Felix d'Hérelle announced the discovery of bacteriophages. Many people immediately recognized phage therapy as a critical step forward in the fight against pathogenic bacterial infections. George Eliava, a Georgian, made similar discoveries. He visited the Pasteur Institute in Paris, where he met d'Hérelle, and in 1923 he established the Eliava Institute in Tbilisi, Georgia, dedicated to phage therapy research. In Russia, Georgia, and Poland, phage therapy is used.

While knowledge of phage biology and how to use phage cocktails properly grew, early phage therapy methods were frequently unreliable. Research into the development of viable therapeutic antibiotics has been ongoing since the early twentieth century. By 1942, the antibiotic penicillin G had been purified and was in use during WWII. The drug proved to be highly effective in treating infected wounds among injured Allied soldiers. Large-scale production of penicillin was possible by 1944, and it became widely available in pharmacies in 1945. Because of the drug's success, it was widely distributed in the United States and Europe, causing Western scientists to lose interest in further research and development of phage therapy for a time.

Despite being cut off from Western advances in antibiotic production in the 1940s, Russian scientists continued to develop phage therapy to treat soldiers' wounds in field hospitals. The Soviet Union used bacteriophages to treat many soldiers infected with various bacterial diseases such as dysentery and gangrene during World War II. Russian scientists continued to develop and improve their treatments, as well as publish their findings. However, due to scientific barriers erected during the Cold War, this knowledge was not translated and did not spread worldwide.

Since the 1950s, there has been renewed interest in phage therapy's ability to eradicate bacterial infections and chronic polymicrobial biofilms due to the development of antibiotic resistance and advances in scientific knowledge (including in industrial situations).

Phages have been studied as a possible way to eliminate pathogens like *Campylobacter* in raw food and *Listeria* in fresh food and bacteria that cause food spoilage. Phages have been used to combat pathogens such as *Campylobacter*, *Escherichia*, and *Salmonella* in farm animals, *Lactococcus* and *Vibrio* pathogens in aquaculture fish, and *Erwinia* and *Xanthomonas* in agricultural plants. Human medicine was, however, the first application. Phages have been used to treat *E. coli*, *Shigella*, and *Vibrio* diarrhea and wound infections caused by facultative pathogens of the skin, such as staphylococci and streptococci. Non-replicating phage and isolated phage enzymes like lysins have recently been added to the antimicrobial arsenal, as has the phage therapy approach to systemic and even intracellular infections. However, there is no actual proof of the efficacy of these phage approaches in the field or the hospital.

Bacteriophages are highly specific, attacking only one or a few bacteria strains. Traditional antibiotics have a broader effect, killing both harmful and beneficial bacteria, including those that aid digestion. However, because bacteriophages are species and strain-specific, they are unlikely to kill harmless or beneficial bacteria while fighting an infection.

Collecting local water samples likely to contain high quantities of bacteria and bacteriophages, such as effluent outlets, sewage, and other sources is the simplest method of phage treatment. First, the samples are taken and applied to bacteria that have been cultured on a growth medium and are to be destroyed. If the bacteria die, as is common, the mixture is centrifuged, and the phages collect on the top and can be drawn off. The phage solutions are then tested to see which ones inhibit the target bacteria's growth (lysogeny) or kill them (lysis). The phage that causes lysis is then amplified on the target bacteria's cultures, filtered to remove everything except the phages, and then distributed.

Because phages are "bacterium-specific," it is often necessary to take a swab from the patient and culture before starting treatment. Isolation of therapeutic phages can take several months in some cases, but clinics typically keep phage cocktails on hand for the most common bacterial strains in a given area.

In eastern countries, phage cocktails are sold in pharmacies. In addition, bacteriophagic cocktails have had their compositions changed regularly to include phages that are effective against emerging pathogenic strains.

In practice, phages are taken orally, applied topically to infected wounds or surfaces, or used during surgical procedures. Because the immune system naturally fights viruses introduced into the bloodstream or lymphatic system, the injection is rarely used, avoiding any risks of trace chemical contaminants present during the bacteria amplification stage.

Without significantly reducing efficiency, phages can usually be freeze-dried and turned into pills. Some types of phages in pill form have been shown to have temperature stability up to 55° C and shelf-lives of 14 months. It is possible to use the product in liquid form, which should be stored in refrigerated vials. When an antacid is added to oral administration, the number of phages that survive passage through the stomach increases. The application of topical medications to gauzes laid on the area to be treated is a common method of topical administration.

Because the bacterial components of such diseases can differ from region to region or even person to person, clinics may need to make different cocktails for treating the same infection or illness due to the high bacterial strain specificity of phage therapy.

7.6 Microbiome

The microbiome is a type of microbial community that lives in a well-defined environment and has distinct physio-chemical properties. The microbiome refers to the microorganisms involved and their activity stage, which results in the formation of ecological niches. The microbiome is integrated into the macro-ecosystems, including eukaryotic hosts, critical for their functioning and health.

The microbiome trend is gaining traction and has the potential to transform the biopharmaceutical industry. Microbiota is an ecosystem of over 100 trillion microorganisms that live inside our bodies or on our skin, coexisting naturally with humans and performing vital functions like vitamin synthesis, digestion, and immune system development. The versatility of microbiota-microbiome genes opens up incredible new possibilities for new drugs.

The microbiota is made up of a variety of microorganisms from different kingdoms (prokaryotes [bacteria, archaea], eukaryotes [e.g., protozoa, fungi, and algae]). Thus, microbial structures, metabolites, mobile genetic elements (such as transposons, phages, and viruses), and relic DNA embedded in the habitat's environmental conditions are all on their radar.

Microbiome research sometimes focuses on the behavior of a specific microbiota group, which is generally concerning or justified by a clear hypothesis. In recent years, terms like bacteriome, archaeome, mycobiome, and virome have begun to appear in scientific publications. These terms refer to biomes (a regional ecosystem with a distinct assemblage of [micro] organisms, and the physical environment often reflects a particular climate and soil), not the microbiome itself.

Bacteria, viruses, fungi, and eukaryotes all live in the human body, a microcosm of diverse microbial communities. Nobody is the same, and neither is their microbiota. The microbiome's role in cellular function and disease regulation has long been recognized and investigated. However, what has changed is the ability to use accurate, sensitive, and non-invasive technologies and assays to dissect the intricate structure, function, types, and location of microbial clusters in the human body. Microbiota can now be studied, characterized, and analyzed in their natural habitats to learn more about how they interact with human cells and clusters. The taxonomic and functional analyses that have resulted reveal a far more complex relationship between the human body and microbial communities than previously thought.

Metagenomics, metatranscriptomics, metaproteomics, and metabolomics have all been used in microbiome research to analyze microbial genes, RNA, proteins, and metabolites, referred to as metagenomics metatranscriptomics, metaproteomics, and metabolomics, respectively. The Human Microbiome Project, MetaHIT, and others have highlighted the diversity and abundance of microbial communities among people from all over the world and across different sites on the same person (skin, gut, and mouth). The microbial signature is affected by age, diet, metabolism, and various states of health.

7.6.1 Impact on Health

Understanding the relationship between human systemic physiology and bacterial symbiosis is being revolutionized by the Human Microbiome Project (www.nature.com/articles/nature06244). This consortium has genetically granularized the gene products that enhance each side of the symbiotic equation, in addition to outlining the number of microbial cells (100 trillion), microbial genes (eight million), and predominant colonization locations. Nutrition, neurobiology, cancer, immunology, cardiovascular disease, biliary function, irritable bowel disorders, and metabolic diseases like obesity and diabetes are all areas where the microbiota is becoming more widely recognized.

Bacterial symbiotes play an important role in carbohydrate metabolism on a chemical level, and glycosyl hydrolases and transferases are abundant in the microbiome. The microbiota is also necessary for the production of several essential vitamins, such as B3, B5, B6, B12, K, biotin, and tetrahydrofolate, and the absorption of iron from the intestinal lumen. Intestinal bacteria's processing of bile acids has been linked to cardiovascular disease. In addition, the gut microbiota produces short-chain fatty acids like acetate and butyrate, which are important for gut epithelial function and the systemic immune system. Surprisingly, it was recently discovered that intestinal bacteria's acetates bind directly to acetylated lysines in mammalian cells and that bacterial-produced butyrates aid this process by inhibiting mammalian lysine deacetylase enzymes. The microbiome appears to evolve quickly and easily as well. In 2010, researchers discovered that the enzyme porphyranase, encoded by marine microorganisms, was acquired by the microbiome of Japanese people who consume porphyrins from red algae in their diet.

7.6.2 Drug Metabolism

It is well known that different people metabolize drugs differently, and it is becoming clear that the microbiome may play a role in some of these differences. Bacteria are the most prevalent and metabolically active of all the microbes found in humans. As a result, the impact of the gut microbiome on drug metabolism is being studied closely, as the large intestine contains the majority of bacteria that metabolize drugs. Antibiotics aren't the only drugs that can affect the microbiome.

Microbiome analysis is being used in early-stage to late-stage clinical trials to improve patient outcomes and success rates. In addition, many marketed drugs are being studied, and their interactions with the human gut microbiota reveal that many of them have antibiotic effects. They are not, however, sold as such. Antipsychotics, anticancer, and antidiabetes drugs, for example, have different effects on the microbiome. In addition, some cholesterol-lowering statins have an impact on the gut microbiome, which changes cholesterol metabolism and causes some patients to receive less or no benefit from the drug.

Aside from sulfa drugs, catalytic functions encoded by mammalian symbiotic bacteria are used to process at least a half-dozen other therapeutic compounds. Because the GI contains the world's largest, most diverse, and variable collection of bacterial species, it has been the subject of previous and likely future studies on microbial drug metabolism. For example, intestinal bacteria have been observed reducing bonds in clinical drugs and other transformations such as hydrolysis, dehydroxylation, acetylation, deacetylation, and deconjugation of glucuronides and sulfates.

The microbiota's drug metabolism reactions can have a significant impact on human health. For example, the bacterial transformation of the antiviral drug sorivudine, which was approved in Japan in 1993, was discovered to be the cause of 18 deaths in 1998, prompting the drug's recall. Sorivudine's key metabolite €-5-(2-bromovinyl)uracil (BVU) is produced by intestinal bacteria, and BVU then travels to the liver, where it inactivates a key liver enzyme that causes a lethal build-up of 5-FU in cancer patients. It's also been recognized that their participation influences drugs' efficacy in enterohepatic recirculation, similar to what bilirubin undergoes. The nonsteroidal anti-inflammatory drug indomethacin, for example, is processed differently by intestinal enzymes in dogs and nonhuman primates than in humans. Thus, drug metabolism, activation, and reactivation are all influenced by the intestinal microbiome.

7.6.3 Drug Toxicity

While the microbiota plays a role in therapeutic mechanisms of action and metabolism, antibiotic overuse and the resulting increase in microbial multidrug resistance strongly support the goal of using chemical approaches that are neither bactericidal nor bacteriostatic.

It is becoming increasingly clear that the human microbiome is an important component of the human genome and that specific microbial enzyme targets can be modulated selectively for scientific and clinical purposes. As we learn more about the microbiota's role in various diseases such as neurobiology, immunology, heart disease, cancer, diabetes, and other metabolic disorders, several new and specific bacterial macromolecules will likely be identified as potential therapeutic targets. However, the ability to "drug" these microbiome members will necessitate the development of new capabilities. Drugs that preferentially remain in the intestinal lumen but can reach their molecular targets within microbial cells, for example, will be required to target bacterial gene products in the GI. These characteristics present drug development and delivery teams with both challenges and opportunities. In the future, the need to target gene products found only in certain GI microbial species and not others may arise, necessitating a better understanding of the species present and their detailed functional genomic and proteomic states.

7.6.4 Biomarkers

Antibiotics, microbial transplants, or dietary changes to eliminate the "bad" microbiota and replace it with "good" ones could all be used to change the microbiome to increase the effectiveness of a drug. Some of these interactions can be tracked by assembling a personalized microbiota collection from a person and analyzing gene, RNA, protein, and metabolite expression over time. In addition, variabilities in health, diet, drug response, and other factors could act as prognostic markers, allowing for prompt intervention and personalized medicine.

Shotgun metagenomics or targeted marker genes are both used in DNA-based microbiome studies. Targeted sequencing of specific genetic markers can quickly identify the types of microbial communities present in a given region or sample by comparing the results to existing reference databases.

7.7 Conclusion

The symbiotic relationship between humans and microbes is still being researched centuries after we first learned of their existence. Because of the inherent diversity of infecting organisms, infection prevention is one of the most diverse sciences. It is still one of the top ten causes of death worldwide, especially in developing countries. The field of genomics has revolutionized how new drugs, such as antibiotics are discovered and developed. We've also learned more about how the microbiome can be manipulated to aid healing. While the focus of new drug development has shifted to biological approaches, antimicrobial drugs will continue to be one of the top research priorities in the future due to the changing nature of infecting organisms. Millions of people's lives are at risk due to rising resistance to essential pathogens like *Mycobacterium tuberculosis*, *Shigella*, and *Streptococcus pneumonia*.

The following three factors require future consideration.

- First, the role of the conjugative DNA transfer of genes within the microbiota, particularly those encoding virulence and antibiotic resistance properties, must be better understood. These processes play critical roles concerning antibiotic resistance genes in the GI microbiome and clinical settings. Thus, mobile plasmids and genetic elements must be appreciated because they will lead to a continually changing field of play. Evidence continues to emerge that conjugative plasmids are, like viruses, regulated by bacterial CRISPR-Cas systems. GI bacterial gene shuffling occurs based on fundamental influences like a diet.
- Second, the role that viruses, fungi, and eukaryotic parasites play in humans—the microbial landscape—is underappreciated to date.
- Third, while our understanding of the microbiome evolves, so does our ability to engineer synthetic microbial cells to serve as therapeutics, as has been demonstrated. Thus, the future of modulating the human microbiome may include the use of designed bacterial cells that deliver the chemicals, genes, or gene.

ADDITIONAL READING

Abandeh FI, Drew ME, Sopirala MM. Carbapenem-hydrolyzing gram-negative bacteria: current options for treatment and review of drugs in development. *Recent Pat Antiinfect Drug Discov.* 2012;7(1):19–27.

Abdalla MA, McGaw LJ. Natural cyclic peptides as an attractive modality for therapeutics: a mini review. *Molecules.* 2018;20;23(8):2080.

Alves MJ, Ferreira IC, Dias J, Teixeira V, Martins A, Pintado M. A review on antimicrobial activity of mushroom (Basidiomycetes) extracts and isolated compounds. *Planta Med.* 2012;78(16):1707–1718.

Anand U, Jacobo-Herrera N, Altemimi A, Lakhssassi N. A comprehensive review on medicinal plants as antimicrobial therapeutics: potential avenues of biocompatible drug discovery. *Metabolites*. 2019;9(11):258.

Annunziato G. Strategies to overcome antimicrobial resistance (AMR) making use of non-essential target inhibitors: a review. *Int J Mol Sci*. 2019 Nov 21;20(23):5844.

Annunziato G, Costantino G. Antimicrobial peptides (AMPs): a patent review (2015–2020). *Expert Opin Ther Pat*. 2020;30(12):931–947.

Augie BM, McInerney PA, van Zyl RL, Miot J. Educational antimicrobial stewardship programs in medical schools: a scoping review protocol. *JBI Evid Synth*. 2020;18(5):1028–1035.

Ayoub Moubareck C. Polymyxins and bacterial membranes: a review of antibacterial activity and mechanisms of resistance. *Membranes (Basel)*. 2020 Aug;10(8):181.

Bai H, Xue X, Hou Z, Zhou Y, Meng J, Luo X. Antisense antibiotics: a brief review of novel target discovery and delivery. *Curr Drug Discov Technol*. 2010;7(2):76–85.

Bansal M, Rastogi S, Vineeth NS. Influence of periodontal disease on systemic disease: inversion of a paradigm: a review. *J Med Life*. 2013;6(2):126–130.

Barker RH, Dagher R, Davidson DM, Marquis JK. Review article: tolevamer, a novel toxin-binding polymer: overview of preclinical pharmacology and physicochemical properties. *Aliment Pharmacol Ther*. 2006;24(11–12):1525–1534.

Bartoszko JJ, Mertz D, Thabane L, Loeb M. Antibiotic therapy for skin and soft tissue infections: a protocol for a systematic review and network meta-analysis. *Syst Rev*. 2018;7(1):138.

Bershad SV. The modern age of acne therapy: a review of current treatment options. Mt Sinai *J Med*. 2001;68(4–5):279–286.

Boisset S, Caspar Y, Sutera V, Maurin M. New therapeutic approaches for treatment of tularaemia: a review. *Front Cell Infect Microbiol*. 2014;4:40.

Carvalho IT, Santos L. Antibiotics in the aquatic environments: a review of the European scenario. *Environ Int*. 2016;94:736–757.

Chandrika NT, Garneau-Tsodikova S. A review of patents (2011–2015) towards combating resistance to and toxicity of aminoglycosides. *Medchemcomm*. 2016;7(1):50–68.

Chaudhary AS. A review of global initiatives to fight antibiotic resistance and recent antibiotics' discovery. *Acta Pharm Sin B*. 2016;6(6):552–556.

Chen M, Wang G, Dai S, Xie L, Li X. [Polyketide antibiotics produced by polyketide synthase in streptomyces – a review]. *Wei Sheng Wu Xue Bao*. 2009;49(12):1555–1563.

Dąbrowska M, Starek M, Skuciński J. Lipophilicity study of some non-steroidal anti-inflammatory agents and cephalosporin antibiotics: a review. *Talanta*. 2011;86:35–51.

de la Morena MT, Nelson RP. Recent advances in transplantation for primary immune deficiency diseases: a comprehensive review. *Clin Rev Allergy Immunol*. 2014;46(2):131–144.

Ducati RG, Ruffino-Netto A, Basso LA, Santos DS. The resumption of consumption – a review on tuberculosis. *Mem Inst Oswaldo Cruz*. 2006;101(7):697–714.

Dudhatra GB, Mody SK, Awale MM, et al. A comprehensive review on pharmacotherapeutics of herbal bioenhancers. *Scientific World Journal*. 2012;2012:637953.

Farzaneh M. Concise review; effects of antibiotics and antimycotics on the biological properties of human pluripotent and multipotent stem cells. *Curr Stem Cell Res Ther*. 2021;16(4):400–405.

Gadakh B, Van Aerschot A. Aminoacyl-tRNA synthetase inhibitors as antimicrobial agents: a patent review from 2006 till present. *Expert Opin Ther Pat*. 2012;22(12):1453–1465.

Heffernan AJ, Sime FB, Lipman J, et al. Intrapulmonary pharmacokinetics of antibiotics used to treat nosocomial pneumonia caused by Gram-negative bacilli: a systematic review. *Int J Antimicrob Agents*. 2019;53(3):234–245.

Kang SJ, Kim DH, Lee BJ. NMR study on small proteins from *Helicobacter pylori* for antibiotic target discovery: a review. *Molecules*. Oct 2013;18(11):13410–13424.

Knoblauch R, Geddes CD. Carbon nanodots in photodynamic antimicrobial therapy: a review. *Materials (Basel)*. 2020;10;13(18):4004.

Koehnke A, Friedrich RE. Review: antibiotic discovery in the age of structural biology – a comprehensive overview with special reference to development of drugs for the treatment of *Pseudomonas aeruginosa* infection. *In Vivo*. 2015;29(2):161–167.

Kosikowska P, Lesner A. Antimicrobial peptides (AMPs) as drug candidates: a patent review (2003–2015). *Expert Opin Ther Pat*. 2016;26(6):689–702.

Kumar R, Ali SA, Singh SK, et al. Antimicrobial peptides in farm animals: an updated review on its diversity, function, modes of action and therapeutic prospects. *Vet Sci.* 2020;18;7(4):20.

Leva-Bueno J, Peyman SA, Millner PA. A review on impedimetric immunosensors for pathogen and biomarker detection. *Med Microbiol Immunol.* 2020;209(3):343–362.

Long DD, Marquess DG. Novel heterodimer antibiotics: a review of recent patent literature. *Future Med Chem.* 2009;1(6):1037–1050.

Lorke DE, Stegmeier-Petroianu A, Petroianu GA. Biologic activity of cyclic and caged phosphates: a review. *J Appl Toxicol.* 2017;37(1):13–22.

Mahajan GB, Balachandran L. Antibacterial agents from actinomycetes – a review. *Front Biosci (Elite Ed).* 2012;4:240–253.

Malathi K, Ramaiah S. Bioinformatics approaches for new drug discovery: a review. *Biotechnol Genet Eng Rev.* 2018;34(2):243–260.

McCaughan JS. Photodynamic therapy: a review. *Drugs Aging.* 1999;15(1):49–68.

Medical College Directory. Yaws. 2021. Retrieved from: https://medicalcollege.directory/yaws

Moore SG, Hasler JF. A 100-Year Review: reproductive technologies in dairy science. *J Dairy Sci.* 2017;100(12):10314–10331.

Office of Infectious Disease and HIV/AIDS Policy. Vaccine types. 2021. Retrieved from: https://www.hhs.gov/immunization/basics/types/index.html

Parenti F, Ciabatti R, Cavalleri B, Kettenring J. Ramoplanin: a review of its discovery and its chemistry. *Drugs Exp Clin Res.* 1990;16(9):451–455.

Petty LA, Gallan AJ, Detrick JA, Ridgway JP, Mueller J, Pisano J. *Candida dubliniensis* pneumonia: a case report and review of literature. *Mycopathologia.* 2016;181(9–10):765–768.

Pires DP, Cleto S, Sillankorva S, Azeredo J, Lu TK. Genetically engineered phages: a review of advances over the last decade. *Microbiol Mol Biol Rev.* 2016;80(3):523–543.

Prideaux L, Kamm MA, De Cruz PP, Chan FK, Ng SC. Inflammatory bowel disease in Asia: a systematic review. *J Gastroenterol Hepatol.* 2012;27(8):1266–1280.

Provenzani A, Hospodar AR, Meyer AL, et al. Multidrug-resistant gram-negative organisms: a review of recently approved antibiotics and novel pipeline agents. *Int J Clin Pharm.* 2020;42(4):1016–1025.

Renwick MJ, Brogan DM, Mossialos E. A systematic review and critical assessment of incentive strategies for discovery and development of novel antibiotics. *J Antibiot (Tokyo).* 2016;69(2):73–88.

Roser M, Ochmann S, Behrens H, Ritchie H, Dadonaite B. Eradication of diseases. 2014. Published online at OurWorldInData.org. Retrieved from: https://ourworldindata.org/eradication-of-diseases [Online Resource].

Salvador-Culla B, Kolovou PE. Keratoprosthesis: a review of recent advances in the field. *J Funct Biomater.* 2016;7(2):13. doi:10.3390/jfb7020013

Scribano M, Prantera C. Review article: medical treatment of moderate to severe Crohn's disease. *Aliment Pharmacol Ther.* 2003;17(Suppl 2):23–30.

Shabir U, Ali S, Magray AR, et al. Fish antimicrobial peptides (AMP's) as essential and promising molecular therapeutic agents: a review. *Microb Pathog.* 2018;114:50–56.

Shi C, Chen J, Kang X, Shen X, Lao X, Zheng H. Approaches for the discovery of metallo-β-lactamase inhibitors: a review. *Chem Biol Drug Des.* 08 2019;94(2):1427–1440.

Sinha MS, Kesselheim AS. Regulatory incentives for antibiotic drug development: a review of recent proposals. *Bioorg Med Chem.* 2016;24(24):6446–6451.

Sun J, Lv PC, Zhu HL. Tyrosyl-tRNA synthetase inhibitors: a patent review. *Expert Opin Ther Pat.* 2017;27(5):557–564.

Tamburrano A, Barbara A, Gentili A, Laurenti P. [Control of antimicrobial resistance in the food chain: a narrative review]. *Ig Sanita Pubbl.* 2018;74(6):565–587.

Tiwari R, Dhama K, Kumar A, Rahal A, Kapoor S. Bacteriophage therapy for safeguarding animal and human health: a review. *Pak J Biol Sci.* 2014;17(3):301–315.

Verderosa AD, Totsika M, Fairfull-Smith KE. Bacterial biofilm eradication agents: a current review. *Front Chem.* 2019;7:824.

Wang W, Wang H, Li A. [Biosynthesis of benzoisochromanequinones antibiotics from streptomycetes – a review]. *Wei Sheng Wu Xue Bao.* 2012;52(5):541–549.

Zhao Y, Li H, Wei S, Zhou X, Xiao X. Antimicrobial effects of chemical compounds isolated from traditional chinese herbal medicine (TCHM) against drug-resistant bacteria: a review paper. *Mini Rev Med Chem.* 2019;19(2):125–137.

8

Therapeutic Proteins

8.1 Background

Biologics are relatively large and complex molecules when compared to conventional chemical drugs. Proteins (and their constituent amino acids), carbohydrates (such as sugars), nucleic acids (such as DNA), and combinations of these substances can all be found in them. Cells or tissues used in transplantation can also be biologics.

A generic drug is chemically identical to the brand-name drug it replaces. A commonly used chemical drug's molecular structure is much smaller than a biologic and, therefore, less complicated and more easily defined. For example, Table 8.1 shows that the chemical drug aspirin contains nine carbon atoms, eight hydrogen atoms, and four oxygen atoms. Remicade, a large biologic drug, has over 6,000 carbon atoms, nearly 10,000 hydrogen atoms, and about 2,000 oxygen atoms in comparison.

Specialty drugs, such as biologics, are expensive. Some biologic medications, such as Soliris (eculizumab) and Vimizim (elosulfase alfa), cost more than $250,000 per patient per year in the United States. In addition, Zolgensma, a new drug approved by the FDA, costs more than $2.1 million per dose. The global spending on biologics exceeded $250 billion in 2019, almost 50% from the United States. By 2026, the biologics market will exceed $700 billion.

8.2 Protein Structure and Properties

Understanding therapeutic proteins begin with understanding proteins, their three-dimensional and fourth-dimensional structures capable of complex interactions with thousands of atoms in the receptor sites, and immune system triggers. The multidimensional character of these molecules differentiates them from small molecule chemical structures that are invariably fixed in their spatial arrangement because of the fixed covalent bonds; in the case of proteins, there is an abundance of hydrogen bonds that form the higher order of structure and the protein activity is determined not just by which functional group is available to react but how it is juxtaposed to other functional groups.

Protein synthesis involves a complex array of cellular machinery, primarily ribosomes. Proteins are synthesized from N-terminus to the C-terminus in a sequential manner at a rate of 50–300 amino acids per minute; the folding begins once the chain has acquired 50–60 amino acids—co-translational protein folding that constraints and limits the pathways a protein can take into HOS, and this may explain why Levinthal calculations come short. Theoretically, the protein folding process into the lowest activation energy status is paradoxical wherein from 0.1 to 1,000 seconds. The protein folds to correct form given the millions of folding possibilities—it is called the Levinthal paradox, for it would otherwise take thousands of years of hit and miss to reach that state of lowest energy. It appears as if there is almost a brain and a central control mechanism—something we do not understand today, but in the future, we might.

Some proteins have no well-defined higher-order structure and stay disordered or unstructured as random coils, like the synthetic polymer chains or denatured proteins. This state may be a transitory state during the binding process and may be responsible for many protein actions in the cell.

It is essential to understand the difference between a dimension and the order of structure. For example, a fixed chemical molecule can have a multidimensional structure. Still, it is fixed, while a protein will have a primary, secondary, tertiary, and quaternary structure that can be further affected by a fourth-dimensional interaction with the milieu in which it is placed.

DOI: 10.1201/9781003146933-8

TABLE 8.1
Relative Size of Chemical and Biologic Drugs

Drug (Nonproprietary Name)	Molecular Formula
Chemical drugs	
Aspirin	$C_9H_8O_4$
Tylenol (acetaminophen)	$C_8H_9NO_2$
Sovaldi (sofosbuvir)	$C_{22}H_{29}FN_3O_9P$
Small biologic drugs	
Lantus (insulin glargine)	$C_{267}H_{404}N_{72}O_{78}S_6$
Epogen (epoetin alfa)	$C_{809}H_{1301}N_{229}O_{240}S_5$
Neupogen, Zarxio (filgrastim)	$C_{845}H_{1339}N_{223}O_{243}S_9$
Growth hormone (somatropin)	$C_{990}H_{1528}N_{262}O_{300}S_7$
Large biologic drugs	
Enbrel, Erelzi (etanercept)	$C_{2224}H_{3472}N_{618}O_{701}S_{36}$
Remicade, Inflectra (infliximab)	$C_{6428}H_{9912}N_{1694}O_{1987}S_{46}$

Source: Drugs@FDA, www.accessdata.fda.gov/scripts/cder/daf/, and Drugs.com.

Notes: The nonproprietary name of a drug product is used in drug labeling, drug regulation, and scientific literature to identify a pharmaceutical substance or active pharmaceutical ingredient. C = carbon; H = hydrogen; O = oxygen; N = nitrogen; F = fluorine; P = phosphorus; S = sulfur.

Proteins and antibodies have a primary structure; the primary structure consists of a specific amino acid sequence. Its resulting peptide chain twists into an α-helix, which is one type of secondary structure. This helical segment is then incorporated into a tertiary structure resulting from the folding of the polypeptide chain. Thus, the quaternary structure is formed of multiple polypeptide chains. Another aspect of this structure is the fourth-dimensional structure that involves protein groups' interaction with the formulation components that can alter the protein structure.

Figure 8.1 shows the four types of possible protein structures.

8.2.1 Primary Structure

During protein synthesis, polypeptide chains are formed on the ribosome during protein synthesis (called the translational phase). The chemical bond formed between the amino acid groups is a covalent bond called a peptide (or amide) bond. Each amino acid's specific characteristics are derived from its side chain that directs how it is placed within the protein structure. This structuring is determined by how the functional groups on amino acid components interact with water around the protein molecule; water is bipolar molecules, and the amino acids are classified as hydrophilic or hydrophobic and the unique classification when there is no side chain such as glycine, which is found at the surface of proteins, often within loops, where it provides high flexibility to the structure. On the other hand, proline provides rigidity to the protein structure by imposing certain torsion angles on the polypeptide chain segment. As a result, these two residues are highly abundant since they are essential for establishing the three-dimensional structure.

The first protein level is the amino acid sequence, comprising only naturally occurring 20 essential amino acids (Figure 8.2).

The chemical link between amino acids is called a peptide bond. It is formed between the carbonyl oxygen and carbon, α-carbons on each side of the peptide bond, and the amide nitrogen and hydrogen due to the partial double bond character between the amide nitrogen and the carbonyl (Figure 8.3). The peptide bond has a planar structure that produces restrictions in the angular range of bond rotation around the Cα-N expressed by ϕ (phi), and C-Cα expressed as Ψ (psi) bonds. These restrictions are

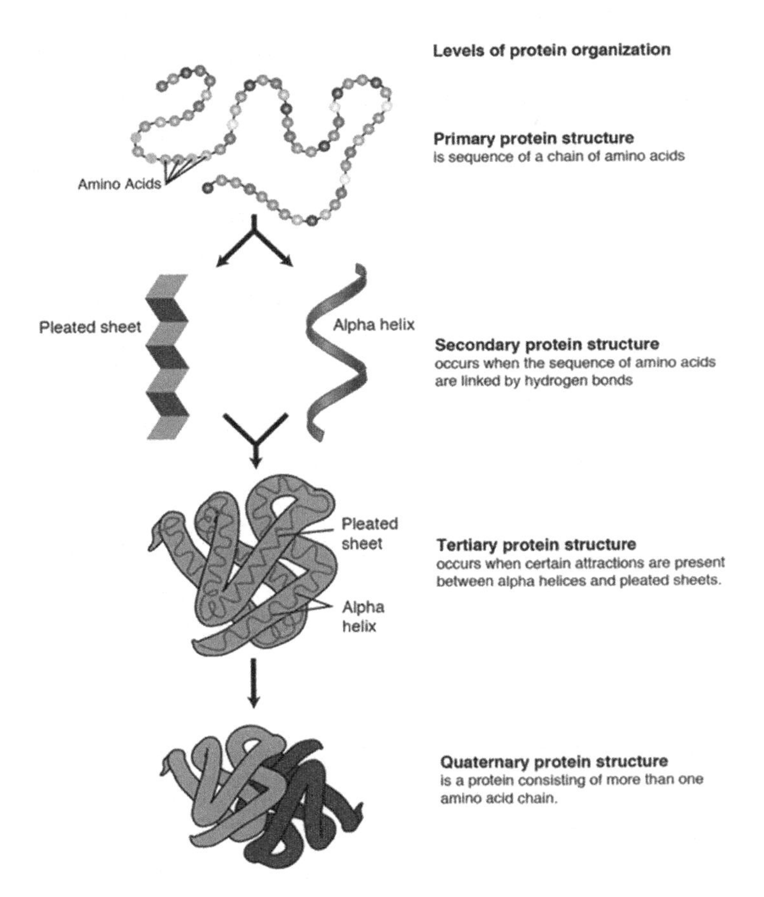
Levels of protein organization
Amino Acids
Primary protein structure
is sequence of a chain of amino acids
Pleated sheet
Alpha helix
Secondary protein structure
occurs when the sequence of amino acids
are linked by hydrogen bonds
Pleated
sheet
Alpha
helix
Tertiary protein structure
occurs when certain attractions are present
between alpha helices and pleated sheets.
Quaternary protein structure
is a protein consisting of more than one
amino acid chain.

FIGURE 8.1 Four elements of possible protein structures. Source: www.genome.gov/genetics-glossary/Protein.

summarized in a two-dimensional graphical plot called the Ramachandran plot that shows how certain structural features of proteins can only exist within limited ranges of angles, e.g., α-helix.

The repeating structural pattern in helices results from repeating phi and psi values, observed as clustering of the torsion angles within a specific Ramachandran plot region. A Ramachandran plot (also known as a Ramachandran diagram or a [φ, ψ] plot), is a way to visualize backbone dihedral angles ψ against φ of amino acid residues in protein structure. The ω angle at the peptide bond usually is 180° since the partial-double-bond character keeps the peptide planar. Because dihedral angle values are circular and 0° is the same as 360°, the Ramachandran plot edges "wrap" right to left and bottom to top (Figures 8.4).

Two electronegative atoms (in the case of α-helix, the amide N and the carbonyl O) must interact with the same hydrogen to form a hydrogen bond. The hydrogen is covalently attached to one atom (the hydrogen-bond donor), but it interacts with the other atoms electrostatically (the hydrogen bond acceptor, O). The ω angle at the peptide bond usually is 180° since the partial-double-bond character keeps the peptide planar.

Most amino acids are found in polar or hydrophobic states (Table 8.2).

The primary structure, a string of amino acids, forms the three-dimensional structure wherein the folding results from the distribution of polar and non-polar side chains. The folding is driven by hydrophobic side chains' burial into the molecule's interior to reduce contact with the aqueous environment and reduce the carbon molecule's free energy. This results in proteins having a hydrophobic core that is surrounded by hydrophilic residues. Peptide bonds are polarized in a hydrophobic environment by hydrogen bonds, giving rise to polypeptide regions to form standard 3D patterns called secondary structures; there are two types of these structures: α-helices and β-sheets.

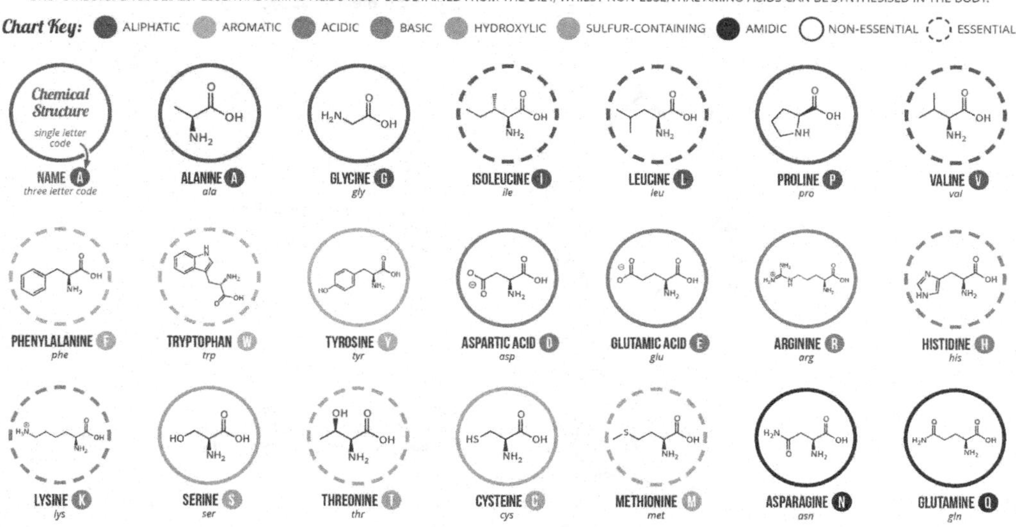

FIGURE 8.2 Essential amino acids. Source: https://fitnesswithana.com/what-are-essential-and-non-essential-amino-acids/.

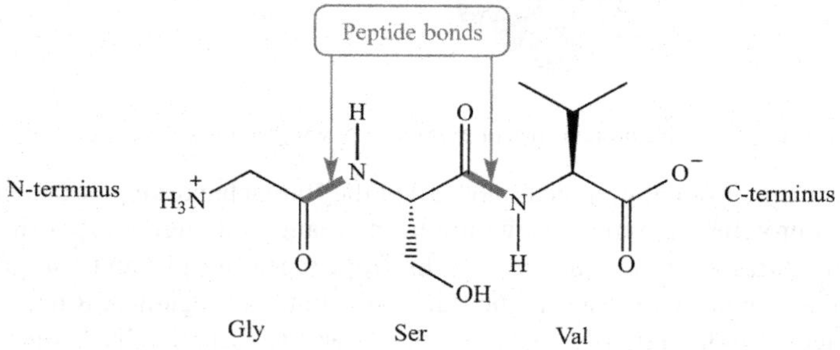

Peptide bonds

N-terminus $H_3\overset{+}{N}$ … O^- C-terminus

Gly Ser Val

FIGURE 8.3 Peptide-bond; the double bond character is about 40% due to resonance. Source: www.chem.ucla.edu/~harding/IGOC/P/peptide_bond.html.

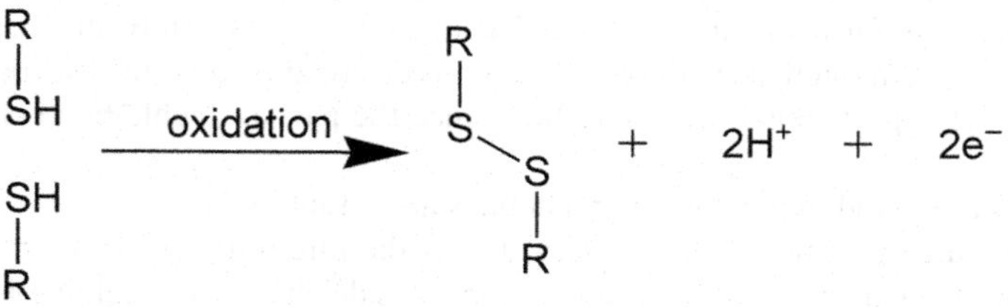

R–SH + HS–R —oxidation→ R–S–S–R + $2H^+$ + $2e^-$

FIGURE 8.4 Formal depiction of disulfide bond formation as oxidation. Source: www.wikidoc.org/index.php/Disulfide_bond.

TABLE 8.2
Physical Properties of Essential Amino Acids

Property	Amino Acids
Charged amino acids	Arginine, lysine, aspartic acid, glutamic acid
Polar (that may participate in hydrogen bonds)	Glutamine, asparagine, histidine, serine, threonine, tyrosine, cysteine, methionine, tryptophan
Hydrophobic (normally buried inside the protein core)	Alanine, isoleucine, leucine, phenylalanine, valine, proline, glycine

8.2.2 Secondary Structure

The secondary structure of proteins is based on the specific sequence of these amino acids in a polypeptide chain; this is the second level of organization that creates structural motifs and folds, creating the third level of organization.

In a three-dimensional structure along with alpha-helix, beta-sheet, beta turns, and other non-covalent interactions, the protein folds to form a motif (a recurring element) that determines the final structure.

A carboxylic group and an amine group are part of every amino acid that is linked to another amino acid to form a chain by a dehydration reaction by joining one amino acid through its carboxyl group to another amino acid, forming a polypeptide chain that has an end with an unbound carboxyl group, the C-terminus, and beginning with an amine group, the N-terminus.

A structural motif is a super-secondary structure, and several motifs pack together to form compact, local, semi-independent units called domains. Prediction of biological functions is not possible from motifs in proteins and enzymes with different functions. An independent folding unit of the three-dimensional protein structure is called a domain, a conserved part of a specific protein sequence and (tertiary) structure that could evolve, operate, and exist independently of the protein string's remainder. Each domain forms a streamlined structure that is three-dimensional and can be folded and stable. Proteins are composed of domains. One domain may look at many different proteins that are distinct. Domains are used by molecular development, and these might be recombined to make proteins. Domains change in duration from between approximately 25 amino acids up to 500 amino acids in length. Metal beams or disulfide bridges stabilize the domain names like zinc fingers. Domains form operational units, like calmodulin's EF-hand domain.

The domain can be "swapped" by genetic engineering between one protein and another to make chimeric proteins independent. Since domains can be cloned, expressed, and purified independently of the rest of the protein, they may even show activity if any known activity is associated with them. Some proteins contain only one domain, a type of fold, but the same folds do not relate (PDB; www.wwpdb.org/index).

The polypeptide chain's tertiary structure forms an individual hydrophobic core built from the secondary structure connected to loop regions.

Core residues are more conserved than residues in the loops. Therefore, the tertiary structure is described in secondary structure as:

- The α domains are built exclusively from α-helices with small folds, often simple bundles with helices running up and down.
- The β domains with antiparallel β-sheets core commonly comprise two sheets that are packed against each other, resulting in patterns that appear as an arrangement of strands.
- The α + β comprise a combination of α and β motifs. Since it is difficult to classify proteins into this class due to the other three classes' overlaps, they are not used in the CATH domain database (www.cathdb.info).
- The α/β domains are made from a combination of β-α-β motifs that predominantly form a parallel β-sheet surrounded by amphipathic α-helices.

Domains have limitations on dimensions and changes by 36 residues in E-selectin into 692 residues in lipoxygenase-1; however, 90% have less than 200 residues with a mean of about 100 residues. Disulfide bonds usually stabilize short domain names, significantly less than 40 residues. More prominent domain names, more extensive than 300 residues, are likely to include multiple hydrophobic cores. Figure 8.4 shows the average disulfide bonds at the creation of domain names.

When two domains are covalently bonded, they represent a functional and structural advantage since there is an increase in stability compared with the same non-covalently associated structures.

8.2.2.1 Alpha Helix

The most common type of secondary structure in proteins is the α-helix (Figure 8.5).

All functional groups in proteins can form H-bonds no matter if the residues are inside a secondary arrangement or not; those are H-bonded with each other or with water molecules. The bipolarity of water enables it to take two hydrogen bonds and stabilize protein structure by creating hydrogen bonds between the side chain and the main chain and side chain groups linking distinct protein groups collectively. Additionally, water is shown to be involved in ligand binding to proteins, mediating charged groups' interactions. The power of a hydrogen bond, based on the angle between the two and the space between the donor and the acceptor, is in the order of 2–10 kcal/mol.

8.2.2.2 Beta-Sheet

Hydrogen bonds also stabilize the secondary structure in proteins, namely beta-sheets. An example of a beta-sheet with the stabilizing hydrogen bonds is shown as dashed lines in Figure 8.9. These hydrogen bonds are not necessarily formed between adjacent residues, as in α-helices. Instead, different amino acid sequence segments, called beta-strands, come together to form a beta-sheet. Thus, the beta-sheet consists of several beta-strands kept together by a network of hydrogen bonds. The organization is described in beta-sheets and α helices that can be repeated and alternate along the amino acid sequence.

8.2.3 Tertiary Structure

Polypeptide chains often fold naturally into tertiary protein structures giving stable structure. However, the forces driving the folding are not fully understood; chaperones are proteins that help other proteins fold correctly using the proteolytic apparatus available in the cells.

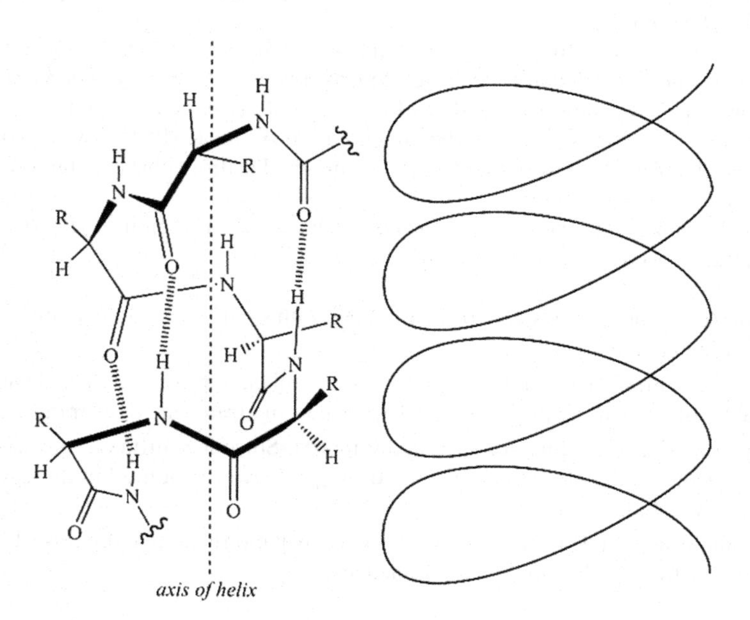

FIGURE 8.5 Two representations of α-helix.

The arrangement of large proteins from structural domains signifies an edge for protein fold. Every domain can independently fold, hastening the folding procedure, and reduce a possibly big blend of residue connections. Additionally, given that the observed arbitrary distribution of hydrophobic residues in proteins, domain creation seems to be the best solution for a vast protein to bury its hydrophobic residues while still retaining the hydrophilic residues on the surface.

Figure 8.4 shows the 3D structure of proteins.

8.2.4 Quaternary Structure

The fourth degree is quaternary construction. The quaternary arrangement consists of many polypeptide chains (subunits), similar (homo-oligomer), or alternative (hetero-oligomer). The subunits interact with each other, interact with the same complex target protein, contribute to an active site, and target proteins.

8.2.5 Post-Translational Modification (PTM)

A protein is characterized by its primary quaternary structure and by its additional characteristics acquired during the cellular process of protein synthesis. These are called "post-translational modifications" because they occur once the gene (nucleic acid sequence) has been translated into the corresponding protein sequence (the amino acid chain). These modifications are also designated as the "maturation phase" essential before the secretion of cell proteins. These modifications consist of the grafting of defined amino acids of one or several chemical groups such as phosphate or sulfate groups or sugars (when it will be termed glycosylation) that modify the global charge and physicochemical or biological characteristics of "mature" proteins as the final active forms (Figure 8.6).

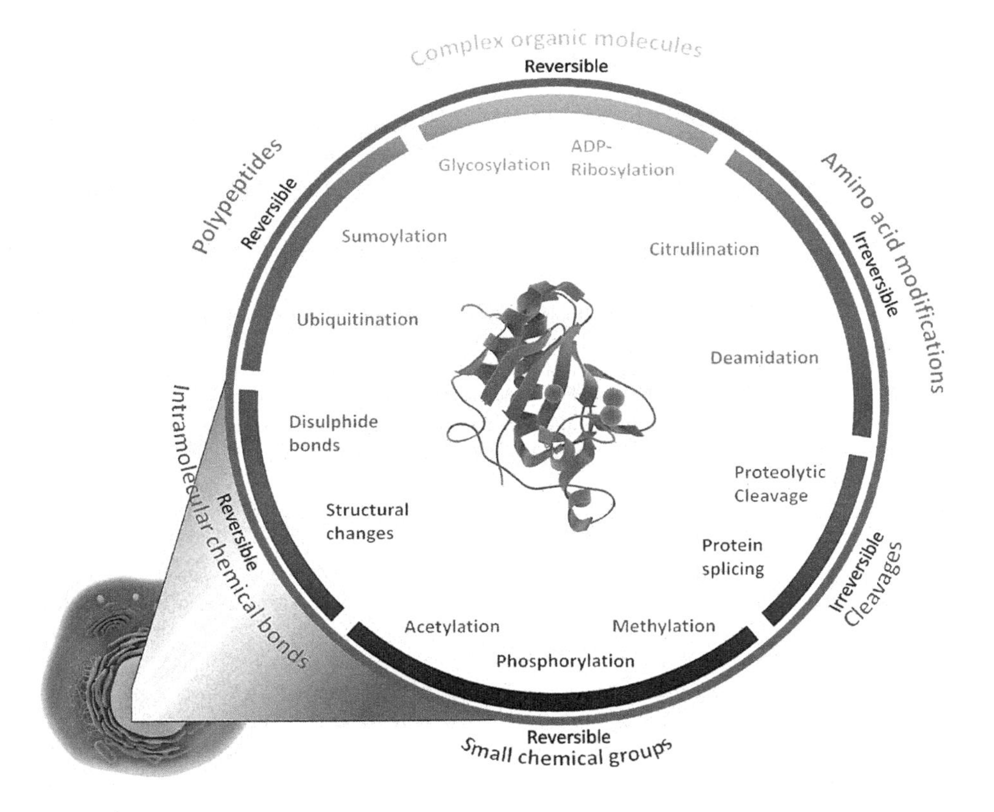

FIGURE 8.6 Post-translation types. Source: www.degruyter.com/view/s/bchm/400/7/article-p895.xml?language=en.

These post-translational modifications take place on specific sites of the protein that are not controlled by the gene that expresses the protein sequence; instead, it is specific to each cellular kind that presents a unique combination of milieu interior such as the presence of enzymes and the thermodynamic conditions during the reaction; it is, for this reason, that often these complex chemical reactions are not controllable by any alteration of the gene sequence, but only by optimizing the production conditions during expression. However, this is not relevant to expression inside prokaryotic organisms (bacteria) or very simple inside inferior eukaryotes such as yeasts. Still, these are indigenous to "mammalian" cells like CHO cells, making upstream processes for these cells complex, requiring significant development effort, especially if the goal is to match the post-translation modification profile, such as in the case of biosimilars.

Table 8.3 lists common PTMs by specific amino acids. Modifications occur on the sidechain unless indicated otherwise.

The ten most common modifications are listed in Table 8.4.

The effect of PTMs on protein activity are well documented, as shown in Table 8.5.

One of the more important post-translation modifications is glycosylation that is a cotranslational and post-translational modification. Glycans serve a variety of structural and functional roles in the membrane and secreted proteins. Most proteins synthesized in the rough endoplasmic reticulum undergo glycosylation.

Glycosylation is the most frequent post-translational modification. IUPAC terms glycan and polysaccharide as synonyms meaning "compounds consisting of a large number of monosaccharides linked glycosidically." However, in practice, the term glycan may also refer to the carbohydrate portion of a glycol-conjugate, such as a glycoprotein, glycolipid, or a proteoglycan, even if the carbohydrate is only an oligosaccharide. Glycans usually consist solely of O-glycosidic linkages of monosaccharides. For example, cellulose is a glycan (or, to be more precise, a glucan) composed of β-1,4-linked D-glucose, and chitin is a glycan composed of β-1,4-linked N-acetyl-D-glucosamine.

TABLE 8.3
Common PTMS by Specific Amino Acid Residues

Amino Acid	Abbrev.	Modification
Alanine	Ala	N-acetylation (N-terminus)
Arginine	Arg	Deimination to citrulline, methylation
Asparagine	Asn	Deamidation to Asp or iso(Asp), N-linked glycosylation
Aspartic acid	Asp	Isomerization to isoaspartic acid
Cysteine	Cys	The disulfide-bond formation, oxidation to sulfenic, sulfinic, or sulfonic acid, palmitoylation, N-acetylation (N-terminus), S-nitrosylation
Glutamine	Gln	Cyclization to pyroglutamic acid (N-terminus), deamidation to glutamic acid, or isopeptide bond formation to a lysine by a transglutaminase
Glutamic acid	Glu	Cyclization to pyroglutamic acid (N-terminus), gamma-carboxylation
Glycine	Gly	N-myristoylation (N-terminus), N-acetylation (N-terminus)
Histidine	His	Phosphorylation
Isoleucine	Ile	
Leucine	Leu	
Lysine	Lys	Acetylation, ubiquitination, SUMOylation, methylation, hydroxylation
Methionine	Met	N-acetylation (N-terminus), N-linked ubiquitination, oxidation to sulfoxide or sulfone
Phenylalanine	Phe	
Proline	Pro	Hydroxylation
Serine	Ser	Phosphorylation, O-linked glycosylation, N-acetylation (N-terminus)
Threonine	The	Phosphorylation, O-linked glycosylation, N-acetylation (N-terminus)
Tryptophan	Trp	Mono- or di-oxidation, the formation of kynurenine
Tyrosine	Tyr	Sulfation, phosphorylation
Valine	Val	N-acetylation (N-terminus)

TABLE 8.4

Frequency of Most Common Modifications in Protein Structure Derived from Reported Protein Structures

Frequency	Modification
58,383	Phosphorylation
6,751	Acetylation
5,526	N-linked glycosylation
2,844	Amidation
1,619	Hydroxylation
1,523	Methylation
1,133	O-linked glycosylation
878	Ubiquitylation
826	Pyrrolidone carboxylic acid
504	Sulfation

Glycans can be homo- or heteropolymers of monosaccharide residues and can be linear or branched. The chemical modifications introduced are very complex due to the glycan structures added to the protein skeleton. The protein glycosylation step consists of the endoplasmic reticulum and Golgi apparatuses. Glycosylation consists of branching on the protein, on determined amino acids (for instance, for N-glycosylation, Asn, which is in the Asn-X-Thr sequence), and sugar groups mannose, fructose, or galactose following a well-determined order. These glycosylation chemical reactions lead to the making of "sugar chains," complex and diversified, considering all the possible attaching combinations (number of an antenna[e] on a glycosylation site, and the nature of sugars making up this antenna), even if some mandatory sequences are found in each structure.

Finally, the end of the sugar chain is most often capped by a sialic acid in the form of neuraminic N-acetyl acid (NANA) in human cells, when for many mammals, a part of the sialic acid is in the form of neuraminic N-glycolyl acid (NGNA) because the gene which codes for the enzyme that allows the NANA form to become NGNA, is muted and inactive in humans. This species specificity is essential when choosing systems involving carbohydrate expression of the recombinant protein of interest to ensure that the sialylation is as close as possible to the human form. The mature protein, so "glycosylated" and more or less "sialylated," gets some characteristics that are acidic with a changed isoelectric point (pI). Consequently, at the end of post-translational modifications, the protein appears not as a single entity but as a mix, a molecular population with the same basic protein structure (primary sequence imposed by gene sequence) on which various types of sugar chains are attached, giving each protein molecule its unique pI, allowing their separation based on their charge in analytical testing (isoelectric focusing).

There are four types of glycosylation links:

- N-linked glycosylation: The most common type of glycosidic bond is necessary to fold eukaryotic proteins and extracellular matrix attachment for cell-cell and cell attachment. Though it rarely occurs in bacterial, the N-linked glycosylation process can occur in eukaryotes and the endoplasmic reticulum archaea lumen, but very rarely in bacteria.
- O-linked glycosylation: A form of glycosylation occurs in eukaryotes in the Golgi apparatus and occurs in archaea and bacteria. Other glycans include xylose, fucose, mannose, and GlcNAc phosphoserine glycans.
- C-mannosylation: In this link, a mannose sugar is added to the first tryptophan residue in the sequence W-X-X-W (W indicates tryptophan, where X is any amino acid). It is a rather unusual reaction because the sugar is linked to carbon rather than nitrogen.
- Formation of GPI anchors (glypiation): A special form of glycosylation is forming a GPI anchor. In this kind of glycosylation, protein is attached to a lipid anchor via a glycan chain.

TABLE 8.5

Effect of PTMs on Protein Function and Physiological Processes

Function	Phosphorylation	Glycosylation	S-nitrosylation	Methylation	N-acetylation	Palmitoylation	N-myristoylation	Prenylation	Sumoylation	Ubiquitination
Apostosis			X		X		X			
Protein stability		X	X		X				X	X
Protein–protein	X	X					X	X		
Protein–membrane						X	X	X		
Protein trafficking	X	X				X				
Thermodynamic, kinetic		X								
Activity		X	X							
Extracellular export							X		X	
Cell signaling			X			X	X		X	
Transcription				X	X					
DNA repair					X				X	
Cell cycle division	X									X
Immune response	X									X
Chromosome maintenance				X						
Chromosome assembly									X	

Source: Martina Audagnotto and Matteo Dal Peraro, www.ncbi.nlm.nih.gov/pmc/articles/PMC5397102/, CC BY-SA 4.0, https://commons.wikimedia.org/w/index.php?curid=75125453.

8.2.6 Association and Aggregation

The higher-order structures of proteins are stabilized through many weak and strong bonds, including weak noncovalent bonds, formed ionic, dipoles (hydrogen bonds), non-polar (hydrophobic), and van der Waals interactions. These bonds involve the interaction of amino acid side chains and the polypeptide chain. Since the transition from a polypeptide chain to a higher-order structure requires a significant loss of structuring, it must be compensated by enthalpy released from the forming of the bond (energy is released when a bond is formed); as a result, the protein structure can remain in a dynamic state of structuring that may affect its activity as well as its stability. In most instances, the changes are transitory, and the protein returns to its native structure. However, the possibility of dynamic changes to protein structure makes it possible for a molecule to have a different activity if its physicochemical properties are altered; additionally, if there is aggregation, this may lead to loss of activity likely increase in the immunogenicity of the protein.

Protein aggregation is caused by two factors: colloidal and conformational instability. The attractions on the surface of proteins can make colloidal dispersions that can be dynamic and significantly affect the safety and efficacy of proteins under stress conditions; the conformational changes are brought about by the buried functional groups' hydrophobic interactions. There is a likelihood of both types of aggregates and, in some instances, one leading to another. So far, the regulatory authorities have not focused on these differentiations. Over time, these would likely be included as part of the risk analysis of the manufacturing process.

There is also a likelihood of aggregation due to molecular crowding when the drug is exposed to the high concentration and high plasma protein concentration. Recently, therapeutic proteins have been formulated in higher concentration formulations to reduce the injection volume to change the route of administration from intravenous administration to subcutaneous administration such as MabThera (rituximab).

8.3 Non-Antibody Therapeutic Proteins

Human body cells exploit an enormous array of proteins, approximately two thousand, to perform nearly every functional and structural role to stay alive. These proteins are expressed inside each of our body cells by coding in the DNA molecules. The genes are DNA portions carrying a message that ultimately leads to the production of proteins. They are present in all living creatures' genomes and are sequences of nucleotides (A, T, G, and C). Each of these genes' sequences is specific for a protein (Figure 8.7).

For many reasons, the body cells may become deficient in producing the required proteins, including genetic mutations that reduce or stop the production of proteins, leading to many life-threatening conditions. The types of proteins that are affected include hormones, enzymes, antibodies, and many more. There are two ways to fix this cellular abnormality. First, administer the deficient proteins, and second, retrain the cells to produce the required proteins. The first category comprises complex therapeutic proteins with considerable molecular weight and variable structures. It is not possible to synthesize these proteins, not only because of lacking technology but also because of their variable structure—essentially, these molecules are a group of molecules—and it is not possible to replicate their variability. As a result, we have two choices: extracting them from healthy subjects or producing them in living entities whose genetic code has been altered to produce these molecules.

The training of cells is the subject of gene therapy and cell therapy technology. In addition to the naturally occurring proteins, we can also design proteins as antibodies to alleviate diseases where a protein-receptor binding is involved in the body. This area of monoclonal antibodies is one of the essential categories of biological medicine products.

Based on their pharmacological activity, therapeutic proteins are classified into the following:

- Those replacing a deficient or abnormal protein.
- Those providing a novel role.
- Those interfering with another molecule.

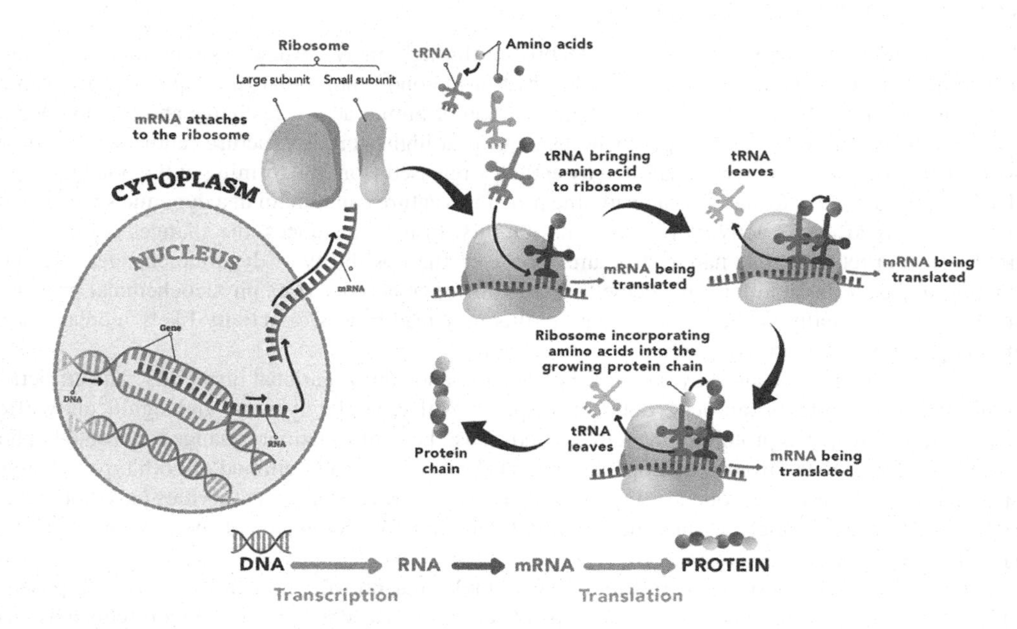

FIGURE 8.7 Structure of DNA and protein production in cells. Source: www.technologynetworks.com/applied-sciences/articles/essential-amino-acids-chart-abbreviations-and-structure-324357.

- Those delivering the cytotoxic drug, effector protein, or a radionuclide.
- Those augmenting a pathway.

Another classification of therapeutic proteins is based on the types of molecules such as enzymes, hormones, interleukins, antibodies, anticoagulants, Fc proteins, growth factors, interferons, etc.

Another classification is based on the molecular mechanism of action:

- Binding non-covalently to target, e.g., mAbs.
- Affecting covalent bonds, e.g., enzymes.
- Showing activity without specific interactions, e.g., serum albumin.

The upcoming engineered proteins include bispecific mAbs and multi-specific fusion proteins, mAbs conjugated with small molecule drugs, and proteins with optimized pharmacokinetics.

8.3.1 Hormone Peptide Drugs

Hormone's definition also includes the autocrine and intracrine signaling chemicals produced in cells; and paracrine signaling with nearby cells. Hormones are produced by glands and sent to the circulatory system; they signify that target organs regulate their physiology. Hormones have diverse chemical structures, including eicosanoids, steroids, amino acid derivatives, peptides, and proteins. The glands that secrete hormones include the endocrine signaling system.

The mRNA that comes from DNA inside the cell nucleus provides the synthesis of hormones, starting with pro-hormones and precursors in the endoplasmic reticulum. The N-terminal signal sequence and often glycosylation are removed. The secretory vesicles in the membrane then receive prohormones from where it is secreted by exocytosis to attend to stimulation, such as an increase in the cAMP concentration of Ca2+ in the cytoplasm.

Amino acid residues that were superfluous are contained in the prohormones to guide the hormone receptor's folding into its active configuration but have no function once the hormone folds. Instead, endopeptidases in the prohormone's cleaving just before it is released into the bloodstream generate the molecule's hormone type. Peptide hormones then proceed through the blood to reach their body cells, where they interact with receptors.

- Human insulin applies to diabetes.
- Growth hormone deficiency, along with development issues and AIDS, requires the use of growth hormone.
- Infertility, ovulation regulation, menopause osteoporosis, and others require the use of follicle-stimulating hormone and other hormones; however, this application is not yet widely used.

8.3.2 Human Hematopoietic Factor

Recombinant human erythropoietin applies to anemia.

- GM-CSF is used in the treatment of cancer and cancer chemotherapy-induced immunity alteration that may lead to infections.
- Hematopoietic factors are also used in children with dysplasia, malignant hematological disease, or complications in diabetes.

8.3.3 Human Cytokines

Cytokines are small proteins (~5–20 kDa) known for their cell signaling ability. Cytokines affect the behavior of body cells as they are involved in the autocrine systems. Examples of cytokines include interferons, chemokines, lymphokines, interleukins, and tumor necrosis factors but generally not hormones or growth factors.

A wide range of cells produce cytokines that comprise B lymphocytes, macrophages, T lymphocytes, endothelial cells, mast cells, stroma cells, and fibroblasts. Multiple cells can produce each cytokine acting by receptor interaction and modulate balancing between humor and cell-based responses. Cytokines further regulate growth, responsiveness, maturation. Cytokines are also known to inhibit or enhance other cytokines. A major difference between the hormones and the cytokines is that while both are cell signaling, the hormones are made by only specific cells and present in a much lower concentration.

- Alpha interferon for chronic viral hepatitis and certain cancers.
- Beta interferon for multiple sclerosis (MS).
- Interleukins 1, 2, and 11, for renal cell carcinoma, chemotherapy-induced thrombocytopenia, and chronic granulomatous diseases.

8.3.4 Human Plasma Protein Factor

- Recombinant human coagulation factor VIII applies to hemophilia A.
- Recombinant human coagulation factor VII (only NovoSeven [Novo Nordisk] is on the market) applies to hemophilia and hemostasis.
- Recombinant human coagulation factor IX (only Renefix [Genetics] is on the market) applies to hemophilia B.
- Tissue plasminogen activator tPA (the earliest product in Activase [Genetech]) applies to acute myocardial infarction.
- C-reactive protein applies to severe sepsis (only has Xigris [Eli Lilly]).
- Recombinant human antithrombin (ATryn) was approved in 2006, the first recombinant drug from transgenic animals.

8.3.5 Human Bone Formation Protein

- Recombinant human bone morphogenetic proteins (rhBMP-x; x = 1 – 15 + 8a 8b) for acute tibial fractures and bone healing.
- Spinal healing, Plexin-B2.

8.3.6 Enzymes

- Applies to congenital enzyme deficiency replacement therapy.
- Fusion protein is a small number of recombinant drugs whose mechanism is inhibition.
- Exogenous recombinant proteins: exogenous proteins can be used to treat human disease, which has been validated during the development of monoclonal antibody drugs. However, only recombinant hirudin was approved on the market, which applies to thrombotic disease.

8.4 Antibody Therapeutic Proteins

Paul Ehrlich first proposed the idea of "magic bullets" in 1900 that if a compound could be made that selects target disease-causing organisms, then a toxin for that organism could be used to kill the organism. Paul Ehrich and Élie Metchnikoff received the 1908 Nobel Prize. In the 1970s, the B cell in cancer multiple myeloma was shown to produce a single type of antibody (a paraprotein: a protein found in the body only in the precancer) and applied to study the structure of antibodies. Jerrold Schwaber first described the production involving human–mouse hybrid cells in 1973; in 1975, Georges Köhler and César Milstein succeeded in making fusions of myeloma cell lines with B cells to create hybridomas to produce antibodies, specific to known antigens, making them immortalized (because of fusion with myeloma cells). They, and Niels Kaj Jerne in 1914, shared the Nobel Prize. Further, Greg Winter and his team pioneered the techniques to humanize mAbs, eliminating the untoward reactions; a Nobel Prize was awarded to Jam Allison and Tasuku Honjo in 2018 to discover cancer therapy through negative immune regulation inhibition using mAbs that prevent inhibitory linkages.

Antibodies or immunoglobulin are glycoprotein molecules that reside in our blood and tissue fluids to help fight infection. Antibody molecules are available in a variety of shapes and sizes. The basic structure, however, is a "Y" shape, with the two tips designed to recognize and bind (Figure 2.1) foreign agents (for example, bacteria, viruses, or harmful cells). The remaining parts of the molecule are known as "effector functions," which allow the antibody to interact with other immune cells or serum proteins. Monoclonal antibodies are obtained from cells grown in the laboratory to bind to specific targets. The definition of antibodies includes antibody fragments, bispecific antibodies, multi-specific antibodies, and antibody fusion products.

Polyclonal antibodies detect a multiplicity of epitopes and therefore recognize antigens from different orientations; this may be important in specific assays where the detection of an analyte would be compromised using a single epitope. B cell hybridomas' continuous culture offers a reproducible and potentially inexhaustible supply of antibodies with high specificity. Several other methods for producing antibodies, including the "display" systems, chemical synthesis, and extracting from B cells (Figure 8.8).

Antibodies are created to find a solution for:

- Neutralizing infecting organisms.
- Binding to receptors to elicit a pharmacologic response.
- Binding to endogenous chemicals to alleviate a disease.
- Creating analytical methods of separating and identifying a large molecule.

A clear understanding of antibodies begins with an understanding of the immune system that produces antibodies. When an immunogen provokes a humoral immune response, many antibodies are produced against different parts or regions of the immunogen termed antigenic determinants, or epitopes, which

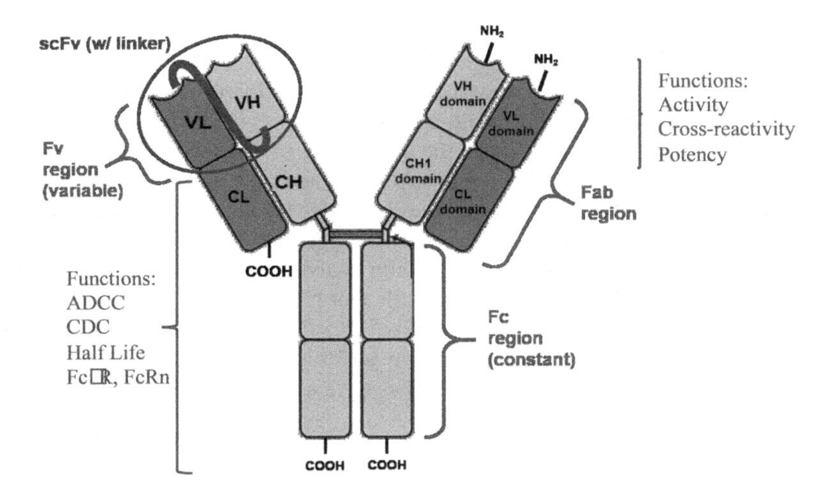

FIGURE 8.8 Schematic of IgG antibody structure. Antibodies (Ab) comprise immunoglobulin (Ig), which is a large (~150 kDa) Y-shape proteins that identify and neutralize pathogens. A paratope, also called an antigen-binding site, is an antibody that recognizes and binds to an antigen. It is a small region (five to ten amino acids) of the antibody's Fab region, part of the fragment antigen-binding (Fab) region. In addition, it contains parts of the antibody's heavy and light chains.

usually comprise six to eight amino acids. Antibodies recognize and interact with three-dimensional shapes (discontinuous epitopes) in folded proteins and recognize linear stretches of amino acids or continuous epitopes. Each antibody molecule recognizes only one epitope, and each antibody is produced by a single B cell clone. Monoclonal antibodies are antibodies that have a single specificity and are derived from a single B cell clone.

Therapeutic antibodies are divided into two broad categories. The naked antibody is the first type of antibody that can work via various mechanisms, including mediated pathways (e.g., ADCC/CDC), direct cancer cell targeting to induce apoptosis, targeting the tumor microenvironment, and targeting immune control points. By recruiting natural killer cells or other immune cells, the antibodies kill cancer cells in mediated pathways.

It is possible to enhance ADCC or CDC therapeutic effects, such as antibody Fc point mutations or glycosylation modification, to enhance cancer cells' ability to destroy cancer cells. The traditional preference mechanism of therapeutic antibodies is the channel-mediated apoptosis of cancer cells. To attack the tumor microenvironment, antibodies can prevent tumorigenesis by containing factors that are involved in the growth of cancer cells; one such example is that the bevacizumab targets the vascular endothelial growth factor (VEGF) to suppress the growth of the blood vessels surrounding the tumor, shutting down the nutritional supply needed for the growth of cancer cells.

Antibodies are made by the body's immune system in reaction to antigens, including bacteria, fungi, parasites, viruses, chemicals, and other substances the immune system identifies as harmful. At times the body mistakenly identifies normal cells as foreign and produces antibodies against the entities. This is the root cause of autoimmune conditions such as rheumatoid arthritis and multiple sclerosis. Antibodies are naturally produced by the immune system to the immune system. The synthetic antibodies are produced by introducing human genes in mice to produce the targeted antibody that similarly neutralizes the body's proteins; several other methods produce antibodies. Monoclonal antibodies come from an identical monoclonal cell and have only one type of antigen; the polyclonal antibodies come from several cells producing multiple antigens.

Most of the antibodies produced as part of the normal immune response are polyclonal, which means that several specific B lymphocytes form them. As a result, each has a slightly different antigen specificity (e.g., by binding different epitopes or binding the same epitope with different affinities). A single B cell clone, on the other hand, can produce large quantities of antibodies.

Monoclonal antibodies (mAbs) are proteins produced by immune cell clones of a single parent cell. They, therefore, have a monovalent affinity in that they bind to the same epitope. Since it is possible to produce monoclonal antibodies that specifically bind to any substance, they can also detect or purify that substance, making antibodies an essential tool in biochemistry, molecular biology, and medical research. In contrast, polyclonal antibodies are produced naturally by the B cells and bind to multiple epitopes. Thus, bispecific monoclonal antibodies target two multi-specific antibodies that can target several epitopes.

Many molecular immunology studies require the use of monoclonal antibodies. Monoclonal antibodies enable antigenic profiling and macromolecular surfaces when used in conjunction with epitope mapping and molecular modeling. Monoclonal antibodies have also become essential components of a wide range of clinical laboratory diagnostic tests. The exquisite specificity of these unique reagents has led to their widespread use in detecting and identifying serum analytes, cell markers, and pathogenic agents. Furthermore, the continuous culture of hybridoma cells that produce these antibodies could provide an endless supply of reagents. In contrast to the relatively limited supply of polyclonal antibody reagents, the ability to standardize both the reagent and the assay technique is enabled by the feature of a continuous supply. Both polyclonal and monoclonal antibodies have advantages and disadvantages in terms of generation, cost, and general applications.

8.4.1 Mode of Action

The variable region of the antibody Fab (antigen-binding fragment) (Figure 2.4) is the smallest unit of an antibody, which has antigen-binding capability resulting in conformational changes in the contact surface areas of both the antibody and the antigen, in a lock and key fit model that minimizes changes in the surface conformation of the unbound and bound states. So, in unbound and bound states, the antibody and antigen's backbone conformations are the same. Conversely, in the induced mode, the antibody and antigen's conformational changes may be quite extensive. After binding, both the side chain and the backbone atoms in the contact region may undergo conformational changes, especially in the CDR (complementarity-determining regions). The antigen samples a population of specific conformational states in the conformational selection model before binding. Antibody binding may depend on the antigen's pre-activation states, which may be affected by the antigen's microenvironment. Sorting out the target interaction kinetics also guides how their pharmacology is optimized.

The antibody recognizes an antigen via its variable region. The tips of the "Y" contain a paratope (an antigen-binding site, which recognizes and binds to an antigen) specific to an epitope (the part of an antigen molecule to which an antibody attaches itself), just like a critical fit, only one lock. This interaction results in the antibody tagging a pathogen or infected cell, neutralizing the target by locking a part of a pathogen required for body invasion. Antibodies communicate with the immune system through its Fc region that is a glycosylation site (Figure 8.2).

The monoclonal antibodies produced in laboratories serve as a substitute to innate antibodies that can restore, enhance, or mimic the immune system's attack on infectious organisms or cancer cells, the two most common therapeutic uses of monoclonal antibodies. As an example, monoclonal antibodies used to treat cancer demonstrate multiple active roles:

- Marking cancer cells. Antibodies are used by some immune system cells to locate the attack's target. Cancer cells that have been coated with monoclonal antibodies may be easier to detect and destroy.
- Destroying cell membranes. Some monoclonal antibodies can activate an immune response that destroys the outer layer of a cancer cell (membrane).
- Stopping the growth of cells. Some monoclonal antibodies prevent cancer cells from interacting with proteins that promote cell growth, which is necessary for tumor growth and survival.
- Preventing the growth of blood vessels. A blood supply is required for a cancerous tumor to grow and survive. Unfortunately, some monoclonal antibody drugs interfere with protein-cell interactions, which are necessary to form new blood vessels.
- Blocking immune system inhibitors. Certain proteins that bind to immune system cells act as regulators, preventing the system from becoming overactive. Cancer-fighting cells can work with fewer inhibitions thanks to monoclonal antibodies that bind to these immune system cells.

- Taking direct aim at cancer cells. Even though they were designed for a different purpose, some monoclonal antibodies may attack the cell more directly. In addition, when some of these antibodies bind to a cell, a cascade of events within the cell may cause the cell to self-destruct.
- Providing radiation therapy. A monoclonal antibody is engineered as a delivery vehicle for other treatments because of its ability to connect with cancer cells. When a monoclonal antibody is attached to a small radioactive particle, it transports the therapy directly to cancer cells, potentially reducing the effect of radiation on healthy cells. Radioimmunotherapy is a type of cancer treatment that differs from standard radiation therapy.
- Administering chemotherapy. Like monoclonal antibodies, some chemotherapeutic drugs are attached to monoclonal antibodies to deliver the treatment directly to cancer cells while avoiding healthy cells.
- Binding cancer and immune cells together. For example, some drugs combine two monoclonal antibodies, one that binds to a cancer cell and the other that binds to a specific immune cell. This link could encourage the immune system to attack cancer cells.

8.4.2 Types of Antibodies

Because non-linear epitopes bind to conventional antibodies, they are monospecific and typically recognize only one antigen. Some antibodies have multi-specificity, which occurs when a very similar epitope is found on multiple antigens. Antibodies that recognize orthologous proteins in different species or antibodies that interact with different conserved protein families are examples of species cross-reactive antibodies. Antibody utility as a therapeutic agent in various animal models has often been hampered by species specificity. Antibody cross-reactivity is modified using the same combinatorial techniques that are used to improve antibody affinity. In silico design strategies and the availability of experimental structural information are also crucial in specificity engineering (Figure 8.9).

8.4.2.1 Recombinant Antibodies

Monoclonal antibodies produced in vitro using synthetic genes are known as recombinant antibodies. Recombinant antibody technology entails extracting the antibody genes from source cells, amplifying

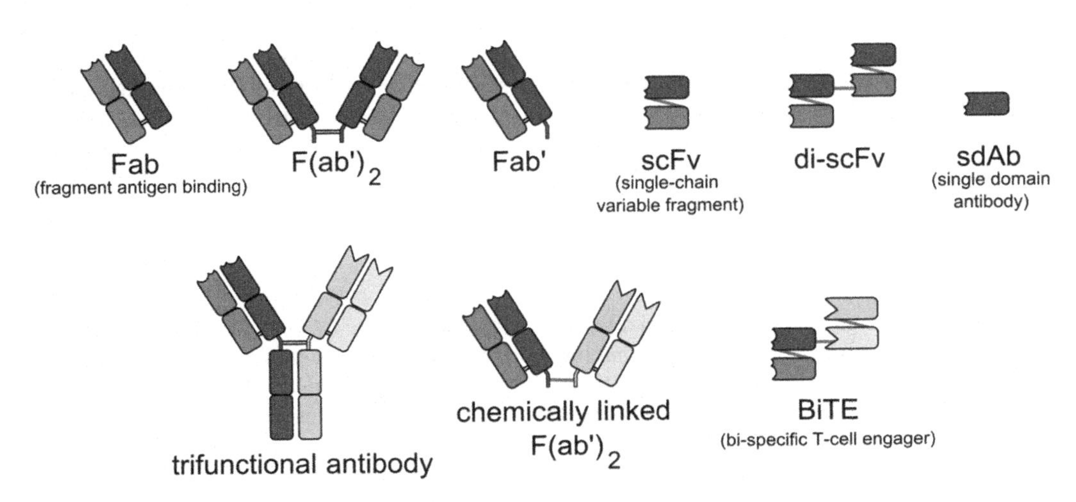

FIGURE 8.9 Types of monoclonal antibodies with other structures than naturally occurring antibodies. Top row: monospecific antibodies (fragment antigen-binding, F[ab']2 fragment, Fab' fragment, single-chain variable fragment, di-scFv, single-domain antibody). Bottom row: bispecific antibodies (trifunctional antibody, chemically linked F[ab']2, bi-specific T cell engager). Legend: heavy chains have a darker shade, light chains have a lighter one. Parts of antibodies with different targets are colored differently. Constant regions are shown as regular round-edged boxes, variable regions as boxes with an irregularly shaped end. Artificial links between fragments are colored red.

and cloning them into a suitable vector, inserting the vector into a host, and producing a functional antibody. If the appropriate oligonucleotide primers or hybridization probes are available, recombinant antibodies can be cloned from any antibody-producing animal species. In vitro generation of new antibodies and antibody fragments, such as Fab fragments and scFv, is possible thanks to the ability to manipulate antibody genes. This can be accomplished by combining sites at the site level and creating new H and L chain combinations. Individual CDRs can be mutated to achieve this as well. In addition, antibody sequence changes can be used to select desirable characteristics using display libraries, which are commonly expressed in phage or yeast.

8.4.2.2 Synthetic Antibodies

Synthetic antibodies are affinity reagents that are manufactured entirely in vitro, without the use of animals. Recombinant antibodies, nucleic acid aptamers, and non-immunoglobulin protein scaffolds are examples of synthetic antibodies. Synthetic antibodies' antigen-recognition sites can be engineered to any desired target thanks to their in vitro manufacturing method. Thus, it could go beyond what natural antibodies can do in terms of the immune repertoire. In addition, synthetic antibodies have many advantages over animal-derived antibodies, including lower production costs, reagent reproducibility, increased affinity, specificity, and stability across a wide range of experimental conditions.

Synthetic antibodies derived from non-immunoglobulins usually have a different structure than antibodies. Aptamers are made from nucleic acids, while non-immunoglobulin protein scaffolds/peptide aptamers are made from non-immunoglobulin protein scaffolds/peptide aptamers non-immunoglobulin protein scaffolds/peptide aptamers are made from non-immunoglobulin. The antigen-binding site is formed by inserting hypervariable loops. The binding affinity and specificity of the synthetic antibody are improved to levels comparable to or exceeding those of a natural antibody by constraining the hypervariable binding loop at both ends within the protein scaffold. These molecules have several advantages over traditional antibody structures, including a smaller size, improved tissue penetration, faster generation times (weeks vs. months for natural and recombinant antibodies), and lower costs.

8.4.2.3 Affimer Proteins

Affimer proteins have a molecular weight of 12–14 kDa and are small, robust affinity reagents. Synthetic antibodies are proteins that have been engineered to bind to their target proteins with high affinity and specificity. The cysteine protease inhibitor family of cystatins provides the basis for the Affimer protein scaffold. Two-variable peptide loops within the protein scaffold and a variable N-terminal sequence provide a high-affinity binding surface for the specific target protein. Affimer binders have been produced for many targets, including ubiquitin chains, immunoglobulins, and C-reactive protein for several molecular recognition applications.

8.4.2.4 Structural Protein Scaffolds

In the cytoskeleton and extracellular matrix, the molecules such as type IV collagen provide a mechanical scaffold; there's an increased focus on making more robust proteins so they may be formulated and used in long-acting dosage forms. There are fundamental stability problems with mAbs, more particularly in the hinge region. Engineered protein scaffolds are protein families with non-IgG architecture that have been developed with novel binding. A scaffold is often described as a single chain polypeptide framework that contains a highly structured core associated with various elements of high conformational tolerance permitting insertions, deletions, and other substitutions. Scaffolds have reduced molecular weight compared to mAbs, and while they have similar features as antibodies, scaffolds have also been described that are unrelated to mAbs. Protein scaffolds possess enhanced solubility and thermal equilibrium, and better tissue penetration. The scaffolds include a single polypeptide chain structure and provide high bacterial expression. Scaffolds can be IgG- (e.g., scFv, single domain names) or non-IgG-like molecules (antibodies, anticline, DARPins, dual-affinity retargeting molecules). These groups

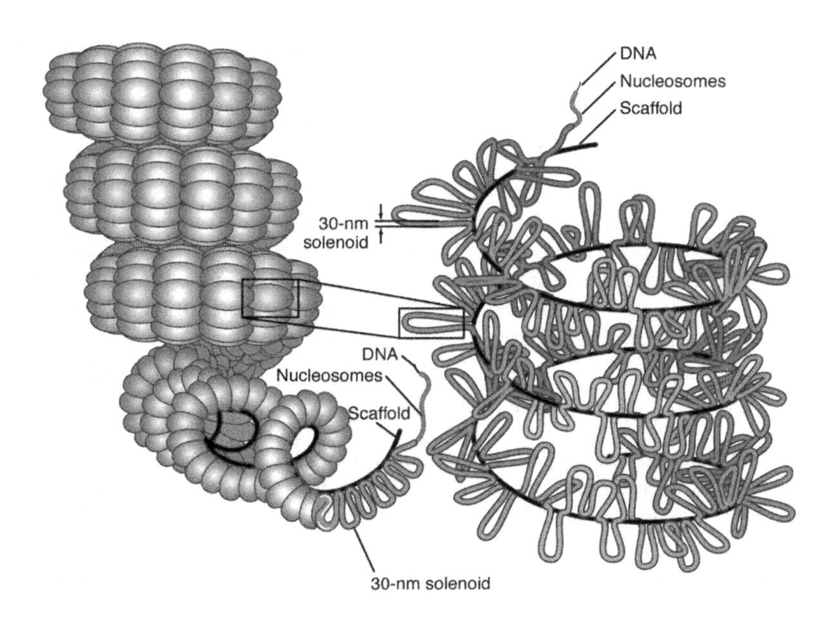

FIGURE 8.10 Protein scaffold structure. Source: www.mun.ca/biology/scarr/Histone_Protein_Structure.html.

provide smaller molecules with epitope binding and specificity properties of mAbs. As an example, non-IgG-like molecules have higher stability, cysteine-free strings, and elastic pharmacokinetic properties (Figure 8.10).

8.4.2.5 Bispecific Antibodies (BsAbs)

If single components' targeting is unsuccessful, an improved therapeutic approach includes more than one target linked to a single action mechanism. However, there are drawbacks to using monospecific antibody formats in that certain patients won't respond to such treatment after a period. In addition, because there may be crosstalk between signaling pathways, resistance can emerge during the diseased tissue growth. Therefore, the use of BsAbs is made to improve the therapeutic profile where multiple diseases are involved.

BsAbs can bind to different antigens or epitopes by combining two antibodies' specificities, especially where spatial-temporal relationships cannot be exploited by combining or overlapping antibodies. Theoretical advantages in the use of BsAbs include assigning different immune cells to tumor cells to boost the killing of tumors; BsAbs also enable simultaneous blocking of two different mediators or pathways that exert unique or overlapping functions in pathogenesis and potentially increase the binding specificity by dealing with two different antigens on the cell surface instead of one.

Antibodies targeting two receptors are intended to improve therapeutic effects for bispecific antibodies further. The functions of antibody-engaged effector cells enhance the therapeutic effectiveness of bispecific antibodies. In the case of immunoliposomes, the antibody's binding site (scFv or Fab) is cleaved from the constant region and then conjugated to different areas.

CAR-T involves inserting the gene into T cells for a chimeric T cell receptor-antibody attacking a cancer antigen. The modified cells recognize and kill cancer cells. Antibodies targeting two receptors are engineered to improve therapeutic effects for bispecific antibodies further. The functions of antibody-engaged effector cells can enhance the therapeutic effectiveness of bispecific antibodies. In immunoliposomes, the antibody's binding site (scFv or Fab) is cleaved from the constant region and then conjugated to different regions. nano-drug delivery systems, such as liposomal drugs, to provide more specific targeting. It offers attractive new possibilities for developing novel protein therapies.

There are three approved BsAbs: catumaxomab, which can bring T cells or T lymphocytes via CD3 binding closer to cells expressing EpCAM (Trion Pharma); blinatumomab, which also has a CD3-binding arm to B lymphomas with CD19 (Micromet/Amgen); and Helimbra or emicizumab-kxwh (Roche/Chugai) that mimics the cofactor VIII for patients with hemophilia A.

8.4.2.6 Multi-Specific Antibodies (MsAbs)

A natural extension of BsAbs is to have an increased number of binding arms to create MsAbs that can effectively engage more epitopes on a target. There is no lack of protein engineering opportunities, with the ability to mix in cytokines and enzymes. There is a dire need to have rapidly neutralized antibodies against highly variable pathogens such as infectious viruses. The Fc region is designed to optimize effector function, clustering, and interaction with Fc receptors. In general, antibody engineering is an essential part of the Fab and Fc regions' drug development process.

8.4.2.7 Fab Fragments and Single-Chain Antibodies

The use of antibody fragments instead of full-length antibodies can improve pharmacokinetics and penetration efficiency in tissues or tumor masses (because fragments are smaller). In addition, fragments typically have a single valence for the antigen (binding site) rather than two valences characteristic of full-length antibodies.

Fragment antigen-binding (Fab), also known as Fab fragments, consists of a variable domain and the first constant region of each heavy and light chain.

The single-chain variable fragment (scFv)–scFv consists of a light chain and heavy chain variable region linked by a single-domain antibody linker peptide (sdAb)–sdAb, which is an antibody fragment consisting of a light chain variable region, or hFab fragments, which lack the antibody Fc portion (the remainder of the heavy chain). They are thus unable to interact with Fc receptors or activate complement.

As a result, they are typically not appropriate for indications that rely on cell killing when used alone. The following are some examples of clinical applications:

- Caplacizumab is a single-domain antibody (sdAb) made up of a bivalent variable-domain-only mAb fragment with a high affinity for the von Willebr and factor X receptors (VWF). Its binding prevents VWF from interacting with platelets, which is important in microvascular thromboses like those seen in thrombotic thrombocytopenic purpura patients (TTP).
- Ranibizumab is a humanized Fab fragment of a recombinant monoclonal antibody that binds to and inhibits human vascular endothelial growth factor A (VEGF-A). Ranibizumab prevents VEGF from binding to its receptors, preventing neovascularization and slowing vision loss. Abciximab is a Fab antibody fragment derived from a chimeric human-murine mAb (7E3) that binds to platelet IIb/IIIa receptors and inhibits platelet aggregation by causing steric hindrance.

8.4.2.8 Humanized and Chimeric mAbs

A variety of non-human species, including rats, pigs, and rabbits, are used to produce antibodies to human targets. All these non-human antibodies require humanization. The most straightforward approach is constructing a chimera by combining non-human antibodies' variable domains with constant human domains to produce 70% human material molecules. Chimeric antibodies have shown reduced immunogenicity in many cases but have still elicited some human anti-therapeutic response to the antibody. A CDR-grafting technique to further minimize immunogenicity involves transferring CDRs from a non-human (very often murine) "parental" antibody to a human antibody's scaffold. In addition to CDR grafting, alternative humanization methods include resurfacing, super-humanization, or optimization of the human string material. These require amino acid sequence analysis to assess the potential effect of substitutions of the amino acids their structure and function antibodies.

The mAbs initially derived from a non-human species (e.g., mouse, rat) are "humanized" to various degrees by engineering amino acid substitutions that make them more like the human sequence. This is done using recombinant DNA technologies. In principle, the more similar a mAb is to human-derived sequences shared among many individuals, the less likely it is to get an immune reaction to the mAb.

Potential adverse reactions of immunogenicity include infusion reactions, and reduced efficacy, although these are not easily predicted.

However, the immunogenicity of not all amino acid residues or groups of residues is the same. Furthermore, defining what constitutes a chimeric antibody versus a humanized antibody (e.g., how many amino acid residues must be changed for an antibody to qualify as humanized) has become increasingly difficult, and definitions have evolved. Humanized mAbs are those with non-human-derived small but critical parts of the complementarity-determining region (CDR), but human-derived large constant regions of the immunoglobulin heavy and light chains.

Chimeric antibodies are those in which the Fc portion of the immunoglobulin molecule is human (but not the CDR). Chimeric mAbs and humanized antibodies, in general, contain between 65% and 90% human sequence. As a result, there are several methods for producing fully humanized antibodies.

The fully human mAbs technique is based on phage display, in which a library is composed of various exogenous genes inserted into filamentous bacteriophages. The library proteins are then introduced as fusions with a phage coat protein on the phage surface, allowing for selecting specific binders and characterization of affinities.

The first CDR-grafted humanized mAb approved by the US FDA came in 1997 for daclizumab, which activates the IL-2 receptor and prevents transplants' rejection in addition to reducing the loss of antigen recognition. Daclizumab uses CDR grafting and the human structure, which is maximally homologous to the murine system. In some cases, certain amino acids are necessary for the murine system to support an antibody's binding activity. Such residues often cooperate with CDRs to present a paratopic antibody or interact directly with antigens. Such essential matrix residues are identified by studying x-ray crystallography, cryo-electron microscopy, and computer-aided protein homology modeling of the antibody-antigen complex structure. The amino acid positions in the framework can then be considered for restoration in CDR-grafted humanized antibodies by "human back to mouse" mutations, thereby improving affinity and end-product stability.

Many processes are available to quantify the humanness of the variable region of mAbs. A tool called "H-score" assesses the "degree of humanization" of the antibody sequences, determining the mean sequence identity compared to the human vector field database sequences subset. A germinal index defines after assist germline humanization of a macaque antibody. G-score derived from the H-score improves the classification of the germline framework sequence. The T20 score analyzer (a tool that calculates the humanization of monoclonal antibody variable region sequences; the analyzer has the ability to consistently differentiate human antibody variable region sequences from the antibody sequences of other species, such as murine sequences) is established in a large database of approximately 38,700 natural antibody variable region sequences to separate human sequences. It is used to show differences between humanized antibodies and antibodies that are fully human.

The use of humanized antibodies is instrumental in improving clinical tolerance to mAb therapy. Half of all mAbs used for human treatment today are chimeric or humanized. Approved in 1998, trastuzumab (Herceptin) is one of the most well-known humanized antibodies. Trastuzumab is used to treat patients with receptor 2 (HER2)-positive metastatic breast cancer and adenocarcinoma gastroesophageal junction with human epidermal growth factor, the only drug identified in the WHO List of Essential Drugs. Murine antibodies are no longer used. The last one was produced in 2003, the same year that adalimumab was created as the first fully human antibody.

8.4.2.9 Affinity Maturation

Antibodies found from humanized, phage, or transgenic methods are often further developed, including residues' substitution in the binding region. Antibody gene diversification is the initial step of in vitro affinity maturation, and this step is accomplished with different strategies, such as random mutations, targeted mutations, or chain shuffling. Mutations are spontaneously introduced by error-pronounced PCR in mutator E in the variable regions of antibody genes of *E. coli*. Chain shuffling methods are those in which one of two chains, VH, and VL, is fixed and recombined to create a next-generation library with a set of partner chains. Also, mutations are added to specific regions of the antibody gene. This method of targeting the mutation approach helps diversify CDR resides to improve antibody affinity. Therefore, this approach is more applicable to in vivo somatic mutations during B cell evolution, as mutations accumulate expeditiously in the CDR than residues in the system.

Natural antibodies, human and non-human, often lack the binding properties needed for their therapeutic uses. Increasing binding affinity is an important step in lead candidate development since it is related to the dose required for treatment and therapeutic effectiveness. Different approaches, tools, and strategies in the engineering of antibodies are directed against different antigens and divided into two groups according to the antibody variant generation process. One is the variants' logical existence, followed by their representation within the system of choice. The other is building a library of variants where multiple positions are diversified, followed by displaying them in a choice system with the appropriate selection method. The latter method is most commonly used for affinity maturation due to many variants in a library covering the entire combinatorial space. In cases where only a few positions and a few amino acids are tested, the former approach may fulfill the task, as it is fast and cheap. Whatever method is used, structure-based computational design can facilitate the process by assessing the candidates in silico to minimize the library's size or the number of mutants to express.

8.4.2.10 Antigenized Antibodies

Antigenization is an investigational approach in which a mAb is engineered to deliver an antigen (e.g., a vaccine). It is accomplished by replacing part of the antibody polypeptide with a fragment of a microbial antigen. In various parts of the antibody molecule, any sequence can be inserted. Antigenized mAbs have a longer serum half-life than isolated antigen fragments and may be better tolerated than some microbial fragments, making them potentially useful as vaccines.

The successful presentation of microbial peptides in antibody molecules is shown in various animal systems (e.g., for influenza viruses in mice). However, this potentially revolutionary technology has only been tested on animals. A bovine herpesvirus B cell epitope, for example, was grafted onto a bovine immunoglobulin molecule using recombinant DNA methods. Cows were immunized with this antigenized antibody, and antibodies were generated against the virus.

8.4.2.11 IgG1 Fusion Proteins

IgG1 fusion proteins (also known as Fc-fusion proteins) are therapeutic proteins that take advantage of some of the immunoglobulin Fc region's properties, such as increased half-life. Antigen-binding complementarity is not determined in IgG1 fusion proteins (CDR). Thus, they do not have a biological target in the same sense that mAbs do, although the protein to which Fc is fused often has a specific biologic function manipulated. Some of these fusion proteins are identified by the suffix "-cept"; others contain "Fc" in their names.

The following are examples of IgG1 fusion proteins in clinical use:

- Etanercept is a fusion of two soluble TNF-alpha receptors with the Fc portion of an IgG molecule. It is bivalent because it has two TNF receptors (i.e., one etanercept molecule binds two TNF molecules). It is used to treat a variety of immunologic and rheumatologic conditions by inhibiting TNF-alpha.
- In people with hemophilia A, recombinant human factor VIII fused to the Fc portion of IgG (rFVIII-Fc) is a type of factor VIII supplementation. For hemophilia B, a similar product is available (FIX-Fc). These fusion proteins have longer half-lives than factor proteins that aren't fused to Fc.

8.4.2.12 Drug or Toxin Conjugation

An antibody-drug conjugate (ADC), a humanized or human monoclonal antibody combined through chemical linkers with highly cytotoxic small molecules (payloads), is a novel therapeutic format with great potential for a paradigm shift in cancer chemotherapy. A new molecular platform based on antibodies allows selective delivery of a potent cytotoxic load to cancer cells, leading to improved effectiveness, reduced systemic toxicity, and preferred pharmacokinetics (PK)/pharmacodynamics (PD) biodistribution compared to traditional chemotherapy. Building on the successes of the FDA-approved Adcetris® and Kadcyla®, this class of drugs has increased, with about 60 ADCs currently in clinical trials.

Examples include:

- Moxetumomab pasudotox is a humanized mouse monoclonal antibody (mAb) that targets CD22 and is conjugated to a *Pseudomonas* exotoxin A toxic fragment.
- Polatuzumab vedotin is a CD79b-targeting humanized monoclonal antibody (the B cell antigen receptor complex-associated protein beta chain). It is linked to the monomethyl auristatin E (MMAE), a dolastatin analog, by a protease-cleavable linker that improves plasma stability.
- Brentuximab vedotin is a CD30-targeting monoclonal antibody that is linked to MMAE via a cleavable linker.

The binding to internalizing receptors is also beneficial for many ADCs, which takes the conjugate into the cell, and allows the active moiety to cause its effects. The first approved ADC was gemtuzumab ozogamicin, which demonstrated an ablation of the cells with acute myeloid leukemia (AML). To form the ADC, gemtuzumab (anti-CD33) is connected to N-acetyl-ÿ-calicheamicin dimethyl hydrazide by non-specific lysine conjugation and a butanoic acid spacer of 4-(4-acetylphenoxy). The average ratio of a drug to an antibody (DAR) is between two and three. Toxins were also conjugated or fused to antibodies to produce tumor-targeting immunotoxins, in addition to natural products. Radionuclides represent an additional class of antibody-radionuclide conjugates (ARCs) that is bound to antibodies.

8.4.2.13 Future Antibodies

- There are several options for developing new antibodies.

  Increase the affinity of antibodies. When a naive antibody repertoire is exposed to an antigen, the primary reaction selects the binder with the best affinity for that antigen from among the nave antibody repertoire. The chosen chains are then subjected to an affinity maturation process to increase their affinity. However, as our understanding of the antibody maturation process grows, so does our ability to replicate it in the lab. To achieve in vitro affinity maturation, random or targeted mutagenesis on the complementarity determining region (CDR) loops of an antibody can be used. These efforts are guided by computational approaches that use protein structure and protein interaction databases to predict which iterations will be more beneficial. And display technologies are used to screen acceptable candidates (i.e., phage, yeast, mammalian cell display). The typically time-consuming and technically demanding approach to in vitro affinity maturation may soon change, thanks to the advent of next-generation sequencing technologies and in silico methods.
- Engineer the region of the Fc. The crystallizable fragment (Fc) of monoclonal antibodies determines the effector function and half-life of these biomolecules. As a result, point mutations and Fc glycoengineering are used to modulate these characteristics. Compared to small drugs and antibody fragments, natural monoclonal antibodies have a much longer half-life in our bodies (at least one week). However, suppose the half-life of these molecules was extended. In that case, a given monoclonal antibody therapy potency could be significantly increased, providing the benefits of passive immunization for more extended periods. In addition, by extending the half-life of these molecules, it would be possible to reduce the number of injections given to patients and, as a result, lower the current high production costs of these biopharmaceuticals. Furthermore, changing the way monoclonal antibodies interact with specific cell receptors could change the type of immune response elicited by these molecules in our bodies. Specific mutations and glycoengineering of the Fc region, for example, could help enhance (or eliminate) common effector responses like antibody-mediated cellular cytotoxicity (ADCC) and antibody-dependent cellular phagocytosis (ADCP), which kill targeted cells by producing cell-death-inducing molecules or phagocytosis, respectively.

- Create antibody cocktail treatments. Monoclonal antibody therapies for cancer and autoimmune diseases have shown to be effective. However, for other applications, such as infectious diseases, there is still a lot of room for improvement. Antibody cocktails are often referred to as the next generation of biopharmaceuticals as a result of this. Antibody cocktails are made up of two or more monoclonal antibodies mixed. They are a middle ground between traditional monoclonal antibody therapies and our body's natural polyclonal immune response. The use of these mixtures is a reasonable effort to overcome monoclonal and polyclonal therapies' inherent limitations. When escape mutants arise during treatment, the former's high specificity may result in reduced efficiency. The high sensitivity of the latter is frequently offset by the low productivity, low scalability, lack of specificity, and high variability of the corresponding production techniques. According to the researchers, antibody cocktails may be less susceptible to mutations than traditional monoclonal antibody therapies and less risky and more robust than traditional polyclonal antibody therapies. This theory has already been proven to work in treating two well-known infectious diseases: rabies and the Ebola virus. RabiMabs (TwinrabTM), a combination of two anti-rabies murine monoclonal antibodies, was approved in India in 2019, and the FDA granted it orphan drug status. This cocktail is at the cutting edge of rabies prevention. It's a better alternative to the current plasma therapy with human and equine antiserum, putting patients at risk of contracting additional human or zoonotic infections.

  REGN-EB3 is another outstanding example. This cocktail is made up of three fully human monoclonal antibodies currently being evaluated by the FDA to treat Ebola virus infections. The frequency of escape mutants is reduced because this cocktail targets non-overlapping epitopes of the same antigen. In late-stage clinical trials conducted in the epicenter of the most recent Ebola virus outbreak, the treatment was more effective than another well-known monotherapy—remdesivir (a nucleotide analog).
- Diffusion within cells should be increased. Antibody therapy has traditionally been limited by the limited diffusion of these molecules across tissues and membranes (e.g., the blood–brain barrier). As a result, the majority of therapeutic antibodies target either extracellular space components or membrane-bound antigens. However, because the cytosol contains at least 20% of the proteome, scientists are increasingly turning their attention to the cytosol, searching for novel targets. However, this approach necessitates developing strategies to improve antibody diffusion across tissues, which is currently limited. Conjugation of antibodies with naturally diffusible molecules like cell-penetrating peptides is one of the most intriguing approaches to increasing antibody diffusion (CPPs). Antibodies fused with CPPs have long been thought to be a viable solution.
- Make precision medicine a part of your overall strategy. Precision medicine takes into account a patient's genetic diversity. In contrast to personalized medicine, this approach aims to divide patients into different "genetic" groups. The concept that different patients respond to the same treatment in different ways is not new. In 2005, the Food and Drug Administration (FDA) approved the first pharmacogenetic test. Artificial intelligence and bioinformatics are at the heart of precision medicine. These tools analyze patients' genetic data and categorize them into different genetic groups. Furthermore, this strategy could be bolstered by incorporating immunomonitoring techniques that take advantage of flow cytometry's high throughput and specificity and fluorescent-labeled antibodies to understand better how a given treatment affects disease progression in different patients.
  - Cytokines and other secreted molecules provide the most effective protection for the body.
  - Products with synergistic effects of antibodies and chemotherapeutic drugs, radiotherapy, or other biological agents are examples of novel therapeutic proteins.
  - The development of new biomarkers would improve the efficacy and specificity of antibody-based therapy for human diseases.
  - Treatment of immune cytokine antibody–drug conjugates, antibody–radionuclide conjugates, bispecific antibodies, immunoliposomes, and T cell (CAR-T) chimeric antigen receptors are common ways to improve antibody efficacy. To enhance delivery specificities, a cytokine is fused with an antibody to create an immunocytokine.

- Antibody–drug conjugates are made up of an antibody targeting a cancer-specific antigen and a small molecule drug; the antibody improves transmission to the tumor site, increasing the small molecule's effectiveness while reducing non-specific toxicity to non-target tissues reducing side effects. The antibody can also be conjugated to a radionuclide to direct radiotherapy closer to the tumor site.

8.4.3 Development of Antibodies

Suppose the molecular mechanisms of disease are elucidated, and the relevant molecules involved in pathogenesis are identified. In that case, antibodies can provide an effective therapeutic choice, as demonstrated by several antibodies in clinical use:

- Anti-CGRP receptor antibodies (erenumab, galcanezumab, or fremanezumab): migraine prevention.
- Anti-protein convertase subtilisin/kexin type 9 (PCSK9) antibodies (evolocumab or alirocumab): hypercholesterolemia.
- Anti-fibroblast growth factor 23 (FGF23) antibody (burosumab): X-linked hypophosphatemia (XLH).
- Anti-IL6R antibodies (sarilumab and tocilizumab): rheumatoid arthritis.
- Anti- IXa/Xa factor antibody (emicizumab): hemophilia A.
- Anti-Willebr, and antibodies factor (caplacizumab): purpura thrombocytopenic.

Recent new classes of therapies include anticancer monoclonal antibodies that work on several mechanisms, rituximab acts by opsonization (making cancer cells more recognizable by the body immune system; ADCC, CDC), cetuximab by blocking epidermal growth signals, bevacizumab by stopping blood vessel formation, and ibritumomab is used to deliver radiation to cancer cells.

Since the affinity of mAbs for the target antigen is determined by the variable region and complementarity-determining region (CDR), antibodies with greater affinity are readily identified. The association constant for binding between the antibody and a single monovalent antigen in vitro is used to determine affinity. This affinity is amplified (e.g., 1,018 [a virtually irreversible binding reaction] rather than 109 L/mol) when the antibody is bivalent (e.g., full-length). Antibody affinities are frequently in the 105 to 1,011 L/mol range (picomolar to nanomolar affinity). Another critical attribute of mAbs is their ability to recruit other immune cells and molecules (such as complement), both of which can destroy target cells, mediated by the antibody's Fc portion.

The desired effect of a mAb directed toward a cell surface antigen includes blocking a cell surface receptor function or killing the target cell. In some cases, the target antigen is a cell surface receptor, and mAb binding can disrupt the receptor's normal or physiological function, preventing cell proliferation or survival. Examples include mAbs targeted against the epidermal growth factor (EGFR) or the receptor tyrosine kinase erbB-2 (also called HER2).

In other cases, a tumor cell or a B cell clone that produces an autoantibody could be the target (e.g., an antiplatelet antibody in immune thrombocytopenia [ITP]). Complement proteins, phagocytes, and natural killer (NK) cells may be enlisted in the cell-killing mechanism, resulting in immune-mediated destruction of the cell(s) expressing the target antigen on their surface.

Interactions with the Fc portion of the mAb are commonly used to recruit immune mediators.

Fc receptors can affect antibody-dependent cellular cytotoxicity (ADCC) or antibody-mediated phagocytosis by monocytes/macrophages by recruiting effector cells, which can modulate the cell-killing effects of mAbs. Fc receptors can also cause cell death through complement-dependent cytotoxicity (CDC), which occurs when a mAb binds to a target cell and activates the complement cascade. On CDC and ADCC, complement activation can have both agonistic and antagonistic effects, and it's unclear which mechanisms are responsible for killing cancer cells. Some antibodies combine ADCC and CDC features, and in some cases, mAbs are engineered to change their Fc binding to improve cell death. Using an antibody as a vehicle to deliver a toxin or cytotoxic drug directly to the target cell using a mAb-drug or mAb-toxin conjugate can also improve target cell killing.

In other cases, a tumor cell or a B cell clone that produces an autoantibody could be the target (e.g., an antiplatelet antibody in immune thrombocytopenia [ITP]). Complement proteins, phagocytes, and natural killer (NK) cells may be enlisted in the cell-killing mechanism, resulting in immune-mediated destruction of the cell(s) expressing the target antigen on their surface.

Interactions with the Fc portion of the mAb are commonly used to recruit immune mediators.

Fc receptors can affect antibody-dependent cellular cytotoxicity (ADCC) or antibody-mediated phagocytosis by monocytes/macrophages by recruiting effector cells, which can modulate the cell-killing effects of mAbs. Fc receptors can also cause cell death through complement-dependent cytotoxicity (CDC), which occurs when a mAb binds to a target cell and activates the complement cascade. Some antibodies combine ADCC and CDC features, and in some cases, mAbs are engineered to change their Fc binding to improve cell death. On CDC and ADCC, complement activation can have both agonistic and antagonistic effects, and it's unclear which mechanisms are responsible for killing cancer cells. Using an antibody as a vehicle to deliver a toxin or cytotoxic drug directly to the target cell using a mAb-drug or mAb-toxin conjugate can also improve target cell killing.

Examples of plasma proteins that are targeted by mAbs include:

- Tumor necrosis factor (TNF)—adalimumab, afelimomab, certolizumab pegol, golimumab, infliximab, and others.
- Vascular endothelial growth factor (VEGF)—bevacizumab.

Examples of drugs include:

- Dabigatran (anticoagulant)—idarucizumab.
- Digoxin (antiarrhythmic agent)—digoxin immune Fab.

These drugs are effectively neutralized when bound to the mAb because they cannot interact with normal targets. Through Fc-mediated uptake and lysosomal degradation, macrophages eventually clear them from the body.

The method by which a therapeutic mAb protects against infectious diseases is like natural humoral immunity, although it does not fully describe the nature of microbe elimination. Potential uses include the treatment or detection of infections. Most mAbs target proteins on a virus's surface, thus neutralizing the virus from getting into cells. Palivizumab is an antibody against the fusion (F) glycoprotein from the respiratory syncytial virus (RSV); it prevents viral entry into host cells. The antiviral preventive mAbs that act on Hemophilus influenza's conserved hemagglutinin A platform. Such treatment may be of help in situations where vaccination produces inadequate humoral immunity. Most mAbs against bacteria can function both prophylactically and therapeutically (e.g., attacking *Bacillus anthracis*' protective antigen domain or one of the *Clostridioides difficile* toxins).

The COVID-19 brought many new development technologies to the surface; one of them uses an antibody cocktail administered to President Trump within hours of his testing positive for COVID-19. A cocktail of two potent neutralizing antibodies (REGN10987 + REGN10933) targeting non-overlapping epitopes on the SARS-CoV-2 spike protein seems to hold promise for a new class of therapeutic antibody proteins.

Therapeutic antibodies are divided into two broad categories. The naked antibody is the first type of antibody that can work via various mechanisms, including mediated pathways (e.g., ADCC/CDC), direct cancer cell targeting to induce apoptosis, targeting the tumor microenvironment, and targeting immune control points. The antibodies kill cancer cells in mediated pathways by recruiting natural killer cells or other immune cells.

It is possible to enhance ADCC or CDC therapeutic effects, such as antibody Fc point mutations or glycosylation modification, to enhance cancer cells' ability to destroy cancer cells. The traditional preference mechanism of therapeutic antibodies is the channel-mediated apoptosis of cancer cells. To attack the tumor microenvironment, antibodies can prevent tumorigenesis by containing factors that are involved in the growth of cancer cells; one such example is that the bevacizumab targets the vascular endothelial growth factor (VEGF) to suppress the growth of the blood vessels surrounding the tumor, shutting down the nutritional supply needed for the growth of cancer cells.

Immune thresholds are important targets for treating cancer. The endogenous method uses a single B cell. An existing antibody against a target antigen is isolated from a patient. This method is especially applicable to cancer therapeutics because removing a tumor and regional lymph nodes are often used in routine treatment. These tissues are used to harvest tumor-infiltrating lymphocytes. Existing antibodies are also isolated from peripheral blood, bone marrow, or other lymphoid tissues such as the spleen or tonsils. Various investigational mAbs against viruses such as the human immunodeficiency virus (HIV) and the hepatitis C virus (HCV) are examples of this method.

This approach to developing monoclonal antibodies from single human B cells is based on an analysis of the immunoglobulin gene's repertoire and reactivity at the single-cell level by applying reverse transcription-polymerase chain reaction (RT-PCR) expression vector cloning.

Up to now, this method has not developed any therapeutic mAbs approved by the US FDA.

8.4.4 Exogenous Methods

Different influenza viruses cause epidemics every year, and the most useful measure to prevent seasonal influenza is the influenza vaccines. Single B cell isolation has become a common undertaking to produce potent and widely neutralizing anti-influenza antibodies.

The primary techniques involved in developing antibodies are immunizing an animal, using a phage display, or using a single B cell from humans to identify the antibody (Figure 8.11). Two techniques are

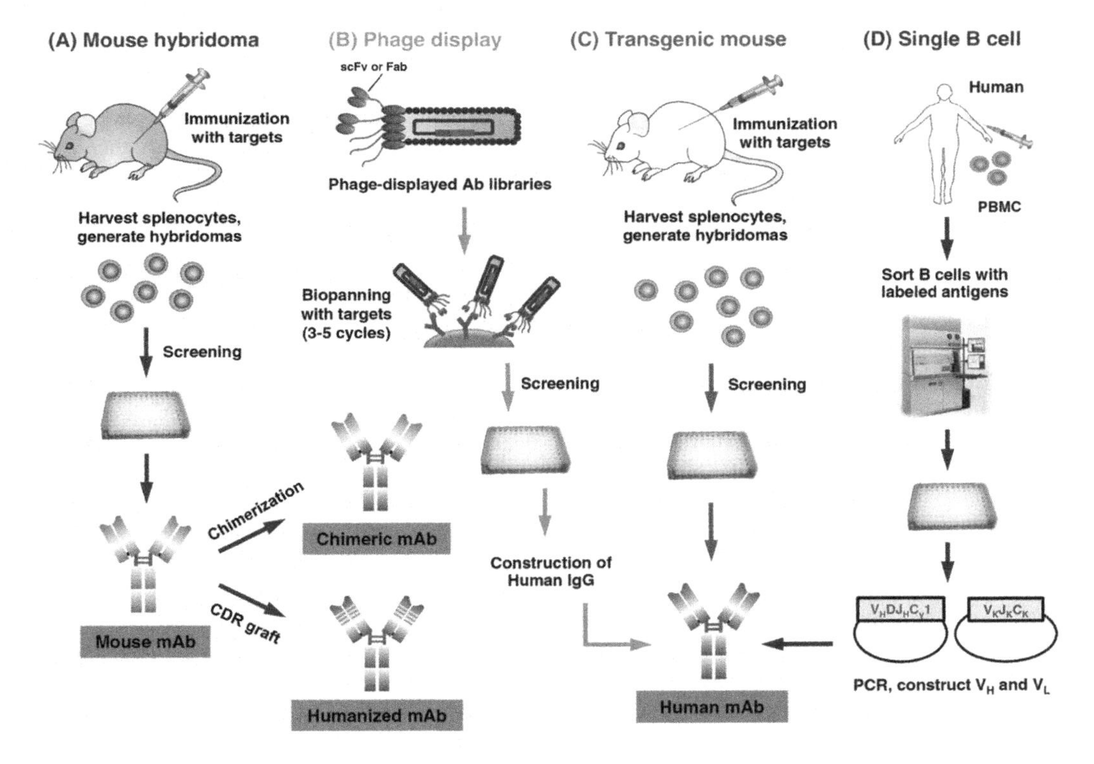

FIGURE 8.11 Approaches to therapeutic antibodies develop. (A) The traditional mouse hybridoma technique begins with mice's immunization with appropriate antigens to cause an immune response. Harvested splenocytes are fused to create hybridoma cells that persistently secrete antibodies with myeloma cells. Selected leads are used after the screening to produce chimeric or humanized antibodies. (B) view of a phage. A human antibody collection shown in phage is used to identify antigens of interest. ELISA screens immune-positive phage clones after 3–5 rounds of biopanning; then, DNA sequences are processed to build, and human IgGs are released. (C) The mouse is transgenic. Compared to the strategy of mouse hybridoma or single B cell approaches. (D) Methodology with a single B cell. PBMCs are prepared for the separation by flow cytometry of suitable B cells from contaminated or vaccinated donors. Following the RT-PCR, each B cell's VH and VL details tell about the generation of human mAbs.

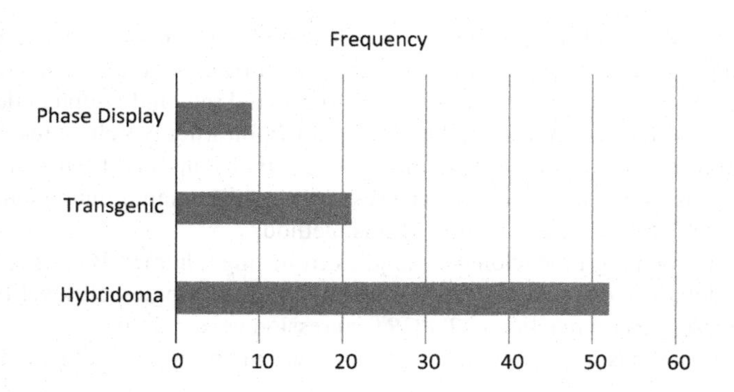

FIGURE 8.12 Method of producing antibodies for identification and testing for structure elucidation for approved antibodies.

used to commercialize an identified antibody: the classic mouse hybridoma technology and recombinant manufacturing, regardless of how they were identified.

Of the approved antibodies, the distribution of technologies to produce the antibody to establish its structure and activity, the most common method is hybridoma (Figure 8.12).

8.4.4.1 Mouse Hybridoma

In 1975 monoclonal antibodies were first developed using a hybridoma technique in mice (Köhler and Milstein). Generating hybridomas involves immunizing a certain species against a specific epitope on an antigen and removing the B-lymphocytes from the animal's spleen. The B-lymphocytes are then fused (by chemical or virus-induced methods) with an immortal myeloma cell line, which lacks the gene hypox anthine-guanine-phosphoribosyltransferase (HGPRT) and does not contain any other cells producing immunoglobulins. These hybridoma cells are then cultivated in vitro in a selective medium (i.e., hypox anthine-aminopterin-thymidine-containing medium) where only hybridomas (i.e., primary fusion) are present. B-lymphocytes and the myeloma cells survive as they inherit immortality from the myeloma cells and selective resistance from the primary B-lymphocytes (since the myeloma cells lack HGPRT, they cannot synthesize the myeloma cells (Figure 8.13).

A majority of approved antibodies were first created in a hybridoma, but only antibody muromonab-CD3 (Orthoclone OKT3) continues to be manufactured in a hybridoma; all other antibodies are produced in a recombinant cell line, primarily the CHO cells. Because some people exposed to mouse antibodies develop an immune response to the mouse antibody sequence, hybridoma technology is no longer used for commercial manufacturing. As a result, methods for engineering changes to the immunoglobulin molecule, such as humanizing the antibody or creating a chimeric antibody, have been developed. These are used in the majority of mAbs that were initially selected in animals. In addition, human immunoglobulin loci have been engineered into mice in place of endogenous mouse sequences, resulting in the generation of human antibodies in mice.

The initial hybridoma culture contains a mixture of antibodies produced from many different primary B-lymph cyclones. Each secretes its specific antibody into the culture medium (i.e., the antibodies are still polyclone). Every single clone is separated into different wells of culture by dilution. It follows screening the cell culture medium for the specific antibody activity required from many additional wells. The correct B-lymphocytes grown from the positive wells were then recloned and retested for growth. The developed positive hybridomas and monoclonal antibodies can then be stored away in liquid nitrogen.

For example, laboratory animals (mammals, for example, mice) are first exposed to the antigen against which an antibody should be developed. Usually, this is done over several weeks through a series of injections of the antigen in question. Usually, these injections are followed using in vivo electroporation, which significantly increases the immune response. After isolation of splenocytes from the patient's spleen, the B cells are mixed with immortalized myeloma cells. Finally, the B cells are combined with

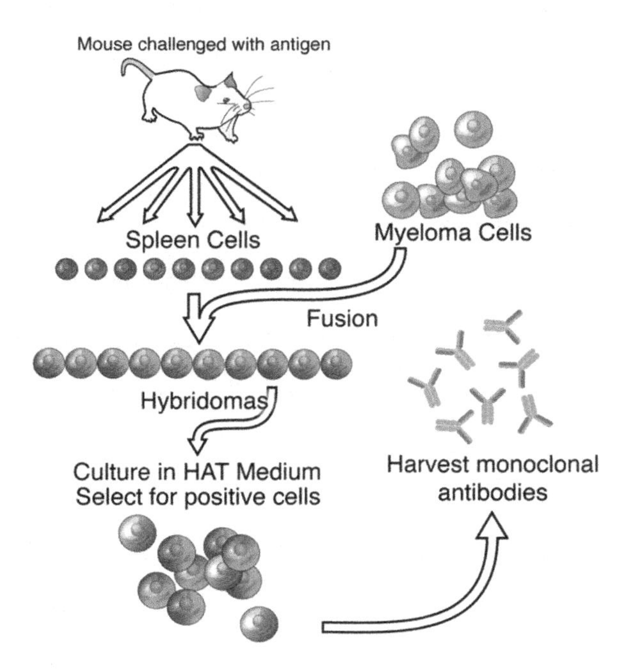

FIGURE 8.13 Hybridoma technology.

myeloma cells using electrofusion. Electrofusion causes the B cells and myeloma cells to align and fuse with the application of an electric field. Alternatively, chemical procedures can make the B cells and myelomas fuse using polyethylene glycol most of the time. The myeloma cells are chosen to ensure that they do not secrete the antibody themselves and lack the gene of hypoxanthine-guanine phosphoribosyltransferase (HGPRT), which renders them immune to the HAT (hypoxanthine-aminopterin-thymidine) medium.

The fused cells are incubated for approximately ten to 14 days in the HAT medium. Aminopterin blocks the pathway, which allows the synthesis of nucleotides. Unfused myeloma cells then die. They are not capable of producing nucleotides through a new or salvaged pathway because they lack HGPRT. It is necessary to remove the unfused myeloma cells because they can outgrow other cells, especially the weakly developed hybridomas. Unfused B cells die because their life span is short. Only the B cell–myeloma hybrids thus survive since the HGPRT gene from the B cells is functional. These cells produce antibodies (a B cell property) and are immortal (a myeloma cell property). The incubated medium is then diluted to such an extent into multi-well plates that each well contains only one cell. Because the antibodies in a well are produced by the same B cell, they are directed to the same epitope and are, therefore, monoclonal antibodies.

The next stage is a rapid primary screening process that identifies and selects only those hybridomas that produce specific antibodies. The method used for the first test is called ELISA. The supernatant hybridoma culture, secondary enzyme-labeled conjugate, and chromogenic substrate are then incubated, and the formation of a colored product indicates a positive hybridoma. Alternatively, immunocytochemical, western blot, and immunoprecipitation–mass spectrometry screening may also be used. In contrast to western blot assays, immunoprecipitation–mass spectrometry allows the screening and rating of clones that bind to the native (non-denatured) protein types.

To generate multiple identical daughter clones, other media containing interleukin-6 is required. When a hybridoma colony is established, it will continue to develop and produce antibodies in a culture medium containing antibiotics and fetal bovine serum. Multi-well plates are initially used to grow the hybridomas and are moved to larger tissue culture flasks after selection. It preserves the integrity of hybridomas and provides appropriate cells for cryopreservation and supernatant for subsequent investigations. The supernatant culture can yield 1 to 60 μg/ml of a monoclonal antibody, kept at –20° C or less until needed. Then, more analysis of a possible monoclonal antibody-forming hybridoma is performed for reactivity, specificity, and cross-reactivity by using culture supernatant or a pure immunoglobulin preparedness.

One of the major limitations of this technology was the sequence. The post-translational modifications of a monoclonal antibody generated in this method were of rodent origin, thereby rendering the molecule immunogenic in human patients, leading to the formation of human anti-mouse antibodies (HAMA). This led to significant advances in genetic engineering, leading to chimeric and humanized antibodies using phage display technology or transgenic mice. The mouse variable light and heavy chain sequences were grafted onto a human IgG scaffold or the exact complementarity determining regions (CDR) to yield chimeric antibodies and humanized antibodies.

The high-affinity human antibodies are obtained by further selecting hybridoma clones created from immunized transgenic mice, depending on the immunization protocol. The development of human neutralizing antibodies from human B cells has also yielded promising results for infectious disease therapies using a potentially similar approach.

8.4.4.2 Transgenic Mice

Several transgenic animals, including fully humanized mice and second-generation human chimeric mice, improve antibody drugs' quality. Human antibodies are acquired with a high affinity depending on the immunization regimen by selecting the animals' clones. Transgenic animals are further developed to achieve fully human mAbs. In 2006 the FDA approved the first human antibody developed in a transgenic mouse, panitumumab, an anti-epidermal growth factor receptor (EGFR). The number of entirely human antibodies made from transgenic mice increased, with the number of drugs currently approved at 19 (Table 3.1).

Transgenic animals provide a robust platform for the development of antibody drugs. Transgenic animals have several advantages over other human antibody production technologies, i.e., no need for humanization, more variety, maturation of in vivo affinity, and clonal selection to optimize the antibody. Nevertheless, the large size of human Ig loci is a problem in developing the transgenic mouse. Also, repertoire production in transgenic mice is comparable to those in humans includes diverse rearrangements combined with high expression of human segments V, D, and J. Different methods are used to generate animals that transmit human antibodies' repertoires to overcome these significant challenges. Given here is a listing of transgenic mice used in commercial products.

- Tetravalent Bispecific Tandem lg (TBTI) (similar to DVD-lg™) transgenic mice.
- Abgenix's XenoMouse® transgenic mice.
- Medarex's HuMAb-Mouse® transgenic mice.
- Medarex's UltiMAb® transgenic mice.
- Veloclmmune® transgenic mice.

8.4.5 Surface Display Libraries

According to surface display technology, exogenous proteins or peptides are expressed on the host (from the most straightforward virus to mammalian cells) by fusing exogenous genes with membrane protein genes or modifying proteins or peptides to be anchored by host surface elements. The main benefit of this technology is that it provides a quick way to link genotype and phenotype. It facilitates the research of proteins and peptides' affinity for their targets and protein functions as enzymes by saving the protein purification process. It is a handy drug discovery tool by high throughput screening for the proteins and peptides binding to a specific ligand and blocking their activities. Figure 8.14 shows the four types of libraries that can be constructed to produce antibodies. While Figure 8.14 shows that a library as a phage library can be produced using yeast, mRNA, and ribosomes, only the phage display has been used to develop currently approved antibodies. Each of these technologies has its advantages and disadvantages, as described in the following sections.

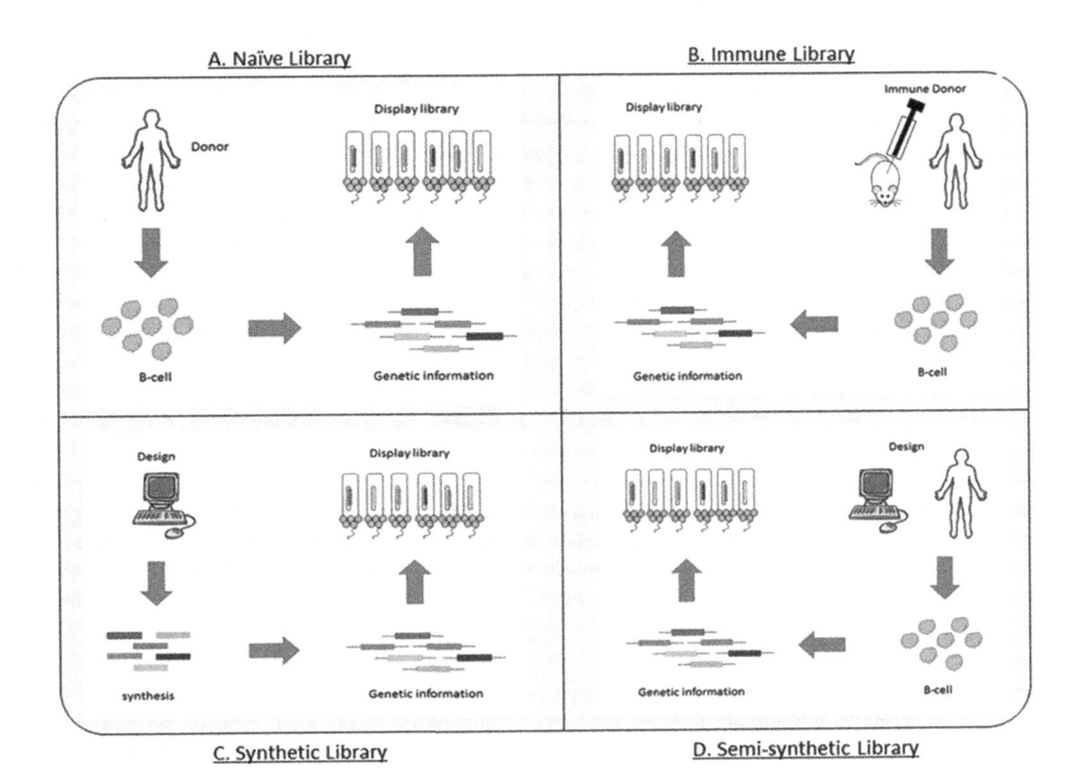

FIGURE 8.14 Types of libraries for making antibodies.

8.4.5.1 Phage Display

The invention of antibody phage displays revolutionized antibody drug discovery. Phage display has been widely used in protein or antibody characterization and, most importantly, antibody discovery since the invention of phage display technology in 1985 by G Smith and the publication of the first collection of antibody libraries displayed on phages in 1990. The conventional generate antibodies require immunization of host animals and subsequent complicated purification steps. Also, the antibodies in clinical applications must be of human origin. It is not practical to immunize humans with specific antigens, so downstream sequencing and humanization of animal-origin antibodies are required, which are usually costly and bring unpredictable results (Figure 8.15).

Alternatively, phage display-based antibodies screening can circumvent these problems but requires the establishment of antibody libraries. The libraries' sources include nonimmunized human B cells, antigen immunized human or animal B cells, and in vitro gene synthesis by randomizing various V(D)J genes of humans. Recombination is the somatic recombination mechanism that occurs only in developing lymphocytes during the early stages of T and B cell maturation. Thus, it results in the highly diverse repertoire of antibodies or immunoglobulins and T cell receptors found in B cells and T cells, respectively. The gene pool is then subcloned into phage display vectors and transformed into appropriate bacteria to harvest the phage libraries. Afterward, the library is subject to several rounds of affinity panning for collecting the specific antigen-binding antibodies displayed on the phage. Then, the monoclonal antibodies are identified by ELISA, sequenced, and cloned into mammalian cells such as CHO for large-scale production.

These libraries consist of variable heavy and light chains and antibody fragments' single event variables (scFv- wherein the V_H and V_L are connected using a polypeptide linker). The antibody fragments fuse to the surface protein (e.g., PIII or PVIII) and are displayed on the bacteriophage (e.g., M13). The antibodies are selected by a process called panning (based on the affinity for the antigen). Multiple

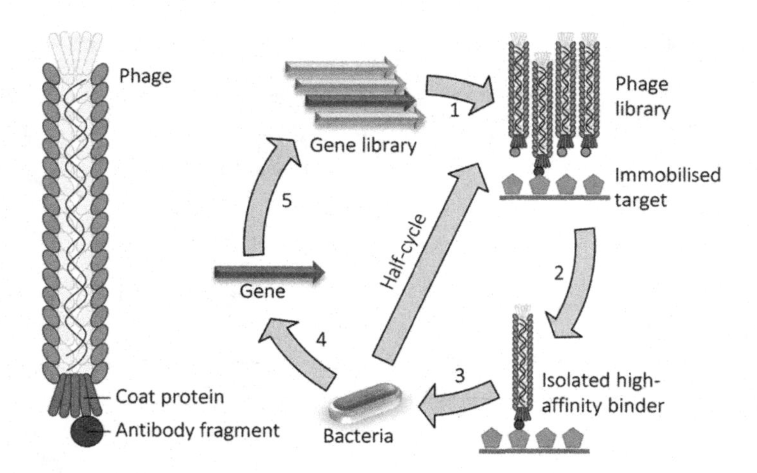

FIGURE 8.15 Phage display library. Phage or bacteriophage is a kind of virus with DNA or RNA encapsulated by coat proteins. They can infect bacteria as a host to insert their genes into the bacteria genome and produce coat proteins and genes to reform phage particles in the cytoplasm followed by secretion into the periplasm. The plasmid that can produce phages after transformation into bacteria is called phagemid. When exogenous genes are inserted into a phagemid and transform into bacteria, phages with exogenous proteins/peptides displayed on the capsid will be produced. A phagemid is a plasmid with an f1 replication origin from an f1 phage. When combined with filamentous phage M13, it can be used as a type of cloning vector. A phagemid can be replicated as a plasmid and packaged as single-stranded DNA in viral particles. The common phages used are *E. coli* filamentous bacteriophages (f1, fd, M13), through T4, T7, and λ phage. Bacteriophage (phage) is a virus capable of infecting and replicating bacteria and archaea by injecting it into the host (bacteria). Phage is made up of proteins that encapsulate a genome of DNA or RNA and can have relatively simple or complicated structures.

rounds of panning may be performed to enrich antigen-specific antibody fragment phages. The selected monoclonal Ab is then cloned into an appropriate vector followed by transfection into a suitable host cell to produce antibodies.

Phage display involves isolating B-lymphocytes from human blood, isolating the mRNA, and converting it to cDNA using PCR to amplify all VH and VL segments. These portions are then be cloned into a vector next to a bacteriophage's PIII protein (usually as scFv) before infecting *E. coli* to build a library containing approximately 10^{10} cells inoculating the library with a supplementary support phage. The most common bacteriophages used in phage displays are M13 and fd filamentous phage, T4, T7, and λ phage. *E. coli* can then secrete the bacteriophage that includes VH and VL segments as part of the bacteriophage coat. Different segments of VH and VL may then be selected against the antigen used to re-inoculate *E. coli.* Then cells that contain the plasmid are isolated and sequenced. Once the library is built, it is used to generate new antibodies. Thus, it does not need to be rehabilitated. No immunizations are needed as the entire process is performed in vitro. Antibodies are generated much faster than traditional hybridoma technology, particularly where toxic antigens cannot be used to vaccinate.

Gene repertoires are obtained from naïve or immunized animals for phage display libraries, or the libraries are constructed synthetically using randomized CDR sequences within fixed frames. Phage display naive antibody libraries are built from IgM repertoires with rearranged V genes. Because the gene sequences are derived from human donor B cells, the naive libraries are relatively close to the human antibody's germline with a low risk of immunogenicity. An immunized library's key advantage over a naïve library is that in vivo antibody genes have undergone natural affinity maturation in the immunized library, allowing the development of high-affinity antibodies against the target. However, this approach requires that the antigen of interest successfully induce immunogenic responses to prepare new libraries for each new target. Single and naïve, and synthetic libraries have yielded high affinity (sub-nanomolar size) antibodies against many targets.

Below is a general protocol followed in phage display screening to identify polypeptides that bind with high affinity to the desired target protein or DNA sequence:

1. Immobilized proteins or DNA sequences are immobilized in microtiter plate wells.
2. In a bacteriophage library, many genetic sequences are expressed fused with the bacteriophage coat protein. They are visible on the viral particle's surface. The protein on display corresponds to the phage's genetic sequence.
3. The phage-display library is added to the dish, and the dish is washed after the phage has had time to bind.
4. All but the phage-displaying proteins that interact with the target molecules stay on the dish while the rest is washed away.
5. The attached phage are eluted and used to infect suitable bacterial hosts to produce more phage. The new phage forms an enriched mixture, with far fewer non-binding (i.e., irrelevant) phages than the original mixture.
6. Steps 3 to 5 can be repeated one or more times to increase the phage library's binding protein content.
7. The DNA of the interacting phage is sequenced after more bacterial-based amplification to identify the interacting proteins or protein fragments.
8. To produce a protein or antibody in large quantities, the gene encoding the binding to a target protein is sequenced and inserted into a recombinant expression system such as CHO.

Antibody libraries displaying millions of different antibodies on phage are used in the pharmaceutical industry to isolate highly specific therapeutic antibody leads for developing antibody drugs primarily as anticancer or anti-inflammatory therapeutics. For example, Adalimumab is the first fully human antibody that is an anti-tumor necrosis factor α (TNFα) antibody approved by the FDA in 2002 for rheumatoid arthritis. Until now, the FDA has approved nine human antibody drugs generated by phage display.

Databases and computational tools for mimotopes are an important part of the phage display study. Databases, programs, and web servers are widely used to exclude target-unrelated peptides, characterize small molecules–protein interactions, and map protein–protein interactions. Developers use a three-dimensional structure of a protein and the peptides selected from the phage display experiment to map conformational epitopes. Many of the fast and efficient computational methods are available online.

A list of selected libraries includes:

- ADAPTIR™ Bispecific Platform and ADAPTIR™ Monospecific Platform antibody phage display libraries.
- Cambridge Antibody Technology (CAT) human antibody phage display library.
- Dyax human antibody phage display library.
- MorphoSys's HuCAL® phage library.
- Azymetric™ human G1-kappa Fab combinatorial phage display library.
- POTELLIGENT® technology (afucosylation) phage display guided selection.

Table 8.6 lists commercial platforms available for phase display development.

Developing drugs depends heavily on obtaining patent protection for products and technologies while avoiding patents issued to others. Consequently, intellectual property rights for sites for phage-display antibody discovery form a changing landscape that significantly affects drug development. All patents relating to phage display technologies have expired, including the critical patents of Breitling/Dübel (EP0440147), McCafferty/Winter (EP0774511, EP0589877), phage antibody libraries for Dyax, and Cambridge Antibody Technologies.

8.4.5.2 Yeast Display

Yeast display, bacterial display, ribosome display, and mRNA display are competing methods for in vitro protein evolution.

Exogenous proteins or peptides are expressed on the cell surface by being linked or anchored to the yeast cell wall composition, as shown in the yeast display. Exogenous genes are fused with cell

TABLE 8.6

Commercial Display Phage Platforms

ABDEG™
Affinity matured from palivizumab
BiTE® (Bispecific T Cell Engager) technology
Chimeric antigen receptor (CAR) T cell engineering
CrossMAb technology
DARPin®
Dual Variable Domain Immunoglobulin (DVD-lg™)
Dual-Affinity Re-Targeting (DART®)
EBV immortalization GPEx®
GlycoExpress™ GlycoMAb®
Glutamine synthetase GS Gene Expression System™ i-body
Glymax technology (defucosylation)
Human hybridoma
Humaneering® technology
Humanization by CDR grafting
Hybridoma of BALB/c
LAPSCOVERY™
MORPHODOMA®
n-CoDeR®
Nanobody®
No glycosylation site CH2 N84.4>A
PENTRA® stable scFv
PETizationTM
SIMPLE antibody ™
Triomab® (Trifunctional Ab)
Trustworthy Human™ antibody discovery platform
VelociGene®
XOMA Metabolism (XMet) platform
XmAb® Antibody Engineering Technology
YB2/0 cell line: low fucosylation (www.groupe-lfb.com/en/innovation/technology-platforms/emabling/)
ZMapp™

wall protein genes to accomplish this, with Aga2p being the most commonly used for antibody display. Aga2p, a member of the yeast agglutinins protein family involved in mating, is anchored to the cell surface by two disulfide bonds with Agalp. Aga2p is relatively far from the cell wall because it is one advantage of using it as the fusion protein. Thus, the fused antibodies are more flexible in space, preventing steric hindrance from reducing activity. Another benefit is that Aga2p is expressed after cell growth under the control of the GAL1 promoter, protecting yeast cells from potentially toxic antibodies and ensuring that all antibodies in the library are displayed. Antigen-coated magnetic beads are used to screen yeast with antibodies or other proteins displaying, followed by several rounds of FACS screening to find antibody/proteins with desirable properties.

Yeast display is widely used in the fermentation industry, in addition to its use in antibody discovery. In the fermentation system, yeast cells with the entire enzyme or the enzyme activity site are used. Yeast display aided fermentation has advantages over traditional methods that use purified enzymes, such as lower enzyme costs, easier fermentation control, and a simpler downstream purification step.

Yeast display has advantages over phage display in some respects, while it also has some drawbacks.

1. Yeast display is suitable for FACS (fluorescence-activated cell sorting) in the screening/panning step, allowing precise sorting of antibodies with desired binding properties. However, by adjusting the washing buffer compositions, antibodies' affinity for antigens in phage display can only be roughly stratified.

2. Because of its eukaryotic expression system, yeast-displayed antibodies can be folded correctly and modified, such as through glycosylation, closer to their native structure in mammals than phage-displayed antibodies.
3. Due to yeast's low transformation efficiency, the diversity of displayed antibodies may be lower than that of phages (107–109 for yeast, up to 1,011 for phages).
4. The yeast display system can select low-affinity antibodies based on antibody avidity because of many more antibodies on the yeast's surface (104–105) than on that of a phage.

8.4.5.3 Ribosome Display

Ribosome display is a technique for in vitro protein evolution that results in proteins that can bind to a specific ligand. The process produces translated proteins and their mRNA progenitor, which are used together in a selection step to bind to an immobilized ligand. The mRNA-protein hybrids that bind well are reverse-transcribed to cDNA, and their sequences are amplified using PCR. The result is a nucleotide sequence that can be used to make proteins that bind tightly. A native library of polypeptide-coding DNA sequences is used to start ribosome display. In vitro, each sequence is transcribed and converted to a polypeptide. The DNA library coding for a library of binding proteins, on the other hand, is genetically fused to a spacer sequence that ends without a stop codon. The absence of a stop codon prevents release factors from binding and triggering the disassembly of the translational complex. As a result, the spacer sequence remains attached to the peptidyl tRNA and occupies the ribosomal tunnel, allowing the protein of interest to protrude and fold. A complex of mRNA, ribosome, and protein binds to a surface-bound ligand as a result. The addition of cations like Mg2+ and lowering the temperature stabilizes this complex.

The complex is introduced to a surface-bound ligand during the subsequent binding or panning, stages. This can be done in various ways, including using an affinity chromatography column with a ligand-containing resin bed, a 96-well plate with an immobilized surface-bound ligand, or magnetic beads coated with the ligand. First, the well-binding complexes are immobilized. The binders are then eluted with high salt concentrations, chelating agents, or mobile ligands that complex with the protei's binding motif, allowing the mRNA to be dissociated. The mRNA can then be reverse transcribed into cDNA, mutated, and fed back into the process, increasing selective pressure to isolate even better binders.

Because the protein progenitor is attached to the complex, the ribosome display processes avoid the microarray, peptide bead, or multiple-well sequence separation that is common in nucleotide hybridization assays, and provide a ready way to amplify the proteins that do bind without having to decrypt the sequence until it is needed. Simultaneously, this method relies on creating large, concentrated pools of sequence diversity with no gaps and preventing these sequences from degrading, hybridizing, or reacting with one another in ways that would result in sequence-space gaps.

The coupling of genotype (RNA, DNA) and phenotype is required for selecting proteins from libraries (protein). This link is established in ribosome display by stabilizing the complex consisting of the ribosome, the mRNA, and the nascent correctly folded polypeptide during in vitro translation. As a result, the ribosomal complexes can bind to a target that has been immobilized on the surface. Non-bound complexes are washed away, but mRNA from complexes that have a binding polypeptide can be recovered. As a result, the binding polypeptides' genetic information is available for analysis.

8.4.5.4 mRNA Display

In vitro protein and peptide evolution using mRNA, the display is used to create molecules that can bind to the desired target. The process produces puromycin-linked translated peptides or proteins that are linked to their mRNA progenitor. In a selection step, the complex binds to an immobilized target (affinity chromatography). The mRNA-protein fusions that bind well are reverse transcribed to cDNA, and their sequences are amplified using a polymerase chain reaction. As a result, a nucleotide sequence is generated that encodes a peptide with a high affinity for the target molecule.

Puromycin is a tyrosyl-tRNA analog with a part of its structure that resembles an adenosine molecule. The other half looks like a tyrosine molecule. Puromycin has a non-hydrolyzable amide bond, unlike the cleavable ester bond in tyrosyl-tRNA. Puromycin interferes with translation. As a result, causing translation products to be released prematurely.

Puromycin is present at the 3' end of the mRNA templates used in mRNA display technology. The ribosome moves along the mRNA template as translation progresses. The fused puromycin will enter the ribosome's A site and be incorporated into the nascent peptide once it reaches the 3' end of the template. The ribosome then releases the mRNA-polypeptide fusion.

Making an mRNA-polypeptide fusion requires more than just adding fused puromycin to the mRNA template. Puromycin must be recruited along with oligonucleotides and other spacers for puromycin to enter the A site with enough flexibility and length.

Even though both ribosome display and mRNA display are in vitro selection methods, mRNA display has a few advantages over ribosome display. mRNA display makes use of puromycin-linked covalent mRNA-polypeptide complexes, whereas ribosome display makes use of stalled, noncovalent ribosome-mRNA-polypeptide complexes. Because ribosome-mRNA-polypeptide complexes are noncovalent, ribosome-mRNA-polypeptide complexes must be kept in a complex for ribosome display. This could make reducing background binding during the selection cycle more difficult. In a ribosome display system, polypeptides are attached to a massive rRNA-protein complex, a ribosome with a molecular weight of more than 2,000,000 Da. It's possible that the selection target and the ribosome will interact unpredictably, resulting in the loss of potential binders during the selection cycle.

The puromycin DNA spacer linker used in mRNA display technology, on the other hand, is a fraction of the size of a ribosome. As a result, this linker may have a lower chance of interacting with a selection target that is immobilized. As a result, mRNA display technology is more likely to produce less skewed results.

8.4.6 Recombinant Expression

Once the antibody has been identified, its commercial manufacturing platform is primarily recombinant expression with one exception (Figure 8.16).

Recombinant DNA technology comprises these steps:

1. Clone heavy chain and light chain and generate the full-length cDNA from the respective mRNA (e.g., cDNA libraries, synthetic gene synthesis).
2. Ligate the gene of interest into the expression vector (expression vector is designed to have elements that will enable expression in the host cell).
3. Then produce the plasmid in competent *E. coli* cells (via transformation).
4. Extract and purify the recombinant plasmid DNA to transfer it into a suitable host cell for production (CHO, HEK, etc.).
5. In the presence of a selectable marker, select positive clones and further screen them for productivity, protein quality, etc., to establish the cell line for producing the protein of interest.

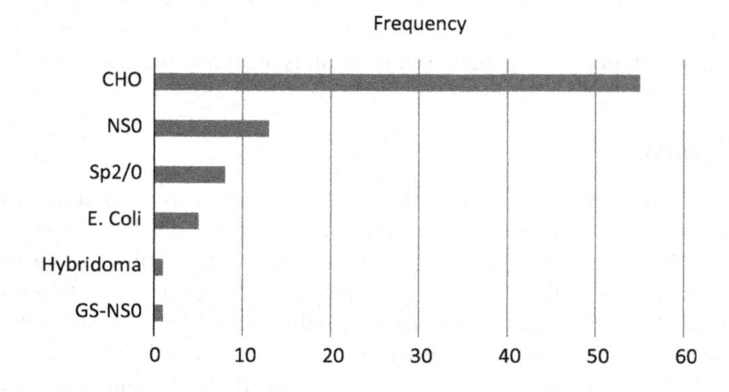

FIGURE 8.16 Expression system used for commercial manufacturing of approved antibodies.

The development of monoclonal antibodies from single human B cells is based on analysis of the immunoglobulin gene's repertoire and reactivity at the single-cell level by applying reverse transcription-polymerase chain reaction (RT-PCR) and expression vector cloning. mAbs are large multimeric proteins (typical molecular weight, approximately 150 kilodaltons, and their proper functioning require several post-translational modifications, including glycosylation and disulfide bond formation. As a result, a eukaryotic production system is used, which includes normal eukaryotic post-translational modifications.

The use of cultured cells, such as CHO cells, is the most common method of producing mAb. However, alternative eukaryotic cell lines for mAb production, such as yeast, which grows faster than mammalian cells, are considered.

8.5 Immunogenicity

Every living species is endowed with a system of protecting it against foreign agents and those that can cause harm. This is part of our internal pharmacy that has helped us survive millions of years of evolution. The immune system comprises an innate system and an adaptive system, both containing humoral and cellular activity.

The humoral system or antibody-mediated beta cellular immunity involves macromolecules in extracellular fluids—antibodies, complement proteins, and antimicrobial peptides—("Humor" refers to body fluids). Humoral immunity involves antibodies, activation of cytokines, isotype switching, germinal center formation, cell generation, and affinity maturation. Additionally, it includes the effector function of antibodies, including toxic and pathogen neutralization, opsonin promotion of phagocytosis, and complement activation.

The word "antigen" means an *anti*body *gen*erator molecule, which provokes an adaptive immune response. Antigens are structural molecules or fragments of molecules that bind specifically to antibodies and are recognized by adaptive immune system antigen receptors (B cell receptor or T cell receptor). Antigens bind to the immune response components such as lymphocytes and their receptors, antibodies, and T cell receptors. Antigens do not elicit the immune response without the help of an immunologic adjuvant. Most commonly, antigens are proteins or polysaccharides, and less often, lipids coming from the cell walls, coats, capsules, flagella, toxins, or fimbriae of pathogens. Nucleic acids and lipids become antigenic only when they are combined with proteins and polysaccharides. Besides the sources being pathogens, antigens can be egg white, pollen, proteins from transplanted tissues, or elements of the surface of transfused blood cells. An excellent example of antigens is vaccines administered to induce an immune response. Antibodies are designed or produced to interact with antigens based on the antibody's complementary determining region.

T cell receptor (TCR) recognition must be processed into small fragments inside the cell and presented to a T cell receptor by a major histocompatibility complex (MHC). For example, a hapten is a small molecule attached to a large carrier molecule, such as a protein, to become antigenic.

The immune system is generally not reactive against the antigens produced in the body called self or endogenous but primarily against the non-self or exogenous sources. However, there are many exceptions to the differentiation between exogenous or endogenous proteins. An excellent example of this is found in the body's autoimmune response in treating type 1 diabetes, resulting from an autoimmune reaction that develops against pancreatic β-cells.

Cells present their antigenic structures through a histocompatibility molecule to the immune system, activating several immune cells. Other attributes of antigens and immunogens are their high molecular weight, molecular complexity, and the degradability of antigens to fragments that can bond "MHC" ("major histocompatibility complex") proteins (or MHC antigens) on the surface of the APC ("antigen-presenting cell") and this whole complex then binds to T cells. Carbohydrate antigens are not processed or presented as they can bind to B cells directly and activate them to produce antibodies. The route of immunization determines the nature of responses; for instance, antigens that encounter mucous membranes generally induce one type of antibodies, whereas intramuscular and intravenous immunization often induces a different type.

8.5.1 Protein Immunogenicity

A therapeutic protein, recombinant or otherwise, can be immunogenic because the human immune system categorizes it as non-self. A protein injected into patients will be taken up by antigen-presenting cells and processed into smaller peptides. T cells generated in the thymus can bind to the peptides presented in the grooves of major histocompatibility complex molecules on the surface of antigen-presenting cells. When the T cells recognize these peptides as foreign, they induce B cell proliferation. B and T cells are both parts of the adaptive immune system; however, B cells interact directly with the protein owing to the immunoglobulins present on their cell surfaces. After binding to the protein's specific three-dimensional structure, activated B cells recruit the complement system and macrophages from the innate immune system to destroy and remove the antigen. Such an immune response against a foreign protein is called a classical immune response, which typically leads to the production of high-affinity antibodies of different isotypes and memory cells responsible for an enhanced response upon repeated challenge with the antigen (the principle behind vaccination).

This immune response may have severe consequences, from a simple tolerance reaction to therapeutic inefficiency when the antibodies are neutralizing type. Antibodies produced against therapeutic proteins like erythropoietin (EPO), hematopoietic growth factors (GM-CSF), and thrombopoietin and megakaryocyte (TPO/MGDF) may have big consequences to the point of blocking not only the exogenous protein's activity but also of the endogenous protein with the serious complications inherent in these actions.

The production of antibodies against biotechnology-derived proteins like insulin, factor VIII or IX, or interferons, does not have the same severe consequences, and treatments continue in the presence of the antibodies, adapting the doses of a therapeutic protein. Generally, if the immunogenicity is not related to any change in the disposition (PK/PD) profile, there is no change to the dose.

The consequences of antibodies produced against monoclonal antibodies have been observed since their first use, mainly when derived from animal or bacterial proteins. The reactions observed could be of a general order, such as systemic reactions during these products' injection, local reactions, or reactions of acute hypersensitivity (generally not due to the antibodies). The immune reactions of anaphylactic type or allergic reactions are rare because of the better purification of proteins produced by recombinant DNA technology and the humanization of monoclonal antibodies' protein skeletons. The production of neutralizing antibodies may correspond to several types of mechanisms like direct bonding to a biological activity site or a site that is not directly related but impedes its activity by a changed structural conformation. The non-neutralizing antibodies bind to the therapeutic protein site without affecting the biological activity site. Suppose they don't directly neutralize the biological target. In that case, they may change the drug's bioavailability by increasing the bonding complex's clearance identical to biological activity neutralization.

When a biological medicine product is immunogenic, its repeated administration to patients over an extended period generally enhances the risk of raising antibodies that can induce anaphylaxis, alter the protein's pharmacokinetic properties, or inhibit binding the drug to its target receptor rendering the protein ineffective. Anaphylaxis is caused by an immediate allergic reaction mediated by immunoglobulin E (IgE) antibodies against the product. An immune response with high titers of neutralizing IgG antibodies strongly decreases the therapeutic activity of the protein. Another possible life-threatening clinical consequence of antibody formation is cross-reactivity with the endogenous protein produced by the patient.

Immunogenicity is a problem only when it is clinically relevant—when it influences the therapeutic protein's safety or efficacy. Clinically relevant immunogenicity includes when antibodies change how the drug reacts in the body, when antibodies make the protein less therapeutically effective, when antibodies change natural proteins in the body, or when antibodies trigger a severe allergic reaction rare. Clinically relevant immunogenicity is not common but must be monitored for all therapies.

The safety of drugs is one of the main concerns and considerations in their development. These concerns have arisen because of the inherent nature of proteins that can cause pronounced effects like immunogenicity responses. However, not all biological drugs demonstrate immune response, and in fact, many have less risk of immunogenicity than even food proteins. Nevertheless, in all regulatory filings, the developer must demonstrate that manufacturing does not produce any structural changes that can be immunogenic; one such factor is the aggregation of proteins, which is a common outcome of these drugs' manufacturing.

The standards used by the regulatory agencies have changed over the last few decades, tightening the safety requirements significantly. If aspirin were discovered today, it would likely not be approved for headaches. The regulatory agencies provide specific definitions for adverse drug reactions and side effects. According to MHRA (the UK agency), the adverse drug reactions (ADRs) or adverse drug effects (ADEs) are a noxious and unintended response to a drug that occurs at normal therapeutic doses used in humans for prophylaxis, diagnosis, or therapy of disease, or the modification of physiologic function. The word "effect" is used interchangeably with "reaction." There are several types of ADRs:

- Type A: Exaggerated pharmacological response, such as pharmacodynamics effect (e.g., bronchospasm from beta-blockers) or toxic response (e.g., deafness from aminoglycoside overdose).
- Type B: Non-pharmacological, often allergic, response, drug-induced diseases (e.g., antibiotic-associated colitis), allergic reactions (e.g., penicillin anaphylaxis), idiosyncratic reactions (e.g., aplastic anemia with chloramphenicol).
- Type C: Continuous or long-term (time-related), such as osteoporosis with oral steroids.
- Type D: Delayed (lag time), teratogenic effects such as with anticonvulsants or lisinopril.
- Type E: Ending of use (withdrawal), such as withdrawal syndrome with benzodiazepines.
- Type F: Failure of efficacy (no response), such as resistance to antimicrobials.

Generally, the side effects are expected responses at normal doses related to the pharmacology of the molecule. Such effects may be well known and even expected and require little or no change in patient management. Drug reactions include all adverse events related to drug administration, regardless of etiology. They can be classified into two groups: immunologic etiology and non-immunologic etiology. Unpredictable effects cause about 20–25% of adverse drug reactions, both immune- and non-immune-mediated, whereas predictable non-immunological events cause 75–80% of adverse reactions.

8.5.2 Immunogenicity Testing

The most practical and commonly used approach for testing unwanted immunogenicity is detecting, measurement, and characterizing antibodies generated specifically against the product. It is anticipated that better models for evaluating immunogenicity will become available in the future and may include DNA microarrays. Generally, no single assay can provide all the necessary information on a biological product's immunogenicity profile. As a result, a panel of carefully selected and suitable assays for detecting and measuring antibodies is used. These antibody responses are then correlated with the PK/PD and clinical effects when evaluated to determine if the antibodies create a "meaningful difference" in determining their safety and efficacy. The testing plans are based on the risk assessment that goes through multiple stages, starting with a screening assay to determine the binding of biological medicine in serum samples of animals and humans. At this point, we are detecting anti-drug antibodies. This evaluation is then subjected to confirmation to ensure there are no false positives. Once established, anti-drug antibodies are characterized.

The human immune system has evolved with robust defense against infection and diseases in two different types: the innate immune system and the adaptive immune system, comprising many cell types from the hematopoietic stem cells located in the bone marrow. Lymphocytic and myeloid progenitors are produced by hematopoietic stem cells.

A mechanism for lymphocytes, inflammatory cells, and hematopoietic cells to communicate with one another is required to mount and coordinate an effective immune response. This function is carried out by cytokines. Cytokines are a large family of small proteins or glycoproteins with a wide range of functions (usually smaller than 30 kDa). Although they were first discovered for their immunomodulatory abilities, they have since been discovered to play other roles in developmental processes, such as cell differentiation and directed migration. Helper T cells (Th cells) and macrophages are the two main producers of cytokines, which influence both innate and adaptive immune responses. They can, however, be induced and secreted transiently by virtually all nucleated cells.

A particular cytokine's downstream effects occur through the high-affinity binding of its receptor expressed on a target cell's surface. This action may occur in an autocrine (acts on the same cell), paracrine (acts on nearby cell), or endocrine (acts on the distant cell; not the normal manner for cytokine responses) manner. Receptor engagement triggers intracellular signaling cascades leading to altered gene expression in the target cell, which leads to a biological effect. After cytokine stimulation, the target cell undergoes differentiation, proliferation, and activation, among other things.

Hematopoietic stem cells produce self-renewal cytokines SCF and TPO and expansion

Basophils are the largest granulocytes, with bi-lobed nuclei and histamine-rich granules, despite being the least common. Basophils play a role in a wide range of inflammatory reactions, including those that cause allergic symptoms. Skin, lungs, and intestines come into contact with the environment outside the body. DCs are the most efficient APCs because they process, present, and cross-present antigens to T and B cells. They can also secrete cytokines like IL-6, IL-10, and IL-12 when activated.

Macrophages are phagocytic scavengers that ingest and process a wide range of unwanted materials that are not found in healthy cells, such as cellular debris, pathogens, and cancer cells. They are tissue residents who have been given unique names based on their location.

Skin, lungs, and intestines come into contact with the environment outside the body. DCs are the most efficient APCs because they process, present, and cross-present antigens to T and B cells. When activated, they can also secrete cytokines like IL-6, IL-10, and IL-12.

Macrophages are phagocytic scavengers that ingest and process a wide range of unwanted materials that are not found in healthy cells, such as cellular debris, pathogens, and cancer cells. They are tissue residents who have been given unique names based on their location. M1 and M2 are the two major activated macrophages. M1 macrophages are pro-inflammatory, whereas M2 macrophages play a role in wound healing and tissue regeneration, and anti-inflammatory properties.

NK cells are cytotoxic cells with perforins and granzymes in their cytoplasm that kill their target cells. They are B and T lymphocytes produced from the common lymphoid progenitor, but they are part of the innate immune system. NK cells kill cancerous and infected cells in a flash, with no need for antigen-specific recognition or activation (Figure 8.17).

8.5.3 Innate System

The body's first line of defense, the innate immune system, provides a quick and broad immune response. On the other hand, the adaptive immune system works by detecting and eliminating specific pathogens that pose a threat to the body. While both systems work to combat infection, the adaptive immune system takes much longer than the innate immune system to respond.

Neutrophils, eosinophils, basophils (named after their staining characteristics), mast cells, and monocytes are all produced by myeloid progenitors, which can then be differentiated into dendritic cells (DCs) and macrophages. Mast cells are tissue-resident granulocytes that secrete histamine and heparin, and other substances involved in parasite defense, wound healing, and angiogenesis. Activated macrophages are divided to help heal wounds and protect against bacteria and viruses.

The cytotoxic NK cells have small granules in their cytoplasm that contain perforins and granzymes that kill their target cells. They come from the same lymphoid progenitor that gives rise to B and T lymphocytes.

8.5.4 Adaptive System

The ability to provide long-term memory is a feature of the adaptive immune system. In future encounters with a specific pathogen, this feature allows for a faster and more efficient immune response.

When activated, mature B cells differentiate into memory cells and plasma cells, which secrete pathogen-specific antibodies and play a key role in the protective immune response (Figure 8.18). (While B cells are generally considered B because of their sourcing from bone, the term was first used to refer to the bursa of Fabricius, the hematopoiesis site necessary for B cell [part of the immune system] development

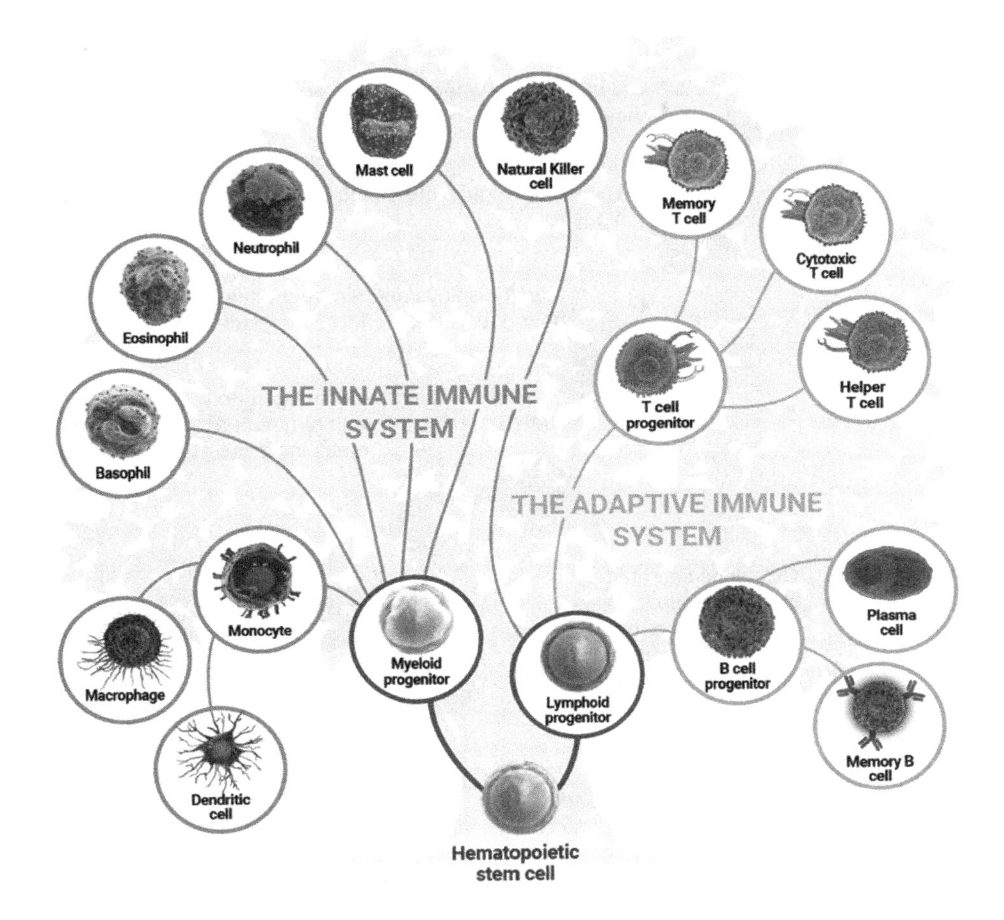

FIGURE 8.17 Innate and adaptive immune system cells. Source: lab-a-porter.com/2019/12/cells-of-the-immune-system/.

in birds.) B cells are one of three types of antigen-presenting cells in the body (APCs). The MHC (major histocompatibility complex) class I proteins are found on the surfaces of all nucleated cells in the body. On the other hand, MHC class II proteins and a variety of co-stimulatory molecules are commonly expressed on the surfaces of APCs such as macrophages, B cells, and dendritic cells. Class II MHC (major histocompatibility complex) cells activate T cells by displaying processed antigen peptide fragments.

Cellular crosstalk plays a vital role in the adaptive immune response, such as naïve B cells that require stimulation by CD4+ Th cells to mount an effective response to antigens. Activated cells, such as neutrophils secrete chemokines and cytokines, which cause crosstalk in the innate immune system. This activity has an impact on DC recruitment and activation.

Thus, the immune system's two arms work together via cellular crosstalk and chemical signals in the form of a comprehensive defense armamentarium.

8.6 Pharmacokinetics of Therapeutic Proteins

Pharmacokinetic profiling is an essential step in estimating therapeutic proteins' efficacy since this profile is subject to many physicochemical and biological factors that are not pertinent in the case of chemical drugs (Table 8.7).

The variances listed in Table 8.4 lead to disposition properties that are highly interdependent among the formulation, pharmacokinetics, and immunogenicity (Figure 8.19).

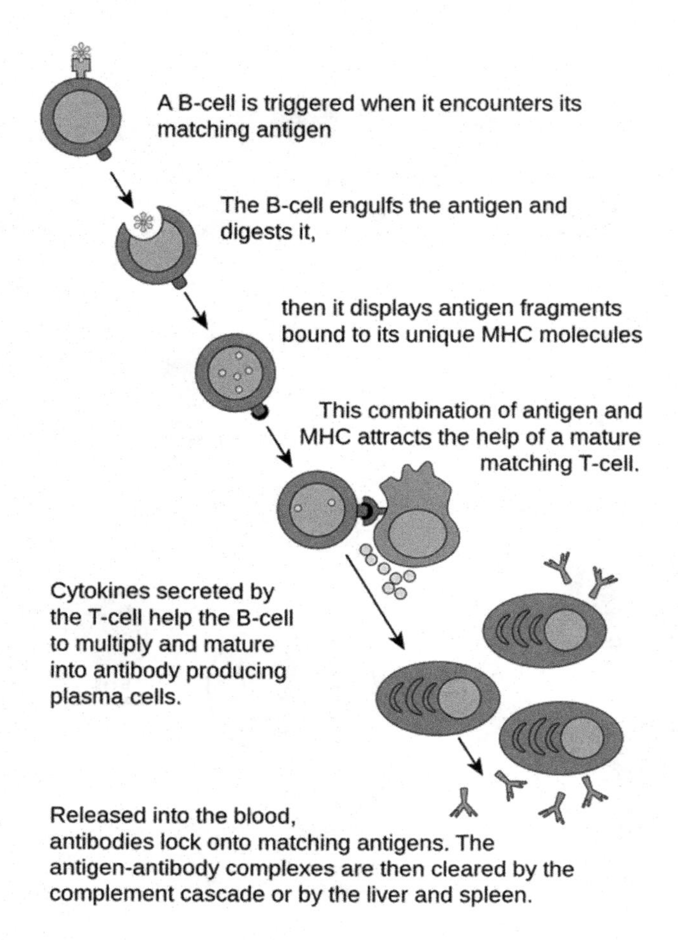

A B-cell is triggered when it encounters its matching antigen
The B-cell engulfs the antigen and digests it,
then it displays antigen fragments bound to its unique MHC molecules
This combination of antigen and MHC attracts the help of a mature matching T-cell.
Cytokines secreted by the T-cell help the B-cell to multiply and mature into antibody producing plasma cells.
Released into the blood, antibodies lock onto matching antigens. The antigen-antibody complexes are then cleared by the complement cascade or by the liver and spleen.

FIGURE 8.18 B cell activation and antibody production.

TABLE 8.7
Comparative Properties of Monoclonal Antibodies and Chemical Drugs Pertinent to PK and PD Profiles

mAb	New Chemical Entity
150,000 dalton	200–500 dalton
Biological production process—heterogeneous (post-translation modifications)	Chemical production process—homogeneous
High species selectivity (affinity/potency)	Generally less selective
Multi-functional—target binding, Fc effector function, FcRn binding	Single target
Toxicity—largely "on target" mediated "exaggerated pharmacology"	Toxicity—often "off target" mediated
Slow clearance; long half-life (days)—infrequent design (weekly/monthly)?	Rapid clearance; short half-life (hours)—frequent dosing (daily)
Target can affect PK behavior (target-mediated drug disposition)	Mostly linear PK; non-linearity from saturation of metabolic pathways
Drug–drug Interaction—few examples and mostly PD related	DDI—many examples and metabolic and/or PD related
Immunogenicity sometimes observed	Immunogenicity rarely observed

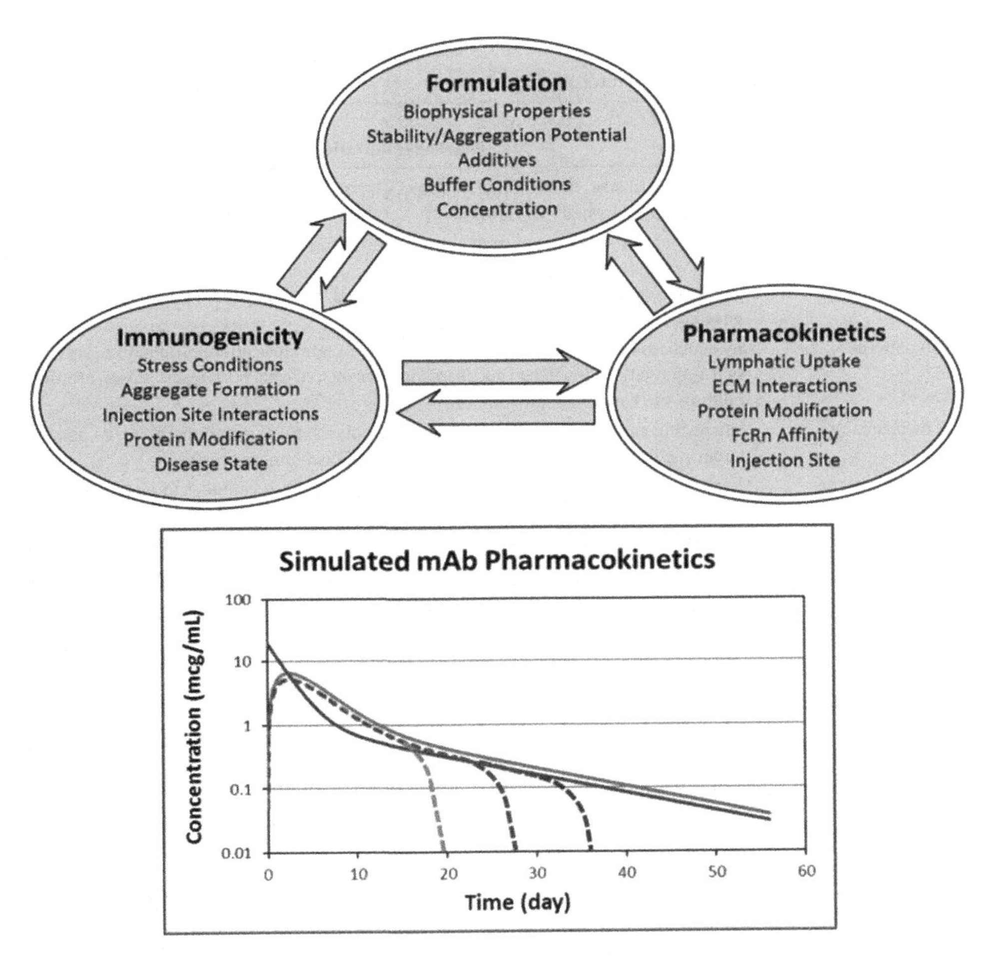

FIGURE 8.19 Interdependence of formulation and immunogenicity factors for monoclonal antibodies.

A summary of how pharmacokinetic parameters are affected is presented in Table 8.8.

8.6.1 Absorption

A comparison of the biological molecule and a chemical molecule's absorption is shown in Figure 8.20. While biological drugs are not administered orally, at least now, the comparison of entry into the body is limited to either subcutaneous or intravenous injection; many products are developed for inhalation therapy and other routes of administration. In subcutaneous administration, there is the possibility of interactions with extracellular materials and forming aggregates at the administration site, where the molecule can also undergo catabolism (conversion to smaller molecules) or metabolism. From this interstitial space, the molecules move into the lymphatic system, where they can further metabolize. For molecules less than 1,000 Da, the route is through capillaries, and for molecules with a molecular weight greater than 16,000, the route is strictly lymphatic. Finally, the molecules enter the circulation and to the tissue sites and interact with various receptors, some of which can prolong the half-life. As a general principle, the higher the molecular weight, the more delayed is the time to peak in the blood.

The lymphatic system is a one-way transport system for fluid and protein coming from interstitial space; the net flow rate of lymph is 100–500 times less than that of blood, resulting in delayed time for the peak concentration of the blood (Figure 8.20).

TABLE 8.8

ADME-Related Consideration and Key Determining Factors

ADME-Related Considerations	Key Determination Factors
Physicochemical properties	Large Mw and size, hydrophilicity, shape, charge, limited solubility, GI degradation, stability, heterogeneity in isoforms
Absorption mechanisms	Route of administration, convective transport through lymphatic vessels, diffusion across blood vessels, dose, injection site and volume, species differences, subject characteristics, pre-systemic metabolism/catabolism, FcRn- and target-dependent mechanisms, physicochemical properties
Distribution patterns	Physicochemical and binding properties, route of administration, production process, FcRn- and target-dependent mechanisms, convective transport, transcytosis, affinity, binding site barrier, inflamed tissues
Metabolic mechanisms	Nonspecific endocytosis, degradation by proteolysis, local metabolism, FcγR- and target-mediated clearance, ICs formation, physicochemical properties
Elimination mechanisms	Metabolism/catabolism, excretion, proteolysis, RES, Fc-receptor- and target-mediated clearance, nonspecific endocytosis and Ics formation followed by complement- or Fc receptor-mediated clearance, protection from catabolism via FcRn mechanism, binding affinities, physicochemical properties

Notes: ADME = absorption, distribution, metabolism, and excretion; MW = molecular weight; GI = gastrointestinal; FcRn = neonatal Fc receptor; ICs = immune-complexes; RES = reticuloendothelial system.

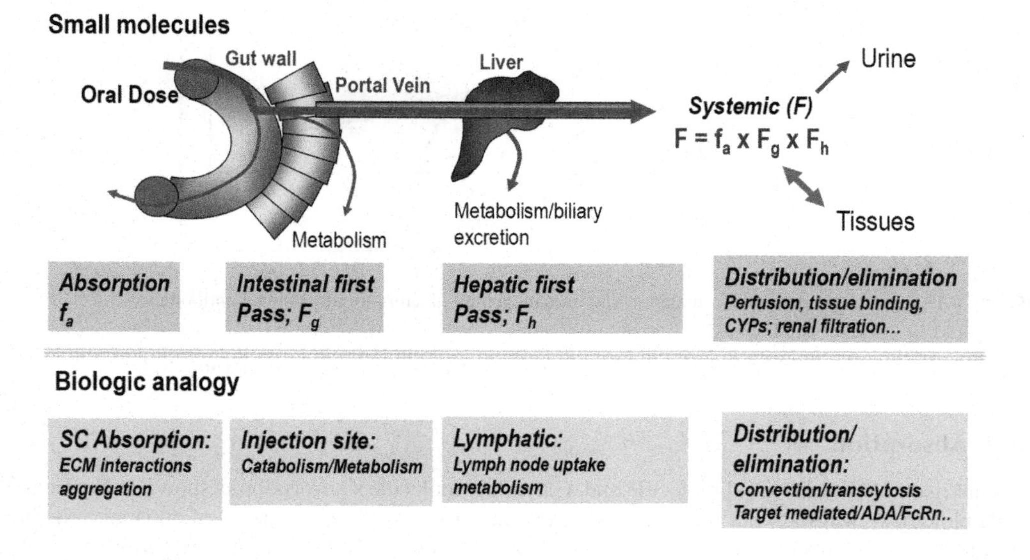

FIGURE 8.20 Uptake of small and large molecules.

Intravenous administration avoids all the steps before the distribution cycle.

Since the larger molecules can demonstrate immunogenicity during the absorption phase, the chances of immunogenicity are the highest for subcutaneous, followed by intramuscular and least with intravenous administration. For this reason, developing a drug with multiple routes of administration and the regulatory agencies require testing in the highest immunogenicity potential site first (Figure 8.21).

While they are administered by a parenteral route, their bioavailability can vary significantly (Table 8.9).

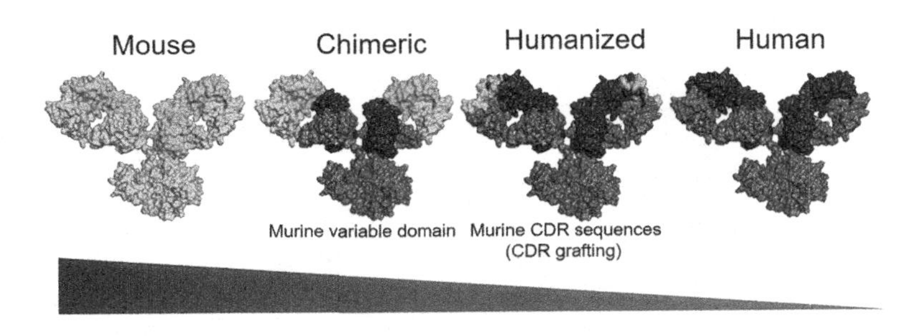

FIGURE 8.21 Types of antibodies and their immunogenicity potential. Source: www.scielo.br/scielo.php?script=sci_arttext&pid=S1984-82502018000700406.

TABLE 8.9
Immunogenicity and Bioavailability of Antibodies

Description/Target	BA (%)	Immunogenicity Rate (%)/ADA Development
Adalimumab	64%	SC 1–12%/NA
Infliximab	N/A	IV 10–27%/NA; SC 5–27%/low-titer
Rituximab	65%	IV 3–4% ADA, SC 2–18% non-nADA
Trastuzumab	77.1%	IV 8.1%/< 1% nADA; SC 14.9%/1–2% nADA
Alemtuzumab	N/A	IV 30–85%/ nADA; SC N/A
Interferon beta	27–50%	2–47% IV nADA; 45% SC; 5.3% IV vs. 16.3% SC nADA
Darbepoetin	30–50%	4%/non-nADA
Factor VIIa	20–30%	11%/non-nADA
Emicizumab	102.3%	4.2%/non-IgE
Etanercept	76%	6%/non-nADA
Abatacept	78.6%	5.8%/67% of those nADA
Insulin	40–100%	SC 14–44%/non-nADA

8.6.2 Distribution

The distribution of biological molecules is slow in tissues, involving two steps: extravasations from the blood circulation into interstitial space and then diffusion through the extracellular matrix to the cell surface target. The key mechanism of transport includes diffusion, convection, pinocytosis, and transcytosis that can be active or facilitated. Most pharmacokinetics estimate Vss (distribution volume at steady state) in a non-compartmental or mammillary model, but these calculations are not appropriate for biological drugs because of the complexity of the binding properties that do not create a steady state at any time. A linear pharmacokinetic profile is anticipated if there is no tissue metabolism; otherwise, the non-linear distribution and more common tissue metabolism require studies of physiology-based pharmacokinetic modeling.

In many diseases like cancer, tissues' vascularization is altered, affecting the distribution and disposition kinetics of biological drugs.

8.6.3 Elimination

The elimination kinetics is often nonlinear because of immune-mediated immunogenicity unique to biological drugs altering the disposition profile. One unique mechanism involved is the FcRN salvaging, a process of recirculating the antibodies, as shown in Figure 8.22. B lymphocytes, follicular dendritic

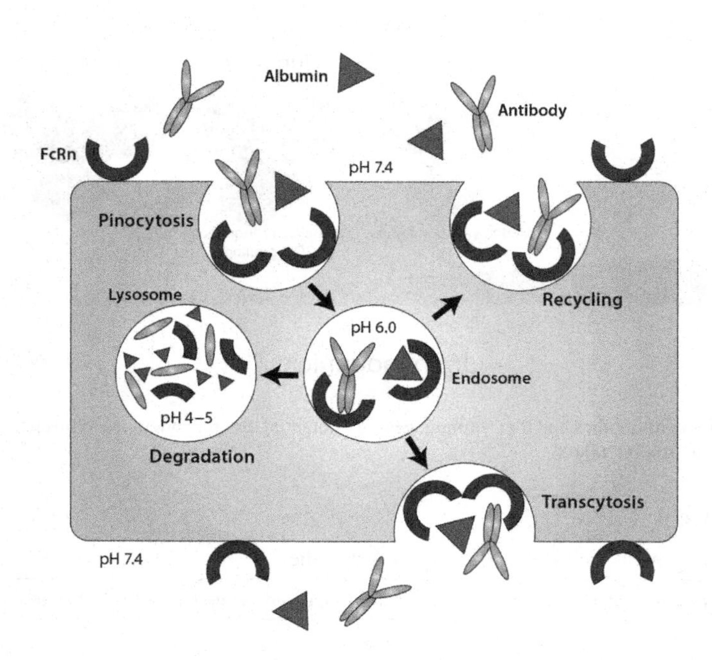

FIGURE 8.22 FcRn-mediated recycling of IgG and albumin in vascular endothelial cells; IgG and albumin are internalized into vascular endothelial cells through pinocytosis. The pH of the endosome is 6.0, facilitating association with membrane-bound FcRn. Endosomes' contents can be processed in two ways: either recycling back to the apical cell membrane or transcytosis from the apical to the basolateral side. In the case of saturated receptors, excess IgG and albumin are degraded by lysosomes. Top, apical side; bottom, basolateral side. Source: Weimer, T et al. *Recombinant Albumin Fusion Proteins: Fusion Protein Technologies for Biopharmaceuticals*. Schmidt S, ed. Hoboken, NJ: John Wiley and Sons; 2013; 163–178.

TABLE 8.10

Methods of Extending Residence of Antibodies in the Body

Strategy	Mechanism	Effect
Fc-fusion, monomeric Fc and CH domains, and albumin fusion	Hijacking FcRn recycling, increasing molecular weight	Half-life extension by reducing catabolism and renal clearance
IgG-Fc or albumin engineering	Increased mAb/albumin affinity for FcRn at pH 6	Half-life extension by reducing catabolism
Fusion to alternate FcRn binding ligands	Hijacking FcRn recycling	Half-life extension by reducing catabolism

cells, natural killer cells, macrophages, neutrophils, eosinophils, basophils, human platelets, and mast cells all have Fc receptors on their surfaces, which help the immune system protect itself.

Several techniques can be used to exploit this property to prolong the stay of the drug in the body (Table 8.10).

The primary receptors mediating hepatic uptake of proteins include the following receptors internalizing ligands through the endocytic pathway for lysosomal degradation.

- Asialoglycorotein receptors (ASGPRs) recognize galactose and N-acetylgalactosamine and primarily express on hepatocytes (used for targeting).
- Mannose receptors recognize terminal mannose, glucose, and N-acetylglucosamine and express on Kupfer cells and macrophages, and endothelial and dendritic cells.

Renal elimination is primarily filtration, and since the glomerular filter is negatively caged, anionic molecules and repelled and not filtered. However, it applies only to molecules smaller than 69 kDa, and

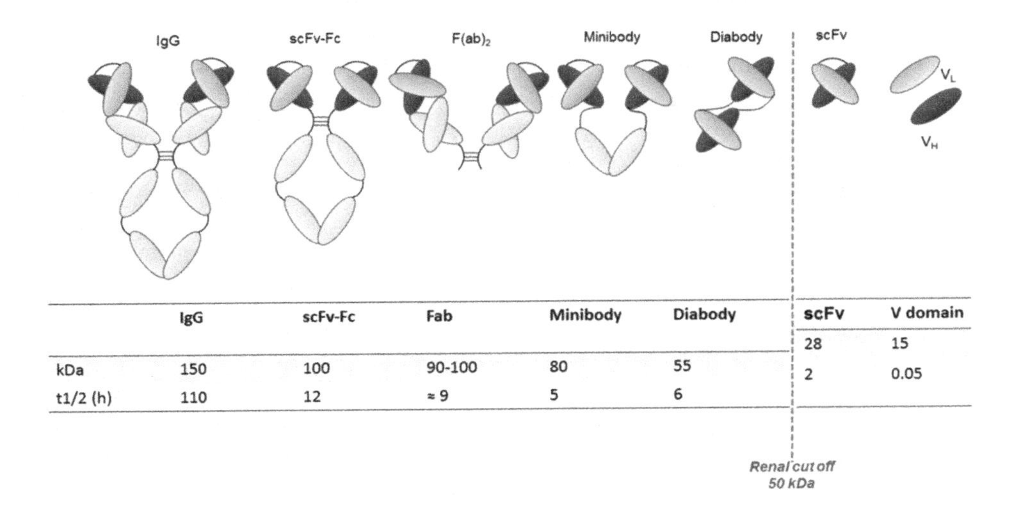

	IgG	scFv-Fc	Fab	Minibody	Diabody	scFv	V domain
kDa	150	100	90-100	80	55	28	15
t1/2 (h)	110	12	≈ 9	5	6	2	0.05

FIGURE 8.23 Antibody formats and half-life. Source: www.mdpi.com/2073-4468/8/2/33/htm.

the glomerular sieving coefficient is the hydrodynamic volume. There is also brush-border catabolism as well as reuptake, section plus catabolism (Figure 8.23).

8.6.4 Pharmacokinetic Manipulations

Therapeutic proteins have a short life in the body that is prolonged by FcN-mediate recycling—changing the half-life from hours to days. Monoclonal antibodies have restricted penetration into tissue because of their large size; they are transported from blood circulation to peripheral tissues by passive transfer through fenestrae pores in capillary walls or by transcellular pathways of endothelial cells; the latter pathway can be an active transport in surrounding tissues like a fluid by fluid-phase pinocytosis, receptors through receptor-mediated endocytosis (FcγR-mediated) and into immune cells by phagocytosis. Passive diffusion depends on the size, hydrophobicity, and charge of the molecule. In the subcutaneous route, macromolecules are restricted to the interstitial space and reach blood through capillaries or lymphatic vessels. Transport through capillaries is passive and limited to molecular weight no more than 16 kDa leaving most large molecule protein drugs dependent on the lymphatic system through the thoracic duct for entry and distribution. Their distribution is also limited to plasma rather than body tissues for the same reasons.

The elimination of antibodies can be affected by their immunogenicity and anti-drug antibodies that can competitively bind to the active portions of the therapeutic proteins, such as receptor binding sites, to make the antibody less effective and alter its pharmacokinetic profile. Aggregation of antibodies enhances their clearance, primarily when used in high doses, promoting phagocytosis in the reticuloendothelial system. Endocytosis is a receptor-mediate process where receptor saturation influences bioavailability targeting surface receptors—antigen sink.

8.6.4.1 Protein Modification to Increase Duration of Action

Therapeutic proteins are widely modified chemically or by recombinant methods to prolong their half-life, as shown in Figure 8.24 using albumin, Fc fusion, and pegylation as major reactions.

8.6.4.1.1 Albumin–Protein Fusions

Albumin has three domains, each having two subdomains connected by a flexible loop leading to seven binding sites for fatty acids. It has a half-life of 19–22 days prolonged because of its FcRn-mediated recycling like the antibodies. Albiglutide (Tanzeum®), a recombinant fusion protein fused to albumin, has been approved for only one product.

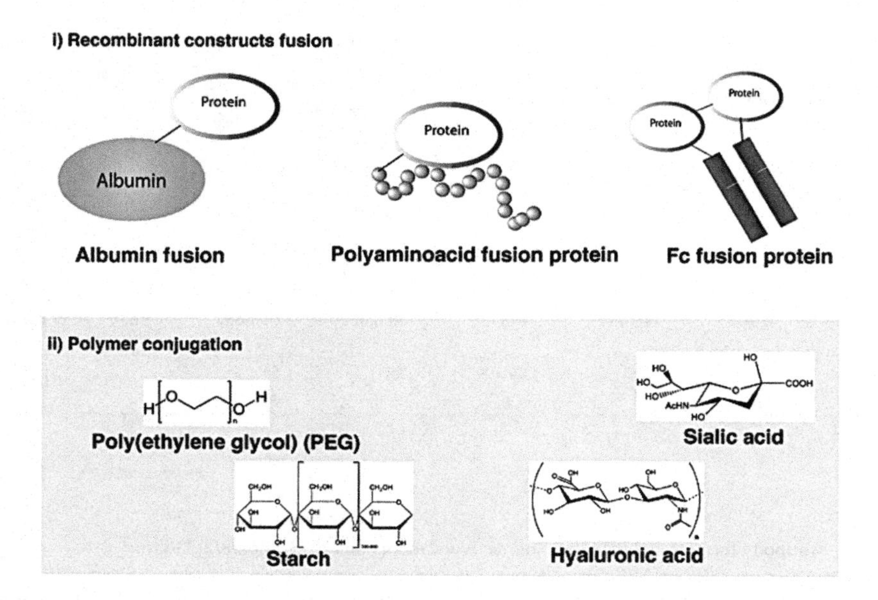

FIGURE 8.24 Methods to increase the duration of action of proteins. Source: www.mdpi.com/1999-4923/10/3/83/htm.

8.6.4.1.2 Fc Fusion Proteins

Fc fusion is proteins or peptides fused with the Fc found in antibodies altering the pharmacokinetics properties. The Fc fusion proteins target receptor–ligand interactions either as antagonists to block receptor binding or as agonists to stimulate receptor functions. A wide range of fusion products have been approved, including etanercept (Enbrel®, Amgen/Pfizer), Alefacept (Amevive®), abatacept (Orencia®), rilonacept (Arcalyst®), romiplostim (Nplate®), belatacept (Nulojix®), aflibercept (Eylea®), and ziv-aflibercept (Zaltrap®). Biobetter fusion proteins include denileukin diftitox (Ontak®), corifollitropin-α (Elonva®), eftrenonacog-α (Alprolix®), albiglutide (Tanzeum®), efraloctocog-α (Eloctate®), and dulaglutide (Trulicity®).

8.6.4.2 Protein Pegylation

Pegylation involves polyethylene binding covalently to proteins forming a conjugate that is considered a new drug; the new product has a long half-life as the higher molecular weight reduces glomerular excretion while reducing immunogenicity and the protein molecule is covered under the PEG molecule. The first pegylated product that was approved is pegademase (Adagen®); other approved products are mainly protein conjugates except for peginesatide (Omontys®) which is a peptide, and pegaptanib (Macugen®) which is an RNA aptamer.

8.6.4.3 Unnatural Construction

Proteins can be labeled as "unnatural" construction—the fusion proteins or the conjugate (e.g., pegylated) proteins and huge assembly of virus particles or nanoparticle delivery systems. The fusion of an Fc (fragment crystallizable) part of an antibody (typically an IgGI antibody) with another pharmaceutically relevant protein through recombinant genetic technology results in fusion proteins. The Fc portion of an antibody increases circulation time just as does the pegylation; examples include Fc fusion to the blood-clotting factor VIII and factor IX. The fusion of two relatively large proteins, each being over 5.0 kDa, raises the question of whether this would impact either protein? While there is potential variance possible, the existing science reveals no significant impact. At present, eleven Fc-fusion proteins have been approved by the FDA.

When a biologically active protein is combined with a long-acting protein, the resulting product has a longer half-life based on several techniques that combine:

- Elastin-like peptide.
- XTEN—recombinant peptide with protein/polymer properties.
- Immunoglobulin Fc fragment.
- Recombinant serum albumin.
- Transferring.
- Carboxy-terminal peptide.

Pegylation is one of the more popular for prolonging the half-life for drugs used to treat hepatitis, multiple sclerosis, cancer, hemophilia, chronic kidney disease, and many more. The first pegylated product approved by the FDA was pegylated ademase bovine in 1990; many more drugs have been approved, as listed in Table 8.7. It's worth mentioning that all the FDA-approved drugs contain methoxypoly (ethylene glycol) or mPEG. The pegylated molecules have a longer half-life and are often less immunogenic because of the protection of protein structural domains. Table 8.11 lists the currently approved pegylated products.

Another class of proteins involves combining a drug with an antibody. With the approvals of antibody-drug conjugates, such as Kadcyla®, Adcetris®, and Besponsa®, and an increasing number of such products are entering clinical trials, the targeted delivery of cytotoxic agents to cancer cells is proving to be a powerful approach.

All living entities produce proteins inside their cells based on the same process of gene coding. Therefore, it is possible to modify the gene code of living entities to produce a target protein. As the genetic code is universal, it will be read the same way by all cellular systems of the animal, plant, or bacterial kingdom (even as dominant codons per cell system is known). This technology is labeled recombinant protein expression. This universality of gene coding is based on the production of recombinant therapeutic proteins of the human sequence into heterologous host systems (bacteria, yeast, plant, a mammalian cell, transgenic animals) to make that host system "produces" a protein of a given sequence.

8.7 Conclusion

Biological medicines comprise a broad category of products, primarily recombinant therapeutic proteins and, more particularly, biosimilars, where this chapter's teachings will be helpful. Given the high cost of developing therapeutic proteins, intellectual property considerations are essential and require understanding by scientists at all levels of development and manufacturing designed and executed based on regulatory regulations across the globe. Understanding therapeutic proteins starts with studying the molecular structure and how the molecules interact with receptors in various classes of therapeutic proteins, hormones, hematopoietic factors, cytokines, plasma protein factors, bone formation factors, recombinant enzymes, and antibodies. Detailed understanding of the primary, secondary, tertiary, and quaternary structure of proteins, including post-translational modifications, is needed to design a robust manufacturing process. Structural designs for pharmacokinetic modulation and increased action duration, such as through pegylation, fusion proteins, and unnatural construction, are essential to new drug development. Most critical for therapeutic proteins is their immunogenicity and how to control it in designing the product and the manufacturing conditions and practices. Recombinant expression requires an understanding of DNA and RNA. The new science of gene and cell therapies is also part of the field of therapeutic proteins.

TABLE 8.11
Currently Approved Pegylated Biological Medicine Products

Brand	INN	Indication	Functionalized PEG	PEG Size (kDa)	Number of PEGs	Year
Adagen	Pegademase bovine	Combined immunodeficiency disease associated with adenosine deaminase	mPEG succinimidyl succinate	5	11–17	1990
Oncaspar	Pegaspargase	Precursor cell lymphoblastic leukemia	mPEG succinimidyl succinate	5	69–82	1994
Pegasys	Peginterferon alfa-2a	Hepatitis B, C	mPEG succinimidyl carbonate	40	1	2001
Neulasta	Pegfilgrastim	Cancer neutropenia	mPEG aldehyde	20	1	2002
Somavert	Pegvisomant	Acromegaly	mPEG succinimidyl succinate	5	4–6	2003
Macugen	Pegaptanib	Age-related macular degeneration	mPEG amino	40	1	2004
Mircera	Methoxy polyethylene glycol epoetin	Anemia associated with chronic kidney disease	mPEG succinimidyl succinate	30	1	2007
Cimzia	Certolizumab pegol	Rheumatoid arthritis	mPEG maleimide	40	1	2008
Kristexxa	Pegloticase	Chronic gout	mPEG p-nitrophenyl carbonate	10	36	2010
Palynziq	Pegvalise	Phenyketonuria	mPEG succinimidyl succinate	20	9	2010
Movantik	Naloxegol	Opioid-induced constipation	mPEG7 (hepaethylene glycol)	0.339	1	2014
PegIntron	Peginterfeon alfa-2b	Hepatitis C	mPEG succinimidyl carbonate	12	1	2014
Plegridy	Peginterferon beta-1a	Multipls sclerosis	mPEG aldehyde	20	1	2014
Adynovate	Rurioctocog alfa pegol	Hemophilia A	—	20	2	2016
Rebinyl	Nonacog beta pegol	Hemophilia B	—	40	1	2017
Asparlas	Calaspargase pegol	Acute lymphoblastic leukemia	mPEG succinylimidyl carbonate	5	31–39	2018
Revcovi	Elapegademase	Adenosine deaminase severe combined immunodeficiency	mPEG succinimidyl carbamate	5.6	13	2018

ADDITIONAL READING

Alfaleh, MA, Jones ML, Howard CB, Mahler SM. Strategies for selecting membrane protein-specific antibodies using phage display with cell-based panning. *Antibodies* (Basel). 2017 Sep;6(3):10.

Arora R, C.A.B. International. *Medicinal plant biotechnology*. Cambridge, MA: CABI; 2010.

Atun RA, Sheridan DJ. *Innovation in the biological medicine industry*. Singapore, NJ: World Scientific Pub.; 2007.

Bawa R, Szebeni J, Webster TJ, Audette GF. *Immune aspects of therapeutic proteins and nanomedicines*. Singapore: Pan Stanford Publishing; 2018.

Beck A. *Glycosylation engineering of therapeutic proteins: methods and protocols*. New York: Humana Press; 2013.

Beck-Sickinger AG. [Directed evolution in drug and antibody development: From the Nobel] Prize to broad clinical application. *Internist (Berl)*. 2019 Oct;60(10):1014–1020.

Behera BK. *Biological medicines: challenges and opportunities*. First edition. Boca Raton, FL: CRC Press; 202 8.

Bharati SL, Chaurasia PK. *Research advancements in pharmaceutical, nutritional, and industrial enzymology*. Hershey, PA: Medical Information Science Reference (an imprint of IGI Global); 2018.

BioDrugs: clinical immunotherapeutics, therapeutic proteins, and gene therapy. In Mairangi Bay. Langhorn, PA: Auckland, N.Z.: Adis International Ltd.; 1997.

Biological medicines. Austin, TX: Landes Bioscience; 1997.

Bluemel J. *The nonhuman primate in nonclinical drug development and safety assessment*. Amsterdam: Elsevier/Academic Press; 2015.

Bolton GR, Mehta KK. The role of more than 40 years of improvement in protein A chromatography in the growth of the therapeutic antibody industry. *Biotechnol Prog*. 2016;32(5):1193–1202.

Buyel JF, Twyman RM, Fischer R. Very-large-scale production of antibodies in plants: The biologization of manufacturing. *Biotechnol Adv*. 2017;35(4):458–465.

Canadian Agency for Drugs and Technologies in Health. Pharmacoeconomic review report. AbobotulinumtoxinA (Dysport therapeutic): (Ipsen Biological medicines Canada, Inc.). In: CADTH common drug review. 8.0. ed. Ottawa, ON: Canadian Agency for Drugs and Technologies in Health; 2017: https://www.ncbi.nlm.nih.gov/books/NBK534676/.

Castilho A. *Glyco-engineering: methods and protocols*. New York: Humana Press; 2015.

Center for Biologics Evaluation and Research. *What is a biological product?* US. Food and Drug Administration; 2010. Retrieved 2014-02-09.

Centers for Disease Control. Vaccines acronyms and abbreviations. https://www.cdc.gov/vaccines/terms/vacc-abbrev.html.

Chahar DS, Ravindran S, Pisal SS. Monoclonal antibody purification and its progression to commercial scale. *Biologicals*. 2020;63:1–13.

Chan SK, Lim TS. Immune human antibody libraries for infectious diseases. *Adv Exp Med Biol*. 2017;1053:61–78.

Chan SK, Rahumatullah A, Lai JY, Lim TS. Naïve human antibody libraries for infectious diseases. *Adv Exp Med Biol*. 2017;1053:35–59.

Chen G, Sidhu SS, Nilvebrant J. Synthetic antibodies in infectious disease. *Adv Exp Med Biol*. 2017;1053:79–98.

Costantino HR, Pikal MJ, American Association of Pharmaceutical Scientists. *Lyophilization of therapeutic proteins*. Arlington, VA: AAPS Press; 2004.

Das TK. *Biophysical methods for biotherapeutics: discovery and development applications*. Hoboken, NJ: Wiley; 2014.

Donini M, Marusic C. Current state-of-the-art in plant-based antibody production systems. *Biotechnol Lett*. 2019;41(3):335–346.

Drake PM, Szeto TH, Paul MJ, Teh AY, Ma JK. Recombinant biologic products versus nutraceuticals from plants – a regulatory choice? *Br J Clin Pharmacol*. 2017;83(1):82–87.

Dumont J, Euwart D, Mei B, Estes S, Kshirsagar R. Human cell lines for biological medicine manufacturing: history, status, and future perspectives. *Crit Rev Biotechnol*. 2016;36(6):1110–1122.

Dutton RL, Scharer JM. *Advanced technologies in biological medicine processing*. First edition. Ames, IA: Blackwell Pub.; 2007.

Elgundi Z, Reslan M, Cruz E, Sifniotis V, Kayser V. The state-of-play and future antibody therapeutics. *Adv Drug Deliv Rev*. 2017;122:2–19.

EMA. Questions and answers on biosimilar medicines (similar biological medicinal products). European Medicines Agency; 2008. Retrieved 2014-10-1.

Faye Lc, Gomord Vr. *Recombinant proteins from plants: methods and protocols*. New York: Springer; 2009.

FDA. Cellular and gene therapy guidances. https://www.fda.gov/BiologicsBloodVaccines/GuidanceComplianceRegulatoryInformation/Guidances/CellularandGeneTherapy/default.htm

Flynne WG. *Biotechnology and bioengineering*. New York: Nova Biomedical Books; 2008.

Foltz IN, Gunasekaran K, King CT. Discovery and bio-optimization of human antibody therapeutics using the XenoMouse® transgenic mouse platform. *Immunol Rev*. 2016;270(1):51–64.

Foster, L. *Patenting in the biological medicine industry—comparing the US with Europe*. Archived from the original on 2006-03-16. Retrieved 2006-06-23.

Franks F, Auffret T. *Freeze-drying of pharmaceuticals and therapeutic proteins: principles and practice*. Cambridge: RSC Publishing; 2008.

Frenzel A, Kügler J, Helmsing S, et al. Designing human antibodies by phage display. *Transfus Med Hemother*. 2017;44(5):312–318.

Frenzel A, Schirrmann T, Hust M. Phage display-derived human antibodies in clinical development and therapy. *MAbs*. 2016;8(7):1177–1194.

Gao W, Zhang J, Xiang J, et al. Recent advances in site-specific conjugations of antibody drug conjugates (ADCs). *Curr Cancer Drug Targets*. 2016;16(6):469–479.

Gaughan CL. The present state of the art in expression, production, and characterization of monoclonal antibodies. *Mol Divers*. 2016;20(1):255–270.

Geigert J. *The challenge of CMC regulatory compliance for therapeutic proteins*. Third edition. Cham: Springer; 2019.

Ghosh C, Sarkar P, Issa R, Haldar J. Alternatives to conventional antibiotics in the era of antimicrobial resistance. *Trends Microbiol*. 2019;27(4):323–338.

Glick BR, Patten CL. *Molecular biotechnology: principles and applications of recombinant DNA*. Fifth edition. Washington, DC: ASM Press; 2017.

Grindley JN, Ogden JE. *Understanding therapeutic proteins: manufacturing and regulatory issues*. Denver, CO: Interpharm Press; 2000.

Gupta SK, Shukla P. Glycosylation control technologies for recombinant therapeutic proteins. *Appl Microbiol Biotechnol*. 2018;102(24):10457–10468.

Günther C, Hauser A, Huss R. *Advances in pharmaceutical cell therapy: principles of cell-based therapeutic proteins*. Newark, NJ: World Scientific; 2016.

Hefferon KL. *Biological medicines in plants: toward the next century of medicine*. Boca Raton, FL: CRC Press/Taylor & Francis; 2010.

HHS, Vaccines Glossary https://www.vaccines.gov/resources/glossary/index.html

Hill RG, Rang HP. *Drug discovery and development: technology in transition*. Second edition. Edinburgh: Churchill Livingstone/Elsevier; 2013.

Ho RJY, Gibaldi M. *Biotechnology and therapeutic proteins: transforming proteins and genes into drugs*. Second edition. Hoboken, NJ: Wiley-Blackwell; 2013.

Holtz BR, Berquist BR, Bennett LD, et al. Commercial-scale biotherapeutics manufacturing facility for plant-made pharmaceuticals. *Plant Biotechnol J*. 2015;13(8):1180–1190.

Houde DJ, Berkowitz SA. *Biophysical characterization of proteins in developing therapeutic proteins*. Waltham, MA: Elsevier; 2015.

Huxsoll JF. *Quality assurance for therapeutic proteins*. New York: Wiley; 1994.

Igawa T. [Next generation antibody therapeutics using bispecific antibody technology]. *Yakugaku Zasshi*. 2017;137(7):831–836.

Ito Y. [Development of a rapid identification method for a variety of antibody candidates using high-throughput sequencing]. *Yakugaku Zasshi*. 2017;137(7):823–830.

IUPAC International Union of Pure and Applied Chemistry. Compendium of chemical terminology: recommendations, compiled by Alan D. McNaught and Andrew Wilkinson, Blackwell Science, 1997. "Gold Book" http://goldbook.iupac.org/

IUPAC. Glossary of terms related to pharmaceutics. *Pure and Applied Chemistry* 2009;81:971–999. thttps://www.iupac.org/publications/pac/81/5/0971/

Jafari B, Hamzeh-Mivehroud M, Morris MB, Dastmalchi S. Exploitation of phage display to develop anticancer agents targeting fibroblast growth factor signaling pathways: new strategies to tackle an old challenge. *Cytokine Growth Factor Rev.* 2019;46:54–65.

Jameel F, Hershenson S. *Formulation and process development strategies for manufacturing therapeutic proteins.* Hoboken, NJ: Wiley; 2010.

Jin Y, Lei C, Hu D, Dimitrov DS, Ying T. Human monoclonal antibodies as candidate therapeutics against emerging viruses. *Front Med.* 2017;11(4):462–470.

Joubert S, Dodelet V, Béliard R, Durocher Y. [Biomanufacturing of monoclonal antibodies]. *Med Sci* (Paris). 2019;35(12):1153–1159.

Jørgensen L, Nielsen HM. *Delivery technologies for therapeutic proteins: peptides, proteins, nucleic acids and vaccines.* Chichester: Wiley; 2009.

Kelley B, Kiss R, Laird M. A different perspective: how much innovation is needed for monoclonal antibody production using mammalian cell technology? *Adv Biochem Eng Biotechnol.* 2018;165:443–462.

Kennedy PJ, Oliveira C, Granja PL, Sarmento B. Monoclonal antibodies: technologies for early discovery and engineering. *Crit Rev Biotechnol.* 2018;38(3):394–408.

Kim MG, Kim D, Suh SK, Park Z, Choi MJ, Oh YK. Current status and regulatory perspective of chimeric antigen receptor-modified T cell therapeutics. *Arch Pharm Res.* 2016;39(4):437–452.

Kingham R, Klasa G, Carver K (2014). *Key regulatory guidelines for the development of biologics in the United States and Europe (PDF).* John Wiley & Sons, Inc. pp. 75–88.

Kiss B, Gottschalk U, Pohlscheidt M, Abraham E. *New bioprocessing strategies: development and manufacturing of recombinant antibodies and proteins.* Cham: Springer; 2018.

Knäblein Jr. *Modern therapeutic proteins: design, development, and optimization.* Weinheim: Wiley-VCH; 2005.

Knäblein Jr. *Modern therapeutic proteins: recent success stories.* Weinheim: Wiley-Blackwell; 2013.

Komives C, Zhou W. *Bioprocessing technology for production of therapeutic proteins and bioproducts.* First edition. Hoboken, NJ: John Wiley & Sons, Inc.; 2019.

Kumar R, Parray HA, Shrivastava T, Sinha S, Luthra K. Phage display antibody libraries: a robust approach for generating recombinant human monoclonal antibodies. *Int J Biol Macromol.* 2019;135:907–918.

Kunert R, Reinhart D. Advances in recombinant antibody manufacturing. *Appl Microbiol Biotechnol.* 2016;100(8):3451–346 8.

Lai JY, Lim TS. Infectious disease antibodies for biomedical applications: a mini review of immune antibody phage library repertoire. *Int J Biol Macromol.* 2020;163:640–648.

Lamanna WC, Holzmann J, Cohen HP, Guo X, Schweigler M, Stangler T, Seidl A, Schiestl M. Maintaining consistent quality and clinical performance of therapeutic proteins. *Expert Opinion on Biological Therapy.* 2018;18(4):369–379.

Lazarus AH, Semple JW. *Immunoglobulin therapy.* Bethesda, MD: AABB Press; 2010.

Lill JR, Sandoval WN. *Analytical characterization of biotherapeutics.* Hoboken, NJ: Wiley; 2017.

Liu C, Morrow J. *Biosimilars of monoclonal antibodies: a practical guide to manufacturing, preclinical, and clinical development.* Hoboken, NJ: John Wiley & Sons, Inc.; 2017.

Lu RM, Hwang YC, Liu IJ, et al. Develop therapeutic antibodies for the treatment of diseases. *J Biomed Sci.* 2020;27(1): 8.

Lushova AA, Biazrova MG, Prilipov AG, Sadykova GK, Kopylov TA, Filatov AV. [Next-generation techniques for discovering human monoclonal antibodies]. *Mol Biol* (Mosk). 2017;51(6):899–906.

Mandenius C-F, Titchener-Hooker NJ. *Measurement, monitoring, modelling and control of bioprocesses.* Heidelberg: Springer; 2013.

Marks L, Royal Society of Chemistry (Great Britain). *Engineering health: how biotechnology changed medicine.* London: The Royal Society of Chemistry; 2018.

Marschall AL, Dübel S, Böldicke T. Recent advances with er targeted intrabodies. *Adv Exp Med Biol.* 2016;917:77–93.

Mastrangeli R, Palinsky W, Bierau H. Glycoengineered antibodies: towards the next-generation of immunotherapeutics. *Glycobiology.* 2019;29(3):199–210.

Ministro J, Manuel AM, Goncalves J. Therapeutic antibody engineering and selection strategies. *Adv Biochem Eng Biotechnol.* 2020;171:55–86.

Mire-Sluis AR, Center for Biologics Evaluation and Research (U.S.). State of the art analytical methods for the characterization of biological products and assessment of comparability. Natcher Building, National Institutes of Health (NIH), Bethesda, MD, June 10–13, 2003: proceedings of a conference. Basel: Karger; 2005.

Morbidelli M, Wolf M, Bielser J-M. *Perfusion cell culture processes for therapeutic proteins: process development, design, and scale-up.* New York: Cambridge University Press; 2020.

Nagano K. [Challenge to the development of molecular targeted therapy against a novel target candidate identified by antibody proteomics technology]. *Yakugaku Zasshi.* 2016;136(2):145–149.

Nature. Biologics: latest research and review. https://www.nature.com/subjects/biologics. 2020.

Nicolini F, Bocchini M, Angeli D, et al. Fully human antibodies for malignant pleural mesothelioma targeting. *Cancers* (Basel). 2020;8;12(4):915.

Neves Jd, Sarmento B. *Mucosal delivery of therapeutic proteins: biology, challenges and strategies.* New York: Springer; 2014.

NFCR Center for Therapeutic Antibody Engineering Glossary, National Foundation for Cancer Research, Dana Farber Cancer Institute. http://research.dfci.harvard.edu/nfcr-ctae/research/tech_glossary.php

Niazi S, Brown JL. *Fundamentals of modern bioprocessing.* Boca Raton, FL: CRC Press; 2016.

Niazi S. *Biosimilarity: the FDA perspective.* Boca Raton, FL: CRC Press; 2019.

Niazi S. *Biosimilars and interchangeable biologics. Strategic elements.* Boca Raton, FL: CRC Press/Taylor & Francis; 2016.

Niazi S. *Biosimilars and interchangeable biologics. Tactical elements.* Boca Raton, FL: Taylor & Francis/CRC Press; 2016.

Niazi S. *Handbook of bioequivalence testing.* Second edition. Boca Raton, FL: CRC Press/Taylor & Francis Group; 2015.

Niazi S. *Handbook of biogeneric therapeutic proteins: regulatory, manufacturing, testing, and patent issues.* Boca Raton, FL: Taylor & Francis; 2006.

Niazi S. *Handbook of pharmaceutical manufacturing formulations.* Third edition. Boca Raton, FL: CRC Press; 2019.

Niazi S. *Handbook of preformulation: chemical, biological, and botanical drugs.* Second edition. Boca Raton, FL: CRC Press; 2019.

Niazi S. *Textbook of biopharmaceutics and clinical pharmacokinetics.* New York: Appleton-Century-Crofts; 1979.

Nick C. The US Biosimilars Act: challenges facing regulatory approval. *Pharm Med.* 2012;26(3):145–152. doi:10.1007/bf03262388

Paine Webber Inc., Industrial Biotechnology Association (U.S.). Meeting. *Biological medicines in transition.* Woodlands, TX: Portfolio Pub. Co.; 1990.

Pandit NK. *Introduction to the pharmaceutical sciences.* First edition. Baltimore, MD: Lippincott Williams & Wilkins; 2007.

Pathak Y, Benita S. *Antibody mediated drug delivery systems: concepts, technology, and applications.* Hoboken, NJ: Wiley; 2012.

Pham PV. *Stem cell drugs: a new generation of therapeutic proteins.* Cham: Springer; 2018.

Prazeres DMF. *Plasmid therapeutic proteins: basics, applications, and manufacturing.* Hoboken, NJ: John Wiley & Sons; 2018.

Primrose SB, Twyman RM. *Genomics: applications in human biology.* Malden, MA: Blackwell Pub.; 2004.

Pugsley MK, Curtis MJ. *Principles of safety pharmacology.* Heidelberg: Springer; 2015.

Rader RA. (Re)defining biological medicine. *Nature Biotechnology.* 2008;26(7):743–758. doi:10.1038/nbt0708-743. PMID 18612293.

Rathore AS, Mhatre R. *Quality by design for therapeutic proteins: principles and case studies.* Hoboken, NJ: Wiley; 2009.

Rathore AS, Sofer GK. *Process validation in manufacturing of therapeutic proteins: guidelines, current practices, and industrial case studies.* Boca Raton, FL: Taylor & Francis; 2005.

Rathore AS, Sofer GK. *Process validation in manufacturing of therapeutic proteins.* Third edition. Boca Raton, FL: Taylor & Francis/CRC Press; 2012.

Razinkov VI, Kleemann GR. *High-throughput formulation development of therapeutic proteins: practical guide to methods and applications.* Amsterdam: Elsevier/Woodhead Publishing; 2017.

Reader RH, Workman RG, Maddison BC, Gough KC. Advances in the production and batch reformatting of phage antibody libraries. *Mol Biotechnol.* 2019;61(11):801–815.

Rehbinder E. *Pharming: promises and risks of therapeutic proteins derived from genetically modified plants and animals.* Berlin: Springer; 2009.

Rojanasakul Y, Wu-Pong S. *Biological medicine drug design and development.* Second edition. Totowa, NJ: Humana Press; 2008.

Schiestl M, Stangler T, Torella C, Cepeljnik T, Toll H, Grau R. Acceptable changes in quality attributes of glycosylated therapeutic proteins. *Nature Biotechnology.* 2011;29(4):310–312. doi:10.1038/nbt.1839. PMID 21478848.

Schmidt SR. *Fusion protein technologies for therapeutic proteins: applications and challenges.* Hoboken, NJ: John Wiley & Sons; 2013.

Shim H. Antibody phage display. *Adv Exp Med Biol.* 2017;1053:21–34.

Shire SJ, American Association of Pharmaceutical Scientists. *Current trends in monoclonal antibody development and manufacturing.* New York: Springer: AAPS Press; 2010.

Shukla AA, Wolfe LS, Mostafa SS, Norman C. Evolving trends in mAb production processes. *Bioeng Transl Med.* 2017;2(1):58–69.

Somasundaram R, Choraria A, Antonysamy M. An approach towards developing monoclonal IgY antibodies against SARS CoV-2 spike protein (S) using phage display method: a review. *Int Immunopharmacol.* 2020;85:106654.

Thomaz-Soccol V, Pandey A, Resende RR. *Current developments in biotechnology and bioengineering. Human and animal health applications.* Boston, MA: Elsevier; 2017.

Tovey MG. *Detection and quantification of antibodies to therapeutic proteins: practical and applied considerations.* Hoboken, NJ: Wiley; 2018.

Ubah O, Palliyil S. Monoclonal antibodies and antibody like fragments derived from immunised phage display libraries. *Adv Exp Med Biol.* 2017;1053:99–117.

Unkauf T, Miethe S, Fühner V, Schirrmann T, Frenzel A, Hust M. Generation of recombinant antibodies against toxins and viruses by phage display for diagnostics and therapy. *Adv Exp Med Biol.* 2016;917:55–76.

Van Hoecke L, Roose K. How mRNA therapeutics are entering the monoclonal antibody field. *J Transl Med.* 2019;17(1):54.

Viardot A, Bargou R. Bispecific antibodies in haematological malignancies. *Cancer Treat Rev.* 2018;65:87–95.

Voigt A, Semenova T, Yamamoto J, Etienne V, Nguyen CQ. Therapeutic antibody discovery in infectious diseases using single-cell analysis. *Adv Exp Med Biol.* 2018;1068:89–102.

Walsh G. Biological medicines: Biochemistry and Biotechnology. Second edition. New York: John Wiley & Sons Ltd.; 2003.

Walsh G, Murphy B. *Biological medicines, an industrial perspective.* Boston, MA: Kluwer Academic; 1999.

Walsh G. *Biological medicines: biochemistry and biotechnology.* Second edition. Hoboken, NJ: John Wiley; 2003.

Wang W, Manmohan S. *Biological drug products: development and strategies.* Hoboken, NJ: John Wiley & Sons; 2014.

Wei B, Berning K, Quan C, Zhang YT. Glycation of antibodies: modification, methods and potential effects on biological functions. *MAbs.* 2017;9(4):586–594.

Wittrup KD, Verdine GL. *Protein engineering for therapeutics. Part B.* First edition. San Diego, CA: Academic; 2012.

Yusibov V, Kushnir N, Streatfield SJ. Antibody production in plants and green algae. *Annu Rev Plant Biol.* 2016;67:669–708.

Zhao A, Tohidkia MR, Siegel DL, Coukos G, Omidi Y. Phage antibody display libraries: a powerful antibody discovery platform for immunotherapy. *Crit Rev Biotechnol.* 2016;36(2):276–289.

9

Manufacturing Trends

9.1 Background

Therapeutic protein manufacturing is based on either unmodified or genetically modified living entities, bacteria, mammalian cells, viruses, yeasts, etc., to produce large molecules. In naturally produced products like penicillins, the systems are straightforward and not included in this chapter.

A clear understanding of the therapeutic proteins manufacturing platform begins understanding DNA and RNA's role in our body. The manufacturing processes are tightly connected at each unit operation of upstream and downstream processing. Yield variation, impurity diversity, and potency achieved are the factors that significantly affect all steps. As a result, the manufacturing process is carefully laid out in a lengthy process definition and development process, a flow chart that identifies sizing issues.

The manufacturing train creates a modified genetically modified cell culture to express the desired therapeutic protein in a bioreactor. (A bioreactor is a device to grow any type of living entity, while a fermenter terminology refers to a bioreaction that results in the production of gases and heat; in many cases, these terms are used interchangeably. The correct term for therapeutic proteins is bioreactors.)

Once the living entities have expressed (meaning products) a desire therapeutic protein, the next step is to remove the expressed protein from the culture media either by filtration (if the therapeutic protein is in solution) or by first disrupting the cells such as bacteria and then removing the protein through a multistep process.

The next steps involve purification of the therapeutic proteins and, in some cases, first inducing proper folding. There is a need to remove any viral contaminations, mainly where the expression entities are mammalian cells that carry viruses.

Finally, the therapeutic protein came to the stage of being labeled as a drug substance when diluted in a buffer and stored at –20° C.

The next steps are formulating the drug substance into a drug product, either as a solution in a vial or a prefilled syringe or as a lyophilized powder. As of now, therapeutic proteins are administered parenterally, but there is hope that we may be able to administer them orally, transdermally, via inhalation, or other routes in the future.

Therapeutic protein manufacturing is an expensive process and subject to strict regulatory controls because even subtle changes in the structure of these molecules can alter their immunogenicity and efficacy. More recent single-use technologies, continuous manufacturing, and online monitoring are fast changing the manufacturing risk profile. They offer many long-term advantages in the planning of manufacturing facilities, as described in this chapter.

9.2 Process Optimizations

9.2.1 Cell Line Development

Traditional cell line development starts with a time-consuming. A critical step in early-stage manufacturing can take around 40+ weeks from concept to creation in establishing a high yielding and quality clone. This includes choosing a suitable cell line, constructing an expression vector, transfection, cell sorting, and clone selection and evaluation based on cell growth and productivity. Single-cell isolation

DOI: 10.1201/9781003146933-9

and screening are critical in the cell line development workflow from a regulatory perspective. The conventional screening approach involves placing a single cell per well in a 96-well plate and then screening multiple such plates to choose a high producer.

Several tools are available today to accelerate some of the cell line development steps that help compress overall timelines. Cell line developers can effectively use a targeted process for transfection, allowing the gene insertion into "hot spots" compared to random transfection events that have been used in the past. This specific manipulation allows creating a high-producing cell line and significantly reduces the follow-on screening process. Additionally, instead of screening each clone individually, placing cells into mini-pools and selecting a high-performing pool of cells gives a smaller population to choose the final single clone rather than screening multiple plates (50–100 in traditional processes). Coupling fluorescence-activated cell sorting (FACS) with glutamine synthetase (GS) can also quicken the clone screening steps. Today microfluidics-based technology is being widely used by cell line developers. These systems can sort and deposit single cells providing evidence of clonality while also providing proliferation rates and specific productivities in a short span (as little as five days). When combined, these technologies can significantly reduce the overall timelines for cell line development to about eight to ten weeks helping the process development progress faster towards early-stage deliverables.

Several manufacturers continue to use outdated techniques like plating into semi-solid media and determining a clone's protein titer during the static phase, which does not correlate well with fed-batch results. Novel approaches including enrichment for potentially higher producers but equally pre-selection by fluorescence-activated cell sorting (FACS) or vector optimization to sort.

One of the myths of bioprocess technology is that the cell line must be pushed to produce higher yields. However, there is a limit to how far this can be done before the cell line becomes unstable; it will produce a high titer. If it is a monoclonal antibody, the variations in glycosylation of other DNA-based changes will be inevitable. Developers must calculate their cost based on media cost that provides the carbon source needed for production before switching over to higher-yielding cell lines. In many cases, a higher-yielding cell line helps reduce the bioreactor's size but not necessarily the cost of goods.

9.2.2 Media

Cell culture media is the primary raw material with over 100 different formulations containing varying critical components, including amino acids, vitamins, fatty acids, and lipids. Chemically defined media, its formulation, and its concentration are crucial factors determining the media's suitability to support cell growth, cellular metabolism, productivity, and protein quality. Cell culture media developments significantly impact cell density, increased specific productivity, and product quality (less variability). This section will present some of the media optimization strategies and challenges that can enhance process intensification.

Media optimization approaches cannot be universally applied across cell lines or even clones; a media that may enhance productivity in one clone may not necessarily do the same for another clone. Likewise, product quality can also be impacted. A platform approach, particularly using single basal media, is always not likely to yield satisfactory results. While there may advantage to using an available media (example: ease of sourcing media components, a fixed and validated approach to preparation) for all mAb products using the same host cell line, variations in the product quality (example: glycosylation, charge variants) may be necessary for the functionality of the final product, and as such having unique solutions, even with a finite number of compounds is highly recommended.

A traditional approach to media development and studying its suitability for a particular cell line involves changing one component in the media at a time. A DoE approach allows interaction and effects between components to be studied to optimize the composition. Depending on the number of components being used, multiple iterations are possible, making it relatively time-consuming. Media blending, an alternative to traditional, DoE approaches, is becoming common practice, allowing for simultaneous media optimization of several components. Additionally, successful media formulation requires reliable analytical methods to quantify metabolites for the entire culture's entire duration. For this purpose, Capillary Electrophoresis (CE), HPLC coupled with MS and GC are commonly used.

Several cell culture media manufacturers offer high throughput technologies to work with drug manufacturers for media optimization (e.g., Millipore Sigma, Sartorius). However, today's newer technology, for example, high throughput microarray analysis, takes a holistic approach towards media analysis rather than measuring these metabolites and ions individually. With the microarray analysis (offered by EMD Millipore Sigma), media components to which cells respond are identified, removing the need for random testing. Because of its ability to replace additional research or even experimental analysis, modeling presents the media development field with many opportunities to reduce time and cost significantly. With such stoichiometric models and kinetic models, online or inline analysis during cell culture can provide valuable inputs to these models to optimize media or even feed solutions to create a more robust process. This can lead to companies creating their platform cell culture media specific to their cell lines.

Most cell culture media optimization is catered to fed-batch processes that utilize intermittent feeding (mostly concentrates on specific media components). However, given the high volumes of media requirements, having a cost-effective solution for media gains paramount importance with perfusion culture. A concentrate on cell culture media is one option to reduce operational footprint. Media at concentrated levels of three to four times its components will be equivalent to approximately 60,000–70,000 L, which can easily support a perfusion process and provide significant space and resource savings. Another option to meet the perfusion process media demands is to have media explicitly designed for the perfusion process. This will be more suitable to support high-cell densities, improve the volumetric productivity, and reduce costs (lower perfusion rates) rather than adapt media used for a fed-batch process (Table 9.1).

9.2.3 High Cell Density Cryopreservation

The cell bank generation process presents an optimal opportunity for process intensification. A typical cell banking process starts with a vial thawing to inoculate at least a 25 mL culture. The culture is subsequently expanded to generate enough cells that can be banked. An industry-wide practice has generally been to have approximately one million cells per vial. Compared to the scale of a production bioreactor for a commercial scale, the scale-up factor or the number of seed trains required to generate sufficient inoculum from the vial to the production bioreactor is high. This is time-consuming and may require additional resources and measures to ensure no failure during the seed generation stage. A seed expansion stage can take about 20–30 days from a low-density bank to a production bioreactor. To negate this additional time and processing, a high cell density bank that accelerates the process by providing a larger working volume at thaw is becoming a recent trend. Using a high cell density cell bank to inoculate the first seed train bioreactor (N-3 bioreactor) can significantly reduce the time. For example, using a 100–150 mL high-density cell bag (cryopreserved) at $50–100 \times 10^6$ cells/mL can reduce the seed expansion process by ten days to two weeks. This innovative process eliminates the need for handling multiple vials, the variability in the cell density is minimized, contamination risks are minimized, and most importantly, the time to start a production bioreactor is significantly reduced. In high cell density cryopreservation, a specific media capable of supporting high cell density while ensuring no cell damage due to freeze-thaw is preferable. Additionally, modern technologies are under development to design single-use bag assemblies that can handle large volumes for cell freezing and banking (fluoropolymer 2D bags).

9.2.4 Cell Culture Operations

While perfusion systems are available, the industry is not widely adopted, primarily due to the need for a high volume of media and vessel capacity to support high cell densities and increased productivity. The last few decades have predominantly focused on fed-batch cultures. Even though the cell densities achievable with fed-batch are relatively low compared to perfusion, the advancements made towards increasing productivities have kept the fed-batch process going for a long. With the need to drive down manufacturing costs and facilities to become more flexible, steady-state perfusion and perfusion-based processes, including concentrated fed-batch, are now being fostered by the increasing adoption of single-use technologies. Perfusion processes in both seed train and production phases can result in a three-fold increase in volumetric productivity. Upstream process intensification can be achieved via

TABLE 9.1

Decision Matrix to Address Bottlenecks and Develop Next-Generation Process

Technology Solutions	Pros	Cons	Comment
Bottleneck: limited facility footprint			
Perfusion	High volumetric productivity	Operational complexity	Needs more process development than fed-batch
Bottleneck: limited CAPEX			
Perfusion	Smaller bioreactor	Operational complexity	Needs more process development than fed-batch
Bottleneck: limited capacity in production bioreactor			
N-1 perfusion	Cell expansion time shifts to N-1; shorter N time with same titer	Operational complexity, possible impact on process performance	Ensure capacity for the shorter turnaround times
Perfusion	High volumetric productivity	Operational complexity	Identify a separation technique that will suit your process
Bottleneck: QC/QA release			
Online sensors and PAT implementations	Reduce number of release methods through tighter process control	Resource demanding to develop	E.g., spectral methods combined with multivariant analysis can offer several process parameters
Multi-attribute release methods	Drastic reduction of release methods	Resource demanding to develop	Still in development
Bottleneck: low-yield process			
Perfusion	High volumetric productivity	Operational complexity	Identify a separation technique that will suit your process
Concentrated fed-batch	High volumetric productivity	Operational complexity	
Bottleneck: several products and process			
Perfusion	Higher level of flexibility	Operational complexity	Scale-out depending on batch volume needed

Source: www.genengnews.com/magazine/324/supplement-next-generation-bioprocess-techniques/.

perfusion-based operations. This includes compressing the seed train duration by reducing the size and number of bioreactors required, maximizing the bioreactor utilization, increasing volumetric productivity, reducing the overall footprint, thereby maximizing facility utilization and efficiency.

N-1 perfusion is a type of seed train intensification that refers to the acceleration of cell growth before the production bioreactor (N). The process is intensified by attaching a cell retention device to the N-1 bioreactor to achieve high cell density and viability. This increases the starting cell density of the production bioreactor and reduces the run time of the production bioreactor. This can significantly increase facility output without requiring any changes to the core manufacturing process. A strong cell retention device is required to achieve a high cell density inoculum for the production bioreactor.

Benefits of N-1 perfusion include:

- Increased fed-batch process efficiency.
- Time and cost savings.
- Reduced operational risk.
- Smaller bioreactor footprint.

N-1 perfusion can help optimize fed-batch production in two ways:

- High cell density seeding of the production bioreactor (N) with the cell retention device attached to the N-1 bioreactor.

- Removal of the N-1 bioreactor with the cell retention device attached to the N-2 bioreactor, if the N-2 bioreactor can provide enough cells for the production bioreactor (N).

The most widely used application for perfusion has been with the N-1 bioreactor. Increasing the N-1 bioreactor's cell density allows for starting the production bioreactor with a high seeding density and possibly reducing the production bioreactor's overall cycle time to achieve the desired titers. Higher productivity and the possibility of inoculating multiple production bioreactors from the single N-1 bioreactor can increase overall upstream capacity and production volumes. This increase in production can also be achieved with a reduced footprint; for example, a traditional process requiring a 20,000 L bioreactor can now be fitted with a 2,000 L perfusion bioreactor. Furthermore, the use of single-use components eliminates the need for cleaning validation, CIP/SIP. Additionally, the perfusion-based process can be extended further down to the N-3 seed train and high cell density cryopreservation, as discussed previously. A single-use bag with approximately 150 mL to 500 mL high cell density culture can be frozen and used to inoculate a seed bioreactor eliminating shake flasks and a lengthy seed expansion step.

Perfusion can dramatically increase the cell density of the N-1 bioreactor and accelerate the production process to achieve efficiency gains. The introduction of perfusion culture within the seed train to increase cell density can reduce the number of bioreactors needed or the time required to reach the desired titer at harvest.

Another application that allows for process intensification is an intensified fed-batch mode or a concentrated fed-batch. A concentrated fed-batch process is much like a perfusion process, except for the cells recirculated here and the product. In combination with a hollow-fiber filter and an ATF pump, the production bioreactor, much like in perfusion, is also used for the concentrated fed-batch process. However, the filter size here should be able to retain both the cells and the product. For an antibody production process, a 30 kDa filter is used. The process typically starts as a fed-batch process, and the cells and product recirculation begin only towards the end of the production cycle. In addition to the high cell densities, an advantage with a concentrated fed-batch process is that the harvest process can be performed in a single operation and does not result in the titer being diluted, as is the case with perfusion. The most widely reported example of the concentrated fed-batch application has been PERCIVIA, a collaboration between Crucell and DSM. The results showed significantly high yields of 27 g/L using PER.C6 cells from the concentrated fed-batch process.

This increased productivity allows for smaller facilities and makes the process efficient when coupled with SUT. A drug manufacturer can leverage these advantages into existing infrastructure while increasing the capacity to remain competitive.

9.2.5 Bioreactor Cycle

A significant limitation of production in a facility is the production bioreactor. The production bioreactor process duration (commonly about two weeks for a fed-batch process) is frequently a rate-limiting step in an industrial facility, given that all other upstream and downstream process steps require only up to a few days. Consequently, there is a need to investigate utilizing perfusion in the bioreactor immediately preceding production. The typical net result is higher densities at the production stage's inoculation, shorter process durations, and similar titer and product quality. Thus, the production process is even more productive with higher overall facility volumetric productivity. The additional challenge lies in optimizing the perfusion medium to generate the necessary cells for the production bioreactor without creating new burdens infrequent, large volume medium preparation in a facility. The cell densities achieved over time and cell-specific productivity are the most critical parameters because they determine the overall cell and product mass generated in the cell culture process.

Another application of upstream process intensification is found in the seed train. Here, an emerging strategy is to use perfusion instead of the batch in the scale-up process. Briefly, the principle is that a perfusion culture can be grown to a very high cell density, enabling inoculation of a production-scale reactor with very few intermediate scale-up steps. For example, a 10 L perfusion culture at 60 million cells/mL can be used for direct inoculation of a 2,000 L reactor at a start cell density of 0.3 million cells/mL. A more conventional scale-up process with batch cultures would have included intermediate vessels of, for example, 50 L, 200 L, and 500 L scale. Another aspect is that a high-density seed culture enables inoculation of the production culture at a high start cell concentration. This can minimize the production lag phase and shorten the production process considerably. A shorter process can enable more production batches annually and better facility utilization. Perfusion to intensify the seed-train is described. Specially designed cryo bags eliminate open cell culture operation steps, lead to better reproducibility in seed train expansion, and decouple cell expansion and batch production, allowing for global distribution of cells to production facilities from a central expansion facility.

9.3 Single-Use Technology (SUT)

The initial resistance to SUT has rapidly shifted towards a broad recognition of the multiple advantages that disposables bring, including increased flexibility and a decreased upfront investment. Manufacturing suites and production plants entirely based on production with single-use are becoming more common, and agile and flexible facilities with disposable technology are being constructed in less time.

These upstream technologies should balance media and single-use costs while considering processing times in the timelines and the annual number of batches produced. Also, the application of smaller bioreactors using SUT could provide flexibility. With fewer limitations on changeover time and cleaning verification, running more lots and products in a facility becomes possible.

Single-use technology has evolved significantly over the last few years and continually undergoes innovation. A facility incorporating SUT or a process using single-use components enables rapid configuration for different processes and changeover between batches—this smart implementation presents drug manufacturers with increased capacity and enhanced flexibility.

While SUT revolves around equipment, the facility and its design are also highly essential. The footprint, ease of operation are key features, and today integrating a modular facility has become popular, particularly when manufacturers want to retain some features of a classic facility. Preconfigured setups allow for a faster establishment of a manufacturing site.

SUT provides the capability to develop a process in one manufacturing location and easily transfer/relocate it to a second location upon establishing the facility. This is accomplished by coupling platform processes with single-use components, resulting in reduced process development times, time, and effort for equipment specifications, suitability, and parallel activities.

SUT suppliers are constantly improvising on existing systems, e.g., multi-use of one equipment for several operations. Examples include the Smart Flexware systems from EMD Millipore. These systems are compatible with both chromatography and TFF operations, thereby reducing footprint and investment. Study comparisons have been reported to show at least a 15% overall cost reduction with SUT versus stainless steel. The new technologies in single-use components increase process robustness, better process control due to automation, flexibility, overall cost reduction, and lower COGS.

A key concern of regulatory agencies in biopharmaceuticals manufacturing is to ensure no cross-contamination of the batches. This cGMP concern is difficult to resolve in the manufacturing of biological products since it is not possible to rely on cleaning validation to ensure that minute traces of substances from previous batches; since even a small number of contaminants can affect the proteins' structure, the issue of cleaning validation is much bigger than for chemical drugs. Additionally, the increase in demand has also necessitated a need for simple yet faster and low-cost production systems.

Single-use technologies (SUT) have addressed some of these challenges compared to conventional stainless-steel systems. This technology has developed over the past three decades with such significant suppliers as Pall, Sartorius, and Millipore taking the lead and developing disposable products pre-sterilized and gamma-irradiated, eliminating the need to conduct cleaning validation exercises.

The earliest SUT products in this category were as simple as filters. Disposable filters have quickly become standard components, accounting for more than 95% of all filters used in bioprocessing. The focus then shifted to other process components leading to bioreactors and chromatography technologies for purification. Additional improvements made on the process, including high titers, process intensification, have provided the ability to run at a relatively smaller scale (10,000 L stainless steel versus 2,000 L single-use bioreactors). The cost savings, a smaller and efficient facility, a faster turnaround between batches, and the elimination of CIP and SIP have added to the SUT's acceptance as the significant revolution in biopharmaceutical manufacturing.

SUT components support various production stages of biopharmaceutical manufacturing, including clone selection, cell banking, upstream and downstream process development, GMP production, formulation, and fill-finish. The combination of SUT with platform processes makes it possible to go from clone selection to GMP products quickly. The adoption of SUT is picking pace, particularly in small-scale or clinical-scale production. Until recently, single-use systems could not handle a large batch size, but newer systems, including TFF, chromatography systems, can offer the capacity.

While the regulatory agencies do not require single-use or disposable items in manufacturing, it is the manufacturer's responsibility to ensure compliance with cross-contamination limits. However, one of the foremost challenges with single-use technologies has been the lack of regulatory guidance on these systems' qualification requirements. When the cost and time needed to meet those requirements become onerous, the cost of single-use or disposable items becomes a serious consideration. The FDA and EMEA strongly urge manufacturers to create environments that would keep the contaminants out rather than clean them and show by validation protocols the effectiveness of cleanliness. This regulatory authorities' stance became sterner in the 1970s as viral contamination came to the surface to prepare human and animal tissue-derived drugs. A large number of manufacturers were forced to close due to their inability to meet the new requirements. The outbreak of TSE added to the complexity, and it became prohibitively expensive to manufacture biological drugs in cGMP-compliant facilities.

The advantages of SUT are apparent: it is safer, greener, cheaper (particularly regarding capital costs), and has greater flexibility. However, there are challenges in the mainstream of manufacturing for a variety of reasons, including lingering questions about the quality of materials used, scalability, operating costs, level of automation possible with these components, reliance on supplier chain, extractable and leachable testing, and the training of staff required to assimilate these components in an established bioprocessing system.

While the EMA has approved a vaccine manufactured using SUT, the FDA has yet to approve a product manufactured using SUT, though several applications are pending approval.

9.3.1 Containers and Mixing Systems

Disposable or single-use bag systems are well adopted as alternates to hard-walled containers. Historically, this is because pharmaceutical products, such as sterile intravenous solutions, blood, plasma, plasma expanders, and hyperalimentation solutions have been stored and dispensed in these types of bags. A disposable bag would typically have a one-layer film made from polyvinyl chloride (PVC) or ethylene-vinyl acetate (EVA) for blood storage. In biomanufacturing, single-use containers are widely used for media storage (bottles, 2D, 3D bags, two-ply, and three-ply bioprocess bags), cryopreservation bags, tank liners for buffers, solutions, as mixing bags, microcarrier filter bags. Typical process steps with mixing include dissolving components of a buffer, culture media, refolding solution, dispersion of cell culture in bioreactors, and heating or cooling of liquids

9.3.2 Drums, Containers, and Tank Liners

Tank liners are simple, single-use (disposable) bags used to line containers and transportation systems. In most cases, they are generally not gamma sterilized since these are used in open systems most of the time, such as in the preparation of buffer solutions and culture media at the first stage of preparation. However, these tank liners are also offered as pre-sterilized versions. Tank liners are a cost-effective alternative to dedicated stainless steel or poly tanks and totes. The container within which the liner is inserted is there only to provide mechanical support. Contour liners reduce cleaning validation and sterilization of traditional containers. Most importantly, because they are single-use, the potential of cross-contamination between different products is reduced.

For smaller volumes, single-use containers of 50 mL to 20 L capacity with integrated handle, integrated hanging capability, and needle-free sampling port are available. These containers may be used with a sterile welder and are known as the manifold system.

For cylindrical tanks, liners for cylindrical tanks of 50 to 750 L capacity are available in 2D and 3D designs, top or bottom drain, and fit most industry standard cylindrical tanks. These tank liners are generally constructed under cGMP conditions in an ISO classified cleanroom to minimize bioburden and other particulate matter. Tank liners eliminate the need for pre-cleaning and post-cleaning, thereby reducing cycle times. These are widely used for the hydration of powdered media, buffer preparation, and other non-sterile solutions.

Commercially available overhead mixers can readily be integrated with most tank liners because these systems are open. However, tank liners are suitable to operate only with specific mixing systems wherein the impeller is powered from the bottom. Generally, the mixing systems that do not involve any mechanical parts inside the bag (either 2D or 3D) are preferred to reduce the cost, the risk of damage to the bag from rotating devices, the grinding of the bag, or the stirrer inside the bag; those stirring systems that use a magnetic field provide better sterility compared to those who are magnetically coupled.

Mixing systems may also be integrated with a load cell, temperature sensor. Additionally, the tank liners may have provisions for pH measurements (reusable and single-use) and sampling ports. The weight measurement (load cell) is of the most significant importance. While most manufacturers would use a floor scale, large-scale production requires installing load cells in the outer containers to avoid moving the containers for weighing. It is noteworthy that the more expensive systems come with programming elements that might make the PAT work easier. Still, at the stage of buffer and media preparation, the challenges are few and readily overcome by implementing the most straightforward and cheapest systems.

Several major equipment suppliers provide a complete line of mixing systems. While these offer an advantage in handling large volumes consistently, one can readily put together a system from off-the-shelf components at a substantially lower cost. A broad choice of low-density polyethylene liners is available from vendors; Thermo Scientific's Hyperforma™ line, EMD Millipore's Mobius® Single-Use Mixing Systems, and Sartorius are some of the popular choices today that supply to several industries.

9.3.2.1 2D Bags

For smaller volumes, 2D bags are available sterile and ready to use, in volumes from 5 mL to 50 L, before they become difficult to handle. These bags are designed for storage, sampling, filtration, and transportation with compatibility for media, buffer, clarified harvest, intermediate product, drug, and drug product. Additionally, these bags are also equipped with ports connected sterilely to other sterile single-use systems. In some instances, it may be necessary to use bags to store powders (such as buffer salts, API, and excipients): these bags have a funnel shape and are equipped with large sanitary fittings or aseptic transfer systems, and are antistatic and free of additives.

9.3.2.2 3D Bags

The 2D bags present the design problem that, at a larger scale, it becomes difficult to maintain their integrity, creating handling and transportation issues. The seals in 2D bags, when filled to their maximum capacity, may not hold since the weight of the fluid inside is transferred to the seams of these bags. This becomes particularly problematic when the 2D bags are rocked or shaken, adding further stress to the seams.

The 3D bags as liners in hard-walled containers obviate the integrity problems of 2D bags; today, these bags are available in varying sizes. The 3D design also provides an additional surface to install ports with complex functions. The 3D bags are made by welding films and are mostly offered in cylindrical, conical, or cube shapes. Often, the shape is determined by how these containers are stored or stacked in outer containers with the same shape, which allows a snug fitting of the 3D bags. These 3D bags are designed for storage and shipping a large volume of solutions. They are supplied sterile and ready to use for quick process implementation.

Single-use bags can be readily used to transport or store frozen products, from cell culture as WCB for direct introduction into a bioreactor to shipping biological API. In contrast, flexible bags can survive temperature variations; often, it is difficult to detect damage to them during transportation and, thus, require a protective surface around them to prevent this risk.

Plastic disposable containers offer the best solution in disposable components utilization as they remove the cleaning and validation requirements. Low-density PE liners in a hard-walled plastic container and a standard mixer make the cheapest combination of pieces to prepare buffers and media. More complex mixing systems are unnecessary, and neither are the expensive proprietary containers to hold these PE liners.

9.3.3 Advantages

The adoption of single-use or hybrid systems represents a faster, more flexible, and less capital-intensive route. Each option's cost and benefits should be weighed against existing infrastructure, technical constraints, and production volume requirements. Single-use manufacturing systems offer multiple advantages versus traditional stainless-steel equipment:

- Increased speed to market.
- Reduced capital—higher equipment and facility utilization, increased number of batches.
- Reduction/elimination of cleaning and validation costs—a biologic manufacturing facility can consume approximately 800,000 gallons of water per day, most of which is used to perform SIP/CIP and operate autoclaves—none of these would be needed with the new generation of single-use systems.
- Elimination of carryover.
- Increased flexibility for facilities with multi-products and batch sizes and faster turnaround—lower cost and flexible capacity to easily adapt to changing scales and accommodate new modalities. SUT allows for a plug-and-play approach when coupled with modular facilities.
- Reduce cross-contamination risks—allows unit operations to be connected, eliminating open processing. This allows concurrent step processing or even potentially multiple product processing.

Evaluation of the cost–benefit of considering a single-use option for a particular process step should include its impact on the other process steps (e.g., previous and subsequent steps). The cost analysis should include end-to-end process manufacturing costs and compare them against the fixed costs of a stainless-steel process. Perhaps the greatest impediment in the wider acceptance of single-use items comes from manufacturers' inability to discard their large investments made, relatively recently (the 1970s and 1980s), in fixed equipment and systems. As a result, smaller businesses, research organizations, and contracting firms are seeing changes. This, however, is about to change dramatically. As patents on blockbuster recombinant drugs have begun to expire, allowing smaller companies to compete on price, the high cost of production acceptable to large pharmaceutical companies must now be challenged—the biosimilar business should persuade the industry to embrace the future of bioprocessing. There are also environmental factors to consider.

Integrating an innovative single-use approach in upstream and downstream processing provides an opportunity to develop a flexible and small-footprint facility, which ultimately is advantageous in manufacturing cost-effective and affordable drugs. A start to finish facility built entirely on disposable and single-use systems. Several analyses have reported that a single-use facility has a lesser operating cost (approximately 22%; Levine 2013) in comparison to stainless steel facility. Figure 9.1 presents a schematic for all manufacturing operations built from start to finish with single-use systems.

9.3.4 Single-Use Bioreactors (SUBS)

The science and the art of bioprocessing date back thousands of years, incorporating newer modalities for biologics, a diverse range of products, more particularly biopharmaceuticals. It took two decades of trials and tribulations to bring cell culture from a benching technique at milligram scales to industrial

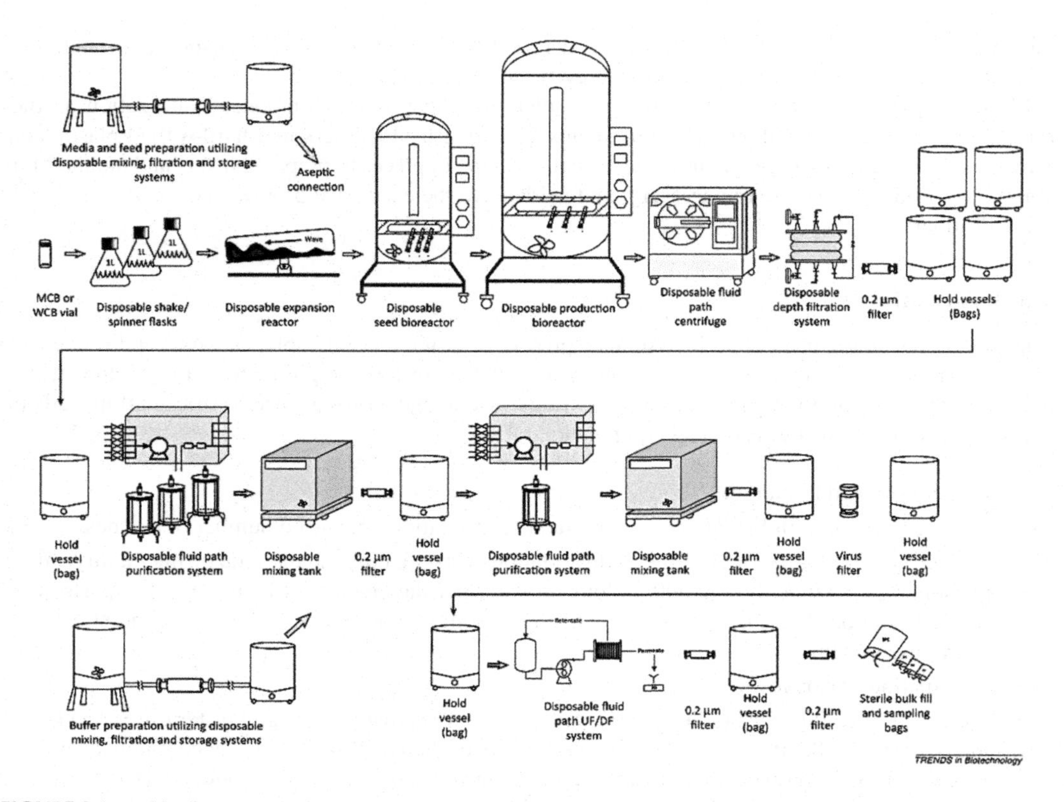

FIGURE 9.1 A biopharmaceutical manufacturing process built with single-use systems.

production at kilogram scales. The current era of biopharmaceuticals is manifested in producing large quantities of biologics in stainless-steel bioreactors. Today those large-scale stirred-tank bioreactors (10,000 L–100,000 L in scale) represent modern mammalian cell culture technology, a significant workhorse of the biopharmaceutical industry.

Stainless-steel bioreactors have been used for centuries. The essential elements, a vessel to contain culture and media with sufficient mixing and aeration, are readily provided in bioreactors' traditional designs. Today, we have a multitude of options in the design of bioreactors. These came about once bioreactors expanded in manufacturing biological drugs requiring many control features that were not needed or required in other industries. With the use of animal, human, and plant cells and viruses to produce therapeutic proteins, vaccines, antibodies, etc., there arose a need to modify the traditional bioreactors to accommodate the growing needs of these new production engines: recombinant engineering put these new engines in the forefront of biological drug production. One major recent change in bioreactors' design is using single-use bioreactors to avoid cleaning validation challenges, reducing the regulatory barriers in drug production. Hundreds of new molecules are under development using disposable bioreactors, and in many instances, disposable bioreactors are used to manufacture clinical supplies.

Almost all the recombinant drugs in the market today were developed by large pharmaceutical companies starting about 40 years ago when the only choice available was the traditional bioreactor; even though their process may be less efficient, it was not worth the effort to switch over to another manufacturing method because of the prohibitive cost of changeover protocols that need to be completed.

The dramatic decrease in changeover time with increased flexibility has been a significant benefit experienced with single-use bioreactors. For example, a change over time for a 200 L bioreactor has been reduced to just two to three hours instead of over 24–48 hours as with a stainless steel reactor.

SUBS have varied designs and purposes, but all of them are made of Class VI plastic films, are sterilized by gamma radiation, and are disposed of after use; they may come with several attachments that allow the filtration of media, monitoring of pH, DO, OD, pCO_2, temperature, and other PAT-related parameters. Using stirrers, paddles, shaking, and rocking the bags by mechanical or hydraulic means achieve mixing and aeration inside the bag, just as effectively as in the traditional stainless-steel tank and, in some instances, lesser stress culture.

SUBS come in many sizes, from mLs to thousands of liters; they can be equipped with control systems from very simple to very complex; they can be manual or highly automated; they can be as inexpensive as a plastic bag to as expensive as the high-end traditional hard-walled bioreactors. The disposable bioreactor industry is still evolving, with new inventions surfacing almost routinely. Examples include replacing glass Petri dishes, T flasks, roller bottles, and glass flasks with plastic plates, polypropylene, and Teflon bags for small-scale bacterial and yeast culturing, disposable hollow fiber systems, WAVE Bioreactors, and stirred 3D reactors.

Types of stirring mechanisms include a mechanical stirrer attached to a motor; a stirrer magnetically levitating, without contact with the motor; a magnetic stirrer at the bottom that rubs off the surface; and a mechanical stirrer inserted from the top. A rocking wave motion is the most commonly used; pioneered by WAVE Bioreactor, several equipment suppliers have adopted this system. The stationary bioreactor concept differs significantly from the usual wave motion that requires moving the plate; the bag stays stationary. A flapper instead pushes down one edge of the disposable bag.

The 3D single-use stirred tank reactor systems have been successfully able to mimic conventional stainless-steel reactors. The dimensions, proportions, sparging systems, and mixing systems are similar to the classical stainless-steel systems (reusable). The single-use bioreactors are equipped with a sparger ring or a microsparger and two axial flow three-blade-segment impellers or one axial flow three-blade-segment and one radial flow six-blade segment impeller. The centered stirring system achieves homogeneous mixing in the bag. All SUBs are equipped to provide mixing, sparging, venting, temperature monitoring. The bioreactor bags have provisions for pH, DO monitoring (single-use and reusable), sampling, liquid transfer, inoculation ports, and harvest ports. SUBs have a plug-and-play setup and operation through standard sterile connections, coupled with easy integration with most control platforms predominantly used industry-wide. The SUBs minimize cleaning, need for sterilization, reduce the risk of cross-contamination. The wide volume range makes these SUBs suitable for process development, clinical manufacturing, and large-scale cGMP manufacturing (Figure 9.2).

The 2D single-use bioreactors such as the CellBag specific to the WAVE systems have also been successfully used. These bioreactor bags use a rocking motion for agitation. These bags are produced from two-layer films, which are welded together at their ends. The result is a flat chamber, which has ports either face welded or end welded. With limitations on volume and challenges with agitation and aeration

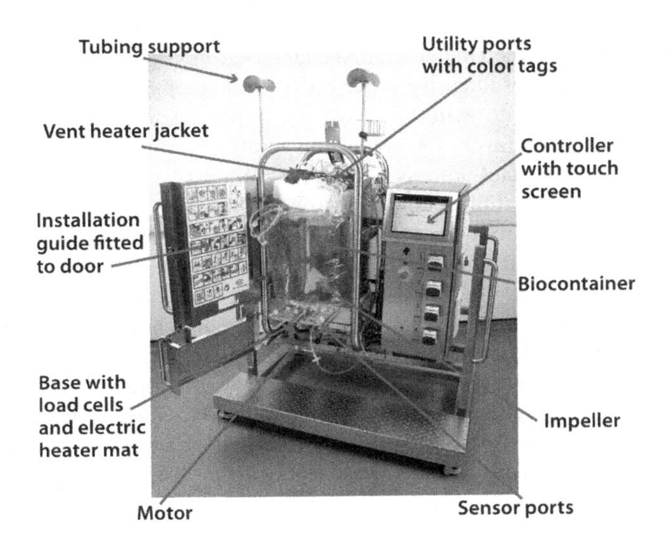

FIGURE 9.2 Single-use bioreactor. Source: https://bioprocessintl.com/2016/design-performance-single-use-stirred-tank-bioreactors/.

at a large scale, these WAVE bioreactors are predominantly used for the seed train steps. Furthermore, they displace the first disposable bioreactors such as roller bottles, cell factories, and hollow fiber bioreactors. This is because most animal and human cells grow serum-free and in suspension and because cell culture bioreactor volumes are currently shrinking due to increased product titers.

Applying non-invasive optical sensor technology to transparent cultivation containers for animal cells has resulted in highly automated or precisely monitored and controlled disposable micro-bioreactor systems. This has paved the way for a change in early-stage process development from being unmonitored to being well characterized and controlled and has made an important contribution to the accurate replication of larger-scale conditions.

It is assumed that the pharmaceutical industry's current drive toward safe, individualized medicines (e.g., personalized antibodies, functional cells for cancer, immune and tissue replacement therapies) will contribute to the continuing growth of disposable bioreactors. When optimized cell densities and product titers must be achieved in the shortest possible time, cell culture technologists need to be willing to move away from their gold standard, that is, the use of stirring systems. In addition to highly instrumented, scalable wave-mixed, and stirred single-use bioreactors, shaken disposable bioreactors and novel approaches such as the PBS or the BayShake are increasing.

Bioreactor manufacturers (Thermo Fisher, Cytiva Life Science [formerly GE Life Sciences], Eppendorf, Sartorius) have demonstrated the successful application of SUBs for cultivating bacteria, supporting high cell density mammalian culture.

9.3.5 Other Components

According to the FDA Guidance for Industry (www.fda.gov/media/71012/download), process analytical technology (PAT) is intended to support innovation and pharmaceutical development efficiency. The PAT is a system for designing, analyzing, and controlling manufacturing by measuring critical quality and performance attributes of raw and in-process materials and processes in real-time (i.e., during processing) to ensure final product quality. It's worth noting that in PAT, the term "analytical" refers to all types of analyses, including chemical, physical, microbiological, mathematical, and risk assessment.

Single-use sensors, which are either integrated into the single-use bioreactor or included in the cover and are disposed of with the bioreactor, must fulfill process requirements. They provide a continuous signal and allow information about the cell culture's status to be gathered at any time.

Because disposable bioreactors are new to the industry, the traditional biosensors used in hard-walled systems to measure bioreactor temperature, dissolved oxygen (DO), pH, conductivity, and osmolality were used as the first attempt to monitor the bioreactor's product. These probes must first be sterilized (via autoclaving) before being welded to penetration adapter fittings in bioreactor bags. Not surprisingly, this is a time-consuming and labor-intensive process that could jeopardize the integrity and sterility of single-use bioreactor bags. However, with the innovation in technology and advancements with SUBs, this has been largely discarded in favor of genuinely disposable sensors. Pressure, pH, DO, cell density, and UV absorbance are all important process parameters frequently monitored. Traditional monitoring technologies are not usually compatible with or effective when integrated into single-use assemblies for various reasons, including cost, cross-contamination, inability to maintain a closed system, and system incompatibility with gamma irradiation. Some of the measurements are done offline due to these difficulties.

The adoption of disposable sensors requires a keen understanding of their need and utilization. Many bioprocess unit operations are either pressure-controlled or have serious pressure-related safety concerns. For example, a sanitary, autoclavable pressure transducer qualified for a certain number of autoclave cycles and required recalibration may be more expensive to use than a single-use pressure sensor.

There are two options in using disposable sensors: one where the sensors are placed in situ in contact with the liquid, and the other where the external sensors contact the medium either optically (ex situ) or via a sterile (and disposable) sample removal system (online). Single-use sensors must be sterilizable or be available pre-sterilized if they contact media and must also be cost-effective and reliable. Better designs use inexpensive sensing elements located inside a disposable bioreactor and combined with reusable (and more expensive) analytical equipment outside the reactor. Inexpensive, single-use sensors can also be placed on transistors and placed either in the headspace, inlet, outlet, or cultivation broth for liquid-phase analysis (temperature, pH, pO_2). These can also be optical sensors, which allow noninvasive monitoring through a transparent window.

9.3.5.1 Optical Sensors

Optical sensors work on the principle of the effect of electromagnetic waves on molecules. It is an entirely non-invasive method and can provide continuous results of many parameters at the same time. It is relatively easy to use them through a transparent window in the bioreactors. The detector part of the system can be physically separated, allowing the utilization of expensive analytical devices allowing optical sensors to be used in situ or online.

Fluorescence sensors can be optimized for nicotinamide adenine dinucleotide phosphate (NADPH) measurements and are used for both biomass estimation and differentiating between aerobic and anaerobic metabolism. The two-dimensional process fluorometry enables several analytes' simultaneous measurement by scanning through a range of excitation and emission wavelengths, including proteins, vitamins, coenzymes, biomass, glucose, and metabolites such as ethanol adenosine-5'-triphosphate (ATP) and pyruvate. Thus, it is possible to use fluorometry to characterize the upstream process. Generally, a fiber-optic light attached to the bioreactor and shining the light through a glass window in the bioreactor works very well. An example of this is the fluorometers from the BioView system (www.bioview.com). The BioView sensor is a multichannel fluorescence detection system for biotechnology, pharmaceutical, chemical, food production, and environmental monitoring. It detects specific compounds and the state of microorganisms and their chemical environment without interfering with the sample. The BioView system measures fluorescence online directly in the process. Interference with the sample is eliminated, reducing the risk of contamination. However, given the complexity of the spectra of multiple components, high-level resolution programming is required.

Many metabolic products in a bioreactor can be readily detected by IR spectroscopy. Still, a water-absorbed IR beam can only be NIR or SIR for biomass analysis when used in transmission mode. NIR transmission probes and ATR-IR probes for bioreactors are now commercially available. These are connected through silver halide fibers or radio frequency connectors.

In addition to IR and fluorescence, optical methods based on photoluminescence, reflection, and absorption are also used. The optical electrodes or *optodes* can be attached using glass fibers leaving the measurement equipment outside of the bioreactor as discussed above for fluorescence detectors, allowing them to use these chemosensors in situ or online.

Oxygen sensors work by quenching fluorescence by molecular oxygen; measurement requires a fluorescent dye (metal complexes) immobilized and attached to one end of an optical fiber. The other end of the fiber is interfaced with an excitation light source. The duration and strength of fluorescence depending on the oxygen concentration in the environment around the dye. The emitted fluorescence light is collected and transmitted for reading outside of the bioreactor. These electrodes work better than the traditional platinum probe electrodes to detect oxygen, working in both liquid and gas phases. PreSens (www.presens.de), for example, are noninvasive oxygen sensors that measure the partial pressure of dissolved and gaseous oxygen. These sensor spots detect glassware and disposables. The sensor spots are permanently attached to the inner surface of the glass or transparent plastic material. Therefore, the oxygen concentration can be measured non-invasive and non-destructive manner from outside through the vessel's wall. Different coatings for different concentration ranges are available. It offers online monitoring of concentration ranges from 1 ppb to 45 ppm DO, with dependence on flow velocity and measuring oxygen in the gas phase. These can be autoclaved.

Ocean Optics (www.oceanoptics.com) offers the world's first miniature spectrometer with a wide array of sensors for oxygen, pH, and the gas phase.

The pH sensors work by fluorescence or absorption, and for fiber-optic pH measurements, both fluorescence-and absorbance-based pH indicators can be applied. For fluorescence, the most common dyes are 8-hydroxyl1,3,6-pyrene trisulfonic acid and fluorescein derivatives, while phenol red and cresol red are used for absorption type measurements. Fluorescent dyes are sensitive to ionic strength limiting their use for broad pH measurement, more than three units.

Carbon dioxide sensors work on the principle of measuring the pH of a carbonate buffer embedded in a CO_2-permeable membrane. The sensors' reaction time is long, and quaternary ammonium hydroxide gives a faster response.

Fluorescence-based sensors are attractive as they facilitate the development of portable and low-cost systems that can be easily deployed outside the laboratory environment. Unlike unreferenced fluorescence intensity measurements, these measurements are unaffected by changes in dye concentration, leaching, and photobleaching of the fluorophore, as well as instrument fluctuations. The sensor system's performance is characterized by a high degree of repeatability, reversibility, and stability.

9.3.5.2 Biomass Sensors

Information about the biomass concentration can also be obtained via turbidity sensors. Generally, these sensors are based on the principle of scattered light. Most turbidity sensors have the disadvantage that there is only a linear correlation for low particle concentrations. But sensors that use backscattering light (180°) also have linear properties for high particle concentrations. A translucent window for the desired wavelength in the IR region is necessary for disposable reactors. The S3 Mini-Remote Futura line of biomass detectors (www.applikonbio.com) incorporates sensors inside disposable bioreactors. This system incorporates an ultra-lightweight pre-amplifier for connecting to the ABER disposable probe (www.bioprocess-eng.co.uk/product/aber-futura-pico/).

9.3.5.3 Electrochemical Sensors

Electrochemical sensors include potentiometric, conductometric, and voltammetry sensors. Thick and thin-film sensors and chemically sensitive field-effect transistors (ChemFETs) possess potential potentiometric disposable sensors in bioprocess control. They can be produced inexpensively and in large quantities.

Many pH sensing systems rely on amperometry methods, but they require constant calibration due to instability or drift. Most amperometry sensors' setups are based on the pH-dependent selectivity of membranes or films on the electrode surface.

While turbidity sensors detect the total biomass concentration, capacitance sensors provide information specifically about the viable cell mass. Electrical capacitance and conductance generally characterize the electrical properties of cells in an alternating electrical field. The integrity of the cell membrane exerts a significant influence on the electrical impedance to estimate only viable cells. The Biodis series for monitoring viable biomass in disposables applications is available from Hamilton (www.hamiltoncompany.com) and Aber (www.aberinstruments.com), and an integrated version is available from Eppendorf (www.eppendorf.com).

9.3.5.4 Pressure Sensors

Another critical process parameter frequently monitored during bioprocess unit operations like filtration, chromatography, and many others is pressure. Using a traditional stainless-steel pressure gauge in conjunction with a single-use experimental setup is possible but has the drawback that the pressure gauge must be sterilized separately. Furthermore, the connection of the sensor to the previously gamma-radiated single-use assembly can be problematic.

Many bioprocess unit operations are either pressure-controlled or have serious pressure-related safety concerns. Traditional stainless-steel reactors are monitored and controlled for pressure, as pressure is used to influence mass transfer and prevent contamination. Also, a high-pressure event is a potentially hazardous situation. A clogged vent filter on a bioreactor can easily rupture bags, spilling the reactor's contents and exposing the operators to unprocessed bulk.

Depth and sterile filtration is another application where pressure monitoring is critical to process performance. The capacity of a filter is primarily determined by flow decay or pressure increases. However, adding reusable traditional pressure transducers to a process train defeats the purpose of a single-use process setup. Depending on the process application, a traditional device's product contact surface requires either sanitization or moist heat sterilization.

Traditional devices are compatible with steam in place (SIP), which exposes only the product contact surface to steam, and autoclavable devices, which expose the entire device to steam. However, because many single-use process components are incompatible with moist heat sterilization temperatures, the stainless-steel device may need to be sterilized separately, resulting in a less-than-ideal connection to a pre-sterilized single-use assembly.

In both development and early-phase clinical manufacturing, single-use pressure sensing allows for rapid product contact parts. PendoTECH's (www.pendotech.com) single-use pressure sensors, for example, were created to enable pressure measurement with single-use assemblies that use flexible tubing as the fluid path. The fluid path materials meet USP Class VI guidelines and are also compliant with EMEA 410 Rev 2 guidelines, and the single-use pressure sensors are gamma compatible (up to 50 KGy).

The USP Class VI designation is the strictest and, as a result, the most useful for medical applications. It entails the following three in vivo biological reactivity tests, which are usually carried out on mice or rabbits to mimic human use.

- Acute Systemic Toxicity (Systemic Injection) Test: Determines the toxicity and irritation of a compound when taken orally, applied to the skin, or inhaled.
- Topical Toxicity Test: When the sample comes into contact with live subdermal tissue, it is tested for toxicity and localized irritation (specifically, the medical device's tissue to contact).
- Implantation Test: Determines the toxicity, infection, and irritation of a compound injected intramuscularly into a test animal over several days.

In addition to demonstrating an extremely low level of toxicity bypassing these three tests, the material will be subjected to several temperature assessments for set periods. Materials that meet USP Class VI standards are thought to have a higher level of quality and are more likely to be accepted by the FDA and USDA because they are thought to reduce the risk of patients being harmed by a toxic material's reaction.

However, USP Class VI Testing is only one method of determining biocompatibility. Some biocompatibility requirements for medical devices, which are not limited to a limited set of tests, may exceed the testing performed in USP Class VI. ISO-10993 is a more rigorous standard for the biological evaluation of medical devices.

Systemic toxicity and intracutaneous reactivity testing are both used in ISO-10993. It does, however, include more extensive cytotoxicity, genotoxicity, chronic toxicity, hemocompatibility tests, and systemic toxicity testing. The different levels of ISO-10993 testing are primarily required for medical devices implanted into a patient permanently or semi-permanently. As a result, ISO-10993 testing may be more extensive than necessary for devices that are not intended to be implanted or have limited contact with patients.

In a single-use bioreactor, a sensor can be installed on a vent line to measure headspace pressure. The core sensor is accurate in the low-pressure range required for a single-use bioreactor, even though the sensors are qualified for use up to 75 psi.

9.3.5.5 Sampling Systems

Continuous sampling from a bioreactor can be accomplished using a sterile filter and a peristaltic pump to obtain a cell-free sample. A pre-sterilized sampling container, including a needleless syringe that can be welded to the bag bioreactor's sampling module, is available for use. A sample is pumped into the container for these assemblies, and these sampling containers can be removed, and the tube is heat-sealed. Other sampling systems involve connecting a pre-sterilized Leuer connection, including a one-way valve, to prevent the sample from flowing back into the reactor. The sample is withdrawn from the reactor by a syringe and directed through a sample line into a reservoir. For example, Cellexus Biosystems (https://cellexus.com) and Millipore (www.sigmaaldrich.com) use this approach. The Cellexus system connected to the sample line can have up to six sealed sample pouches. The reservoir sample can then be pushed into the pouches separated by a mechanical sealer, resulting in sealed, sterile samples. Several sampling manifolds with a customizable option are offered by bioreactor manufacturers/suppliers.

The proprietary Millipore system comprises a port insert that can be fitted to several bioreactor side ports and several flexible conduits that can be opened and closed individually for sampling and are connected to flexible, single-use sampling containers. Sampling is limited to the number of available conduits in each module.

These sampling systems allow aseptic sampling but are limited by the number of samples taken per module and the lack of automation. And while these methods help create good validation data, the risk of contamination is not removed since the bioreactor is breached every time a sample is withdrawn. There is a need to develop other methods that will not require contact with the media.

9.3.5.6 Connectors

The complexity of bioprocessing makes it difficult to design systems without any weak links; contamination is a risk that requires all connectors, tubing, and implements to join various steps of a process and perform sampling in a sterile environment. Single-use components came into use first in connectors and lines, as it was difficult to clean them. Flexible tubing used in single-use transfer lines, unlike hard piping, does not require costly and time-consuming cleaning and validation. Innovative manufacturers are now incorporating single-use tubing assemblies throughout the bioprocess from seed trains to final fill applications. This enables manufacturers to change process steps or switch to a new product quickly. This is a significant benefit for multiple manufacturing facilities where process requirements vary depending on the manufactured drug. Reduced labor, chemical, water, and energy demands associated with cleaning and validation result in additional cost savings.

Still, in hard-walled systems, SIP (steam-in-place) systems are used only because there is steam for CIP (clean-in-place)/SIP operations. Even then, the risk of contamination remains. Since much of the SUT in these applications has come from the biomedical field, the device industry had always been ahead of the regulatory requirements. Biocompatibility issues have long been resolved, and vendors can provide detailed information on their devices that regulatory agencies might need. Since the manufacturing of these devices is complex, it is unlikely for a user to request custom devices; however, today's diversity of choices is enough to modify any system that would use an off-the-shelf item. As before, the emphasis on the importance of an off-the-shelf item over custom designs remains. The tube connectors and sealers are a newer entry as single-use bags for mixing and bioreactors have become more popular; still, there is a limited choice of suppliers, mainly Cytiva LifeSciences Sartorius-Stedim. This equipment's cost is still high, but the alternative comes down to using expensive aseptic connectors. Generally, if a good choice of aseptic connectors is available, that should be preferred over tube connectors since it is always possible to make a poor connection using the heat-activated systems; also, the use of aseptic connectors allows connecting tubes that may not be thermolabile.

Inoculum is scaled up from a few million cells in a few milliliters of culture to thousands of liters in modern bioprocessing facilities. At each point along the seed train, an aseptic transfer is required. Scaling up in traditional bioprocessing facilities is done with a dedicated series of stainless-steel bioreactors connected by valves and rigid tubing. A CIP system is built into each bioreactor, vessel, and piping line in these systems to remove any residual materials and prevent contamination between production runs. These CIP and SIP systems' valves and piping require extensive validation testing, and the valves and piping can present additional validation challenges.

Advances in SUT allow bioprocess engineers to replace most storage vessels and fixed piping networks with single-use storage systems and tubing assemblies. By eliminating expensive vessels, valves, and sanitary piping assemblies, single-use components eliminate the need for CIP validation for many components and lower maintenance and capital costs.

For volumes ranging from 20 to 2,500 L, single-use media storage systems are commonly used. When they arrive at the bioprocess facility sterilized by gamma irradiation, media storage systems are frequently equipped with integrated filters, sampling systems, and connectors. Using single-use digital-to-analog connectors (DACs) or even tube welders and sealers with compatible tubing allows operators to make sterile connections between these pre-sterilized single-use systems bioreactors for aseptic transfer of media, cells, and any other liquid additions. These aseptic connectors can be used for high flow and high-pressure applications. The DACs are also suitable for downstream applications.

Similarly, customized pre-sterilized single-use tubing assemblies are used to transfer inoculum between bioreactors using either a peristaltic pump or headspace pressure. Flexible tubing with aseptic connectors is used as transfer lines between each reactor in the process. Such transfer lines reduce the number of reusable valves required for transfer and eliminate problem areas for CIP and SIP validation. Terminating each pre-sterilized transfer line with a single-use SIP connector provides sterility assurance equal to traditional fixed piping at lower capital costs.

There are also instances when liquids are transferred from a higher ISO environment to a lower ISO environment, and assurance is needed that it does not result in cross-contamination; to assure this, a conduit can be installed in the walls connecting the two areas, with the cleaner room having a higher pressure. A pre-sterilized tube is then inserted from the lower ISO class side to the higher ISO class side and connected to the vessels between which the liquid is transferred by a peristaltic pump; upon completion of the transfer, the tube is pulled into the higher ISO class area and discarded. This method allows the connection between downstream and upstream areas without the risk of transferring any contamination to a lower ISO class area, such as a downstream area.

9.3.5.7 Tubing

Flexible tubes are an essential part of all single-use systems and are subject to the safety concerns described in an earlier chapter about the leachable and extractable. Several attributes of flexible tubing require evaluation, such as their heat resistance, operating temperature range, chemical resistance, color, density, shore hardness, flexibility, elasticity, surface smoothness, mechanical stability, abrasion resistance, gas permeability, visible and ultraviolet (UV) light sensitivity, the composition of layers, weldability, sealability, and sterilizability by gamma radiation or in an autoclave.

All tubes used in bioprocessing conform to USP Class VI classification, FDA 21 CFR 177.2600, and EP 3A Sanitary Standard. For cGMP manufacturing, these are classified as bulk pharmaceuticals.

9.3.5.8 Pumps

Pumps are used for fluid transfer by creating hydrostatic pressure or differential pressure; the maximum allowed pressure would be determined by the weakest part of the bioprocess component exposed to the pressure. In some unit operations like harvesting, tangential flow filtration (TFF), and chromatography, the molecule is highly sensitive to any pumping changes. The pulsing can either impact the fluid being pumped or even damage the pump parts. The pump must have the following capabilities for suitability with the intended use:

- Low volume and surface area exposure.
- Low levels of leachable and extractable.
- Controlled flow and pressure.
- Low shear and pulsation.
- No mechanical spalling/shedding of contact materials.
- Self-priming.
- No heat buildup.
- Sterility.
- High volumetric efficiency.

Permanent stainless-steel process lines are expensive to install, complex, and require extensive cleaning and validation. Some pumps use mechanical seals that cannot maintain constant flow or compromise the sterility, making them less suited for handling biologics.

Peristaltic pumps, syringe pumps, and diaphragm pumps are all currently used to provide single-use pumping solutions. Single-use positive displacement quaternary diaphragm pumps are one of the best options for bioprocessing applications. These are volume displacement pumps, easy to use and avoid contact with the product; however, they can produce stress on the tubing, primarily when the operations are conducted for an extended period. The tube's stress may produce particles from erosion of the tube and contaminate the fluids being passed through. Many biological drugs are shear-sensitive, and peristaltic pumps protect them by applying low pressure and providing gentle handling. In contrast, a piston pump's valve system generates fast flow through small orifices, potentially damaging biological products. Even valveless piston pumps apply high pressures and high shear factors that could harm a biological product.

High-end peristaltic dispensing pumps have benefited from improved pulsation-free pump head design, a precise drive motor, and a state-of-the-art calibration algorithm. They are exceptionally accurate at microliter fill volumes. Peristaltic pumps that incorporate single-use tubing eliminate cross-contamination and do not require cleaning because the tubing is the only part that contacts the product. Likewise, the cleaning validation of peristaltic pumps with single-use tubing is significantly easier than for piston pumps. On the other hand, viscous products can be problematic for peristaltic pumps. The pumps apply only approximately 1.3 bar of pressure, and their accuracy suffers when they handle products more viscous than 100 cP. There have been several improvements made with pumps meant for downstream processing, including high-performance liquid chromatography (HPLC), tangential flow filtration (TFF), and virus filtration (VF) applications, enable high process yields throughout the pressure range (e.g., Quantum; www.watson-marlow.com/us-en/range/watson-marlow/single-use-pumps/quantum/). Single-use pumps usually consist of bags instead of stainless-steel vessels and use special agitators, single-use tubing, coupling, and valves. The single-use components reduce the cost of cleaning and eliminate extensive validation. Plug and play options are available for TFF applications. These pumps provide a liner flow across the pressure range required for the process; they induce ultra-low shear, increasing the downstream process yield.

A diaphragm pump is a positive displacement pump that uses the reciprocating action of a rubber, thermoplastic, or Teflon diaphragm and non-return check valves to pump a fluid. Quaternary diaphragm pumps are driven one after another by connector plates that move back and forth. These pumps are ideal for all liquid biologics handling, including viscous liquids. Some pumps also can self-prime, run dry, and be operated at a constant flow, with low shear, pulsation, and without any heat buildup.

9.3.5.9 Tube Welder and Sealers

When using a thermoplastic tube, welding offers an easy, inexpensive, and very secure solution. Examples of thermoplastic tubes include C-Flex, PharMed, and Bioprene. Both thermoplastic tubes must be aseptic, have the same dimensions (inner diameter and OD), and have their ends capped. The tubes are place parallel in opposite directions while a heated blade cuts through them and seals them simultaneously. Preheating the blade is necessary to achieve the welding temperature and sterilize and depyrogenate the blade before the welding process. The depyrogenate procedure normally lasts 30 s at 250° C or 3 s at 320° C. After being cut, the tubes are moved against each other so that each tube's ends connected to the aseptic systems are positioned directly opposite each other on either side of the blade. A welding cycle can be between 1 and 4 min, depending on the material and the tubes' diameter. The main welding systems available today include Sterile Tube Fuser (GE Healthcare), BioWelder (Sartorius-Stedim), Aseptic Sterile Welder 3960 (SEBRA), TSCD (Terumo), and SCD 11B (Terumo). Terumo supplies its equipment mainly to the blood transfusion industry. Both GE Healthcare and Sartorius-Stedim lead the installations in the bioprocessing industry.

When disconnecting an aseptic connection, the ends must be capped with aseptic caps. This can be done under a laminar hood or by using tube sealers, the examples of which include offerings from PDC (www.pdcbiz.com), Saint-Gobain (www.Saint-Gobain.com), Sartorius-Stedim (www.sartorius-stedim.com), GE Healthcare (www.GELifesciences.com), Terumo (www.terumotransfusion.com), and SEBRA (www.sebra.com). Most of these sealers can seal from 0.25 to about 1.5 in tubes and take from 1–4 min to complete the seal. Most operate on the electrical heating element but electrical, and radio frequencies are also used for sealing tubes. There is no need to use a laminar flow hood for these operations. In most instances, applying a crimper in two places and cutting the tube between the crimps offers the cheapest solution.

9.3.6 Sampling

Sampling is a routine during manufacturing to assure compliance by obtaining these in-process parameters like pH, DO, OD, pCO_2, etc. Most single-use systems have one or more integrated sampling lines, partly equipped with special sampling valves, sampling manifolds, or special sampling systems. A popular single-use sample valve is the Clave connector from ICU-Medical (www.icumed.com), which is also used in intravascular catheters for medical applications. It allows a sample to be taken with a Luer-Lok syringe. A dynamic seal inside the valve guarantees that the sample is not taken until the syringe is connected, thereby ensuring the sample only contacts the valve's inner aseptic parts. However, the samples drawn do not remain sterile.

Manifolds consisting of sampling bags, sampling flasks, or syringes are appropriate for taking aseptic samples in single-use systems. These manifolds can be connected to the systems via aseptic connectors or tube welding. Only one connection has to be made to allow several bags to be filled. Sampling manifolds allow multiple sampling for quality purposes over a given period. The main feature of the manifold is that the number of manipulations in a process is significantly reduced. The manifold systems are delivered ready for process use, preassembled, and sterile.

Also used for sampling are manifold systems where sample containers of a manifold are arranged in parallel, whereby the last one is used as a waste container. The initial flow and the subsequent sample are guided to the appropriate containers using Y-, T-, or X-hose barbs and tube clamps. SIP connections, of course, also allow the connection of manifold systems to conventional stainless-steel processing equipment.

9.3.7 Downstream Processing

Single-use technology is an attractive solution for minimizing downtimes between batches, the additional burden on cleaning, validating these procedures, and, most importantly, reducing the risk of contamination between batches. Single-use technologies also facilitate easy switching between product lines in a multiproduct facility. SUTs have been successfully used for the upstream process and become an integral part of evolution with downstream processes., such as columns, other disposable hardware systems, and single-use flow paths.

Single-use liquid chromatography systems, such as the ÄKTA ready XL chromatography systems with disposable flow paths and prepacked columns, can support large-scale commercial manufacturing and conveniently meet the capacity from single-use 2,000 L upstream processes with high titer. These systems have shown to be very useful in both technology transfer and process scale-up operations.

There is an increased emphasis on supporting therapeutic drugs to be more affordable. Single-use systems and continuous manufacturing operations are critical drivers in bringing down the overall manufacturing and investment cost to make this a possibility.

Adopting single-use components in downstream bioprocessing has been an evolutionary process with a few revolutionary peaks here and there. It started with buffer bags and devices for normal flow filtration, including virus filtration and guard filters for chromatographic columns. Still, gradually, more complex concepts have been introduced, including single-use devices for tangential flow filtration and chromatography in the downstream processing. Today, the consensus of the industry is that while many of the upstream operations can be converted to fully single-use systems, at least some elements of downstream processing will remain traditional, and the reasons quoted for this assertion is that columns and resins will always be too expensive to throw away and, since columns can be of very large size, it will be difficult to find a suitable single-use substitution. However, as history tells, these were the same arguments presented just 15 years ago, opposing bioreactors' conversion to single-use devices. Today, the downstream processing science is developing more rapidly than upstream science; more recently, the use of membrane adsorbs has been recommended for large-scale purification of antibodies. These membranes are much cheaper than classical resins.

9.3.7.1 Cell Harvest

For cell harvesting and debris removal, filtration is an alternative to conventional centrifugation. Single-use filtration systems are available, and these offer flexibility and scalability of operations. Benefits include the ease of scale-up and the availability of pre-sterilized filter capsules that can be integrated directly into production lines. Though this stage is generally completed by centrifugation or lenticular filtration, the depth filter systems (for example, Millipore's POD Filtration) provided the first available alternative in single-use lenticular filters combining two distinct separation technologies in an adsorptive depth filter to enhance filter capacity and retention while compressing multiple filtration steps into one efficient operation. Depth filters employ a porous filtration medium that allows particles to be retained throughout the medium rather than on its surface. Depth filters are made of fibers spread out on a substrate to make a mesh; special additives activated carbon, ceramic fibers, and other such specific components are embedded with a binder's help to form the filter. Depth filters use their entire depth to retain particulate based on sieving compounded by adsorption effects, unlike retentive filters where the filtered material is concentrated on the surface. These filters are commonly used when the fluid to be filtered a high load of particles because, relative to other types of filters, they can retain a large mass of particles before becoming clogged.

Scale-up is achieved by inserting multiple pods into a holder, with formats allowing 1–5 or 5–30 pods as required. Further single-use depth filter formats include the Stax-System from Pall Life Science, encapsulated Zeta Plus from Cuno, and the L-Drum from Sartorius-Stedim, as well as Millipore's Clarisolve, DOHC, and XOHC adsorptive depth filters for primary and secondary clarification. These filters allow efficient cell clarification by reducing the cell biomass, HCP, and host DNA and removes most of the cell debris to enable easy load in the chromatographic column.

The performance of depth filters is dependent on the colloid content of the bioreactor offload and the cell debris removal capacity of the upstream centrifuge. Usually, depth filters are operated with a constant flow of 100–200 L/(m^2 h) and up to 150 L feed/m^2 of filter depending on the feed stream's composition. The Millipore Millistak+ Pod system has a maximum 33 m^2 filter area capacity, resulting in a 3 L to 5,000 L batch capacity. The Millipore Mobius FlexReady process equipment supports a larger 55 m^2-filter area. Since the washing of these filters requires huge buffers, appropriate size holding tanks can be lined with single-use PE liners.

In some instances, for high volumes of clarified harvest, crossflow filtration is performed to reduce the volume for subsequent purification; however, debris buildup extends the time for filtration. While this process is not sterile, the use of a single-use filter prevents the problem of cross-contamination.

A single-use continuous centrifugation device such as kSep® is proposed for processing several recombinant proteins and vaccines. The kSep® is a closed constant centrifuge and works by creating centrifugal force and feed flow force. This system offers the benefit of efficient processing without impacting recovery due to its low shear and continuous operation.

Each technology has its advantages and drawbacks, so testing each option and choosing a specific method and cell type is recommended. The above single-solution performance depends on the USP performance, cell density, viability, and the extent of the cell debris present in the bioreactor broth.

9.3.7.2 Purification

For capturing and polishing, a steel column is packed with a resin (stationary phase) comprising porous beads made of a polysaccharide, mineral, or synthetic matrix conjugated to specific functional groups exploiting different separative principles. The protein mixed with other components is loaded onto the column slowly. Once it is bound to resin, the resin is eluted with appropriate pH and electrolyte solutions to separate the mixture's target protein. The resin is cleaned and sanitized for repeated use that may involve dozens or perhaps hundreds of cycles.

Several vendors now offer columns such as GE's ReadyToProcess systems for use in ÄKTA machines to overcome the time needed to pack resin and operate a column. GE offers a wide range of resins and offers custom resins as well. These are high-performance bioprocessing columns that come prepacked, prequalified, and pre-sanitized. The ReadyToProcess columns and the use of single-use or single-use flow paths eliminate the risk for cross-contamination. The ÄKTA ready system has a sanitary design and is well-suited for use in a cGMP-regulated environment. The simple procedures and low downtime between products and batches of ÄKTA ready enable improved economy and productivity. Other prepacked columns offered like the ReadyToProcess include Opus (Repligen) and GoPure (Life Technologies).

The ÄKTA system is designed for seamless scalability, delivering the same performance level as conventional processing columns such as AxiChrom™ and BPG™. Currently available with a range of BioProcess™ media in four different sizes, 1, 2.5, 10, and 20 L, these are designed to purify biopharmaceuticals for clinical phase I and II studies. Depending on the scale of operations, they can also be used for full-scale manufacturing and preclinical studies. The columns can be used in a wide range of chromatographic applications to separate various compounds such as proteins, endotoxins, DNA, plasmids, vaccines, and viruses.

ÄKTA ready chromatography systems built for process scale-up and manufacturing. Single-use chromatography solutions such as ÄKTA XL systems are offered with prepacked columns, single-use flow paths, plug-and-play chromatography columns, and membranes, as well as pre-sterilized filters and tubing to eliminate cleaning and validation activities. Operates with ready-to-use, single-use flow paths eliminating cleaning and validation between products and batches.

Purification of proteins from complex mixtures is a key process in pharmaceutical research and production. But chromatography based on particulate matrices involves lengthy procedures and separation times.

There are several available ligands, shown in Table 9.2.

A special advantage in using membrane adsorbers is removing high-molecular-weight contaminants such as DNA and viruses in monoclonal antibody manufacturing. Such molecules do not readily diffuse into traditional resins; thus, most polishing steps relying on column chromatography require dramatically oversized columns. These hydrodynamic benefits provide the opportunity to operate membrane adsorber at much greater flow rates than columns, considerably reducing buffer consumption and shortening the overall process time by up to 100-fold. Commercially used membrane adsorbers are Mustang® (Pall), Sartobind® (Sartorius), Chromasorb® (Millipore), and Adsept® (Natrix). These membranes are commonly used for process-related impurities such as DNA, endotoxin removal in flow-through mode.

The accelerated seamless antibody purification (ASAP) process is an entirely single-use continuous mAb downstream process, based on ÄKTA periodic counter-current chromatography (PCC) protein A, mixed-mode, and anion exchange resin columns where the three columns are cycled simultaneously. These systems offer both single-use and continuous processing in a single application while providing flexibility and ease of operation with an increased capacity.

When selecting single-use consumables, it is crucial to ensure that the supply chain is strong. Ensuring the right documentation and testing for extractable and leachable is following the regulatory compliance.

Single-use systems provide great flexibility to handle several products in a facility; the fast turnaround time between batches or products results in a quicker product release.

9.3.7.3 Virus Removal

Virus contamination can occur in any biotechnology product derived from human or animal cell lines. Contamination of a product by endogenous viruses from cell banks or adventitious viruses spread by

TABLE 9.2

Different Types of Membranes and Ligands.

Membrane Type	Description	Ligand	Pore Size (µm)
Sulfonic acid (S)	Strong acidic cation exchanger	$R\text{-}CH_2\text{-}SO_3\text{-}$	> 3
Quaternary ammonium (Q)	Strong basic anion exchanger	$R\text{-}CH_2\text{-}N^+(CH_3)_3$	> 3
Carboxylic acid(C)	Weak acidic cation exchanger	R-COO-	> 3
Diethylamine (D)	Weak basic anion exchanger	$R\text{-}CH_2\text{-}N(C_2H_5)_2$	> 3
Phenyl	Hydrophobic interaction (HIC)	Phenyl	> 3
IDA	Metal chelate	Iminodiacetic acid	> 3
Protein A	Affinity	Protein A	0.45
Epoxy-activated	Coupling	Epoxy group	0.45
Aldehyde-activated	Coupling	Aldehyde group	0.45

Source: Sartorius-Stedim.

employees can have serious clinical consequences. Three complementary approaches assure the viral safety of licensed biological products are:

- Testing for viral contaminants in the cell line and all raw materials.
- Determining the capacity of downstream processing to remove infectious viruses.
- Testing the product for contaminating viruses at appropriate stages.

The FDA requires a demonstration of virus clearance by two methods. A combination of methods inactivation, adsorption, and size exclusion are available. Examples of inactivation procedures are solvent and detergent, chemical treatments, low pH, or microwave heating. Methods of adsorption utilize chromatography, and removal by mechanical or molecular size exclusion uses normal (forward) and tangential flow filtration methods.

Ion exchange and protein A chromatography are widely used to remove viruses, and several key studies have been conducted in collaboration with the FDA. Yet, the responsibility of proving the suitability of any method remains the responsibility of the developer. Membrane filtration has been used for viral clearance in mAb processes for many years. Hollow fiber membrane cartridges and even surface-modified, hydrophilic membranes with high void volume and minimal fouling capable of high viral titer reduction are some of the recent single-use options for viral clearance. Adsorptive filters can be used to end the purification process in line with the viral filtration step. These filters combine size exclusion and adsorptive properties to retain aggregates by hydrophobic interactions while increasing viral filtration efficiency. Several manufacturers like Sartorius, Pall, and Millipore offer single-use virus filtration solutions to remove large enveloped viruses and small non-enveloped viruses. They are frequently employed in the removal of viruses. The most common retention ratings for these filters are 20 or 50 nm.

9.3.7.4 Filtration—UF/DF and TFF

Filtration applications are well suited for single-use processing. Ultrafiltration and diafiltration steps are used to concentrate and change the buffer of a solution. During the final formulation, ultrafiltration, and diafiltration transfer the active pharmaceutical ingredient to a stabilizing environment and achieve the correct concentration. Up to 300–5,000 L may need to be processed, depending on whether the column eluates can be fractionated. Membranes with a 30 kDa molecular weight cutoff are often used to retain antibodies, and the process intermediate is concentrated and washed with 5× volumes. Modules of up to 3 m^2 are available that can process 200 L/(h m^2). Several single-use systems are available (Scilog, Millipore) for a limited filter area (up to 2.5 m^2), but larger systems that might replace existing reusable systems with 14 m^2 because there are already single-use modules and pumps available, its logical to carry the filtration steps in a closed system.

Single-use TFF modules are available as ready-to-use cassettes to be used in TFF setups. These systems provide quick turnaround and increased flexibility. Single-use systems are available as preassembled units with gamma-irradiated flow paths and sensors, reducing setup time. A peristaltic pump or a four-piston diaphragm pump is used. Pre-packaged cassettes that are pre-sanitized are also an available option as a single-use component. Cleaning a TFF system and cassette is an important step in the downstream process, particularly for multi-product use. It is essential to minimize cross-contamination risk while also ensuring that the flux rates are well maintained. Cleaning procedures must be well-validated, even for each product's dedicated systems, to ensure no product carryover from previous batches. A completely single-use TFF system can be built together with off-the-shelf components (including valves, sensors, and 2D bags for liquid). Technology improvements and integration of single-use components can allow automated single-use systems to be applied conveniently for large-scale manufacturing.

9.3.7.5 General Filtration Applications

Except for steel meshes in bulk manufacturing of nonsterile dosage forms, filters are rarely reused in the pharmaceutical industry. Single-use filter devices in biological manufacturing were the earliest changes that went single-use, mainly because of the problems with cleaning them; these parts' cost has always been reasonable.

The biopharmaceutical industry employs a wide variety of filter designs and mechanisms. Pleated or wound filter fleeces made from melt-blown random fiber matrices are commonly used as prefilters. These filters are used to filter fluids with a high contaminant content. Prefilters come in a wide range of retention ratings and can be tailored to fit any application. Prefilters are most commonly used to protect membrane filters, which are more precise and selective than prefilters. Fluids are polished or sterilized using membrane filters. To determine whether or not these filters meet the performance criteria, they must be integrity tested. Micro or ultrafiltration membranes can be used for crossflow filtration. The fluid sweeps over the membrane layer, preventing it from becoming clogged. The diafiltration or concentration of fluid streams is also possible with this filtration mode.

Dead-end filtration is one of the simplest modes of operation for filters. Dead-end filtration operates on the principle of passing a fluid feed stream through a filter device using a pressure drop, usually applied by either a pump or compressed gas pressure before the filter device. All contaminants larger in size than the filter media's pore size are retained by the filter material and will finally cause a filter blockage by plugging its channels or pores. The setup uses minimum accessories such as tubing/piping, tanks, controls. Dead end filters using microporous membranes manufactured out of synthetic polymers such as polyethersulfone, polyamide, cyanoacrylate, and polyvinylidene fluoride are used extensively for sterile processing. They are used for media filtration into sterile bags and containers, bioburden reduction during cell harvest clarification, chromatography column protection, and final filtration of the purified bulk drug substance. These filters often come attached to single-use bags and are pre-sterilized by gamma irradiation.

9.3.8 Fill Finish Operations

Fill-finish, the final process step DS and DP require tight control of aseptic operations without compromising the sterility and integrity while ensuring safety and efficiency. As such, fill-finish operations typically require sophisticated equipment and technology. The traditional fill-finish setup uses fixed systems with complex components that require extensive cleaning and sterilization, assembly, and disassembly. A time-pressure system and a piston pump are widely used for dosing and filling operations. However, these require assembly, validated CIP, and SIP to ensure the final product meets the sterility specifications. Using single-use components for these critical process steps is more likely to ensure that the final product is not compromised while reducing cross-contamination risk. Additionally, SUT in fill-finish can reduce the turnaround time between batches and increase flexibility, particularly for a multiple-product facility.

A traditional, fixed system can adopt single-use solutions. The figure depicts a single-use fill finish with installed hardware, hard-piped connections, and limited operational flexibility. This setup combined Millipore's expertise in single-use fluid-path management to ensure sterility and integrity of operation (Figure 9.3).

Successful implementation of a single-use system goes beyond assembling single-use components. Using suppliers with experience in validating such systems and understanding the need of the manufacturer's requirements to integrate and offer customized solutions, ensure compatibility, perform assessments will be critical to the success of single-use implementation and assurance of sterility. SUT's flexibility is applicable for single and multi-product filling facilities, increasing facility efficiency and utilization due to ease of installation, operation, and CIP/SIP elimination.

9.3.9 Safety

Biologics manufacturers must comply with regulatory requirements. This includes ensuring the supplier is reliable, can provide the necessary documentation supporting suitability (product contact material), qualification, and validation of the single-use systems supports audits by the end-user. The end-user must have a user requirements specification and perform a technical evaluation with multiple vendors to

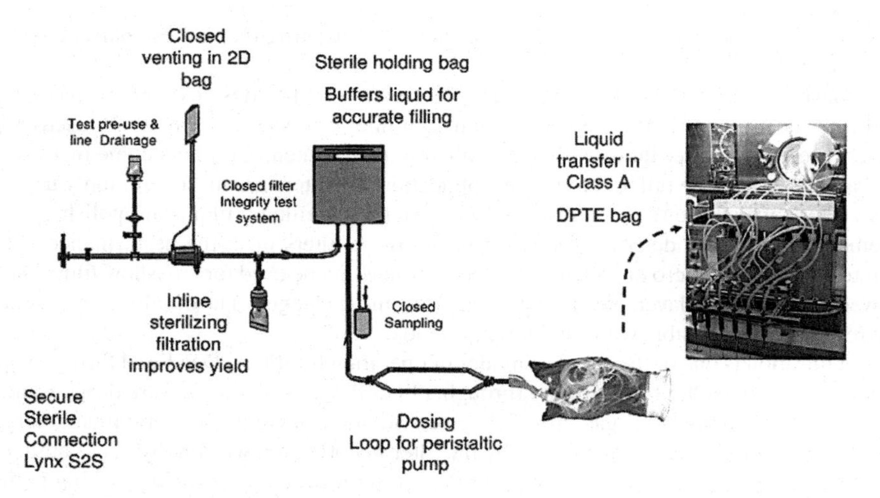

FIGURE 9.3 Closed system filling transfer set to isolator. Source: www.emdmillipore.com.

determine suitability with their process. Single-use components must be qualified in conjunction with the equipment for the intended use. Additionally, these should also be included in the process validation exercise.

Plastic materials or elastomer systems are widely used in single-use devices, ranging from filter housings to the lining of bioreactors. The controversy over the possibility of contamination of the product from the chemicals in the plastic film is perhaps the most significant impediment to the wider acceptance of single-use systems today. All final containers and closures must be made of a material that will not accelerate the deterioration of the product or make it less suitable for its intended use in any way (21CFR600.11 Biologics) (h).

The effect of leachable on the three and four-dimensional structure of protein drugs, which can render the drug more immunogenic if not less effective, is a risk unique to biological drugs. These side effects are thus of greater importance to the bioprocessing industry. Leachable are chemicals that migrate from single-use processing equipment into various components of the drug product during manufacturing. Extractables are chemical entities (organic and inorganic) extracted from single-use components using common laboratory solvents in controlled experiments. They represent the worst-case scenario and predict the types of leachable that may be encountered during pharmaceutical production.

It should be noted that the leaching is not only peculiar to plastics, but even stainless-steel leaches chemicals. 316 L stainless steel, commonly used in biopharmaceutical applications, is an alloy made up primarily of iron, nickel, and chromium, with minor amounts of manganese and vanadium. Stainless steel is a significant metal leachable source, particularly if the surface of the equipment or tank has not been properly treated. Iron, chromium, and nickel are the most easily leachable elements. Un-passivated stainless-steel vessels have been shown to leach several times more metals such as iron and nickel into a liquid formulation after storage at room temperature than passivated stainless-steel vessels.

9.3.9.1 Polymers and Additives

Rather than traditional metal or glass, polymers such as plastic or elastomers (rubber) are commonly used to fabricate single-use processing equipment for biopharmaceutical manufacturing. Polymers are more versatile than their traditional counterparts because they are lighter, more flexible, and more durable. Plastic and rubber are also single-use components that are not cleaned or validated. To clarify glass or add color to labels or code parts, additives can be incorporated into polymers. Additives are also used to control polymer degradation (stabilizers).

When a plastic resin is processed, it is frequently melted at high temperatures in an extruder. Its stability is influenced by its molecular structure, polymerization process, residual catalysts, and production finishing steps. Extrusion processing conditions (such as temperature, shear, and extruder residence time) can significantly impact polymer degradation. End-use conditions that expose a polymer to excessive heat or light (for example, outdoor applications or medical sterilization techniques) can cause premature failure of polymer products, resulting in a loss of flexibility or strength. If left unchecked, the plastic component's total failure is often the result.

Extractable and leachable analyses are extremely complex and challenging due to the complexity of chemical reactions in plastics manufacturing. Those lesser-known minor chemical species may leach into a drug product during extractable and leachable testing, but this is not predictable because it is, to a greater extent, a function of the product's characteristics. All polymer byproducts and additives (stabilizers, fillers, and elastomers) can leach into a drug product.

Despite the risks associated with using additives added to polymers, the utility of polymers in single-use bioprocess equipment (as well as in all medical and pharmaceutical applications) far outweighs the risks. These risks can be effectively managed by following three steps: material selection, implementation of a proper testing program, and vendor collaboration.

9.3.9.2 Material Selection

The type of plastic used should match the needed physical and chemical properties and compatibility of its additives. The amount of leaching that can occur is often reduced by ensuring compatibility. It's also crucial to use polymers and additives that have been approved by regulatory authorities for the specific application. Because these compounds have already undergone extensive analytical and toxicological testing, a wealth of information is often available. As a result, most manufacturers are likely to keep using these additives, and the user does not change the composition at a later stage because of these compounds. Because significant changes in the process must be reported back to the FDA, the art of using them is likely to survive, obviating the need for a change control step.

Commercially available plastic films are made up of proprietary formulas and arrangements; for example, Advanced Scientific uses two films to make its bags. A 5.0 mm polyethylene fluid contact film is used. The outer layer is a five-layer, seven-millimeter co-extrusion film that offers barrier and durability. A typical test report is given in Table 9.3.

9.3.9.3 Testing

Polymers used in medical and pharmaceutical applications should follow USP guidelines, and USP Class VI testing, as documented in USP 88, is recommended. Appropriate extractable and leachable testing programs must be implemented for all bioprocessing materials that directly contact the drug.

The BPSA provides the best-practice guidelines for conducting such testing as a two-part technical guideline for evaluating the risk associated with extractable and leachable, specifically for single-use processing equipment. This organization is dedicated to encouraging the use of single-use systems and provides excellent support and assistance; the reader is highly encouraged to visit their website for newer information and participate in their many seminars and conventions to stay abreast of the developments in this fast-changing field.

The testing for leachable does not end once the materials have been qualified. It is necessary to have a quality control program instead of testing the product or equipment alone. The level of quality control testing will depend on risk tolerance. The manufacturing of recombinant drugs involves extensive purification steps that are likely to remove most of these leachable. Also, the final medium used for protein solutions is aqueous, and many of the leachables are not soluble in water, further reducing the risk. A greater risk also comes from the final packaging components; for example, rubber stoppers used in packaging the final dosage form are more likely to risk the protein formulation than any other component in the chain of a single-use drug manufacturing process. Biologics manufacturers need to work with suppliers to ensure regulatory requirements adhere to a product safety standpoint.

A vital specification or testing requirement that the DP should meet is for particulate matter—visible and subvisible. The contamination of drug products with particulate matter is typically well controlled by filtration and visual inspection performed during filling. The single-use components must also be manufactured under controlled conditions that can reduce particulate matter to a minimum in the final product.

TABLE 9.3
Summary of the Tests Carried Out and Results Obtained for a Plastic Film to Produce Bioreactor Bags

Biocompatibility			
USP Acute Systemic Injection Test	Pass		USP <88>
USP Intracutaneous Injection Test	Pass		USP <88>
USP Intramuscular Implantation Test	Pass		USP <88>
USP MEM Elution Method	Non-cytotoxic		USP <87>
Physicochemical Test for Plastics	Pass		USP <661>
Extractables			
	TOC after 90 days (ppm)		pH shift after 90 days
Purified water (pH = 7)	< 2		–0.79
Acidic water (pH < 2)	< 3		+0.01
Basic water (pH > 10)	< 4		+0.87
Physical Data			
Water vapor transmission rate (g/100 in^2/24 h)	0.017		ASTM F-1249
Carbon dioxide transmission rate (cc/100 in^2/24 h)	0.129		ASTM F-2476
Oxygen transmission rate (cc/100 in^2/24 h)	0.023		ASTM F-1927
Average force	Average MOE	Average elongation	
Tensile 32.73 lbs	25,110 psi	1,084%	ASTM D882-02
Min force	Average force	Max force	
Tear 6.77 lbs Resistance	7.21 lbs	7.74 lbs	ASTM D1004-03
Puncture 16.42 lbs Resistance	18.61 lbs	19.51 lbs	FTMS 101C

9.3.9.4 Regulatory

Extractable and leachable from single-use bioprocessing materials are not covered by any specific standards or guidelines. Many relevant references were written with processing materials and equipment in mind, rather than construction materials.

9.3.9.4.1 The United States and Canada

Extractables and leachables from single-use bioprocessing materials are not mentioned in any specific standards or guidelines. Many applicable references were written with processing materials and equipment in mind, rather than construction materials.

9.3.9.4.2 Europe

The rules governing the manufacture of medicinal products in the European Union contain a similar statement to the US 21 CFR 211.65. In a good manufacturing practice document, according to the EU, the production equipment should not harm the products. Parts of the production equipment that come into contact with the product must not be reactive, additive, or absorptive to the point where they compromise the product's quality or pose a hazard.

The European Medicines Evaluation Agency (EMEA) published a guideline on plastic immediate packaging materials (www.ema.europa.eu/en/documents/scientific-guideline/guideline-plastic-immediate-packaging-materialsen.pdf) that covers container-closure systems and has been used to guide single-use process contact materials. Data for extractable and leachable components comes from extraction studies (worst-case leachables), interaction studies, and migration studies (which are similar to leachable information for those components). Determine what additional information or testing is needed, and then devise and implement a strategy to fill in the gaps.

9.4 Online Monitoring

Online monitoring is widely used for upstream processes, such as temperature, pH, pCO2 or pO2, and other chemistry indicators. This allows adjustments to feed, pH modulation, and other changes continuously. However, online monitoring of the downstream process has not been possible. First, it is not established the optimal parameters to monitor, optimize the observed properties, and alter downstream processing.

However, in recent years, much emphasis has been placed on creating methodologies for online monitoring to alter the process to modify the yield, molecular structure, and safety elements of the product. It is now the fastest emerging technology, yet it is adopted slowly because of the technical and regulatory complexities of reliance on online data. Table 9.4 shows how online monitoring can affect downstream processing, and Table 9.5 shows the status of technology.

9.5 Continuous Manufacturing

Continuous manufacturing is a version of highly intensified processing with brief downtimes compared to the typical time used for traditional batch production. Process intensification, therefore, becomes a prerequisite to continuous manufacturing technologies that can increase tier, manage high media volumes, buffers, and in general, intensify the process to extract more from the entire production process.

The advantages of intensification and continuous processing are mostly concerned with increasing productivity and reduced need to invest in conventional, highly costly manufacturing facilities. Businesses can synergistically use single-use and intensification facilities that lead to reduced facility footprints and costs. Continuous manufacturing is a crucial step in promoting drug quality and enhancing production efficiency, resulting in lower drug prices.

One of the key drivers to the successful incorporation of continuous manufacturing is the principle of connected manufacturing, where unit processes are connected both physically and, most notably, even digitally integrated (automated). This helps streamline the process from start to finish using a fully integrated, connected system that can control and monitor product quality.

The benefit of improving product quality is that the product spends less time on some of the unit operations that can potentially cause degradation or more variations, such as bioreactor process and chromatography separation that can effectively resolve its other variants (isoforms). An example of a continuous biomanufacturing process can include a perfusion bioreactor coupled to a multi-column chromatography capture step, followed by flow-through virus inactivation, multi-column intermediate purification, a flow-through membrane adsorber polishing step, continuous virus filtration, and a final ultrafiltration step operated in continuous mode. Continuous capture steps gain a lot of traction, mostly due to modern multi-column chromatography ideal for commercial-scale manufacturing.

Continuous manufacturing operations are a step towards reducing waste and streamlining operations to be more efficient. While the concept may be relatively new or more underutilized in the biological medicine industry, other downstream operations such as UF/DF must also be adapted to this concept. Despite this being a challenge, using sterile UF capsules, which allows for easy assembly and operation of closed systems with minimized contamination risks or reduced bioburden, is one solution. Additionally,

TABLE 9.4

The Potential Impact of Monitoring Critical Properties, Factors, and Conditions in Downstream Processing

Critical Properties, Factors, and Conditions	Purpose/Motivation	Product Quality	Production Economy	Regulatory Compliance
Product-related properties				
Product activity	Immediate information on product activity during DSP	↗	↗	↗
Product variants	Evaluation and separation of different product variants	↗	↗	↗
Impurities	Assurance of sufficient removal of impurities (HCP, DNA)	↗	↗	↗
Contaminants	Detection of possible fungal, microbial, yeast bioburden	↗	↗	↗
USP media components and introduced chemicals, resin leakage	Assurance of sufficient removal of USP media components and introduced chemicals	↗	↗	↗
Economic factors				
Investment costs of instrumentation	—	—	↘	—
Operational and maintenance costs	—	—	↘	—
Training costs of personnel	—	—	↘	—
Productivity	Productivity improvement based on monitoring	—	↗	—
Direct batch release after formulation	Batch release after final DSP step, no storage	—	↗	↗
Process endpoint monitoring	Facilitation to determine the endpoint of each DSP step	↗	↗	↗
Lifetime of instrument	Usage for an extended period	—	↗	↗
Monitoring of batch-to-batch variations	Determination of batch variations and comparison to previous results (batch trajectory)	↗	↗	↗
Conditions by regulatory demands				
Online monitoring and process control	Possibility to fine-tune each DSP step promptly and take corrective actions	↗	↗	↗
Robustness of monitoring system	Adoption to changing process environment	↗	↗	↗
Identification of critical quality attributes	Increase process understanding and impact of CQAs in DSP steps	↗	↗	↗
Process automation	Improve process efficiency	—	↗	↗
Risk assessment	Evaluations of risks and risk-based product development	↗	↗	↗
Fulfillment of final product specifications	Ensuring quality criteria of each batch	↗	↗	↗

Source: based on Roch, P and Mandenius, C-F. Online monitoring of downstream bioprocesses. *Current Opinion in Chemical Engineering*. 2016;14:112–120. http://dx.doi.org/10.1016/j.coche.2016.09.007.

Note: ↗ indicates a positive impact, a negative impact is indicated by ↘ and — shows no influence

incorporating automation for process monitoring and data acquisition combined with single-use technologies is considered to design UF/DF operations to a continuous approach. Single-pass TFF systems are gaining a lot of attention and are indeed favorable single-use alternatives. Still, there is undoubtedly a lot of scope for improving these skids available for commercial-scale and formulations requiring high product concentration.

TABLE 9.5

Status of Technology to Implement Online Monitoring Downstream

Techniques	Biological Relevance	Sensitivity	Selectivity	Response Time	Precision	Reproducibility	Readiness for Implementation
Temperature and pressure sensors	•	•••	•	•••	•••	•••	•
pH sensor	•	•••	•	•••	•••	••	•
Optical density	•	••	•	•••	••	••	•
Mass flowmeters	•	•	•	•••	••	••	•
Dipsticks for antigens	•••	•	••	••	•	••	•
Flow injection analysis	••	••	••	••	••	••	••
HPLC online	••	••	••	••	•••	••	•••
Capacitive immunosensors	••	•••	•••	••	••	••	•••
Advanced mass spectrometry	•••	•••	•••.	••	••	••	••
Multi fluorescence spectroscopy	••	•••	•••	•••	•••	••	••
UV/VIS spectroscopy	••	••	•••	•••	•••	••	••
Near-infrared spectroscopy	••	••	••	•••	•••	••	••
Mid-infrared spectroscopy	••	••	•••	•••	•••	••	••
Raman spectroscopy	•••	••	•	•••	•••	••	••
Surface plasmon resonance	•••	•••	•••	••	••	•	•••
Capillary electrophoresis online	••	••	••	••	(••		••
Flow cytometry online	••	••	••	••	••	••	••
NMR online	•••	••	•••	•	•••	••	••
Offline biosensors	•••	•••	•••	••	••	••	•••
Circular dichroism	•••	•••	•••	••	••	••	••
Light scattering	••	•••	•	••	••	••	••

Source: based on Roch, P and Mandenius, C-F. Online monitoring of downstream bioprocesses. *Current Opinion in Chemical Engineering*. 2016;14:112–120. http://dx.doi.org/10.1016/j.coche.2016.09.007.

The first step towards adopting the concept starts with recognizing the need for continuous processing and sketching out specifics on how the batch process can be transformed or adapted into a continuous one. It may not be easy right away to convert a batch operation into a continuous operation at the outset, for it must be understood that not all batch processes are designed to be continuous. Batch processing involves multiple steps, using online and offline analyses to define the control strategy and support the process. Hence, only a few steps may be initially easier to convert, but any changes made should only be done if it increases or maintains productivity and has no negative impact on product quality.

A hybrid approach to continuous biomanufacturing, such that only the upstream or part of the downstream process is operated continuously, is a more logical and sounder step towards adopting continuous manufacturing. This can be operating upstream as a perfusion operation combined with batch mode purification or having a fed-batch process with a constant chromatography capture step.

Continuous manufacturing is also seeing increase support from the regulators. The FDA's recommendation for continuous unit operations is confirmation that biological medicine processing is progressing towards a future that promotes emerging technologies. The need is driven to reduce product failure, increase quality, and improve efficiency. This works to supplement further efforts towards automation, intensifying processes, and effectively utilizing resources (facility and equipment).

9.5.1 Continuous Chromatography Operations

Continuous chromatography systems are designed for continuous processing, mainly when the purification stage is linked to upstream bioreactor perfusion or even a simple fed-batch process. With a batch chromatography mode of operation, a single large column for each purification step is used. In a continuous multi-column setup, multiple smaller columns are operated in series over numerous cycles, effectively managing activities across these columns in a simultaneous manner. When product loading happens on one column, the other column(s) can be prepped up or in the wash, elution, and regeneration stages. Alternatively, the loading step can be split across two columns set up in series.

Continuous chromatography attracts a lot of interest in advancing the process towards clinical development and making it more likely for commercial-scale production, particularly with regulators' support and encouragement. Continuous chromatography operations can help minimize facility footprint by using smaller bioreactors (that can support high productivity), small-mid size columns, reduced buffer consumptions coupled with options to perform inline dilutions. Multi-column chromatography helps realize these potential benefits and provides an opportunity for better utilization in protein A resin capacity. A fed-batch process can be connected to a continuous chromatography capture step, reducing costs and possibly improving product quality. However, with the greater sophistication of hardware systems and certain perceived regulatory complexities, there are still obstacles to address.

Implementing a continuous end-to-end system may not be an immediate possibility, and an easy switch from batch processing to continuous processing is not always possible. However, emerging technologies such as straight-through processing (STP), simulated moving bed (SMB), and periodic countercurrent chromatography (PCC) can be used as alternatives to traditional batch processing, as a continuous or a semi-continuous processing option. Nonetheless, before deciding if continuous chromatography is the best alternative, a detailed review is performed for each project based on the protein's operational scale, properties, and other process requirements.

9.5.1.1 Straight Through Processing (STP)

In STP, two or more chromatography steps are connected in series, with inline adjustment of process conditions between columns to ensure optimized loading conditions during the next step. The need for intermediate conditioning steps in conventional batch processes would be removed by this setup, requiring little to no intermediate hold-up tanks, improving efficiency, and minimal equipment requirements (Figure 9.4).

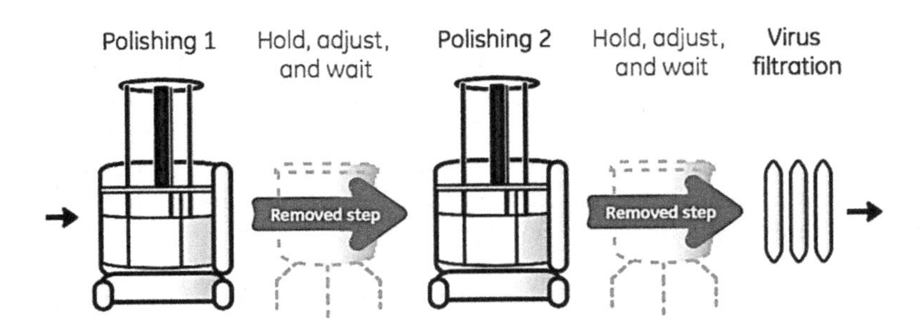

FIGURE 9.4 The total equipment footprint can be reduced by connecting the purification and filtration systems in a series and moving adjustments in line. Source: Cytiva Life Sciences.

9.5.1.2 *Periodic Countercurrent Chromatography (PCC)*

PCC is a multi-step approach to maximizing chromatography resin capacity utilization (in turn, reducing resin volume) and minimizing process time. PCC uses three or more column chromatography operations to completely capitalize on the resin capacity. Column 1 is loaded up to 60–80% breakthrough, then disconnected to perform the wash and elution and equilibration steps. In the meantime, the process is switched to column 2, which is also loaded up to breakthrough, followed by disconnecting, wash, elution, and equilibration operations, and then the same sequence of operations with column 3 is performed. At this point, column 1 is ready to come back online to repeat these steps, thus creating continuous processing. This increases the available resin utilization while allowing for a smaller equipment footprint and effective time management.

9.5.1.3 *Simulated Moving Bed (SMB) Chromatography*

Simulated moving bed (SMB) chromatography has been in use in the petrochemical and food industries. It is characterized by allowing processes to achieve high productivity relative to batch methods resulting from the efficient utilization of the solid and liquid phases required for separation.

The basic concept of simulated moving bed chromatography is to use multiple smaller columns containing the solid adsorbent (beds) and to move the beds in the opposite direction of the fluid (feed, eluent, and product) to achieve a countercurrent flow. The "simulated movement" is typically carried out through multiport valves interspersed between the columns, such that the input and output fluid streams (feed, eluent, product) can be periodically switched from column to column in the direction of fluid flow. The valves' arrangement and control help strategize the sample and solvent's movement, allowing various separation stages to be carried out simultaneously by different columns as a continuous cycle.

9.6 Conclusion

Several regulatory advances include 3D printing of solid dosage forms, continuous batch manufacturing, and online in-process control in place of release testing. The role of artificial intelligence and machine learning will be heavily embedded in all manufacturing operations. SUT will eventually replace the hard-lined systems once the regulatory agencies begin approving products manufactured by SUT. More particularly, the startups will adopt this trend.

Appendix: Databases Relevant to Antibodies

GenBank(R) is a comprehensive database of publicly available DNA sequences for more than 205,000 named species. More than 60,000 within the embryophyte, collected by submissions from individual laboratories and batch submissions from large-scale sequencing projects. The NIH genetic sequence database is an annotated list of all DNA sequences open to the public (Nucleic Acids Research, 2013 Jan;41(D1): D36–42). GenBank is part of the International Nucleotide Sequence Database Collaboration, which includes Japan's DNA DataBank (DDBJ), the European Nucleotide Archive (ENA), and NCBI's GenBank. These three organizations make the daily exchange of data. A release of GenBank happens every two months and is accessible from the FTP site. The release notes for GenBank's current version provide detailed information regarding the release and notice of future changes to GenBank. There are several ways to search GenBank for and retrieve data.

Search GenBank for sequence identifiers and annotations with Entrez Nucleotide (www.ncbi.nlm.nih.gov/nucleotide/]).

Search and align GenBank sequences to a query sequence using BLAST (Basic Local Alignment Search Tool) (www.ncbi.nlm.nih.gov/blast).

Search, link, and download sequences programmatically using NCBI e-utilities (www.ncbi.nlm.nih.gov/s/NBK25501/).

The ASN.1 and flat file formats are available at NCBI's anonymous FTP servers: ftp://ftp.ncbi.nlm.nih.gov/ncbi-asn1 and ftp://ftp.ncbi.nlm.nih.gov/genbank.

The Protein Data Bank (PDB) (www.rcsb.org) includes more than 164,840 antibody fragment structures (Fabs, Fvs, scFvs, and Fcs), and a small number of complete antibody structures as of May 2020. The structural data includes the complexes of these proteins, other macromolecules, peptides, and haptens molecules. The Drug Bank database (www.drugbank.ca/drugs/) is a unique resource in bioinformatics and cheminformatics that combines detailed data on drugs with comprehensive information about drug targets. DrugBank's latest release (version 5.8.6, published 4/22/2020) includes 13,577 entries of drugs, including 2,634 approved small molecule drugs, 1,377 approved biologics (proteins, peptides, vaccines, and allergens), 131 nutraceuticals, and more than 6,375 experimental (discovery phase) drugs. Additionally, these drug entries are linked to 5,229 non-redundant protein (i.e. drug target/enzyme/transporter/carrier) sequences. Each entry contains over 200 data fields, half of which are dedicated to drug/chemical data, and the other half to drug target or protein data.

IMGT/mAb-DB is part of IMGT®, the international immunogenetics information system, an integrated information system specializing in immunoglobulins (IG), T cell receptors (TR), major histocompatibility complexes (MHC) of humans and other vertebrate species, immunoglobulin superfamily (IgSF), MHC superfamily (MhcSF), and related proteins of the immune system (RPI) of vertebrate and invertebrate species (www.imgt.org/mAb-DB/).

European Collection of Cell Cultures is a cell culture collection service for the research community that holds over 40,000 cell lines, including 450+ antibodies (www.hpacultures.org.uk/collections/ecacc.jsp).

The Hybridoma Databank (HDB) holds data on various aspects of hybridomas and their immunoreactive products. Information on a hybridoma's construction and the reactivity and non-reactivity of its secreted product is included. Also, information on the availability of an individual hybridoma and its Mab product are included. Information in the HDB is derived from literature, catalogs, and survey forms (www.atcc.org/).

The Monoclonal Antibody Index is a biotechnology database with yearly updated information on more than 9,000 monoclonal antibodies produced for the diagnosis and therapy of cancer, transplant, infection, heart-related disorders, etc. (www.gallartinternet.com/mai/index.htm).

ADDITIONAL READING

Application Note 293-I. Huether-Franken CM, et al. Scalability of parallel E. coli fermentations in BioBLU® f single-use bioreactors. Juelich, Germany: Eppendorf AG; 2013; https://www.eppendorf.com/product-media/doc/en/70274/DASGIP_Fermentors-Bioreactors_Application-Note_293_BioBLU-f_Scalability-Parallel-E-coli-Fermentations-BioBLU-f-Single-Bioreactors.pdf.

Application Note CO29180. Brown J, et al. Scale-up of microbial fermentation using recombinant E. coli in HyPerforma 30 L and 300 L single-use fermentors. San Jose, CA: Thermo Fisher Scientific; 2014; https://www.thermofisher.com/content/dam/LifeTech/Documents/PDFs/CO29180-SUF-Launch-AppNotes-Scale-Up%20of%20Microbial-Global-FLR_V2.pdf.

Arnold L, Lee K, Rucker-Pezzini J, Lee JH. Implementation of fully integrated continuous antibody processing: effects on productivity and COGm. *Biotechnol J.* 2019;14(2):e1800061. doi:10.1002/biot.201800061

Baeshen MN, Al-Hejin AM, Bora RS, et al. Production of biological medicines in E. coli: current scenario and future perspectives. *J Microbiol Biotechnol.* 2015;25(7):953–962. doi:10.4014/jmb.1412.12079

Baghban R, Farajnia S, Rajabibazl M, et al. Yeast expression systems: overview and recent advances. *Mol Biotechnol.* 2019;61(5):365–384. doi:10.1007/s12033-019-00164-8

Bakeev KA. *Process Analytical Technology: Spectroscopic Tools and Implementation Strategies for the Chemical and Pharmaceutical Industries.* 2nd edition. John Wiley & Sons Inc.; 2010.

Baur D, Angelo JM, Chollangi S, et al. Model assisted comparison of protein A resins and multi-column chromatography for capture processes. *J Biotechnol.* 2018;285:64–73. doi:10.1016/j.jbiotec.2018.08.014

Belongia B, Blanck R, Tingley S. Single-use disposable filling for sterile pharmaceuticals. *Pharm Eng.* 2003;23:26–134.

Beni V, Nilsson D, Arven P, Norberg P, Gustafsson G, Turner APF. Printed electrochemical instruments for biosensors. *ECS J Solid State Sc.* 2015;4:3001–3005.

Berlec A, Strukelj B. Current state and recent advances in biological medicine production in Escherichia coli, yeasts and mammalian cells. *J Ind Microbiol Biotechnol.* 2013;40(3–4):257–74. doi:10.1007/s10295-013-1235-0

Berrie DM, Waters RC, Montoya C, Chatel A, Vela EM. Development of a high-yield live-virus vaccine production platform using a novel fixed-bed bioreactor. *Vaccine.* 2020;38(20):3639–3645. doi:10.1016/j.vaccine.2020.03.041

Biopharmaceutic Market: https://www.alliedmarketresearch.com/biologicalmedicine-market#:~:text=Biologicalmedicines%20Market%20Overview%3A,13.8%25%20from%202018%20to%202025.

Bisschops M, Frick L, Fulton S, Ransohoff T. Single-use, continuous countercurrent, multicolumn chromatography. *BioProcess Int.* 2009;7:S18–S23.

Boedeker B, Goldstein A, Mahajan E. Fully single-use manufacturing concepts for clinical and commercial manufacturing and ballroom concepts. *Adv Biochem Eng Biotechnol.* 2018;165:179–210. doi:10.1007/10_2017_19

Bohonak D, Mehta U, Weiss ER, Voyta G. Adapting virus filtration to enable intensified and continuous mAb processing. *Biotechnol Prog.* 2020:e3088. doi:10.1002/btpr.3088

Bracewell DG, Brown RA, Hoare M. Addressing a whole bioprocess in real-time using an optical biosensor-formation, recovery and purification of antibody fragments from a recombinant E-coli host. *Bioprocess Biosyst Eng.* 2004;26:271–282.

Brestrich N, Briskot T, Osberghaus A, Hubbuch J. A tool for selective inline quantification of co- eluting proteins in chromatography using spectral analysis and partial least squares regression. *Biotechnol Bioeng.* 2014;111:1365–1373.

Brestrich N, Sanden A, Kraft A, McCann K, Bertolini J, Hubbuch J. Advances in inline quantification of co-eluting proteins in chromatography: process-data-based model calibration and application towards real-life separation issues. *Biotechnol Bioeng.* 2015;112:1406–1416.

Broschard TH, Glowienke S, Bruen US, et al. Assessing safety of extractables from materials and leachables in pharmaceuticals and biologics – Current challenges and approaches. *Regul Toxicol Pharmacol.* 2016;81:201–211. doi:10.1016/j.yrtph.2016.08.011

Brower M, Hou Y, Pollard D. Monoclonal antibody continuous processing enabled by single-use. In Subramanian G, ed. *Continuous Processing in Pharmaceutical Manufacturing.* Wiley VCH; 2015:255–296.

Buyel JF, Fischer R. Downstream processing of biopharmaceutical proteins produced in plants: the pros and cons of flocculants. *Bioengineered.* 2014;5(2):138–142. doi:10.4161/bioe.28061

Capito F, Skudas R, Kolmar H, Stanislawski B. Host cell protein quantification by fourier transform mid infrared spectroscopy (FT-MIR). *Biotechnol Bioeng.* 2013;110:252–259.

Carrondo MJT, Alves PM, Carinhas N, Glassey J, Hesse F, Merten O-W, Micheletti M, Noll T, Oliveira R, Reichl U, et al. How can measurement, monitoring, modeling and control advance cell culture in industrial biotechnology? *Biotechnol J.* 2012;7:1522–1529.

Chemmalil L, Prabhakar T, Kuang J, et al. Online/at-line measurement, analysis and control of product titer and critical product quality attributes (CQAs) during process development. *Biotechnol Bioeng.* 2020. doi:10.1002/bit.27531

Chen PH, Cheng YT, Ni BS, Huang JH. Continuous cell separation using microfluidic-based cell retention device with alternative boosted flow. *Appl Biochem Biotechnol.* 2020;191(1):151–163. doi:10.1007/s12010-020-03288-9

Contreras-Gómez A, Sánchez-Mirón A, García-Camacho F, Molina-Grima E, Chisti Y. Protein production using the baculovirus-insect cell expression system. *Biotechnol Prog.* 2014;30(1):1–18. doi:10.1002/btpr.1842

De Luca C, Felletti S, Lievore G, et al. Modern trends in downstream processing of therapeutic proteins through continuous chromatography: the potential of multicolumn countercurrent solvent gradient purification. *Trends Analyt Chem.* 2020;132:116051. doi:10.1016/j.trac.2020.116051

Dhara VG, Naik HM, Majewska NI, Betenbaugh MJ. Recombinant antibody production in CHO and NS0 cells: differences and similarities. *BioDrugs.* 2018;32(6):571–584. doi:10.1007/s40259-018-0319-9

Dorival-García N, Bones J. Monitoring leachables from single-use bioreactor bags for mammalian cell culture by dispersive liquid-liquid microextraction followed by ultra high performance liquid chromatography quadrupole time of flight mass spectrometry. *J Chromatogr A.* 2017;1512:51–60. doi:10.1016/j.chroma.2017.06.077

Dumont J, Euwart D, Mei B, Estes S, Kshirsagar R. Human cell lines for biological medicine manufacturing: history, status, and future perspectives. Crit Rev Biotechnol. 2016;36(6):1110–1122. doi:10.3109/07388551.2015.1084266

Dyson MR. Fundamentals of expression in mammalian cells. *Adv Exp Med Biol.* 2016;896:217–24. doi:10.1007/978-3-319-27216-0_14

Elich T, Goodrich E, Lutz H, Mehta U. Investigating the combination of single-pass tangential flow filtration and anion exchange chromatography for intensified mAb polishing. *Biotechnol Prog.* 2019;35(5):e2862. doi:10.1002/btpr.2862

Eibl R, Eibl D, eds. New single-use sensors for online measurement of glucose and lactate: the answer to the PAT initiative. *Single-Use Technology in Biopharmaceutical Manufacture.* New York: John Wiley & Sons Inc; 2011:295–299.

Esbensen K, Kirsanov D, Legin A, Rudnitskaya A, Mortensen J, Pedersen J, Vognsen L, Makarychev-Mikhailov S, Vlasov Y. Fermentation monitoring using multisensor systems: feasibility study of the electronic tongue. *Anal Bioanal Chem.* 2004;378:391–395.

Feidl F, Vogg S, Wolf M, et al. Process-wide control and automation of an integrated continuous manufacturing platform for antibodies. *Biotechnol Bioeng.* 2020;117(5):1367–1380. doi:10.1002/bit.27296

Fernández FJ, Vega MC. Choose a suitable expression host: a survey of available protein production platforms. *Adv Exp Med Biol.* 2016;896:15–24. doi:10.1007/978-3-319-27216-0_2

Fisher AC, Kamga MH, Agarabi C, Brorson K, Lee SL, Yoon S. The current scientific and regulatory landscape in advancing integrated continuous biological medicine manufacturing. *Trends Biotechnol.* 2019;37(3):253–267. doi:10.1016/j.tibtech.2018.08.008

Flickinger MC. Upstream industrial biotechnology. In Flickiner MC, ed. *Equipment, Process Design, Sensing, Control, and cGMP Operations.* John Wiley & Sons Inc.; 2013.

Fuller M, Pora H. Introducing disposable systems into biomanufacturing: a CMO case study. *BioProcess Int.* 2008;6:30–36.

Gagnon M, Nagre S, Wang W, Coffman J, Hiller GW. Novel, linked bioreactor system for continuous production of biologics. *Biotechnol Bioeng.* 2019;116(8):1946–1958. doi:10.1002/bit.26985

Gagnon M, Nagre S, Wang W, Hiller GW. Shift to high-intensity, low-volume perfusion cell culture enabling a continuous, integrated bioprocess. *Biotechnol Prog.* 2018;34(6):1472–1481. doi:10.1002/btpr.2723

Gallihere PM, Hodge G, Guertin P, Chew L, Deloggio T. Single use bioreactor platform for microbial fermentation. In Eibl R, Eibl D, eds. *Single-Use Technology in Biopharmaceutical Manufacture.* John Wiley & Sons Inc; 2011:241–250.

Ge X, Hanson M, Shen H, et al. validation of an optical sensor-based high-throughput bioreactor system for mammalian cell culture. *J Biotechnol.* 2006;122(3):293–306. doi:10.1016/j.jbiotec.2005.12.009

Goussen C, Goldstein L, Brèque C, et al. Viral clearance capacity by continuous protein A chromatography step using sequential multicolumn chromatography. *J Chromatogr B Analyt Technol Biomed Life Sci.* 2020;1145:122056. doi:10.1016/j.jchromb.2020.122056

Grilo AL, Mantalaris A. Apoptosis: a mammalian cell bioprocessing perspective. *Biotechnol Adv.* 2019;37(3):459–475. doi:10.1016/j.biotechadv.2019.02.012

Gupta SK, Shukla P. Microbial platform technology for recombinant antibody fragment production: a review. *Crit Rev Microbiol.* 2017;43(1):31–42. doi:10.3109/1040841x.2016.1150959

Gupta SK, Shukla P. Sophisticated cloning, fermentation, and purification technologies for an enhanced therapeutic protein production: a review. *Front Pharmacol.* 2017;8:419. doi:10.3389/fphar.2017.00419. PMID: 28725194; PMCID: PMC5495827.

Hacker DL, Balasubramanian S. Recombinant protein production from stable mammalian cell lines and pools. *Curr Opin Struct Biol.* 2016;38:129–136. doi:10.1016/j.sbi.2016.06.005

Hansen SK, Jamali B, Hubbuch J. Selective high throughput protein quantification based on UV absorption spectra. *Biotechnol Bioeng.* 2013;110:448–460.

Health USD, Services H. Pharmaceutical CGMPs: Guidance for Industry PAT – A Framework for Innovative Pharmaceutical Development, Manufacturing and Quality Assurance. Food and Drug Administration; 2004.

Heidemann R, Lünse S, Tran D, Zhang C. Characterization of cell-banking parameters for the cryopreservation of mammalian cell lines in 100-mL cryobags. *Biotechnol Prog.* 2010;26(4):1154–1163.

Helal NA, Elnoweam O, Eassa HA, et al. Integrated continuous manufacturing in pharmaceutical industry: current evolutionary steps toward revolutionary future. *Pharm Pat Anal.* 2019;8(4):139–161. doi:10.4155/ppa-2019-0011

Hilbold NJ, Le Saoût X, Valery E, et al. Evaluation of several protein a resins for application to multi-column chromatography for the rapid purification of fed-batch bioreactors. *Biotechnol Prog.* 2017;33(4):941–953. doi:10.1002/btpr.2465

Hogwood CE, Bracewell DG, Smales CM. Measurement and control of host cell proteins (HCPs) in CHO cell bioprocesses. *Curr Opin Biotechnol.* 2014;30:153–160.

Hughson MD, Cruz TA, Carvalho RJ, Castilho LR. Development of a 3-step straight-through purification strategy combining membrane adsorbers and resins. *Biotechnol Prog.* 2017;33(4):931–940.

Ichihara T, Ito T, Gillespie C. Polishing approach with fully connected flow-through purification for therapeutic monoclonal antibody. *Eng Life Sci.* 2019;19(1):31–36. doi:10.1002/elsc.201800123

Jacquemart R, Vandersluis M, Zhao M, Sukhija K, Sidhu N, Stout J. A single-use strategy to enable manufacturing of affordable biologics. *Comput Struct Biotechnol J.* 2016;14:309–318. doi:10.1016/j.csbj.2016.06.007

Jazayeri SH, Amiri-Yekta A, Bahrami S, Gourabi H, Sanati MH, Khorramizadeh MR. Vector and cell line engineering technologies toward recombinant protein expression in mammalian cell lines. *Appl Biochem Biotechnol.* 2018;185(4):986–1003. doi:10.1007/s12010-017-2689-8

Jordi MA, Khera S, Roland K, et al. Qualitative assessment of extractables from single-use components and the impact of reference standard selection. *J Pharm Biomed Anal.* 2018;150:368–376. doi:10.1016/j.jpba.2017.12.029

Kadlec P, Gabrys B, Strandt S. Data-driven soft sensors in the process industry. *Comput Chem Eng.* 2009;33:795–814.

Kamga MH, Cattaneo M, Yoon S. Integrated continuous biomanufacturing platform with ATF perfusion and one column chromatography operation for optimum resin utilization and productivity. *Prep Biochem Biotechnol.* 2018;48(5):383–390. doi:10.1080/10826068.2018.1446151

Kateja N, Agarwal H, Hebbi V, Rathore AS. Integrated continuous processing of proteins expressed as inclusion bodies: GCSF as a case study. *Biotechnol Prog.* 2017;33(4):998–1009. doi:10.1002/btpr.2413

Kateja N, Tiwari A, Thakur G, Rathore AS. Complete or periodic continuity in continuous manufacturing platforms for production of monoclonal antibodies? *Biotechnol J.* 2021;16:e2000524. doi:10.1002/biot.202000524

Kelley B, Kiss R, Laird M. A different perspective: how much innovation is really needed for monoclonal antibody production using mammalian cell technology? *Adv Biochem Eng Biotechnol.* 2018;165:443–462. doi:10.1007/10_2018_59

Kelly PS, Dorival-García N, Paré S, et al. Improvements in single-use bioreactor film material composition leads to robust and reliable Chinese hamster ovary cell performance. *Biotechnol Prog.* 2019;35(4):e2824. doi:10.1002/btpr.2824

Krämer O, Klausing S, Noll T. Methods in mammalian cell line engineering: from random mutagenesis to sequence-specific approaches. *Appl Microbiol Biotechnol.* 2010;88(2):425–436. doi:10.1007/s00253-010-2798-6

Kreyenschulte D, Paciok E, Regestein L, Bluemich B, Buechs J. Online monitoring of upstream processes via non-invasive low-field NMR. *Biotechnol Bioeng.* 2015;112:1810–1821.

Krishnan R, Chen H. Overview of single-use technologies for biologics production. *Am Pharm Rev.* 2012;15(3):15–19.

Kuczewski M, Schirmer E, Lain B, Zarbis-Papastoitsis G. A single-use purification process for the production of a monoclonal antibody produced in a PER.C6 human cell line. *Biotechnol J.* 2011;6(1):56–65. doi:10.1002/biot.201000292

Kunert R, Reinhart D. Advances in recombinant antibody manufacturing. *Appl Microbiol Biotechnol.* 2016;100(8):3451–61. doi:10.1007/s00253-016-7388-9

Lacki KM. High throughput process development in biomanufacturing. *Curr Opin Chem Eng.* 2014;6:25–32.

Łącki KM, Riske FJ. Affinity chromatography: an enabling technology for large-scale bioprocessing. *Biotechnol J.* 2020;15(1):e1800397. doi:10.1002/biot.201800397

Lalonde ME, Durocher Y. Therapeutic glycoprotein production in mammalian cells. *J Biotechnol.* 2017;251:128–140. doi:10.1016/j.jbiotec.2017.04.028

Laukel M, Rogge P, Dudziak G. Single-use downstream processing for clinical manufacturing. Current capabilities and limitations. *BioProcess Int.* 2011;S2:14–21.

Levine HL. Efficient, flexible facilities for the 21st century. *Bioprocess Int.* 2013. https://bioprocessintl.com/manufacturing/facility-design-engineering/efficient-flexible-facilities-for-the-21st-century-337813/

Li F, Vijayasankaran N, Shen AY, Kiss R, Amanullah A. Cell culture processes for monoclonal antibody production. *MAbs.* 2010;2(5):466–479. doi:10.4161/mabs.2.5.12720

Lin H, Leighty RW, Godfrey S, Wang SB. Principles and approach to developing mammalian cell culture media for high cell density perfusion process leveraging established fed-batch media. *Biotechnol Prog.* 2017;33(4):891–901. doi:10.1002/btpr.2472

Luitjens A, Lewis J, Pralong A. Single-use biotechnologies and modular manufacturing environments invite paradigm shifts in bioprocess development and biopharmaceutical manufacturing. In Subramanian G, ed. *Biopharmaceutical Production Technology.* Wiley VCH; 2012:817–857.

Lute S, Kozaili J, Johnson S, Kobayashi K, Strauss D. Development of small-scale models to understand the impact of continuous downstream bioprocessing on integrated virus filtration. *Biotechnol Prog.* 2020;36(3):e2962. doi:10.1002/btpr.2962

Luttmann R, Bracewell DG, Cornelissen G, Gernaey KV, Glassey J, Hass VC, Kaiser C, Preusse C, Striedner G, Mandenius CF. Soft sensors in bioprocessing: a status report and recommendations. *Biotechnol J.* 2012;7:1040–1048.

Mahajan E, Ray-Chaudhuri T, Vogel JD. Standardization of single-use components extractable studies for industry. *Pharm Eng.* 2012;32(3):1–3.

Mahalik S, Sharma AK, Mukherjee KJ. Genome engineering for improved recombinant protein expression in Escherichia coli. *Microb Cell Fact.* 2014;13:177. doi:10.1186/s12934-014-0177-1

Merhar M, Podgornik A, Barut M, Jaksa S, Zigon M, Strancar A. High performance reversed-phase liquid chromatography using novel CIM RP-SDVB monolithic supports. *J Liq Chrom & Rel Technol.* 2001;24:2429–2443.

Minow B, Rogge P, Thompson K. Implementing a fully disposable MAb manufacturing facility. *BioProcess Int.* 2012;10:48–57.

Mire-Sluis A. Extractables and leachables. *Bioprocess Int.* https://bioprocessintl.com/business/cmc-forums/extractables-and-leachables-311844/ 2011.

Munro TP, Mahler SM, Huang EP, Chin DY, Gray PP. Bridging the gap: facilities and technologies for development of early stage therapeutic mAb candidates. *MAbs.* 2011;3(5):440–452. doi:10.4161/mabs.3.5.16968

National Academies of Sciences Eg, and Medicine, Studies DoEaL, Technology BoCSa. Continuous Manufacturing for the Modernization of Pharmaceutical Production: Proceedings of a Workshop; 2019.

Nicholson P, Storm E. Single-use tangential flow filtration in bioprocessing – an approach to design and development. *BioProcess Int.* 2011;9:38–47.

Noui L, Hill J, Keay PJ, Wang RY, Smith T, Yeung K, Habib G, Hoare M. Development of a high resolution UV spectrophotometer for at-line monitoring of bioprocesses. *Chem Eng Process.* 2002;41:107–114.

Odman P, Johansen CL, Olsson L, Gernaey KV, Lantz AE. Online estimation of biomass, glucose and ethanol in Saccharomyces cerevisiae cultivations using in-situ multi-wavelength fluorescence and software sensors. *J Biotechnol.* 2009;144:102–112.

Oh SK, Yoo SJ, Jeong DH, Lee JM. Real-time estimation of glucose concentration in algae cultivation system using Raman spectroscopy. *Bioresour Technol.* 2013;142:131–137.

Omasa T, Onitsuka M, Kim WD. Cell engineering and cultivation of chinese hamster ovary (CHO) cells. *Curr Pharm Biotechnol.* 2010;11(3):233–40. doi:10.2174/138920110791111960

Oosterhuis NM, van den Berg HJ. How multipurpose is a single-use bioreactor? *BioPharm Int.* 2011;24:51–56.

Ötes O, Flato H, Vazquez Ramirez D, Badertscher B, Bisschops M, Capito F. Scale-up of continuous multi-column chromatography for the protein a capture step: from bench to clinical manufacturing. *J Biotechnol.* 2018;281:168–174. doi:10.1016/j.jbiotec.2018.07.022

Ötes O, Flato H, Winderl J, Hubbuch J, Capito F. Feasibility of using continuous chromatography in downstream processing: comparison of costs and product quality for a hybrid process vs. a conventional batch process. *J Biotechnol.* 2017;259:213–220. doi:10.1016/j.jbiotec.2017.07.001

Pais DA, Carrondo MJ, Alves PM, Teixeira AP. Towards real-time monitoring of therapeutic protein quality in mammalian cell processes. *Curr Opin Biotechnol.* 2014;30:161–167.

Papathanasiou MM, Quiroga-Campano AL, Steinebach F, Elviro M, Mantalaris A, Pistikopoulos EN. Advanced model-based control strategies for the intensification of upstream and downstream processing in mAb production. *Biotechnol Prog.* 2017;33(4):966–988. doi:10.1002/btpr.2483

Pegel A, Reiser S, Klein S. Evaluating disposable depth filtration platforms for MAb harvest clarification. *BioProcess Int.* 2011;9:52–56.

Pidgeon T. Single-use technologies for fill-finish of clinical trials materials. *Pharm Technol.* 2010;Suppl 34:s22–s25.

Pollock J, Ho SV, Farid SS. Fed-batch and perfusion culture processes: economic, environmental, and operational feasibility under uncertainty. *Biotechnol Bioeng.* 2013;110(1):206–219.

Porowińska D, Wujak M, Roszek K, Komoszyński M. Prokariotyczne systemy ekspresyjne [Prokaryotic expression systems]. *Postepy Hig Med Dosw* (Online). 2013;67:119–129. doi:10.5604/17322693.1038351

Rajendran A, Paredes G, Mazzotti M. Simulated moving bed chromatography for the separation of enantiomers. *J Chromatogr A.* 2009;1216(4):709–738. doi:10.1016/j.chroma.2008.10.075

Rathore AS, Kumar D, Kateja N. Recent developments in chromatographic purification of biological medicines. *Biotechnol Lett.* 2018;40(6):895–905. doi:10.1007/s10529-018-2552-1

Rawlings B, Pora H. Environmental impact of single-use and reusable bioprocess systems. *BioProcess Int.* 2009;7:18–26.

Riesen N, Eibl R. Single-use bag systems for storage, transportation, freezing and thawing. In Eibl R, Eibl D, eds. *Single-Use Technology in Biopharmaceutical Manufacture.* Hoboken, NJ: JohnWiley & Sons Inc; 2011:14–20.

Ritacco FV, Wu Y, Khetan A. Cell culture media for recombinant protein expression in Chinese hamster ovary (CHO) cells: history, key components, and optimization strategies. *Biotechnol Prog.* 2018;34(6):1407–1426. doi:10.1002/btpr.2706

Roque ACA, Pina AS, Azevedo AM, et al. Anything but conventional chromatography approaches in bioseparation. *Biotechnol J.* 2020;15(8):e1900274. doi:10.1002/biot.201900274

Saeed AF, Wang R, Ling S, Wang S. Antibody engineering for pursuing a healthier future. *Front Microbiol.* 2017;8:495. doi:10.3389/fmicb.2017.00495

Sanchez-Garcia L, Martín L., Mangues R, Ferrer-Miralles N, Vázquez E, Villaverde A. Recombinant pharmaceuticals from microbial cells: a 2015 update. *Microbial Cell Factories.* 2016;15(1):9.

Schofield M. Current state of the art in continuous bioprocessing. *Biotechnol Lett.* 2018;40(9–10):1303–1309. doi:10.1007/s10529-018-2593-5

Shukla AA, Gottschalk U. Single-use disposable technologies for biopharmaceutical manufacturing. *Trends Biotechnol.* 31:147–154.

Shukla AA, Hubbrard B, Tressel T, Guhan S, Low D. Downstream processing of monoclonal antibodies. *J Chromatogr B.* 2007;848:28–39.

Sinclair A, Leveen L, Monge M, Lim J, Cox S. The environmental impact of disposable technologies – can disposables reduce your facility's environmental footprint? *BioPharm Int.* 2008;6:4–15.

Sonnleitner B. Automated measurement and monitoring of bioprocesses: key elements of the M(3)C strategy. *Adv Biochem Eng Biotechnol.* 2013;132:1–33.

Stanke M, Hitzmann B. Automatic control of bioprocesses. In Mandenius CF, Titchener-Hooker N, eds. *Measurement, Monitoring, Modelling and Control of Bioprocesses.* Springer; 2013:35–63.

Stepper L, Filser FA, Fischer S, Schaub J, Gorr I, Voges R. Pre-stage perfusion and ultra-high seeding cell density in CHO fed-batch culture: a case study for process intensification guided by systems biotechnology. *Bioprocess Biosyst Eng.* 2020;43(8):1431–1443. doi:10.1007/s00449-020-02337-1

Sugimoto MAA, Toledo VPCP, Cunha MRR, et al. Quality of bevacizumab (Avastin®) repacked in single-use glass vials for intravitreal administration. *Arq Bras Oftalmol.* 2017;80(2):108–113. doi:10.5935/0004-2749.20170026

Tao Y, Shih J, Sinacore M, Ryll T, Yusuf-Makagiansar H. Development and implementation of a perfusion-based high cell density cell banking process. *Biotechnol Prog.* 2011;27(3):824–829.

Thorne BA, Waugh S, Wilkie T, LaBreck M. Implementing a single-use TFF system in a cGMP biomanufacturing facility. *BioPharm.* 2012;25:s20–s26.

Tripathi NK, Shrivastava A. Recent developments in bioprocessing of recombinant proteins: expression hosts and process development. *Front Bioeng Biotechnol.* 2019;7:420. doi:10.3389/fbioe.2019.00420

Türkanoğlu Özçelik A, Yılmaz S, Inan M. Pichia pastoris promoters. *Methods Mol Biol.* 2019;1923:97–112. doi:10.1007/978-1-4939-9024-5_3

Ullrich KK, Hiss M, Rensing SA. Means to optimize protein expression in transgenic plants. *Curr Opin Biotechnol.* 2015;32:61–67. doi:10.1016/j.copbio.2014.11.011

Vachette E, Fenge C, Cappia JM, Delaunay L, Greller G, Magali B. Robust and convenient single-use processing: superior strength and flexibility of flexsafe bag. *Bioprocess Int.* 2014;12(5):23–25.

Walther J, Hwang C, Konstantinov K, Godawat R, Abe Y, Sinclair A. The business impact of an integrated continuous biomanufacturing platform for recombinant protein production. *J Biotechnol.* 2015;213:3–12.

Warikoo V, Godawat R, Brower K, Jain S, Cummings D, Simons E, Johnson T, Walther J, Yu M, Wright B, McLarty J, Karey KP, Hwang C, Zhou W, Riske F, Konstantinov K. Integrated continuous production of recombinant therapeutic proteins. *Biotechnol Bioeng.* 2012;109(12):3018–3029. doi:10.1002/bit.24584. Epub 2012 Aug 6. PMID: 22729761.

Wells E, Robinson AS. Cellular engineering for therapeutic protein production: product quality, host modification, and process improvement. *Biotechnol J.* 2017;12(1). doi:10.1002/biot.201600105

Westbrook A, et al. Application of a two-dimensional single-use rocking bioreactor to bacterial cultivation for recombinant protein production. *Biochem. Eng. J.* 2014;88:154–161. doi:10.1016/j.bej.2014.04.011.

Wolton D, Heaven L, McFeaters S, Kodilkar M. Standardization of disposables design: the path forward for a potential game changer. *Bioprocess Int.* 2015;2015;2.

Xiao-Jie L, Hui-Ying X, Zun-Ping K, Jin-Lian C, Li-Juan J. CRISPR-Cas9: a new and promising player in gene therapy. *J Med Genet.* 2015;52(5):289–296. doi:10.1136/jmedgenet-2014-102968

Xu J, Xu X, Huang C, et al. Biomanufacturing evolution from conventional to intensified processes for productivity improvement: a case study. *MAbs.* 2020;12(1):1770669. doi:10.1080/19420862.2020.1770669

Xu S, Gavin J, Jiang R, Chen H. Bioreactor productivity and media cost comparison for different intensified cell culture processes. *Biotechnol Prog.* 2017;33(4):867–878. doi:10.1002/btpr.2415

Yilmaz D, Mehdizadeh H, Navarro D, Shehzad A, O'Connor M, McCormick P. Application of Raman spectroscopy in monoclonal antibody producing continuous systems for downstream process intensification. *Biotechnol Prog.* 2020;36(3):e2947. doi:10.1002/btpr.2947

Yongky A, Xu J, Tian J, et al. Process intensification in fed-batch production bioreactors using non-perfusion seed cultures. *MAbs.* 2019;11(8):1502–1514. doi:10.1080/19420862.2019.1652075

Zhao M, Vandersluis M, Stout J, Haupts U, Sanders M, Jacquemart R. Affinity chromatography for vaccines manufacturing: finally ready for prime time? *Vaccine.* 2019;37(36):5491–5503.

Zhao R, Natarajan A, Srienc F. A flow injection flow cytometry system for online monitoring of bioreactors. *Biotechnol Bioeng.* 1999;62:609–617.

Zhou Y, Lu Z, Wang X, Selvaraj JN, Zhang G. Genetic engineering modification and fermentation optimization for extracellular production of recombinant proteins using Escherichia coli. *Appl Microbiol Biotechnol.* 2018;102(4):1545–1556. doi:10.1007/s00253-017-8700-z

Zhu J, Hatton D. New mammalian expression systems. *Adv Biochem Eng Biotechnol.* 2018;165:9–50. doi:10.1007/10_2016_55

10

Therapeutic Protein Delivery Systems

10.1 Background

Therapeutic proteins' development requirements are different from those of the small chemical molecule drugs because of the molecular size and the variability of molecular structure and how these properties impact the body's immune systems.

The formulation of therapeutic proteins is a broad field of study with several peculiarities compared to small molecule drugs.

First, most protein drugs are administered by parenteral routes, and, as a result, most of the science of protein drug formulation deals with the art of injectable formulations. The choice of delivery route is restricted because of 1) instability of the protein structures in many sites of administration environment, such as the acidity in the gastrointestinal tract, 2) the large molecular size and high hydrophilicity preventing absorption across some biological membranes, leading to faster elimination, and 3) high dose-response sensitivity that does not allow significant variation in the bioavailability.

Second, there are several common structural features of proteins, such as 1) functional groups methionine, cysteine, histidine, tryptophan, and tyrosine, all of which are subject to oxidation, requiring some common approaches to stabilize, 2) conformational changes, and aggregation, properties peculiar to large molecules, requiring the inclusion of product-specific formulation components to prevent aggregation, and 3) inactive components having a greater impact on the bioavailability and conversion to more immunogenic forms with a possibility of altered pharmacokinetic profile that may change the effectiveness of the drug.

Third, all proteins are sensitive to temperature, light, and agitation during storage, shipping, and handling. In some instances, the label includes a caution not to shake the product. With so many variables that can affect the quality and efficacy, the formulation challenges are heightened to address many aspects not generally considered in small molecule drugs.

Therapeutic proteins' formulations largely vary depending on the delivery route, mostly parenteral, but recent advances extend the routes to many other non-invasive routes. The choice of administration route is made based on the practicality and probability factors requiring a detailed understanding of the interaction of therapeutic proteins with the administration's environment. Over the past two decades, many computation tools have become available that allow the fast creation of decision matrices to optimize the formulations.

The administration route selection faces unique biological barriers due to the administration's anatomical and physiological characteristics. Many formulation approaches have been developed to overcome these barriers, including the advances in information technology, biotechnology, and nanotechnology, combined with sophisticated medical devices, electric or magnetic forces, or sonic waves to maximize non-invasive drug effectiveness delivery systems.

A formulation is intended to deliver a biological product active to the administration site, crossing biological barriers, entering the bloodstream, and finally, the site of action that may or may not be known. Given the high likelihood of the degradation of products during the shelf-life, a large volume of proprietary technology has been developed, including thousands of patents, to enable a dosage form to deliver the drug to the site of action.

Appendix 10.1 at the end of this chapter details the physicochemical properties of the proteins and peptides approved by the FDA, an essential information source in designing formulations.

DOI: 10.1201/9781003146933-10

Since therapeutic proteins' development is costly, scientists inevitably get engaged with evaluating the intellectual property relating to the biological product manufacturing and delivery system. Chapter 15 provides details about intellectual property and its management. It forms a required reading for the scientists engaged in the formulation of the therapeutic protein, whose stability is managed by either chemically modifying the molecule or selecting from a large variety of excipients. These combinations will assure stability without affecting the safety or efficacy of the product. Structure modifications include creating protein scaffolds and pegylate the molecules and other technologies elaborated in Chapter 1.

10.2 Route Selection

The formulation composition of therapeutic proteins, like other products, depends on the route of administration and the physicochemical properties of the product. However, the high molecular mass and the large size of drug molecules result in poor membrane permeability limits the choice of delivery routes. For example, drugs with a relatively small molecular mass of < 500 Da readily penetrate through membranes in the gastrointestinal tract and the skin through passive diffusion. In terms of ocular delivery, the human retina's inner and outer plexiform layers limit the diffusion of macromolecules larger than 76 kDa, and macromolecules larger than 150 kDa are unable to reach the inner retina. For molecules larger than 1 kDa, the membrane permeability of the nasal mucosa is also low. Given that proteins larger than 3–5 kDa are considered peptidyl molecules, and antibodies more significant than 150 kDa are considered antibodies, therapeutic proteins' hydrophilicity eliminates several routes of administration.

Most protein drugs are highly hydrophilic, with a log P value less than zero, which makes drug permeation across biological membranes difficult and complicates protein drug delivery to intracellular targets (see Appendix 10.1). Proteins' large size and hydrophilic nature limit their diffusion and passage through paracellular pathways due to the lipophilic nature of biological membranes and the 3–10 paracellular space. As a result, active transport or endocytosis controls the cellular uptake of hydrophilic proteins rather than passive diffusion. One of the major drawbacks of the endocytic pathway for proteins is endosome entrapment, which leads to lysosomal enzyme degradation.

The surface charge of a biological product derived from the amino acid sequence of the protein and its surroundings' pH is another physicochemical drug property that influences absorption. This complex and heterogeneous physicochemical property is typically caused by deamination, isomerization, or post-translational modification, resulting in a change in the net charge of a protein and acidic and basic variants. In addition, protein drugs may interact with molecules on cell surfaces or tissue components due to their surface charge, affecting protein absorption, distribution, and elimination in the body.

10.2.1 Selection

Depending on anatomical size and position, microclimate, specific physiological conditions, and formulations, each administration route has its own set of limitations. Drug absorption may also be affected by the volume and viscosity of the fluid in the rectum.

The ionization, chemical instability, and absorption of protein-based drugs and their delivery systems can be affected by pH conditions in various biological environments. Protein drugs, for example, are frequently unstable at physiological pH. The strongly acidic gastric environment (pH 1–3) causes protein drug destabilization in the stomach, but chemical degradation in the ileum and colon is significantly reduced due to higher pH. The buffering agent in an ocular delivery system is critical because hyperosmotic solutions cause transient dehydration of anterior chamber tissues, while hypotonic solutions can cause edema.

The gastrointestinal tract's enzyme degradation is a formidable barrier to oral protein delivery and low bioavailability. While the enzymatic activity of proteases is high in the small intestine, it is much lower in the colon; as a result, colon-targeted delivery systems have gotten a lot of attention as a viable delivery system for protein drugs. Additionally, colon-targeted drug delivery can result in longer drug absorption and residence time. Thus, colon-targeted drug delivery systems help treat local bowel diseases such as colon cancer, ulcerative colitis, Crohn's disease, and amoebiasis, in addition to systemic delivery of protein drugs. Even though non-oral routes of administration avoid the hepatic first-pass effect, enzymatic barriers may cause a "pseudo-first-pass effect." For example, even low metabolic enzyme activity may be a barrier to protein drug delivery via nasal and pulmonary routes.

Non-injectable drug administration is thwarted by mucus and epithelial cell layers, which act as a significant absorption barrier. Mucus coats all mucosal epithelia, acting as the first line of defense against mechanical damage and the entry of harmful substances at the surfaces of the eye, respiratory tract, and gastrointestinal tract. The mucus layer also acts as a physical barrier for large molecules. Because of its hydrophilic nature and negative charge, the drug interacts with mucus components, slowing drug diffusion and limiting drug absorption in the intestine (Figure 10.1).

Secreted mucin-type glycoproteins are important components of mucus, and the thickness of the mucus layer varies greatly throughout the body. For example, airway mucus can be anywhere from 5 to 55 microns thick, but the nasal tract has a thin mucus layer. As a result, it is more permeable than other mucosal surfaces. In the eye, the secreted precorneal mucin gel covering the conjunctiva can be as thick as 30–40 um. The mucus layer thickness in the gastrointestinal tract varies significantly depending on the location and digestive activity. For example, the mucus layer is thickest in the stomach and colon, but it varies in thickness between 10 and more than 170 um in the ileum and stomach. As a result, while the lack of proteolytic activity in the colon makes it a good absorption site for proteins, drugs must pass through a thicker mucus layer.

10.2.2 Excipients and Properties

Preformulation involves understanding the biological product amino acid sequence that determines the biochemical and biophysical characterization as a function of pH, ionic strength, and excipients. Preformulation also involves developing stability-indicating assays and defining a few lead excipients using (preferably) a systematic approach such as the design of experiment (DOE) or the empirical phase diagram (EPD) as examples. Structural changes (e.g., secondary, tertiary, etc.) and functional changes (e.g., movement, potency, binding wherever possible) occur in the presence of stress.

Excipients that are used in biological product formulations are not approved alone as part of the finished products. They vary from well-known organic or inorganic molecules to biological product structures that are more complex and difficult to characterize. The excipient selection also depends on the regulatory requirements of the respective jurisdictions. In the United States, the Food and Drug Administration (FDA) maintains a searchable database (IID) with approved concentrations, dosage forms, and routes of

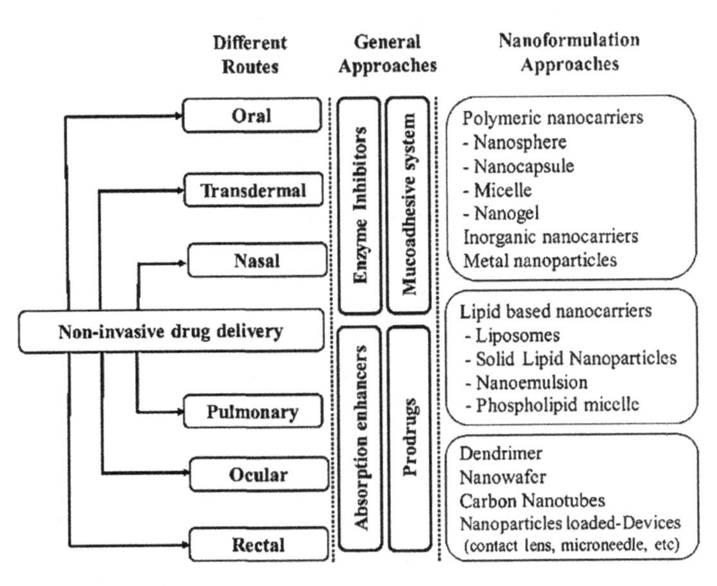

FIGURE 10.1 Barriers to absorption in various routes of administration.

administration (www.accessdata.fda.gov/scripts/cder/iig/index.cfm). In Japan, the Japanese Prescription Excipients Council (JPEC) compiles excipients in the Japanese Pharmaceutical Excipients Dictionary (JPED) detailing approved products, route of administration, and patient treatment (www.yakuji.co.jp/wpyj-002/wp-content/uploads/2020/05/jpe2018_order_form.pdf).

Health Canada publishes a list of acceptable non-medicinal agents. However, the European Medicines Agency does not provide an equivalent list or database for European products.

Categories and examples of some commonly used pharmaceutical excipients in biological products are listed in Table 10.1 (see also Table 10.2).

The dosing requirements determine the number of active components in the composition, and the concentration depends on the product's solubility. Protein solubility is the average amount of protein in the presence of co-solutes where the solution remains visibly clear (i.e., it does not reveal precipitated proteins, crystals, or gels). The dependence of protein solubility on ionic strength, salt form, pH, temperature, and certain excipients is well demonstrated by changes in bulk water surface tension and protein binding to water and ions versus self-association. Protein binding to different excipients or salts influences solubility by modifying the protein conformation or masking certain amino acids involved in self-interaction. Proteins are also preferentially hydrated by certain salts, amino acids, and sugars (and stabilized as more compact conformations), contributing to their altered solubility.

Several common excipients are used to stabilize protein formulations optimization of formulation variables for product stability is the most critical part of protein formulation development. Various formulation excipients and buffers (Table 10.1) can be utilized. They must, therefore, be chosen to maximize the pharmaceutical quality of the product (i.e., stability and activity) without introducing significant side effects.

TABLE 10.1

Categories and Examples of Some Commonly Used Pharmaceutical Excipients in Biological Product Formulations

Category	Example
Buffers	Acetate, succinate, citrate, histidine, phosphate, tris
Amino acids	Arginine, aspartic acid, glutamic acid, lysine, proline, glycine, histidine, methionine
Stabilizers/bulking agents	Lactose, trehalose, dextrose, sucrose, sorbitol, glycerol, albumin, gelatin, mannitol, dextran
Surfactants	Tween 20, Tween 80, Pluronic F68
Preservatives	Benzyl alcohol, m-cresol, phenol, 2-phenoxyethanol
Cyclodextrins	Hydroxypropyl beta cyclodextrin
pH	Buffers
Stabilizer	Surfactants, sugars, salts, antioxidants
Solubilizer	Salts, amino acids, surfactants
Buffer	Phosphate, acetate, histidine, glutamate
Tonicity, bulk modifier	Sodium chloride, sorbitol, mannitol, glycine, polyanions, salts

TABLE 10.2

General Ranges of Formulation Components

Component	General Range
Buffer	5–100 mM
pH	4–8
Stabilizers	1–10%
Salts	0–300 mM
Surfactants	0.01–0.1% (w/v)

Note: While formulations vary widely in their composition, Table 10.2 lists the most common ranges of quantities used.

An analysis of common components of biological product drugs formulations shows that most ingredients are used as:

- Buffering agents to assure that the pH is maintained at the most stable level, and these include phosphates, citrates, and acetates.
- Stabilizers such as surfactants and sugars, and sorbates, albumin, mannitol, sucrose, and sorbitol.
- Tonicity and conductivity adjusting ingredients, including some sugars and electrolytes like sodium chloride.

Of the approximately 200 biological product injectable drugs, the percentage of the most prevalent components used is given in Figure 10.2.

10.2.2.1 pH

Among the listed formulation variables, the most important one is the pH. Problems associated with the physical properties, e.g., precipitation due to solubility and stability, are generally very difficult to manage by other formulation means. Optimization of pH is a simple but beneficial solution for such problems. Most chemical reactions also are affected by pH, e.g., deamidation, cyclic imide formation, disulfide scrambling, peptide bond cleavage, and oxidation. Other functional excipients should also be carefully evaluated for the benefit of the product (e.g., sucrose used to stabilize protein during lyophilization and storage in the dried solid).

Usually, a protein solution can be stabilized against oxidation and precipitation by controlling the solution's pH and ionic strength, adding sugars, amino acids, and polyols, and using surfactants. A comprehensive evaluation of optimal pH and osmotic conditions is a critical element of formulation development to prevent protein aggregation or precipitation—irreversible aggregation arising from denaturation that can be prevented with surfactants, polyols, or sugars.

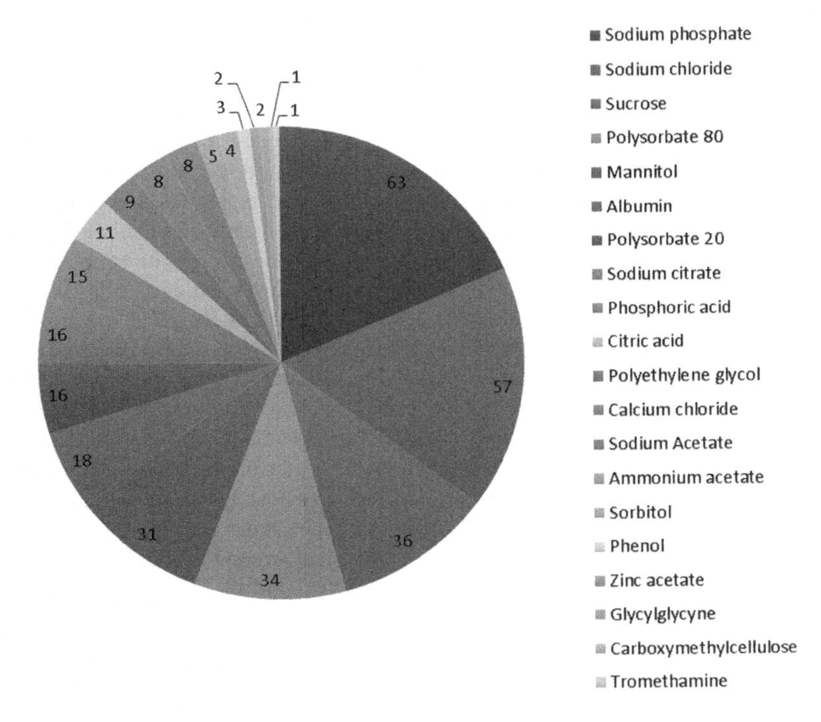

FIGURE 10.2 Percentage occurrence of common formulation components in biological product drugs.

10.2.2.2 Surface Tension

Surfactants are surface-active molecules containing both a hydrophobic portion (e.g., alkyl chain) and a hydrophilic portion (e.g., carboxyl and carboxylate groups). Thus, the surfactant can be used in the invention's formulations. For example, polysorbates are one type of surfactant that can be used in the formulations of the present invention (e.g., polysorbates 20 or 80); poloxamers (e.g., poloxamer 188); sorbitan esters and derivatives; Triton; sodium lauryl sulfate; sodium octyl glycoside; lauryl-, myristyl-, linoleyl-, or stearyl-sulfobetadine; lauryl-, linoleyl-, or stearyl-sarcosine; linoleyl-, myristyl-, or cetyl-betaine; lauramidopropyl-cocamidopropyl-, linoleamidopropyl-, myristamidopropyl-, palmidopropyl-, or isostearamidopropylbetaine (e.g., lauroamidopropyl); myristamidopropyl-, palmidopropyl-, or isostearamidopropyl-dimethylamine; sodium methyl cocoyl- or disodium methyl oleyl-taurate; and the MONAQUAT™ series (Mona Industries, Inc., Paterson, NJ), polyethylene glycol, polypropyl glycol, and copolymers of ethylene and propylene glycol (e.g., Pluronics, PF68, etc.).

In many cases, the addition of nonionic detergents (surfactants) increases stability and prevents aggregation. The protein–surfactant interaction is hydrophobic, so these compounds stabilize proteins by lowering the surface tension of their solution and binding to hydrophobic sites on their surfaces, thus reducing the possibility of protein-protein interactions that could lead to aggregate formation. The nonionic detergents Tween 20 and Tween 80 can prevent the formation of soluble protein aggregates at concentrations of surfactants below the critical concentrations of micelles (CMC). Added to IgG solutions, polysorbate (Tween) 80 stabilizes small aggregates and prevents them from growing into larger particles

10.2.2.3 Tonicity

An "isotonic" formulation is one, which has the same osmotic pressure as the human blood essentially. Isotonic formulations will generally have an osmotic pressure from about 250 to 350 mOsmol/kg H_2O. When added to an aqueous solution, buffering agents are one or more components that can protect the solution against variations in pH that can result when adding acid or alkali or upon dilution with a solvent. In addition to phosphate buffers, glycinate, carbonate, citrate buffers can be used, in which case, sodium, potassium, or ammonium ions can serve as a counterion.

10.2.2.4 Protectants

The limited degree of protein stabilization achieved by commonly used excipients prompted the evaluation of uncommon excipients/substances in improving protein/peptide stability. These include resveratrol, a natural phenol, hydroxybutyrate, polyamines, octanoic acid, and quinone-tryptophan derivatives. Among these, hydrophobic salts, such as a salt of pentane-1,5-diamine and camphor-10-sulfonic acid, have been shown to reduce mAb solutions' viscosity by tenfold. Uncommon excipients, on the other hand, may require extensive safety testing, which could include in vivo studies.

Lyoprotectants include molecules that prevent or reduce the protein's chemical and physical instability upon lyophilization and subsequent storage when combined with a protein of interest.

Preservatives include an agent that reduces bacterial action and may be optionally added to the formulations herein. For example, adding a preservative can ease the development of a multi-use (multiple doses) formulation. Examples of potential preservatives include octadecyl-dimethyl-benzyl ammonium chloride, hexamethonium chloride, benzalkonium chloride (a mixture of alkyl benzyl dimethylammonium chlorides in which the alkyl groups are long-chain compounds), and benzethonium chloride. Other types of preservatives include aromatic alcohols such as phenol, butyl, and benzyl alcohol, alkyl parabens such as methyl or propylparaben, catechol, resorcinol, cyclohexanol, 3-pentanol, and m-cresol.

A typical approach to mitigating aggregation is to limit protein mobility to reduce the number of collisions. Excipients usually inhibit aggregation and protect the protein by adsorbing to the air-liquid interface; for example, the use of surfactants (e.g., polysorbate 20 and 80), carbohydrates (e.g., cyclodextrin derivatives), and amino acids (e.g., arginine and histidine) can help prevent aggregation by this mechanism. However, polysorbate 80 can lead to micelle formation and hence, increase the chance of immunogenicity. Cyclodextrin stabilizes commercially available antibody-based drugs in a hydrogel formulation. Some commonly recognized excipients regarded as safe (GRAS) include Pluronic F68, trehalose, glycine, and amino acids such as arginine, glycine, and glutamate histidine found in several commercial proteins therapy products. Avastin® (bevacizumab, 25 mg/mL), for instance, contains trehalose dehydrate, sodium phosphate, and polysorbate 20. Histidine hydrochloride, histidine, trehalose dehydrate, polysorbate 20, methionine, and water for injection are excipients in subcutaneous Herceptin® (trastuzumab, 600 mg). Chelating agents also can be used to prevent metal-induced protein aggregation.

10.2.2.5 Stabilizers

The use of a large polymeric excipient/material was found to be effective in protein stabilization. As crowding agents, neutral polymers stabilize a protein because of the volume effect (steric repulsion) removed. Many neutral polymers, such as PVP, Ficoll70, hydroxyethyl (heta) starch, or PEG 4000, also stabilize proteins. Newer entities include functionalized trehalose-containing dextrans and glycopolymers as the side chain units for improved process and storage stability. Glycopolymers made from modified trehalose monomers achieve stabilization. Due to the delicate formation of protein-polyion interactions such as heparin and dextran sulfate, pentosan polysulfate, polyphosphoric acid, poly-L-glutamic acid, poly (acrylic acid), poly (methacrylic acid), polyanions/polycations are potential stabilizers. Activity between polycationic chitosan and negatively charged lactate dehydrogenase (LDH) during air-jet nebulization leads to significant stabilization. In contrast, negative heparin and keratinocyte growth factor 2 (KGF-2) activity promote protein aggregation during agitation. It is evident that strong interactions, as shown by the preferential mechanism of interaction, can lead to protein destabilization.

The fibrillation process involves interactions between crystalline and non-native protein species. A particular case is recombinant hyaluronidase enzyme in protein formulation to promote the rapid distribution of tissue and, thus, the administration of a larger than normal injection amount. But, again, using polymers or proteins to formulate proteins increases the formulation's complexity and complicates protein formulations' characterization and stability studies.

10.2.3 Liquid Formulations

Liquid formulations require the study of electrostatic interactions, Van der Waals interactions, hydrogen bonding, and hydrophobicity. For example, the native conformation of biologics can be stabilized by high concentrations of saccharides such as sucrose, trehalose, lactose, etc., as well as by polyhydrated alcohols such as sorbitol, mannitol, polyethylene glycol, etc. due to the preferential exclusion from the protein surface, thus providing stabilization. Saccharose is excluded because of increased surface tension. The solubility of proteins can often be increased by adding small salt concentrations, a phenomenon called "salting in." Salts are also used as tonicity modifiers; however, they may negatively impact conformational stability in some cases. So, the option of counterions (referring to the Hofmeister series) and their concentration can be used to modify the biological product's stability profile. In pre-formulation screening, this is considered critical. For example, the same pH condition can be obtained with different buffer species at different concentrations (i.e., at different ionic strengths) and can thus modify the protein's stability. Ligand binding may also support the native protein state, as seen, for example, by binding Zn2+ to the growth hormone in humans.

Surface-active agents are often used to prevent the adsorption, denaturation, and aggregation of proteins at interfaces (both air-water and solid-water) and affect stability by differential binding to the protein's native or denatured states. Agitation and freeze-thaw stress experiments are often used to demonstrate surface denaturation mechanisms and the addition of low surfactant concentrations such as polysorbate 20, polysorbate 80, Pluronic F68, or others can be effective in minimizing both soluble and insoluble aggregates. Leachates such as metal ions, barium from glass vials, vulcanizing agents from stoppers, tungsten oxide from prefilled syringes, and silicone oil penetration are additional concerns related to the primary contact surfaces to be addressed during excipient selection. For example, EDTA can be used for removing metal leachates from stoppers. So, the option of counterions (referring to the Hofmeister series) and their concentration can be used to modify the biological product's stability profile. This is considered critical during screening before formulation. For example, the same pH state can be obtained with different buffer species at different concentrations (i.e., at different ionic strengths) and can alter protein stability. Ligand binding, as seen, for example, with the binding of Zn^{2+} to human growth hormone, can also support the native state of proteins.

One-third of biological products are available as multidose, and these typically require antimicrobial preservatives to be added. By inducing protein aggregation, the preservatives may present additional stabilization challenges for therapeutic proteins. The common preservatives include m-cresol, benzyl alcohol or phenol, phenoxyethanol, and chlorobutanol. Screening of different preservatives is recommended before use, either alone or in combination.

10.2.4 Lyophilized Formulations

By reducing protein mobility and restricting conformational flexibility, lyophilization with appropriate excipients can improve protein stability against aggregation, with the added benefit of reducing hydrolytic reactions. The addition of suitable excipients, including lyoprotectants, can prevent aggregates' formation during the lyophilization process and final product storage. The lyoprotectant's molar ratio to the protein is called protection. In general, molar ratios of 300:1 or higher are required for adequate stability, especially when stored at room temperature. However, such ratios can result in an undesirable increase in viscosity.

The protein's instability requires appropriate storage requirements, and shipping is better met with a lyophilized product than a liquid formulation, especially for highly thermolabile products and live virus vaccine products. The lyophilization process requires freezing, followed by primary and secondary drying under vacuum; the drying process presents a new set of challenges. Denaturation can occur during freezing, either in the freeze-concentrate state, frozen surface interfaces, or through cold-denaturation. Formulations should also address the impact of local salt and buffer concentrations and increase the concentration of trapped oxygen during the freeze-concentrate process.

Similarly, changes in pH due to buffer crystallization have to be considered for lyophilized products during the formulation design space. For example, buffering at physiological pH conditions with a low concentration (including 10 mM) of potassium phosphate over sodium phosphate buffer is preferable; this can be due to the pH change to increase buffer concentration a large pH shift during freezing for sodium phosphate. On the other hand, due to minimal pH changes during freezing, citrate, tris, and histidine are good choices for the buffer if at the correct pH range. Likewise, antioxidants (e.g., ascorbates) and scavengers (e.g., thiourea) may be added to reduce oxidation.

External stabilizers known as lyoprotectants may be required in addition to cryoprotectants. For example, liquid pre-formulation screening could suggest that sorbitol is a good stabilizer; however, sorbitol is not preferred in dried formulations because of its low glass transition temperature. It should be noted that the two key attributes of lyoprotectants are high glass transition temperatures to reduce molecular mobility while maintaining the native state in the dried state by acting as a strong water replacement (e.g., sucrose, trehalose). Therefore, the use of reduced sugars (e.g., lactose) must be specifically measured in the risk assessment analysis. Nevertheless, the possibility of phase separation (especially for a multi-stabilizer system) can limit some combinations of excipients (for example, PEG-dextran). Likewise, low pH acid hydrolysis capacity makes trehalose a better option for sucrose.

Bulking agents are also added to the lyophilized product to avoid product "blowout" for products with a low concentration (including 1% solid). Excipients can function as amorphous bulking agents (e.g., sucrose, trehalose, lactose, raffinose, dextran, hydroxyethyl starch (HES), or as crystalline bulking agents (e.g., glycine, mannitol) for amorphous excipients (such as HES) or high eutectic temperatures (T_{eu}) for crystalline excipients (such as glycine and mannitol). Nonetheless, the presence of mannitol hydrate form and the risk of glass breakage during manufacture (be it due to high fill volume, incorrect freezing procedure, and high concentration) can restrict mannitol selection during excipient screening.

Administration, reducing pain when given, may be beneficial. Isotonicity of a lyophile is difficult to achieve due to the concentration of both the protein and the excipients during the reconstitution cycle. In the excipient, a 500:1 protein molar ratio may result in hypertonic preparations if the protein is targeted at > 100 mg/mL.

While freeze-drying is one of the most widely used processes for protein drugs, this method has several disadvantages, and several alternative drying methods are developed that include spray-drying, spray-freezing, supercritical drying of fluids, supercritical fluid drying, and foam drying applied to proteins, including insulin, trypsin, human growth hormones, and monoclonal antibodies.

10.3 Delivery Routes

Parenteral means all routes except by mouth or the alimentary canal (e.g., rectal). The most common administration route for therapeutic proteins is a parenteral injection that includes intravenous bolus, intravenous infusion, subcutaneous injection, and intramuscular injection. However, parenteral injection is not always the preferred delivery system for being invasive, causing pain, risk of infection, high cost, and low patient compliance.

The noninvasive drug delivery routes such as oral, nasal, pulmonary, ophthalmic, rectal, or transdermal routes are challenging to develop due to the large molecular size, hydrophilicity, low permeability, and chemical/enzymatic instability of therapeutic proteins. With the alternative methods of drug delivery, there are two significant problems. The site, or route, of administration of the drug is frequently hostile to polypeptides, e.g., orally delivered proteins are subjected to harsh conditions before absorption through the gastrointestinal tract or absorption through the nasal mucosa, a considerable metabolism may occur. The second problem, the absorption of sufficient amounts of the drug through the respective barrier layers after administration, can significantly achieve a pharmacological response. Strategies to improve absorption of usually hydrophilic (hence poorly absorbed) compounds include encapsulation into hydrophobic carriers, combination with penetration enhancers, active electrical transport, or chemical modification to increase hydrophobicity. Advancements in nanotechnologies promote novel nano-formulations with controlled particle size and surface modification, which improves the target selectivity, systemic half-life, and bioavailability of protein drugs.

10.3.1 Intravenous

The most common routes to deliver biopharmaceutics include intravenous bolus, intravenous infusion, and subcutaneous. The intravenous route administers most drugs that would have either low or highly variable bioavailability to get exact dosing, like oncology drugs. Intravenous injections are also preferred for drugs that might irritate subcutaneous tissue. However, this route cannot be recommended for self-administration of drugs, a significant cost element of drug therapy. There are not many formulation concerns except that the drug must be either in a solution form or extremely fine emulsion to prevent veins' blockage. Recently, some therapeutic proteins that were initially developed as intravenous injection or infusion are reformulated for subcutaneous administration to enable self-administration.

10.3.2 Subcutaneous

The first biological product, insulin, was approved as a subcutaneous product. Intravenous bolus or infusion is the common route for drugs where a dose must be calculated, such as in the use of oncology drugs and administered by professionals. However, recently there has been a shift taking place from intravenous to subcutaneous administration for economic reasons. After subcutaneous formulations of trastuzumab and rituximab were introduced in Europe in 2013 and 2014, respectively, several drugs were reformulated in a subcutaneous dosage form, shifting from intravenous, allowing self-injection for rheumatoid arthritis, multiple sclerosis, or primary immunodeficiency therapies, where mixed dosing (not calculated based on body weight) is recommended (Table 10.3).

The biological product pharmacokinetic profile administered through the subcutaneous route is distinct from that of the intravenous form. A biotherapeutic intravenous infusion or injection directly into the bloodstream usually results in immediate maximum serum concentrations (C_{max}), whereas the pharmacokinetic profile of biological products subcutaneously injected is typically characterized by a sluggish rate absorption from the subcutaneous extracellular matrix with C_{max} levels below those achieved with

TABLE 10.3

Examples of Therapeutic Proteins Delivered in Subcutaneous Dosage Forms

Molecule	Brand Name (Originator)	Dosing Frequency	Injection Volume	Device
Abatacept	Orencia (Bristol-Myers Squibb)	q1w	1 ml	Prefilled syringe, prefilled pen/autoinjector
Adalimumab	Humira (AbbVie)	q2w	0.4–0.8 ml	Prefilled syringe, vial, prefilled pen
Anakinra	Kineret (Swedish Orphan Biovitrum GmbH)[a]	q1d or q2d	0.67 ml	Prefilled syringe
Certolizumab pegol	Cimzia (UCB-Euronext and BEL20)[a]	q2w and q4w	1 ml	Prefilled syringe, vial, prefilled pen
Etanercept	Enbrel (Amgen)	q1w or twice weekly	0.5–1 ml	Prefilled syringe, vial, prefilled pen/autoinjector, prefilled cartridge for reusable autoinjector
Glatiramer acetate	Copaxone (Teva)	q1d or three times per week	1 ml	Prefilled syringe, pen/autoinjector
Golimumab	Simponi (Janssen)	q1m	0.5–1 ml	Prefilled syringe, prefilled pen/autoinjector
Insulin	Several	PRN	Variable	Vials, prefilled pen, syringes
Interferon-beta-1a	Rebif (EMD Serono/Pfizer)	Three times per week	0.2–0.5 ml	Prefilled syringe, prefilled pen/autoinjector, electronic injection system
Interferon beta-1b	Betaseron/Betaferon (Bayer)	q2d	0.25–1 ml	Prefilled syringe. vial, autoinjector
Interferon beta-1b	Extavia (Novartis)	q2d	0.25–1 ml	Prefilled syringe, vial, autoinjector
Peg-interferon beta-1a	Plegridy (Biogen)	q2w	0.5 ml	Prefilled syringe, prefilled pen/autoinjector
Rituximab	MabThera/Rituxan Hycela (Roche)	q3w–q3mc	11.7–13.4 ml	Vial and syringe
Sarilumab	Kevzara (Sanofi-Aventis)	q2w	1.14 ml	Prefilled syringe, prefilled pen
Tocilizumab	Actemra (Roche)	q1w and q2w	0.9 ml	Prefilled syringe, prefilled pen
Trastuzumab	Herceptin (Roche)	q3w	5 ml	Vial and syringe

intravenous dosing. This absorption of macromolecules into the blood results from their reduced permeability across the vascular endothelial; hence lymphatics provide an alternative absorption pathway into the circulation system. Nonetheless, lymphatic absorption has also been identified as a barrier for the full infiltration of molecules injected subcutaneously. Such factors contributing to the incomplete bioavailability of subcutaneously injected molecules may include the dose formulation structure, duration, pH, viscosity, interactions with interstitial glycosaminoglycans, and proteins and enzyme degradation.

Following subcutaneous injection, molecules reach the systemic circulation via either the blood capillaries or the lymphatic system. Unlike small molecules, biological products with molecular weights of > 20 kDa exhibit limited transport into the blood capillaries and cross into the circulation system predominantly via the lymphatics. Such increased exposure to the lymphatic system has led to the suggestion that biotherapeutic subcutaneous administration may be more immunogenic than intravenous dosing. In this context, it is necessary to consider the production of anti-drug antibodies (ADAs) with the various routes of administration per se and their effect on the biotherapeutic's exposure, efficacy, and safety. The regulatory agencies currently require immunogenicity testing of the subcutaneous dosage form over intravenous if there is an option.

A drawback of subcutaneous administration of biological products is the incomplete bioavailability of the injected molecule, ranging widely from 50% to 80% for mAbs and even more for other biological products. As for the enzymes involved and their translation through organisms, the underlying pre-systemic catabolism at the subcutaneous administration site or the lymphatic system is still poorly understood. For mAbs, subcutaneous bioavailability appears to be inversely correlated with clearance after intravenous dosing, so that mAbs with a lower intravenous clearance exhibit higher subcutaneous bioavailability. This correlation may be due to hematopoietic cells (e.g., macrophages or dendritic cells) in both subcutaneous first-pass clearance and systemic clearance after intravenous dosing. Since inadequate bioavailability typically leads to the need for a higher dose for subcutaneous infusions than for intravenous infusions, the cost of goods for subcutaneous formulations can be modified in an attempt to increase the subcutaneous bioavailability of a biotherapeutic; subcutaneous infusions can be co-administered (or produced as coformulations) with the dispersion-enhancer hyaluronidase. This enzyme facilitates the spreading of an injected fluid in the subcutaneous tissue. This increased dispersion in the interstitial tissue can result in the higher bioavailability of a co-injected molecule.

Subcutaneous injections are often formulated in a buffered aqueous solution, some of which can be irritating, like the citrate buffer. In an interesting example, the best-selling biological product drug, Humira, was launched in a citrate buffer that causes smarting upon injection; once the patent on the gene sequence expired, Abbvie reformulated the product by removing the buffer and justified it by stating that the large proteins themselves have a buffering effect. Therefore, there is no need for a citrate buffer. The new formulation is more concentrated, reducing the injection volume, less irritation, and allowed Abbvie another patent that now protects the product for decades. Some sustained-release subcutaneous therapeutics have been available for several decades, such as insulin glargine precipitating subcutaneous injection to allow prolonged release. Recent advances in polymer science have resulted in hydrogels that provide sustained drug release, have high tissue biocompatibility, and enable patient self-administration. Hydrogels provide a deformable drug depot that slowly elutes a high drug concentration to surrounding tissue for an extended period. However, because most hydrogels only physically bind to the drugs rather than forming covalent bonds, rapid drug release occurs over a few hours to days, limiting their utility for long-term drug delivery.

10.3.3 Oral

Oral delivery is the most preferred dosage form. Still, the significant molecular weight of protein drugs makes it almost impossible due to permeability issues and complexity due to the instability. The inconsistency of bioavailability common to oral formulations that bring dose-response challenges is often very narrow for protein drugs. However, efforts are made, including using lipophilic derivatives of insulin and thyrotropin-releasing hormone by fatty acylation with palmitic or lauric acid. The modified drug molecules spontaneously form vesicle-like structures (Prosome®, Pharmacosome®), which greatly increase the bioavailability and circulation time of the drug in patients (Table 10.4).

Encapsulation involves the polypeptide drug's entrapment within a polymeric, phospholipid, or carbohydrate particulate delivery system such as microspheres, liposomes, and nanoparticles.

TABLE 10.4

Orally Administered Therapeutic Proteins

Product	Drug	Route	Indications
Minirin	Desmopressin	Oral, nasal	Cranial diabetes insipidus or nocturia associated with multiple sclerosis
Sandimmune	Cyclosporine A	Oral	Immunosuppressants
Colomycin	Colistin	Oral	Intestinal infection (caused by sensitive Gram-negative organisms)
Cytorest	Cytochrome C	Oral	Leucopenia
Cachexon®	Glutathione	Oral	AIDS-related cachexia
Ceredist OD	Taltirelin	Oral	Spinocerebellar ataxia
Anginovag	Tyrothricin	Oral	Pharyngitis
Vancocin	Vancomycin	Oral	Infection, *Clostridium difficile*–associated diarrhea
Oral-Lyn	Insulin	Buccal	Diabetes mellitus

10.3.4 Nasal

The nasal route has some advantages, such as increased bioavailability and ease of administration, but it also allows drugs to be delivered directly to the brain through the nose. Similarly, the lungs are exceptionally permeable to macromolecules; thus, pulmonary delivery can be an effective noninvasive route for protein delivery. Inhaled insulin was more quickly absorbed than subcutaneously injected insulin, resulting in a better physiological response to a meal. However, an inhalation insulin product was recalled because of the inconsistency of the dose delivered. A list of nasally administered products appears in Table 10.5.

The blood–brain barrier controls the passage of most therapeutics, including proteins, into the central nervous system and represents a significant hurdle in drug delivery to treat many neuronal degenerative disorders. In this context, the nasal route can be the most reliable alternative to oral and parenteral routes. The incorporation of absorption enhancers promotes permeation through the membrane, mucoadhesive formulations to improve nasal residential time, and prodrug approaches to optimize absorption. The use of absorption enhancers such as bile salts, surfactants, fluidic acid derivatives, phosphatidylcholines, fatty acids (tauro dihydro fusidate), cyclodextrins (CDs), cationized polymers, chelators, and cell penetration peptides facilitate drug permeation across the nasal membrane. In addition, mucoadhesive systems extend nasal retention time because protein bioavailability can be limited by a short residence time in the nasal cavity. As a result, it appears that using Carbopol 941 and carboxymethyl cellulose, improved nasal bioavailability of calcitonin and insulin is possible. Mucoadhesive polymers also act as permeation enhancers by opening the nasal epithelium's tight junctions. As a result, mucoadhesive micro-/nanoparticles can be useful carriers for protein drug delivery through the nose because they have a longer residence time and better permeation across the membrane.

10.3.5 Transdermal

Many cytokines can be used topically; for example, applying a human epidermal growth factor in liposomes significantly improves the effect. Niosomes (liposomes made of nonionic surfactants) may also be useful for peptide drug delivery through the skin's pilosebaceous route. For example, vesicles composed of glyceryl dilaurate cholesterol and polyoxyethylene-10-stearyl ether enhance the absorption of interferon-alpha and cyclosporine. Another type of liposome preparation, transfersomes (a phosphatidylcholine/sodium cholate mixture), can be used to deliver insulin through topical application in vivo.

TABLE 10.5

Nasally Administered Therapeutic Proteins

Product	Drug	Route	Indications
Suprifact	Buserelin	Nasal	Prostate cancer, endometriosis
Suprecur	Buserelin	Nasal	Prostate cancer, endometriosis
Synarel	Nafarelin	Nasal	Endometriosis
Kryptocur	LHRH	Nasal	Cryptorchism
Miacalcin	Salmon calcitonin	Nasal	Hypercalcemia or osteoporosis
Fortical®	Salmon calcitonin	Nasal	Hypercalcemia or osteoporosis
Desmospray	Desmopressin	Nasal	Cranial diabetes insipidus or nocturia associated with multiple sclerosis
Syntocinin	Oxytocin	Nasal	Indicated for the initiation or improvement of uterine contractions
Antepan	Protirelin	Nasal	Hypothyroidism and acromegaly
FluMist® Quadrivalent	Vaccine	Nasal	Influenza
Minirin	Desmopressin	Oral, nasal	Cranial diabetes insipidus or nocturia associated with multiple sclerosis

The approaches to delivering peptides through the skin utilize methods that temporarily compromise the skin's integrity or physicochemical characteristics, including the use of penetration enhancers such as *N*-alkylazacycloheptanones (Azone) for desglycinamide arginine vasopressin. In addition, the non-ionic surfactant n-decyl methyl sulphoxide enhances the penetration of leu-enkephalin through hairless mouse skin in vitro, and a urea/ethanol/menthol/camphor/methyl salicylate hydroxypropyl cellulose gel enhanced absorption of the nonapeptide leuprolide (a luteinizing-hormone-releasing-hormone analog) through hydration and keratolytic effect.

Iontophoresis, a method based on electrical stimulation of skin permeability for mostly ionized molecules, has been employed by many researchers in the last few years for the enhancement of delivery of short peptides (model tripeptides, vasopressin), growth-hormone-releasing factor (amino acids 1–44), insulin, and luteinizing-hormone-releasing hormone. In addition, ultrasonic vibration was tried for delivery in vivo of insulin, with some success.

Microneedles are extremely small needles that can pass through the stratum corneum to create microchannels. Their lengths range from 50 to 900 um. As a painless device, microneedles improve patient compliance and provide a versatile platform for hydrophilic and high molecular weight drugs, including protein drugs, to overcome the skin barrier. Silicon, metals, biodegradable polymers, and carbohydrates can all be used to make them. Solid microneedles were used in the first generation of microneedles to perforate the skin membrane and increase drug permeability. Although solid microneedles appeared to deliver insulin effectively, their use is limited due to low delivery efficiency, complicated administration, a lack of precise dosing, and infection risk. Solid microneedles have recently been modified by coating the drug payload directly onto the microneedle surface. Coating the microneedles is done in a variety of ways, including dip-coating, casting, and deposition. Following the hydrolysis of the biodegradable polymer matrix, biodegradable microneedles provide sustained drug release. When making these microneedles, polymers with a high molecular weight and crosslinking density are preferred.

Ultrasound waves are used in sonophoresis to increase drug permeability in the skin. Ultrasound waves cause the air pockets in the stratum corneum to expand and oscillate, disrupting the lipid bilayer and forming cavities that improve drug permeability through the skin. The degree of drug delivery by sonophoresis is determined by the drug's physicochemical properties, as well as the net ultrasound exposure time and the pulse "on" duration. Although sonophoresis can improve therapeutic protein transdermal delivery, the potential for protein instability caused by ultrasound should be carefully considered. Drug delivery through the skin can be effectively enhanced by combining sonophoresis with other enhancement methods such as chemical enhancers, electroporation, and iontophoresis.

Electroporation, which uses ultra-short pulses lasting a few milliseconds and intensity of a few hundred volts to induce changes in the skin and allow hydrophilic compounds to pass, is the most recent approach to transdermal delivery of proteins and peptides. Electroporation and iontophoresis use an electric field to propel a drug into the skin; however, electroporation works primarily on the skin to alter membrane permeability to improve drug penetration, whereas iontophoresis works directly on it the drug to propel it into the skin.

10.3.6 Pulmonary

The lung allows rapid and high drug absorption due to its large surface area (approximately 80–140 m^2), very thin alveolar epithelium thickness (0.1–0.5 mm), and large blood supply. Pulmonary drug delivery is advantageous because it avoids the hepatic first-pass effect, and it is also noninvasive, efficacious at lower doses, and applicable for local or systemic delivery. Lung tissue has relatively low enzymatic activity than the gastrointestinal tract; the pulmonary epithelium has many immunological properties. However, pulmonary delivery has some drawbacks, such as a short duration of action due to the drug's rapid removal. After deposition in the lungs, inhaled drugs can be swept from the airways toward the mouth and removed via phagocytosis by alveolar macrophages. As a result, a significant slow-drug release necessitates a way to avoid or suspend the lungs' natural clearance mechanisms until the encapsulated drugs are effectively delivered. Proteins with molecular weights of 6,000 to 50,000 D have good bioavailability after inhalation in general. As a result, pulmonary administration has attracted a lot of attention as a promising delivery method for protein drugs.

Many drugs under development for pulmonary delivery include interleukin-1 receptor (asthma therapy), heparin (blood clotting), human insulin (diabetes), -1 antitrypsin (emphysema and cystic fibrosis), interferons (multiple sclerosis and hepatitis B and C), and calcitonin and other peptides (osteoporosis). Gene therapy can be delivered through inhalation delivery methods that target specific tissues or organs. Many patients who previously received injections will be able to independently and painlessly inhale medicine into the deep lung, where it will be absorbed naturally and efficiently into the bloodstream, thanks to Inhale's novel dry powder formulation, processing, and filling, combined with aerosol device technology.

The selection of a delivery device is critical in the formulation design for pulmonary drug delivery because it plays a critical role in the effectiveness of pulmonary drug administration. Nebulizers (e.g., jet nebulizers, ultrasonic nebulizers, and vibrating mesh nebulizers), metered-dose inhalers, and dry powder inhalers are the most common devices to deliver therapeutics as aerosols.

Various nanotechnology-based formulation approaches for effective protein delivery via the pulmonary route have been thoroughly investigated. Nanoparticles, in general, appear to be promising as a protein delivery carrier in the lungs because of their targeting ability and controlled drug release. Furthermore, nanoparticles smaller than 200 nm may avoid detection by alveolar macrophages, resulting in more effective uptake and drug action. Other types of nanocarriers, such as liposomes and solid lipid nanoparticles, have been used for the pulmonary delivery of protein drugs in addition to polymeric nanoparticles. The sections that follow provide a more in-depth look at these nanocarriers.

Inhalable insulin is a powdered form of insulin, delivered with an inhaler into the lungs where it is absorbed. In general, inhaled insulins have been more rapidly absorbed than subcutaneously injected insulin, with a faster peak concentration in serum and more rapid metabolism. Exubera, developed by Inhale Therapeutics (later named Nektar Therapeutics), became the first inhaled insulin product to be marketed in 2006 by Pfizer, but poor sales led Pfizer to withdraw it in 2007. Afrezza, a monomeric inhaled insulin developed by Mannkind, was approved by the FDA in 2014. Dypreza, an inhaled insulin developed by Highlands Pharmaceuticals, was approved for sale in Europe in 2013 and the United States in 2016. The critical issue with inhalable insulin comes from the need to control the dosing accurately; that is not always possible when using a device to administer the drug.

10.3.7 Ocular

The blood–retinal barrier and efflux transporters expressed in the posterior segment obstruct protein delivery to the eye. Ocular drug delivery is also affected by the viscosity of formulations. High viscosity extends when the cornea is in contact with the surface of the eye, but it also causes reflex tearing and blinking, which changes the viscosity of the formulation.

Ocular delivery is fast growing with at least two products already approved: the anti-vascular endothelial growth factor (anti-VEGF) aptamer and monoclonal antibody (Lucentis; Ranibizumab). Since topically applied conventional dosage forms, such as eye drops, have the main drawbacks of low bioavailability and subsequent low therapeutic efficiency, various new strategies have been developed to overcome the ocular delivery barriers and enhance the bioavailability of proteins ocular route of administration. For example, the utilization of chemical chaperones and coadministration of recombinant human hyaluronidase have been attempted to facilitate protein delivery through the ocular route. Since protein aggregation is one of the primary concerns in the formulation of proteins for ocular diseases, a novel strategy to utilize chemical chaperones (protein aggregation inhibitors) was developed to prevent protein misfolding and/or inhibit the self-assembly of aggregation-prone sequences in native protein structures. The coadministration of recombinant hyaluronidases has also been used for decades to increase the penetration of biological product drugs across ocular tissue barriers. Hyaluronidases catalyze the degradation of hyaluronic acid, a critical structural component of tissues. Furthermore, various nanocarriers, including polymeric micelles, liposomes, nanospheres, nano wafers, and dendrimers, are extensively

TABLE 10.6
Ocular Biological Products

Product	Drug	Route	Indications
Cenegermin	Oxervate	Eye drop	Neurotrophic keratitis
Eylea	Aflibercept	Ocular	Wet age-related macular degeneration (WAMD), diabetic macular edema (DME) or diabetic retinopathy (DR) in DME, macular edema following retinal vein occlusion (MEtRVO) WAMD, DME or DR in DME, MEtRVO, myopic choroidal neovascularization (mCNV)
Lucentis	Ranibizumab	Ocular	

evaluated for their controlled and targeted delivery of proteins via the ocular route. Table 10.6 lists the drugs administered through ocular routes.

Nano wafers are tiny transparent circular or rectangular membranes that contain arrays of drug-loaded nano reservoirs that release drugs in a highly controlled manner and for a longer duration than eye drops (a few hours to several days). They are composed of various polymers such as polyvinyl alcohol, polyvinyl pyrrolidone, hydroxypropyl methylcellulose, and carboxymethyl cellulose. Nano wafers are applied by the patient's fingertip, can withstand constant blinking without removal, release the drug slowly, enhance drug resident time and absorption into ocular tissues, and improve therapeutic efficacy. Furthermore, during drug release, the nano wafer slowly dissolves, rendering ocular surfaces free of polymers.

Drug-loaded contact lenses could also be used to deliver and treat ocular drugs. Longer drug residence time on the eye with contact lenses improves drug permeation through the cornea. Drug molecules diffuse slowly from the lens matrix, allowing for long-term drug release. Entrapping the drug in nano-carriers and dispersing the drug-loaded nanocarriers in the lens matrix can improve the residence time and drug release rate even more. To achieve the desired therapeutic goals, the use of drug-loaded contact lenses as an ocular delivery system for macromolecules needs to be further investigated. However, limitations such as drug leaching during storage and distribution and surface roughness-related safety concerns must be addressed.

10.3.8 Rectal

Rectal drug delivery can improve the bioavailability of protein drugs, which are very vulnerable to physicochemical and enzymatic destabilization; the approaches include the utilization of absorption enhancers, protease inhibitors, prodrugs, and nanoformulations. In general, absorption enhancers are required to increase macromolecules' rectal absorption, such as insulin, heparin, calcitonin, recombinant human granulocyte colony-stimulating factor (rhGCSF), and human chorionic gonadotrophin. Although several absorption enhancers can be used in rectal drug delivery, some cause membrane damage and irritation. Similarly, protease inhibitors are also effective at improving rectal bioavailability by reducing the degradation of proteins and enhancing the enzymatic stability of protein drugs. Prodrug approaches are being pursued to strengthen proteins and peptides' absorption by protecting them against degradation from peptidases and other mucosal enzymes. In addition to those approaches, nanotechnology-based formulation approaches are available for improving protein drug delivery via rectal administration.

10.4 Formulation Technologies

10.4.1 Hydrogels and In Situ Forming Gels

Hydrogels are three-dimensional polymeric networks made up of crosslinked hydrophilic and biocompatible polymers that swell in aqueous media due to their thermodynamic compatibility with water. Contact lenses, biosensors, tissue engineering materials, and drug delivery carriers are examples of clinical applications for hydrogels. Hydrogels can also be used to deliver protein drugs more effectively and conveniently. 2-hydroxyethyl methacrylate is one of many polymers.

A hydrogel system releases the protein in its active form while maintaining the therapeutic concentration for at least three months, a possible alternative to associated particulate formulations. Hydrogels are polymeric materials that, under physiological conditions, do not dissolve in water and that swell considerably in an aqueous medium. They are networks of covalently linked polymer leading chains, known as crosslinking, and sometimes the polymer crosslinks can be non-covalent solid interactions. The crosslinking of polymer chains prevents the polymer from dissolving entirely. Therefore, hydrogels made of hydrophilic polymers can imbibe water into the structure and swell of their network. The hydrogel's high-water content properties make them biocompatible and are therefore being studied in tissue regeneration applications. However, hydrogels' high water content is a problem in developing extended formulations for drug release, although there are potential advantages of hydrogels compared to other drug delivery systems.

For pharmaceutical applications, they're also crucial. To achieve the desired mechanical properties, hydrogel crosslinking must be adjusted, as a higher degree of crosslinking results in a stronger but more brittle structure. Copolymerization can also be used to make hydrogels that are both strong and elastic.

Physiological stimuli such as pH, ionic strength, and temperature are frequently used to design hydrogels. However, such hydrogels can change their swelling behavior, network structure, permeability, and mechanical strength dramatically in response to environmental stimuli.

Nanogels are water-swollen, cross-linked polymer nanoparticles with hydrodynamic sizes ranging from 10 to 100 nanometers that can be dispersed in an aqueous medium while maintaining their fixed conformation. Natural and synthetic polymers can be used to make them. Nanogels have the advantage of being able to control and tailor their size, surface charge, network density, and chemical functional groups to achieve the desired structural and functional properties.

For nasal delivery, insulin molecules have been covalently attached to soft, highly hydrophilic, and multifunctional nanogels. Compared to free-insulin, poly (N-vinyl pyrrolidone)-based nanogels covalently attached to insulin cross the blood-brain barrier after intranasal administration and exhibit neuroprotection against amyloid ß-induced dysfunction.

10.4.2 Nanoparticles

Nanotechnology was discussed in depth in Chapter 6. By encapsulating proteins in a polymeric matrix with a size range of 10–1,000 nm, nanoparticles improve protein physicochemical stability in the gastrointestinal tract. Nanoparticles should be non-toxic and non-immunogenic when used as an oral protein carrier. Also, nanoparticles play a crucial role in intestinal absorption, distribution, elimination, and in vivo activity. For instance, nanoparticles < 100 nm can be well absorbed across the intestinal mucosa, but intestinal absorption is dramatically reduced for nanoparticles > 500 nm. The surface of nanoparticles can be decorated with specific ligands for targeting the receptor-mediated transport pathways.

10.4.3 Liposome

Liposomes are widely used to improve protein drugs' membrane permeability by encapsulating proteins inside the aqueous core. Liposomes' structural similarity to the cellular membrane aids in intestinal absorption. On the other hand, liposomes have some drawbacks as an oral protein carrier, such as gastrointestinal chemicals and enzymatic instability. Because surface modification of liposomes using ligands that interact with specific receptors on the cellular membrane should be advantageous for oral drug delivery in liposomes, various approaches have been tried to modify liposomes' surfaces using ligands that interact with specific receptors cellular membrane. Lectins, a type of glycoprotein found in plants, are a promising ligand for specific binding to carbohydrate receptors on the mucosal surface.

Liposomes are bilayer vesicles composed of phospholipids containing hydrophilic and hydrophobic compounds encapsulated in the vesicle's aqueous core or intercalated into the bilayer structure. The formation of liposomes comes from the molecular arrangement of phospholipids in water. Hydrophilic phosphate head groups are exposed to the aqueous environment due to their amphiphilic structure. The hydrocarbon chains bind with each other, forming a lipid film. Upon adding water and stirring, the lipid layer converts into covered vesicles. Liposomes can contain one bilayer (unilamellar) or multiple bilayers (multilamellar), with the former vesicles varying in size from about 20–100 nm (small unilamellar vesicles) to larger vesicles at about 100–1,000 nm (large unilamellar vesicles). Some techniques used to prepare liposomes include dry lipid hydration, freeze-thawing extrusion, reverse evaporation, and double emulsification. In short, it all involves lipid film hydration, subsequent mechanical dispersion to form liposomes, and removal of solvents. Vigorous shaking is widely used for the dispersal of liposomes but produces polydispersed multilamellar vesicles. Thus, to obtain mono-dispersed small unilamellar vesicle liposomes, liposomes' size can be managed and reduced by extrusion through a small orifice. However, many physical stresses (e.g., heat, organic solvents, and agitation) are involved during liposome preparation and may affect proteins' stability.

Unlike polymeric particles, proteins in liposomal structures are less likely to have prolonged release in the capsulated form. The effect of pH on bilayer destabilization will account for liposome breakdown and hence the release of encapsulated agents. Processes such as protonation of the phospholipid head group and acid-catalyzed bilayer hydrolysis can result in vivo breakdown of biolayers. Modification of the lipid bilayer may alter the drug kinetic profile, such as the type of s or the cholesterol incorporation into the layers. Functionalizing the liposomal surface with PEGylation can prevent liposomes aggregation, enhancing stability by decreasing the protein's interactions with biological fluids.

Archaeosomes are a lipid-based oral delivery system made from the polar lipids of different Archaeobacteria. They have unique structural features that allow them to maintain stability at high temperatures, low or high pH, and in the presence of phospholipases and bile salts, which could lead to better gastrointestinal stability. As a result, they've gotten a lot of press as carriers for proteins, genes, and vaccines.

Because it allows direct nose-to-brain drug delivery via nanoparticles, nasal administration of drug-loaded liposomes has been shown to treat CNS disorders effectively. In addition, liposomes can be used to deliver therapeutic proteins and peptides intranasally.

Liposomes are effective carriers for therapeutics delivery into the skin. Liposomes are easily absorbed by the epidermis and reach the deepest layers of the skin because their components are similar to skin lipids. Hydration layers improve absorption by molecular mixing of the liposome bilayer with intracellular lipids in the stratum corneum, in addition to delivering higher concentrations of a drug into the skin.

Protein encapsulation in liposomes has been used to develop a non-invasive macromolecule transdermal delivery system. In addition, many advanced forms of liposomes have been used to improve macromolecules' skin permeation through the stratum corneum, which limits drug delivery efficiency through the skin to overcome the limited success of conventional liposomes.

Liposomal formulations are incorporated into a dissolving microneedle array for more effective macromolecule delivery into the skin.

Liposomes are the most effective pulmonary carrier for protein drugs because they provide enhanced and sustained drug release, biocompatibility, biodegradability, and non-immunogenicity. In addition, liposomes can improve drug permeation through the alveolar epithelium by changing the drug's physicochemical properties (making it hydrophobic) and decreasing mucociliary clearance (due to their surface viscosity). As a result, liposomal formulations for protein drug delivery to the lungs have been developed. Solid lipid nanoparticles (SLN) have also been studied as carriers of therapeutic proteins to deliver through the lung epithelium, in addition to liposomes. The development of spray-dried powders containing SLNs, for example, has solved the issue of low inertia, which can prevent nanoparticles from settling in the lungs.

10.4.4 Higher Concentration Formulations

High concentrations are often needed to accommodate the low management volume combined with their practical applications for subcutaneous administration. Sadly, with growing protein concentrations, the physical behavior of such a substance will change dramatically. Such properties may include substantially improving opalescence, viscosity, and protein aggregation/immunogenicity of the solution. Such altered properties challenge processes for the manufacture of drug products, product administration, and marketability.

Treatments with high doses of more than 1 mg/kg or 100 mg per dose often allow formulations to be formulated at concentrations exceeding 100 mg/mL due to the small volume (< 1.5 mL) that the subcutaneous routes may provide. Achieving these high concentration formulations is a developmental challenge for proteins that have the potential to accumulate at higher concentrations. Even for the intravenous delivery route where large quantities can be managed,

The interaction between proteins at higher concentration formulation may result in reversible self-association, which may further progress towards the formation of insoluble aggregates; at a higher concentration, the probability of one molecule bumping into other increases, enhancing the probability of formation of reversible oligomers such as a dimer, tetramers, etc. The formation of aggregates occurs through multiple mechanisms, including forming covalent linkages (e.g., disulfide exchange). Even minor conformational changes in the native structure may lead to the formation of aggregates. The probability of such an occurrence is greater in higher concentrations.

High concentration is defined by the solution where the solutes occupy a significant portion (≥ 0.1). Another description of a high concentration solution is when the molecular size and the distance between the Van der Waals' surfaces are of the same magnitude. Regardless of the meaning, high concentration refers to the molecular proximity intermolecular space. The primary challenge in achieving a high concentration formulation is the solubility of the target protein. Solubility is controlled by its molecular property (sequence, charge distribution, etc.), as well as by the solution condition, such as pH, ionic strength, excipient concentration, etc. A protein's solubility is defined by the maximum amount of the protein present in a solution, without the appearance of any visible aggregates, precipitates, etc. A more technical definition will be the full amount of protein that remains in the solution, following 30 min of centrifugation at 30,000 g in the presence of co-solute. Besides solubility, there are other issues associated with the development of high concentration mAb formulation. These include opalescence, viscosity, and aggregation. Opalescence is commonly expressed by the turbidity unit with nephelometry. Although opalescence is not a major issue and may occur independently of aggregation, it remains a major concern as it may fail to satisfy patient compliance due to its appearance. Reversible protein–protein and liquid–liquid phase separation may also lead to opalescence. Protein–protein interaction at high concentration is a significant factor that may influence opalescence and viscosity. When molecules are near, they can interact with each other, resulting in reversible self-association, an increase in viscosity, opalescence, and even aggregation.

The increase in viscosity at high concentration has a significant impact on manufacturability and injectability. Tangential flow filtration (TFF) is one of the leading technologies used for buffer exchange and concentrating proteins during large-scale manufacturing (clinical and commercial). The increase in viscosity at high concentration may create back pressure high enough to exceed the pump's capacity inducing considerable stress to the mAb. Rapid pumping and continuous circulation through the narrow tubing create significant cavitation shear stress. The increase in viscosity may further increase the backpressure that can be more destabilizing to the protein. At a minimum, this increases the processing time, and in turn, the cost of manufacture. The increase in viscosity has a significant impact on the administration of subcutaneous dosage form. The glide force describes the ease of subcutaneous injection or extrusion force, which refers to the force required to push the liquid through the syringe. While various factors, including needle gauge, the needle's length, and glide force, one of the main contributing factors is solution viscosity. Viscosity has been reported to be directly correlated to glide force for subcutaneous injection. The increase in viscosity increases the injection site and the injection site's pain, leading to decreased patient compliance.

One of the latest emerging concepts for addressing protein stability and high viscosity issues is forming "nanoclusters"—densely packed protein molecules formed in the presence of a crowder such as trehalose. Protein molecules were shown to be crowded into colloidally stable dispersions of distinct nanoclusters (35–80 nm), exhibiting hydrodynamic diameters of equilibrium at very high concentrations (up to 320 mg/mL), without gelation. An IgG protein's nanoclusters are in harmony with monomers, which can be less than 2%. One dispersion of the nanocluster at 220 mg/mL in the presence of 70 mg/trehalose showed a viscosity of 36 cP, which is syringeable through a 25 G needle. Subcutaneous injection of these preparations for nanoclusters resulted in indistinguishable pharmacokinetics against a standard solution for the antibody in mice.

The distances between protein molecules in nanoclusters could be smaller than in bulk solutions. The shorter distance between proteins may improve protein-protein interactions, but it may also cause stability issues. In addition, the nanocluster concept is new and needs to be tested further.

10.5 Examples of Formulation

The drug product formulation is a crucial step; most therapeutic proteins are either packaged in a liquid form or in lyophilized form, requiring a certain minimum volume to contain the final drug product. As a result, it may be necessary to include a size-exclusion or desalting step to reduce the volume. While upstream and downstream processes get more attention, the formulation step can significantly affect these lyophilized products' safety and efficacy. There to be no added ingredients, but it could have several common ingredients. Examples in liquid formulations include albumin, sucrose, polysorbates, buffer salts, etc. Given here is the composition of a few such examples:

10.5.1 Oprelvekin Injection (Interleukin IL-11)

Bill of Materials (Batch Size 1 L):					
Scale/mL		Item	Material	Quantity	UOM
1.00	mg	1	Oprelvekin (interleukin IL-11)	1.00	g
4.60	mg	2	Glycine	4.60	g
0.32	mg	3	Dibasic sodium phosphate heptahydrate	0.32	g
0.11	mg	4	Monobasic sodium phosphate monohydrate	0.11	g
qs	mL	5	Water for injection, qs to	1.00	L

10.5.2 Interleukin Injection (IL-2)

Bill of Materials (Batch Size 1 L):					
Scale/mL		Item	Material	Quantity	UOM
0.25	mg	1	IL-2	0.25	g
0.70	mg	2	Sodium laurate	0.70	g
10.00	mM	3	Disodium hydrogen phosphate	10.00	M
50.00	mg	4	Mannitol	50.00	g
Qs	mL	5	Hydrochloric acid for pH adjustment 1 M	qs	—
qs	mL	6	Water for injection, qs to	1.00	L

10.5.3 Interferon Alfa-2a Injection

Bill of Materials (Batch Size 1 L):					
Scale/mL		Item	Material	Quantity	UOM
3MM	IU	1	Interferon alfa-2a	3B	IU
7.21	mg	2	Sodium chloride	7.21	g
0.20	mg	3	Polysorbate 80	0.20	g
10.00	mg	4	Benzyl alcohol	10.00	g
0.77	mg	5	Ammonium acetate	0.77	g
qs	mL	6	Water for injection, qs to	1.00	L

10.5.4 Interferon Beta-1b

Bill of Materials (Batch Size 1 L):					
Scale/mL		Item	Material	Quantity	UOM
0.30	mg	1	Interferon beta-1b	0.30	g
15.00	mg	2	Albumin (human)	15.00	g
15.00	mg	3	Dextrose	15.00	g
5.40	mg	4*	Sodium chloride	5.40	g
qs	mL	5	Water for injection, qs to	1.00	L

This item is packaged separately as 0.54% solution (2 mL diluent for the product).

10.5.5 Interferon Beta-1a Injection

Bill of Materials (Batch Size 1 L):					
Scale/mL		Item	Material	Quantity	UOM
*33.00	mcg	1	Interferon beta-1a	33.00	mg
15.00	mg	2	Albumin (human)	15.00	g
5.80	mg	3	Sodium chloride	5.80	g
5.70	mg	4	Dibasic sodium phosphate	5.70	g
1.20	mg	5	Monobasic sodium phosphate	1.20	g
qs	mL	6	Water for injection, qs to	1.00	L

10.5.6 Interferon Alfa-n3 Injection

Bill of Materials (Batch Size 1 L):					
Scale/mL		Item	Material	Quantity	UOM
5 MM	U	1	Interferon-alpha-n3	5B	U
3.30	mg	2	Liquefied phenol	3.30	g
1.00	mg	3	Albumin (human)	1.00	g
8.00	mg	4	Sodium chloride	8.00	g
1.74	mg	5	Sodium phosphate dibasic	1.74	g
0.20	mg	6	Potassium phosphate monobasic	0.20	g
0.20	mg	7	Potassium chloride	0.20	g
qs	mL	8	Water for injection, qs to	1.00	L

10.5.7 Interferon Alfacon-1 Injection

Bill of Materials (Batch Size 1 L):					
Scale/mL		Item	Material	Quantity	UOM
0.03	mg	1	Interferon alfacon-1	0.03	g
5.90	mg	2	Sodium chloride	5.90	g
3.80	mg	3	Sodium phosphate	3.80	g
qs	mL	4	Water for injection, qs to	1.00	L

10.5.8 Interferon Gamma-1b Injection

Bill of Materials (Batch Size 1 L):					
Scale/mL		**Item**	**Material**	**Quantity**	**UOM**
200.00	mcg	1	Interferon gamma-1b*	200.00	mg
40.00	mg	2	Mannitol	40.00	g
0.72	mg	3	Sodium succinate	0.72	g
0.10	mg	4	Polysorbate 20	0.10	g
qs	mL	5	Water for injection, qs to	1.00	L

10.5.9 Infliximab for Injection

Bill of Materials (Batch Size 1 L):					
Scale/mL		**Item**	**Material**	**Quantity**	**UOM**
10.00	mg	1	Infliximab	10.00	g
50.00	mg	2	Sucrose	50.00	g
0.05	mg	3	Polysorbate 80	0.05	g
0.22	mg	4	Monobasic sodium phosphate monohydrate	0.22	g
0.61	mg	5	Dibasic sodium phosphate dihydrate		
qs	mL	6	Water for injection, qs to	1.00	L

10.5.10 Daclizumab for Injection

Bill of Materials (Batch Size 1 L):					
Scale/mL		**Item**	**Material**	**Quantity**	**UOM**
5.00	mg	1	Daclizumab	5.00	g
3.60	mg	2	Sodium phosphate monobasic monohydrate	3.60	g
11.00	mg	3	Sodium phosphate dibasic heptahydrate	11.00	g
4.60	mg	4	Sodium chloride	4.60	g
0.20	mg	5	Polysorbate 80 (Tween®)	0.20	G
qs	mL	6	Water for injection, qs to	1.00	L
Qs	mL	7	Sodium hydroxide for pH adjustment	qs	—
Qs	mL	8	Hydrochloric acid for pH adjustment	qs	—
Qs	Cu ft	9	Nitrogen gas	qs	—

10.5.11 Coagulation Factor VIIa (Recombinant) Injection

Bill of Materials (Batch Size 1,000 Vials):					
Scale/Vial		**Item**	**Material**	**Quantity**	**UOM**
*1.20	mg	1	rFVIIa	1.20	g
5.84	mg	2	Sodium chloride	5.84	g
2.94	mg	3	Calcium chloride dihydrate	2.94	g
2.64	mg	4	Glyclyglycine	2.64	g
0.14	mg	5	Polysorbate 80	0.14	g
60.00	mg	6	Mannitol	60.00	g

10.5.12 Reteplase Recombinant for Injection

Bill of Materials (Batch Size 1,000 Vials):					
Scale/Vial		Item	Material	Quantity	UOM
18.10	mg	1	Reteplase	18.10	g
8.32	mg	2	Tranexamic acid	8.32	g
136.24	mg	3	Dipotassium hydrogen phosphate	136.24	g
51.27	mg	4	Phosphoric acid	51.27	g
364.00	mg	5	Sucrose	364.00	g
5.20	mg	6	Polysorbate 80	5.20	g

10.5.13 Alteplase Recombinant Injection

Bill of Materials (Batch Size 1,000 Vials):					
Scale/Vial		Item	Material	Quantity	UOM
58MM	IU	1	Alteplase	100.00	g
3.50	g	2	L-Arginine	3.50	kg
1.00	g	3	Phosphoric acid	1.00	kg
11.00	mg	4	Polysorbate 80	11.00	g
qs	mL	5	Water for injection, qs to	1.00	L

10.6 Conclusion

Delivery of drugs requires a dosage form that can deliver the active molecule to the site of action at a pre-determined rate and concentration. Biological products are large molecules that are inherently unstable in the environment of many routes of administration, leaving the parenteral route as the only possibility. Unlike chemical products, therapeutic proteins' safety and efficacy can be significantly altered based on the formulation and manufacturing technology applied. While scientists in the development teams undertake formulations, the teams responsible for manufacturing need to learn a lot about the sensitivity of formulations to manufacturing factors to ensure that each batch of the product is equally safe and effective. Many novel routes of administration are developed to create new applications of therapeutic proteins. This chapter provides several model formulations for various classes of therapeutic proteins.

Appendix 10.1 Physicochemical Properties of Proteins and Peptides Approved by the FDA

Name	MOA	MW	Formula	IEP	Hydrophobicity	MP	Half-Life
Abarelix	IIIc	1,416	C72H95ClN14O14	NA	NA	NA	13.2 ± 3.2 d
Abatacept	IIa	92,300	C3498H5458N922O1090S32	NA	NA	NA	12–23 d
Abciximab	IIa	145,651	C6462H9964N1690O2049S48	6.16	–0.424	71	0.5 hrs
Adalimumab	Ic	144,190	C6428H9912N1694O1987S46	8.25	–0.441	NA	240–480 hrs
Aflibercept	Ib	115,000	C4318H6788N1164O1304S32	NA	NA	NA	7.13 d
Agalsidase beta	Ia	45,352	C2029H3080N544O587S27	5.17	–0.307	NA	45–102 min
Albiglutide	Ib	72,970	C3232H5032N864O979S41	NA	NA	NA	4–7 d
Aldesleukin	Ib	15,315	C690H1115N177O202S6	7.31	–0.192	NA	0.22–1.42 hrs
Alefacept	IIa	51,801	C2306H3594N610O694S26	7.86	–0.432	NA	270 hrs
Alemtuzumab	IIa	145,454	C6468H10066N1732O2005S40	8.76	–0.431		288 hrs
Alglucerase	Ia	55,597	C2532H3854N672O711S16	7.41	–0.168	NA	3.6–10.4 min
Alglucosidase alfa	Ic	105,271	C4435H6739N1175O1279S32	NA	NA	NA	2.3 ± 0.4 hrs
Alirocumab	Ic	146,000	C6472H9996N1736O2032S42	NA	NA	NA	17–20 d
Aliskiren	IIa	552	C30H53N3O6	NA	NA	NA	24 hrs
Alpha-1-proteinase inhibitor	IIa	44,325	C2001H3130N514O601S10	5.37	–0.302	59	NA
Alteplase	Ib	59,042	C2569H3928N746O781S40	7.61	–0.516	60	NA
Anakinra	IIa	17,258	C759H1186N208O232S10	5.46	–0.412	NA	4–6 hrs
Ancestim	Ib	18,500	NA	NA	NA	NA	NA
Anistreplase	Ic	59,042	C2569H3928N746O781S40	7.61	–0.516	60	NA
Anthrax immune globulin (human)	IIa	NA	NA	NA	NA	NA	24.3 d
Anti-inhibitor coagulant complex	Ia	NA	NA	NA	NA	NA	4–7 hrs
Anti-thymocyte globulin (equine)	IIIb	NA	NA	NA	NA	NA	1.5–13 d
Anti-thymocyte globulin (rabbit)	IIIb	NA	NA	NA	NA	61	2–3 d
Antihemophilic factor	Ia	264,726	C11794H18314N3220O3553S83	6.97	–0.533	NA	8.4–19.3 hrs
Antithrombin alfa	Ia	57,215	C2191H3457N583O656S18	NA	NA	NA	11.6 –17.7 hrs
Antithrombin III (human)	Ia	58,000	NA	NA	NA	NA	2.5–4.8 d
Antithymocyte globulin	IIa	NA	NA	NA	NA	61	2–3 d
Aprotinin	IIa	6,511	C284H432N84O79S7	NA	NA	>100	10hrs

(Continued)

Name	MOA	MW	Formula	IEP	Hydrophobicity	MP	Half-Life
Arcitumomab	IIb	144,483	C6398H9900N1714O1995S54	8.26	–0.423	61	1 hr
Asfotase alfa	Ia	180,000	C7108H11008N1968O2206S56	NA	NA	NA	5 d
Asparaginase	Ic	31,732	C1377H2208N382O442S17	4.67	0.059	NA	8–30 hrs
Asparaginase erwinia chrysanthemi	Ic	140,000	C1546H2510N432O476S9	NA	NA	NA	16 hrs
Atezolizumab	IIa	145,000	NA	NA	NA	NA	27 d
Autologous cultured chondrocytes	Ia	NA	NA	NA	NA	NA	NA
Basiliximab	IIa	143,801	C6378H9844N1698O1997S48	8.68	–0.473	61	7.2 ± 3.2
Becaplermin	Ib	12,294	C532H892N162O153S9	9.38	–0.16	NA	NA
Belatacept	IIa	92,300	C3508H5440N922O1096S32	NA	NA	NA	9.8 d
Belimumab	IIa	147,000	C 6358 H 9904 N 1728 O 2010 S 44	NA	NA	NA	19.4 d
Beractant	Ia	NA	NA	NA	NA	NA	20–30 hrs
Bevacizumab	IIa	149,000	C6538H10034N1716O2033S44	NA	NA	61	NA
Bivalirudin	Ia	2,180	C98H138N24O33	3.91	–0.985	NA	0.42 hrs
Blinatumomab	IIIc	54,100	C2367H3577N649O772S19	NA	NA	NA	2.11 hrs
Botulinum toxin type A	Ic	149,323	C6760H10447N1743O2010S32	6.06	–0.368	NA	NA
Botulinum toxin type B	Ic	150,804	C690H1115N177O202S6	NA	NA	NA	NA
Brentuximab vedotin	IIb	149,200–151,800	C6476H9930N1690O2030S40	NA	NA	NA	4–6 d
Brodalumab	IIa	144,000	C6372H9840N1712O1988S52	NA	NA	NA	NA
Buserelin	IIIc	NA	C62H90N16O15	NA	NA	NA	50–80 min
C1 esterase inhibitor (human)	Ia	105,000	NA	NA	NA	NA	56 hrs
C1 esterase inhibitor (recombinant)	IIa	67,000	NA	NA	NA	NA	2.4–2.7 hrs
Canakinumab	IIIb	145,200 (deglycosylated)	C6452H9958N1722O2010S42	NA	NA	NA	26 d
Canakinumab	IIa	145,200	C6452H9958N1722O2010S42	NA	NA	NA	26 d
Capromab	IV	NA	NA	NA	NA	NA	NA
Certolizumab pegol	IIb	91,000	C2115H3252N556O673S16	NA	NA	NA	14 d
Cetuximab	IIIc	145,782	C6484H10042N1732O2023S36	8.48	–0.413	71	114 hrs
Choriogonadotropin alfa	Ib	25,720	C1105H1770N318O336S26	8.61	–0.258	55	29 ± 6 hrs
Chorionic gonadotropin (human)	Ia	25,719	C1105H1770N318O336S26	NA	NA	NA	NA
Chorionic gonadotropin (recombinant)	Ia	25,720	C1105H1770N318O336S26	8.61	–0.258	55 °C	4.5 ± hrs
Coagulation factor ix	Ia	46,548	C2041H3136N558O641S25	5.2	–0.431	54	19.4 4 hrs
Coagulation factor VIIa	Ib	45,079	C1972H3076N560O597S28	6.09	–0.311	58	NA
Coagulation factor X human	Ib	NA	NA	NA	NA	NA	NA

(Continued)

Name	MOA	MW	Formula	IEP	Hydrophobicity	MP	Half-Life
Coagulation factor XIII A-subunit (recombinant)	Ia	NA	NA	NA	NA	NA	5.1 d
Collagenase	Ic	112,023	C5028H7666N1300O1564S21	5.58	–0.714	NA	NA
Conestat alfa	Ia	NA	NA	NA	NA	NA	2.4–2.7 hrs
Corticotropin	IV	4,541	C207H308N56O58S	NA	NA	NA	15 min
Cosyntropin	IV	2,933	C136H210N40O31S	NA	NA	NA	15 min
Daclizumab	Iia	142,612	C6332H9808N1678O1989S42	8.46	–0.437	61	11–38 d
Daptomycin	IIa	1,621	C72H101N17O26	NA	NA	NA	7 d
Daratumumab	IIIc	148,000	NA	NA	NA	NA	18 d
Darbepoetin alfa	Ib	18,396	C815H1317N233O241S5	8.75	–0.188	53	NA
Defibrotide	NA	NA	NA	NA	NA	NA	A few hrs
Denileukin diftitox	IIb	57,647	C2560H4042N678O799S17	5.45	–0.301	NA	1.16–1.3 hrs
Denosumab	IIIc	144,700	C6404H9912N1724O2004S50	NA	NA	NA	25.4 d
Desirudin	Ib	6,964	C287H440N80O110 S6	NA	NA	NA	2–3 hrs
Digoxin immune fab (ovine)	IIa	47,302	C2085H3223N553O672S16	8.01	–0.343		15–20 hrs
Dinutuximab	IIIc	145,000	C6422H9982N1722O2008S48	NA	NA	NA	10 d
Dornase alfa	Ib	29,254	C1321H1999N339O396S9	4.58	–0.083	67	NA
Drotrecogin alfa	Ib	55,000	C1786H2779N509O519S29	6.78	–0.291	NA	5.5 hrs
Dulaglutide	Ib	59,670	C2646H4044N704O836S18	NA	NA	NA	5 d
Eculizumab	Ia	148,000	NA	NA	NA	NA	272 hrs
Efalizumab	IIa	150,000	NA	NA	NA		5 d
Efmoroctocog alfa	Ib	NA	NA	NA	NA	NA	NA
Elosulfase alfa	Ia	110,800	C5020H7588N1364O1418S34	NA	NA	NA	7.52– 35.9 min
Elotuzumab	IIIc	148,100	C6476H9982N1714O2016S42	NA	NA	NA	NA
Enfuvirtide	IIa	4,492	C204H301N51O64	4.3	–0.875	NA	3.8 hrs
Epoetin alfa	Ib	18,396	C815H1317N233O241S5	8.75	NA	53	NA
Epoetin zeta	Ib	18,200	C809H1301N229O240S5	NA	NA	NA	7.37 hrs
Eptifibatide	NA	832	C35H49N11O9S2	NA	–2.3	NA	29 ± 6 hrs
Etanercept	IIa	51,235	C2224H3475N621O698S36	7.89	–0.529	71	102 ± 30 hrs
Evolocumab	Iia	141,800	C6242H9648N1668O1996S56	NA	NA	NA	NA
Exenatide	Ib	4,187	C184H282N50O60S	NA	NA	NA	2.4 hrs
Factor IX complex (human)	Ib	NA	NA	NA	NA	NA	11–28

(Continued)

Name	MOA	MW	Formula	IEP	Hydrophobicity	MP	Half-Life
Fibrinogen concentrate (human)	Ia	340,000	NA	NA	NA	NA	78.7 ± 18.13 hrs
Fibrinolysin aka plasmin	Ic	88,400	C3848H5912N1096O1185S60	NA	NA	NA	24 hrs
Filgrastim	1b	18,800	C845H1343N223O243S9	5.65	0.209	60	3.5 hrs
Filgrastim-sndz	IIIc	NA	NA	NA	NA	NA	3.5 hrs
Follitropin alpha	Ib	NA	NA	NA	NA	NA	24–53 hrs in females
Follitropin beta	Ib	22,673	C975H1513N267O304S26	7.5	–0.33	55	35–40 hrs
Galsulfase	Ia	56,013	C2534H3851N691O719S16	NA	NA	NA	6–40 min
Gastric intrinsic factor	Ib	NA	NA	NA	NA	NA	NA
Gemtuzumab ozogamicin	IIb	151,000–153,000	NA	NA	NA	61	NA
Glatiramer acetate	IIa	5,000–9,000	C254H422N70O72	NA	NA	NA	NA
Glucagon (recombinant)	IV	3,767	C165H249N49O51S1	9.52	–1.197	NA	NA
Glucarpidase	Ic	44,017	C1950H3157N543O599S7	NA	NA	NA	5.6 hrs
Golimumab	IIb	146,943	C6530H10068N1752O2026S44	NA	NA	NA	2 weeks
Gramicidin D	IIa	1,882	C99H140N20O17	NA	NA	229	NA
Hepatitis A vaccine	IIIa	NA	NA	NA	NA	NA	
Hepatitis B immune globulin	IIIa	NA	NA	NA	NA	NA	22–25 d
Human calcitonin	Ib	NA	NA	NA	NA	NA	NA
Human clostridium tetani toxoid immune globulin	IIIb	NA	NA	NA	NA	NA	NA
Human rabies virus immune globulin	IIIa	NA	NA	NA	NA	NA	NA
Human rho(D) immune globulin	IIIb	NA	NA	NA	NA	NA	24 – 30.9 d
Human serum albumin	Ia	66,472	C2936H4624N786O889S41	5.67	–0.395	62	NA
Human varicella-zoster immune globulin	IIIa	NA	NA	NA	NA	NA	26.2 d
Hyaluronidase	Ic	53,871	C2455H3775N617O704S21	5.73	–0.117	NA	NA
Hyaluronidase (human recombinant)	Ib	61,000	NA	NA	NA	NA	NA
Ibritumomab	IIb	143,376	C6382H9830N1672O1979S54	7.91	–0.359		0.8 hrs
Ibritumomab tiuxetan	IIIc	143,376	C6382H9830N1672O1979S54	7.91	–0.359	61 °C	0.8 hrs
Idarucizumab	Ib	47,766	C2131H3299N555O671S11	NA	NA	NA	4.5 – 10.8 hrs
Idursulfase	Ia	76,000	C2654H4000N688O774S14	NA	NA	NA	44 ± 19 min
Imiglucerase	Ia	55,597	C2532H3854N672O711S16	7.41	–0.168	NA	0.06–0.173 hrs
Immune globulin (human)	IIIb	142,682	C6332H9826N1692O1980S42	NA	NA	NA	> 20 hrs

(*Continued*)

Name	MOA	MW	Formula	IEP	Hydrophobicity	MP	Half-Life
Infliximab	IIa	144,190	C6428H9912N1694O1987S46	8.25	–0.441		9.5 d
Insulin aspart	Ia	582,580	C256H381N65O79S6	NA	NA	NA	81 min
Insulin (beef)	Ia	5,734	C254H377N65O75S6	NA	NA	NA	NA
Insulin degludec	Ia	6,104	C274H411N65O81S6	NA	NA	NA	25 hrs
Insulin detemir	Ia	5,917	C267H402N64O76S6	NA	NA	NA	425 ± 78 min
Insulin glargine	Ia	6,063	C267H404N72O78S6	6.88	0.098	81	30 hrs
Insulin glulisine	Ib	5,823	C258H384N64O78S6	NA	NA	NA	42 min
Insulin lispro	Ia	5,808	C257H387N65O76S6	5.39	0.218	81	1 hr
Insulin (pork)	Ia	5,796	C257H387N65O76S6	5.39	0.218	NA	NA
Insulin (regular)	Ia	5,808	C257H383N65O77S6	5.39	0.218	81	NA
Insulin (porcine)	Ia	5,796	C257H387N65O76S6	5.39	0.298	NA	NA
Insulin, isophane	Ia	5,808	C257H383N65O77S6	9	NA	NA	NA
Interferon alfa-2a (recombinant)	Ib	19,241	C860H1353N227O255S9	5.99	–0.336	NA	6–8 hrs
Interferon alfa-2b	Ib	19,271	C860H1353N229O255S9	5.99	–0.339	61	2–3 hrs
Interferon alfa-n1	Ib	19,241	C860H1353N227O255S9	5.99	–0.336	61	1.2 hrs
Interferon alfa-n3	Ib	NA	NA	5.99	NA	61	NA
Interferon alfacon-1	Ib	19,271	C860H1353N229O255S9	5.99	0.339	61	2–3 hrs
Interferon beta-1a	Ib	20,027	C908H1408N246O252S7	8.93	–0.427	NA	10 hrs
Interferon beta-1b	Ib	20,011	C908H1408N246O253S6	9.02	–0.447	NA	10–20 min
Interferon gamma-1b	Ib	17,146	C761H1206N214O225S6	9.54	–0.823	61	NA
Intravenous immunoglobulin	Ia	142,682	C6332H9826N1692O1980S42	8.13	–0.331	61	20 hrs
Ipilimumab	IIIc	148,000	C6572H10126N1734O2080S40	NA	NA	NA	14.7–15.4 d
Ixekizumab	Ic	146,158	NA	NA	NA	NA	13 d
Laronidase	Ia	69,899	C3160H4848N898O881S12	9.09	–0.3	NA	1.5–3.6 hrs
Lenograstim	Ib	18,668	C840-H1330-N222-O242-S8	NA	NA	NA	2.3–3.3 hrs
Lepirudin	Ia	6,963	C287H440N80O110S6	4.04	–0.777	65	1.3 hrs
Leuprolide	IIa	1,209	C59H84N16O12	NA	0.1	NA	3 hrs
Liraglutide	Ib	3,751	C172H265N43O51	NA	NA	NA	13 hrs
Lucinactant	Ib	2,470	C126H238N26O22	NA	NA	NA	NA
Lutropin alfa	Ib	30,000	C1014H1609N287O294S27	8.44	–0.063	55	4.4 hrs
Mecasermin	Ib	7,649	C331H518N94O101S7	NA	NA	NA	2 hrs
Menotropins	Ib	23,390	C1014H1609N287O294S27	8.44	–0.063	55	NA

(Continued)

Name	MOA	MW	Formula	IEP	Hydrophobicity	MP	Half-Life
Mepolizumab	Ib	149,000		NA	NA	NA	16–22 d
Methoxy polyethylene glycol-epoetin beta	Ib	60,000	NA	NA	NA	NA	134 ± 65 hrs
Metreleptin	Ib	16,155	C714H1167N191O221S6	NA	NA	NA	3.8–4.7 hrs
Muromonab	IIa	146,190	C6460H9946N1720O2043S56	8.31	–0.513	61	0.8 hrs
Natalizumab	IIa	NA	NA	NA	NA	61	11 ± 4 d
Natural alpha interferon OR multiferon	IIa	19,300–22,100	NA	NA	NA	NA	NA
Necitumumab	IIIc	144,800	NA	NA	NA	NA	14 d
Nesiritide	Ib	3,464	NA	NA	NA	NA	18 mins
Nivolumab	IIIc	143,597	C6362H9862N1712O1995S42	NA	NA	NA	26.7 d
Obiltoxaximab	IIIa	148,000	NA	NA	NA	NA	NA
Obinutuzumab	IIb	146,100	C6512H10060N1712O2020S44	NA	NA	NA	28.4 d
Ocriplasmin	Ic	272,500	C1214H1890N338O348S14	NA	NA	NA	NA
Ofatumumab	IIIc	146,100	C6480H10022N1742O2020S44	NA	NA	NA	2.3–61.5 d
Omalizumab	IIa	145,058	C6450H9916N1714O2023S38	7.03	–0.432	61	624 hrs
Oprelvekin	Ib	19,047	C854H1411N253O235S2	11.16	–0.07	NA	6.9 hrs
OspA lipoprotein	IIIa	27,743	C1198H2012N322O422S2	6.72	–0.652	NA	1.2 hrs
Oxytocin	Ib	1,007	C43H66N12O12S2	5.51	–2.7	NA	1–6 min
Palifermin	Ib	16,193	C721H1142N202O204S9	9.47	–0.65	NA	NA
Palivizumab	IIIa	NA	NA	NA	NA	61	18–20 d
Pancrelipase	Ia	131,126	C5850H8902N1606O1739S49	6.44	NA	48-50	NA
Panitumumab	IIa	NA	NA	NA	NA	NA	7.5 d
Pegademase (bovine)	Ia	40,788	C1821H2834N484O552S14	5.33	–0.428	NA	NA
Pegaptanib	IIa	NA	NA	NA	NA	NA	10 ± 4 d
Pegaspargase	Ic	31,732	C1377H2208N382O442S17	4.67	0.059	NA	NA
Pegfilgrastim	Ib	18,803	C845H1343N223O243S9	5.65	0.209	60	15–80 hrs
Peginterferon alfa-2a	Ib	60,000	NA	5.99	NA	61	80 hrs
Peginterferon alfa-2b	Ib	31,000	C130H219N43O42	5.99	NA	61	40 hrs
Peginterferon beta-1a	Ia	20,000	NA	NA	NA	NA	78 hrs
Pegloticase	Ib	34,193	C1549H2430N408O448S8	NA	NA	NA	14 d
Pegvisomant	IIa	22,129	C990H1532N262O300S7	5.27	–0.411	76	6 d
Pembrolizumab	IIIc	146,286	C6504H10004N1716O2036S46	NA	NA	NA	28 d

(Continued)

Name	MOA	MW	Formula	IEP	Hydrophobicity	MP	Half-Life
Pertuzumab	IIIc	148,000	NA	NA	NA	NA	18 d
Poractant alfa	Ia	NA	NA	NA	NA	NA	NA
Pramlintide	Ia	3,949	C171H267N51O53S2	NA	NA	NA	48 min
Preotact	Ib	9,420	C408H674N126O126S2	NA	NA	NA	1.5 hrs
Protamine sulfate	Ib	NA	NA	NA	NA	NA	4.5 min.
Protein S (human)	Ib	69,000	NA	5.05.5	NA	NA	NA
Prothrombin complex concentrate	Ia	NA	NA	NA	NA	NA	48–60 hrs
Ragweed pollen extract	IIIa	NA	NA	NA	NA	NA	NA
Ramucirumab	IIIc	143,600	C6374H9864N1692O1996S46	NA	NA	NA	15 d
Ranibizumab	IIa	48,350	C2158H3282N562O681S12	NA	NA	NA	9 d
Rasburicase	Ic	34,110	C1521H2381N417O461S7	7.16	–0.465	NA	18 hrs
Raxibacumab	IIa	142,845	C6320H9794N1702O1998S42	NA	NA	NA	16–19 d
Reteplase	Ib	39,590	C1736H2671N499O522S22	6.86	–0.435	60	NA
Rilonacept	IIa	251,000	C9030H13932N2400O2670S74	NA	NA	NA	8.6 d
Rituximab	IIa	143,860	C6416H9874N1688O1987S44	8.68	–0.414	61	0.8 hrs
Romiplostim	Ib	59,000	C2634H4086N722O790S18	NA	NA	NA	3.5 d
Sacrosidase	Ia	100,000	NA	NA	NA	NA	NA
Salmon calcitonin	Ib	3,432	C145H240N44O48S2	8.86	–0.537	NA	0.83–1.33 hrs
Sargramostim	Ib	14,435	C639H1006N168O196S8	5.05	NA	NA	NA
Satumomab pendetide	IV	141,479	C6268H9708N1666O1971S48	7.02	–0.427	61	0.80 hrs
Sebelipase alfa	Ia	55,000	C1968H2945N507O551S15	NA	NA	NA	5.4–6.6 mins
Secretin	IV	3,056	C130H219N43O42	9.45	–0.463	NA	NA
Secukinumab	IIa	147,940	C6584H10134N1754O2042S44	NA	NA	NA	NA
Sermorelin	Ia	3,358	C149H246N44O42S	9.99	–0.33	NA	11–12 min
Serum albumin	IV	66,472	C2936H4624N786O889S41	5.67	–0.395	62	NA
Serum albumin iodonated	IV	66,472	C2936H4624N786O889S41	5.67	–0.395	62	NA
Siltuximab	Iia	145,000	C6450H9932N1688O2016S50	NA	NA	NA	20.6 d.
Simoctocog alfa	Ia	170,000	NA	NA	NA	NA	14.7 hrs
Sipuleucel-T	IIIc	NA	NA	NA	NA	NA	NA
Somatotropin (recombinant)	Ib	22,129	C990H1532N262O300S7	5.27	–0.411	76 at pH 3.5	NA
Somatropin (recombinant)	Ib	22,129	C990H1532N262O300S7	5.27	–0.411	76	NA
Streptokinase	Ic	47,287	C2100H3278N566O669S4	5.12	–0.728	NA	NA

(Continued)

Name	MOA	MW	Formula	IEP	Hydrophobicity	MP	Half-Life
Sulodexide	IIIc	5,000–8,000	NA	NA	NA	NA	11.7 ± 2.0 hrs
Susoctocog alfa	Ib	NA	NA	NA	NA	NA	~17 hrs
Taliglucerase alfa	Ia	56,638	C2580H3918N680O727S17	10.54	NA	NA	NA
Teduglutide	Ia	3,752	C164H252N44O55S	NA	NA	NA	2 hrs
Teicoplanin	IIa	1,880	C88H97Cl2N9O33	NA	NA	NA	70–100 hrs
Tenecteplase	Ib	58,951	C2561H3919N747O781S40	7.61	–0.528	60	1.9 hrs
Teriparatide	Ib	4,118	C181H291N55O51S2	NA	NA	NA	NA
Tesamorelin	Ib	5,136	C221H366N72O67S	NA	NA	NA	38 min
Thrombomodulin alfa	Ib	52,124	C2230-H3357-N633-O718-S50	NA	NA	NA	2–3 d
Thymalfasin	Ib	3,108	C129H215N33O55	NA	NA	NA	2 hrs
Thyroglobulin	Ib	660	NA				65 hrs
Thyrotropin alfa	IV	22,673	C975H1513N267O304S26	7.5	–0.33	55	5 ± 10 hrs
Tocilizumab	IIa	148,000	C6428H9976N1720O2018S42	NA	NA	NA	11 d
Tositumomab	IIb	143,860	C6416H9874N1688O1987S44	8.68	–0.4144		0.8 hrs
Trastuzumab	IIa	145,532	C6470H10012N1726O2013S42	8.45	–0.415	61	28.5 d
Tuberculin purified protein derivative	IV	NA	NA	NA	NA	NA	NA
Turoctocog alfa	Ia	NA	NA	NA	NA	NA	NA
Urofollitropin	Ib	980	C42H65N11O12S2	7.5	–0.33	55	35–40 hrs
Urokinase	Ib	31,127	C1376H2145N383O406S18	8.66	–0.466	76	12 min
Ustekinumab	IIIb	14,690	NA	NA	NA	NA	NA
Vasopressin	Ib	1,050	C43H67N15O12S2	NA	–4.9	NA	10–20 min
Vedolizumab	IIa	146,837	C6528H10072N1732O2042S42	7.6	NA	NA	336–362 hrs
Velaglucerase alfa	Ia	63,000	C2532H3850N672O711S16	NA	NA	NA	11–12 min

Notes: MOA (mode of action): Group Ia—replacing a protein that is deficient or abnormal; Group Ib—augmenting an existing pathway; Group Ic—providing a novel function or activity; Group IIa—interfering with a molecule or organism; Group IIb—delivering other compounds or proteins; Group IIIa—protecting against a deleterious foreign agent; Group IIIb—treating an autoimmune disease; Group IIIc—treating cancer; Group IV—protein diagnostics.

ADDITIONAL READING

Abramovich RA, Bykov VA, Elagina IA, Papazova NA, Vorob'ev AN. [Scientific approaches to development of medicinal formulation based on biotechnological substance]. *Antibiot Khimioter.* 2012;57(1–2):13–16.

Agersø H, Møller-Pedersen J, Cappi S, Thomann P, Jesussek B, Senderovitz T. Pharmacokinetics and pharmacodynamics of a new formulation of recombinant human growth hormone administered by ZomaJet 2 Vision, a new needle-free device, compared to subcutaneous administration using a conventional syringe. *J Clin Pharmacol.* 2002;42(11):1262–1268.

Agrawal G, Wakte P, Shelke S. Formulation optimization of human insulin loaded microspheres for controlled oral delivery using response surface methodology. *Endocr Metab Immune Disord Drug Targets.* 2017;17(2):149–165.

Alebouyeh M, Tahzibi A, Yaghoobzadeh S, et al. Rapid formulation assessment of filgrastim therapeutics by a thermal stress test. *Biologicals.* 2016;44(3):150–156.

Allison AC, Byars NE. An adjuvant formulation that selectively elicits the formation of antibodies of protective isotypes and of cell-mediated immunity. *J Immunol Methods.* 1986;95(2):157–168.

Ameri M, Kadkhodayan M, Nguyen J, et al. Human growth hormone delivery with a microneedle transdermal system: preclinical formulation, stability, delivery and PK of therapeutically relevant doses. *Pharmaceutics.* 2014;6(2):220–234.

Anderson PM, Sorenson MA. Effects of route and formulation on clinical pharmacokinetics of interleukin-2. *Clin Pharmacokinet.* 1994;27(1):19–31.

Andya JD, Maa YF, Costantino HR, et al. The effect of formulation excipients on protein stability and aerosol performance of spray-dried powders of a recombinant humanized anti-IgE monoclonal antibody. *Pharm Res.* 1999;16(3):350–358.

Anish C, Upadhyay AK, Sehgal D, Panda AK. Influences of process and formulation parameters on powder flow properties and immunogenicity of spray dried polymer particles entrapping recombinant pneumococcal surface protein A. *Int J Pharm.* 2014;466(1–2):198–210.

Aubin Y, Hodgson DJ, Thach WB, Gingras G, Sauvé S. Monitoring effects of excipients, formulation parameters and mutations on the high order structure of filgrastim by NMR. *Pharm Res.* 2015;32(10):3365–3375.

Balasubramanian SV, Bruenn J, Straubinger RM. Liposomes as formulation excipients for protein pharmaceuticals: a model protein study. *Pharm Res.* 2000;17(3):344–350.

Bednarek E, Sitkowski J, Bocian W, et al. Structure and pharmaceutical formulation development of a new long-acting recombinant human insulin analog studied by NMR and MS. *J Pharm Biomed Anal.* 2017;135:126–132.

Bei R, Guptill V, Masuelli L, et al. The use of a cationic liposome formulation (DOTAP) mixed with a recombinant tumor-associated antigen to induce immune responses and protective immunity in mice. *J Immunother.* 1998;21(3):159–169.

Bello-Rivero I, Garcia-Vega Y, Duncan-Roberts Y, et al. HeberFERON, a new formulation of IFNs with improved pharmacodynamics: perspective for cancer treatment. *Semin Oncol.* 2018;45(1–2):27–33.

Bellomi F, Muto A, Palmieri G, et al. Immunogenicity comparison of interferon beta-1a preparations using the BALB/c mouse model: assessment of a new formulation for use in multiple sclerosis. *New Microbiol.* 2007;30(3):241–246.

Bhambhani A, Kissmann JM, Joshi SB, Volkin DB, Kashi RS, Middaugh CR. Formulation design and high-throughput excipient selection based on structural integrity and conformational stability of dilute and highly concentrated IgG1 monoclonal antibody solutions. *J Pharm Sci.* 2012;101(3):1120–1135.

Bittner B, Richter WF, Hourcade-Potelleret F, et al. development of a subcutaneous formulation for trastuzumab-nonclinical and clinical bridging approach to the approved intravenous dosing regimen. *Arzneimittelforschung.* 2012;62(9):401–409.

Bogard WC, Dean RT, Deo Y, et al. Practical considerations in the production, purification, and formulation of monoclonal antibodies for immunoscintigraphy and immunotherapy. *Semin Nucl Med.* 1989;19(3):202–220.

Boven K, Stryker S, Knight J, et al. The increased incidence of pure red cell aplasia with an Eprex formulation in uncoated rubber stopper syringes. *Kidney Int.* 2005;67(6):2346–2353.

Brückl L, Hahn R, Sergi M, Scheler S. A systematic evaluation of mechanisms, material effects, and protein-dependent differences on friction-related protein particle formation in formulation and filling steps. *Int J Pharm.* 2016;511(2):931–945.

Bush L, Webb C, Bartlett L, Burnett B. The formulation of recombinant factor IX: stability, robustness, and convenience. *Semin Hematol.* 1998;35(2 Suppl 2):18–21.

Bye JW, Platts L, Falconer RJ. Biological product liquid formulation: a review of the science of protein stability and solubility in aqueous environments. *Biotechnol Lett.* 2014;36(5):869–875.

Bysted BV, Scharling B, Møller T, Hansen BL. A randomized, double-blind trial demonstrating bioequivalence of the current recombinant activated factor VII formulation and a new robust 25 degrees C stable formulation. *Haemophilia.* 2007;13(5):527–532.

Chang BS, Hershenson S. Practical approaches to protein formulation development. *Pharm Biotechnol.* 2002;13:1–25.

Chang BS, Reeder G, Carpenter JF. Development of a stable freeze-dried formulation of recombinant human interleukin-1 receptor antagonist. *Pharm Res.* 1996;13(2):243–249.

Chen BL, Arakawa T, Hsu E, Narhi LO, Tressel TJ, Chien SL. Strategies to suppress aggregation of recombinant keratinocyte growth factor during liquid formulation development. *J Pharm Sci.* 1994;83(12): 1657–1661.

Chen FM, Zhao YM, Sun HH, et al. Novel glycidyl methacrylated dextran (Dex-GMA)/gelatin hydrogel scaffolds containing microspheres loaded with bone morphogenetic proteins: formulation and characteristics. *J Control Release.* 2007;118(1):65–77.

Chen S, Guo D, Guo B, et al. Investigation on formulation and preparation of adenovirus encoding human endostatin lyophilized powders. *Int J Pharm.* 2012;427(2):145–152.

Cun D, Wan F, Yang M. Formulation strategies and particle engineering technologies for pulmonary delivery of therapeutic proteins. *Curr Pharm Des.* 2015;21(19):2599–2610.

Davio SR, Hageman MJ. Characterization and formulation considerations for recombinantly derived bovine somatotropin. *Pharm Biotechnol.* 1993;5:59–89.

Dawson PJ. Effect of formulation and freeze-drying on the long-term stability of rDNA-derived cytokines. *Dev Biol Stand.* 1992;74:273–282; discussion 282–274.

Devrim B, Bozkir A, Canefe K. Preparation and evaluation of PLGA microparticles as carrier for the pulmonary delivery of rhIL-2 : I. Effects of some formulation parameters on microparticle characteristics. *J Microencapsul.* 2011;28(6):582–594.

Di Minno G, Cerbone AM, Coppola A, et al. Longer-acting factor VIII to overcome limitations in haemophilia management: the PEGylated liposomes formulation issue. *Haemophilia.* 2010;16 Suppl 1:2–6.

Eng M, Ling V, Briggs JA, et al. Formulation development and primary degradation pathways for recombinant human nerve growth factor. *Anal Chem.* 1997;69(20):4184–4190.

Engler H, Machemer TR, Schluep T, et al. Development of a formulation that enhances gene expression and efficacy following intraperitoneal administration in rabbits and mice. *Mol Ther.* 2003;7(4):558–564.

Fabregas B. [New formulation of recombinant coagulation factor: simplicity, rapidity and manageability]. *Soins.* 2008(725):22–23.

Fatouros A, Sjöström B. Recombinant factor VIII SQ--the influence of formulation parameters on structure and surface adsorption. *Int J Pharm.* 2000;194(1):69–79.

Frokjaer S, Otzen DE. Protein drug stability: a formulation challenge. *Nat Rev Drug Discov.* 2005;4(4):298–306.

García-García I, Hernández-González I, Díaz-Machado A, et al. Pharmacokinetic and pharmacodynamic characterization of a novel formulation containing co-formulated interferons alpha-2b and gamma in healthy male volunteers. *BMC Pharmacol Toxicol.* 2016;17(1):58.

Giannos SA, Kraft ER, Zhao ZY, Merkley KH, Cai J. Formulation stabilization and disaggregation of bevacizumab, ranibizumab and aflibercept in dilute solutions. *Pharm Res.* 2018;35(4):78.

Gibbons A, McElvaney NG, Cryan SA. A dry powder formulation of liposome-encapsulated recombinant secretory leukocyte protease inhibitor (rSLPI) for inhalation: preparation and characterisation. *AAPS PharmSciTech.* 2010;11(3):1411–1421.

Gietz U, Arvinte T, Häner M, Aebi U, Merkle HP. Formulation of sustained release aqueous Zn-hirudin suspensions. *Eur J Pharm Sci.* 2000;11(1):33–41.

Gombotz WR, Pankey SC, Bouchard LS, Phan DH, MacKenzie AP. Stability, characterization, formulation, and delivery system development for transforming growth factor-beta 1. *Pharm Biotechnol.* 1996;9:219–245.

Gourbatsi E, Povey JF, Smales CM. The effect of formulation variables on protein stability and integrity of a model IgG4 monoclonal antibody and translation to formulation of a model ScFv. *Biotechnol Lett.* 2018;40(1):33–46.

Govardhan C, Khalaf N, Jung CW, et al. Novel long-acting crystal formulation of human growth hormone. *Pharm Res.* 2005;22(9):1461–1470.

Grumetto L, Prete AD, Ortosecco G, Borrelli A, Prete SD, Mancini A. A gel formulation containing a new recombinant form of manganese superoxide dismutase: a clinical experience based on compassionate use-safety of a case report. *Case Rep Ophthalmol Med.* 2016;2016:7240209.

Guo P, Yu C, Wang Q, Zhang R, Meng X, Feng Y. Liposome lipid-based formulation has the least influence on rAAV transduction compared to other transfection agents. *Mol Ther Methods Clin Dev.* 2018;9:367–375.

Gurny R, Friess W. Unmet needs in protein formulation science. *Eur J Pharm Biopharm.* 2011;78(2):183.

Hahn SK, Kim JS, Shimobouji T. Injectable hyaluronic acid microhydrogels for controlled release formulation of erythropoietin. *J Biomed Mater Res A.* 2007;80(4):916–924.

Hahn SK, Kim SJ, Kim MJ, Kim DH. Characterization and in vivo study of sustained-release formulation of human growth hormone using sodium hyaluronate. *Pharm Res.* 2004;21(8):1374–1381.

Hamizi S, Freyer G, Bakrin N, et al. Subcutaneous trastuzumab: development of a new formulation for treatment of HER2-positive early breast cancer. *Onco Targets Ther.* 2013;6:89–94.

Hancock GE, Heers KM, Smith JD. QS-21 synergizes with recombinant interleukin-12 to create a potent adjuvant formulation for the fusion protein of respiratory syncytial virus. *Viral Immunol.* 2000;13(4):503–509.

Heller MC, Carpenter JF, Randolph TW. Protein formulation and lyophilization cycle design: prevention of damage due to freeze-concentration induced phase separation. *Biotechnol Bioeng.* 1999;63(2):166–174.

Herman AC, Boone TC, Lu HS. Characterization, formulation, and stability of Neupogen (Filgrastim), a recombinant human granulocyte-colony stimulating factor. *Pharm Biotechnol.* 1996;9:303–328.

Hofer C, Göbel R, Deering P, Lehmer A, Breul J. Formulation of interleukin-2 and interferon-alpha containing ultradeformable carriers for potential transdermal application. *Anticancer Res.* 1999;19(2C):1505–1507.

Hora MS, Rana RK, Wilcox CL, et al. Development of a lyophilized formulation of interleukin-2. *Dev Biol Stand.* 1992;74:295–303; discussion 303–296.

Hughes HP, Rossow S, Campos M, et al. A slow release formulation for recombinant bovine interferon alpha I-1. *Antiviral Res.* 1994;23(1):33–44.

Huyghebaert N, Vermeire A, Rottiers P, Remaut E, Remon JP. Development of an enteric-coated, layered multi-particulate formulation for ileal delivery of viable recombinant *Lactococcus lactis. Eur J Pharm Biopharm.* 2005;61(3):134–141.

Iglesias E, Franch O, Carrazana Y, et al. Influence of aluminum-based adjuvant on the immune response to multiantigenic formulation. *Viral Immunol.* 2006;19(4):712–721.

Iyer LK, Phanse R, Xu M, et al. Pulse proteolysis: an orthogonal tool for protein formulation screening. *J Pharm Sci.* 2019;108(2):842–850.

Jaber A, Driebergen R, Giovannoni G, Schellekens H, Simsarian J, Antonelli M. The Rebif new formulation story: it's not trials and error. *Drugs R D.* 2007;8(6):335–348.

Jacobsen LV, Rolan P, Christensen MS, Knudsen KM, Rasmussen MH. Bioequivalence between ready-to-use recombinant human growth hormone (rhGH) in liquid formulation and rhGH for reconstitution. *Growth Horm IGF Res.* 2000;10(2):93–98.

Kamat MS, Tolman GL, Brown JM. Formulation development of an antifibrin monoclonal antibody radiological medicine. *Pharm Biotechnol.* 1996;9:343–364.

Kapoor R, Shome D. Intradermal injections of a hair growth factor formulation for enhancement of human hair regrowth-safety and efficacy evaluation in a first-in-man pilot clinical study. *J Cosmet Laser Ther.* 2018;20(6):369–379.

Karsdal MA, Henriksen K, Bay-Jensen AC, et al. Lessons learned from the development of oral calcitonin: the first tablet formulation of a protein in phase III clinical trials. *J Clin Pharmacol.* 2011;51(4):460–471.

Kim SJ, Hahn SK, Kim MJ, Kim DH, Lee YP. Development of a novel sustained release formulation of recombinant human growth hormone using sodium hyaluronate microparticles. *J Control Release.* 2005;104(2):323–335.

Kim SJ, Kim CW. Characterization of recombinant human growth hormone variants from sodium hyaluronate-based sustained release formulation of rhGH under heat stress. *Anal Biochem.* 2015;485:59–65.

Kim SJ, Kim CW. Development and characterization of sodium hyaluronate microparticle-based sustained release formulation of recombinant human growth hormone prepared by spray-drying. *J Pharm Sci.* 2016;105(2):613–622.

Kim SY, Lee SJ, Lim SJ. Formulation and in vitro and in vivo evaluation of a cationic emulsion as a vehicle for improving adenoviral gene transfer. *Int J Pharm.* 2014;475(1–2):49–59.

Kraiem H, Zouari F, Abderrazek RB, et al. Two-dimensional isoelectric focusing OFFGEL, micro-fluidic lab-on-chip electrophoresis and FTIR for assessment of long-term stability of rhG-CSF formulation. *IEEE Trans Nanobioscience.* 2017;16(8):694–702.

Krasner A, Pohl R, Simms P, Pichotta P, Hauser R, De Souza E. A review of a family of ultra-rapid-acting insulins: formulation development. *J Diabetes Sci Technol.* 2012;6(4):786–796.

Kumar PS, Ramakrishna S, Saini TR, Diwan PV. Influence of microencapsulation method and peptide loading on formulation of poly(lactide-co-glycolide) insulin nanoparticles. *Pharmazie.* 2006;61(7):613–617.

Kumar V, Sharma VK, Kalonia DS. In situ precipitation and vacuum drying of interferon alpha-2a: development of a single-step process for obtaining dry, stable protein formulation. *Int J Pharm.* 2009;366(1–2):88–98.

López M, González LR, Reyes N, Sotolongo J, Pujol V. Stabilization of a freeze-dried recombinant streptokinase formulation without serum albumin. *J Clin Pharm Ther.* 2004;29(4):367–373.

Lv BH, Tan W, Zhu CC, Shang X, Zhang L. Properties of a stable and sustained-release formulation of recombinant human parathyroid hormone (rhPTH) with chitosan and silk fibroin microparticles. *Med Sci Monit.* 2018;24:7532–7540.

Lynch JM, Barbano DM, Bauman DE, Hartnell GF, Nemeth MA. Effect of a prolonged-release formulation of N-methionyl bovine somatotropin (sometribove) on milk fat. *J Dairy Sci.* 1992;75(7):1794–1809.

Macdougall IC. Pure red cell aplasia with anti-erythropoietin antibodies occurs more commonly with one formulation of epoetin alfa than another. *Curr Med Res Opin.* 2004;20(1):83–86.

Mach H, Arvinte T. Addressing new analytical challenges in protein formulation development. *Eur J Pharm Biopharm.* 2011;78(2):196–207.

Maeda H, Nakagawa T, Adachi N, et al. Design of long-acting formulation of protein drugs with a double-layer structure and its application to rhG-CSF. *J Control Release.* 2003;91(3):281–297.

Mahjoubi N, Fazeli MR, Dinarvand R, et al. Preventing aggregation of recombinant interferon beta-1b in solution by additives: approach to an albumin-free formulation. *Adv Pharm Bull.* 2015;5(4):497–505.

Malek-Sabet N, Masoumian MR, Zeinali M, Khalilzadeh R, Mousaabadi JM. Production, purification, and chemical stability of recombinant human interferon-γ in low oxygen tension condition: a formulation approach. *Prep Biochem Biotechnol.* 2013;43(6):586–600.

Malyala P, Singh M. Micro/nanoparticle adjuvants: preparation and formulation with antigens. *Methods Mol Biol.* 2010;626:91–101.

Mandal A, Pal D, Agrahari V, Trinh HM, Joseph M, Mitra AK. Ocular delivery of proteins and peptides: challenges and novel formulation approaches. *Adv Drug Deliv Rev.* 2018;126:67–95.

Mattern M, Winter G, Kohnert U, Lee G. Formulation of proteins in vacuum-dried glasses. II. Process and storage stability in sugar-free amino acid systems. *Pharm Dev Technol.* 1999;4(2):199–208.

Maurice T, Mustafa MH, Desrumaux C, et al. Intranasal formulation of erythropoietin (EPO) showed potent protective activity against amyloid toxicity in the $A\beta_{25-35}$ non-transgenic mouse model of Alzheimer's disease. *J Psychopharmacol.* 2013;27(11):1044–1057.

Mitragotri S, Burke PA, Langer R. Overcoming the challenges in administering therapeutic proteins: formulation and delivery strategies. *Nat Rev Drug Discov.* 2014;13(9):655–672.

Mizoguchi M, Nakatsuji M, Inoue H, et al. Novel oral formulation approach for poorly water-soluble drug using lipocalin-type prostaglandin D synthase. *Eur J Pharm Sci.* 2015;74:77–85.

Mizoguchi M, Nakatsuji M, Takano J, Ishibashi O, Wada K, Inui T. Development of pH-independent drug release formulation using lipocalin-type prostaglandin D synthase. *J Pharm Sci.* 2016;105(9):2735–2742.

Mordenti J, Thomsen K, Licko V, et al. Intraocular pharmacokinetics and safety of a humanized monoclonal antibody in rabbits after intravitreal administration of a solution or a PLGA microsphere formulation. *Toxicol Sci.* 1999;52(1):101–106.

Murányi A, Bartoš P, Tichý E, Lazová J, Pšenková J, Žabka M. Development of gel-forming lyophilized formulation with recombinant human thrombin. *Drug Dev Ind Pharm.* 2015;41(9):1566–1573.

Naito M, Hainz U, Burkhardt UE, et al. CD40L-Tri, a novel formulation of recombinant human CD40L that effectively activates B cells. *Cancer Immunol Immunother.* 2013;62(2):347–357.

Naughton CA, Duppong LM, Forbes KD, Sehgal I. Stability of multidose, preserved formulation epoetin alfa in syringes for three and six weeks. *Am J Health Syst Pharm.* 2003;60(5):464–468.

Nguyen TH, Ward C. Stability characterization and formulation development of alteplase, a recombinant tissue plasminogen activator. *Pharm Biotechnol.* 1993;5:91–134.

Norbury LJ, Basałaj K, Zawistowska-Deniziak A, et al. Intranasal delivery of a formulation containing stage-specific recombinant proteins of *Fasciola hepatica* cathepsin L5 and cathepsin B2 triggers an anti-fecundity effect and an adjuvant-mediated reduction in fluke burden in sheep. *Vet Parasitol.* 2018;258:14–23.

Osterberg T, Fatouros A, Mikaelsson M. Development of freeze-dried albumin-free formulation of recombinant factor VIII SQ. *Pharm Res.* 1997;14(7):892–898.

Osterberg T, Fatouros A, Neidhardt E, Warne N, Mikaelsson M. B-domain deleted recombinant factor VIII formulation and stability. *Semin Hematol.* 2001;38(2 Suppl 4):40–43.

Page C, Dawson P, Woollacott D, Thorpe R, Mire-Sluis A. Development of a lyophilization formulation that preserves the biological activity of the platelet-inducing cytokine interleukin-11 at low concentrations. *J Pharm Pharmacol.* 2000;52(1):19–26.

Panjwani N, Hodgson DJ, Sauvé S, Aubin Y. Assessment of the effects of pH, formulation and deformulation on the conformation of interferon alpha-2 by NMR. *J Pharm Sci.* 2010;99(8):3334–3342.

Park K. Significance of handling, formulation and storage conditions on the stability and bioactivity of rhBMP-2. *J Control Release.* 2012;162(3):654.

Patro SY, Freund E, Chang BS. Protein formulation and fill-finish operations. *Biotechnol Annu Rev.* 2002;8:55–84.

Pellequer Y, Ollivon M, Barratt G. Formulation of liposomes associated with recombinant interleukin-2: effect on interleukin-2 activity. *Biomed Pharmacother.* 2004;58(3):162–167.

Pereira P, Kelly SM, Cooper A, Mardon HJ, Gellert PR, van der Walle CF. Solution formulation and lyophilisation of a recombinant fibronectin fragment. *Eur J Pharm Biopharm.* 2007;67(2):309–319.

Peters EE, Ameri M, Wang X, Maa YF, Daddona PE. Erythropoietin-coated ZP-microneedle transdermal system: preclinical formulation, stability, and delivery. *Pharm Res.* 2012;29(6):1618–1626.

Piedmonte DM, Treuheit MJ. Formulation of Neulasta (pegfilgrastim). *Adv Drug Deliv Rev.* 2008;60(1):50–58.

Rasmussen T, Tantipolphan R, van de Weert M, Jiskoot W. The molecular chaperone alpha-crystallin as an excipient in an insulin formulation. *Pharm Res.* 2010;27(7):1337–1347.

Remmele RL, Nightlinger NS, Srinivasan S, Gombotz WR. Interleukin-1 receptor (IL-1R) liquid formulation development using differential scanning calorimetry. *Pharm Res.* 1998;15(2):200–208.

Richard J, Prang N. The formulation and immunogenicity of therapeutic proteins: product quality as a key factor. *IDrugs.* 2010;13(8):550–558.

Ruiz L, Reyes N, Sotolongo J, et al. Long-term stabilization of a new freeze-dried and albumin-free formulation of recombinant human interferon alpha 2b. *PDA J Pharm Sci Technol.* 2006;60(1):72–78.

Ruiz L, Rodriguez I, Baez R, Aldana R. Stability of an extemporaneously prepared recombinant human interferon alfa-2b eye drop formulation. *Am J Health Syst Pharm.* 2007;64(16):1716–1719.

Santana H, García G, Vega M, Beldarraín A, Páez R. Stability studies of a freeze-dried recombinant human epidermal growth factor formulation for wound healing. *PDA J Pharm Sci Technol.* 2015;69(3):399–416.

Senet P, Mons B, Aractangi S, Tilleul P. Evaluation of the stability and efficacy of rhGM-CSF as a topical agent in a gel formulation. *J Wound Care.* 2002;11(4):132–134.

Shire SJ. Stability characterization and formulation development of recombinant human deoxyribonuclease I [Pulmozyme, (dornase alpha)]. *Pharm Biotechnol.* 1996;9:393–426.

Singh M, Shirley B, Bajwa K, Samara E, Hora M, O'Hagan D. Controlled release of recombinant insulin-like growth factor from a novel formulation of polylactide-co-glycolide microparticles. *J Control Release.* 2001;70(1–2):21–28.

Sønderby P, Bukrinski JT, Hebditch M, Peters GHJ, Curtis RA, Harris P. Self-interaction of human serum albumin: a formulation perspective. *ACS Omega.* 2018;3(11):16105–16117.

Steiner S, Hompesch M, Pohl R, et al. A novel insulin formulation with a more rapid onset of action. *Diabetologia.* 2008;51(9):1602–1606.

Stote R, Marbury T, Shi L, Miller M, Strange P. Comparison pharmacokinetics of two concentrations (0.7% and 1.0%) of Nasulin, an ultra-rapid-acting intranasal insulin formulation. *J Diabetes Sci Technol.* 2010;4(3):603–609.

Stote R, Miller M, Marbury T, Shi L, Strange P. Enhanced absorption of Nasulin™, an ultrarapid-acting intranasal insulin formulation, using single nostril administration in normal subjects. *J Diabetes Sci Technol.* 2011;5(1):113–119.

Takeshita A, Saito H, Toyama K, et al. Efficacy of a new formulation of lenograstim (recombinant glycosylated human granulocyte colony-stimulating factor) containing gelatin for the treatment of neutropenia after consolidation chemotherapy in patients with acute myeloid leukemia. *Int J Hematol.* 2000;71(2):136–143.

Thompson CA. New interferon alfa formulation licensed for treatment of hepatitis C. *Am J Health Syst Pharm.* 2001;58(6):452.

Vemuri S, Yu CT, Roosdorp N. Formulation and stability of recombinant alpha 1-antitrypsin. *Pharm Biotechnol.* 1993;5:263–286.

Volkin DB, Middaugh CR. The characterization, stabilization, and formulation of acidic fibroblast growth factor. *Pharm Biotechnol.* 1996;9:181–217.

Wang S, Zhang X, Wu G, Tian Z, Qian F. Optimization of high-concentration endostatin formulation: harmonization of excipients' contributions on colloidal and conformational stabilities. *Int J Pharm.* 2017;530(1–2):173–186.

Wei Y, Wang Y, Kang A, et al. A novel sustained-release formulation of recombinant human growth hormone and its pharmacokinetic, pharmacodynamic and safety profiles. *Mol Pharm.* 2012;9(7):2039–2048.

Wright JF, Qu G, Tang C, Sommer JM. Recombinant adeno-associated virus: formulation challenges and strategies for a gene therapy vector. *Curr Opin Drug Discov Devel.* 2003;6(2):174–178.

Yatuv R, Dayan I, Carmel-Goren L, et al. Enhancement of factor VIIa haemostatic efficacy by formulation with PEGylated liposomes. *Haemophilia.* 2008;14(3):476–483.

11

Gene and Cell Therapy

11.1 Background

Gene and cell therapy constitute the recent advances in the field of DNA-based medicines. An overview of the diseases, risks, development, and ethical issues is introduced in this chapter, along with a comprehensive list of currently approved products. Gene therapy and cell therapy, including the DNA and mRNA vaccines and CAR-T techniques, are introduced. Gene editing technologies define the methodologies and their relative advantages. Upstream and downstream technologies for gene and cell therapy products and allogenic products are described, including understanding regulatory controls, characterization of the cell population, release testing, and radioisotope tagging. Issues related to vectors and vector preparation are provided. Finally, preclinical evaluation methods of evaluation and challenges in commercializing gene and cell therapy products are pointed out.

Somatic (relating to the body and not mind) cell therapy is the administration of autologous (cells obtained from the same person), allogeneic (same type of tissue cells from another person), or xenogeneic (foreign) living cells that have been manipulated or processed ex vivo. Ex vivo propagation, expansion, selection, or pharmacologic treatment of cells and other biological changes are part of the manufacturing process for somatic cell therapy products. These cellular products could also be used for diagnosis or prevention.

The cells used in cell therapy are pluripotent cells that convert into every cell in the body or multipotent cells that can turn into one or other types of cells. Cells are implanted as an in vivo source of a molecular species like an enzyme, cytokine, or coagulation factor. lymphokine-activated killer cells and tumor-infiltrating lymphocytes are among the activated lymphoid cells that can be infused. and implantation of manipulated cell populations such as hepatocytes, myoblasts, or pancreatic islet cells, all examples of somatic cell therapies.

Cells for therapeutic purposes are delivered by infusion, injection at various sites, or surgically implanting in aggregated form or along with solid supports or encapsulating materials. The matrices, fibers, beads, or other materials used in addition to the cells are listed as excipients, additional active components, or medical devices. Blood transfusion is the most common type of cell therapy.

Gene therapy is a clinical intervention based on the addition, removal, or modification of living cells' genetic material. Cells are modified ex vivo for subsequent administration to humans or are altered in vivo by gene therapy given directly to the subject—similar to cell therapy. Genetic manipulation can be therapeutic, preventative, or used to mark cells for later identification. Recombinant DNA materials used to transfer genetic material for gene therapy are considered components of gene therapy and are regulated accordingly (Figure 11.1).

Gene therapy decreases or increases a protein's levels and produces new and modified proteins by transferring genetic material in a carrier or vector and integrating it into the relevant body cells. The alteration and administration of somatic cells were the first approaches to gene therapy.

Gene therapy and cell therapy are often used together, where stem cells are removed from the patient, genetically modified in tissue culture to produce a new gene, expanded to sufficient numbers, and then returned to the patient to relieve the underlying cause of genetic diseases and acquired diseases by replacing the defective protein(s) or cells that trigger the symptoms of the disease, to reverse the symptoms.

Gene and cell therapy aim to produce a lifetime treatment to avoid frequent treatment that will be impractical. Like the immune system's muscle cells, most cells, stem cells, neurons, and memory cells

DOI: 10.1201/9781003146933-11

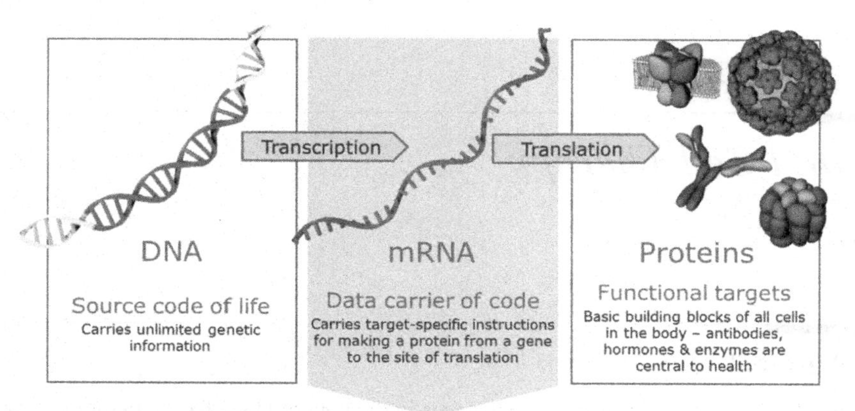

FIGURE 11.1 Genome translation and transcription process. Source: https://en.wikipedia.org/wiki/Protein_biosynthesis.

are long-lived and may last the patient's lifetime. Stem cells provide gene and cell therapy with two significant benefits. First, they provide a type of cell that can regenerate and last the patient's lifetime. Second, stem cells offer daughter cells that mature in the tissue's specialized cells. These segregated daughter cells replace the affected diseased cells. Thus, gene and cell therapy utilizing the stem cells also potentially enhance the treatment as far as the modified stem cells live, hopefully, the patient's lifetime.

In its broadest sense, gene therapy is the introduction, removal, or alteration of a person's genetic code to treat or cure a disease. The transferred genetic material alters the cell's ability to produce a single protein or a group of proteins. Thus, gene therapy can be used to lower levels of a disease-causing protein, boost the production of disease-fighting proteins, or create new/modified proteins.

Cell therapy is the injection of healthy, living cells into a patient to help treat or cure a disease. The cells may come from the patient (autologous cells) or a donor (allogeneic cells). The ability of cells used in cell therapy to transform into different cell types can be classified. Multipotent cells can transform into other cell types, while pluripotent cells can transform into any cell type in the body. Nonetheless, they have a smaller repertoire than pluripotent cells. Primary cells, whether differentiated or undifferentiated, are of a fixed type. The treatment determines the type of cells used.

Gene therapy and cell therapy are both used in some protocols. In this case, the patient's stem cells are isolated, genetically modified in tissue culture to express a new gene, expanded to a sufficient number, and then returned to the patient.

Gene therapy and cell therapy offer a promising alternative or adjunct treatment for many acquired diseases, including cancer, rheumatoid arthritis, diabetes, Parkinson's disease, Alzheimer's disease, etc. The most common disease in gene therapy clinical trials is cancer. Cancer gene therapy focuses on killing cancer cells, preventing tumor vascularization, and increasing the immune response to tumor antigens.

The types of gene therapies are listed here.

- Gene addition entails inserting a new copy of a gene into target cells to increase protein production. A modified virus such as an adeno-associated virus (AAV) is frequently used to carry the gene into the cells. Adenosine deaminase severe combined immunodeficiency (ADA-SCID), congenital blindness, hemophilia, Leber's congenital amaurosis, lysosomal storage diseases, X-linked chronic granulomatous disease, and other diseases are all being treated with gene addition therapies.
- Using recently developed gene-editing technology (e.g., CRISPR-Cas9, TALEN, or ZFN) to remove repeated or faulty gene elements or replace a damaged or dysfunctional region of DNA, gene correction can be accomplished. The goal of gene correction is to create a protein that

functions normally rather than in a disease-causing manner. Recent experimental work has used gene editing technologies to extract HIV from the genomes of affected laboratory mice and excise the expanded region responsible for Huntington's disease from the human gene, suggesting that gene correction could be used to treat a wide range of diseases.

- Gene silencing prevents the production of a specific protein by directing messenger RNA (mRNA; a precursor to protein expression from a gene) to be degraded, resulting in no protein being produced. Human and animal cells have single-stranded mRNA, whereas viruses have double-stranded RNA. Double-stranded RNA is recognized by human and animal cells as viral in origin, and it is destroyed to prevent its spread. Small RNA sequences are used in gene silencing to bind unique sequences in the target mRNA and double-strand it. This causes the mRNA to be destroyed by the same cellular machinery that destroys viral RNA. Gene silencing is an effective gene therapy for diseases characterized by excessive protein production. Too much tumor necrosis factor (TNF) alpha, for example, is frequently found in the afflicted joints of rheumatoid arthritis patients. Because TNF alpha is only required in trace amounts throughout the body, gene silencing reduces TNF alpha levels only in the affected tissue.
- Reprogramming is the process of changing the characteristics of cells by adding one or more genes to them. This technique works well in tissues with various cell types, as long as a malfunction in one of them causes the disease. Type 1 diabetes, for example, is caused by damage to the pancreas' insulin-producing islet cells. At the same time, the pancreatic cells that make digestive enzymes are unaffected. Reprogramming these cells to produce insulin would aid in the recovery of type 1 diabetic patients.
- Cell elimination strategies typically target the overgrowth of benign (non-cancerous) tumor cells while destroying malignant (cancerous) tumor cells. For example, the introduction of "suicide genes," which enter tumor cells and release a prodrug that causes cell death in those cells, can be used to eliminate tumor cells. In addition, viruses can be genetically modified to have a preference for tumor cells. These oncotropic viruses can carry therapeutic genes that make tumor cells more toxic, stimulate the immune system to attack the tumor, or stop the growth of blood vessels that feed the tumor.

Gene therapy is delivered by the following methods.

- Electroporation, passive delivery, and ballistic delivery are examples of non-vector methods. Using high voltage electroporation, simple strands of naked DNA or RNA can be pushed into cells. In the lab, this is a common technique. Using a normal cellular process called endocytosis and the medium surrounding the cells, naked DNA or RNA can also be taken up by target cells. Finally, a device is known as a "gene gun" can be used to introduce genetic material using sheer mechanical force. Vesicles that are attached to a membrane. Liposomes (fluid-filled sacs surrounded by a fatty membrane) can be used to package genetic material to be more easily absorbed by cells than naked DNA/RNA. Different types of liposomes are being developed to bind to specific tissues more effectively. Recent research has used an endogenously produced and released subtype of membrane vesicles (extracellular vesicles or "exosomes") to transport small RNA sequences into specific tissues.
- Vectors of viral infection are another method. Viruses are born with the ability to enter cells. For example, a cold virus enters the upper respiratory tract cells and hijacks the cell's machinery to manufacture more viruses, resulting in symptoms. After removing the virus's ability to divide, viral vectors for gene therapy are modified to use the virus's ability to enter cells. Viruses of various types have been engineered to serve as gene therapy vectors. The gene(s) of interest and control signals replace all essential viral genes in adeno-associated virus (AAV) and retrovirus/lentivirus vectors, preventing the viral vector from replicating. Fewer viral genes are replaced in oncolytic viruses like adenovirus and herpes simplex virus, and the virus can still replicate in a limited number of cell types. Thus, viral vectors preferentially enter a subset of tissues, express genes at different levels, and interact with the immune system differently.

- Gene therapy and cell therapy can be used together. First, purified and expanded in vitro cells are taken from the patient or a matched donor. Scientists and clinicians then use one of the three methods described above to deliver the gene to the cells. The patient is then re-administered with the cells that express the therapeutic gene.
- Gene therapy is classified according to whether it is given to cells inside or outside the body. In vivo gene therapy refers to treatment that is administered directly to the patient. As a result, the patient's body retains the targeted cells. Ex vivo gene/cell therapy entails removing the patient's targeted cells and administering gene therapy to them in vitro before reintroducing them into the body.
- Somatic cell gene therapy is a type of gene therapy that targets cells in the body that aren't involved in reproduction. The cells that make up the retina, liver, and heart are examples. Somatic cell gene therapies are being developed for various diseases, but the FDA has not yet approved most gene therapies for widespread use. Patients who are currently receiving somatic gene therapy do so as part of FDA-approved clinical trials.

Types of cell therapies include the following.

- Red blood cell, white blood cell, and platelet transfusions from a donor are all examples of blood transfusions. Another common cell therapy is the over 40-year-old procedure of transplanting hematopoietic stem cells to create bone marrow. Cell therapy subtypes, like gene therapy, can be classified in a variety of ways. There is no formal classification system for cell therapies at the moment. Cell potency has been used to classify the various types of cells used in cell therapy. The authors describe four pluripotent stem cells and four types of multipotent stem cells derived from adult tissue.
- Embryonic stem cells are a type of stem cell that can be used (ESCs). Pluripotent stem cells (PSCs) are pluripotent stem cells derived from embryos. Embryos used to isolate stem cells are usually unused embryos from assisted reproduction procedures such as in vitro fertilization (IVF). Because ESCs are pluripotent, they can self-renew and form any type of cell in the body. Because of their pluripotency, ESCs are versatile, but using embryos to develop therapeutic strategies raises ethical concerns. Furthermore, stem cell lines derived from embryos are not genetically matched to the patient, increasing the likelihood that the patient's immune system will reject the transplanted cell.
- Pluripotent stem cells that have been induced (iPSCs) can also be used. Reprogramming a differentiated adult (somatic) cell, such as a skin cell, returns to a pluripotent state. Thus, these cells have the benefit of pluripotency without the ethical issues associated with embryonic stem cells. Immune rejection can also be avoided by using iPSCs derived from the patient. Adult cells are transformed with a cocktail of genes delivered via a viral vector to produce iPSCs. While the process efficiency has improved dramatically since its inception, the low reprogramming rate continues to be a source of concern. Another issue is that iPSCs are derived from adult cells, making them "older" than embryonic stem cells, as evidenced by a higher rate of programmed cell death, lower rates of DNA damage repair, and a higher rate of point mutations.
- Embryonic stem cell nuclear transfer (ntESCs) is another type of therapy. The nucleus of an adult cell obtained from the patient is transferred to an oocyte (egg cell) obtained from a donor to produce pluripotent cells. The process of transferring the nucleus to the egg cell transforms it into a pluripotent cell. The derived cells, like iPSCs, are genetically identical to the patient's nuclear genome and are unlikely to be rejected by the body. The main advantage of this technique is that the resulting ntESCs carry the patient's nuclear DNA and mitochondria from the donor, making it particularly suitable for diseases involving damaged or dysfunctional mitochondria. One disadvantage of ntESCs is that the generation process is time-consuming and requires a donor oocyte. Only lower mammals have been shown to produce stem cells using this technique at the time of writing.

- Embryonic stem cells that are parthenogenetic (pES) can be used. Unfertilized oocytes are the final option for obtaining pluripotent cells. The oocyte is treated with chemicals that cause parthenogenesis (embryogenesis without sperm), and ESCs are extracted from the developing embryo. ESCs that are genetically identical to the female patient are created using this method. However, this method is still in its early stages of development, and it is unknown whether parthenogenesis-derived cells and tissues develop normally.
- HSCs (hematopoietic stem cells) are multipotent blood stem cells that can differentiate into any type of blood cell. Adult bone marrow, peripheral blood, and umbilical cord blood all contain HSCs.
- MSCs are multipotent cells found in various tissues, including the umbilical cord, bone marrow, and fat tissue. MSCs promote adipose marrow tissue by generating bone, cartilage, muscle, and adipocytes (fat cells).
- NSCs (nervous stem cells) are another therapy option. In the mammalian brain, adult neural stem cells are found in small numbers in specific areas. These multipotent cells replenish the brain's neurons and supporting cells. On the other hand, adult neural stem cells cannot be obtained from patients because of their location in the brain. As a result, iPSCs or ESCs are used to make neural stem cells for cell therapies.
- Epithelial stem cells are cells that originate from the epithelia of the skin. Epithelial cells are taken from the epidermis and the gastrointestinal tract's lining, as well as other body surfaces and linings. These areas contain multipotent epithelial stem cells, whereas unipolar stem cells only differentiate into one cell type. For example, the corneal epithelium of the eye has been successfully regenerated using epithelial stem cells.
- Immunotherapy is a type of cell therapy that uses the body's immune cells, blood cells, and skin cells, which reproduce rapidly in the body and can usually be produced ex vivo under the right conditions. This enables the use of differentiated adult immune cells in cell therapy. Before returning to the body, the cells can be removed from the body, isolated from a mixed cell population, modified, and expanded. Adult self-renewing T lymphocytes that have been genetically modified to increase their immune potency to kill disease-causing cells are being used in a newly developed cell therapy.

11.2 Gene Therapy

Gene therapy modifies a patient's genetic code to treat a disease; the transferred genetic material controls how proteins are produced by cells. Cell therapy is administering live cells into a patient to treat wherein the cells can originate from the patient (autologous cells) or a donor (allogeneic cells). These transferred cells can give rise to any cell type and the multipotent cells into other cell types with pluripotent limitations. Figure 11.2 describes the gene and cell therapy design; the product introduced in the patient is the biological product.

Viruses are used as vectors of gene delivery and as oncolytic viruses in gene therapy after they are modified. Viral vectors defend the new gene from blood-borne enzymes that can kill it and deliver it to the relevant cells. Effectively, viral vectors force the cells to take over the new gene from the virus to their nucleus. The transduced cells then start using the latest gene to synthesize a new protein, to perform its normal function. Viral vectors are genetically modified to remove most essential genes, preventing unchecked virus replication and allowing gene injection.

Viral vector selection for use in gene therapy is based on 1) the size of the DNA or gene that is packed, 2) the quality of the absorption by the desired therapy cells, 3) the length of gene expression, 4) the impact on the immune response, 5) the ease of manufacturing, and 6) the ease of incorporation into the DNA or the capacity to remain as a stable DNA.

Viruses of oncolytic origin are engineered to replicate in cancer cells and not in normal human cells. As oncolytic viruses multiply in cancer cells, the cancer cells explode, allowing more oncolytic viruses to infect the cancer cells around them.

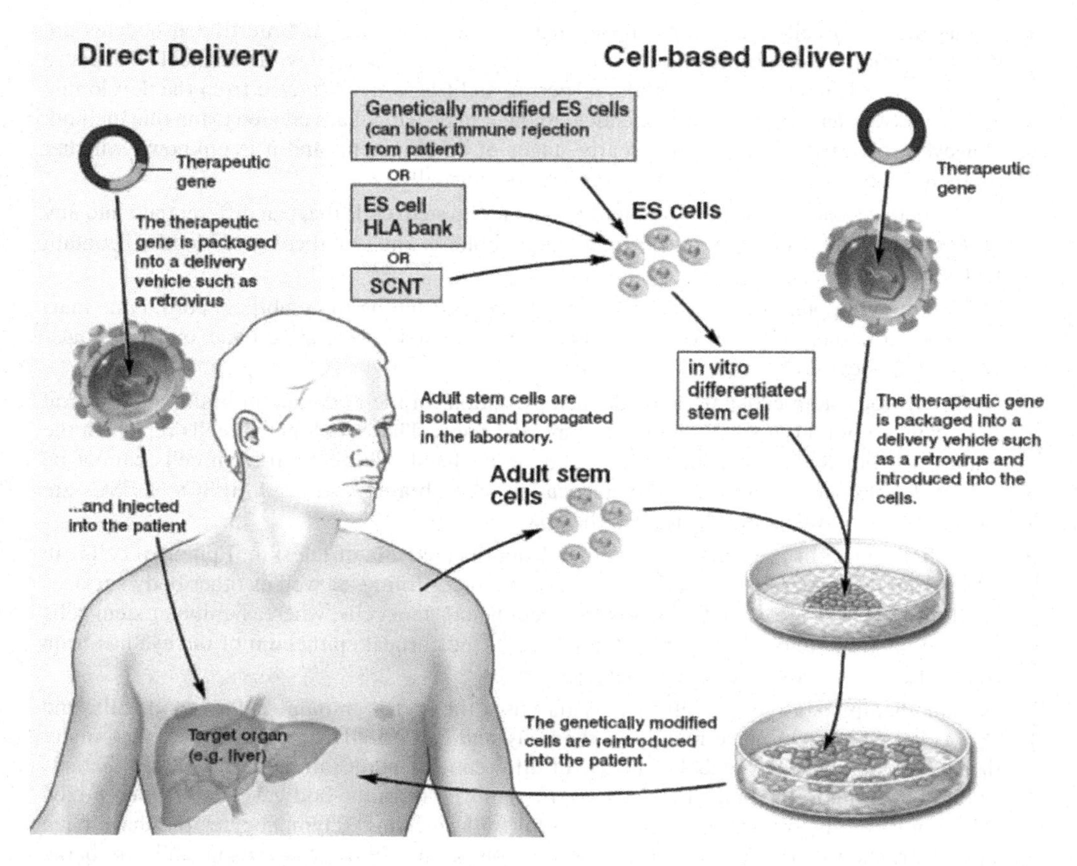

FIGURE 11.2 Strategies for delivering therapeutic transgenes to patients. Source: Zwaka, T. Use of genetically modified stem cells in experimental gene therapies. 2006;4. DOI:10.1201/9780849387999.ch34

Historically, more focus has been placed on retroviral and adenoviral vectors; however, vectors derived from adeno-associated virus (AAV) and lentiviral vectors have advanced in evolution protection and improved target tissue expression profiles. In addition, herpes simplex virus and pox/vaccinia vectors are also promising as oncolytic vaccines for their efficacy.

The AAV is the most commonly used genetic modification vector in vivo and can target different tissues within the body using several serotypes (naturally occurring or recombinant). In addition, the AAV is not known to be pathogenic and is thought to be well-tolerated, resulting in a lower inflammatory response. Therefore, unlike other viral vectors such as lentivirus, which integrate into the host cell's genome, AAV is thought to remain primarily episomal.

Table 11.1 summarizes the physical properties of the various viruses that are used for gene therapy.

11.2.1 Viral Vector Manufacturing

There are several potential systems available for producing viral vectors. The system's choice depends on tissue tropism, ability to incorporate or non-integrated alteration, in vivo or ex vivo phase, previous immune response, and whether the target cell replicates. In addition, high-efficiency transduction and stable transgenic expression levels are desirable outcomes in viral vector applications.

Typically, viral vectors are formed using multiple expressible units to significantly reduce the possibility of producing a wild-type particle by recombination. Usually, the expressible units are individual plasmids (a genetic structure in a cell that can replicate independently of the chromosomes, typically a small circular DNA strand in the cytoplasm of a bacterium or protozoan) injected into producer cells

TABLE 11.1
Overview of Common Viruses Used for Generating Gene Therapy Viral Vectors

Parameter	Retrovirus	Lentivirus	AAV	Adenovirus
Coat	Enveloped	Enveloped	Non-enveloped	Non-enveloped
Packing capacity (Kb)	8	8	~4.5	7.5
Inflammatory, infection	Dividing cells	Broad	Broad excluding hematopoietic cells	Broad
Hot genome interaction	Integrating	Integrating	Integrating, non-integrating	Non-integrating
Transgene expression	Long-lasting	Long-lasting	Potentially long-lasting	Transient or long-lasting depending on immunogenicity
Size	~90–120 nm	~90–120 nm	~20 nm	~90 nm
Stability	Low	Low	High	High
Buoyant density	1.16 CsCl (sucrose)	1.16 CsCl (sucrose)	1.41 CsCl	1.34 CsCl

either by transfection or by virus-transducing "helper." Usually, the expression units are further updated with mutations to deactivate the wild-type virus's role should a recombination event impact them. Newer HIV lentiviral vectors, for example, lack genes for virulence factors tat, vpr, vpu, nef, and have gag and pol on different plasmids from rev and env1and/or bear other mutations such as deletions in the 3' LTR.

The goal in the design of viral vectors is to effectively bundle the therapeutic gene or nucleotides into infectious viral particles to prevent wild-type particles or empty particles from being produced. Therefore, many vector systems are manufactured either for safety, convenience, or requirement through transient co-transfection of multiple plasmids to avoid the toxicity of a vector component in producer cells (Figure 11.3).

The elements of the AAV vector and the therapeutic gene are transfected, usually as separate cassettes of expression from different plasmids. Expression cassettes are expressed inside the cell, resulting in viral proteins and a genetic DNA containing the therapeutic gene(s) expression cassette. Viral particles that contain the transgene assemble in the cytoplasm in the AAV system. Particles are released via cellular lysis for further purification and characterization to the public (https://cellculturedish.com/genetherapybook/).

Viral vector production requires multiple fabrication steps or platforms. The materials needed to produce the therapeutic viral vector include plasmids encoding helper-virus and the therapeutic gene, cell lines used to make the vector, and other products. In some cases, plasmids are replaced by helper transducing viruses. Additionally, to reduce or eliminate the transfection and transduction steps and optimize the production process, reliable producer cell lines are developed.

The next step in the manufacture of vectors involves generating an infectious viral vector (Figure 3.5). To establish the viral vector, which is collected, cells are transfected with plasmids. The AAV viral particles concentrate in the media and the cytoplasm, optimizing total yield by lysing the cells. It is then distilled, filtered, titrated, characterized, and stored for later use ex vivo or in vivo. Next, host cells are collected and modified by the viral vector in ex vivo transduction (Figure 11.4). Upon modification and pre-transplantation, the cells are harvested, characterized, and formulated. In some methods, transduced cells are extended before re-infusion into the patients in cell culture.

While there are significant increases in hollow fiber and fixed-bed bioreactor systems, the variety is currently limited. Another alternative for adherent cells is microcarriers' use in rocking bioreactors or stirring tank bioreactors, providing a large surface area for cell attachment. Rocking bioreactors with a microcarrier or single-cell suspension culture are an option to produce smaller vector volumes for research or clinical trials, as their current capacity at low cell density is 500 L maximum. Rocking bioreactors are reusable and are used to supply cell seed to larger bioreactors as well. Virus processing in the vaccine industry is successfully scaled up to 2,000+ L using microcarriers in the stirred tanks' bioreactors. A single 2,000 L bioreactor operating at a microcarrier density of 10 cm^2/mL has a surface area of 2,000 m^2. Microcarrier drawbacks are developmental factors that maximize cell attachment,

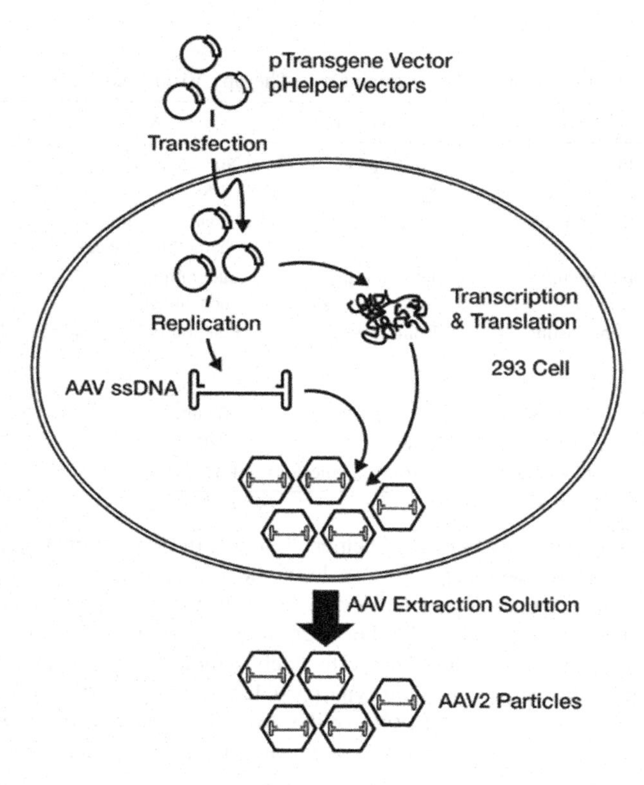

FIGURE 11.3 Schematic of AAV vector development through transfection. The elements of the AAV vector and the therapeutic gene are transfected, usually as separate cassettes of expression from different plasmids. Expression cassettes are expressed inside the cell, resulting in viral proteins and a genetic DNA containing the therapeutic gene(s) expression cassette. Viral particles that contain the transgene assemble in the cytoplasm in the AAV system. Particles are released via cellular lysis for further purification and characterization to the public. Source: https://cellculturedish.com/genetherapybook/.

growth, and viability. The ability to transfect/transduce cells that grow on a microcarrier must be recognized early in development. Bioreactors with a stirred tank are the most prevalent bioreactor used to commercialize mAbs and recombinant proteins. As a result, the system is very well defined, and its implementation is well known to both industry and regulatory authorities. These are the most effective ways to produce large volumes.

Bioreactors are best adapted to the growth of suspension cells. The culture of single-cell suspension has a significant advantage over adherent cells. It is easily scaled from spinner to bioreactor on a laboratory scale to bioreactor development without cell detachment. Because of the reduced risk of adventitious agents and the reduced purification, animal-free media is a desirable feature for production. Nonetheless, it is time-consuming to adapt custom cells to the suspension culture and prolong process development times.

Selecting the upstream production process will affect the efficiency of downstream purification. For instance, shear forces can increase cell debris on adhered cells on microcarrier systems or other fluid-motion systems. Another explanation is that sometimes a fixed-bed bioreactor may benefit by bringing fewer impurities into the bed.

11.2.2 Downstream Manufacturing

The downstream processing is intended to separate the viral vector from the different impurities created in the upstream processing and get the virus into the appropriate state to formulate for administration to patients.

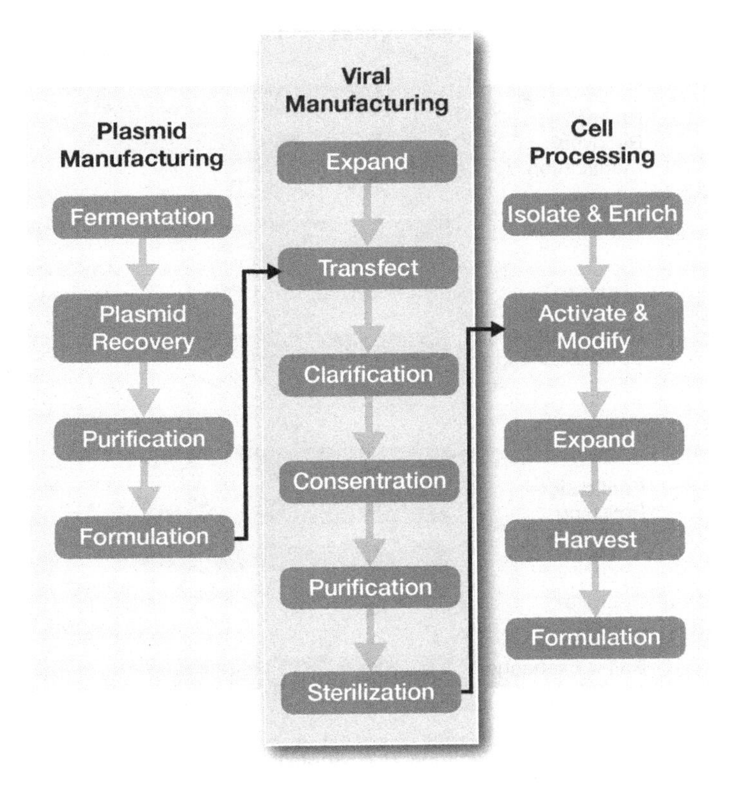

FIGURE 11.4 Example of three manufacturing platforms for the generation of modified cells for ex vivo gene therapy via viral vectors produced by transfection. Source: https://cellculturedish.com/genetherapybook/.

Traditional steps of purification are based on ultracentrifugation, flocculation, and other techniques of various complexities. Recent advances have allowed the same degree of impurity removal as more traditional methods using highly scalable chromatography and tangential flow filtration.

The differences in physical characteristics between different vectors present various purification challenges, resulting in various techniques and solutions needed for the industry. For example, AAV has also been collected in the media and is partly extracted from cells through a lytic process. In general, AAV viruses are harvested by cell lysis to improve yield. Cell lysis will produce substantial amounts of pollutants in host cells, including DNA and protein, increasing the purification burden. AAV vectors will contain up to 95% of total particles to a significant portion of "soft" particles devoid of the transgene. Despite the ongoing controversy about a potential benefit from empty particles in AAV treatments, these are still regarded as major contaminants. Downstream processing of RV/LV vectors presents unique challenges of their own.

Other specific vector purification challenges are created by the upstream manufacturing process chosen.

Notwithstanding differences in physical characteristics between vectors, existing downstream protocols typically have a common workflow involving a confirmation stage (which may include cell lysis), purification (centrifugation or chromatography of ion exchange/affinity), and polishing step (additional step/size exclusion) (Figure 11.5). Typically, in addition to the above, filtration/dialysis/centrifugation steps are used to concentrate, switch filters, or final formulation.

The clarification stage includes eliminating the initial crude suspension of large debris and macromolecular complexes and may consist of cell lysis to increase viral yield (AdV, AAV). Nucleases (for example, benzonase) are typically added during or after cell lysis to destroy nucleic acids and disrupt the macromolecular complexes. Every cell lysis method requires optimization since lysis depends on

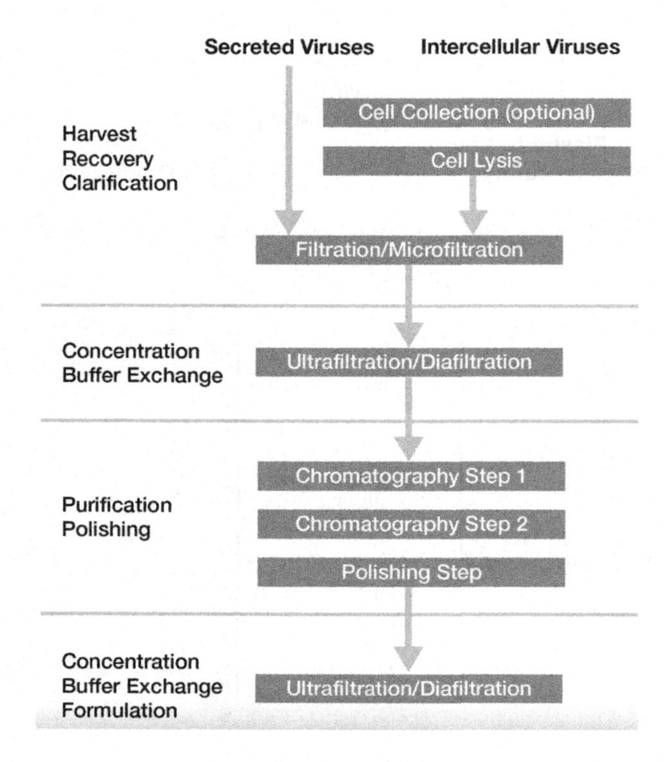

FIGURE 11.5 Downstream process for secreted viruses (lentivirus/retrovirus) and viruses released by cell lysis. Source: https://cellculturedish.com/genetherapybook/.

cell concentration, incubation time, incubation temperature, type of cell, and the virus produced. During clarification, the initial elimination of cell debris and impurities usually involves using multiple filters with decreasing pore size down to 0.2 μm, which acts as an integral part of an overall bioburden control strategy.

The purification of small amounts of virus for study or limited clinical studies has relied heavily on ultracentrifugation methods. Viral particles are usually pelleted and condensed in these methods through a matrix, followed by resuspension and purification using gradient ultracentrifugation through the buoyant mass. To further purify the particles, multiple rounds of gradient ultracentrifugation are required. In the past, CsCl was commonly used for the ultracentrifugation of AAV and AdV. However, iodixanol is now preferred to CsCl because it is less toxic, requires less dialysis, decreases oxidation, and shortens run times from 24 h to a few hours. Because enveloped viruses such as RV/LV have limited stability, sucrose is widely used to reduce this concern.

Chromatography has been commonly used to purify vaccines and vectors for gene therapy and is applied in various downstream stages, including selection, concentration, purification, and polishing. The use of chromatography for vector purification is an established method that can purify the vector by its physical property of net charge, hydrophobicity, ligand affinity, size, or other properties. Chromatography is considered significantly more flexible and cost-effective than centrifugation. Columns are used repeatedly, and columns are used in different strategies in parallel or combination. Furthermore, chromatography is an effective means of eliminating potential adventitious forces, an essential aspect of late-stage development.

Ion exchange chromatography (IEC) is a simple and cost-effective technique applied to many types of viruses. Both anion or cation exchanges are used to bind viruses, which are charged either positively or negatively. Theoretically, IEC will require separating empty particles from all AAV serotypes; nevertheless, resins and conditions would also need to be optimized for each serotype. One downside to the separation with empty particles is that it takes a long time to develop, often more than two months, since the gradients necessary for separation are shallow. In addition, anything that influences a vector charge, such as serotype, vector height, or transgene insert length, may require redevelopment of the gradient conditions.

Hydrophobic reaction chromatography (HIC) has been used in the vector and recombinant protein industry for viral capture/clearance years. In addition, HIC has been used in purification procedures for the purification of both AdV and AAV2. However, its use with AAV with different serotypes has not been extensively documented. Likewise, IEC solutions with high ionic strength during binding can affect the stability of some viruses.

Affinity chromatography (AC) relies on the viral particle interaction to a ligand. Chromatography of heparin affinity was used to purify LV and other viruses and is also handles larger volumes. Mild salt solutions can help preserve the integrity of the vectors. However, there are drawbacks, including non-specific impurity binding that requires additional purification steps. One problem in AC arises when using the AAV that complete particles cannot be isolated from empty particles, resulting in additional measures for that purpose, such as ion-exchange chromatography or ultracentrifugation. One issue is the leakage of the ligand into the vector preparation in affinity chromatography. Ligand leakage can require additional analytical steps, as well as possible further purification steps.

The size exclusion chromatography exclusion (SEC) separates virus particles from contaminants based on size and mass. Since there is no binding or elution, SEC has benefits because it is highly flexible; nonetheless, SEC may not be suitable for large-scale processing because it has low throughput, requires low flow rates, which increases processing time, and it may dilute the sample and result in requiring additional concentration steps. As a result, SEC is commonly thought not to scale well beyond 1,000 L. SEC has nonetheless made use of many viruses, including AAV and LV, as final polishing.

Pelleting the virus by ultracentrifugation can provide higher effective concentrations and high vector yields. However, pelleting has potential disadvantages, such as loss of functional vector particles due to shear stress and impurity enhancement. A gentler approach is the use of low-speed centrifugation for a longer duration. However, the methods of centrifugation have limited scalability. For concentration or buffer transfer, TFF has advantages in that it is typically flexible, enabling mild processing conditions for less stable vectors. Many options are available in various configurations based on the cutoff of molecular weight, the membranes' geometry, or the bottle's composition. Although the possible concentration factors are often lower than centrifugation methods, there is an additional benefit during the concentration process. All impurities are removed.

Bioburden control is critical for products with a GMP regulatory requirement to reduce the end product's risk of microbial contamination. In most protocols, the vector's final preparation is filtered as a control component by 0.2 μm filtration, although there are differences in its positioning in downstream protocols. Some vector products are not filtered to sterilize because of their size. Sterile filtration is skipped if the process is accredited as completely aseptic; however, this requires validation and operations that must be carried out in a cleanroom.

11.2.3 Risks of Gene Therapy

- Gene therapy or cell therapy may not be as effective as intended, potentially prolonging or aggravating symptoms or complicating the disease with adverse therapy effects.
- The genetic material expression or stem cell survival is insufficient. As a result, it is too short-lived to heal or improve the disease altogether, or the replacement of proteins causes a robust immune response to the protein.
- The immune response becomes unregulated and results in attacks on normal proteins or cells, as in autoimmune diseases.
- Cancer or viral/fungal/bacterial infections are involved, causing an inadequate immune response inducing therapy resistance.
- There is no way to "switch off" gene expression with the current generation of vectors in clinical trials if it seems to cause harmful effects.

- The integration of the genetic material into DNA might occur alongside a gene involved in regulating cell growth from the retroviral or lentiviral vectors. The insertion induces a tumor over time through the insertion mutagenesis.
- There is little data on affecting the embryo in pregnancy.
- There is a lack of tight control over the stem cell division resulting in transplanted stem cells gaining growth advantage and advance to a type of cancer or teratomas.

11.2.4 Gene Editing

Gene editing changes an organism's DNA by adding, removing, or altering a genome's particular location. A variety of technologies are available, as shown in Figure 11.6. Today's most important technology is CRISPRs (clustered regularly interspaced short palindromic repeats), which bacteria use to create immunity against viruses. It comprises short sequences coming from the viral genome that gets incorporated into the bacterial genome. The Cas (CRISPR-associated proteins) cuts the matching viral DNA sequences, so by introducing plasmids containing Cas genes, the eukaryotic genome is cut at any desired position. The FDA has not yet approved any gene-editing product; recently, a CRISPR-based diagnostic kit was approved for COVID-19 monitoring. The 2020 Noble Prize in Chemistry went to Emmanuelle Charpentier of the Max Planck Unit for the Science of Pathogens, Berlin, Germany, and Jennifer A. Doudna of the University of California, Berkeley, USA, for the discovery of the CRISPR technology.

Cells are the basic building blocks of all living things; the human body is composed of trillions. Within our cells, thousands of genes provide the information to produce specific proteins and enzymes that make muscles, bones, and blood, supporting most of our body's functions, such as digestion, making energy, and growing. When cells become defective or turn nonfunctional, they are supplemented

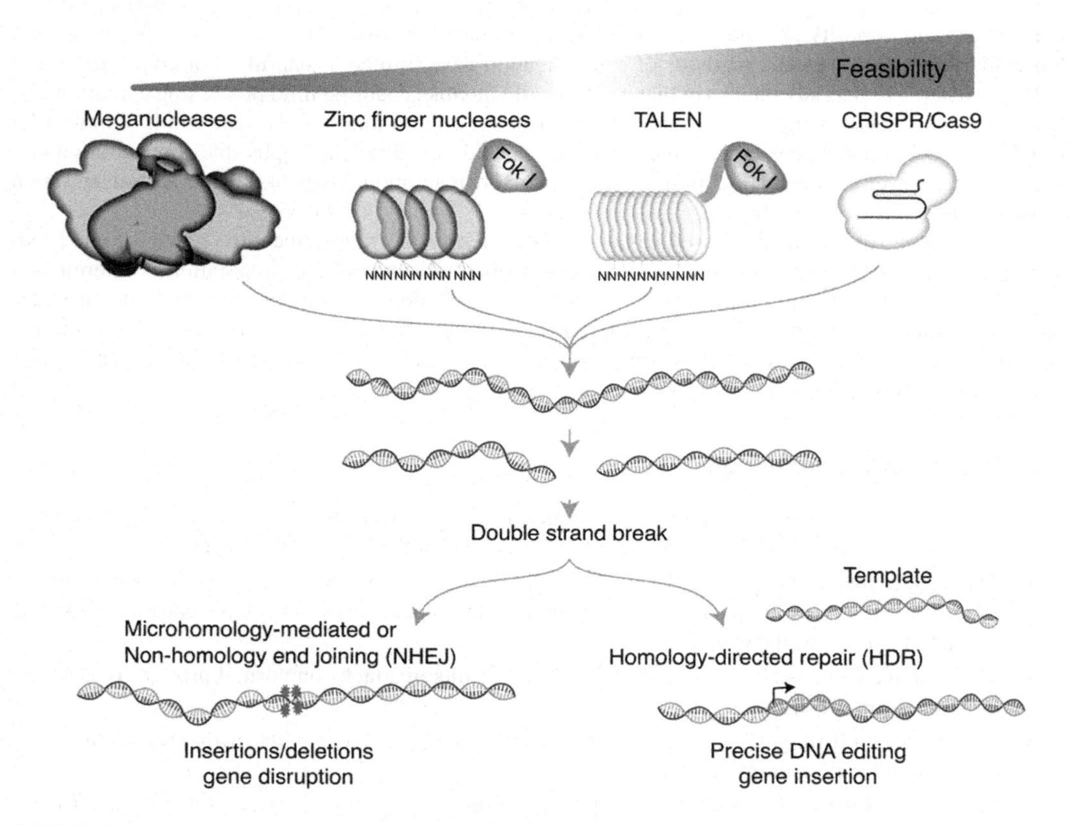

FIGURE 11.6 Comparison of four gene-editing technologies. Source: https://en.wikipedia.org/wiki/Genome_editing.

with cells; the best example of cell therapy is blood transfusion, but that doesn't constitute a biological product. Somatic (relating to the body and not mind) cell therapy is the administration of autologous (cells obtained from the same person), allogeneic (same type of tissue cells from another person), or xenogeneic (foreign) living cells that have been manipulated or processed ex vivo. Ex vivo propagation, expansion, selection, or pharmacologic treatment of cells and other biological changes are part of the manufacturing process for somatic cell therapy products. These cellular products could also be used for diagnosis or prevention.

In gene therapy, we replace a gene that causes a disease with one that doesn't add genes to help the body fight or treat disease or turn off genes that produce disease. To insert new genes directly into cells, the vehicle is a "vector," genetically engineered to deliver the gene. For example, viruses have a natural ability to deliver genetic material into cells and are used as vectors. Before a virus can carry therapeutic genes into human cells, it is modified to remove its ability to cause infectious disease.

When a cell is genetically modified, this is a combination of cell-gene therapy.

Gene therapy is performed both inside and outside the body. A gene can be defective or missing in whole or part from birth or change or mutate during adulthood. Any of these variations can cause problems with protein synthesis, resulting in disease (Figure 11.7).

Gene therapy requiring genetic modification outside of the body needs a vector injected carrying the gene directly into the part of the body with defective cells. In gene therapy used to modify cells outside of the body, blood, bone marrow, or another tissue is taken from a patient, and specific types of cells are separated in the lab. The vector containing the desired gene is introduced into these cells. The cells can multiply in the lab before being injected back into the patient, continuing to multiply until the desired effect is achieved (Figure 11.8).

11.2.5 Techniques

The key methods used to prevent or treat diseases in gene therapy include the following.

- The insertion of genes entails injecting a new copy of a gene into the target cells to produce more protein. A mutated virus such as an adeno-associated virus (AAV) is most commonly used that brings the genome into the cells. Gene-added treatments are applied to many diseases, including extreme combination immunodeficiency adenosine deaminase (ADA-SCID), hemophilia, Leber's congenital amaurosis, congenital blindness, lysosomal storage diseases, X-linked chronic granulomatous disease, and many more.
- Gene repair is accomplished by altering part of a gene using a recently developed gene-altering technique (e.g., CRISPR-Cas9, TALEN, or ZFN) to delete repetitive or abnormal gene elements or replace an impaired or faulty DNA region. Gene correction produces a protein that

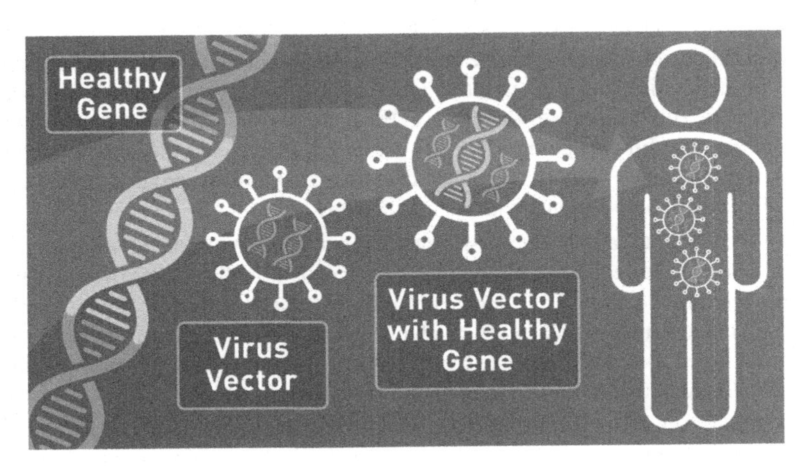

FIGURE 11.7 Mechanism of gene therapy. Source: www.flickr.com/photos/fdaphotos/39151355192/in/photostream/.

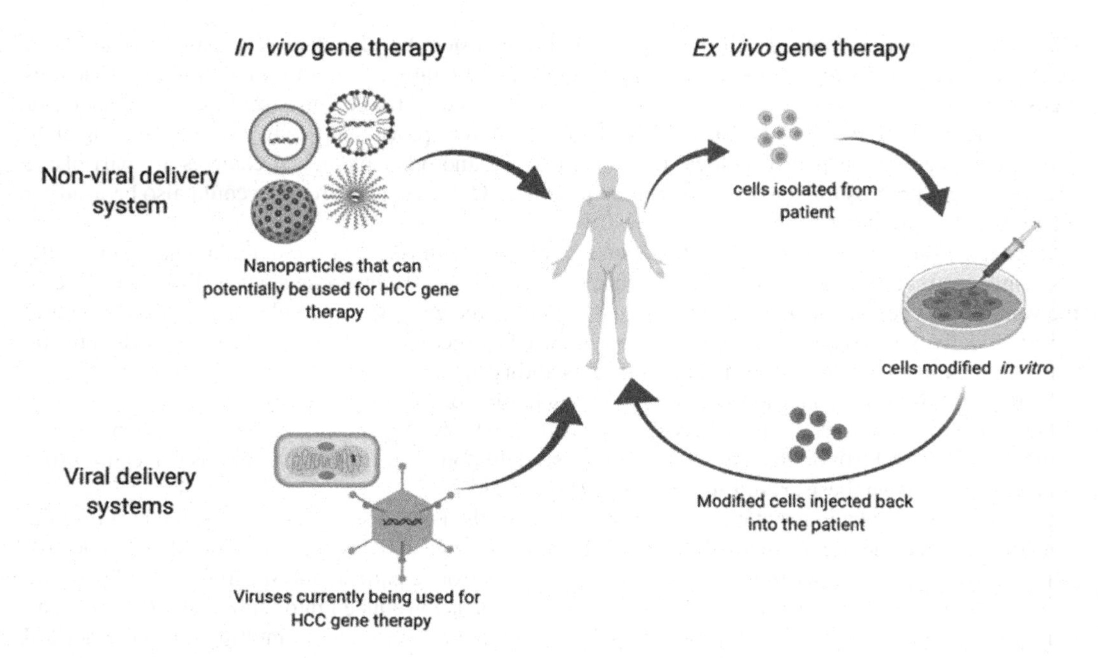

FIGURE 11.8 Comparison of in vivo and ex vivo gene therapy. Source: Reghupaty, SC and Sarkar, D. Current Status of Gene Therapy in Hepatocellular Carcinoma. ***Cancers***. 2019;11:1265.

functions naturally to treat the disease. Gene repair is used to diagnose a wide variety of diseases; recent scientific research has used gene editing techniques to remove HIV from the genome of infected laboratory mice and eliminate from the human gene the enlarged area responsible for Huntington's disease.

- Gene silencing stops a specific protein from being created by targeting messenger RNA (mRNA). The mRNA occurs in both human and animal cells in a single-stranded form, whereas viruses have double-stranded RNA. Human and animal cells identify and kill double-stranded RNA as being viral to prevent it from spreading. Genome silencing uses limited RNA sequences to bind to double-strand special sequences in the target mRNA. It allows mRNA degradation using the cellular machinery that kills viral RNA. Gene silencing is useful for treating disorders. There is an overproduction of protein; for example, in rheumatoid arthritis, the alpha tumor necrosis factor is abundant (TNF) in the joints. Cell silencing targets only the affected tissue to reduce the TNF alpha levels.
- Reprogramming involves adding single or multiple genes to a specific cell to change its properties. This procedure is especially effective in tissues where several types of cells occur, and a disruption in one cell type causes the disease. For example, diabetes type happens when many of the pancreas' insulin-producing islet cells get damaged. Around the same time, no damage is done to the pancreatic cells that produce digestive enzymes. Reprogramming such cells to produce insulin will help patients with type 1 diabetes.
- Cell removal techniques are used to destroy malignant (cancer) tumor cells and target the overgrowth of healthy (non-cancer) tumor cells. Tumor cells are eliminated by inserting "suicide genes" into the tumor cells and releasing a prodrug that causes cell death in those cells. Viruses are designed to have tumor cell affinity. Such oncotropic viruses can carry therapeutic genes to enhance tumor cell toxicity to activate the immune system to fight the tumor or prevent blood vessels' development that provides nutrients for the tumor.
- In 2015, Chinese scientists published a paper outlining the use of a CRISPR-Cas9 for editing the gene responsible for β-thalassemia in embryos. The germline gene therapy is an experimental procedure that modifies the reproductive cells (eggs or sperm) or pregnancy cells to

establish heritable genetic modification. The germ cells from sperm or egg cells are modified by inserting activated genes into their genomes in germline gene therapy (GGT). Altering a germ cell causes the modified gene to be present in all cells of the organism. Thus, the alteration is heritable and passes on to later generations. Many countries, including Australia, Canada, Germany, Israel, Switzerland, and the Netherlands, ban GGT for human use, citing potential threats to future generations and higher risks than SCGT. The US does not have any federal laws explicitly targeting human genetic engineering (over and above FDA therapy regulations).

11.2.6 Gene Editing Technologies

Genome engineering came into existence in the 1970s, when it was shown that yeast and bacteria could take up exogenous DNA and be randomly integrated into the genome. A variety of techniques are currently used for gene editing.

- Cre-Lox recombination is a site-specific recombinase technique to conduct deletions, insertions, translocations, and cell DNA reversals at specific sites. This technique requires altering the DNA to be targeted to a particular cell or activated by an external stimulus. It is applied in both eukaryotic and prokaryotic systems.
- LoxP (locus of X[cross]-over locus in P1) sites are 34-base-pair long recognition sequences consisting of two 13-bp long palindromic repeats, separated by an asymmetric core spacer sequence 8-bp.
- FLP-FRT recombination is a site-driven recombination technique similar to the recombination of Cre-Lox. It involves recombining sequences between the short flippase recognition target (FRT) sites by recombinase flippase (Flp) produced from the saccharomyces cerevisiae baker's yeast 2μ plasmid.
- Homologous recombination is a type of genetic recombination in which nucleotide sequences are shared between two similar or identical double-stranded or single-stranded nucleic acid molecules (usually DNA, as in cellular organisms, but is RNA, in viruses).
- Zinc finger nucleases (ZFNs) are artificial restriction enzymes created by fusing a zinc finger's DNA-binding domain to a DNA cleavage.
- Transcription activator-like effector nucleases (TALEN) are restriction enzymes programmed to sever specific DNA sequences. They are made by fusing a DNA-binding domain of the TAL effector to a DNA cleavage domain (a nuclease that breaks DNA strands).
- The Sleeping Beauty transposon is a synthetic DNA transposon designed to introduce accurately defined DNA sequences into vertebrate animal chromosomes to introduce new traits and discover new genes and functions.
- Recombineering (recombination-mediated genetic engineering) is a genetic and molecular biology technique focused on homologous recombination systems, in contrast to the older/more common method of mixing DNA sequences in a specified order using restrictive enzymes and leagues.

11.2.7 CRISPR

The CRISPR-Cas system is a prokaryotic immune system that protects foreign genetic elements such as those found in plasmids and phages that provide a source of immunity gained. RNA harboring the spacer gene allows us to recognize and split foreign pathogenic DNA by Cas (CRISPR-associated) proteins. Specific Cas proteins that are directed by RNA break international RNA. CRISPR is present in about 50% of sequenced bacterial genomes and almost 90% of sequenced archaea. Cas9 (or CRISPR-associated protein 9) is an enzyme that uses CRISPR sequences as a tool for identifying and cleaving specific DNA strands complementing the CRISPR gene. With CRISPR sequences, Cas9 enzymes form the basis of a technology known as CRISPR-Cas9, which is used to modify genes within humans. This

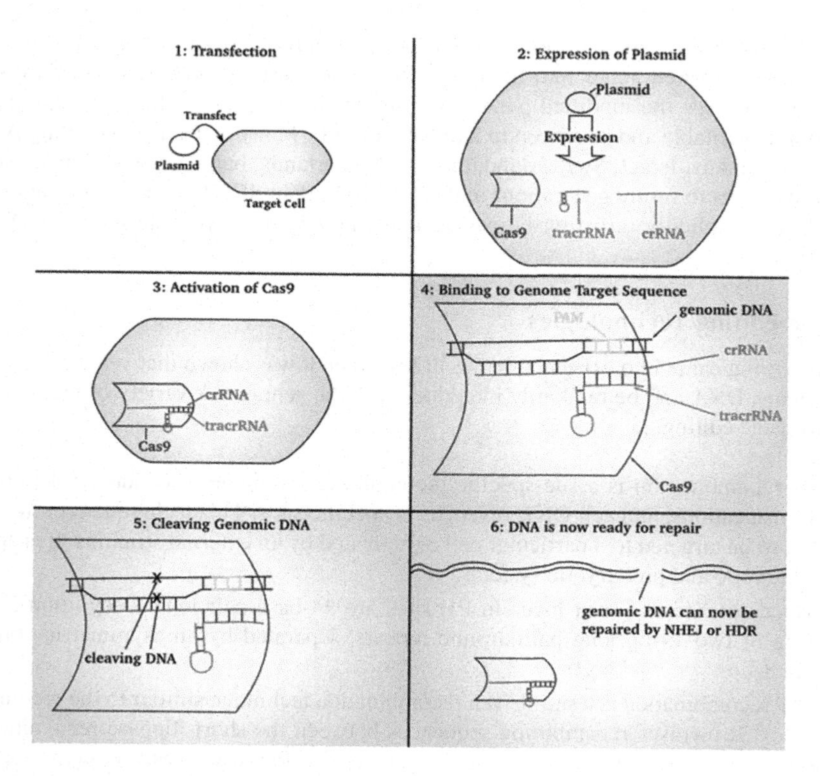

FIGURE 11.9 CRISPR system. Source: By Nielsrca—own work based on figures in ***Nature Protocols***, CC BY-SA 4.0, https://commons.wikimedia.org/w/index.php?curid=45011253.

editing process has a wide range of fundamental biological research, biomedical product development, and disease treatment (Figure 11.9). The ability to modify different DNA sequences gives it an instrument to repair mutations that cause disease.

CRISPR's impact is also proving disruptive and revolutionary, with the potential to irreversibly alter drug discovery and pre-clinical development in a variety of ways. For example, disease-relevant cellular reporter models manipulated to reflect disease phenotypes are one set of CRISPR applications that should be on every drug hunter's radar. While the move away from in vitro and immortalized cell assay systems has been underway for a decade, the pace has accelerated by introducing easily manipulated stem cells for creating fit-for-purpose biochemical and high content, high throughput screens. In addition, the use of CRISPR editing to create organotypic and disease-specific models, as well as the direct use of patient-sourced cells and assembled organoids (disease and control) as platforms for drug SAR and efficacy testing, has been a significant advance.

Such cells are generated in sufficient numbers to perform whole-genome genetic screens to identify molecular and cellular mechanisms of disease and therapeutic targets and high throughput drug screening to identify compounds that can revert the disease phenotype. In addition, differences between patient-derived and control cells are used to identify potential therapeutic targets or agents. A compelling example in an underserved area of research lies in developing CRISPR-driven new assays for glioblastoma. CRISPR manipulation is ineffective for knocking in or knocking out traits/phenotypes targeted and modulated by candidate drugs via activation (CRISPRa) or interference (CRISPRi) (Figure 11.10). The technology is also extensible to organoids, deriving additional informational value from this more physiologically meaningful cell platform.

CRISPR-based cell reporter assays are notable for avoiding the inconsistencies (or outright impossibility) of either stable or transient transfection in attaching the reporter to a target regulatory element at specific gene loci. With benchmark methodology, representative implementations include tagging with luciferases and luminescent proteins for high throughput and high content imaging assays.

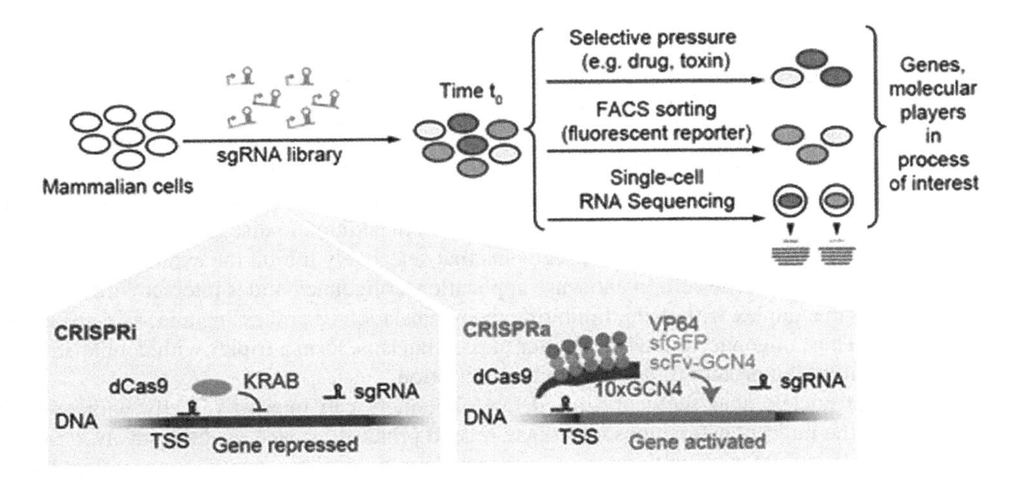

FIGURE 11.10 Elucidating drug targets and mechanisms of action by genetic screens in mammalian cells. Source: Kampmann, *Chem. Comm.* 2016 (not O/A), http://rsc.li/2jlNTRa.

The CRISPR-Cas9 system, which allows for targeted genome editing, holds great promise for the future of medicine. CRISPR (clustered regularly interspaced short palindromic repeats) is a system made up of two key molecules: Cas9, a "molecular scissors" capable of cutting the two strands of DNA at a specific location in the genome, and gRNA, a pre-designed RNA sequence within a larger RNA scaffold. The latter's job is to direct Cas9's "scissors" to the desired location in the DNA. The CRISPR-Cas9 gene-editing technique has forever changed biomedical research. The CRISPR-Cas9 system is more straightforward, more precise, and relatively cheaper than its "predecessors," such as zinc finger nucleases (ZFNs) and transcription activator-like effector nucleases (TALENs), making it an ideal vehicle for "playing with the genome."

CRISPR stands for clustered regularly interspaced short palindromic repeats, and the CRISPR-Cas9 gene-editing system is a huge step forward in our ability to edit DNA efficiently and precisely. Short guide RNAs (sgRNA) are used in this technique to target and edit a specific DNA location. However, the guide RNA can fit multiple DNA locations, resulting in unintended consequences (off-target effects). Thus, a significant bottleneck in applying the CRISPR system is the careful selection of guide RNA with the fewest dangerous side effects. For predicting the degree of both guide-target interactions and off-target effects for a given sgRNA, machine learning models have been shown to produce the best results. This could hasten the development of guide RNA for every segment of human DNA.

Human gene therapy is defined as the introduction of new genetic material into the cells of an individual to produce a therapeutic benefit. Several human diseases are genetic in origins, such as Huntington's chorea, cystic fibrosis, and many heredity connections. Replacing the defective gene(s) with a normal healthy gene (gene therapy) is the most potent future technology using DNA as a drug to restore a function, not correct it. Drugs approved for somatic gene therapy do not alter the genetic makeup of offspring. It is possible in germline gene therapy to target the gametes (sperm and ova) unborn subjects. Gene transfer at an early stage of embryonic development can alter somatic and germline cells—the germline gene therapy.

Nucleic acid-based drugs offer selective recognition of molecular targets and pathways, making it most specific and include plasmids, oligonucleotides for antisense and antigene applications, DNA aptamers, and DNAzymes. In gene therapy, gene transfer technologies are DNA delivery systems for nucleic acid-based therapeutics. Examples include cancer, AIDS, neurological disorders such as Parkinson's disease and Alzheimer's disease, and cardiovascular disorders. The elucidation of the human genome has also accelerated the identification of human genes involved in diseases, potentially leading to DNA and RNA-based drugs for gene replacement or potential gene ablation targets. The Human Genome Project will aid in the discovery of genetic markers responsible for drug response, drug interactions, and potential side effects in patients.

11.2.8 DNA-Based Therapeutics

Plasmids are double-stranded DNA constructs with high molecular weight transgenes that encode specific proteins. Plasmid DNA molecules are considered pro-drugs because they use the cell's DNA transcription and translation apparatus to biosynthesize the therapeutic entity, the protein, after being internalized. The plasmid DNA mechanism requires that plasmid molecules gain access to the nucleus after entering the cytoplasm. The efficiency of gene expression is ultimately controlled by nuclear access or lack thereof. Plasmids are used as DNA vaccines for genetic immunization in addition to disease treatment.

Oligonucleotides are single-stranded DNA segments that selectively inhibit the expression of a single protein when internalized by the cell. In antisense applications, oligonucleotides interact with mRNA or pre-mRNA and form a duplex with them, inhibiting their translation or processing and, as a result, protein biosynthesis. Thus, oligonucleotides must enter the cell nucleus, form a triplex with double-stranded genomic DNA, and inhibit protein translation and transcription.

Double-stranded nucleic acid segments called DNA-aptamers can interact directly with proteins. Aptamers disrupt the molecular functions of disease-related proteins, as well as those involved in transcription and translation. Because of their specificity, non-immunogenicity, and pharmaceutical formulation stability, aptamers are preferred over antibodies in protein inhibition. HIV-1 integrase enzyme DNA-aptamers have shown promise in the intervention of pathogenic protein biosynthesis.

DNAzymes are analogs of ribozymes with more excellent biological stability. DNA motifs replace the RNA backbone chemistry, resulting in increased biological stability.

11.2.9 Gene Transfer Technologies

Gene transfer technologies or DNA delivery methods are classified into three general types; electrical techniques, mechanical transfection, and vector-assisted delivery systems.

11.2.9.1 Mechanical and Electrical Techniques

Mechanical and electrical strategies of introducing naked DNA into cells include microinjection, particle bombardment, pressure, and electroporation. Microinjection is highly efficient since one cell is targeted for DNA transfer; however, this precision is achieved at the expense of time. Ballistic transfer of gold micro-particles is achieved using particle bombardment equipment such as the gene gun used to transfer gold microparticles. To facilitate DNA transfer, electroporation employs a high-voltage electrical current.

11.2.9.2 Vector-Assisted Delivery Systems

Vector-assisted DNA/gene delivery systems are classified as biological viral DNA delivery systems and chemical nonviral delivery systems. Nonpathogenic attenuated viruses, particularly plasmids, are used as delivery systems for genes/DNA molecules in viral delivery systems. Both RNA and DNA viruses are used as viral DNA delivery vectors. The viruses used as gene therapy vectors include retroviruses, adenoviruses, adeno-associated viruses, and herpes simplex viruses. Gene expression using viral vectors successfully delivered to the kidney, heart muscle, eye, and ovary.

Retroviral vectors used in gene therapy are replication-deficient, such that they are unable to replicate in the host cell and can infect only one cell, and are widely used. For example, adenoviruses deliver therapeutic DNA to patients suffering from metastatic breast, ovarian, and melanoma cancer. The gutless adenoviral vectors, which lack all viral genes, have facilitated adenoviral delivery of up to 30 Kb of a therapeutic DNA sequence with decreased toxicity.

The use of adeno-associated viral (AAV) vectors for gene therapy provides an alternative to adenoviral vectors and a method for long-term gene expression with a lower risk of adverse reactions after vector administration. AAV viruses are single-stranded DNA parvoviruses with a linear genome that cause no disease in humans. The chromosome is where AAV viral DNA is integrated into humans. Most of the AAV genome is replaced with the therapeutic gene in AAV vector engineering, which reduces adverse reactions. Despite this, the therapeutic gene is only about 5 kilobytes in size.

Herpes simplex virus (HSV) vector is a large and relatively complex enveloped, double-stranded DNA virus that can encode large therapeutic genes. Like AAV, it can remain latent in infected cells providing the potential for long-term expression of the therapeutic gene. However, HSV vectors are currently limited in their use due to vector toxicity, despite their ability to infect a wide range of cell types.

Non-viral delivery systems have the most significant advantage over viral delivery systems in the lack of immune response and ease of formulation and assembly. Commonly used non-viral vectors for delivering DNA-based therapeutics are naked DNA delivery systems, polymeric delivery systems, and liposomal delivery systems.

Naked DNA is administered either by ex vivo or in vivo delivery. The naked DNA delivery method has successfully introduced DNA into endothelial and smooth muscle cells ex vivo. However, its reliance on the culture of harvested cells renders it unsuitable for many cell types. In vivo delivery of naked DNA using particle bombardment technology enables localized DNA delivery readily into skin or muscle. Another technique for the delivery of naked DNA directly into target cells is electroporation.

Cationic polymers are used in polymeric delivery systems to deliver genes because they can easily complex with anionic DNA molecules. These poly-complexes' mechanism of action is based on the generation of a positively charged complex due to the electrostatic interaction of these cationic polymers with anionic DNA. Commonly used polymers include polyethyleneimine (PEI), poly-L-lysine (PLL), chitosans, and dendrimers. Agents such as folates, transferrin, antibodies, or sugars such as galactose and mannose are also incorporated for tissue targeting. Synthetic polymers such as protective interactive non-condensing polymers (PINC), poly-L-lysine, cationic polymers, and dendrimers offer an alternative to cationic lipids as a vehicle for DNA delivery into target cells. The encapsulation of a DNA molecule or even a therapeutic viral vector within a biodegradable polymer allows for weeks or months of controlled DNA release in a targeted cell. However, some polymers have pharmacological properties that make them unsuitable for specific applications (for example, chitosans cause hypercholesterolemia).

Liposomes are one of the most versatile tools for the delivery of DNA therapeutics. Liposome and drug/lipid complexes have been used to deliver the anticancer drugs doxorubicin and daunorubicin. Liposomes are used as DNA drug delivery systems by encasing DNA-based therapeutics inside the aqueous core or complexing them with phospholipid lamellae. Liposomes are also used for specialized gene delivery, such as long circulation half-life, sustained delivery, and targeted delivery.

As an alternative to cationic lipids, the potential of anionic lipids for DNA delivery is also possible but not practical inefficient entrapment of DNA molecules within anionic liposomes caused by electrostatic repulsion between these negatively charged species.

pH-sensitive liposomes, immunoliposomes, and stealth liposomes are examples of specialized liposomal delivery platforms. Liposomes containing 1,2-dioleoyl-3-phosphoethanolamine (DOPE) are made by mixing them with acidic lipids like cholesteryl hemisuccinate or oleic acid.

It's also possible to use pH-sensitive liposomes. These lipids have a typical bilayer structure at neutral cellular pH 7. Still, upon endosomal compartmentalization, they undergo protonation and collapse into a non-bilayer structure, causing the endosomal bilayer to be disrupted and destabilized, allowing for the rapid release of DNA into the cytoplasm. Citraconyl-DOPE, a chemical derivative of DOPE, is used to deliver DNA-based therapeutics to cancer cells, combining the targeting and rapid endosome-releasing characteristics of specialized liposomal delivery systems.

11.2.10 Approved Products

As of the end of 2020, the gene and cell therapy products approved by global regulatory agencies are listed in Table 11.2. Readers can update the information by visiting www.fda.gov/vaccines-blood-biologics/cellular-gene-therapy-products/approved-cellular-and-gene-therapy-products.

11.3 Cell Therapy

Cell therapy is a substitution of cells within a patient to treat diseases to produce specialized cells continuously. Cell therapy originated in the 19th century when scientists experimented with preventing

TABLE 11.2

Approved Gene Therapy and Cell Therapy Products

Product	Treatment/Indication
Allogeneic cultured keratinocytes and fibroblasts in bovine collagen (Gintuit)	An allogeneic cellularized scaffold product indicated for topical (non-submerged) application surgically created vascular wound bed to treat mucogingival conditions in adults.
Autologous CD34+ enriched cell fraction (Strimvelis)	The first ex vivo stem cell gene therapy treats a rare disease ADA-SCID (severe combined immunodeficiency adenosine deaminase deficiency).
Autologous cultured chondrocytes on a porcine collagen membrane (MACI)	Indicated for repairing single or multiple symptomatic, full-thickness cartilage defects of the knee with or without bone involvement in adults. MACI is an autologous cellularized scaffold product.
Azficel-T (Laviv)	A medication for improving the appearance of moderate to severe nasolabial fold wrinkles in adults.
Betibeglogene autotemcel (Zynteglo)	A treatment for beta-thalassemia, a rare and potentially debilitating blood disorder.
Axicabtagene ciloleucel (KTE-C19, Axi-cel, Yescarta)	Treatment for large B cell lymphoma that has failed conventional treatment. The patient T cells are genetically engineered and returned to the patient to populate the bone marrow.
Eteplirsen (Exondys 51)	Treats types of Duchenne muscular dystrophy (DMD) caused by a specific mutation. Eteplirsen is a form of antisense therapy.
Gendicine	A recombinant adenovirus engineered to express wildtype-p53 (rAd-p53) designed to treat patients with mutated p53 genes.
Glybera (alipogene tiparvovec)	Reverses lipoprotein lipase deficiency (LPLD), a rare inherited disorder that can cause severe pancreatitis.
Macugen (pegaptanib sodium injection)	An anti-angiogenic treatment of neovascular (wet) age-related macular degeneration (AMD).
Mipomersen (Kynamro)	Used to treat homozygous familial hypercholesterolemia and administered by subcutaneous injection.
Neovasculgen cambiogen plasmid	Treatment of peripheral artery disease, including critical limb ischemia; delivers the gene encoding for a vascular endothelial growth factor (VEGF). It was developed by the Human Stem Cells Institute in Russia and approved Russia in 2011.
Nusinersen (Spinraza)	Treats spinal muscular atrophy (SMA), a rare neuromuscular disorder.
Onasemnogene abeparvovec (Zolgensma)	Treats spinal muscular atrophy (SMA).
Patisiran (Onpattro)	A double-stranded small interfering ribonucleic acid (siRNA) formulated for targeted delivery to hepatocytes, the primary source of transthyretin (TTR) protein production
Provenge (Sipuleucel-T)	To treat asymptomatic or minimally symptomatic metastatic castrate-resistant (hormone-refractory) prostate cancer.
Single-stranded oligonucleotide (Defitelio)	A mixture of single-stranded oligonucleotides purified from the intestinal mucosa of pigs. It is used to treat the liver's Veno-occlusive disease, having had a bone marrow transplant.
Talimogene laherparepvec (Imlygic)	Indicated in the local treatment of unresectable cutaneous, subcutaneous, and nodal lesions in patients with recurrent melanoma after the initial surgery.
Tisagenlecleucel (Kymriah)	A treatment of B cell acute lymphoblastic leukemia (ALL) uses the body's T cells to fight cancer (adoptive cell transfer). It is a genetically engineered herpes virus (an oncolytic herpes virus). Two genes were removed—one that shuts down an individual cell's defenses and another that helps the virus evade the immune system, and a gene for human GM-CSF was added.
Voretigene neparvovec (Luxturna)	Treats Leber's congenital amaurosis. It is the first in vivo gene therapy approved by the FDA. Leber's congenital amaurosis, or biallelic RPE65-mediated inherited retinal disease, is an inherited disorder causing progressive blindness.

and treating disease by injecting animal tissue. Although such efforts yielded little positive benefit, subsequent studies showed in the mid-20th century that human cells could be used to help prevent donor organs from being rejected by the human body, leading in time to successful bone marrow transplantation as it is now a common practice in treating patients having damaged bone marrow following disease, infection, radiation or chemotherapy. However, in recent decades, researchers have gained significant interest in stem cell-and cell transplantation as a potential new therapeutic strategy for a wide range of diseases, particularly for degenerative and immunogenic pathologies.

Blood transfusion is the most common cell therapy and donor transfusion of red blood cells, white blood cells, and platelets. Another popular cell therapy is hematopoietic stem cell transplantation, to produce bone marrow has been performed for over 40 years.

Somatic (relating to the body and not mind) cell therapy is the administration of autologous (cells obtained from the same person), allogeneic (same type of tissue cells from another person), or xenogeneic (foreign) living cells that have been manipulated or processed ex vivo. Ex vivo propagation, expansion, selection, or pharmacologic treatment of cells and other biological changes are part of the manufacturing process for somatic cell therapy products. These cellular products could also be used for diagnosis or prevention.

The cells used in cell therapy are pluripotent cells that convert into all types of cells in the body or multipotent cells that can convert into only or other types of cells. Implantation of cells as an in vivo source of a molecular species such as an enzyme, cytokine, or coagulation factor; implantation of manipulated cell populations such as hepatocytes, myoblasts, or pancreatic islet cells to perform a complex biological function; and infusion of activated lymphoid cells, such as lymphokine-activated ki67 cells, are all examples of somatic cell therapies.

Cells for therapeutic purposes are delivered by infusion, injection at various sites, or surgically implanting in aggregated form or along with solid supports or in encapsulated materials. The matrices, fibers, beads, or other materials used in addition to the cells are listed as excipients, additional active components, or medical devices. The most common type of cell therapy is blood transfusion.

Gene therapy and cell therapy are often used together, where stem cells are removed from a patient, genetically modified in tissue culture to produce a new gene, expanded to sufficient numbers, and then returned to the patient to relieve the underlying cause of genetic diseases and acquired diseases by replacing the defective protein(s) or cells that trigger the symptoms of the disease, to reverse the symptoms.

Genetic and cell therapy progress shares many ethical problems with other therapies, including prosthetics, medications, organ transplantation, and protein replacement. The issue of contamination of the human genome with novel DNA sequences has two concerns. First, there's the question of unintended genome interference when conducting gene or cell therapy on somatic (adult) cells. To remove this risk, all vectors are tested in laboratory animals to guarantee that they do not enter the germline, and sperm from human males are tested in clinical trials to ensure that the gene is not integrated into the genome. Second, there is the question of deliberate germline manipulation to alleviate disease. While new gene-editing techniques have now the process simpler, there remains much controversy about the ethics of editing or not editing.

The use of embryonic stem cells as a source of stem cells, or human fetal tissue, remains a major ethical issue.

11.3.1 Types of Cell Therapies

There is no standardized system for classifying cell therapies. However, a classification is made based on cell types by cell potency.

- Embryonic stem cells (ESCs). These are pluripotent embryonic stem cells. The embryos involved in isolating stem cells are usually unused embryos produced for assisted reproduction by in vitro fertilization (IVF). Because ESCs are pluripotent, they retain self-renew and shape any cell in the body. Owing to their pluripotency, ESCs have the benefit of flexibility in designing therapeutic strategies posing ethical concerns. Furthermore, the stem cell lines generated from embryos are not genetically suited to the patient, as they increase the risk of the patient's immune system rejecting the transplanted cell.

- Pluripotent induced stem cells (iPSCs). A separated (somatic) adult cell is reprogrammed to return to a pluripotent state, such as a skin cell. These cells give the pluripotency advantage but without embryonic stem cell ethical concerns. Likewise, iPSCs are derived from the patient and therefore avoid immune rejection problems. The iPSCs are developed by transforming an adult cell with a cocktail of genes generally transmitted via a viral vector. While the process efficiency has improved considerably, the relatively low rate of reprogramming is an issue. One issue is that the iPSCs are derived from adult cells and are thus "older" than embryonic stem cells, as demonstrated by a higher rate of programmed cell death, lower rates of DNA damage repair, and increased occurrence of point mutations.
- Embryonic stem cells for nuclear transfer (ntESCs). These pluripotent cells are generated by transferring the nucleus from the patient's adult cell to an oocyte (egg cell) derived from a donor. The nucleus transfer process reprograms the egg cell into pluripotency. The derived cells, including iPSCs, fit the patient's nuclear genome and are unlikely to be rejected by the body. The key advantage of this technique is that the resulting ntESCs bear the patient's nuclear DNA alongside the donor mitochondria, making this method especially appropriate for diseases where the mitochondria are weakened or dysfunctional. A disadvantage of ntESCs is that the generation process is cumbersome and requires a donor oocyte.
- Embryonic stem cells with parthenogenesis (pES). Unfertilized oocytes provide the pluripotent cells treated with chemicals that induce the generation of embryos without the addition of sperm (parthenogenesis) and the harvesting of ESCs from the developing embryo.
- Hematopoietic stem cells (HSCs). These are multipotent stem cells in the blood, which give rise to all blood cell types. HSCs are present in adult bone marrow, peripheral blood, and blood from the umbilical cord. MSCs are multipotent tissue cells, including the umbilical cord, bone marrow, and fat tissue. MSCs result in bone, cartilage, muscle, and adipocytes (fat cells), promoting adipose marrow tissue.
- Nervous stem cells (NSCs). In identified regions of the mammalian brain, adult neural stem cells are present in a limited number. These multipotent cells replenish brain neurons and support brain cells. However, owing to its position inside the brain, adult neural stem cells cannot be derived from patients. The neural stem cells are either obtained from the iPSCs or ESCs.
- Epithelial cells. The stem cells are epithelial that form the body's surfaces and linings, including the epidermis and gastrointestinal tract lining. There are multipotent epithelial stem cells and unipolar stem cells that differentiate into only one cell type in such areas. Epithelial stem cells were successfully employed to rebuild the eye's corneal epithelium.
- Immune cell treatment. Cells that replicate rapidly in the body, such as immune cells, blood cells, or skin cells, are worked ex vivo, provided the conditions are conducive. Blood transfusion is the most common cell therapy and donor transfusion of platelets and white and red blood cells.

11.3.2 CAR-T Therapy

Chimeric antigen receptor T cells (also known as CAR-T cells) are the T cells genetically engineered to produce an artificial T cell receptor for immunotherapy use. Chimeric liposomes (fluid sacs surrounded by a fatty membrane) are more easily absorbed by cells than naked DNA/RNA. Various types of liposomes are used to bind preferentially to specific tissues. In addition, a subtype of membrane vesicles formed and endogenously released by cells (extracellular vesicles or "exosomes") has been used to carry small RNA sequences into specific tissues.

Antigen receptors (CARs, also known as chimeric immunoreceptors, chimeric T cell receptors, or artificial T cell receptors) are receptor proteins designed to allow T cells to access a new protein. The receptors are chimeric in that they combine functions that cause both antigen-binding and T cells to bind into a single receptor.

CAR-T immunotherapy is premised on manipulating T cells to more effectively target and kill cancer cells. CAR-T cells are derived from T cells in the patient's own blood (autologous) or derived from other healthy (allogeneic) donor T cells. Once removed from a human, such T cells are genetically engineered to express a specific CAR, which codes them to target an antigen found on the tumor surface. CAR-T cells are designed for protection to be unique to an antigen found on a tumor not expressed in healthy cells. They act as a "living vaccine" against cancer cells after the CAR-T cells are inserted into a patient. Once they contact a cell with their desired antigen, the CAR-T cells bind to it, activate, increase, and become cytotoxic. CAR-T cells kill cells through various mechanisms, including extensive stimulated cell proliferation, increased cytotoxicity (toxicity to other living cells), and increased secretion of factors that affect other cells, such as cytokines, interleukins, and growth factors.

T cells from human blood are isolated as the first step in the production of CAR-T cells. Then, in a process known as leukocyte apheresis, leukocytes are isolated using a blood cell separator. After that, PBMCs (peripheral blood mononuclear cells) are separated and collected. The leukocyte apheresis products are then transported to a cell processing facility. As a result, specific T cells are stimulated to proliferate and expand in large numbers in the cell processing center. The cytokine interleukin 2 (IL-2) and anti-CD3 antibodies are commonly used to promote T cell expansion.

The expanded T cells are processed and then transduced via a retroviral vector, usually either an integrative gamma retrovirus (RV) or a lentiviral (LV) vector, with a programmed CAR gene encoding. These vectors are safe due to the partial deletion of the U3 region. The new gene-editing tool CRISPR-Cas9 can inject the CAR gene into specific sites within the genome instead of retroviral vectors. Before the activation of the modified CAR-T cells, the patient undergoes lymphodepletion chemotherapy. The reduction of the number of circulating leukocytes in the patient upregulates the number of cytokines released. It reduces resource rivalry, which leads to the expansion of the modified CAR-T cells. T cells are genetically modified to express chimeric antigen receptors specific for antigens found in tumor cells and then injected into the patient, where they attack and kill cancer cells.

The first two CAR-T therapies approved by the FDA target the CD19 antigen found on many B cell cancers. Tisagenlecleucel (Kymriah) is approved for the treatment of relapsed/refractory B cell precursor acute lymphoblastic leukemia (ALL) and axicabtagene ciloleucel (Yescarta/Kite Pharma) is approved for the treatment of B cell lymphoma (DLBCL) relapsed/refractory diffuse.

Newer technologies include using a transposon/transposase-based system that uses DNA plasmids and a process called electroporation to transfer genes into T cells. In addition, to reduce the duration of time from genetic modification to infusion to two days or less, cytokines (interleukin 15) are genetically tethered to the T cell membrane during the CAR-T cell production process; membrane-bound IL-15 (mbIL-15). It is also possible to include multiple antigen receptors. Finally, he argued that the use of cells as a donor graft could be extended in the future to an off-the-shelf, allogeneic T cell therapy from donor cells without the need for gene editing.

CAR-T cells are, without question, a breakthrough in treating cancer. However, serious side effects result from introducing CAR-T cells into the body, including cytokine release syndrome and neurological toxicity. In addition, because it is a relatively new treatment, limited data are available on CAR-T cell therapy's long-term effects. Thus, long-term survival of patients and pregnancy complications in female patients treated with CAR-T cells remain the primary concerns.

11.3.3 Allogenic Cell Therapy

The difference between the allogeneic and the autologous is the source of the therapy cells. Allogeneic therapies are produced from different donor tissues (such as bone marrow) in large batches, while autologous drugs are produced from the recipient being treated as a single lot. For some autologous operations in the clinic or hospital, the patient's cells are treated on-site. These therapies are not regarded as biological products and are not produced under cGMP. While both treatments use similar technologies that are important to cell growth, the scale is different. Allogeneic therapies are "off the market" used to treat multiple patients (sometimes thousands), and there is more time available before delivery in quality control of the medication. Autologous therapies are "normal" items for each patient, and the patient sample identification chain is critical to ensuring the patient is provided with the correct product. Scale-up of production to allogeneic cells is like methods used to produce protein drugs and other large-scale cell-derived components. In contrast, autologous cells require scale-up, simultaneously producing multiple individual products.

The cell therapy scale-up manufacturing solutions will likely be needing batches of up to 2,000 L in single-use disposable formats with matching downstream process hardware.

The newer allogeneic cell therapies are the modified mesenchymal stem cell (MSC) or fibroblast, which are tested for their capacity for lineage differentiation and their effects on immunomodulation and paracrine signaling. A limited number of approved MSC-based products include Prochymal and stem cells for graft versus host disease (GvHD) diagnosis and Cartistem for osteoarthritis. In addition, therapies derived from a pluripotent stem cell (PSC) are currently under development for retinal pigment epithelium (RPE) for macular degeneration treatment, neural lineage cells for spinal cord injury, and pancreatic beta cells insulin-dependent diabetes treatment. So far, the PSC-derived cell drugs are usually grown on a small scale using traditional manual tissue culture approaches. Also emerging is the preclinical development of cardiomyocytes, neurons, and hepatocytes produced from PSC, potentially supplying large markets.

Requirements for cell dosing for these PSC therapies remain uncertain; however, dosing estimates require up to 10^9 cells/patient. With market sizes expected to be in the tens to hundreds of doses for some therapies, it is expected that manufacturing on a commercial scale will require batch sizes between 200 and 2,000 L.

Several factors make the manufacturing of cell therapy unique. These include criteria for properly preserving or regulating cell identification and viability, the need to recover functional cells instead of soluble components at the end of fermentation, and the failure to make the final drug product sterile.

Downstream processing of products for cell therapy is probably the most significant distinction from the traditional bioprocessing field. While upstream cultivation of cell therapy products is performed in equipment initially designed to produce bacterial or CHO cells with relatively minor hardware adaptation, many of the cell harvests, wash, which formulation needs are very different. The cells themselves are the drug product most critical for cell therapeutics and must be recovered consistently with high viability and quality and potency maintenance. In comparison, the protein and virus processing equipment can retain the culture media product, leading to cell death, disruption, or pre-recovery. However, the culture's biological conditions may create additional problems, such as the need to disaggregate normally adherent cells before harvesting. Enzymes are commonly used to dissociate aggregates in the culture vessels, but available harvesting solutions typically require that cells be reduced to a single cell suspension before harvesting. It raises problems around incorporating enzymes, mixing, adequate post-incubation destruction, and removing or inactivating enzymes within a short time.

11.4 Regulatory Considerations

As of June 2020, there were around 3,300 interventional clinical trials undergoing gene therapy. Since every gene in the human genome is targeted, the potential for new therapies is immense. However, no federal legislation lays out the human genetic engineering recommendations or limits. The subject is regulated by local and federal authorities' concurrent legislation, including the Department of Health and Human Services, the Recombinant DNA Advisory Committee of the FDA, and NIH. The NIH serves as the primary agent of gene therapy for federally funded research. Privately funded work is recommended to abide by these rules. The NIH also provides funding for research that advances or enhances genetic engineering techniques and reviews current research ethics and performance. A set of guidelines on gene manipulation has been issued by an NIH advisory committee. The recommendations address the health of laboratories and human test subjects and different types of experiments that involve genetic changes. Before any clinical trials begin, the protocol for a clinical trial of gene therapy must be accepted by the NIH's Recombinant DNA Advisory Committee; this is different from any other form of clinical research.

The FDA provides an extensive list of guidelines for gene and cell therapy at www.fda.gov/vaccines-blood-biologics/biologics-guidances/cellular-gene-therapy-guidances.

The WHO also guides gene therapy products (www.who.int/ethics/topics/human-genome-editing/WHO-Commissioned-Governance-1-paper-March-19.pdf).

Biological products are frequently complex mixtures that are difficult to define. The manufacturing process, as well as the final product, require quality control. Poor production process control can result in the introduction of adventitious agents or other contaminants, as well as accidental changes in the biological product's properties or stability that may not be detectable in final product testing. As a result, the methods and reagents used in the manufacturing process must be defined. Quality control should also be applied to cell banks and key intermediates in the manufacturing process. The lot-to-lot reproducibility of both the final product and critical materials such as vector-containing supernatants should be examined. Existing general regulations (21 CFR 210, 211, 312, and 600) are relevant and should be consulted for guidance.

Phase I of the investigation trial for somatic cell and gene therapy products should be based on data that provide reasonable assurance of safety and rationale. Fewer data are submitted to support beginning exploratory trials than is presented at later stages of product development, especially in severe or life-threatening diseases. The review of data to support the start of phase I trials is primarily concerned with safety, though some evidence of rationale should also be provided.

At a later stage of product development, data from additional product testing should be available. A quantitative potency assay that reflects bioactivity in vivo should be developed to ensure product integrity, and product stability should be investigated. For licensure, evidence of clinical efficacy is required in addition to safety.

If a product's formulation is changed during development, quantitative biological potency assays and when appropriate, preclinical safety evaluation should be used to compare the different formulations. Suppose the product used in later phase trials differs significantly from that used in earlier trials, and the results of earlier trials are critical to the final product evaluation. In that case, product comparability should be demonstrated, or the sponsor should consider whether earlier trials should be repeated.

Manufacturing information is submitted in a master file for vectors used in multiple INDs to make the filing process more accessible. There is no such thing as an "approved" or "disapproved" master file or the product it describes. The master file, on the other hand, contains information and data that support the IND. Using the same product for different patient populations may raise different issues or indicate acceptable risk levels. Still, the master file can help identify common issues and facilitate their efficient resolution. Multiple IND sponsors are authorized to cross-reference a master file, reducing redundant submissions and retaining desired confidentiality.

11.4.1 Development and Characterization of Cell Populations for Administration (https://www.fda.gov/media/72402/download)

11.4.1.1 Collection of Cells

The following information should be provided:

- Cell types: The origin of the cells used should be classified as autologous, allogeneic, or xenogeneic. The source of the tissue, as well as any other pertinent identifying information, should be provided.
- Donor selection criteria: Any relevant characteristics of the donor(s), such as age and gender, should be specified. Allogeneic donors should meet the standards for blood donors (21 CFR 640.3), the testing and acceptance procedures should be described, and any deviations should be justified, according to the "Points to Consider in the Collection, Processing, and Testing of Ex-Vivo-Activated Mononuclear Leukocytes for Administration to Humans." Additional Public Health Service recommendations about organ and tissue donors should be incorporated where applicable. The presence or likelihood of HIV-1 and HIV-2, hepatitis B and C viruses, HTLV-1, and other infectious agents should be used as exclusion criteria. Donor data such as serological, diagnostic, and clinical history should be specified. In some cases, it will be necessary to provide for donor follow-up, and methods for securing donor data and maintaining records should be thoroughly described.

If autologous cells are used, additional guidance on adventitious agent testing and labeling can be found in "A Proposed Approach to the Regulation of Cellular and Tissue-Based Products," February 28, 1997 (62 FR 9721). Suppose animal species other than humans are used. In that case, a description should be provided of the origin, relevant genetic traits, husbandry, and health status of the herd or colony (more information is available in the "PHS Guidelines on Infectious Disease Issues in Xenotransplantation," August 1996 (61 FR 49920) and January 1997 (62 FR 3563) (FDA 1998).

11.4.1.2 Tissue Typing

If allogeneic donors are to be used, polymorphisms such as blood type should be typed when necessary. In addition, the importance of histocompatibility antigen matching between donor and recipient (HLA classes I and II, and possibly minor antigens in some cases) should be discussed, and typing procedures and acceptance criteria.

Suppose it is necessary or indicated to use cell mixtures from multiple donors. In that case, special attention should be paid to potential cell interactions that could result in immune responses or other changes that could affect the cells' performance.

Multiple-donor cell mixtures are challenging to characterize. Multiple-donor cell mixture products would not meet the criteria for regulation as human cellular or tissue-based products under section 361 of the Public Health Service Act, as outlined in the "Proposed Approach to the Regulation of Cellular and Tissue-Based Products," February 28, 1997 (62 FR 9721) (the PHS Act). The Federal Food, Drug, and Cosmetic Act and section 351 of the Public Health Service Act would apply to such products (FDA 1998).

11.4.1.3 Procedures

The procedures for collecting cells, including the facility's location, and any devices or materials used, should be submitted (FDA 1998).

11.4.1.3.1 Cell Culture Procedures

- Procedures for quality control: Cell culture operations should be carefully managed in terms of material quality, manufacturing controls, and equipment validation and monitoring in general.
- For all media and components, including serum additives and growth factors, validation of serum additives and growth factors and freedom from adventitious agents should be established. It's essential to keep track of the culture media components, including their sources and lot numbers. As medium components that can cause sensitization, certain animal sera, selected proteins, and blood group substances, for example, should be avoided. To ensure the reproducibility of cell culture characteristics, identity, purity, and potency, measures for growth factors should be established. Because of the risk of severe hypersensitivity reactions in patients, it is recommended that penicillin and other beta-lactam antibiotics be avoided during production.
- Cell cultures with adventitious agents: Documentation should be provided that cells are handled, propagated, and subjected to laboratory procedures under conditions that minimize adventitious agent contamination. Cells should be tested for contamination regularly during long-term culturing. Bacteria, yeast, mold, mycoplasma, and adventitious viruses should all be tested for in cells.
- Monitoring cell identity and heterogeneity: Manufacturing and testing procedures should be implemented to ensure cell culture identity and heterogeneity are controlled.

Practices and facilities for cell culture should be designed to prevent contamination of one cell culture with another.

Extensive drift in a cell population's properties, or overgrowth by a different cell type previously present in low numbers, can occur during cell culturing. Cell identity should be assessed quantitatively to detect such changes by monitoring cell surface antigens or biochemical markers. The identification method should detect contamination or replacement by other cells in use in the facility. Limits for acceptable culture composition should be established. Quantitative functional potency assays can sometimes be used to phenotype populations. When cells are manipulated, the desired function should be monitored, and tests should be performed regularly to ensure that the desired trait is retained. In some cases, identity testing should include donor-recipient matching and immunological phenotyping.

- Suppose the intended therapeutic effect is based on a specific molecular species synthesized by cells. In that case, sufficient structural and biological data should be provided to show that an appropriate and biologically active form exists.
- Culture longevity: The essential characteristics of the cultured cell population should be defined (phenotypic markers such as cell surface antigens, functional properties, and bioassay activity, as appropriate). In culture, the stability of these characteristics has been established over time. This profile should be used to define the cultural period's boundaries (FDA 1998).

11.4.1.3.2 Cell Banking System Procedures

Cell banking systems are appropriate for some somatic cell therapy products made repeatedly from the same cells. Bacterial cells produce plasmids, while mammalian cells produce recombinant viral vectors when packaging or producer cells make gene therapy vectors. A formal cell banking system should manage these cell stocks (often a two-tiered system).

The cell bank system used should be described as follows:

- Contaminating organisms should be tested: MCBs should be free of contaminating biological agents such as fungi, viruses other than vectors, mycoplasma, and bacteria other than the intended bacterial host strain.

In MCBs consisting of bacteria carrying plasmids of interest, testing for bacteriophage is not required. Still, the possible presence of bacteriophage should be considered since it could adversely affect stability and yield.

- Expiration dating: As part of the product development process, data should be gathered to show how long and under what conditions cells can be frozen and usable when thawed.
- Tests on thawed cells: After thawing and expansion, viability, cell identity, and function tests should be repeated. Before freezing, compare the yield of viable cells and quantitative functional equivalents to those values. Using aliquots of the frozen cells, sterility should be confirmed.

If working cell banks are used, they should be subjected to limited phenotypic or genotypic testing for identity. Restriction mapping or an assay of secreted protein activity, as in MCBs, should be used to confirm vector retention and identity. They should be free of microbial and viral contamination as well.

Extended culture of end-of-production cells for producer cells should be done only once to see if growth conditions induce new contaminants or if vector integrity is compromised. Sponsors should propose a testing schedule that includes the most informative and sensitive steps.

With cell therapies explicitly made for each patient, such as autologous cells to treat individual patients, it may not be possible to use cell banking practices. However, consideration should be given to testing the final cellular product for crucial characteristics (FDA 1998).

11.4.1.3.3 Materials Used During Manufacturing

Materials used during in vitro manipulation procedures, such as antibodies, cytokines, serum, protein A, toxins, antibiotics, other chemicals, or solid supports such as beads, can affect the final therapeutic product's safety, purity, and potency. These components should be identified, and a qualification program with specific specifications for each component should be established to determine whether it is acceptable for use in the manufacturing process. The qualification program should include testing for the component's safety, purity, and potency when using reagent-grade material, as needed. For the use of clinical-grade features, abbreviated testing is appropriate. In some cases, materials of animal origin will need to be tested for adventitious agents. When there is a risk of transmissible agents causing spongiform encephalopathy, the country of origin should be certified.

All production components that may persist in the final product should have concentration limits established. The methods used to remove them and quantitative testing (including a description of the methods and sensitivity) should be provided to demonstrate the effectiveness of their removal. When cells are administered by binding or uptake, some additional components are present in measurable amounts. Testing the toxicity of these components in animals or other appropriate systems should be considered in such cases (FDA 1998).

11.4.2 Characterization and Release Testing of Cellular Gene Therapy Products

These requirements apply to cellular products, including ex vivo transduced cells for gene therapy.

Quality control testing should be performed on the final biological product and the manufacturing process and materials used. The specifications for the final product and other production elements and the range of acceptable values for each should be specified.

A quantity of material that has been thoroughly mixed in a single vessel is considered one lot of a biological product. This concept is used in the planning of lot testing procedures for somatic cell and gene therapy. This means that appropriate lot release testing should be performed on each cell population, vector preparation, or other product for such therapies prepared as a unique final mixture. Individually prepared preparations differ from large-batch preparations, and appropriate lot release criteria should be chosen to fit each protocol's practical constraints. Lot-to-lot variation is a measure of the procedures' reproducibility (FDA 1998).

11.4.2.1 Cell Identity

Quantitative testing by phenotypic and chemical assays should be used to confirm cell identity and assess heterogeneity (21 CFR 610.14) (FDA 1998).

11.4.2.2 Potency

The cells' relevant function, if known, and relevant products biosynthesized by the cells should be defined and quantitated as a measure of potency (21 CFR 610.10) (FDA 1998).

11.4.2.3 Viability

The viability of the cells should be determined, and an acceptable lower limit set (FDA 1998).

11.4.2.4 Adventitious Agent Testing

According to the tests, bacteria, fungi, mycoplasma, and viruses should not be found in the cells. In addition, the FDA will soon allow for validation of a mycoplasma-free manufacturing process in cases where the final cell therapy product is too short-lived to complete adequately sensitive testing before administration to patients (FDA 1998).

11.4.2.5 Purity

Endotoxin testing should be validated by LAL or other acceptable assays to ensure purity (21 CFR 610.13). On a case-by-case basis, the suitability and appropriateness of endotoxin testing methods should be considered. The test should be validated to demonstrate that cell preparation does not affect endotoxin detection (FDA 1998).

11.4.2.6 General Safety Test

The general safety test (21 CFR 610.11) must be performed on the final product. When appropriate, modified procedures are developed according to 21 CFR 610.9 (FDA 1998).

11.4.2.7 Frozen Cell Banks

Lot release testing on thawed cells is required when cell populations frozen for later administration are thawed, expanded, and then administered to patients (FDA 1998).

11.4.3 Additional Applications: Addition of Radioisotopes or Toxins to Cell Preparations

Therapeutic or diagnostic applications are proposed involving cells modified by radiolabeling or preloading with bioactive materials such as toxins. Thus, the cell implant is used as a delivery system for its products, functions, and other products. Novel safety concerns may arise related to cell implantation and localization of the radionuclide or toxin or the cells' metabolic properties. Wherever possible, these should be anticipated and addressed. The use of radiolabeled or toxin-conjugated antibodies has raised similar special issues in the past (FDA 1998).

11.4.4 Production, Characterization, and Release Testing of Vectors for Gene Therapy

The types of information needed to ensure adequate safety vary depending on the proposed clinical trial's nature, such as the administration route and frequency and the patient population. The information requested below is challenging to acquire in some systems. Sponsors may present alternative methods and data to CBER staff for review (FDA 1998).

11.4.4.1 Vector Construction and Characterization

Source materials for vectors should be thoroughly characterized and documented. Confirmatory identity tests should be performed on viral vectors or plasmids generated from cloned and characterized constructs. The information provided should include vector derivation, including descriptions of any vectors, helper viruses, and producer cell lines used to prepare the final construct. Within the construct, known regulatory elements such as promoters and enhancers should be identified.

Vector characterization, consisting of sequence data from appropriate portions of vectors and an indication mapping supplemented by protein characterization, is acceptable early in the product development process. More detailed sequencing information should be provided for later stages of product development and licensure. When sequencing the entire vector is not possible due to the construct's size, sequencing the genetic insert plus flanking regions and any significant modifications to the vector backbone or sites known to be vulnerable to change during molecular manipulations are sufficient. If known, vector sequences that modulate vector–host interactions should be described, and the host cell/vector system's stability should be considered (FDA 1998).

11.4.4.2 Vector Production System

The vector production system comprises the host cell, the final gene construct, and, when necessary, the vector intermediate (for example, retroviral producer cell), the method of transferring the gene construct into the host cell, and the procedure for selecting the final gene construct. The recombinant host cell clone's selection and characterization, including vector copy number and the final vector's physical state, construct inside the host cell (i.e., integrated or extra-chromosomal) should be described in detail. It is necessary to provide a detailed description of the procedures for propagating and expanding the recombinant host cell clone, establishing the seed stock, and qualifying the seed stock (FDA 1998).

11.4.4.3 Master Viral Banks

It is recommended that a Master Viral Bank be created and characterized when a virus, with or without a therapeutic gene, is used as a seed in the manufacture of a therapeutic vector. This category includes vectors derived from adenovirus, adeno-associated virus, herpes virus, poxviruses, and other lytic and non-lytic viruses. The sponsor should describe the source materials (plasmids, vectors, oligomers, etc.) and molecular methods used to create the source or seed vector. The seed vector's genetic integrity and stability (i.e., identity) should be confirmed, as well as the vector seed's bioactivity. In the absence of bioactivity data, the gene's expression should be evaluated.

Master seed stocks should also be demonstrated to be free of adventitious agents, including viruses, bacteria, fungi, and mycoplasma. In the case of replication-defective or replication-selective vectors, Master Viral Banks should be demonstrated to be free of replication-competent viruses, which may arise due to contamination or recombination during the generation of the MVB. Testing for other inappropriate viruses will depend upon the vector and feasibility of assays in the vector virus presence (FDA 1998).

11.4.4.4 Lot-to-Lot Release Testing and Specifications for Vectors

General testing recommendations are given below. Not all tests listed will apply to every vector class. Sponsors should choose appropriate testing protocols and consult CBER if there are questions about a specific test's applicability. For example, suppose drug substance (defined as the bulk product not necessarily in final formulation) and drug product (defined as a product in its final formulation) are the same. In that case, only a single set of tests is necessary.

Any standard assays for the properties listed below can measure quantitative and adequate specificity and sensitivity. Assay methods should be validated by testing known amounts of reference lots, spiked samples, other appropriate measures, and data documenting assay performance submitted to the IND.

Tests of drug substance (bulk product not necessarily in final formulation) include:

- Purity (21 CFR 610.13).
  - Test for total DNA or RNA content if appropriate to vector composition, e.g., A260/A280.
  - Test for homogeneity of size and structure, supercoiled versus linear, e.g., agarose gel electrophoresis.
  - Test for contamination with RNA or with host DNA, e.g., gel electrophoresis, including a test with the bacterial host-specific probe.
  - Test for proteins if present as a contaminant, e.g., silver-stained gel.
  - Test for the non-infectious virus in cases that would be a contaminant, such as empty capsids.
  - Tests for toxic materials involved in the production.
- Identity (21 CFR 610.14).
  - Test for vector identity by methods such as restriction enzyme mapping with multiple enzymes or PCR should be performed on the drug substance. It should be verified that identity testing can distinguish between constructs and detect cross-contamination if a facility produces multiple constructs (FDA 1998).

11.4.4.5 Adventitious Agents

As testing methods for adventitious agents become increasingly sensitive and specific over time, sponsors are encouraged to accumulate data validating testing methods other than those indicated to permit future updating of this policy. In cases in which a vector product interferes with appropriate assays, for example, a lytic viral vector that kills indicator cells in an assay for an adventitious virus, some information is obtained by parallel mock cultures using the same media and other reagents to allow outgrowth of a contaminant, or by assays in the presence of neutralizing antibody. In addition, the following tests should be performed:

- Sterility test (21 CFR 610.12) for aerobic and anaerobic bacteria and fungi.
- Mycoplasma testing, as specified in the "Points to Consider in the Characterization of Cell Lines Used to Produce Biologicals (1993)," Attachment #2 (58 FR 42974), which specifies the procedures for detecting mycoplasma contamination.

Testing for adventitious viruses, in some cases, source materials or cell lines used in vector production, introduce the risk of contamination with adventitious viruses. In other cases, the adventitious virus is introduced during product manufacture. Therefore, testing for an appropriate range of possible contaminating viruses is recommended.

- Potency assays should be validated during the product development process. Expression of the inserted gene is determined by the transfection of appropriate cells and the demonstration of an active gene product by an appropriate assay, characterized as to its sensitivity and specificity.
- Whenever possible, a potency assay should measure the expressed gene product's biological activity, not merely its presence. For example, if the enzymatic activity is the basis of the proposed therapy, an enzyme activity assay detecting substrate conversion to the product would be preferred over an immunological assay detecting epitopes on the enzyme. If no quantitative potency assay is available, then a qualitative potency test should be performed.
- Tests of the drug product (product in its final formulation). The vector product in the final container form should be tested for quantitative, validated assays for the properties listed below. Tests for endotoxin and general safety, if performed on a drug product (final product), need not be performed on a drug substance (bulk product).
- Validation of endotoxin testing by LAL or another acceptable assay. As per 21 CFR 610.11, general safety is not needed for therapeutic DNA plasmid products because they are among the specified biotechnology products., even if liposomes are added (FDA 1998).

11.4.5 Issues Related to Particular Classes of Vectors for Gene Therapy

11.4.5.1 Additional Considerations for the Use of Plasmid Vector Products

Many products and quality control considerations provided above are appropriate for plasmid DNA products. In general, complete sequencing of the plasmid should be performed. Plasmids should be characterized, and specifications set about the presence of RNA, protein, and bacterial host DNA contaminants, quantities of linear and supercoiled DNA in the preparation, and presence of toxic chemicals. Toxic chemicals such as ethidium bromide should be avoided during production.

It is recommended that penicillin and other beta-lactam antibiotics be avoided during production due to the risk of serious hypersensitivity reactions in patients. If antibiotic selection is used during production, it is preferable not to use selection markers that confer resistance to antibiotics in effective clinical use to avoid unnecessary risk of spread antibiotic resistance traits to environmental microbes. Also, the residual antibiotic in the final product should be quantitated when possible and the allergy potential.

Plasmid vectors are administered in conjunction with lipid preparations, local anesthetics, or other chemicals intended to facilitate DNA uptake. If such a facilitating agent is added during formulation, a specification for its amount and identity in the final product should be established. If toxic organic solvents such as chloroform are used in producing a lipid component, then processing should remove them, and lot release specifications should include testing for residual solvent (FDA 1998).

11.4.5.2 Additional Considerations for the Use of Retroviral Vector Products

Testing for replication-competent retrovirus: Alternative assays (e.g., marker rescue) are acceptable if sensitivity is comparable to the PG4 S+L– assay. Testing should be complete before patient administration, particularly if cells are cryopreserved; otherwise, testing should be performed concurrently. To gain biological information about events during production, molecular characterization of any RCR detected in clinical lots is also recommended.

A Master Cell Bank of vector-producing cells (one-time testing) includes:

- Supernatant testing: 5% of the total supernatant from the cells' culture for a master cell bank should be tested by amplification on a permissive cell line (e.g., *Mus dunni*), including several blind passages followed by the PG4 S+L– or alternative assay.

- Producer cell testing: 1% of pooled producer cells, or 108 cells, whichever is fewer, should be cocultured with a permissive cell line (e.g., *Mus dunni*), including several blind passages. Supernatant from the coculture should be tested by PG4 S+L– or alternative assay.

Working cell bank (one-time testing): Either supernatant testing *or* cocultivation of cells is recommended, using conditions described for master cell bank testing.

Lot testing of vector products:

- For clinical-grade supernatant, 5% of the supernatant should be tested by amplification on a permissive cell line (e.g., *Mus dunni*), including several blind passages, followed by the PG4 S+L– or alternative assay.
- Testing of end of production cells, 1% of total pooled end of production cells or 108 cells, whichever is fewer, should be cocultured with a permissive cell line (e.g., *Mus dunni*) and then amplified by several blind passages. Supernatant from the coculture should be tested by S+L– or alternative assay.

Lot testing of ex vivo transduced cells:

- 1% of pooled transduced cells or 108 cells, whichever is fewer, should be cocultured with a permissive cell line (e.g., *Mus dunni*), including several blind passages. Supernatant from the coculture should be tested by PG4 S+L– or alternative assay.
- 5% of the transduced cells' supernatant should be tested by amplifying a permissive cell line (e.g., *Mus dunni*), including several blind passages. Supernatant from the coculture should be tested by PG4 S+L– assay.

Patients given retrovirus-related products should be monitored for RCR exposure following CBER guidance (FDA 1998).

11.4.5.3 Additional Considerations for the Use of Adenoviral Vectors

11.4.5.3.1 Measurement of Particles versus Infectious Units

Patient doses of adenovirus-based gene therapy vectors are presently based upon some method of enumerating viral particles, plaque-forming units (PFU), or infectious units (IU) measured in cell lines complementing the replication defect (not to be confused with measurement of RCA). CBER recommends that patient dosing be based on particle number, given the potential toxicity of the adenoviral particles themselves. This recommendation also reflects that the particle number is readily and reproducibly measured. However, since some outcomes may be a function of the number of infectious units administered, investigators or sponsors need to develop in vitro infectivity assays that are reproducible and informative and to set appropriately tight specifications on the ratio of infectious particles to total viral particles.

Adenovirus particle measurement is commonly based on genomic DNA quantitation. Using the absorbance at 260 nm in the presence of sodium dodecyl sulfate or other virus lysing agents, the maximum number of adenoviral particles is calculated from OD260. The presence of non-adenovirus nucleic acid may yield inaccurate particle numbers and should be minimized during the manufacturing and viral purification process. Electron microscope particle count has also been used for viral particle enumeration.

Presently the titer of an adenovirus vector preparation usually refers to the infectious titer. The cell used for determining the titer is often the producer cell line. Differences in viral vectors may lead to changes in growth properties and kinetics. The plaque method is efficient for adenoviral vectors with an easily complemented replication defect. Vectors with multiple replication defects are more readily tittered by alternative methods such as fluorescent antibodies.

Both assays require optimization for adsorption time, the need for disaggregation of virus, stability, etc. The inclusion of a standard wild-type virus control may facilitate the comparison of titers between various vectors and laboratories.

It is currently recommended that a ratio in viral particles to a biologically active virus of less than 1,001 be employed in phase I studies. This specification aims to ensure consistent recombinant viruses and the highest bioactivity/particle/ patient dose and limit possible toxicity due to viral structural proteins. In addition, as new assays are developed and validated, their comparison to old ones and their use in product characterization is encouraged (FDA 1998).

11.4.5.3.2 Detection of Replication-Competent Adenovirus

The presence of RCA in clinical lots of adenovirus vector raises a variety of safety concerns, including the possibility of adenovirus infection, unintended vector replication due to the presence of wild-type helper function, and exacerbation of host inflammatory responses. The safety risks entailed by these events and other potential adverse events will differ depending on the indication and the patient population. Preclinical safety studies are inherently limited in assessing RCA-related risks since no animal models support extensive replication of human wild-type or replication-competent recombinant adenovirus.

Therefore, adenovirus vectors intended to be replication-defective should be examined for the presence of replication-competent adenovirus (RCA). RCA may arise at multiple steps during the manufacturing process, through recombination with host sequences or contamination. The amount of RCA generated during manufacture will be influenced by the overall design of the vector. The use of replication-selective adenovirus vectors raises additional considerations and may call for additional or different testing strategies. Such cases should be discussed with CBER.

Detection of RCA in the final vector product by a cell culture/cytopathic effect method is preferred. Validation of assay sensitivity by spiking decreasing wild-type adenovirus particles into the test inoculum is recommended. Input multiplicity of infection (MOI) should be carefully chosen because of the toxicity of higher doses of virus inoculum unrelated to RCA. It should also be noted that too high an input MOI may suppress RCA outgrowth by the vector. One- or two-blind passages on cells permissive for growth of the RCA, for example, A549 cells, is performed to amplify RCA before reading out on an indicator cell line. It is also recommended that the assay be quantitative, that is, to determine the number of RCA present in any patient dose.

Previous recommendations from the FDA have been that patient doses should contain no more than one pfu of RCA or equivalent in patients whose adenovirus infection would be considered a potential risk. However, the FDA recognizes that current production techniques may make this recommendation prohibitively burdensome in combination with proposed dosing schemes. Therefore, if sponsors wish to propose a different specification, data should be provided, demonstrating that RCA's level represents an acceptable risk for the intended patient population, administration route, and dose. To gain biological information about events during production, molecular characterization of any RCA present in clinical lots is also recommended at this time. It should be as thorough as it is practical until more is known about the recombination types (FDA 1998).

11.4.5.3.3 Adeno-Associated Virus

Because of AAV's association with adenovirus, AAV testing is currently recommended in the Master Cell Bank, the Master Virus Seed Stock, and the final product (FDA 1998).

11.4.5.3.4 Other Gene Delivery Systems

Other gene delivery systems, including additional viral or nucleic acid vectors, are currently under development. Sponsors using new systems are encouraged to contact CBER early in product development to facilitate a safe and efficient development process (FDA 1998).

11.4.6 Modifications in Vector Preparations

Two aspects of IND submission are affected by considering a product as a modified vector: the decision as to whether a new IND should be submitted and the decision as to what data should be submitted for review. Certain changes, for example, minor modifications in the genetic insert or changes in the antibiotic resistance gene, do not necessarily call for a new IND or full product retesting. In all cases, the derivation of a new vector should be described, and the vector should meet the specifications for release testing. The other data that should be collected will vary with the degree and nature of the vector modifications. The need for additional preclinical testing is determined by the likelihood of altered vector biology, not just the number of nucleotide changes. In some cases, tissue localization, germline alteration, and animal pharmacology/ toxicology studies are optional. Instead, the relevant safety studies could focus on specific safety concerns related to changes in the vector.

When several related vectors involving minor modifications are studied, they are considered members of a panel, analogous to panels of monoclonal antibodies described in the "Points to Consider in the Manufacture and Testing of Monoclonal Antibody Products for Human Use," 1997 revision, 62 FR 9196. As stated, such panels could be studied under a single IND and submitted for approval in a single license application. Therefore, phase III clinical trials should include some experience with all panel members and efficacy established for the overall panel.

Vector modifications should be discussed with CBER case by case. Suppose a sponsor wishes to abbreviate testing and IND submission for a product or product series. In that case, the sponsor should verify with CBER the proposed abbreviated testing scheme's adequacy before initiating clinical trials. Data forthcoming from sponsors can help establish whether particular changes in vectors alter their behavior when compared in vivo, therefore, whether complete testing should continue to be performed (FDA 1998).

11.4.7 Preclinical Evaluation of Cellular and Gene Therapies

11.4.7.1 General Principles

Preclinical studies are intended to define the pharmacologic and toxicologic effects predictive of the human response, not only before the initiation of clinical trials but also throughout drug development. These studies' goals include defining safe starting doses and escalation schemes for clinical trials, identifying target organs for toxicity and parameters to monitor in patients receiving these therapies, and determining populations that are at greater risk for toxicities of a given cellular or gene therapeutics (FDA 1998).

Design of preclinical studies should take into consideration: 1) the population of cells to be administered or the class of vector used, 2) the animal species and physiologic state most relevant for the clinical indication and product class, and 3) the intended doses, route of administration, and treatment regimens. The parameters that should be studied will be discussed in the following (FDA 1998).

Due to the unique and diverse nature of the products employed in cellular and gene therapies, conventional pharmacology and toxicity testing may not always be appropriate to determine these agents' safety and biologic activity. Available animal models mimicking the disease indication may help obtain sufficient safety and efficacy data before entering these agents into clinical trials. Issues such as species specificity of the transduced gene, permissiveness for infection by viral vectors, and comparative physiology should be considered in these studies' designs (FDA 1998).

The ICH Draft Guideline S6, "Preclinical Safety Evaluation of Biotechnology-Derived Pharmaceuticals" (Step 4, approved by ICH, 7/16/1997), is the flexible application of Good Laboratory Practices in testing biotechnology products. Although pivotal safety studies in support of marketing (e.g., carcinogenicity, reproductive toxicology) are expected to be conducted in compliance with the regulations as outlined in 21 CFR part 58, it is recognized that studies in support of entry into clinical trials may not always strictly adhere to GLP. In these cases, the principles of the regulation should be followed as closely as possible. Where deviations occur, they should be evaluated for impact on the expected clinical application and discussed in the report submitted to the FDA (FDA 1998).

If a product is comparable to agents for which there is a wide previous clinical experience or the insertion of a different expression cassette is not expected to influence the toxicity or disseminate the vector, less extensive preclinical testing may suffice. It is recommended that plans for preclinical studies be discussed with representatives from CBER before their initiation. Clinical plans requiring rapid enrollment of patients should be anticipated and preceded by adequate preclinical testing (FDA 1998).

11.4.7.2 Animal Species Selection and Use of Alternative Animal Models

It is recognized that animal models of disease may not be available for every cellular or gene therapy system. Therefore, these agents' preclinical pharmacologic and safety testing should employ the most appropriate, pharmacologically relevant animal model. A suitable animal species would be one in which the therapy's biological response would be expected to mimic the human response. For example, a vector expressing a human cytokine would best be tested in an animal species. That cytokine binds to the corresponding cytokine receptor with an affinity comparable to that seen with human receptors and initiates a pharmacologic response comparable to that expected in humans (FDA 1998).

11.4.7.3 Somatic Cell and Gene-Modified Cellular Therapies

11.4.7.3.1 In Vivo Biological/Pharmacological Activity

The transduction procedure, dose of expanded or genetically modified cells, and administration route planned for the clinical trial should be evaluated preclinically. Pharmacologic studies in animals may provide useful information regarding the in vivo function, survival time, and appropriate trafficking of the modified cells (FDA 1998).

11.4.7.3.2 Toxicologic Testing

Safety testing of expanded, activated, or genetically modified somatic cells should be conducted in an appropriate animal model. Data on distribution, trafficking, and persistence of these cells in vivo mentioned above should be evaluated for safety implications. At a minimum, treated animals should be monitored for general health status, serum biochemistry, and hematologic profiles. Target tissues should be examined microscopically for histopathological changes (FDA 1998).

11.4.7.4 Direct Administration of Vectors In Vivo

Many different vectors are currently in development for direct administration to human subjects. Direct administration of any of these vectors presents many safety concerns that will be addressed here. All toxicity and localization studies, including studies of gonadal tissue described below, should use the final formulated product. Adding materials such as liposomes, or changes in pH or salt content, may alter the toxicity or distribution pattern.

Specific concerns for each vector subclass will generally be handled on a case-by-case basis, and discussion with CBER is encouraged (FDA 1998).

11.4.7.4.1 Route of Administration

The route of administration of vectors can influence toxicity in vivo. Therefore, safety evaluation in the preclinical studies should be conducted by the identical route and method of administration as in the clinical trial whenever possible. When this is difficult to achieve in a small animal species, a method of administration similar to that planned for use in the clinic is advised. For example, intrapulmonary instillation of adenoviral vectors by intranasal administration in cotton rats or mice is an acceptable alternative to direct intrapulmonary administration through a bronchoscope (FDA 1998).

11.4.7.4.2 Selection of Animal Species

The animal species chosen for preclinical toxicity evaluations should be selected for their sensitivity to infection and pathologic sequelae induced by the wild-type virus related to a vector and its utility as a model of biologic activity of the vector construct. Unlike non-human primates, Rodent models are useful if they are susceptible to pathology induced by the virus class. When evaluating a vector's activity in an animal model of the clinical indication, safety data is gathered from the same model to assess the contribution of disease-related changes in physiology or underlying pathology to the vector's response (FDA 1998).

11.4.7.4.3 Selection of Dose to Be Employed

The vectors studied preclinically should be selected based on preliminary activity data from studies in vitro and in vivo. A no-effect level dose, an overtly toxic dose, and several intermediate doses should be determined, and appropriate controls, such as naive or vehicle-treated animals should be included. A maximum feasible dose is administered as the highest level tested in the preclinical studies for products in limited supply or inherently low toxicity. Preclinical safety evaluations should include at least one dose equivalent to and at least one dose escalation level exceeding those proposed for the clinical trial; the multiples of the human dose required to determine adequate safety margins may vary with each class of vector employed and the relevance of the animal model to humans. Scaling doses based on either body weight or total body surface area as appropriate facilitates comparisons across species. The information generated is used to determine the vector's margin of safety for use in the clinical trial and gauge an acceptable dose-escalation scheme (FDA 1998).

11.4.7.4.4 Toxicologic Testing

Treated animals should be monitored for general health status, serum biochemistry, and hematology, and tissues should be examined for pathological changes in histology (FDA 1998).

11.4.7.4.5 Distribution of Vector out of the Site of Administration

Localization studies, designed to determine the vector's distribution after administration to its proposed site, are also recommended. Whenever possible, the intended route of administration should be employed. Other groups of animals are treated intravenously as a "worst-case" scenario representing the effects of widespread vector dissemination. Transferring the gene to normal, surrounding, and distal tissues and the target site should be evaluated using the most sensitive detection methods possible and should include evaluating gene persistence. Dose levels selected should follow those used in toxicity testing. When aberrant or unexpected localization is observed, studies should be conducted to determine whether the gene is expressed and whether its presence is associated with pathologic effects (FDA 1998).

11.4.7.5 Expression of Gene Product and Induction of Immune Responses

Expression of the therapeutic gene product in intended or unintended tissues may result in unexpected toxicities, which should be addressed in preclinical studies. Inflammatory, immune, or autoimmune responses induced by the gene product are of concern. Animal studies should be conducted over a sufficient duration of time to allow the development of such responses. Host immune responses against viral or transgene proteins may limit their usefulness for repeated administration in the clinic (FDA 1998).

11.4.7.6 Vector Localization to Reproductive Organs

With vectors for direct administration, the risk of vector transfer to germ cells should be considered. Animal testicular or ovarian samples should be analyzed for vector sequences by the most sensitive method possible. For example, suppose a signal is detected in the gonads. In that case, further studies should be conducted to determine if the sequences are present in germ cells instead of stromal tissues, using techniques that may include but are not limited to cell separations or in situ PCR, or other methods. Semen samples for analysis are collected from mature animals, including mice, to determine vector incorporation into germ cells (FDA 1998).

11.4.7.6.1 Host Immune Status and Effects on Gene Therapy Vectors

The intended recipients of gene therapy's immune status should be considered in the risk–benefit analysis of a product, particularly for viral vectors. If immunocompromised patients' exclusion unduly restricts a clinical protocol, immune-suppressed, genetically immunodeficient, or newborn animals are used in preclinical studies to evaluate potential safety risks (FDA 1998).

11.5 Conclusion

Biotechnology evolved quickly over the past few decades, allowing the emergence of techniques that revolutionized DNA manipulation to treat and diagnose disease. Cell therapy and gene therapy have transformed the future of medicine. Biologicals overlap the cell and gene therapy fields where recombinant manipulation is involved. Given the complexity and risks of gene manipulation, the regulatory agencies have provided extensive guidance and requirements for developing and manufacturing them. This chapter provides details of cell and gene therapies pertinent to development, manufacturing, and regulatory compliance.

ADDITIONAL READING

CDC and Fort Dodge animal health achieve first licensed DNA vaccine. CDC. 2005-07-18. Archived from the original on 2007-08-20. Retrieved 2007-11-21.

Al-Rubeai M, Naciri M. Stem cells, and cell therapy. In *Cell engineering*. Springer; 2014:viii, 189 pages.

Alarcon JB, Waine GW, McManus DP. DNA vaccines: technology and application as anti-parasite and anti-microbial agents. *Advances in Parasitology*. 1999;42:343–410.

André S, Seed B, Eberle J, Schraut W, Bültmann A, Haas J. Increased immune response elicited by DNA vaccination with a synthetic gp120 sequence with optimized codon usage. *Journal of Virology*. 1998;72(2):1497–1503.

Armbruster N, Jasny E, Petsch B. Advances in RNA vaccines for preventive indications: a case study of a vaccine against rabies. *Vaccines*. 2019;7(4):132.

Barouch DH, Santra S, Steenbeke TD, Zheng XX, Perry HC, Davies ME, Freed DC, Craiu A, Strom TB, Shiver JW, Letvin NL. Augmentation and suppression of immune responses to an HIV-1 DNA vaccine by plasmid cytokine/Ig administration. *Journal of Immunology*. 1998;161(4):1875–1882.

Benteyn D, Heirman C, Bonehill A, Thielemans K, Breckpot K. mRNA-based dendritic cell vaccines. *Expert Review of Vaccines*. 2014;14(2):161–176.

Berkhout B, Ertl HCJ, Weinberg MS, American Society of Gene & Cell Therapy. Gene therapy for HIV and chronic infections. In *Advances in experimental medicine and biology*. Springer; American Society of Gene & Cell Therapy; 2015:xvi, 236 pages.

Boelens JJ, Wynn RF. *Stem cell therapy in lysosomal storage diseases. Stem cell biology and regenerative medicine*. Humana Press; 2013:ix, 171 pages.

Boulis N, O'Connor D, Donsante A. *Molecular and cellular therapies for motor neuron diseases*. Elsevier, Academic Press; 2017:xiii, 321 pages.

Carralot JP, Probst J, Hoerr I, Scheel B, Teufel R, Jung G, et al. Polarization of immunity induced by direct injection of naked sequence-stabilized mRNA vaccines. *Cell Mol Life Sci*. 2004;61:2418–24.24.

Casaroli-Marano RP, Zarbin MA. *Cell-based therapy for retinal degenerative disease. Developments in ophthalmology*. Karger; 2014:xii, 205 pages.

Cathomen T, Hirsch M, Porteus MH, American Society of Gene & Cell Therapy. *Genome editing: the next step in gene therapy. Advances in experimental medicine and biology*. Springer; 2016:xvi, 263 pages.

Chase LG, Vemuri MC. *Mesenchymal stem cell therapy. Stem cell biology and regenerative medicine*. Humana Press; 2013:xii, 453 pages.

Chen J, Lin L, Li N, She F. Enhancement of Helicobacter pylori outer inflammatory protein DNA vaccine efficacy by co-delivery of interleukin-2 and B subunit heat-labile toxin gene encoded plasmids. *Microbiol Immunol*. 2012;56:85–92.

Chen Y, Webster RG, Woodland DL. Induction of CD8+ T cell responses to dominant and subdominant epitopes and protective immunity to Sendai virus infection by DNA vaccination. *Journal of Immunology* 1998 Mar;160(5):2425–32.

Dzau VJ, Liew C-C. *Cardiovascular genetics and genomics for the cardiologist*. Blackwell Futura; 2007:xi, 308 pages.

FDA. Guidance for Industry. 1998. Retrived from: https://www.fda.gov/media/72402/download

Freese A. Principles of molecular neurosurgery. In Freese A, ed. *Progress in neurological surgery*. Karger; 2005:xiv, 659 pages.

Fuster V, *Fundació "La Caixa." International Center for Scientific Debate. New York Academy of Sciences. Evolving challenges in promoting cardiovascular health. Annals of the New York Academy of Sciences.* Published by Blackwell Pub. on behalf of the New York Academy of Sciences; 2012:175 pages.

Fynan EF, Webster RG, Fuller DH, Haynes JR, Santoro JC, Robinson HL. DNA vaccines: protective immunizations by parenteral, mucosal, and gene-gun inoculations. *Proceedings of the National Academy of Sciences of the United States of America.* 1993;90(24):11478–11482.

Galli MC, Serabian M, American Society of Gene & Cell Therapy. Regulatory aspects of gene therapy and cell therapy products: a global perspective. In *Advances in experimental medicine and biology.* Springer; American Society of Gene & Cell Therapy; 2015:xii, 230 pages.

Gao Q, Dong X, Xu Q, et al. Therapeutic potential of CRISPR/Cas9 gene editing in engineered T-cell therapy. *Cancer Med.* 2019;8(9):4254–4264.

Greaves DR, Gordon S. Thematic review series: the immune system and atherogenesis. Recent insights into the biology of macrophage scavenger receptors. *J Lipid Res.* 2005;46:11–20.

Greenwell P, McCulley M. *Molecular therapeutics: 21st century medicine.* John Wiley & Sons; 2007:x, 251 pages.

Grier EV. *Focus on stem cell research.* Nova Biomedical Books; 2004:xi, 233 pages.

Grier EV. *Stem cell therapy.* Nova Biomedical Books; 2006:x, 234 pages.

Hakim NS. *Pancreas, islet, and stem cell transplantation for diabetes.* 2nd ed. Oxford University Press; 2010:xiv, 526 pages.

Harrison RP, Chauhan VM. Enhancing cell and gene therapy manufacture through the application of advanced fluorescent optical sensors (Review). *Biointerphases.* 2017;13(1):01A301.

Hostiuc S. *Clinical ethics at the crossroads of genetic and reproductive technologies.* Elsevier/Academic Press; 2018:xiv, 417 pages.

Huebener N, Fest S, Strandsby A, Michalsky E, Preissner R, Zeng Y, Gaedicke G, Lode HN. A rationally designed tyrosine hydroxylase DNA vaccine induces specific antineuroblastoma immunity. *Molecular Cancer Therapeutics.* 2008;7(7):2241–2251.

Jain KK. *Applications of biotechnology in neurology.* Humana Press; 2013:xxxv, 638 pages.

Kanagavelu SK, Snarsky V, Termini JM, Gupta S, Barzee S, Wright JA, et al. Soluble multi-trimeric TNF superfamily ligand adjuvants enhance immune responses to a HIV-1 Gag DNA vaccine. *Vaccine.* 2012;30:691–702.

Klinman DM, Yamshchikov G, Ishigatsubo Y. Contribution of CpG motifs to the immunogenicity of DNA vaccines. *Journal of Immunology.* 1997;158(8):3635–3639.

Kreiter S, Diken M, Selmi A, Diekmann J, Attig S, Hüsemann Y, et al. FLT3 ligand enhances the cancer therapeutic potency of naked RNA vaccines. *Cancer Res.* 2011;71:6132–6142.

Kuhn AN, Diken M, Kreiter S, Selmi A, Kowalska J, Jemielity J, et al. Phosphorothioate cap analogs increase stability and translational efficiency of RNA vaccines in immature dendritic cells and induce superior immune responses in vivo. *Gene Ther.* 2010;17:961–971.

Kutzler MA, Weiner DB. DNA vaccines: ready for prime time? *Nature Reviews. Genetics.* 2008;9(10):776–788.

Leri A, Anversa P, Frishman WH. *Cardiovascular regeneration and stem cell therapy.* Blackwell Futura; 2007:xii, 229 pages.

Lewis PJ, Babiuk LA. DNA vaccines: a review. In *Advances in virus research.* 54. Academic Press; 1999, pp. 129–188.

Loudon PT, Yager EJ, Lynch DT, Narendran A, Stagnar C, Franchini AM, et al. GM-CSF increases mucosal and systemic immunogenicity of an H1N1 influenza DNA vaccine administered into the epidermis of non-human primates. *PLoS One.* 2010;5:e11021.

Mancini-Bourgine M, Fontaine H, Bréchot C, Pol S, Michel ML. Immunogenicity of a hepatitis B DNA vaccine administered to chronic HBV carriers. *Vaccine.* 2006;24(21):4482–4489.

Mejía Vázquez MdC, Navarro S. *New approaches in the treatment of cancer. Cancer etiology, diagnosis and treatments.* Nova Science Publishers; 2010:217 pages.

Morstyn G, Sheridan W. *Cell therapy: stem cell transplantation, gene therapy, and cellular immunotherapy. Cancer, clinical science in practice.* Cambridge University Press; 1996:xxix, 617 pages.

Ng P, Brunetti-Pierri N. *Therapeutic applications of adenoviruses. Gene and cell therapy series.* CRC Press; 2017:xiv, 242 pages.

Odé Z, Condori J, Peterson N, Zhou S, Krenciute G. CRISPR-mediated non-viral site-specific gene integration and expression in T cells: protocol and application for T-cell therapy. *Cancers* (Basel). 2020;12(6):1704.

Pardi N, Hogan MJ, Porter FW, Weissman D. mRNA vaccines—a new era in vaccinology. *Nature Reviews Drug Discovery*. 2018;17(4):261–279.

Pardi N, Weissman D. Nucleoside modified mRNA vaccines for infectious diseases. In *RNA vaccines*, Springer, New York, 1499, 2016; pp. 109–121.

Pascolo, Steve. Vaccination with messenger RNA. DNA vaccines. *Methods in Molecular Medicine*. 2006;127; 23–40.

Perales M-A, Abutalib SA, Bollard C. *Cell and gene therapies. Advances and controversies in hematopoietic transplantation and cell therapy*. Springer; 2019:vi, 288 pages.

Petite H, Quarto R. *Engineered bone. Tissue engineering intelligence unit*. Landes Bioscience: Eurekah.com; 2005:225 pages.

Polak JM. *Cell therapy for lung disease*. Imperial College Press; 2010:xxiv, 504 pages.

Rees RC. *Tumor immunology and immunotherapy*. First edition. Oxford University Press; 2014:xxvi, 442 pages.

Reichmuth AM, Oberli MA, Jaklenec A, Langer R, Blankschtein D. mRNA vaccine delivery using lipid nanoparticles. *Therapeutic Delivery*. 2016;7(5):319–334.

Robinson HL, Pertmer TM. DNA vaccines for viral infections: basic studies and applications. *Advances in Virus Research*. 2000;55:1–74.

Sedegah M, Jones TR, Kaur M, Hedstrom R, Hobart P, Tine JA, Hoffman SL. Boosting with recombinant vaccinia increases immunogenicity and protective efficacy of malaria DNA vaccine. *Proceedings of the National Academy of Sciences of the United States of America*. 1998;95(13):7648–7653.

Segal BH. *Management of infections in the immunocompromised host*. Springer; 2018:xiv, 445 pages.

Sideman S, Beyar R. *Cardiac engineering: from genes and cells to structure and function*. Annals of the New York Academy of Sciences. New York Academy of Sciences; 2004:xviii, 406 pages.

Sreebny LM, Vissink A. *Dry mouth: the malevolent symptom: a clinical guide*. Wiley-Blackwell; 2010:xxii, 245 pages.

Templeton NS. *Gene and cell therapy: therapeutic mechanisms and strategies*. 2nd ed. Marcel Dekker; 2004:xviii, 875.

Terai S, Suda T. *Gene therapy and cell therapy through the liver: current aspects and future prospects*. Springer; 2016:x, 185 pages.

Tousoulis D. *Coronary artery disease: from biology to clinical practice*. Elsevier/Academic Press; 2018:xxi, 477 pages.

van den Berg JH, Oosterhuis K, Hennink WE, Storm G, van der Aa LJ, Engbersen JFJ, et al. Shielding the cationic charge of nanoparticle-formulated dermal DNA vaccines is essential for antigen expression and immunogenicity. *J Control Release*. 2010;141:234–40.

Verbeke R, Lentacker I, De Smedt SC, Dewitte H. Three decades of messenger RNA vaccine development. *Nano Today*. 2019;28:100766.

Vogel AB, Lambert L, Kinnear E, Busse D, Erbar S, Reuter KC, Wicke L, Perkovic M, Beissert T, Haas H, Reece ST. Self-amplifying RNA vaccines give equivalent protection against influenza to mRNA vaccines but at much lower doses. *Molecular Therapy*. 2018;26(2):446–455.

Wang PJ. *New arrhythmia technologies*. Blackwell Futura; 2005:xiv, 290 pages.

Weiss WR, Ishii KJ, Hedstrom RC, Sedegah M, Ichino M, Barnhart K, Klinman DM, Hoffman SL. A plasmid encoding murine granulocyte-macrophage colony-stimulating factor increases protection conferred by a malaria DNA vaccine. *Journal of Immunology*. 1998;161(5):2325–2332.

Whitehouse D, Rapley R. *Molecular and cellular therapeutics*. Wiley-Blackwell; 2012:xiii, 315 pages.

Widera G, Austin M, Rabussay D, Goldbeck C, Barnett SW, Chen M, Leung L, Otten GR, Thudium K, Selby MJ, Ulmer JB. Increased DNA vaccine delivery and immunogenicity by electroporation in vivo. *Journal of Immunology*. 2000;164(9):4635–4640.

Wiwanitkit, V. Cell, gene, and molecular therapy: new concepts. Nova Biomedical Books; 2009:xv, 187 pages.

Xu H, Zhao G, Huang X, Ding Z, Wang J, Wang X, et al. CD40-expressing plasmid induces anti-CD40 antibody and enhances immune responses to DNA vaccination. *J Gene Med*. 2010;12:97–106.

12

Nucleic Acid Vaccines

12.1 Background

According to the European Medicines Agency (EMA), a gene therapy medicinal product generally consists of a vector or delivery formulation/system containing a genetic construct engineered to express a specific transgene ("therapeutic sequence") for the regulation, repair, replacement, addition, or deletion of a genetic sequence. Nevertheless, a broader perspective is usually accepted from a scientific point of view, and the concept of gene therapy includes the therapeutic application of products containing any nucleic acid. So far, about 17 nucleic acid–based products have been approved worldwide. It is expected that nucleic acid–based products will substantially impact the market in vaccines that have been used to prevent infections for hundreds of years; their therapeutic use, a form of immunomodulation to treat infections and cancer, is relatively new. Nucleotide vaccines, DNA- or mRNA-based (messenger RNA), are the most recent types of vaccines, and only the mRNA vaccines received approval in 2020 (Figure 12.1).

Nucleotide vaccines are safer than other vaccines, and mRNA vaccines are safer than DNA vaccines because of their transient nature and cytosolic location. In contrast, more stable DNA vaccines require nuclear delivery and promoter-driven expression and risk integration within the host genome, which is less desirable. No DNA vaccine has been approved for human use yet (Figure 12.2).

The active component of nucleotide vaccines is treating diseases as a mixture consisting of a protein antigen causing autoimmune disease or the epitope polypeptides thereof. The recombinant eukaryotic vector with an autoantigen's coding genes or the epitope polypeptides thereof is inserted into multiple cloning sites. For a vaccine to prevent diabetes type 1, the autoantigen is insulin, glutamic acid decarboxylase or heat shock protein, myelin oligodendrocyte glycoprotein, myelin antigens, zona pellucida 3, myoglobulin, type II collagen, thyroglobulin, cell membrane surface antigen, type II colloid antigen, acetylcholine receptor, thyrocyte cell surface antigen, salivary gland duct antigen, thyroglobulin, superantigen, or interphotoreceptor retinoid-binding protein. The vaccine can inhibit T cells' proliferation from inducing immune suppression and prevent and treat autoimmune diseases effectively.

12.2 mRNA Vaccine

The year was 1796 when the first vaccine against smallpox was used; now, 225 years later, we have administered a synthetic vaccine to prevent COVID-19 infection developed within months rather than the normal time of decades to bring a new antiviral vaccine. When Sanofi Pasteur tested RNA encoding an influenza antigen in mice nearly three decades ago, the idea of using RNA in vaccines was born. It elicited a response, but the team's lipid delivery system was too toxic to use in humans. It would take another decade for companies researching RNA-interference therapeutics to discover the LNP (lipid nanoparticle) technologies that allowed the COVID-19 vaccines to be developed. Moderna, a DARPA-funded company, created the COVID-19 vaccine within four days of receiving the SARS-CoV-2 genome sequence from NIH, demonstrating the speed with which these vaccines can be developed. It concentrated on the virus's spike protein, a surface protein that allows it to enter cells. Classical approaches to vaccine creation would have taken years.

DOI: 10.1201/9781003146933-12

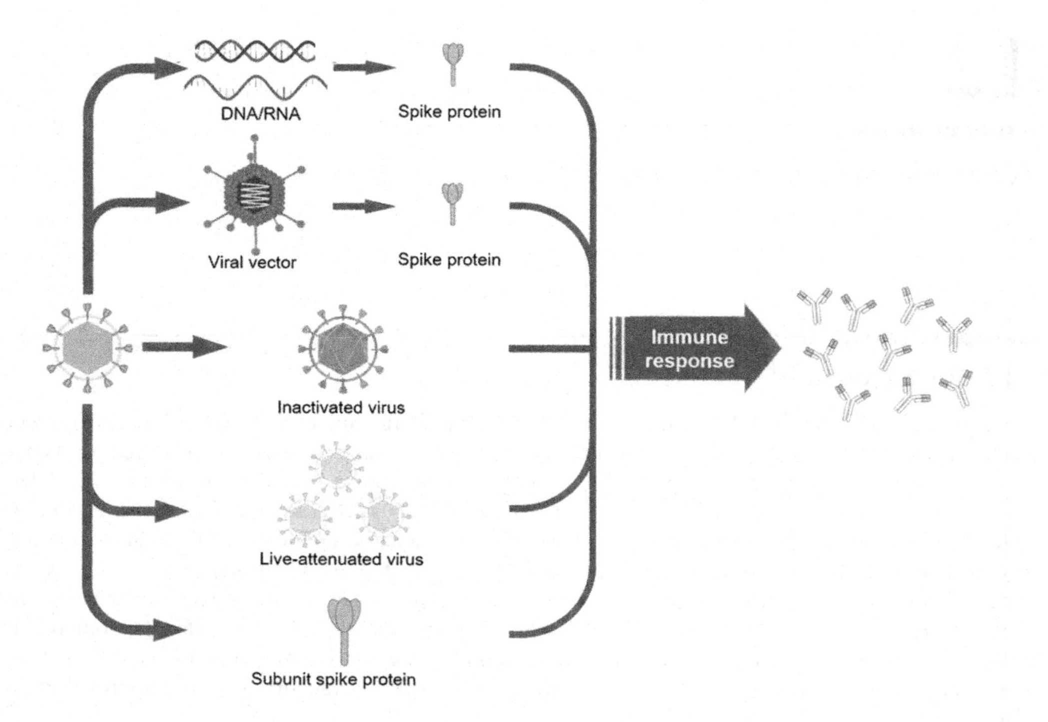

FIGURE 12.1 Types of vaccines. Source: https://theconversation.com/from-adenoviruses-to-rna-the-pros-and-cons-of-different-covid-vaccine-technologies-145454.

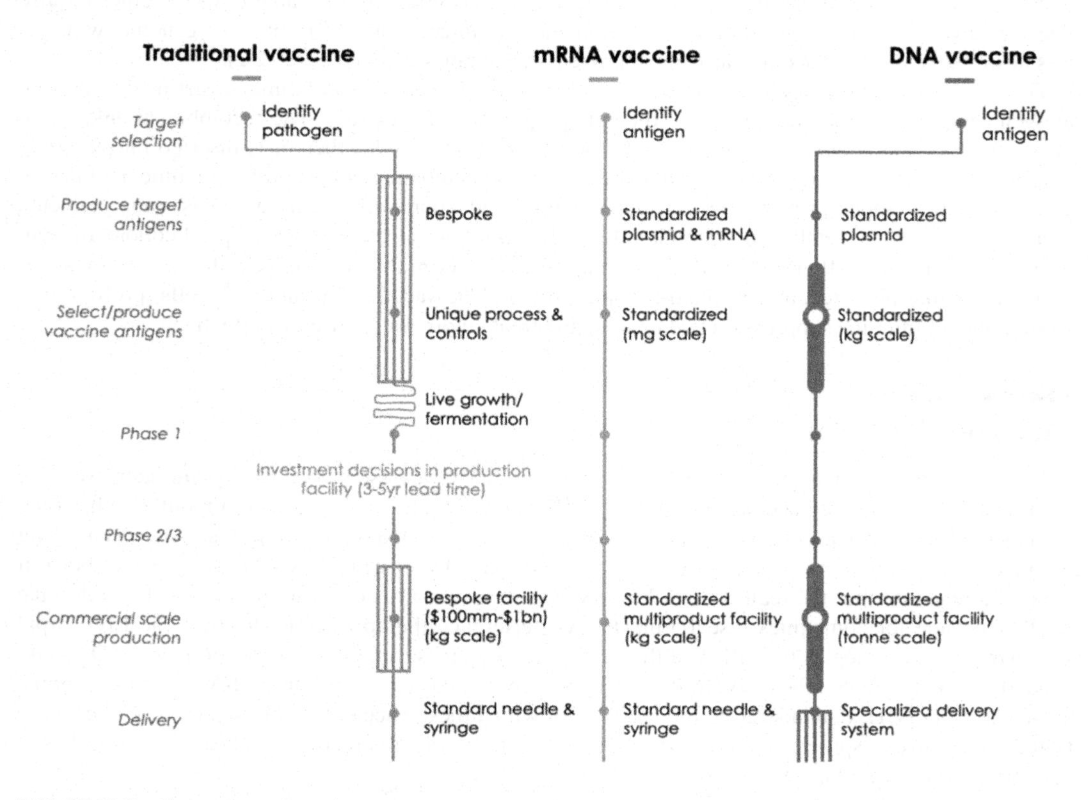

FIGURE 12.2 Comparison of vaccine types. Source: www.genengnews.com/insights/race-for-a-coronavirus-vaccine/.

It is now possible to create a universal flu shot that would work against any strain of the virus without being redesigned each year; since RNA vaccines can include instructions for multiple antigens, either strung together in a single strand or packaged together in a single nanoparticle—essentially a single vaccine in place of multiple—a combination of sexually transmitted diseases like HPV, HIV, and chlamydia can be combined.

New applications of mRNA vaccines would include:

- Multiple mRNAs, strung or single, in a single nanoparticle for recalcitrant diseases, such as tuberculosis, HIV, and malaria.
- Continuous modulation of the seasonal flu vaccine.
- Monoclonal antibody replaced with innate antibody production.
- Antigens to produce antibodies against rogue antibodies: autoimmune disorders to prevent diabetes 1, Parkinson's disease, Alzheimer's, and others.
- Diabetes protection vaccine against the six strains of the Coxsackie B (CVB) virus and myocarditis and meningitis.

The current issues in mRNA vaccines include contaminants in vaccine synthesis and the LNP delivery system, both of which can be reactogenic, but these are now quickly resolved. In addition, since the dosing of mRNA is small, a large supply of mRNA vaccines can be made within small facilities. For example, at a dose of 30 mcg of mRNA in the Pfizer COVID-19 vaccine, a 1 kg batch of mRNA will provide 33 million doses.

An mRNA vaccine provides acquired immunity through an mRNA containing vectors, such as lipid nanoparticles, wherein the mRNA sequence codes for antigens and identical proteins resembling those of the pathogen. Upon delivering the vaccine into the body, this sequence is translated by the host cells to produce the encoded antigens, which then stimulate the body's adaptive immune system to produce antibodies against the pathogen (Figures 12.3 and 12.4).

MHC molecules' function is to bind peptide fragments derived from pathogens and display them on the cell surface for recognition by the appropriate T cells (Figure 12.5). The consequences are almost always harmful to the pathogen—virus-infected cells are killed, macrophages are activated to kill bacteria living in their intracellular vesicles, and B cells are activated to produce antibodies that eliminate or neutralize extracellular pathogens. Thus, there is strong selective pressure in favor of any pathogen that has mutated in such a way that it escapes presentation by an MHC molecule. Due to two distinct properties of the MHC, pathogens find it difficult to evade immune responses in this way. To begin with, the MHC is polygenic, containing multiple MHC class I and MHC class II genes. Thus, every individual possesses a set of MHC molecules with varying ranges of peptide-binding specificities. Second, the MHC is highly polymorphic; that is, there are multiple variants of each gene within the population. Thus, the MHC genes are the most polymorphic genes known. This section will describe the organization of the genes in the MHC and discuss how the variation in MHC molecules arises. Also discussed is the effect of polygeny and polymorphism on the range of peptides that can be bound to contribute to the immune system's ability to respond to the multitude of diverse and rapidly evolving pathogens.

The difference between the two classes of the MHC is shown in Figure 12.5.

The targeted mRNA vaccines and therapies are among the safest treatment modalities today because of their transient nature and cytosolic location. In addition, the mRNA vaccine can also inhibit T cells' proliferation from inducing the occurrence of immune suppression and preventing or treating autoimmune diseases effectively.

There are two types of RNA vaccines, conventional and self-amplifying, capable of preventing multiple infectious diseases, including influenza, RSV, rabies, Ebola, and HIV-1. Self-amplifying RNAs have enhanced antigen expression at lower doses compared to conventional mRNA (Figure 12.6). The incorporation of chemically modified nucleotides, sequence optimization, and different purification strategies improve the efficiency of mRNA translation efficiency and reduces intrinsic immunogenic properties. On the other hand, antigen expression is proportional to the number of conventional mRNA transcripts delivered successfully during vaccination. Thus, to achieve adequate expression for protection

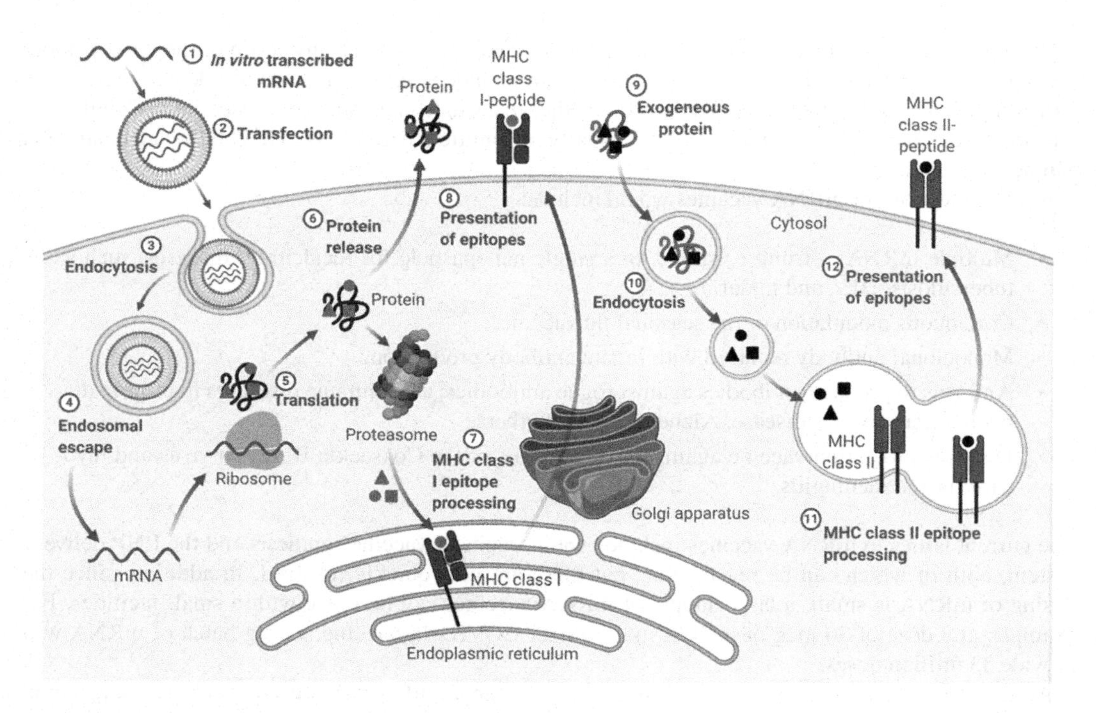

FIGURE 12.3 Mechanism of action of mRNA vaccines. 1) In a cell-free system, mRNA is in vitro transcribed (IVT) from a DNA template. 2) IVT mRNA is then transfected into dendritic cells (DCs) through the process of 3) endocytosis. 4) Endosomal escape allows entrapped mRNA to be released into the cytosol. 5) The mRNA is translated into antigenic proteins using the translational machinery of the host cell (ribosomes). Post-translational modifications are made to the translated antigenic protein. It can act in the cell where it is produced. 6) The protein can also be secreted by the host cell. 7) The proteasome is the cytoplasm that degrades the antigen protein. Antigenic peptide epitopes are synthesized and transported to the endoplasmic reticulum, loaded onto MHC class I molecules (MHC I: cell-mediated). 8) After T cell receptor recognition and appropriate co-stimulation, the loaded MHC I-peptide epitope complexes are presented on the surface of cells, eventually leading to the induction of antigen-specific CD8+ T cell responses. DCs can take up exogenous proteins. 9) They're degraded in endosomes before being presented through the MHC II (antibody-mediated) pathway. Furthermore, the protein should be routed through the MHC II pathway to obtain cognate T cell assistance in antigen-presenting cells. 10) The antigenic peptide epitopes that have been generated are then loaded onto MHC II molecules. 11) The antigen-specific CD4+ T cell responses are induced after the loaded MHC II-peptide epitope complexes are presented on the cell surface. Cross-presentation is a mechanism that allows exogenous antigens to be processed and loaded onto MHC class I molecules (see Figure 12.4). Source: Wadhwa A, Aljabbari A, Lokras A, Foged C, and Thakur A. Opportunities and Challenges in the Delivery of mRNA-Based Vaccines. *Pharmaceutics*. 2020;12(2):102. https://doi.org/10.3390/pharmaceutics12020102.

or immunomodulation, large doses or multiple administrations may be required. This limitation is addressed by saRNA vaccines, genetically engineered replicons derived from self-replicating single-stranded RNA viruses. They are delivered as viral replicon particles (VRPs), containing the saRNA, or as a fully synthetic saRNA produced after in vitro transcription. During production, envelope proteins are provided in trans as defective helper constructs to generate replication-defective VRPs. Following a first infection, the resulting VRPs lack the ability to form infectious viral particles, and only the RNA can be amplified further. Positive-sense and negative-sense RNA viruses both produce VRPs. On the other hand, the latter is more complicated and requires reverse genetics to save the VRPs (Figure 12.6).

5' cap (m7G) and poly-A tail are common to all RNA transcripts (Figure 12.7). Traditional mRNAs encode the vaccine immunogen and flanking 5' and 3' UTRs. The nonreplicating transcript is used to create an antigen or immunotherapy. 5' and 3' conserved sequence elements (CSE) sequences, the nsP1–4 genes, a subgenomic promoter, and the vaccine immunogen are encoded by self-amplifying RNA. The nonstructural proteins 1–4 (nsP1–4) form an RNA-dependent RNA polymerase (RdRP) complex after in situ translation, recognizing flanking CSE sequences and amplifying vaccine-encoding transcripts. As a result, the antigen or immunotherapy accumulates within the cell. To achieve a similar

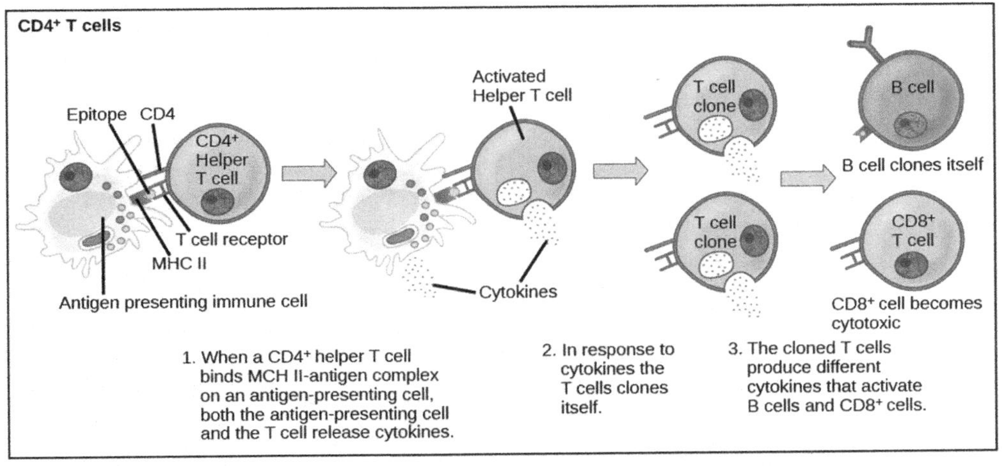

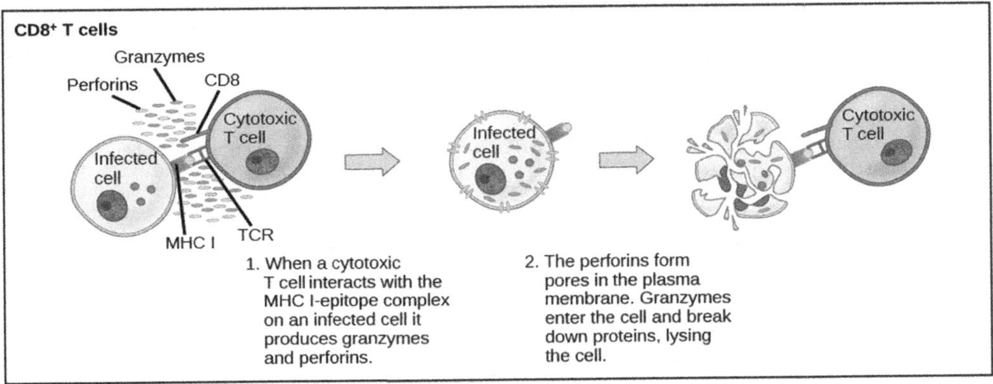

FIGURE 12.4 Role of major histocompatibility complex (MHC) in neutralizing antigens. Source: Silva, M, Cunha, F, Terra, F, and Camara, N. Old Game, New Players: Linking Classical Theories to New Trends in Transplant Immunology. *World Journal of Transplantation*. 2017;7(1). 10.5500/wjt.v7.i1.1.

effect to self-amplifying RNAs, trans-amplifying mRNAs use two different transcripts. A separate transcript encoding the viral CSE sequences, the subgenomic promoter, and the vaccine immunogen is co-delivered with a conventional mRNA encoding the nsP1–4 genes flanked by 5' and 3' untranslated regions (UTRs). The RdRP complex is formed when conventional mRNA is translated in situ, and it then amplifies the vaccine-encoding transcript to accumulate the antigen or immunotherapy.

Another form of the mRNA vaccination can encode fully human IgG antibodies that are identical or resembling the antibodies found in a patient with a prior history of potent immunity. This application can replace antibody therapy and allow the modulation of autoimmune responses. This new research area offers numerous opportunities to treat diseases currently considered not treatable, like Parkinson's disease, Alzheimer's, diabetes, and many rare cancers.

Whereas most early work in mRNA vaccines focused on cancer applications, more emphasis has recently been placed on preventing infectious pathogens, including the influenza virus, Ebola virus, Zika virus, *Streptococcus* spp. *T. gondii*, and coronavirus.

mRNA production avoids the common risks associated with other vaccine platforms, such as live viruses, viral vectors, inactivated viruses, and subunit protein vaccines. It does not require toxic chemicals or cell cultures that could be contaminated with adventitious viruses. Furthermore, the short manufacturing time for mRNA prevents microorganism contamination. The theoretical risks of infection or vector integration into host cell DNA are not a concern for mRNA in the vaccinated population. For the reasons stated above, mRNA vaccines are thought to be a relatively safe vaccine format.

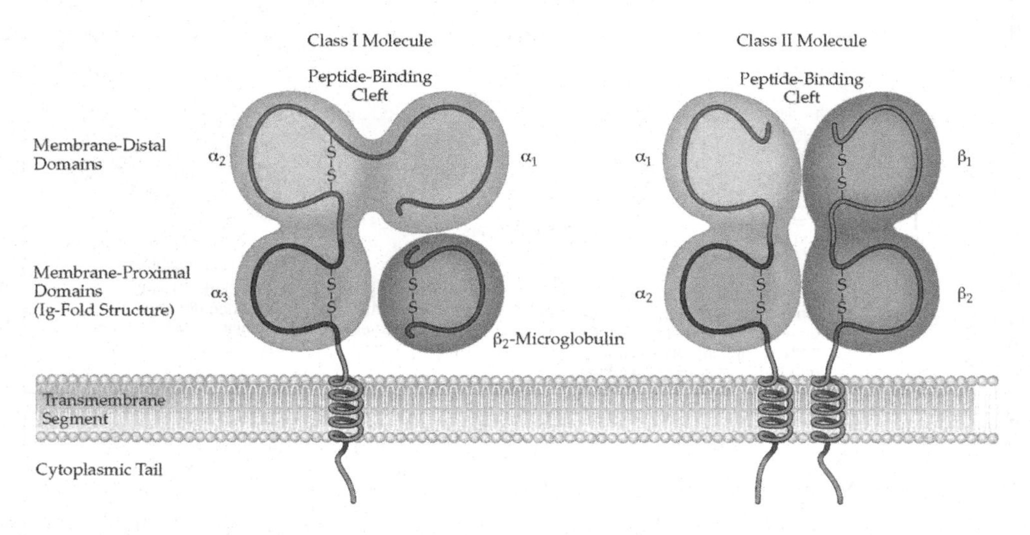

FIGURE 12.5 Difference between MHC Class I and MHC Class II molecules. Source: https://microbenotes.com/differences-between-mhc-class-i-and-class-ii/.

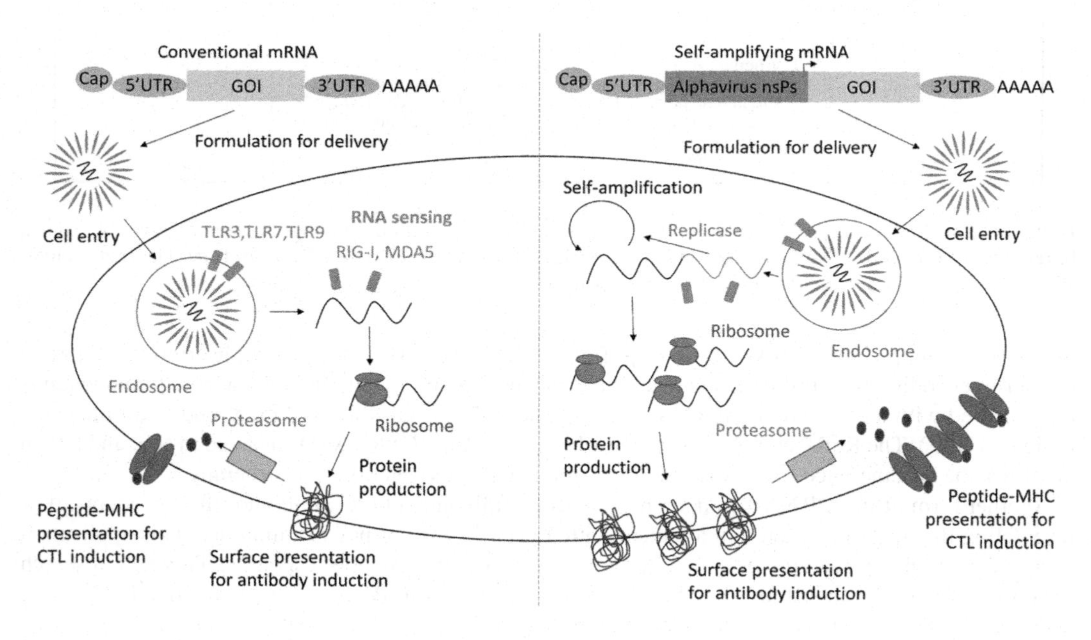

FIGURE 12.6 Two types of RNA vaccines. Source: Sandbrink, JB and Shattock, RJ. RNA Vaccines: A Suitable Platform for Tackling Emerging Pandemics? *Front. Immunol.* 2020. https://doi.org/10.3389/fimmu.2020.608460.

Local and systemic inflammation, biodistribution and persistence of expressed immunogen, stimulation of autoreactive antibodies, and potential toxic effects of non-native nucleotides and delivery system components are investigated in preclinical and clinical studies. Some mRNA-based vaccine platforms have been linked to inflammatory and possibly autoimmunity type I interferon responses, which have been linked to inflammation and possibly autoimmunity. Another potential hazard stemming from the presence of extracellular RNA during mRNA vaccination could be the presence of extracellular RNA.

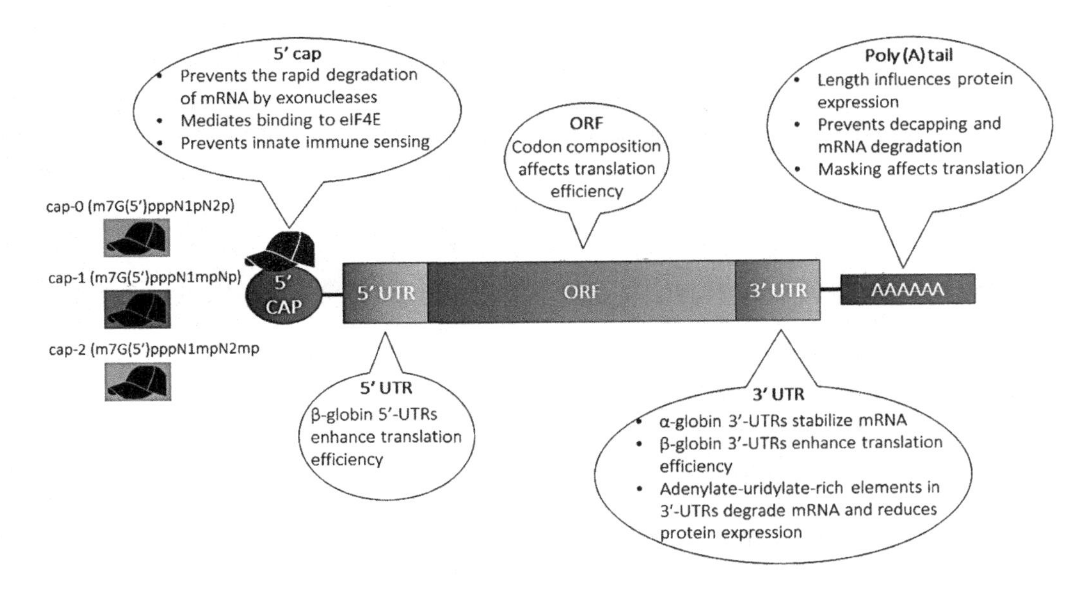

FIGURE 12.7 The structure of in vitro transcribed (IVT) mRNA and the most common modifications. IVT mRNA has a 5' cap, 5' and 3' untranslated regions (UTRs), an open reading frame (ORF) encoding antigen(s), and a 3' poly(A) tail which is based on the blueprint of eukaryotic mRNA. To modulate the protein's duration and kinetic profile expression, the IVT mRNA can be modified at one or more sites, such as the caps, UTRs, and poly(A) tail. The eukaryotic translation initiation factor 4E (eIF4E) is a protein that initiates translation in eukaryotes. Source: *Pharmaceutics*. 2020;12(2):102. https://doi.org/10.3390/pharmaceutics12020102.

Naked RNA from the extracellular environment has been shown to increase the permeability of densely packed endothelial cells, contributing to edema. The extracellular RNA also promotes blood coagulation and pathological thrombus formation. Therefore, safety will need continued evaluation as different mRNA modalities and delivery systems are utilized for the first time in humans and are tested in larger patient populations.

12.2.1 Development Cycle

If the pathogen and antigen(s) genomes are not already known, a combination sequencing, bioinformatics, and computational technique is used to determine the pathogen and antigen(s) genome. Candidate vaccine antigen sequences are deposited online and internationally for in silico mRNA vaccine creation, followed by molecular cloning or synthesis of a plasmid DNA template. In vitro transcription and capping of the mRNA, purification, and formulation with the delivery mechanism are used to make pilot vaccine batches in a cell-free system. To assess the quality of pilot mRNA vaccine batches, in-process analytic and potency testing are done. Pilot mRNA vaccine batches can be examined further in the immunogenicity and illness animal model if necessary. The finished mRNA vaccine is scaled up and manufactured using a generic technique with minor changes, tested quickly, and sent out for usage (see Figure 12.8)

GMP mRNA production begins with creating a DNA template, which is then followed by enzymatic in vitro transcription. To begin the production process, template plasmid DNA produced in *E. coli* is linearized with a restriction enzyme, and runoff transcripts with a poly(A) tract at the 3' end are synthesized. Next, the mRNA is synthesized from nucleoside triphosphates (NTP) by a DNA-dependent RNA polymerase from a bacteriophage (T7, SP6, or T3). After that, DNase is used to degrade the template DNA. Finally, the mRNA is capped, either chemically or enzymatically, to allow for efficient translation in vivo (Figure 12.7).

Alternate methods to replace plasmid DNA are evolving and include PCR-based DNA replication and circular DNA. A polymerase-chain-reaction (PCR)-produced linear DNA offers a cleaner,

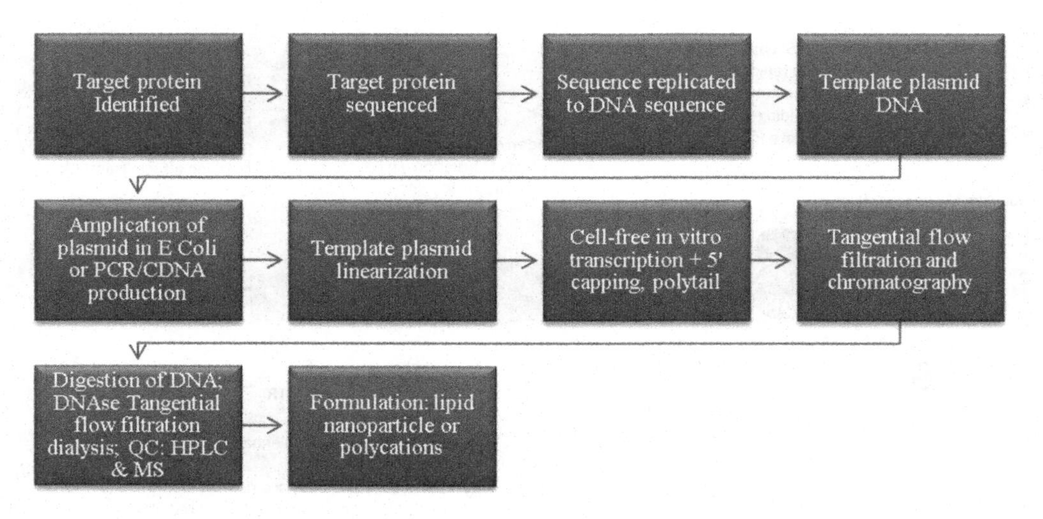

FIGURE 12.8 GMP production of mRNA vaccine.

TABLE 12.1
Comparison of Plasmid DNA and LineaRx PCR-Based Production of mRNA

Attribute	PCR DNA Production	Plasmid DNA Production
Risk of antibiotic resistance transfer	None	Yes
Endotoxin	None	Yes
Cellular purification	None	Required
Yield	Fixed	Variable
Cycle time	Hours	Days to weeks
Chemical modification of DNA by primer modification	Yes	No
Long homogenous poly-A tails (part of mRNA template)	Yes	No

higher-performing alternative to plasmid DNAs that are produced by fermentation in bacteria (https://adnas.com/linearx-pcr-produced-linear-dna/) (Table 12.1).

Another alternate to bacterial-based growth of cDNA clones is in vitro amplification using rolling circle amplification (RCA), an isothermal, high yield method of DNA amplification that uses a highly processive polymerase that amplifies DNA by 70 kb. Importantly, the enzyme replicates DNA with high fidelity due to its 3'-5'exonuclease or proofreading activity (www.biorxiv.org/content/10.1101/2020.06.22.165241v1) (Figure 12.9).

While the in vitro methods described above are attractive, the economics of the construction of mRNA vaccines remains dependent on plasmid DNA.

After mRNA is generated, it is purified to remove reaction components such as enzymes, unbound nucleotides, leftover DNA, and truncated RNA fragments, among other things. While lithium chloride precipitation is commonly employed for laboratory-scale preparation, derivatized microbeads in batch or column formats, which are easier to handle on a large scale, are used for clinical purification. In addition, for some mRNA platforms, removing dsRNA and other contaminants is critical for the final product's potency, as it is a potent inducer of interferon-dependent translation inhibition.

The desired mRNA transcript comprises a complex mixture of nucleotides, oligodeoxynucleotides, short abortive transcripts from abortive cycling during initiation, and protein. These contaminants are removed from the sample by a combination of precipitation and extraction steps.

However, the sample contains additional contaminating RNA species that are difficult to distinguish from the correct transcript using conventional methods: premature termination during elongation results in shorter than expected transcripts. Template DNA linearized with an enzyme that leaves

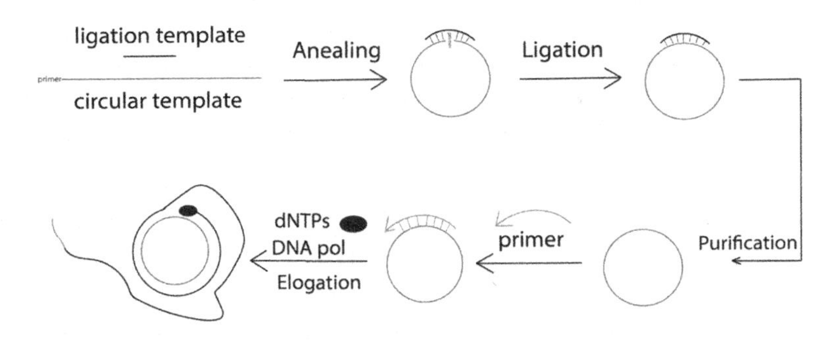

FIGURE 12.9 Rolling circle amplification of DNA.

a 3'-overhang or traces of nonlinearized template DNA results in longer than designated transcripts. The RNA-dependent RNA polymerase activity of bacteriophage polymerases also produces undesirable transcripts. As a result, mRNA will need to be purified further to remove such contaminating transcripts before being used as a drug substance.

A single chromatographic step is all that is required.

A single chromatographic step (e.g., HPLC) that separates mRNA according to size removes both shorter and longer transcripts, yielding a pure single mRNA product. The use of such chromatographic purification in a GMP mRNA production process increases mRNA molecules' activity in terms of protein expression in vivo by several-fold.

Protein expression from in vitro transcribed, enzymatically capped mRNA is further increased by enzymatic 2'-O-methylation of the first transcribed nucleotide, resulting in protein expression from mRNA capped with ARCA co-transcriptionally.

Generally, mRNA synthesis yields more than 2 g/1 of full-length mRNA in multi-gram scale reactions under optimized conditions. The scaleup is also simple since the in vitro processes are not batch-size dependent, as are the upstream processes.

12.2.2 Formulation and Delivery

Additional immunological considerations include delivery formulations, inoculation sites, and adjuvants. For example, RNA therapeutics and vaccines are delivered using nonviral formulations such as cationic lipids, LNPs, polymers, and protamine sulfate, as well as physical methods such as electroporation. In addition, because saRNAs contain the nsP1–4 replicon sequence, they are much longer than conventional RNAs, which is important for formulation.

Newer approaches aimed to improve the delivery of saRNAs include novel bio-reducible polymer formulations with high molecular weight poly(CBA-co-4amino-1-butanol) (pABOL), ornithine dendrimers, mannosylated polyethyleneimine, or multiple linear peptides that help facilitate intracellular trafficking and endosomal release. Manosylation of polyethyleneimine improves delivery of saRNA reporter constructs to human skin explants. Intramuscular (IM) delivery of saRNAs as neutral lipopolyplexes (LPPs) results in an increase in antigen-specific T cells with a concurrent loss of antigen-expressing cells. These LPPs are generated by creating core RNA/polyethyleneimine polyplexes before encapsulation in PEGanionic liposome formulations with mannosylated lipids. The inclusion of mannose improves vaccine delivery to antigen-presenting cells. saRNAs, on the other hand, do not require encapsulation to protect them from RNAse degradation. The exterior of positively charged LNPs formulated with dimethyl dioctadecyl ammonium (DAA) cationic lipids is completely protected from RNase treatment when saRNAs are complexed on the outside.

The Pfizer-BioNTech COVID-19 vaccine includes the following ingredients: mRNA, lipids ([{4-hydro xybutyl}azanediyl]bis[hexane-6,1-diyl]bis[2-hexyldecanoate], 2[{polyethylene glycol}-2000]-N,N-ditetradecylacetamide, 1,2-distearoyl-sn-glycero-3-phosphocholine, and cholesterol), potassium chloride, monobasic potassium phosphate, sodium chloride, dibasic sodium phosphate dihydrate, and sucrose.

The Moderna COVID-19 vaccine contains the following ingredients: messenger ribonucleic acid (mRNA), lipids (SM-102, polyethylene glycol [PEG] 2000 dimyristoyl glycerol [DMG], cholesterol, and 1,2-distearoyl-sn-glycero-3-phosphocholine [DSPC]), tromethamine, tromethamine hydrochloride, acetic acid, sodium acetate, and sucrose.

Both enzymatic and chemical degradation pathways are capable of degrading RNA. Formulation buffers are tested for contaminating RNases and may include buffer components like antioxidants and chelators to reduce the effects of reactive oxygen species and divalent metal ions on mRNA stability. mRNA degrades rapidly by ubiquitous extracellular ribonucleases before being taken up by cells. Thus, the efficacy of mRNA vaccines benefits from complexing agents that protect RNA from degradation. Complexation enhances uptake by cells and improves delivery to the cytoplasm's translation machinery. To this end, mRNA is often complexed with either lipids or polymers. Packaging mRNA products in nanoparticles or co-formulation with RNase inhibitors may also improve their stability. At least six months of stability has been observed for lipid-encapsulated mRNA, but longer-term storage of such mRNA–lipid complexes in an unfrozen form has not yet been reported. The Pfizer mRNA vaccine, the first to be approved by the FDA, requires storage at –90° C while a similar vaccine by Moderna requires –25° C to –15° C (Figure 12.10).

Not all complexing agents that promote DNA transfection are suitable for mRNA's complexation (Figure 12.10). Different large polycations, all proven DNA transfection reagents, strongly inhibit mRNA translation in cell-free translation systems and inside cells. Only much smaller polycations prove useful. If mRNA is bound to large polycations, it is not released in the cytosol, whereas endogenous RNA releases DNA from large polycations.

mRNA encapsulated in liposomes is most common, where cationic lipids are used for the intradermal and intravenous injection of antigen-encoding mRNA. However, mRNA's complexation with protamine, a small arginine-rich nuclear protein that stabilizes DNA during spermatogenesis, also stabilizes mRNA against degradation by serum components.

The vaccine delivery method is broadly classified by whether the RNA transfer to cells happens within (in vivo) or outside (ex vivo) the organism. Dendritic cells are immune cells that display antigens on their surfaces, leading to T cells' interactions to initiate an immune response. Dendritic cells are collected from patients and programmed with the desired mRNA. Then, they are re-administered back into patients to create an immune response.

In vivo approaches offer several advantages over ex vivo methods, particularly by avoiding the cost of harvesting and adapting dendritic cells from patients and by imitating a regular infection. However, to start translation, evolutionary mechanisms that prevent the infiltration of unknown nucleic material and promote RNase degradation must be bypassed. Furthermore, because RNA is too heavy to diffuse inside the cell independently, it is vulnerable to being discovered and eliminated by the host cell.

Non-viral delivery methods have been engineered to achieve similar immunological responses as RNA viruses. Retroviruses, lentiviruses, alphaviruses, and rhabdoviruses are common RNA viruses used as vectors, and each has its structure and function.

The delivery of the vaccine is simply held in a buffer with a naked injection.

Self-amplifying mRNA has different mechanisms and, as a result, is evaluated differently. This is because self-amplifying mRNA is a much larger molecule.

Refining saRNA pharmacokinetics is possible by revising the 5' cap structure, controlling the length of the poly(A) tail, including modified nucleotides, codon, sequence optimization, and altering the 5' and 3' UTRs is used to modify the pharmacokinetics of RNA. For longer saRNA transcripts, balancing the intrinsic and extrinsic immunogenic properties of the synthetic RNA, the vaccine antigen, and the delivery formulation is equally important. The translation is improved, and RNA-associated immunogenicity is reduced by incorporating pseudouridine-modified nucleotides during transcription because saRNAs use host-cell factors to replicate mRNA; adding modified nucleotides is less useful because they are lost during amplification.

One practical approach to improving the translation of saRNA vaccines is through optimization of 5' and 3' UTRs, which is based on the evolution of naturally occurring alphaviruses. The single-stranded RNA genome forms various secondary structures to allow alphaviruses to bypass requirements of

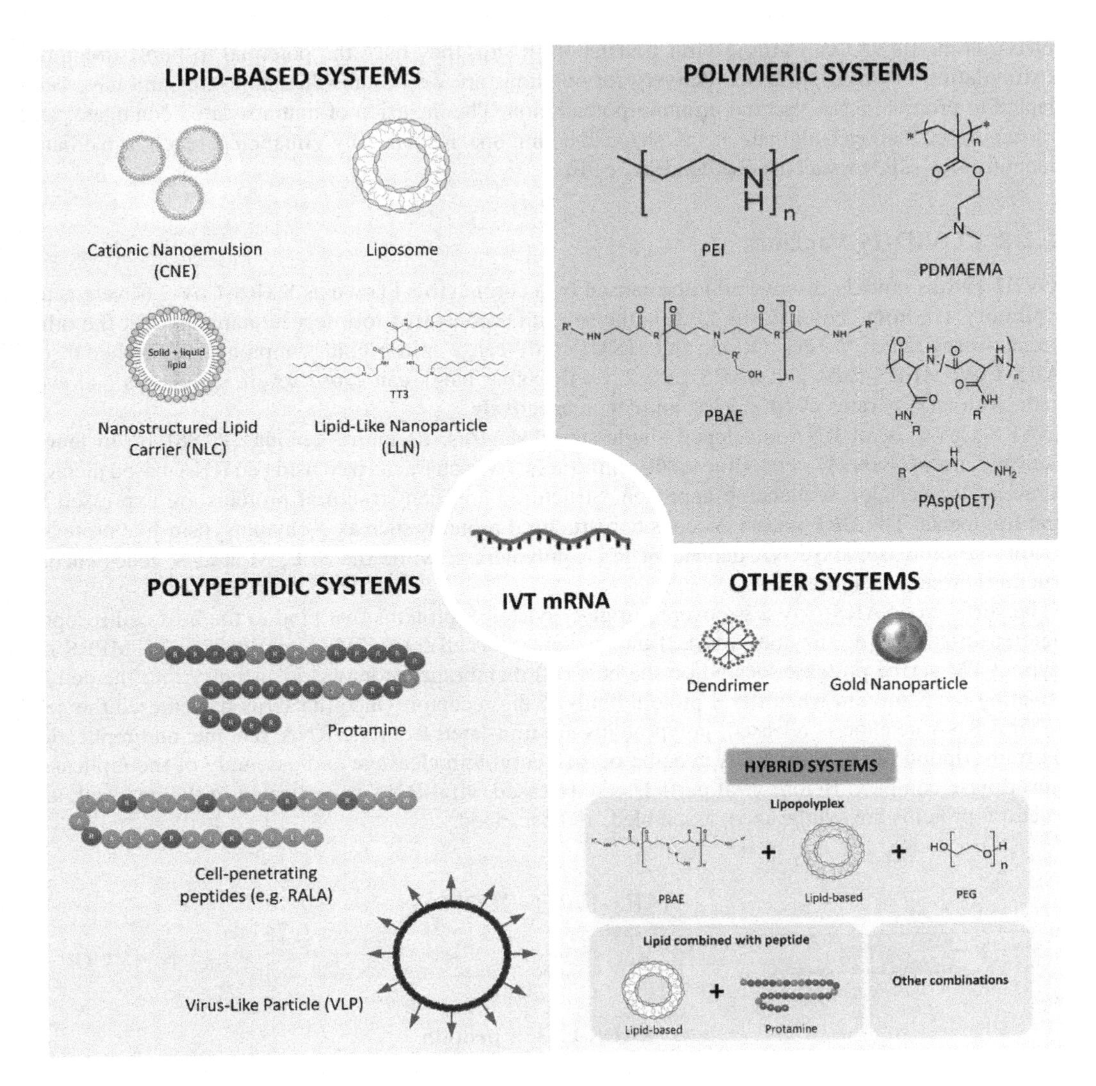

FIGURE 12.10 Types of formulations of mRNA vaccines. Source: Gómez-Aguado, I, Rodríguez-Castejón, J, Vicente-Pascual, M, Rodríguez-Gascón, A, Solinís, MÁ, and del Pozo-Rodríguez, A. Nanomedicines to Deliver mRNA: State of the Art and Future Perspectives. *Nanomaterials.* 2020;10(2):364. https://doi.org/10.3390/nano10020364. http://creativecommons.org/licenses/by/4.0/.

normal host-cell translation processes and evade immune responses. It is also beneficial to review the sequence encoding the nsP1–4 replicon genes.

An approach to protecting in vitro transcribed RNAs from nuclease digestion and augmenting translation is the modification of the synthetic 5' cap structure. By only capping transcripts in the forward orientation, the anti-reverse cap analog and phosphorothioate derivatives improve in situ translation of RNAs. Post-transcription capping enzymes derived from the vaccinia virus have high capping efficiencies, and when combined with 2'-O-methyltransferases, generate Cap 1 structures that mimic natural eukaryotic mRNAs.

Adjuvants have long been used in vaccines to boost adaptive immunity and shape T cell responses. Adjuvants currently used in licensed vaccines include aluminum salts, emulsions, lipid analogs, and virosomes, to name a few. The value of such adjuvants in RNA vaccinology is unknown, and it depends on the types of modifications made during design and production. Clinical trials with conventional mRNA vaccines have so far revealed only a limited level of humoral immunity. Because saRNAs contain native alphavirus motifs and can mimic viral translation in situ, they have the potential to boost immunity by stimulating PRRs. Lipid-based delivery formulations are well-established adjuvants and have been adapted to promote RNA vaccine immuno-potentiation. The inclusion of mannosylated conjugates and chitosan-based nanogel alginate helps shape the immune response by enhancing receptor-mediated endocytosis of saRNA vaccines by dendritic cells.

12.2.3 COVID-19 Vaccine

COVID-19 was quickly discovered to be caused by a coronavirus known as SARS-CoV-2 (severe acute respiratory syndrome coronavirus 2). It is the seventh coronavirus to infect humans; four of the other coronaviruses (229E, NL63, OC43, and HKU1) only cause minor cold symptoms. The other three, SARS-CoV, MERS-CoV, and SARS-CoV-2, on the other hand, can cause severe symptoms and even death, with fatality rates of 10%, 37%, and 5%, respectively.

SARS-CoV-2 is an RNA-enveloped single-stranded virus. Its entire genome, 29,881 bp in length (GenBank no. MN908947), encoding 9,860 amino acids, was characterized using an RNA-based metagenomic next-generation sequencing approach. Structured and non-structural proteins are expressed by gene fragments. The ORF region encodes nonstructural proteins such as 3-chymotrypsin-like protease, papain-like protease, and RNA-dependent RNA polymerase, while the S, E, M, and N genes encode structural proteins (Figure 12.11).

The surface of SARS-CoV-2 is covered in glycosylated S proteins that bind to the host cell receptor angiotensin-converting enzyme 2 (ACE2) and mediate viral cell entry. TM protease serine 2 (TMPRSS2), a type 2 TM serine protease located on the host cell membrane, promotes virus entry into the cell by activating the S protein when the S protein binds to the receptor. Once the virus has entered the cell, the viral RNA genome is released, polyproteins are translated from the RNA genome, and replication and transcription of the viral RNA genome occur via protein cleavage and assembly of the replicase–transcriptase complex. Before viral particles are released, viral RNA is replicated in the host cell, and structural proteins are synthesized, assembled, and packaged.

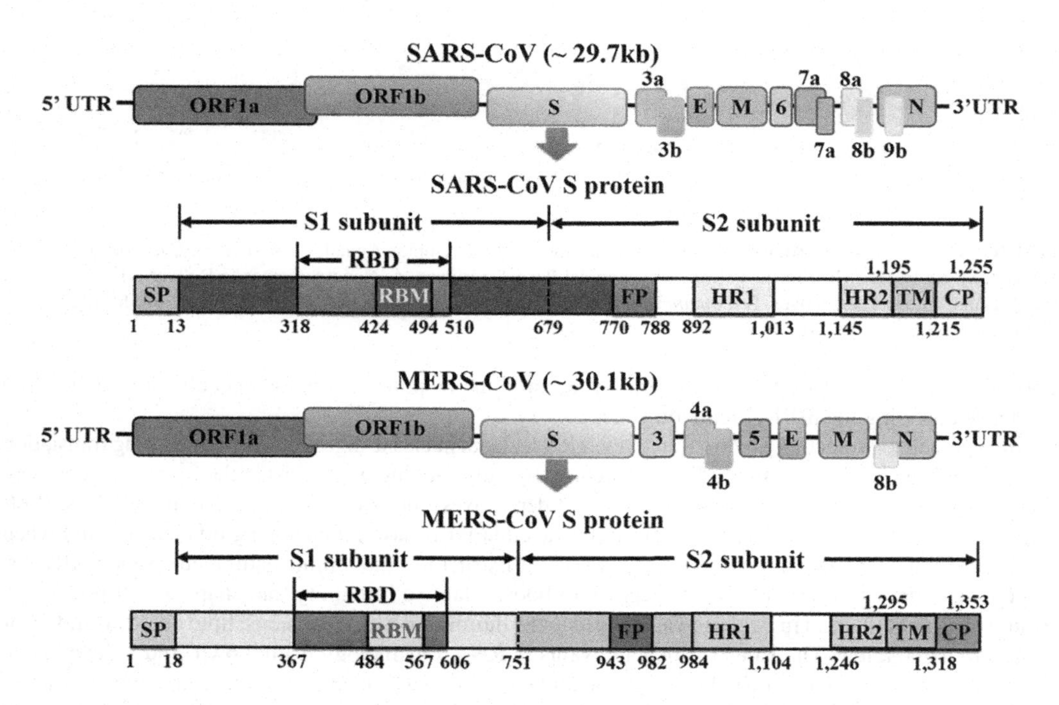

FIGURE 12.11 SARS-CoV protein structure. Source: https://commons.wikimedia.org/w/index.php?curid=88420710 Schematic of the SARS-CoV-2 S protein.

These proteins are essential for the viral life cycle and could be used as drug targets. Experiments have shown that ACE2-based peptides, 3CLpro inhibitors (3CLpro-1), and a novel vinyl sulfone protease inhibitor effectively against SARS-CoV-2. The SARS-CoV-2 S protein is involved in receptor recognition, viral attachment, and entry into host cells and is highly conserved among all human coronaviruses (HCoVs). Its essential functions represent one of the most critical targets for the COVID-19 vaccine and therapeutic research.

The S protein has an extracellular N-terminus, a transmembrane (TM) domain anchored in the viral membrane, and a short intracellular C-terminal segment with a size of 180–200 kDa. S is normally in a metastable prefusion conformation; however, when the virus interacts with the host cell, the S protein undergoes extensive structural rearrangement, allowing the virus to fuse with the host cell membrane. To avoid detection by the host immune system during entry, the spikes are coated with polysaccharide molecules.

The signal peptide (amino acids 1–13) located at the N-terminus, the S1 subunit (14–685 residues), and the S2 subunit (686–1,273 residues) make up the total length of SARS-CoV-2 S. The last two regions are responsible for receptor binding and membrane fusion, respectively.

The initiation of virus infection occurs when virus particles bind to cell receptors on the host cell's surface; thus, receptor recognition is an important determinant of viral entry and a drug design target.

Several mAbs have shown promising results in neutralizing SARS-CoV-2. CR3022, a SARS-CoV-specific human mAb, binds potently with SARS-CoV-2 (KD of 6.3 nM, measured by BLI in OctetRED96), suggesting that CR3022 has the potential to be developed as candidate therapeutic, alone or in combination with other nAbs, for the prevention and treatment of SARS-CoV-2 infection. SARS-CoV-2 and SARS-CoV infections have recently been shown to be neutralized by a mAb targeting S1 prepared from immunized transgenic mice expressing human Ig variable heavy and light chains via an unknown mechanism that is independent of the blockade of RBD–hACE2 interaction. Many human blocking mAbs (311mab-31B5, 311mab- 32D4, 47D11, n3130, n3088, S309, P2C-1F11, P2B-2F6, B38, H4) have been successfully cloned from single memory B cells from recovered COVID-19 patients. These mAbs specifically bind to SARS-CoV-2 S to effectively neutralize infection. Also, sera from SARS patients during rehabilitation or animals specifically immunized with SARS-CoV S1 may cross-neutralize SARS-CoV-2 and reduce S protein-mediated SARS-CoV-2 entry.

12.3 DNA Vaccine

The techniques for developing a DNA vaccine and gene therapy are similar. A DNA vaccine works by infecting an immunized species with a specific antigen DNA-coding sequence (Figure 12.12).

DNA vaccines work by injecting a genetically modified plasmid containing the antigen(s) for which an immune response is desired. As a result, the cells produce the antigen directly, resulting in a protective immune response. As a result, DNA vaccines have theoretical advantages over traditional vaccines, such as eliciting a broader range of immune responses. Several DNA vaccines for veterinary use have been tested. Animals have been protected from disease in some cases, but not all. As of the middle of 2021, no DNA vaccine has been approved.

DNA vaccines contain DNA that codes for specific proteins produced by a pathogen (antigens). The DNA is injected into the body and taken up by cells, which use their normal metabolic processes to produce proteins based on the plasmid's genetic code. Because they contain regions of amino acid sequences that are characteristic of bacteria or viruses, these proteins are recognized as foreign. The immune system is notified when they are processed by the host cells and displayed on their surface, triggering immune responses. The DNA can also be encapsulated in protein to aid cell entry. The resulting vaccine will have the potency of a live vaccine without the risk of reversion if this capsid protein is included in the DNA.

The advantages of DNA vaccines include:

- First, there is no risk of infection.
- Both MHC class I and class II molecules present antigens.

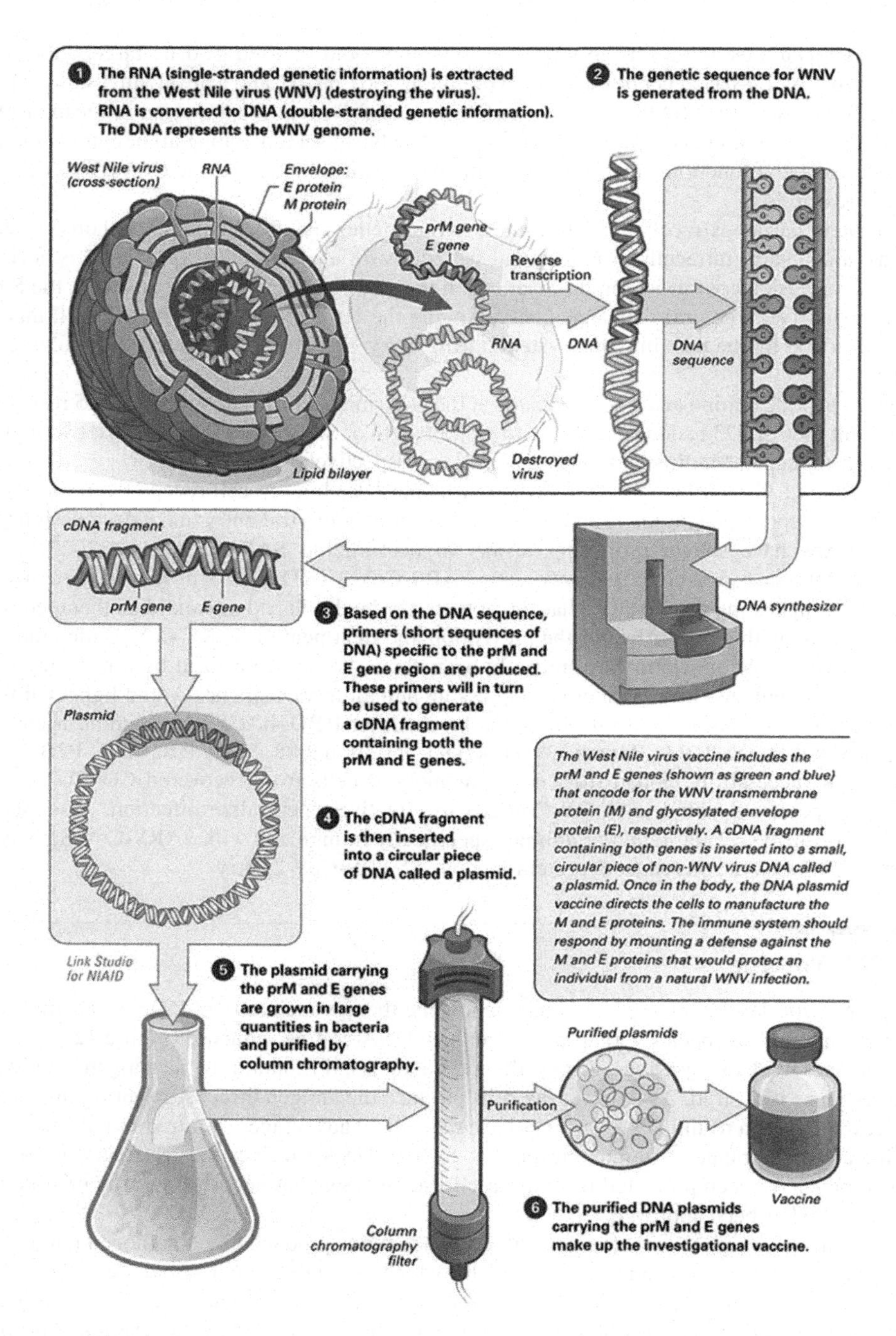

1 The RNA (single-stranded genetic information) is extracted from the West Nile virus (WNV) (destroying the virus). RNA is converted to DNA (double-stranded genetic information). The DNA represents the WNV genome.
2 The genetic sequence for WNV is generated from the DNA.
West Nile virus (cross-section)
RNA
Envelope:
E protein
M protein
prM gene
E gene
Reverse transcription
RNA
DNA
DNA sequence
Lipid bilayer
Destroyed virus
cDNA fragment
prM gene
E gene
DNA synthesizer
3 Based on the DNA sequence, primers (short sequences of DNA) specific to the prM and E gene region are produced. These primers will in turn be used to generate a cDNA fragment containing both the prM and E genes.
Plasmid
4 The cDNA fragment is then inserted into a circular piece of DNA called a plasmid.
The West Nile virus vaccine includes the prM and E genes (shown as green and blue) that encode for the WNV transmembrane protein (M) and glycosylated envelope protein (E), respectively. A cDNA fragment containing both genes is inserted into a small, circular piece of non-WNV virus DNA called a plasmid. Once in the body, the DNA plasmid vaccine directs the cells to manufacture the M and E proteins. The immune system should respond by mounting a defense against the M and E proteins that would protect an individual from a natural WNV infection.
Link Studio for NIAID
5 The plasmid carrying the prM and E genes are grown in large quantities in bacteria and purified by column chromatography.
Purified plasmids
Purification
Column chromatography filter
6 The purified DNA plasmids carrying the prM and E genes make up the investigational vaccine.
Vaccine

FIGURE 12.12 The making of a DNA vaccine. Source: unknown author – NIAID Begins Clinical Trial of West Nile Virus Vaccine on National Institute of Allergy and Infectious Diseases, Public Domain, https://commons.wikimedia.org/w/index.php?curid=3271397.

- T cell response is polarized toward type 1 or type 2.
- The immune response was concentrated on the antigen in question.
- Ease of development and production.
- Storage and shipping stability.
- Cost-effectiveness.

- Removes the need for peptide synthesis, recombinant protein expression, and purification, as well as the use of toxic adjuvants.
- Long-term persistence of immunogen.
- In vivo expression ensures protein more closely resembles standard eukaryotic structure, with accompanying post-translational modifications.

The potential adverse effects include:

- Limited to protein immunogens (not valid for non-protein-based antigens such as bacterial polysaccharides).
- Risk of affecting genes controlling cell growth[citation needed.
- Possibility of inducing anti-DNA antibody production.
- Tolerance to the antigen (protein) produced is a possibility.
- Atypical protein processing by bacteria and parasites is a possibility.
- Potential for transfecting non-target cells, such as brain cells, using plasmid DNA nanoparticles delivered via nasal spray.

12.3.1 Delivery

DNA vaccines are delivered systemically by intravenous injection to reach secondary lymphatic organs, by oral application of (attenuated) bacteria as a vehicle to confer uptake of DNA by intestinal APC, and by pulmonary administration of nebulized DNA to achieve uptake by lung cells. Transdermal delivery primarily addresses LC (Langerhans cells), and both needle-free deliveries of particle-adsorbed DNA vaccines by helium pressure (gene gun, particle mediated epidermal delivery [PMED]) and needle-based administration via microneedles and tattoo devices are clinically tested. Transfection of cutaneous APC (antigen-presenting cells) and non-APC by intradermally injected DNA vaccines is enhanced by immediate electroporation. Subcutaneous injection mainly results in the transfection of fibroblasts and keratinocytes, expressing transgenes and releasing antigen for uptake of APC. Likewise, intramuscular injection of DNA vaccines primarily yields transfection of myocytes that express/release antigen for APC uptake, and myocyte transfection rates are enhanced by electroporation at the site of injection as well (Table 12.2).

Table 12.3 lists the relative advantages of delivery methods.

TABLE 12.2

Summary of Plasmid DNA Delivery Methods

Method of Delivery		Formulation of DNA	Target Tissue	Amount of DNA
Parenteral	Injection (hypodermic needle)	The aqueous solution in saline	IM (skeletal); ID; IV, subcutaneous and intraperitoneal with variable success	Large amounts (approximately 100–200 μg)
	Gene gun	DNA-coated gold beads	ED (abdominal skin); vaginal mucosa; surgically exposed muscle and other organs	Small amounts (as little as 16 ng)
	Pneumatic (jet) injection	Aqueous solution	ED	Very high (as much as 300 μg)
Topical application		Aqueous solution	Ocular; intravaginal	Small amounts (up to 100 μg)
Cytofectin-mediated		Liposomes (cationic); microspheres; recombinant adenovirus vectors; attenuated *Shigella* vector; aerosolized cationic lipid formulations	IM; IV (to transfect tissues systemically); intraperitoneal; oral immunization to the intestinal mucosa; nasal/lung mucosal membranes	Variable

TABLE 12.3

Advantages and Disadvantages of Commonly Used DNA Vaccine Delivery Methods

Method of Delivery	Advantage	Disadvantage
Intramuscular or intradermal injection	No special delivery mechanism Permanent or semi-permanent expression pDNA spreads rapidly throughout the body	Inefficient site for uptake due to morphology of muscle tissue Relatively large amounts of DNA used Th1 response may not be the response required
Gene gun	DNA bombarded directly into cells Small amounts of DNA	Th2 response may not be the response required Requires inert particles as a carrier
Jet injection	No particles required DNA is delivered to cells mm to cm below the skin surface	Significant shearing of DNA after high-pressure expulsion Ten-fold lower expression and lower immune response Requires large amounts of DNA (up to 300 μg)
Liposome-mediated delivery	High levels of the immune response are generated Can increase transfection of intravenously delivered pDNA Intravenously delivered liposome-DNA complexes can potentially transfect all tissues Intranasally delivered liposome-DNA complexes can result in expression in distal mucosa as well as nasal mucosa and the generation of IgA antibodies	Toxicity Ineffectiveness in serum Risk of disease or immune reactions

Source: https://en.wikipedia.org/wiki/DNA_vaccination.

DNA vaccines are introduced by multiple methods. The two most popular approaches were injection of DNA in saline using a standard hypodermic needle or using a gene gun delivery. DNA is delivered to extracellular spaces by injecting saline intramuscularly (IM) or intradermally (ID) into skeletal muscle. This is assisted either 1) by electroporation, 2) by temporarily damaging muscle fibers with mycotoxins such as bupivacaine, or 3) by using hypertonic solutions of saline or sucrose. Immune responses to this method are affected by needle type, needle alignment, injection speed, injection volume, muscle type, age, sex, and the recipient's physiological condition. Delivery of a gene gun plasmid DNA (pDNA) absorbed onto gold or tungsten microparticles is ballistically accelerated into target cells using compressed helium as an accelerant.

Aerosol instillation of naked DNA on mucosal surfaces such as the nasal and lung mucosa and topical administration of pDNA to the eye and vaginal mucosa were two other options. In addition, cationic liposome-DNA preparations, biodegradable microspheres, attenuated *Salmonella*, *Shigella*, or *Listeria* vectors for oral administration to the intestinal mucosa, and recombinant adenovirus vectors have all been used for mucosal surface delivery.

DNA vaccines are also delivered using a hybrid vehicle made up of bacteria cells and synthetic polymers. The inner core of *E. coli* and the outer coat of poly(beta-amino ester) work together to increase efficiency by addressing barriers to antigen-presenting cell gene delivery, such as cellular uptake and internalization, phagosomal escape, and intracellular cargo concentration.

Expression library immunization is another method of DNA vaccination (ELI). This technique can deliver all of a pathogen's genes at the same time, which is useful for attenuating or cultivating problematic pathogens. In addition, ELI is used to identify which genes induce a protective response.

12.3.2 Antibody Response

Multiple factors influence antibody responses elicited by DNA vaccinations, including antigen type, antigen location (intracellular versus secreted), number, frequency, and immunization dose, site, and method of antigen delivery.

TABLE 12.4

Comparison of T-Dependent Antibody Responses Raised by DNA Immunizations, Protein Inoculations, and Viral Infections

	Method of Immunization		
	DNA Vaccine	**Recombinant Protein**	**Natural Infection**
Amount of inducing antigen	ng	µg	? (ng–µg)
Duration of antigen presentation	Several weeks	< 1 week	Several weeks
Kinetics of antibody response	Slow rise	Rapid rise	Rapid rise
Number of inoculations to obtain high avidity IgG and migration of ASC to bone marrow	1	2	1
Ab isotype (murine models)	C'-dependent or C'-independent	C'-dependent	C'-independent

After a single DNA injection, humoral responses are much longer-lived than after a single injection with a recombinant protein. For example, antibody responses to the hepatitis B virus (HBV) envelope protein (HBsAg) have been shown to last for up to 74 weeks in mice after gene gun delivery, while lifelong maintenance of a protective response to influenza haemagglutinin has also been demonstrated. Antibody-secreting cells migrate to the bone marrow and spleen to produce long-term antibodies, and they usually settle down after a year.

The comparison of antibody responses generated by natural (viral) infection, immunization with recombinant protein, and immunization with plasmid DNA is summarized in Table 12.4.

Antibodies induced by DNA immunization have a higher affinity for native epitopes than antibodies induced by recombinant proteins. To put it another way, DNA immunization produces a higher-quality response. Antibodies are induced after one vaccination with DNA, whereas recombinant protein vaccinations generally require a boost. In addition, DNA immunization can bias the immune response's T-helper profile and thus the antibody isotype, which is not possible with either natural infection or recombinant protein immunization.

Antibody responses induced by DNA are also slower to develop than those induced by natural infection or recombinant protein immunization. In mice, peak titers can take up to 12 weeks to reach, though boosting can shorten the time. This is most likely due to the low levels of antigen expressed over a long period, which supports both primary and secondary phases of antibody response. Adults with chronic hepatitis were given a DNA vaccine expressing HBV small and middle envelope proteins. The vaccine resulted in the production of specific interferon-gamma cells. T cells specific for middle envelope protein antigens have also been developed. However, the patients' immune responses were insufficient to control HBV infection.

ADDITIONAL READING

Agrawal AS, Tao X, Algaissi A, Garron T, et al. Immunization with inactivated middle east respiratory syndrome coronavirus vaccine leads to lung immunopathology on challenge with live virus. *Hum Vaccin Immunother.* 2016;12(9):2351–2356, https://www.ncbi.nlm.nih.gov/pmc/articles/PMC5027702/.

Bolles M, Deming D, Long K, Agnihothram S, et al. A double-inactivated severe acute respiratory syndrome coronavirus vaccine provides incomplete protection in mice and induces increased eosinophilic proinflammatory pulmonary response upon challenge. *J Virol.* 2011;85(23):12201–12215, https://www.ncbi.nlm.nih.gov/pmc/articles/PMC3209347/.

Centers for Disease Control and Prevention. Coronavirus disease 2019 (COVID-19) at risk for severe illness, last reviewed May 14, 2020, https://www.cdc.gov/coronavirus/2019-ncov/need-extra-precautions/groups-at-higher-risk.html.

FDA. COVID-19 public health emergency: general considerations for pre-IND meeting requests for COVID-19 related drugs and biological products; guidance for industry, May 2020, https://www.fda.gov/media/137927/download.

FDA. Draft guidance for industry: how to comply with the pediatric research equity act, September 2005, https://www.fda.gov/media/72274/download.*

FDA. Emergency use authorization of medical products and related authorities; guidance for industry and other stakeholders, January 2017, https://www.fda.gov/media/97321/download.

FDA. FDA guidance on conduct of clinical trials of medical products during COVID-19 public health emergency; guidance for industry, investigators, and institutional review boards, March 2020 and updated June 2020, https://www.fda.gov/media/136238/download.

FDA. Guidance for industry: considerations for developmental toxicity studies for preventive and therapeutic vaccines for infectious disease indications, February 2006, https://www.fda.gov/media/73986/download.

FDA. Guidance for industry: considerations for plasmid dna vaccines for infectious disease indications, November 2007, https://www.fda.gov/media/73667/download.

FDA. Guidance for industry: content and format of chemistry, manufacturing and controls information and establishment description information for a vaccine or related product, January 1999, https://www.fda.gov/media/73614/download.

FDA. Guidance for industry: E2E pharmacovigilance planning, April 2005, https://www.fda.gov/media/71238/download.

FDA. Guidance for industry: establishment and operation of clinical trial data monitoring committees, March 2006, https://www.fda.gov/media/75398/download.

FDA. Guidance for industry: postmarketing studies and clinical trials — implementation of section 505(o)(3) of the Federal Food, Drug, and Cosmetic Act, April 2011, https://www.fda.gov/media/131980/download.

FDA. Guidance for industry: process validation: general principles and practices, January 2011, https://www.fda.gov/media/71021/download.

FDA. Postapproval pregnancy safety studies; draft guidance for industry, May 2019, https://www.fda.gov/media/124746/download.*

FDA. Pregnant women: scientific and ethical considerations for inclusion in clinical trials; draft guidance for industry, April 2018, https://www.fda.gov/media/112195/download.*

Haagmans BL, Boudet F, Kuiken T, deLang A, et al. Protective immunity induced by the inactivated SARS coronavirus vaccine, Abstract S 12–1 Presented at the *X International Nidovirus Symposium*, Springs, CO; 2005.

Perlman S, Dandekar AA. Immunopathogenesis of coronavirus infections: implications for SARS. *Nat Rev Immunol* 2005;5:917–927, https://doi.org/10.1038/nri1732.

Tseng C-T, Sbrana E, Iwata-Yoshikawa N, Newman P, et al. Immunization with SARS coronavirus vaccines leads to pulmonary immunopathology on challenge with the sars virus. *PloS One*. 2012;7(4):e35421, https://journals.plos.org/plosone/article?id=10.1371/journal.pone.0035421.

World Health Organization. Guidelines on the nonclinical evaluation of vaccine adjuvants and adjuvanted vaccines, Annex 2, WHO Technical Report Series, 987:59–100, https://www.who.int/biologicals/areas/vaccines/TRS_987_Annex2.pdf?ua=1.

World Health Organization. WHO guidelines on nonclinical evaluation of vaccines, Annex 1, WHO Technical Report Series, 2005; 927:31–63, 2005. https://www.who.int/biologicals/publications/trs/areas/vaccines/nonclinical_evaluation/ANNEX%201Nonclinical.P31-63.pdf.

Yasui F, Kai C, Kitabatake M, Inoue S, et al. Prior immunization with severe acute respiratory syndrome (SARS) – associated coronavirus (SARS-CoV) nucleocapsid protein causes severe pneumonia in mice infected with SARS-CoV. *J Immunol*. 2008;181(9):6337–6348, https://www.jimmunol.org/content/181/9/6337.long.

13

Botanical Products

13.1 Overview

Humanity began treating diseases using the botanicals that were found all around in the foraging communities; all discoveries were anecdotal and based on trial and error with no rationale for determining plants' effectiveness in treating diseases. Many who tried new plants in curiosity also never lived to tell the story. The botanical products are still used as concoctions or concentrated plant extracts without isolation of active compounds. Modern medicine, however, prefers to isolate and purify the active components. However, the isolation of the "active compound" can make the extract ineffective since it is often not possible to identify the active component or how it acts in the presence of other active or inactive components. Recognizing this uniqueness of plant medicines, the regulatory agencies now accept applications for drugs based on plant extracts without declaring the active ingredient (www.fda.gov/media/93113/download).

Drug discovery is a multidiscipline task requiring several scientific approaches from chemistry to pharmacology to clinical testing. Still, it all starts at identifying a target, an approach that has evolved significantly, yet its basic model remains the same. New ways to process complex botanical products and use their structures to create novel drugs have been paved by recent advances in analytical and computational techniques. In the current era, computational molecular design is applied to the development of botanical products. Predictive computational software has contributed to the discovery of molecular targets of botanical products and their derivatives. Quantum computing, computational software, and databases will be used in the future to model molecular interactions and predict features and parameters required for drug development, such as pharmacokinetics and pharmacodynamics, resulting in fewer false-positive leads in drug development. This chapter discusses plant-based natural product drug discovery and how innovative technologies play a role in next-generation drug discovery. This chapter also includes a description of the regulatory requirements relevant to securing approval of new botanical products.

The low rate of drug discovery success necessitates a paradigm shift in drug development strategies. Botanical products for the effective treatment of disease conditions serve as a source of inspiration for innovative drug development. Botanical products' importance in developing innovative drugs to combat communicable and non-communicable diseases cannot be overstated. Technological advancements have made it possible to decipher the profiles of these complex botanical products, potentially leading to the discovery of new drugs. Natural product lead compounds have been used to isolate or synthesize a large number of blockbuster drugs. Natural product drug discovery is thus positioned as a highly successful strategy for developing novel therapeutic drugs. Innovative drug discovery from botanical products can increase the success rate of new therapeutic moieties in this era of rapidly advancing scientific technology. Thus, natural product drug discovery is a critical component of addressing global health challenges and achieving health-related sustainable development goals.

13.2 Complimentary Medicines

The utility of botanicals dates back at least to the hunter-gatherer societies. Based strictly on trial and error, the selection of foods, items of religious significance, or medication, as civilization progressed,

DOI: 10.1201/9781003146933-13

followed a familiar path. Earlier folklore relates many stories of plant medicines. There are references to medicinal herbs and plants in the Bible. There are references to medicinal herbs and plants in the Bible. Every religion implies plant remedies as part of their sacred heritage—the magic potion had the hand of a deity, it was believed. Anecdotal discoveries from digitalis to chloroquine gave scientists reasons to study the chemistry of medicines. In the 1700s and 1800s, botanicals were the only source of drugs for the treatment of disease. The treatment of illness. For a long time, anti-infective agents have been derived from extracts from molds and fungi. The new medicine discovery from plants continues faster, with more modern technologies of isolating and testing plants' chemical components and modifying the structure to improve effectiveness or decrease toxicity. The era of botanicals is not gone by. Although reserpine has been used in India and parts of China for over a thousand years, it was only purified and used as an effective antihypertensive agent in the 1950s.

Phytomedicines, botanical products, botanical products, and other terms describe drugs derived from plants. A botanical product can be a food component (such as a dietary supplement), a drug (such as a biological drug), a medical device (such as gutta-percha), or a cosmetic. Plant materials, algae, macroscopic fungi, and combinations are all included in the term botanical.

Since prehistoric times, botanical products have been used in traditional medicine for defense against insects, fungi, diseases, and herbivorous mammals. Plants synthesize hundreds of chemical compounds. As a result, phytochemicals with biological activity, either potential or established, have been widely identified. However, because a single plant contains such a wide range of phytochemicals, the effects of using the whole plant, a portion of it, or an extract as medicine create numerous permutations and combinations to investigate. Furthermore, many medicinal plants' phytochemical content and pharmacological actions, if any, remain unknown due to a lack of rigorous scientific research to determine efficacy and safety.

Botanical products are widely used in non-industrialized societies, mainly because they are readily available and cheaper than modern medicines. Traditional medicine is unregulated in many countries, but the World Health Organization coordinates a network to promote its safe and rational use.

According to the World Health Organization (WHO), four billion people—or 80% of the global population—use botanical products for some aspect of primary healthcare. Botanical products are a common element in Ayurvedic, homeopathic, naturopathic, traditional oriental, and Native American Indian medicine and are a significant component in all indigenous peoples' traditional medicine. In countries where botanical remedies are used, medical and health professionals have differing opinions on the safety, efficacy, and appropriateness of medicinal herbs. In some countries, professionals consider historical, empirical evidence to be the only criterion for botanical product efficacy. Others would declare all herbal remedies illegal because they are dangerous or of questionable value.

The Baseline Natural Health Products Survey among consumers, conducted by Health Canada in March 2005, is one of the most critical reports on the use of botanical products in North America. According to the survey results, 71% of people have used botanicals, with 38% using them daily, 37% seasonally, and 11% weekly, 57% using vitamins, 15% using echinacea, and 11% using other botanical remedies, algal, and fungal products. Botanical products are believed to be safer by nearly 80% of North Americans, and their use is expected to grow in the future. Regulatory agencies, however, consider botanical products to be anecdotal and ineffective and only allow them to be sold as food supplements, despite their long history of use. However, now there is a formal process of securing regulatory approval of botanical products; however, it has not yet produced any significant number of products. This chapter engages in teaching how a developer can adopt a formal process of securing FDA approval of botanicals.

13.2.1 History

In both health and illness, early humans recognized their reliance on nature. Primitive men and women used plants, animal parts, and minerals that were not normally part of their diet to treat disease, guided by instinct, taste, and experience. Physical evidence of herbal remedies dates back 60,000 years, to a Neanderthal man's burial site discovered in 1960. Plants have a long history of use in folk medicine in all cultures. The invention of writing provided a focal point for the accumulation and growth of botanical knowledge. The Mesopotamian clay tablet writings and the Egyptian papyri, which contain

876 prescriptions made up of over 500 different substances, including many herbs, are the first written records detailing the use of herbs in treating illness. The Greco-Roman era is followed by the writing of the *De Materia Medica*, which contains 950 curative substances, 600 of which are plant products and the rest of which are of animal or mineral origin. The Arab medical system was founded on the Greco-Roman system and the work of Jami of Ibn Baiar (died 1248 AD), which lists over 2,000 substances, many of which are plant products. In addition, 582 herbs are listed in the *Charaka Samhita*, an Ayurvedic book on internal medicine from India. Individual herb descriptions are a focus of the *Classic of the Materia Medica*, which was compiled in China no earlier than the first century AD. There are 252 botanical compounds, 45 mineral compounds, and 67 animal-derived compounds in it. Under Emperor Ingyo (411–453 AD), traditional Chinese medicine was brought to Japan via Korea, and the Japanese adopted Chinese-influenced Korean medicine.

The earliest historical records of herbs can be found on clay tablets from the Sumerian civilization, which list hundreds of botanical products, including opium. Over 850 plant medicines are described in the Ebers Papyrus from ancient Egypt, dating to around 1550 BC. In *De Materia Medica*, c. 60 AD, the Greek physician Dioscorides, who served in the Roman army, documented over 1,000 recipes for treatments using over 600 botanical products; this formed the basis of pharmacopeias 1,500 years later. Ethnobotany is used in drug research to find pharmacologically active substances. In this way, he has discovered hundreds of beneficial compounds in nature. Aspirin, digoxin, quinine, and opium are just a few examples. Plants contain a wide range of compounds, but most belong to one of four biochemical classes: alkaloids, glycosides, polyphenols, and terpenes.

Starting with the *Grete Herball* in 1526, illustrated botanicals flourished across Europe during the Early Modern period. In 1597, based on Rembert Dodoens, John Gerard published *The Botanical or General History of Plants*, and Nicholas Culpeper published *The English Physician Enlarged*. Many new plant medicines arrived in Europe due to Early Modern exploration and the Columbian Exchange, which saw livestock, crops, and technologies exchanged between the Old World and the Americas in the 15th and 16th centuries. Garlic, ginger, and turmeric were among the medicinal herbs that arrived in the Americas, while coffee, tobacco, and coca went the other way. The Badianus Manuscript, written in Mexico in the 16th century, described botanical products available in Central America.

Early explorers in North America exchanged knowledge with Native American Indians. Lafitau, a French explorer, discovered *Panax quinquefolius* L., a ginseng species growing in Iroquois territory in the New World in 1716. This American ginseng quickly became a staple in the global herb trade. The Jesuits dug up much ginseng in the United States, sold it to the Chinese, and used the proceeds to build schools and churches. Even today, American ginseng is a significant crude export from the United States. Unfortunately, with the onslaught of allopathic medicines, Americans have lost touch with botanical products, which once played a significant role in their lives.

13.2.2 Development Innovations

The pharmaceutical industry has its origins in the apothecary shops of Europe in the 1800s, where pharmacists provided customers with local traditional medicines such as morphine, quinine, and strychnine extracts. Two therapeutically important drugs derived from botanical products are Camptothecin (from *Camptotheca acuminata*, used in traditional Chinese medicine) and Taxol (from *Taxus brevifolia*, a Pacific yew). In the 1950s, the anti-cancer Vinca alkaloids vincristine and vinblastine were discovered in the Madagascar periwinkle, *Catharanthus roseus*.

Thanks to technologies like high-performance liquid chromatography, nuclear magnetic resonance spectroscopy, mass spectrometry, microfluidics, and computational algorithms, medicinal chemistry made significant progress in the 20th century. This has made it possible to identify chemical plant components and use them in drug development. Many drugs have been discovered using botanical plant products thanks to high throughput assays using bioreactors and microfluidics systems. Opium and morphine are two of these botanical products. In today's clinics and hospitals, structural analogs of these compounds are used.

Current drug development strategies prefer to use a single compound-based medicine, as the multi-component formulations are generally discouraged by the regulatory agencies. Individual compounds have a better therapeutic effect than taking whole plants or extracts without isolating components, as is done in traditional medicine. This is significant because most plant metabolites are likely to work together to extract the therapeutic effect. Therefore, researchers must research the use of whole plant extracts to determine the molecular basis of the plant extracts' therapeutic effect. For example, an anti-asthma botanical product made from extracts from *Ganoderma lucidum*, *Glycyrrhiza uralensis*, and *Sophora flavescens* alleviates bronchoconstriction in an animal model while restoring cytokines balance, contributing to longer-lasting anti-asthma benefit after treatment. The therapeutic effect is solely due to the synergistic effect of the three botanical ingredients' chemical components.

The regulatory agencies have recently begun to realize the holistic approach's value, allowing drugs based on plant extracts rather than single or multiple compounds. However, the success rate for regulatory approval of botanical products remains, especially in the US, very low due to many scientific challenges in proving their safety and efficacy. New and innovative computational and analytical methods are needed to identify chemical components of crude plant extracts to identify therapeutically effective compounds and optimize their extraction efficiently. More introductions of focus on combinatorial effects of chemicals from plant extracts and not just single compounds are needed. During drug development, available "-omics" platforms, automation, and big data are used to investigate how these combinations affect genes and proteins involved in various cellular processes. Testing allows for the rapid production of drugs from plant-based botanical products using computer-aided drug design.

Developments in microfluidics and computational analysis have also allowed designing and testing plant extract chemicals in drug discovery more efficiently. In addition, technological advancements, such as the development of new analytical and bioinformatic techniques, will aid in designing new structures, their synthesis, and their biological testing.

13.2.3 Technologies

Innovative drug discovery from botanical products necessitates a multidisciplinary approach that uses existing and cutting-edge technologies to package natural product compounds for medical use and drug development (Figure 13.1).

Most medicinal extract components often work synergistically to elicit their therapeutic effects, so isolating individual components may be counterproductive. Innovative approaches are needed to study and harness such compounds that can effectively lead to new drug molecules with a single molecular target and advocate for the complete equilibrium of a physiological system undergoing synchronized mechanisms on multiple molecular targets. The application of available technologies such as genomics, transcriptomics, proteomics, metabolomics, and metabonomics, automation, and computational strategies, combined with a systems biology approach, will pave the way for innovative drug design and better drug candidates. Molecular libraries of lead compounds from botanical products research and development will serve as sources of lead compounds/botanical tinctures for innovative drugs. When using innovative technologies in conjunction with systems biology, the focus should be on the synergistic effects of compounds rather than a reductionist approach of trying to find a single active compound. Understanding the complex molecular mechanisms of botanical products will necessitate a non-reductionist approach.

13.2.4 Genomics and Biomarkers

For successful innovations, the plant species from which the natural product is obtained must be of high quality, have precise identification, and reliability of supply. An incorrect plant species will likely affect the therapeutic properties due to unrelated compounds in the species. Genomic methods are essential in establishing an accurate identification method for plants and natural product species. Genomic techniques such as DNA barcoding rely on sequence diversity in short and standard DNA regions (400–800 bp) for species-level identification. DNA barcoding utilizing genomics will provide a more robust and precise identification than traditional morphological identification and local conventional (vernacular) names. DNA barcoding of botanical products has been applied in biodiversity inventories and authentication of botanical products. Using an integrative approach that included ITS2 or psbA-trnH sequence amplification, plant species such as *Amaranthus hybridus* L. and crude drugs recorded

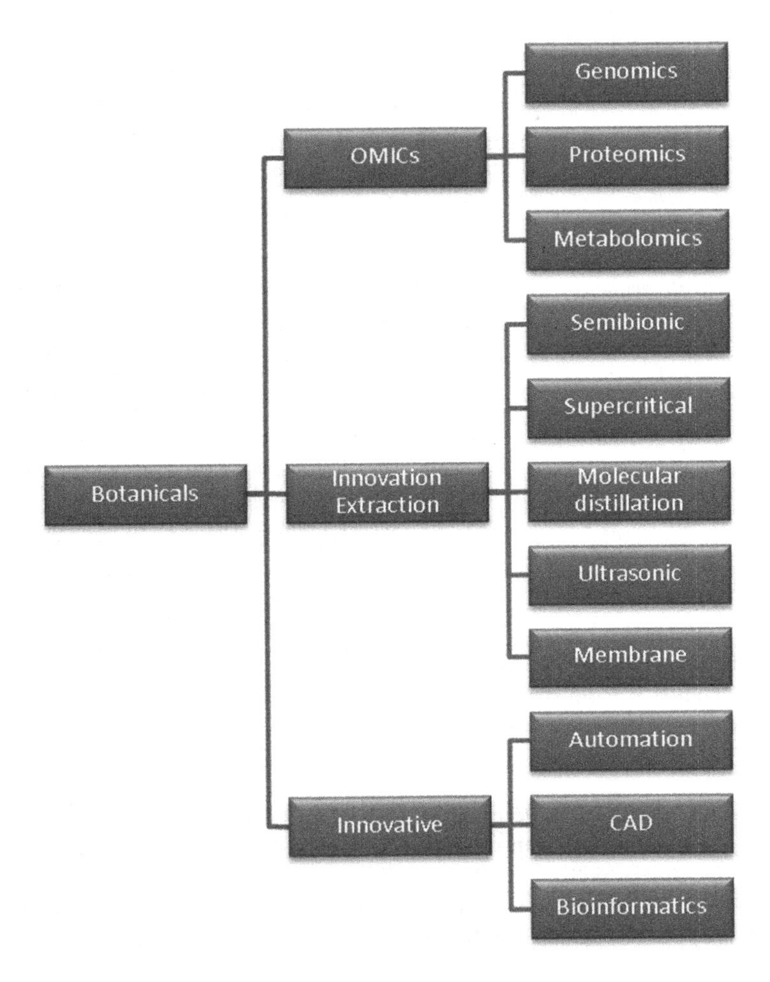

FIGURE 13.1 Innovative technologies for natural product drug discovery.

in the Japanese pharmacopeia were identified. Even though genomic-based techniques are an effective platform for identifying natural products, due to differences in growing conditions, different parts of the same plant with similar sequences may have different qualities, clinical utility, and indications.

Markers derived from species using genomic techniques can be incorporated into DNA chips, resulting in a high-throughput genotyping and plant species authentication tool. Microarray analysis of gene expression is a novel transcriptomic technique that allows for the rapid and accurate analysis of many transcripts. This transcriptomic analysis makes it possible to evaluate variations in multiple gene expressions concurrently. This represents a robust tool for elucidating therapeutic botanical products' molecular mechanisms and biological networks underlying their pharmacological actions.

Genomic analysis can be used for natural or compound targeting, in addition to botanical product identification. Whole-genome sequencing combined with transcriptomic analyses has opened up previously uncharted territory in drug or compound targeting. Transcription factor binding sites, protein modifications, DNA structure changes, and methylation patterns can now be analyzed and measured at the genome level. Several studies, including our own, have found deletions, insertions, copy number variations, splicing variants, and translocations linked to certain cancers, revealing new drug targets in the process. The development of novel and unrivaled technologies, allowing genome-wide analysis, has enabled drug targets' unbiased discovery. These technologies, combined with the availability of vast databases of chemicals or compounds, have allowed for a reduction in the time required for the entire drug discovery process, from drug design to clinical trials.

TABLE 13.1
Systematized Description of Botanical Products

Plant	Link
Atropa belladonna	http://medicinalplantgenomics.msu.edu/33113.shtml
Camptotheca acuminata	http://medicinalplantgenomics.msu.edu/16922.shtml
Cannabis sativa	http://medicinalplantgenomics.msu.edu/3483.shtml
Catharanthus roseus	http://medicinalplantgenomics.msu.edu/4058.shtml
Digitalis purpurea	http://medicinalplantgenomics.msu.edu/4164.shtml
Dioscorea villosa	http://medicinalplantgenomics.msu.edu/330167.shtml
Echinacea purpurea	http://medicinalplantgenomics.msu.edu/53751.shtml
Ginkgo biloba	http://medicinalplantgenomics.msu.edu/3311.shtml
Hoodia gordonii	http://medicinalplantgenomics.msu.edu/197266.shtml
Hypericum perforatum	http://medicinalplantgenomics.msu.edu/65561.shtml
Panax quinquefolius	http://medicinalplantgenomics.msu.edu/44588.shtml
Rauvolfia serpentina	http://medicinalplantgenomics.msu.edu/4060.shtml
Rosmarinus officinalis	http://medicinalplantgenomics.msu.edu/39367.shtml
Valeriana officinalis	http://medicinalplantgenomics.msu.edu/19953.shtml

As of 2020, only 18 botanical products were systematized in the Botanical Product Transcriptomics Database (http://medicinalplantgenomics.msu.edu), including a sequence reference for the transcriptome and links to their chemistry and pharmacology (Table 13.1).

13.2.5 Proteomics

The use of proteomic platforms in describing the mechanism of action of many botanical products is complementary to genomic and transcriptomic approaches to quality control and sample variation. Based on therapeutic effects, proteomic approaches to innovative drug discovery from botanical products can elucidate protein expression, protein function, metabolic, and biosynthetic pathways, resulting in consistency in product quality and profile. Quantitative protein profiling will be aided by techniques such as mass spectrometry with isotope tags and two-dimensional electrophoresis, which generate quantitative data on a scale and sensitivity comparable to that generated at the genomic level. For example, the Chinese botanical product *Panax ginseng* versus *Panax quinquefolium* was successfully identified using proteomics. The therapeutic effects of botanical products can be elucidated using proteomics and imaging techniques to successfully study the metabolism of botanical products and their compounds. Proteomics is an effective way to explain the multi-target effects of complex natural product preparations, discover multiple compounds and fractions, characterize botanical products, and ultimately a molecular diagnostic platform.

It is critical to identify the target proteins of botanical products before they can be used as drugs. Several methods, including affinity chromatography, have been used to successfully identify target proteins. The introduction of technologies that allow for target protein identification without modifying the natural product has resulted in more active botanical products. The cellular thermal shift assay is based on stabilizing target proteins when they bind to their ligand, thermal proteome profiling based on target proteins' stability at high temperatures, bioinformatic-based connectivity analysis, and drug affinity responsive target stability examples of such methods. Botanical products exhibit a wide range of biological activities due to their many structures and complexity. This is owing to their ability to bind to a variety of ligands. Because of its off-target effects, every potential drug will have to be tested for side effects. To identify all of its potential target proteins, complex natural compounds with potential target proteins must be thoroughly evaluated. Affinity chromatography is one of the most widely used methods for identifying target proteins and their biological activities. The natural product is immobilized on solid physical support in this method, which is a pull-down method. Mass spectrometry is used to determine which proteins are bound. Botanical products that have been modified, on the other hand, may have less or no activity. Therefore, the success of target identification depends on the development of novel and innovative approaches that do not require any changes. Using label-free botanical products, several methods have recently been able to identify target proteins. The natural product-target protein complex responses to proteomic and thermal treatment are measured using these new and improved methods. Proteomic analysis can identify several target proteins for a single natural product using this unique approach.

13.2.6 Target Identification of Label-Free Botanical Products

Drug affinity responsive target stability (DARTS) is one of the direct methods to identify target proteins using label-free botanical products that take advantage of the changes in the stability of a natural product-bound protein versus an unbound protein subjected to proteolytic treatment. This method validates several target proteins for compounds such as resveratrol and rapamycin. However, it is challenging to use DARTS to identify low abundance protein targets in cell lysates.

The stability of proteins from oxidation rates (SPROX), which measures the irreversible oxidation of methionine residues on target proteins, is another method that takes advantage of ligand-induced changes to target proteins. A mixture of candidate drug compounds and proteins is incubated with an oxidizing agent and guanidinium hydrochloride to oxidize methionine. The mass spectrometry analysis of the generated peptides is then used to assess selective methionine oxidation. The transition midpoint shift in proteins bound to ligands is larger than in control samples, according to analyses of oxidized and non-oxidized methionine-containing peptides versus guanidinium hydrochloride concentration. SPROX was used to confirm the target proteins of compounds like resveratrol and cyclophilin A. This method, on the other hand, necessitates the analysis of highly concentrated proteins.

Stable isotope labeling with amino acids in cell culture (SILAC)-based SPROX, a modification of the SPROX method, improves the original method and has the advantage of covering more target proteins. However, this method can only be used to identify proteins that contain methionine.

Cellular thermal shift assay (CETSA) is based on stabilizing a target protein by binding to its ligand. Cell lysates and intact cells are heated to various temperatures after being treated with the candidate drug compound. Then, western blot analysis is used to separate the target protein from the destabilized protein. When ligand–target interactions are plotted against temperature, shifts or changes in melting curves are detected. This method identifies target proteins of many anti-cancer therapeutic agents such as raltitrexed and methotrexate. This method's advantage is the apparent use of intact cells with no need for treatments or preparations. In addition, it can be very selective because of the western blot step. However, some target proteins with unfolded binding sites may go undetected. Also, due to the non-specificity of some antibodies used in the western blot step, off-target proteins may be identified as false positives.

Thermal proteome profiling (TPP) is a variation of the CETSA method that identifies target proteins with thermal stability at high temperatures caused by ligand binding and uses mass spectrometry to measure the ligand–target protein interaction cellular level. For high-resolution mass spectrometry, this method employs isobaric mass tagging. Most expressed soluble proteins will have melting curves, allowing both target and off-target proteins to be identified. TPP can be used to investigate the potential side effects of candidate drug compounds by identifying off-targets. However, this method is very costly and is labor-intensive.

Small interfering RNA and short hairpin RNA are clear choices for target gene manipulation to validate target protein and natural product interactions functionally. In addition, it is possible to investigate the off-target effects of candidate compounds by using interfering RNA to knock down target proteins.

The clustered regularly interspaced short palindromic repeats-Cas9 (CRISPR-Cas9) genome editing approach can overcome off-target effects of candidate compounds and delineate how many natural compounds work. DrugTargetSeqR (www.nature.com/articles/nchembio.1551) combines CRISPR-Cas9 genome editing with high-throughput sequencing and computer-based mutation analysis to study drug resistance and validate several anti-cancer therapeutic agents.

13.2.7 Metabolomics and Metabonomics

Metabolomics is the study of small molecules, also known as metabolites, in cells, biofluids, tissues, and organisms on a large scale. The metabolome refers to the collection of small molecules and their interactions

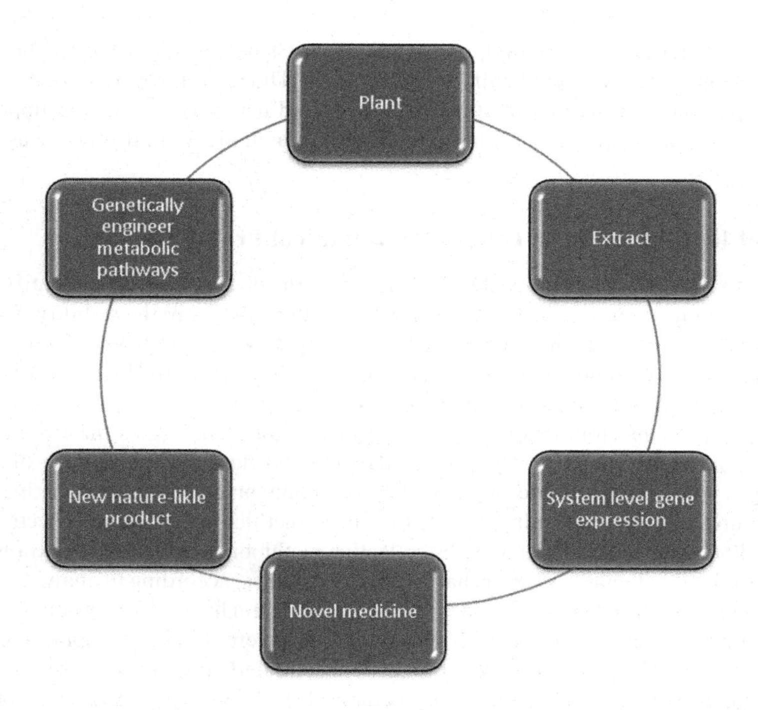

FIGURE 13.2 Exploiting the properties of plant extracts in the development of novel medicines inspired by compounds found in botanical product extracts.

within a biological system. Metabonomics is a subset of metabolomics, defined as the quantitative measurement of multiparametric metabolic responses of living systems to pathophysiological stimuli or genetic modification, emphasizing elucidating differences in population groups due to genetic modification.

Untargeted metabolomic and analgesic approaches to discovering therapeutic interest compounds from botanical products can potentially find innovative drug discovery. The goal of metabolomic profiling of botanical products is to identify and quantify the full range of their metabolites. On the other hand, metabonomics aims to assess the global and dynamic metabolic response of living systems to biological stimuli or genetic manipulation in a broad sense. Although the terms are often used interchangeably, metabonomics is a systems biology-guided approach to studying the functions and perturbations of a biological system due to a pharmacological effect. This elucidates the natural product's complete biological mechanism as well as its impact on a living system (Figure 13.2).

Metabolomic profiling of botanical products using ultra-performance liquid chromatography–quadrupole TOF MS (UPLC–QTOF MS) enables identification of compounds that confer therapeutic properties such as *Newbouldia laevis*, *Cassia abbreviata*, *Hyptis suaveolens*, and *Panax* herbs. As a quality control measure and to show consistency in species usage, metabolomics is used to identify processed *Panax* species (*Panax ginseng* and *Panax quinquefolius*) using nuclear magnetic resonance (NMR)-based metabolomics, UPLC–QTOF MS, and multivariate statistical analysis. The systems biology approach of metabolomics allows the profiling of botanical products in an all-inclusive manner regarding metabolite and biology systems effect. Metabolomic and metabonomics profiling using NMR, MS, and UPLC elucidate the pharmacodynamic, pharmacokinetic, and toxicological value of botanical products.

13.3 Regulatory Plan

13.3.1 Background

A botanical product that is used to maintain health, is administered for a specific condition, or both is considered a drug. In 2002, the Food and Agriculture Organization estimated that more than 50,000 botanical products are used globally. In 2016, the Royal Botanic Gardens, Kew estimated that 17,810 plant species have medicinal uses out of a total of 30,000 plants for which any kind of use is documented is supported by evidence.

Around a quarter of the drugs prescribed to patients in modern medicine are derived from plants. In other medicine systems, botanical products may constitute most often informal attempted treatments, not tested scientifically. The World Health Organization estimates that about 80% of the world's population depends on traditional medicine (including but not limited to plants); perhaps some two billion people are primarily reliant on botanical products. Plant-based materials, including botanical or natural health products with supposed health benefits, increase in developed countries. The World Health Organization established a policy on traditional medicine in 1991 and guidelines and monographs on commonly used botanical products.

A government department, AYUSH, regulates the practice of Ayurveda in India, including the operation of an Ayurvedic pharmacy in Rishikesh. To improve the quality of medical products made from botanical products and their claims, the World Health Organization (WHO) has been coordinating a network called the International Regulatory Cooperation for Botanical Products. In 2015, only around 20% of countries had well-functioning regulatory agencies, while 30% had none, and around half had limited regulatory capacity. According to the WHO, there are four goals for traditional medicines: integrate them as policy into national healthcare systems, provide knowledge and guidance on their safety, efficacy, and quality, increase their availability and affordability, and promote their rational, therapeutically sound use. According to the WHO, countries face seven challenges in implementing the strategy, including developing and enforcing policy, integration, product safety, and quality, particularly in product evaluation and practitioner qualification, advertising regulation, research and development, education and training, and information sharing.

According to the US FDA, the botanical product is intended to diagnose, cure, mitigate, treat, or prevent disease in humans.

- A botanical product consists of vegetable materials, including plant materials, algae, macroscopic fungi, or combinations.
- A botanical product may be available as (but not limited to) a solution (e.g., tea), powder, tablet, capsule, elixir, topical, or injection.
- Botanical product products frequently have distinguishing characteristics, such as complex mixtures, the lack of a distinct active ingredient, and extensive prior human use. In addition, botanical product products do not include fermentation products or highly purified or chemically modified botanical substances.

During the FDA review process, the unique characteristics of a botanical product must be taken into account and adjusted. CDER issued Botanical Drug Development Guidance for Industry, which considers these characteristics and makes it easier to develop new therapies from botanical sources. The guidance covers only botanical products intended for development and uses as drugs (www.fda.gov/media/93113/download).

Hundreds of compounds have been discovered due to ethnobotany research into plants used by indigenous peoples for medicinal purposes. Curcumin, epigallocatechin gallate, genistein, and resveratrol are examples of important phytochemicals that are pan-assay interference compounds, which means that in vitro studies of their activity are often unreliable.

To date (end of 2020), only two botanical products have fulfilled the Botanical Drug Development Guidance for Industry's definition of a botanical product. Both botanical products have been approved for marketing as prescription drugs (sinecatechins as Veregen® and crofelemer as Mytesi™). Some botanical products, including cascara, psyllium, and senna, are included in the over-the-counter (OTC) drug review. There must be published data establishing a general recognition of safety and effectiveness, including the results of adequate and well-controlled clinical studies, for a botanical product substance to be included in an OTC monograph. The approval record of botanicals in the US is abysmal. In the years leading up to 2018, the FDA received over 800 botanical investigational new drug applications (IND) and pre-IND meeting requests (PIND). According to current data, indications for submitted INDs cover nearly every FDA review division. Because of botanicals' chemical and biological complexity, efforts to characterize their pharmacology, demonstrate therapeutic efficacy, and ensure quality consistency are scientific and regulatory challenges.

The Botanical Review Team (BRT) of the CDER is part of the Office of Pharmaceutical Quality (OPQScience)'s Staff. The BRT has scientific knowledge in a wide range of botanical concerns, including the intricacies of natural goods and the inherent challenges of developing natural product drugs. The team also ensures that the Botanical Drug Development Guidance for Industry is interpreted consistently.

About a quarter of all Food and Drug Administration (FDA)- and European Medical Agency (EMA)-approved drugs are plant-based, with well-known drugs such as paclitaxel and morphine isolated from plants. About a third of FDA-approved drugs over the past 20 years are based on botanical products or their derivatives. Following the discovery of penicillin from fungus, many microorganisms were screened for potential antibiotics. Indeed, drug discovery from botanical products revolutionized medicine. Tetracycline, produced by *Streptomyces aureofaciens*, artemisinin, produced by *Artemisia afra*, and doxorubicin, produced by *Streptomyces peucetius*, are among them. Plant extracts have traditionally been used as concoctions containing a variety of ingredients. Some of the ingredients do not have therapeutic properties independently, but their synergistic effects are required.

The following are some of the current obstacles to using botanical products and accepting their therapeutic efficacy: 1) lack of standardization procedures, 2) lack of isolation of pure chemical products or compounds, 3) lack of biological mechanism elucidation and infrequently undergoing so-called controls, and 4) lack of documented clinical trials following "standards."

Historically, scientific evidence on the therapeutic efficacy of botanical products, as previously mentioned, led to the development of some conventional blockbuster medicines. However, searching for new drug candidates from botanical products is often made difficult by the molecular mixtures' complexity. Plant extracts' therapeutic activity is usually due to the synergistic and simultaneous action of several chemicals. Given the complexity of many diseases, such as cancer and degenerative diseases, it's unsurprising that single-compound-based drug discovery has failed to produce effective cures. When evaluating candidate compounds, plant-based drug discovery must start with a combinatorial approach. With the advent of new technologies such as quantum computing, profiling techniques, computational biology techniques, big data, microfluidics, and artificial intelligence, scientists will harness plant-based therapeutic properties of botanical products while also studying their molecular effects in physiological conditions. It's possible, however, that not all plant extract components have detectable effects. One way to improve screening and simplify extracts is to remove potentially interfering components such as polyphenolic tannins. Several reported innovative strategies can be used to achieve this, and these include pre-fractionation and extraction methods. These extraction strategies have indeed resulted in more hit leads during drug development. Innovative extraction technologies, including semi-bionic extraction, supercritical fluid extraction, microwave-assisted, ultrasonic-assisted and enzyme-assisted extraction, molecular distillation methods, and membrane separation technology, can extract natural compounds efficiently from plants. These extraction strategies have been shown to mimic traditional methods, allowing the extraction process to extract the most compounds from the natural product.

The legal process of regulation and legislation of botanical products changes from country to country (Table 13.2). The reason for this variation comes from the historical use of botanical products without any scientific proof for their safety or efficacy, allowing their use on a carte blanche basis. Thus, few botanical preparations have been tested for safety and efficacy. The WHO has published guidelines to define basic criteria for evaluating botanical products' quality, safety, and efficacy to assist national regulatory authorities, scientific organizations, and manufacturers. Furthermore, the WHO has prepared *Pharmacopeia* monographs on botanical products and guidelines for assessing botanical products.

13.3.2 Chemistry

While the current trend towards biological drugs and gene-related technologies seems to overshadow other classic approaches to drug discovery, botanical products remain a robust category of drugs to come in the future. The reason why botanical products remain a significant focus is the nonlinear possibility of finding new cures. The chemistry of plants remains unexplored primarily, and many plant species remain

TABLE 13.2

Botanical Product Approval Rules in Different Countries

Argentina	The sale of *herboristerias* as plant drugs is permitted but not as mixtures. Plant drug mixtures are regulated (Law No. 16.463). The mandatory registration of medicinal herbs was established by a Ministry of Health regulation in 1993. Crude extracts, extracts or fractions of complex chemical composition, and pure active principles were regulated by the *Argentinian National Pharmacopeia*. In Argentina, there are approximately 889 monographs. About 56 refer to pure drugs, while 33 refer to extracts or fractions. Raw materials are uncontrolled, wild plants are uncontrolled, scientific criteria for collecting plants are uncontrolled, and drying, conservation, and grinding methods are uncontrolled.
Australia	The Working Party on Natural and Nutritional Supplements was established by the Australian Parliament to investigate the quality, safety, efficacy, and labeling of botanical and related products (Therapeutic Good Act, 1990). Traditional claims for botanical remedies are permissible under the act, as long as general advertising requirements are met and such claims are supported by literature references.
Brazil	In 1994, the Brazilian Ministry of Health established a commission to assess botanical products. The commission proposed a directive for botanical products based primarily on German and French regulations and WHO guidelines. The phytopharmaceutical product was defined as "a processed drug containing active ingredients exclusively plant material and plant drug preparations" in 1995 by "Directive Number 6," which established the legal requirement to register botanical products. They are used to diagnose, treat, cure, alleviate, and prevent diseases. Unfortunately, laws that aren't well-defined aren't enforced well.
Canada	The Canadian HPB established a special committee (three pharmacists, two botanists, one nutritionist, and one physician) in 1986 to classify botanical products as "Folk Medicine." As long as scientific studies back up the claim, the regulation is based on traditional uses. For example, the HPB issued a list of 64 herbs that were deemed unsafe in 1990. In 1992, the HPB proposed to the Canadian Parliament a regulatory proposal that listed 64 additional herbs as adulterants. The Canadian regulatory system for botanical product evaluation follows WHO guidelines.
Chile	The Unidad de Medicina Tradicional was founded in 1992 to incorporate proven traditional medicine into health programs (Law No. 19.253, October 1993). Botanical products with therapeutic indication claims and dosage recommendations were classified as drugs restricted for sale in pharmacies and drug stores under Directive No. 435/81. Botanical products require registration for marketing authorization. The following legal distinctions apply to botanical products: 1) drugs intended to treat, alleviate, or prevent disease; (2) medicinal and therapeutic food products; and 3) food products for nutritional purposes.
China	Pharmaceuticals and botanical preparations were virtually unregulated in China until 1984. The People's Republic of China implemented the Drug Administration Law in 1984, which stated that traditional botanical preparations were generally considered "old drugs" and were exempt from efficacy and side effect testing, except for new uses. The Chinese Ministry of Public Health would oversee the administration of new botanical products.
England	In England, the prior use rule holds that hundreds of years of use with apparent positive effects and no evidence of harmful side effects are sufficient evidence (rather than other scientific data) that the product is safe. The Ministry of Agriculture, Fisheries, and Food and the Department of Health collaborated to create a database of adverse effects of nonconventional medicines at the National Poisons Unit to promote the safe use of botanical remedies. Labels that read "Traditionally used for..." distinguish these products from approved pharmaceutical drugs. Consumers understand this is understood to mean that the indications are based on historical evidence and have not been confirmed by modern scientific experimentation.
Europe	Drug approval criteria in Europe are identical to those in the United States, where drugs are assessed for safety, efficacy, and quality. Europeans, on the other hand, have a better grasp of the historical value of phytomedicines. As a result, phytomedicine approval is less expensive, particularly if there is a long history of anecdotal use. Drug approval criteria in Europe are identical to those in the United States, where drugs are assessed for safety, efficacy, and quality. Europeans, on the other hand, have a better grasp of the historical value of phytomedicines. As a result, phytomedicine approval is less expensive, particularly if there is a long history of anecdotal use. Recognizing the need to standardize botanical product approval, the EEC developed The Quality of Botanical Remedies Directive (EEC Directive, 75/318/EEC adopted November 1988), a set of guidelines that outlines quality, quantity, and production standards for botanical remedies as well as labeling requirements that member countries must meet. The EEC guidelines are based on the WHO's Botanical Product Assessment Guidelines (1991). In the absence of scientific evidence to the contrary, these guidelines state that a substance's historical use is a proper way to document safety and efficacy. As a starting point for determining product safety, the guidelines suggest the following: • A guiding principle should be that if a product has been used in the past without causing harm, no specific regulatory action should be taken unless new evidence necessitates a revised risk-benefit analysis. Long-term, trouble-free use of a substance usually indicates its safety.

(*Continued*)

TABLE 13.2 (CONTINUED)

Botanical Product Approval Rules in Different Countries

	• The guidelines state that for the treatment of minor disorders and nonspecific indications, some relaxation in the requirements for proof of efficacy is justified, considering the extent of traditional use; the same considerations may apply to prophylactic use (WHO 1991).
WHO	According to the WHO guidelines, approval should be based on existing monographs. If one exists, referring to a pharmacopeia monograph should suffice. However, if no such monograph exists, one must be written and formatted in the same way that an official pharmacopeia is written and formatted.
ESCOP	The ESCOP was founded by the phytotherapy societies of Belgium, France, Germany, Switzerland, and the United Kingdom to further the standardization effort and increase European scientific support. ESCOP's solution to varying quality and therapeutic use within the EEC is to create "European" monographs based on the German scientific monograph system.
	Botanical remedies are divided into three categories in Europe. Prescription drugs, including injectable phytomedicines and those used to treat life-threatening diseases, are the most strictly regulated. The second category is OTC phytomedicines, which are similar to OTC drugs in the United States. Traditional botanical remedies are the third category, which has not undergone extensive clinical testing but has been deemed safe based on generations of use without serious incident.
France	In France, approximately 200 herbs with varying claims have been approved as OTC. The approval of phytomedicines is subject to the same regulations that apply to all drugs. There is only one type of license, but it is granted based on adapted documentation and an abridged application for some plant drugs and preparations. This approval procedure involved 115 herbs and 31 laxatives in 1990. Approximately 205 botanical products are currently listed. Traditional medicines can be sold in France with labeling based on traditional use, but they must be licensed by the French Licensing Committee and approved by the French Pharmacopoeia Committee.
Germany	Commission E (Phytotherapy and Botanical Substances) was founded in 1978 in Germany. It is a separate division of the German Federal Health Agency that gathers data on botanical products and assesses their safety and efficacy. Commission E employs the following methods and criteria: 1) traditional use; 2) chemical data; 3) experimental, pharmacological, and toxicological studies; 4) clinical studies; 5) field and epidemiological studies; 6) patient case records from physician's files; and 8) other studies, including unpublished proprietary data submitted by manufacturers. There are two types of monographs: mono preparations and fixed combinations. Physicians, pharmacists, pharmacologists, toxicologists, industry representatives, and laypeople make up Commission E, which has 24 members. There are three options for marketing botanical products: 1) temporary marking authorization for old botanical products until they are evaluated for safety and efficacy; 2) marketing authorization monographs; and 3) individual marketing authorization. Monographs that approve or disapprove of botanical products for over-the-counter use are published as evaluations. Pharmacies, drug stores, and health food stores all sell botanical products. A physician's prescription is required for some botanical products. About 300 monographs have been published by Commission E, with 200 "positives" and 100 "negatives." In Germany, about 600–700 plants are sold. Approximately 70% of physicians prescribe botanical products that have been approved by the FDA. A portion of the annual sales is covered by government health insurance. Exclusive botanical products are treated as a single active ingredient in Germany, making it easier to define and approve the product. The German Federal Health Office uses a monograph system to regulate products like ginkgo and milk thistle extracts, resulting in standardized potency and manufacturing processes. The monographs are produced under the auspices of the Ministry of Health Committee for Botanical Remedies. They are compiled from the scientific literature on a specific herb in a single report (Kommission E). Approval of such remedies necessitates more scientific documentation than traditional treatments but less than the approval of new pharmaceutical drugs.
India	India has thousands of years of history of using Ayurvedic medicine; almost 70–80% of India's rural population depends on this mode of traditional medicine; no significant control on the quality of drugs of botanical origin exists in India.
Japan	Kampo, or traditional Japanese medicine, is similar to and historically derived from Chinese medicine, including traditional Japanese folklore medicines. Between 1868 and 1912, when Western medicine was introduced, Kampo began to decline, but by 1928, it had begun to recover. Kampo medicines are now prescribed by nearly half of Japan's Western-trained medical practitioners, and they are covered by the Japanese national health insurance system. The Japanese botanical product industry established regulations in 1988 to regulate the manufacture and quality control of extract products used in Kampo medicine. These rules are in line with the Japanese government's Drug Manufacturing Control and Quality Control Regulations.

(Continued)

TABLE 13.2 (CONTINUED)

Botanical Product Approval Rules in Different Countries

The USA.	Since 1994, botanical products have been regulated under the Dietary Supplement Health and Education Act of 1994. Based on this law, botanical products are not evaluated by the FDA, and, most important, these products are not intended to diagnose, treat, cure, or prevent diseases. In August 2000, the United States Food and Drug Administration (FDA) published its first botanical product approval guidelines. The NCCAM's mission includes conducting rigorous research on complementary and alternative medicine practices to evaluate the benefits and risks of CAM agents and optimize their effect on human diseases and conditions. The National Center for Complementary and Alternative Medicine (NCCAM) divides complementary and alternative medicine into five categories: biologically based therapies, manipulative and body-based methods, mind-body interventions, energy therapies, and alternative medical systems. The DSHEA 1994 regulates biologically based complementary and alternative medicine. Botanicals and their constituents, vitamins, minerals, and amino acids are all covered by this regulation. The Food and Drug Administration (FDA) in the United States classifies botanicals and other dietary agents based on their intended use rather than their chemical makeup. If the agent's intended use is to "promote health," it's classified as a dietary supplement; if it's to treat or prevent a disease, it's classified as a drug.

Abbreviations: CAM = complementary and alternative medicine; DSHEA = Dietary Supplement Health, and Education Act; EEC = European Economic Community; ESCOP = European Societies' Cooperative of Phytotherapy; HPB = Health Protection Branch; NCCAM = National Center for Complementary and Alternative Medicine; OTC = over the counter; US FDA = United States Food and Drug Administration; WHO = World Health Organization.

unidentified across the globe and most significantly in the marine world. For example, wood has two primary chemical components: lignin (18–35%) and carbohydrate (65–75%). Both are complex polymeric materials. Minor amounts of extraneous materials, mainly in the organic extractives and inorganic minerals (ash), are also present in wood (usually 4–10%). Trees have existed for over 370 million years. The world's total number of mature trees is estimated to be around three trillion. The majority of tree species are angiosperms. About 1,000 species of gymnosperm trees, including conifers, cycads, ginkgophytes, and Gnetales (*Ephedra*, *Gnetum*, *Welwitschia*).

The chemicals in the plants describe a long evolutionary history of the plant kingdom. All plants produce chemical compounds that have given them an evolutionary advantage, such as defending against herbivores or acting as a hormone in plant defenses, as in salicylic acid. The major classes of pharmacologically active phytochemicals include:

- Alkaloids: These are bitter-tasting chemicals concentrated in plant parts that are most likely to be eaten by herbivores, such as the stem; they may also protect against parasites found in many botanical products and are often toxic. Like drugs, there are several types with various modes of action, both recreational and pharmaceutical. Other classes of medicines include atropine, scopolamine, and hyoscyamine (all from nightshade), berberine (from plants like *Berberis* and *Mahonia*), caffeine (*Coffea*), cocaine (*Coca*), ephedrine (*Ephedra*), morphine (opium poppy), nicotine (tobacco), reserpine (*Rauwolfia serpentina*), quinidine and quinine (*Cinchona*), vincamine (*Vinca minor*), and vincristine (*Catharanthus roseus*). The opium poppy *Papaver somniferum* is the source of the alkaloids morphine and codeine. Morphine and codeine are two types of opiates. Nicotine, an alkaloid found in tobacco, binds directly to nicotinic acetylcholine receptors in the body, which explains its pharmacological effects. Tropane alkaloids, such as atropine, scopolamine, and hyoscyamine, are produced by the deadly nightshade *Atropa belladonna*.
- Glycosides: Botanical products like rhubarb, cascara, and Alexandrian senna contain anthraquinone glycosides. Senna, rhubarb, and aloe are examples of plant-based laxatives made from such plants. The cardiac glycosides are potent drugs derived from plants such as foxglove and lily of the valley. Digoxin and digitoxin, for example, support the heart's beating and act as diuretics. For millennia, *Senna alexandrina*, which contains anthraquinone glycosides, has been used as a laxative. Digoxin, a cardiac glycoside, is found in the foxglove, *Digitalis*

purpurea. Long before glycoside was discovered, the plant was used to treat heart problems. Atrial fibrillation, atrial flutter, and heart failure are all treated with digoxin.

- Polyphenols: Polyphenols come in a variety of classes and provide a variety of defenses against plant diseases and predators. Hormone-mimicking phytoestrogens and astringent tannins are among them. Plants containing phytoestrogens have been used for centuries to treat gynecological issues like infertility, menstrual irregularities, and menopausal symptoms. These plants include *Pueraria mirifica*, kudzu, angelica, fennel, and anise. Many polyphenolic extracts are sold as dietary supplements and cosmetics without proof or legal health claims, such as grape seeds, olives, and maritime pine bark. The astringent rind of the pomegranate, which contains polyphenols called punicalagin, is used as a medicine in Ayurveda. Angelica has long been used to treat gynecological problems because it contains phytoestrogens. Phytoestrogens are polyphenols that mimic animal estrogen.
- Terpenes: Terpenes and terpenoids of various types can be found in various botanical products and resinous plants like conifers. They have a pungent odor that deters herbivores. Essential oils are used in perfumes such as rose and lavender, as well as aromatherapy. Thymol, for example, is an antiseptic and was once used as a vermifuge (anti-worm medicine). The monoterpene thymol, an antiseptic and antifungal, is found in the essential oil of common thyme (*Thymus vulgaris*). Plants contain a variety of terpenes, including thymol.

Several minerals are found in marine flora, and they provide nutraceutical benefits and can be an essential part of the diet. For example, they're a good source of iron that's bioavailable. They also contain the mineral vanadium, which aids in carbohydrate metabolism and blood sugar regulation. In addition, nonflavonoid and noncarotenoid antioxidants, alkaloid antioxidants, and sulfated polysaccharides are found in marine floras and are known to have anti-inflammatory and antiviral properties. They also reduce cholesterol and, as a result, estrogen levels and the risk of breast cancer.

Botanical products or phytomedicines are standardized botanical preparations consisting of complex mixtures of one or more plants used in most countries to manage various diseases. According to the WHO definition, botanical products contain plant parts or plant materials in their raw or processed state and excipients such as solvents, diluents, or preservatives. The active principles that cause their pharmacological action are usually unknown. One essential characteristic of botanical products is that they do not possess an immediate or pharmacological solid action. For this reason, botanical products are not used for emergency treatment. Other characteristics of botanical products are their wide therapeutic use and great acceptance by the population. Botanical products, in contrast to modern medicines, are frequently used to treat chronic diseases. Botanical products do not include combinations with chemically defined active substances or isolated constituents. Homeopathic preparations are not botanical products, even though they frequently contain plants.

Compared with well-defined synthetic drugs, botanical products exhibit some marked differences, namely:

- The active principles are frequently unknown; standardization, stability, and quality control are possible but difficult to achieve; raw material availability and quality are often problematic; and well-controlled double-blind clinical and toxicological studies to demonstrate efficacy and safety are uncommon.
- Undesirable side effects appear to be less familiar with botanical products, but well-controlled randomized clinical trials have revealed that they do exist, and botanical products are typically less expensive than synthetic drugs.

13.3.3 Specifications

The specification of a botanical preparation (botanical substance) and the botanical medicinal product is part of a larger control strategy that includes raw material and excipient control, in-process testing, process evaluation/validation, batch stability testing, and batch consistency testing. When these elements are combined, they ensure that the product maintains its appropriate quality. Because specifications are chosen to confirm rather than characterize a product's quality, the manufacturer should explain why certain quality attributes were included and excluded from testing. In addition, the following considerations should be taken into consideration when establishing scientifically justifiable specifications.

Specifications for botanical substances are linked to:

- Botanical characteristics of the plant (genus, species, variety, chemotype; use of genetically modified organisms).
- Macroscopical and microscopical characterization, phytochemical characteristics of plant part constituents with known therapeutic activity or marker substances, toxic constituents (identity, assay, limit tests).
- The quality of the botanical substance (as previously discussed).
- The definition of the botanical preparation (drug extract ratio, extraction solvents' constituents—constituents with known therapeutic activity or marker substances).
- Other constituents (identification, assay, and limit tests) (safety and efficacy considerations).
- The quality of the botanical substance and botanical preparation.
- The manufacturing process (temperature effects, residual solvents); the profile and stability of the active constituents/formulation in packaging.
- The batches used in preclinical/clinical testing are all factors that influence botanical medicinal product specifications (safety and efficacy considerations).

Data from lots used to demonstrate manufacturing consistency should be used to create specifications. It's critical to link specifications to a manufacturing process, especially when it comes to product-related substances, impurities, and process-related impurities. Where historical batch data are available, these should be used.

Changes in the manufacturing process and degradation of products produced during storage could result in a product that differs from what was used in preclinical and clinical trials. Therefore, it is necessary to assess the significance of these changes.

Due to the inherent complexity of botanical products, there may not be a single stability-indicating assay or parameter that profiles the stability characteristics. As a result, the applicant should propose a series of product-specific, stability-indicating tests, the results of which will ensure that changes in the product's quality over its shelf life are detected. Product-specific criteria will be used to determine which tests should be included. The "Note for Guidance on Stability Testing of New Drug Substances and Products" (committee for proprietary medicinal products [CPMP]/ICH/2736/99), and the "Guideline on Stability Testing of New Veterinary Drug Substances and Medicinal Products" (Committee for Veterinary Medicinal Products [CVMP]/International Cooperation on Harmonisation of Technical Requirements for Regulators) are recommended to applicants.

13.3.4 Standardization

Plants contain hundreds of constituents, some of which are only present in trace amounts. Despite the availability of modern chemical analytical procedures, photochemical investigations are only occasionally successful in isolating and characterizing all secondary metabolites present in the plant extract. Aside from that, plant constituents vary greatly depending on various factors, making quality control of phototherapeutic agents difficult. There are several steps involved in the quality control and standardization of botanical products. However, the source and quality of raw materials are critical in ensuring the quality and stability of botanical preparations. Other factors, such as the use of fresh plants, temperature, light exposure, water availability, nutrients, collection period and time, method of collection, drying, packing, storage, and transportation of raw material, age and part of the plant collected, and so on, can all have a significant impact on the quality and therapeutic value of botanical products. Heat-labile plant constituents necessitate low-temperature drying of plants containing them. Enzymatic processes that continue for long periods after plant collection destroy other active principles. This helps to explain why the composition of botanical products varies so much. As a result, proper standardization and quality control of raw materials and botanical preparations should be carried out continuously. When the active principles are unknown, a marker substance or substances should be identified for analytical purposes. However, in the vast majority of cases, these markers have never been tested to see if they are responsible for the therapeutic effects of botanical products. Apart from these variable factors, others such as the extraction method and contamination with microorganisms, heavy metals, pesticides, and the like can also affect botanical products' quality, safety, and efficacy. Pharmaceutical companies prefer cultivated plants over wild-harvested plants for these reasons, as cultivated plants have fewer variations in their constituents. Furthermore, and perhaps more importantly, when botanical products are produced through cultivation, the primary-secondary metabolites can be monitored, allowing the best harvesting period to be determined.

Recent advances in the purification, isolation, and structure elucidation of naturally occurring substances have made it possible to develop appropriate strategies for quality analysis and standardization of botanical preparations to preserve the homogeneity of the plant extract to the greatest extent possible. Thin-layer chromatography (TLC), gas chromatography (GC), high-performance liquid chromatography (HPLC), mass spectrometry (MS), infrared spectrometry (IRS), ultraviolet/visible (UV/VIS) spectrometry, and other techniques can be used to standardize and control the quality of both raw materials and finished botanical products when used individually or in combination.

13.3.5 Efficacy and Safety

Although clinical trials with botanical products are feasible, few well-controlled double-blind (placebo-controlled) trials have been carried out with botanical products. Several factors might contribute to the explanation of such discrepancies, for example:

- The botanical products used in clinical trials lack standardization and quality control.
- Different dosages of botanical products are used.
- There is inadequate randomization and improper patient selection in most studies.
- The numbers of patients in most trials are insufficient for statistical significance.
- There are difficulties in establishing appropriate placebos due to tastes, aromas, and other factors.
- There are wide variations in the duration of botanical product treatments.

However, a large number of clinical trials have been performed with some botanical products, including:

- *Hypericum perforatum* (St. John's wort), an antidepressant.
- *Ginkgo biloba*, used to treat central nervous system and cardiovascular disorders.
- *Tanacetun parthenium* (feverfew), used to treat migraine headaches.
- *Allium sativum* (garlic), used to lower low-density protein cholesterol and some cardiovascular disturbances.
- *Matricaria chamomilla* (chamomile), recommended as a carminative, anti-inflammatory, and antispasmodic.

13.3.6 Prior Human Use

Plants are often extracted and processed in non-reproducible methods. Therefore, the product produced for a clinical trial must be similar in analysis to the original product used in humans.

Consider the following example of a three-part botanical product. Component 1 is potentially toxic, while components 2 and 3 may be effective at low doses but may be toxic at higher doses. For two lots of

TABLE 13.3

Example of Component Combinations for a Botanical Product

	Component 1 • potentially toxic	Component 2 • low dose: effective • high dose: toxic	Component 3 • low dose: effective • high dose: toxic
Lot 1	1 unit	122 units	48 units
Lot 2	12 units	11 units	10 units

the drug, Table 13.3 shows the number of units of each component. If lot 1 is used, but the previous lots were comparable to lot 2, the higher doses of components 2 and 3 will cause toxicity in the participants. Participants will experience toxicity from the higher dose of component 1, and efficacy will be reduced due to the lower doses of components 2 and 3. If lot 2 is administered, but the lots previously used were comparable to lot 1, participants will experience toxicity from the higher dose of component 1, and efficacy will be diminished due to the lower doses of components 2 and 3.

This example demonstrates the wide range of compositions that can be found in botanical products with identical labels. As a result, if preliminary clinical data is used to justify the proposed trial, analysis of the proposed product for study in a clinical trial must be performed and shown to be similar to the botanical analysis with prior human experience.

Therefore, the following information is needed for products previously used in humans:

- Plant substance:
  - Description of the plant.
  - Genus.
  - Species (cultivar if appropriate).
  - Country(s) of origin.
  - Plant extraction procedure.
- Product of the plant.
- Chemical or biological parameters are used to analyze commonly accepted or alleged active ingredient(s) or analyze a significant chemical component (analytical marker compound).

13.3.7 CMC

In general, chemistry, manufacturing, and control (CMC) requirements for standard synthetic/semisynthetic drugs are:

- Drug synthesis.
- Manufacturing of the product that is administered to the patient.
- Process control.

As a result, the drug and the product are repeatable, ensuring that only active ingredients are given to patients and that toxic contaminants are avoided.

Column 3 of Table 13.3 lists more specific CMC requirements, such as a plant substance that is later transformed into a pure drug (e.g., digitalis for heart failure, artemisinins for malaria).

Botanicals, unlike standard drugs, have been in use for a long time before being studied in a clinical trial. Prior human testing ensures that the product is both safe and effective. For botanical products, some of the CMC information required for a standard drug is also required.

Botanical products, unlike synthetic drugs, are made up of unidentified constituents. A therapeutic advantage is thought to be provided by a mixture. Unknown constituents, for example, may combine with known constituents in an additive or synergistic way to provide greater efficacy than the known constituent alone. Analysis of the active ingredient(s) in botanical products may be best approached by testing for one or more hypothesized active ingredients such as a chemical fingerprint of the total ingredients or a chemical constituent that makes up a significant percentage of the total ingredients. The last two analyses are surrogates for analysis of the unknown constituents that contribute to efficacy.

13.3.7.1 Starting Material

Only a rigorous and detailed definition of the starting materials, particularly the specific botanical identification of the plant material used, can ensure consistent quality for botanical origin products. To ensure consistent quality, it's also important to know the botanical substance's geographical source and the conditions under which it is obtained.

Standardized extracts are botanical preparations that have been adjusted to a given content of constituents with known therapeutic activity within an acceptable tolerance; standardization is accomplished by adjusting the botanical preparations with inert material or blending batches of botanical preparations. "Quantified extracts" are botanical preparations adjusted to a defined range of constituents; adjustments are made by blending botanical preparations batches. "Other extracts" are botanical preparations essentially defined by their production process and their specifications.

The quantity of a botanical substance or a botanical preparation consisting of comminuted or powdered botanical substances shall be given as a range corresponding to a defined quantity of constituents with known therapeutic activity, or the quantity of the botanical substance.

Sennae folium, 415–500 mg, corresponding to 12.5 mg of hydroxyanthracene glycosides, calculated as sennoside B, or *Valerianae radix* 900 mg, are two examples of how the composition is listed.

In the case of a botanical preparation produced by steps that exceed comminution, the nature and concentration of the solvent and the extract's physical state have to be given. Furthermore, the following have to be indicated (European Medicines Agency 2011):

- Standardized extracts: If the constituents with known therapeutic activity are known, the equivalent quantity or ratio of the botanical substance to the botanical preparation must be stated, and the quantity of the botanical preparation may be given as a range corresponding to a defined quantity of these constituents.
- Quantified extracts: If the constituents with known therapeutic activity are known, the equivalent quantity or ratio of the botanical substance to the botanical preparation must be stated, and the quantity of the botanical preparation may be given as a corresponding range. Furthermore, the content of the quantified substance(s) must be specified in a range.
- Other extracts: If constituents with known therapeutic activity are unknown, the equivalent quantity or ratio of the botanical substance to the botanical preparation must be stated.

The added substance must be listed as an "other substance" and the genuine extract as the "active substance" if the preparation is being adjusted to a defined content of constituents with known therapeutic activity or for any other reason. When different batches of the same extract are used to adjust constituents with known therapeutic activity to a defined content or for any other reason, the final mixture is considered the genuine extract and listed as the "active substance" in the unit formula. The dossier must, however, include complete production and control details.

The following are some examples of representation:

- *Sennae folium* 50–65 mg, corresponding to 12.5 mg of dry extract ethanolic 60% (V/V) hydroxyanthracene glycosides, calculated as ([a–b]: 1) Sennoside B.
- *Ginkgo biloba* L. *folium* 60 mg, containing 13.2–16.2 mg of flavonoid dry extract acetonic 60% (V/V) expressed as flavone glycosides ([a–b]: 1) 1.68–2.04 mg ginkgolides A, B, and C and 1.56–1.92 mg bilobalide.
- *Valerianae radix* 125 mg dry extract ethanolic 60% (V/V) or *Valerianae radix* 125 mg dry extract ethanolic 60% (V/V) equivalent to x–y mg *Valerianae radix*.

13.3.7.2 Control of Botanical Substances and Preparations

As a general rule, botanical substances must be tested, unless otherwise justified, for microbiological quality and residue pesticides and fumigation agents, toxic metals, likely contaminants, and adulterants, and so on. The International Conference on Harmonization (ICH) guidelines prohibit ethylne oxide for decontamination of botanical substances. If there are any concerns, radioactive contamination should be tested. Specifications and descriptions of the analytical procedures, as well as the applied limits, must be submitted. To validate analytical procedures not listed in a *Pharmacopoeia*, use the ICH guideline "Validation of Analytical Procedures: Methodology" (CPMP/ICH/281/95) or the corresponding VICH guideline (CVMP/VICH/591/98).

The botanical substances must have reference samples available for use in comparative tests, such as macroscopic and microscopic examination, chromatography, and so on.

If the botanical medicinal product contains a preparation, rather than merely the botanical substance itself, the botanical substance's comprehensive specification must be followed by a description and validation of the manufacturing process for the botanical preparation. The data can be provided as part of a marketing authorization application or through the European Active Substance Master File procedure. If the latter route is chosen, the documentation should be submitted following the "Guideline on Active Substance Master File Procedure" (EMEA/CPMP/QWP/227/02 and EMEA/CVMP/134/02).

A monograph on the preparation has been published by the *European Pharmacopoeia*. To demonstrate compliance with the relevant *European Pharmacopoeia* monograph, the European Directorate for the Quality of Medicines Certification procedure (for Certificates of Suitability, CEPs) can be used.

A detailed specification is required for each botanical preparation. This should be based on recent scientific data and include details about the characteristics, identification, and purity tests. Chromatographic methods that are appropriate should be used. Tests on microbiological quality, pesticide residues, fumigation agents, solvents, and toxic metals should be performed if deemed necessary by analyzing the starting material. If there are any concerns about radioactivity, it should be tested. It's also necessary to perform a quantitative determination (assay) of markers or substances with known therapeutic activity. The content should be indicated with as little tolerance as possible (the narrowest possible tolerance with both upper and lower limits stated). The test methods should be thoroughly described.

Assume that botanical substances containing therapeutically active constituents are standardized (i.e., adjusted to a defined content of constituents with known therapeutic activity). In that case, it should be stated how standardization is achieved. If another substance is to be used for these purposes, the amount that can be added must be specified as a range.

13.3.7.3 Control of Vitamins and Minerals (If Applicable)

Vitamins and minerals, which may be used as ancillary substances in traditional botanical medicinal products for human use, must meet the requirements of the "Guideline on the Summary of Requirements for Active Substances in the Quality Part of the Dossier" (CHMP/QWP/297/97 Rev. 1 corr).

13.3.7.4 Control of Excipients

Excipients should be described following the "Note for Guidance on Excipients in the Dossier for Application for Marketing Authorization of a Medicinal Product" (Eudralex 3AQ 9A) or the "Note for Guidance on Excipients in the Dossier for Application for Marketing Authorization of Veterinary Medicinal Products" (EMEA/CV). The dossier requirements for active substances apply to novel excipients (see Directive 2001/83/EC as amended for human medicinal products and Directive 2001/82/EC as amended for veterinary medicinal products for more information).

The composition of the active substance should be determined qualitatively and quantitatively using control tests on the finished product(s). A specification should be provided, which may include markers where constituents with known therapeutic activity are unknown. These constituents should be specified and quantitatively determined in botanical substances or botanical preparations with constituents of known therapeutic activity. For traditional botanical medicinal products for human use containing vitamins and minerals, the vitamins and minerals should also be specified and quantitatively determined.

Suppose a botanical medicinal product contains several botanical substances or preparations of botanical substances, and a quantitative determination of each active substance is not possible. In that case, several active substances may be done jointly. First, however, the necessity of this procedure must be demonstrated.

Unless otherwise justified, the *European Pharmacopoeia*'s criteria for ensuring microbiological quality should be followed. Testing for microbial contamination should be justified regularly.

13.3.7.5 Stability Testing

Because the entire botanical substance or botanical preparation is considered the active substance, determining the stability of the constituents with known therapeutic activity will not suffice. Other substances present in the botanical substance or botanical preparation should, to the extent possible, be demonstrated as well, for example, using appropriate fingerprint chromatograms. It should also be shown that the proportional content of their contents remains constant.

Suppose a botanical medicinal product contains a mixture of botanical substances or botanical preparations, and it is not possible to determine the stability of each active ingredient. In that case, the medicinal product's stability should be determined using fingerprint chromatograms, overall assay methods, physical and sensory tests, or other appropriate tests. The applicant must demonstrate that the tests are appropriate.

Unless justified, the variation in content in a botanical medicinal product containing a botanical substance or botanical preparation with constituents of known therapeutic activity during the proposed shelf life should not exceed 5% of the initial assay value. In the case of a botanical medicinal product containing a botanical substance or botanical preparation where constituents with known therapeutic activity are unknown, a variation in marker content of 10% of the initial assay value can be accepted if the applicant can justify it.

The vitamins and minerals stability should be demonstrated in traditional botanical medicinal products for human use containing vitamins and/or minerals.

13.3.7.6 Testing Criteria

Implementation of the recommendations in the following section should take into account the ICH/VICH guidelines "Validation of Analytical Methods: Definitions and Terminology" (CPMP/ICH/381/95 and CVMP/VICH/590/98) and "Validation of Analytical Procedures: Methodology" (CPMP/ICH/281/95 and CVMP/VICH/591/98).

13.3.7.7 Botanical Substances

- Description of the plant.
- Procedure by which a part of the plant is extracted.
- Quantity of active ingredients in the extract.
- How the active ingredient is identified.
- Stability of the active ingredient (at least over the time of the trial).

Botanical substances are a diverse range of botanical materials, including leaves, herbs, roots, flowers, seeds, bark, etc. Therefore, a comprehensive specification must be developed for each botanical substance, even if the starting material for the finished product is a botanical preparation. A botanical substance specification is required unless justified in the case of fatty or essential oils used as active substances of botanical medicinal products. The specification should be established based on recent scientific data and should be set out in the same way as the *European Pharmacopoeia* monographs. The general monograph *Botanical Products (Botanical Substances)* of the *European Pharmacopoeia* should be consulted to interpret the following requirements.

A description of the plant, including genus, species (cultivar if appropriate), country(s) of origin, time of harvest, and plant extraction procedure (Table 13.4) is required.

- Botanical description.
- Statement that the plant is cultivated according to Good Agricultural Practices or harvested according to Good Wildcrafting Practices.
- Extraction procedure.
- Quantity and identity of active ingredient(s) and sizeable chemical constituent.
- Statement that extraction and analytic procedures are performed under Good Manufacturing Practices (GMP) (e.g., that the manufacturing processes and their controls provide the appropriate levels of assurance for the product's important quality characteristics).

The following tests and acceptance criteria are generally considered applicable to all botanical substances:

1. Definition: A qualitative statement of the botanical source, plant part used, and its state (e.g., whole, reduced, powdered, fresh, dry). It is also essential to know the geographical source(s) and the conditions under which the botanical substance is obtained.
2. Characteristics: A qualitative statement wherein the organoleptic character(s), including macro and microscopic botanic properties of the botanical substance, is described.
3. Identification: Identifying testing optimally should discriminate between related species and potential adulterants/substitutes, which are likely to be present. Identification tests should be specific for the botanical substance and usually involve three or more of the following: macroscopic, microscopic, chromatographic, and chemical.

TABLE 13.4

Chemistry–Manufacturing–Control Considerations for National Center for Complementary and Alternative Medicine Clinical Trials

Subject of Study	Study Parameters	Study Details	Data Required for {roposed NCCAM Trial	
			Phase I/II Trial	Phase III Trial
Plant substance	Starting material	Botanical description	X	Expanded
		Extraction procedure	X	Expanded
		Quantity of active moiety		X
		Identity: chemical/biologic assay		X
		Stability		X
Plant product	Manufacturing	Reagents/process		X
	Finished product	Quantity of active moiety	X	X
	Product assay	Methods/specifications		X
		Identity: chemical/biologic assay	X	X
		Purity		X
	Storage	Describe conditions	X	X
	Stability	Light/heat/time	X	X
	Excipients	List		X
	Impurities	List/analyze	X	X
	Reference standard	Standard batch		X
	In-process controls	Standard operating procedures		X
	Bioavailability	Disintegration/dissolution rate	X	X
	Microbiology	Contamination		X
	Environmental	Assessment		X

Note: X means applicable.

4. Tests:
   - Foreign matter.
   - Total ash.
   - Ash insoluble in hydrochloric acid.
   - Water-soluble extractive.
   - Extractable matter.
   - Particle size: Particle size can significantly impact dissolution rates, bioavailability, and stability for some botanical substances used in botanical teas or solid botanical medicinal products. In such cases, particle size distribution testing should be performed using an appropriate procedure, with acceptance criteria provided. In addition, the disintegration time of solid dosage forms can also be affected by particle size.
   - Water content: This test is important when the botanical substances are known to be hygroscopic. For non-pharmacopeial botanical substances, acceptance criteria should be justified by data on the effects of moisture absorption. A loss on drying procedure may be adequate; however, in some cases (essential oil–containing plants), a detection procedure that is specific for water is required.
   - Inorganic impurities, toxic metals: The need to include tests and acceptance criteria for inorganic contaminants should be studied during development and based on knowledge of the plant species, its cultivation, and the manufacturing process. Acceptance criteria will ultimately depend on safety considerations. Procedures and acceptance criteria for sulfated ash/residue on ignition should, where possible, be based on pharmacopeia precedents; other inorganic impurities can be determined using other methods, such as atomic absorption spectroscopy.
   - Microbial limits: There may be a need to specify the total count of aerobic micro-organisms, the total count of yeasts and molds, and the absence of specific objectionable bacteria. When considering the inclusion of other pathogens (e.g., *Campylobacter* and *Listeria* species) in addition to those listed in the *European Pharmacopoeia*, the source of the botanical material should be considered. Microbial counts should be determined using pharmacopeial procedures or other validated procedures. The *European Pharmacopoeia* gives guidance on acceptance criteria.
   - Mycotoxins: The potential for mycotoxins contamination should be fully considered. Wherever necessary, suitable validated methods should be used to control potential mycotoxins, and the acceptance criteria should be justified.
   - Pesticides, fumigation agents, and the like: The potential for pesticide residues, fumigation agents, and the like should be fully considered. Wherever necessary, suitable validated methods should be used to control potential residues, and the acceptance criteria should be justified. In the case of pesticide residues, the method, acceptance criteria, and guidance on the *European Pharmacopeia* methodology should be applied unless fully explained.
   - Other appropriate tests (e.g., swelling index).
5. Assay: In the case of botanical substances with known therapeutic activity constituents, assays of their content are required with details of the analytical procedure. Wherever possible, a specific, stability-indicating procedure should be included to determine the botanical substance's content. In cases where the use of a nonspecific assay is justified, other supporting analytical procedures should be used to achieve overall specificity. For example, if essential oil determination is used to assay a botanical substance, the assay can be combined with a suitable test for identification (e.g., fingerprint chromatography). In botanical substances where the constituents responsible for the therapeutic activity are unknown, assays of marker substances or other justified determinations are required. The appropriateness of the choice of marker substance should be justified. For example, a reference to the assay of a marker substance in the *European Pharmacopeia*'s relevant monograph is an appropriate justification.

13.3.7.8 Botanical Product

- How the product is manufactured.
- Quantity of active ingredients in the product.
- How the active ingredient is identified.
- Impurities in the product, including microbial, pesticides, heavy metals, and contaminants.
- Storage circumstances and the active ingredient's physical-chemical stability during storage.
- Bioavailability of the active ingredient (disintegration and dissolution, or breakdown, in physiologic solutions in vitro, absorption in vivo).
- Whether the environment is contaminated, for example, with carcinogens, during the manufacturing process so that each batch is similar to the reference batch.

Extracts, tinctures, oils, and resins are among the botanical preparations available, ranging from simple, comminuted plant material to extracts, tinctures, oils, and resins. As a result, a complete specification based on recent scientific data must be prepared for each botanical preparation. The *European Pharmacopoeia*'s general monograph *Botanical Product Preparations (Botanical Preparations)* should be used to interpret the following requirements.

The testing and approval criteria listed below are typically accepted for all botanical preparations.

1. A declaration of the botanical source and the manner of preparation (e.g., dry or liquid extract). The botanical material to botanical preparation ratio must be specified.
2. Characteristics: A qualitative comment of the botanical preparation's organoleptic characteristics.
3. Identification: Identification tests should be specific to the botanical preparation and, ideally, selective against possible substitutes/adulterants. A mixture of chromatographic tests (e.g., HPLC and TLC-densitometry) or a combination of tests into a single procedure, such as HPLC/UV-diode array, HPLC/MS, or GC/MS, for example, is not considered to be specific.
4. Tests:
   - Residual solvents: For more information, see the *European Pharmacopoeia* general text on residual solvents (01/2005: 50400).
   - Water content: When botanical preparations are known to be hygroscopic, this test is critical. Data on the effects of hydration or moisture absorption could be used to justify the acceptance criteria. A loss on drying approach may be sufficient in some circumstances; but, in others (essential oil–containing formulations), a water-specific detection procedure is necessary.
   - Toxic metals and inorganic impurities: The necessity for inorganic impurity tests and acceptability criteria should be researched during the development phase and based on knowledge of the plant species, cultivation, and manufacturing method. The possibility of harmful substances being concentrated throughout the production process should be thoroughly investigated. The testing with the botanical ingredient may be sufficient if the manufacturing method decreases the burden of harmful residues. Safety issues will eventually determine acceptance requirements. Procedures and acceptability criteria for sulfated ash/residue on ignition should, when possible, be based on pharmacopeial precedents; other inorganic impurities can be evaluated using other methods, such as atomic absorption spectroscopy.
   - Microbial limits: The total count of aerobic microorganisms, the total count of yeasts and molds, and the lack of specific undesirable bacteria may all need to be specified. These restrictions should be in line with the *European Pharmacopoeia.*
   - Mycotoxins: Contamination by mycotoxins should be thoroughly considered. To regulate potential mycotoxins, appropriate validated procedures should be employed wherever possible, and the acceptance criteria should be justified.

- Pesticides, fumigation agents, and other chemicals: Pesticide residues, fumigation agents, and other chemicals should all be taken into account. To control potential residues, appropriate validated procedures should be utilized whenever possible, and the acceptance criteria should be justified. Unless the method, acceptance criteria, and guidance on the *European Pharmacopeia* methodology are adequately stated, the method, acceptance criteria, and guidance on the *European Pharmacopeia* methodology should be used in the event of pesticide residues.

5. Assay: Assays of the composition of botanical preparations with established therapeutic active ingredients are required, together with details of the analytical technique. To determine the botanical substance's content in the botanical preparation, a specific, stability-indicating process should be incorporated wherever possible. Other supporting analytical techniques should be employed to establish overall specificity in circumstances where the use of a nonspecific assay is justified. When testing anthraquinone glycosides with a UV/VIS spectrophotometric assay, for example, a combination of the assay with a relevant test for identification (e.g., fingerprint chromatography) can be utilized. Assays of marker compounds or other justifiable findings are necessary for botanical preparations where the ingredients responsible for the therapeutic efficacy are unclear. The suitability of the marker substance selection should be demonstrated. Analysis of commonly accepted or alleged active ingredient(s) using chemical or biological parameters is required, including:
   - Analysis of a significant chemical constituent (analytical marker compound).
   - Analysis using chemical fingerprints (analytical markers).
   - Analysis for pesticides, heavy metals, and synthetic drug adulterants (e.g., the manufacturing processes and controls provide appropriate assurance for its critical quality characteristics).

13.4 Conclusion

While the new era of drug discovery is inundated with artificial intelligence, gene therapy, mRNA vaccines, and indiviudalized medicine, botanical products remain one of the most important classifications of products that are waiting to be discovered. The reason for this optimism comes from the belief in the symbiosis of nature. We may be able to accurately define the structure of an antibody but we are still far off from predicting the pharmacology of products derived from nature, particularly botanical products. The human race has survived for millions of years depending on what we could find in nature to cure our ailments, and this dependence is not going anywhere.

ADDITIONAL READING

Abbasi AM, Khan SM, Ahmad M, Khan MA, Quave CL, Pieroni A. Botanical ethnoveterinary therapies in three districts of the lesser Himalayas of Pakistan. *J Ethnobiol Ethnomed.* 2013;9:84. doi:10.1186/1746-4269-9-84

Afaq F, Adhami VM, Ahmad N, Mukhtar H. Botanical antioxidants for chemoprevention of photocarcinogenesis. *Front Biosci.* 2002;7:d784–d792. doi:10.2741/afaq

Afaq F, Mukhtar H. Botanical antioxidants in the prevention of photocarcinogenesis and photoaging. *Exp Dermatol.* 2006;15(9):678–684. doi:10.1111/j.1600-0625.2006.00466.x

Afaq F, Mukhtar H. Photochemoprevention by botanical antioxidants. *Skin Pharmacol Appl Skin Physiol.* 2002;15(5):297–306. doi:10.1159/000064533

Álvarez DM, Castillo E, Duarte LF, et al. Current antivirals and novel botanical molecules interfering with herpes simplex virus infection. *Front Microbiol.* 2020;11:139. doi:10.3389/fmicb.2020.00139

Aminimoghadamfarouj N, Nematollahi A. Structure elucidation and botanical characterization of diterpenes from a specific type of bee glue. *Molecules.* 2017;22(7):1185. doi:10.3390/molecules22071185

Amit A, Joshua AJ, Bagchi M, Bagchi D. Safety of a novel botanical extract formula for ameliorating allergic rhinitis. Part II. *Toxicol Mech Methods.* 2005;15(3):193–204. doi:10.1080/15376520590945612

Amit A, Saxena VS, Pratibha N, Bagchi M, Bagchi D, Stohs SJ. Safety of a novel botanical extract formula for ameliorating allergic rhinitis. *Toxicol Mech Methods.* 2003;13(4):253–261. doi:10.1080/713857188

Amit A, Saxena VS, Pratibha N, et al. Mast cell stabilization, lipoxygenase inhibition, hyaluronidase inhibition, antihistaminic and antispasmodic activities of Aller-7, a novel botanical formulation for allergic rhinitis. *Drugs Exp Clin Res.* 2003;29(3):107–115.

Antignac E, Nohynek GJ, Re T, Clouzeau J, Toutain H. Safety of botanical ingredients in personal care products/cosmetics. *Food Chem Toxicol.* 2011;49(2):324–341. doi:10.1016/j.fct.2010.11.022

Arora R, Chawla R, Dhaker AS, et al. Podophyllum hexandrum as a potential botanical supplement for the medical management of nuclear and radiological emergencies (NREs) and free radical-mediated ailments: leads from in vitro/in vivo radioprotective efficacy evaluation. *J Diet Suppl.* 2010;7(1):31–50. doi:10.3109/19390210903534996

Arumugam G, Swamy MK, Sinniah UR. *Plectranthus amboinicus* (Lour.) Spreng: botanical, phytochemical, pharmacological and nutritional significance. *Molecules.* 2016;21(4):369. doi:10.3390/molecules21040369

Baker TR, Regg BT. A multi-detector chromatographic approach for characterization and quantitation of botanical constituents to enable in silico safety assessments. *Anal Bioanal Chem.* 2018;410(21):5143–5154. doi:10.1007/s00216-018-1163-y

Barak-Shinar D, Draelos ZD. A randomized controlled study of a novel botanical acne spot treatment. *J Drugs Dermatol.* 2017;16(6):599–603.

Barhate G, Gautam M, Gairola S, Jadhav S, Pokharkar V. Enhanced mucosal immune responses against tetanus toxoid using novel delivery system comprised of chitosan-functionalized gold nanoparticles and botanical adjuvant: characterization, immunogenicity, and stability assessment. *J Pharm Sci.* 2014;103(11):3448–3456. doi:10.1002/jps.24161

Benelli G, Pavela R, Canale A, Mehlhorn H. Tick repellents and acaricides of botanical origin: a green roadmap to control tick-borne diseases? *Parasitol Res.* 2016;115(7):2545–2560. doi:10.1007/s00436-016-5095-1

Benzie IFF, Wachtel-Galor S. *Herbal Medicine: Biomolecular and Clinical Aspects.* Boca Raton, FL: CRC Press; 2011.

Benzinq DH. The origin and rarity of botanical carnivory. *Trends Ecol Evol.* 1987;2(12):364–369. doi:10.1016/0169-5347(87)90137-6

Bhatia AC, Jimenez F. Rapid treatment of mild acne with a novel skin care system containing 1% salicylic acid, 10% buffered glycolic acid, and botanical ingredients. *J Drugs Dermatol.* 2014;13(6):678–683.

Bigler D, Gulding KM, Dann R, Sheabar FZ, Conaway MR, Theodorescu D. Gene profiling and promoter reporter assays: novel tools for comparing the biological effects of botanical extracts on human prostate cancer cells and understanding their mechanisms of action. *Oncogene.* 2003;22(8):1261–1272. doi:10.1038/sj.onc.1206242

Bonn-Miller MO, ElSohly MA, Loflin MJE, Chandra S, Vandrey R. Cannabis and cannabinoid drug development: evaluating botanical versus single molecule approaches. *Int Rev Psychiatry.* 2018;30(3):277–284. doi:10.1080/09540261.2018.1474730

Bullangpoti V, Visetson S, Milne M, et al. The novel botanical insecticide for the control brown planthopper (*Nilaparvata lugens* Stal.). *Commun Agric Appl Biol Sci.* 2006;71(2 Pt B):475–481.

Callegari PE, Zurier RB. Botanical lipids: potential role in modulation of immunologic responses and inflammatory reactions. *Rheum Dis Clin North Am.* 1991;17(2):415–425.

Carroll SP, Venturino J, Davies JH. A milestone in botanical mosquito repellents: novel PMD-based formulation protects more than twice as long as high-concentration deet and other leading products. *J Am Mosq Control Assoc.* 2019;35(3):186–191. doi:10.2987/19-6824.1

Cheng Y, Chen M, Tong W. An approach to comparative analysis of chromatographic fingerprints for assuring the quality of botanical products. *J Chem Inf Comput Sci.* 2003;43(3):1068–1076. doi:10.1021/ci034034c

Choi SZ, Son MW. Novel botanical product for the treatment of diabetic neuropathy. *Arch Pharm Res.* 2011;34(6):865–867. doi:10.1007/s12272-011-0621-2

Colapietro A, Yang P, Rossetti A, et al. The botanical product PBI-05204, a supercritical CO. *Front Pharmacol.* 2020;11:552428. doi:10.3389/fphar.2020.552428

Dryburgh LM, Martin JH. Using therapeutic drug monitoring and pharmacovigilance to overcome some of the challenges of developing medicinal cannabis from botanical origins. *Ther Drug Monit.* 2020;42(1):98–101. doi:10.1097/FTD.0000000000000698

Echard BW, Talpur NA, Fan AY, Bagchi D, Preuss HG. Hepatoprotective ability of a novel botanical formulation on mild liver injury in rats produced by acute acetaminophen and/or alcohol ingestion. *Res Commun Mol Pathol Pharmacol.* 2001;110(1–2):73–85.

European Medicines Agency. Guideline on quality of herbal medicinal products/traditional herbal medicinal products. 2011. Retrieved from: https://www.ema.europa.eu/en/documents/scientific-guideline/guideline-quality-herbal-medicinal-products-traditional-herbal-medicinal-products-revision-2_en.pdf

Evans JM, Luby R, Lukaczer D, et al. The functional medicine approach to COVID-19: virus-specific nutraceutical and botanical agents. *Integr Med (Encinitas).* 2020;19(Suppl 1):34–42.

Evans S, Dizeyi N, Abrahamsson PA, Persson J. The effect of a novel botanical agent TBS-101 on invasive prostate cancer in animal models. *Anticancer Res.* 2009;29(10):3917–3924.

Falkowski M, Jahn-Oyac A, Odonne G, et al. Towards the optimization of botanical insecticides research: *Aedes aegypti* larvicidal natural products in French Guiana. *Acta Trop.* 2020;201:105179. doi:10.1016/j.actatropica.2019.105179

Fang F, Qi Y, Lu F, Yang L. Highly sensitive on-site detection of drugs adulterated in botanical dietary supplements using thin layer chromatography combined with dynamic surface enhanced Raman spectroscopy. *Talanta.* 2016;146:351–357. doi:10.1016/j.talanta.2015.08.067

Gallo R, Pastorino C, Gasparini G, Ciccarese G, Parodi A. Scutellaria baicalensis extract: a novel botanical allergen in cosmetic products? *Contact Dermatitis.* 2016;75(6):387–388. doi:10.1111/cod.12659

Godlewska K, Pacyga P, Michalak I, et al. Field-scale evaluation of botanical extracts effect on the yield, chemical composition and antioxidant activity of celeriac. *Molecules.* 2020;25(18):4212. doi:10.3390/molecules25184212

Gruenwald J. Novel botanical ingredients for beverages. *Clin Dermatol.* 2009;27(2):210–216. doi:10.1016/j.clindermatol.2008.11.003

Gulati OP, Berry Ottaway P. Legislation relating to nutraceuticals in the European Union with a particular focus on botanical-sourced products. *Toxicology.* 2006;221(1):75–87. doi:10.1016/j.tox.2006.01.014

Guo LX, Li R, Liu K, et al. Structural characterization and discrimination of Chinese medicinal materials with multiple botanical origins based on metabolite profiling and chemometrics analysis: Clematidis Radix et Rhizoma as a case study. *J Chromatogr A.* 2015;1425:129–140. doi:10.1016/j.chroma.2015.11.013

Heinrich M, Scotti F, Booker A, Fitzgerald M, Kum KY, Löbel K. Unblocking high-value botanical value chains: is there a role for blockchain systems? *Front Pharmacol.* 2019;10:396. doi:10.3389/fphar.2019.00396

Hu Z, Wang Z, Liu Y, Wang Q. Leveraging botanical resources for crop protection: the isolation, bioactivity and structure-activity relationships of lycoris alkaloids. *Pest Manag Sci.* 2018;74(12):2783–2792. doi:10.1002/ps.5065

Imai S, Yoshida R, Endo Y, et al. *Rhizobacter gummiphilus* sp. nov., a rubber-degrading bacterium isolated from the soil of a botanical garden in Japan. *J Gen Appl Microbiol.* 2013;59(3):199–205. doi:10.2323/jgam.59.199

James SA, Soltis PS, Belbin L, et al. Herbarium data: global biodiversity and societal botanical needs for novel research. *Appl Plant Sci.* 2018;6(2):e1024. doi:10.1002/aps3.1024

Jiang Y, Gong P, Madak-Erdogan Z, et al. Mechanisms enforcing the estrogen receptor β selectivity of botanical estrogens. *FASEB J.* 2013;27(11):4406–4418. doi:10.1096/fj.13-234617

Johnson BM, Bolton JL, van Breemen RB. Screening botanical extracts for quinoid metabolites. *Chem Res Toxicol.* 2001;14(11):1546–1551. doi:10.1021/tx010106n

Juwita T, Melyani Puspitasari I, Levita J. Torch ginger (Etlingera elatior): a review on its botanical aspects, phytoconstituents and pharmacological activities. *Pak J Biol Sci.* 2018;21(4):151–165. doi:10.3923/pjbs.2018.151.165

Kan J, Cheng J, Guo J, Chen L, Zhang X, Du J. A novel botanical combination attenuates light-induced retinal damage through antioxidant and prosurvival mechanisms. *Oxid Med Cell Longev.* 2020;2020:7676818. doi:10.1155/2020/7676818

Kan J, Velliquette RA, Grann K, et al. A novel botanical formula prevents diabetes by improving insulin resistance. *BMC Complement Altern Med.* 2017;17(1):352. doi:10.1186/s12906-017-1848-3

Kan J, Wang M, Liu Y, et al. A novel botanical formula improves eye fatigue and dry eye: a randomized, double-blind, placebo-controlled study. *Am J Clin Nutr.* 2020;112(2):334–342. doi:10.1093/ajcn/nqaa139

Katoulis AC, Liakou AI, Alevizou A, et al. Efficacy and safety of a topical botanical in female androgenetic alopecia: a randomized, single-blinded, vehicle-controlled study. *Skin Appendage Disord.* 2018;4(3):160–165. doi:10.1159/000480024

Kawamoto T, Fuchs A, Fautz R, Morita O. Threshold of toxicological concern (TTC) for botanical extracts (Botanical-TTC) derived from a meta-analysis of repeated-dose toxicity studies. *Toxicol Lett.* 2019;316:1–9. doi:10.1016/j.toxlet.2019.08.006

Keaney TC, Pham H, von Grote E, Meckfessel MH. Efficacy and safety of minoxidil 5% foam in combination with a botanical hair solution in men with androgenic alopecia. *J Drugs Dermatol.* 2016;15(4):406–412.

Khalil RA. Novel therapies and botanical and mechanical approaches for management of cardiovascular disease. *Recent Pat Cardiovasc Drug Discov.* 2013;8(1):1. doi:10.2174/1574890111308010001

Koo B, Bae HJ, Goo N, et al. A botanical product composed of three herbal materials attenuates the sensorimotor gating deficit and cognitive impairment induced by MK-801 in mice. *J Pharm Pharmacol.* 2020;72(1):149–160. doi:10.1111/jphp.13199

Kortesniemi M, Rosenvald S, Laaksonen O, et al. Sensory and chemical profiles of Finnish honeys of different botanical origins and consumer preferences. *Food Chem.* 2018;246:351–359. doi:10.1016/j.foodchem.2017.10.069

Kosini D, Nukenine EN. Bioactivity of novel botanical insecticide from *Gnidia kaussiana* (Thymeleaceae) against *Callosobruchus maculatus* (Coleoptera: Chrysomelidae) in stored *Vigna subterranea* (Fabaceae) grains. *J Insect Sci.* 2017;17(1):004. doi:10.1093/jisesa/iex004

Kozlowska W, Wagner C, Moore EM, Matkowski A, Komarnytsky S. Botanical provenance of traditional medicines from Carpathian mountains at the Ukrainian-Polish border. *Front Pharmacol.* 2018;9:295. doi:10.3389/fphar.2018.00295

Kuo YL, Chen CH, Chuang TH, et al. Gene expression profiling and pathway network analysis predicts a novel antitumor function for a botanical-derived drug, PG2. *Evid Based Complement Alternat Med.* 2015;2015:917345. doi:10.1155/2015/917345

Lee BA, Lee HS, Jung YS, et al. The effects of a novel botanical agent on lipopolysaccharide-induced alveolar bone loss in rats. *J Periodontol.* 2013;84(8):1221–1229. doi:10.1902/jop.2012.120460

Levine WZ, Samuels N, Bar Sheshet ME, Grbic JT. A novel treatment of gingival recession using a botanical topical gingival patch and mouthrinse. *J Contemp Dent Pract.* 2013;14(5):948–953. doi:10.5005/jp-journals-10024-1431

Liao S, Han L, Zheng X, et al. Tanshinol borneol ester, a novel synthetic small molecule angiogenesis stimulator inspired by botanical formulations for angina pectoris. *Br J Pharmacol.* 2019;176(17):3143–3160. doi:10.1111/bph.14714

Little JG, Marsman DS, Baker TR, Mahony C. In silico approach to safety of botanical dietary supplement ingredients utilizing constituent-level characterization. *Food Chem Toxicol.* 2017;107(Pt A):418–429. doi:10.1016/j.fct.2017.07.017

Liu R, Dobson CC, Foster BC, et al. Effect of an anxiolytic botanical containing *Souroubea sympetala* and *Platanus occidentalis* on in-vitro diazepam human cytochrome P450-mediated metabolism. *J Pharm Pharmacol.* 2019;71(3):429–437. doi:10.1111/jphp.13045

Liu Z. Preparation of botanical samples for biomedical research. *Endocr Metab Immune Disord Drug Targets.* 2008;8(2):112–121. doi:10.2174/187153008784534358

Luo Z, Deng Y, Luo B, et al. Design and synthesis of novel n-butyphthalide derivatives as promising botanical fungicides. *Z Naturforsch C J Biosci.* 2020:0192. doi:10.1515/znc-2020-0192

Lv D, Cao Y, Chen L, et al. Simulation strategies for characterizing Phosphodiesterase-5 inhibitors in botanical dietary supplements. *Anal Chem.* 2018;90(18):10765–10770. doi:10.1021/acs.analchem.8b01609

Ma Z, Gulia-Nuss M, Zhang X, Brown MR. Effects of the botanical insecticide, toosendanin, on blood digestion and egg production by female *Aedes aegypti* (Diptera: Culicidae): topical application and ingestion. *J Med Entomol.* 2013;50(1):112–121. doi:10.1603/me12119

Mangang IB, Tiwari A, Rajamani M, Manickam L. Comparative laboratory efficacy of novel botanical extracts against *Tribolium castaneum*. *J Sci Food Agric.* 2020;100(4):1541–1546. doi:10.1002/jsfa.10162

Maramaldi G, Togni S, Franceschi F, Lati E. Anti-inflammaging and antiglycation activity of a novel botanical ingredient from African biodiversity (Centevita™). *Clin Cosmet Investig Dermatol.* 2014;7:1–9. doi:10.2147/CCID.S49924

Mena P, Tassotti M, Andreu L, et al. Phytochemical characterization of different prickly pear (*Opuntia ficus-indica* (L.) Mill.) cultivars and botanical parts: UHPLC-ESI-MS. *Food Res Int.* 2018;108:301–308. doi:10.1016/j.foodres.2018.03.062

Miller Coyle H, Ladd C, Palmbach T, Lee HC. The Green Revolution: botanical contributions to forensics and drug enforcement. *Croat Med J.* 2001;42(3):340–345.

Moriguchi N, Sato A, Kimura M, Shibata T, Yoneda Y. [A historical review of the therapeutic use of wood creosote based on its botanical origin]. *Yakushigaku Zasshi.* 2007;42(2):110–118.

Moy RL, Levenson C. Sandalwood album oil as a botanical therapeutic in dermatology. *J Clin Aesthet Dermatol.* 2017;10(10):34–39.

Narváez A, Rodríguez-Carrasco Y, Castaldo L, Izzo L, Ritieni A. Ultra-high-performance liquid chromatography coupled with quadrupole orbitrap high-resolution mass spectrometry for multi-residue analysis of mycotoxins and pesticides in botanical nutraceuticals. *Toxins (Basel).* 2020;12(2):114. doi:10.3390/toxins12020114

Osorio MT, Haughey SA, Elliott CT, Koidis A. Identification of vegetable oil botanical speciation in refined vegetable oil blends using an innovative combination of chromatographic and spectroscopic techniques. *Food Chem.* 2015;189:67–73. doi:10.1016/j.foodchem.2014.11.164

Pagnier GJ, Kastanenka KV, Sohn M, et al. Novel botanical product DA-9803 prevents deficits in Alzheimer's mouse models. *Alzheimers Res Ther.* 2018;10(1):11. doi:10.1186/s13195-018-0338-2

Pan H, Yao C, Yang W, et al. An enhanced strategy integrating offline two-dimensional separation and step-wise precursor ion list-based raster-mass defect filter: characterization of indole alkaloids in five botanical origins of Uncariae Ramulus Cum Unicis as an exemplary application. *J Chromatogr A.* 2018;1563:124–134. doi:10.1016/j.chroma.2018.05.066

Patil VM, Masand N, Gupta SP. HCV inhibitors: role of compounds from botanical sources. *Curr Top Med Chem.* 2016;16(12):1402–1409. doi:10.2174/1568026616666151120112802

Patron NJ. Beyond natural: synthetic expansions of botanical form and function. *New Phytol.* 07 2020;227(2):295–310. doi:10.1111/nph.16562

Pavlovič A, Saganová M. A novel insight into the cost-benefit model for the evolution of botanical carnivory. *Ann Bot.* 2015;115(7):1075–1092. doi:10.1093/aob/mcv050

Peng KY, Horng LY, Sung HC, Huang HC, Wu RT. Hepatocyte growth factor has a role in the amelioration of diabetic vascular complications via autophagic clearance of advanced glycation end products: Dispo85E, an HGF inducer, as a potential botanical product. *Metabolism.* 2011;60(6):888–892. doi:10.1016/j.metabol.2010.08.009

Pesek T, Abramiuk M, Garagic D, Fini N, Meerman J, Cal V. Sustaining plants and people: traditional Q'eqchi' Maya botanical knowledge and interactive spatial modeling in prioritizing conservation of medicinal plants for culturally relative holistic health promotion. *Ecohealth.* 2009;6(1):79–90. doi:10.1007/s10393-009-0224-2

Pilegaard K, Eriksen FD, Soerensen M, Gry J. Information on plant foods in eBASIS: what is in a correct botanical scientific name? *Eur J Clin Nutr.* 2010;64 Suppl 3:S108–S111. doi:10.1038/ejcn.2010.220

Pillai L, Burnett BP, Levy RM. Group GSC. GOAL: multicenter, open-label, post-marketing study of flavocoxid, a novel dual pathway inhibitor anti-inflammatory agent of botanical origin. *Curr Med Res Opin.* 2010;26(5):1055–1063. doi:10.1185/03007991003694522

Prada D, Boyd V, Baker ML, O'Dea M, Jackson B. Viral diversity of microbats within the south west botanical province of western Australia. *Viruses.* 2019;11(12):157. doi:10.3390/v11121157

Presley BC, Jansen-Varnum SA, Logan BK. Analysis of synthetic cannabinoids in botanical material: a review of analytical methods and findings. *Forensic Sci Rev.* 2013;25(1–2):27–46.

Qiu LP, Chen KP. Anti-HBV agents derived from botanical origin. *Fitoterapia.* 2013;84:140–157. doi:10.1016/j.fitote.2012.11.003

Reivitis A, Karimi K, Griffiths C, Banayan A. A single-center, pilot study evaluating a novel TriHex peptide- and botanical-containing eye treatment compared to baseline. *J Cosmet Dermatol.* 2018;17(3):467–470. doi:10.1111/jocd.12542

Ruiz P, Ares AM, Valverde S, Martín MT, Bernal J. Development and validation of a new method for the simultaneous determination of spinetoram J and L in honey from different botanical origins employing solid-phase extraction with a polymeric sorbent and liquid chromatography coupled to quadrupole time-of-flight mass spectrometry. *Food Res Int.* 2020;130:108904. doi:10.1016/j.foodres.2019.108904

Sampalis JS, Brownell LA. A randomized, double blind, placebo and active comparator controlled pilot study of UP446, a novel dual pathway inhibitor anti-inflammatory agent of botanical origin. *Nutr J.* 2012;11:21. doi:10.1186/1475-2891-11-21

Sarveswaran S, Ghosh R, Parikh R, Ghosh J. Wedelolactone, an anti-inflammatory botanical, interrupts c-Myc oncogenic signaling and synergizes with enzalutamide to induce apoptosis in prostate cancer cells. *Mol Cancer Ther.* 2016;15(11):2791–2801. doi:10.1158/1535-7163.MCT-15-0861

Schepetkin IA, Quinn MT. Botanical polysaccharides: macrophage immunomodulation and therapeutic potential. *Int Immunopharmacol.* 2006;6(3):317–333. doi:10.1016/j.intimp.2005.10.005

Shaalan EA, Canyon D, Younes MW, Abdel-Wahab H, Mansour AH. A review of botanical phytochemicals with mosquitocidal potential. *Environ Int.* 2005;31(8):1149–1166. doi:10.1016/j.envint.2005.03.003

Shrestha B, Finke DL, Piñero JC. The 'Botanical Triad': the presence of insectary plants enhances natural enemy abundance on trap crop plants in an organic cabbage agro-ecosystem. *Insects.* 2019;10(6):181. doi:10.3390/insects10060181

Simmonds MS. Novel drugs from botanical sources. *Drug Discov Today.* 2003;8(16):721–722. doi:10.1016/s1359-6446(03)02693-x

Siroha AK, Punia S, Kaur M, Sandhu KS. A novel starch from *Pongamia pinnata* seeds: comparison of its thermal, morphological and rheological behaviour with starches from other botanical sources. *Int J Biol Macromol.* 2020;143:984–990. doi:10.1016/j.ijbiomac.2019.10.033

Vaclavik L, Krynitsky AJ, Rader JI. Mass spectrometric analysis of pharmaceutical adulterants in products labeled as botanical dietary supplements or herbal remedies: a review. *Anal Bioanal Chem.* 2014;406(27):6767–90. doi:10.1007/s00216-014-8159-z

Waidyanatha S, Ryan K, Roe AL, et al. Follow that botanical: challenges and recommendations for assessing absorption, distribution, metabolism and excretion of botanical dietary supplements. *Food Chem Toxicol.* 2018;121:194–202. doi:10.1016/j.fct.2018.08.062

Wang CZ, Wan JY, Wan J, et al. Human intestinal microbiota derived metabolism signature from a North American native botanical *Oplopanax horridus* with UPLC/Q-TOF-MS analysis. *Biomed Chromatogr.* 2020:e4911. doi:10.1002/bmc.4911

Wang N, Zhang C, Xu Y, et al. OMICs approaches-assisted identification of macrophages-derived MIP-1γ as the therapeutic target of botanical products TNTL in diabetic retinopathy. *Cell Commun Signal.* 2019;17(1):81. doi:10.1186/s12964-019-0396-5

Wang X, Xu X, Li Y, et al. Systems pharmacology uncovers Janus functions of botanical products: activation of host defense system and inhibition of influenza virus replication. *Integr Biol (Camb).* 2013;5(2):351–371. doi:10.1039/c2ib20204b

Wang X, Zhu HJ, Munoz J, Gurley BJ, Markowitz JS. An ex vivo approach to botanical-drug interactions: a proof of concept study. *J Ethnopharmacol.* 2015;163:149–156. doi:10.1016/j.jep.2015.01.021

Ward L, Pasinetti GM. Recommendations for development of botanical polyphenols as "Natural Drugs" for promotion of resilience against stress-induced depression and cognitive impairment. *Neuromolecular Med.* 2016;18(3):487–495. doi:10.1007/s12017-016-8418-6

Wegiel B, Persson JL. Effect of a novel botanical agent Drynol Cibotin on human osteoblast cells and implications for osteoporosis: promotion of cell growth, calcium uptake and collagen production. *Phytother Res.* 2010;24 Suppl 2:S139–47. doi:10.1002/ptr.3026

Wieser F, Yu J, Park J, et al. A botanical extract from channel flow inhibits cell proliferation, induces apoptosis, and suppresses CCL5 in human endometriotic stromal cells. *Biol Reprod.* 2009;81(2):371–377. doi:10.1095/biolreprod.108.075069

Xiao HH, Lv J, Mok D, Yao XS, Wong MS, Cooper R. NMR applications for botanical mixtures: the use of HSQC data to determine Lignan content in. *J Nat Prod.* 2019;82(7):1733–1740. doi:10.1021/acs.jnatprod.8b00891

Yamaguchi M, Murata T, Shoji M, Weitzmann MN. The flavonoid p-hydroxycinnamic acid mediates anticancer effects on MDA-MB-231 human breast cancer cells in vitro: Implications for suppression of bone metastases. *Int J Oncol.* 2015;47(4):1563–1571. doi:10.3892/ijo.2015.3106

Yang Z, Shao Q, Ge Z, Ai N, Zhao X, Fan X. A bioactive chemical markers based strategy for quality assessment of botanical products: Xuesaitong injection as a case study. *Sci Rep.* 2017;7(1):2410. doi:10.1038/s41598-017-02305-y

Yimam M, Jiao P, Hong M, et al. Repeated dose 28-day oral toxicity study of a botanical composition composed of *Morus alba* and *Acacia catechu* in rats. *Regul Toxicol Pharmacol.* 2018;94:115–123. doi:10.1016/j.yrtph.2018.01.024

Yong EL, Wong SP, Shen P, Gong YH, Li J, Hong Y. Standardization and evaluation of botanical mixtures: lessons from a traditional Chinese herb, epimedium, with oestrogenic properties. *Novartis Found Symp.* 2007;282:173–88; discussion 188–91, 212–218. doi:10.1002/9780470319444.ch12

Yoon J, Lee H, Chang HB, et al. DW1029M, a novel botanical product candidate, inhibits advanced glycation end-product formation, rat lens aldose reductase activity, and TGF-β1 signaling. *Am J Physiol Renal Physiol.* 2014;306(10):F1161–F1170. doi:10.1152/ajprenal.00651.2013

Zareisedehizadeh S, Tan CH, Koh HL. A review of botanical characteristics, traditional usage, chemical components, pharmacological activities, and safety of *Pereskia bleo* (Kunth) DC. *Evid Based Complement Alternat Med.* 2014;2014:326107. doi:10.1155/2014/326107

Zhao X, Xi X, Hu Z, Wu W, Zhang J. Exploration of novel botanical insecticide leads: synthesis and insecticidal activity of β-dihydroagarofuran derivatives. *J Agric Food Chem.* 2016;64(7):1503–1508. doi:10.1021/acs.jafc.5b05782

Zhong G, Hu M, Liu X, Peng C. [Determination of rhodojaponin, a novel botanical insecticide by HPTLC]. *Se Pu.* 2004;22(3):296.

Zhu Q, Cao Y, Chai Y, Lu F. Rapid on-site TLC-SERS detection of four antidiabetes drugs used as adulterants in botanical dietary supplements. *Anal Bioanal Chem.* 2014;406(7):1877–1884. doi:10.1007/s00216-013-7605-7

14

Regulatory Optimization

14.1 Background

A critical component of accessible medicines is their availability at a timely basis and cost. Regulatory approvals take years, reducing the ready availability of newer medicines. Future medicine development plans should include new and novel regulatory approaches based on new and emerging science. Contrary to the popular belief, blockbuster drugs are not always developed by the big pharma, they often come from smaller companies or academia. In the case of many biological medicines, scientists at public-sector research institutions originally discovered some of the best-known biologics, including Remicade, Enbrel, Humira, Avastin. Additionally, about 25% of new molecular entities were developed from publicly funded work.

The following platform technologies were all developed with public funds:

- Recombinant DNA technology (Cohen-Boyer patents).
- Bacterial production methods for recombinant DNA (Riggs-Itakura patents).
- Production and chimerization methods for antibodies (Cabilly patents).
- Methods to produce glycosylated recombinant proteins in mammalian cells (Axel patents).
- Methods of gene silencing with the use of small interfering RNAs (Mello-Fire patents).

Without these platform technologies, many new drugs would not have been developed, resulting perhaps in a vastly different economic outlook for the pharmaceutical industry. As an example, originally called D2E7, Humira, the world's highest-selling product, emerged from a collaboration between BASF Bioresearch Center in Massachusetts and the Cambridge Antibody Technologies in the UK. Abbott acquired BASF and then when Abbott split, Humira went to Abbvie.

The purpose of this chapter is to define:

- Three practical drug discovery and early development paths to advancing new cancer therapies to early-stage clinical trials, including:
- Discovery and early development of a new chemical entity (NCE).
- Discovery of new, beneficial activity currently marketed drugs possess against novel drug targets, also referred to as "drug repurposing."
- Application of novel platform technology to the development of improved delivery of currently marketed drugs.
- Within each of the three strategies, decision stages have been identified along the commercial value chain and the following concepts have been addressed:
- Key data required at each decision stage, targets, and expectations required to support further development.
- An estimate of the financial resources needed to generate the data at each decision stage.

DOI: 10.1201/9781003146933-14

- The opportunities available to outsource activities to optimally leverage strengths within the institution.
- Integration of these activities with the intellectual property management process potential decision stages, which:
- Offers opportunities to initiate meaningful discussions with regulatory agencies to define requirements for the advancement of new cancer therapies to human evaluation.
- Affords opportunities to license technologies to university start-ups, biotechnology, and major pharmaceutical companies
- Defines potential role(s) the National Institutes of Health SBIR programs may play in advancing new cancer therapies along the drug discovery and early development path.

14.2 Scope

This chapter describes an approach to drug discovery and development for the treatment, prevention, and control of cancer. The guidelines and decision stages described herein may serve as the foundation for collaborative projects with other organizations in multiple therapeutic areas.

14.2.1 Assumptions

These guidelines are being written with target identification as the initial decision stage, although the process outlined here applies to a project initiated at any of the subsequent stages. The final decision stage is human and/or clinical proof of concept.

The decision stages in this chapter are specific to the development of a drug for the treatment of relapsed or refractory late-stage cancer patients. Many of the same criteria apply to the development of drugs intended for other indications and therapeutic areas, but each disease should be approached with logical customization of this plan. The development of compounds for the prevention and control of cancer would follow a more conservative pathway as the benefit/risk evaluation for these compounds would be different. When considering prevention of a disease one is typically treating patients at risk, but before the disease has developed in individuals that are otherwise healthy. The development criteria for these types of compounds would be more rigorous initially and would typically include a full nonclinical development program to support the human studies. Similarly, compounds being developed to control cancer suggest that the patients may have a prolonged life expectation such that long-term toxicity must be fully evaluated before exposing a large patient population to the compound. The emphasis of the current chapter is on the development of compounds for the treatment of late-stage cancer patients.

Human and/or clinical proof of concept strategies will differ depending upon the intent of the product (treatment, prevention, or control). The concepts and strategies described in this chapter can be modified for the development of a drug for the prevention or control of multiple diseases.

The cost estimates and decision stages are specific to the development of a small molecule drug. The development of large molecules will require the evaluation of additional criteria and may be very specific to the nature of the molecule under development.

This plan is written to describe the resources required at each decision stage and does not presume that licensing will occur only at the final decision stage. It is incumbent upon the stakeholders involved to decide the optimal stage at which the technology should move outside their institution.

The plan described here does not assume that the entire infrastructure necessary to generate the data underlying each decision criterion is available at any single institution. The estimates of financial resource requirements are based on an assumption that these services can be purchased from an organization (or funded through a collaborator) with the necessary equipment, instrumentation, and trained personnel to conduct the studies.

It is reasonable to assume that variability in the costs and duration of specific data-generating activities will depend upon the nature of the target and molecule under development.

14.2.2 Definitions

At-risk initiation: The decision by the project team to begin activities that do not directly support the next unmet decision stage, but support a subsequent decision stage. At-risk initiation is sometimes recommended to decrease the overall development time.

Commercialization stage: The stage at which a commercial entity is involved to participate in the development of the drug product. This most commonly occurs through a direct licensing arrangement to continue the development of the product.

Counter-screen: A screen performed in parallel with or after the primary screen. The assay used in the counter-screen is developed to identify compounds that have the potential to interfere with the assay used in the primary screen (the primary assay). Counter-screens can also be used to eliminate compounds that possess undesirable properties, for example, a counter-screen for cytotoxicity.

Cumulative cost: This describes the total expenditure by the project team from project initiation to the stage at which the project is either completed or terminated.

Decision stage #1: The latest moment at which a predetermined course of action is initiated. Project advancement based on decision stages optimizes the use of development resources with the requirement to develop the technology to a commercialization stage as quickly as possible. Failure to meet the criteria listed for the following decision stages will lead to a no go recommendation.

False positive: Generally related to the "specificity" of an assay. In screening, a compound may be active in an assay but inactive toward the biological target of interest. For the purposes of this chapter, this does not include activity due to spurious, non-reproducible activity (such as lint in a sample that causes light-scatter or spurious fluorescence and other detection-related artifacts). Compound interference that is reproducible is a common cause of false positives or target-independent activity.

Go decision: The project conforms to key specifications and criteria and will continue to the next decision stage.

High-throughput screen (HTS): A large-scale automated experiment in which large libraries (collections) of compounds are tested for activity against a biological target or pathway. It can also be referred to as a "screen" for short.

Hits: A term for putative activity observed during the primary high-throughput screen, usually defined by percent activity relative to control compounds.

Chemical lead compound: A member of a biologically and pharmacologically active compound series with desired potency, selectivity, pharmacokinetic, pharmacodynamic, and toxicity properties that can advance to IND-enabling studies for clinical candidate selection.

Incremental cost: A term used to describe the additional cost of activities that support decision criteria for any given decision stage, independent of other activities that may have been completed or initiated to support decision criteria for any other decision stage.

Library: A collection of compounds that meet the criteria for screening against disease targets or pathways of interest.

New chemical entity (NCE): A molecule emerging from the discovery process that has not previously been evaluated in clinical trials.

No go decision: The project does not conform to key specifications and criteria and will not continue.

Off-target activity: Compound activity that is not directed toward the biological target of interest but can give a positive read-out, and thus can be classified as active in the assay.

Orthogonal assay: An assay performed following (or in parallel to) the primary assay to differentiate between compounds that generate false positives from those compounds that are genuinely active against the target.

Primary assay: The assay used for the high-throughput screen.

Qualified task: A task that should be considered, but not necessarily required to be completed at a suggested stage in the project plan. The decision is usually guided by factors outside the scope of this chapter. Such tasks will be denoted in this chapter by enclosing the name of the tasks in parentheses in the Gantt chart, e.g. (qualified task).

Secondary assay: An assay used to test the activity of compounds found active in the primary screen (and orthogonal assay) using robust assays of relevant biology. Ideally, these are of at least medium-throughput to allow the establishment of structure–activity relationships between the primary and secondary assays and establish a biologically plausible mechanism of action.

14.3 New Chemical Entities

In Chapter 4, I listed many novel methods of identifying new chemical entities that apply to both chemical and biological entities. Table 14.1 lists a timeline chart from identification to clinical proof.

14.3.1 Decision Stage #1—Target Identification

Target-based drug discovery begins with identifying the function of a possible therapeutic target and its role in the disease. There are two criteria that justify the advancement of a project beyond target identification. These are:

- Previously published (peer-reviewed) data on a particular disease target pathway or target, OR
- Evidence of new biology that modulates a disease pathway or target of interest.

Resource requirements to support this initial stage of drug discovery can vary widely as the novelty of the target increases. In general, the effort required to elucidate new biology can be significant. Most projects will begin with these data in hand, whether from a new or existing biology. We estimate that an additional investment might be needed to support the target identification data that might already exist (Table 14.2). However, as reflected in Table 14.2, if additional target validation activities proceed at risk, the total cost of the project at a "no go" decision will reach approximately $468,500 (estimated).

14.3.2 Decision Stage #2—Target Validation

Target validation requires a demonstration that a molecular target is directly involved in a disease process and that modulation of the target is likely to have a therapeutic effect. There are seven criteria for evaluation prior to advancement beyond target validation. These are:

- Known molecules modulate the target.
- Type of target has a history of success (e.g., ion channel, GCPR, nuclear receptor, transcription factor, cell cycle, enzyme, etc.).
- Genetic confirmation (e.g., knock-out, siRNA, shRNA, SNP, known mutations, etc.).
- Availability of known animal models.
- Low-throughput target validation assay that represents biology.
- Intellectual property of the target.
- Market potential of the disease/target space.

The advancement criteria supporting target validation can usually be completed in approximately 12 months by performing most activities in parallel. In an effort to reduce the overall development timeline, we recommend starting target validation activities at risk (prior to a "go" decision on target identification). Table 14.2 illustrates the dependencies between the criteria supporting the first two decision stages. The incremental cost of the activities supporting decision-making criteria for target validation is approximately $268,500. However, a decision to initiate target validation prior to completion of target initiation (recommended) and subsequent initiation of identification of actives at risk would lead to a total project cost (estimate) of $941,000 if a "no go" decision was reached at the conclusion of target validation.

TABLE 14.1

Composite Gantt Chart Roll-Up Representing Target ID through Clinical Proof of Concept (POC)

		Year 1				Year 2				Year 3				Year 4				Year 5				Year 6				Year 7				Year 8				Year 9			
Task Name	**Cost**	**Q1**	**Q2**	**Q3**	**Q4**	**Q1**	**Q2**	**Q3**	**Q4**	**Q1**	**Q2**	**Q3**	**Q4**	**Q1**	**Q2**	**Q3**	**Q4**	**Q1**	**Q2**	**Q3**	**Q4**	**Q1**	**Q2**	**Q3**	**Q4**	**Q1**	**Q2**	**Q3**	**Q4**	**Q1**	**Q2**	**Q3**	**Q4**	**Q1**	**Q2**	**Q3**	**Q4**
#1 Target identification	$200,000		$200,000																																		
#2 Target validation	$268,500					$468,500																															
#3 Identification of actives	$472,500							$941,000																													
#4 Confirmation of hits	$522,000										$1,463,000																										
#5 Identification of chemical lead	$353,300													$1,816,300																							
#6 Selection of optimized chemical lead	$302,500															$2,118,800																					
#7 Selection of a development candidate	$275,000																	$2,393,800																			
#8 Pre-IND meeting with FDA	$37,000																	$2,430,800																			
#9 File IND	$780,000																		$3,210,800																		
#10 Human proof of concept	$1,000,000																								$4,210,800												
#11 Clinical proof of concept	$5,000,000																															$9,210,800					

TABLE 14.2
Target Identification and Target Validation

		Year 1				Year 2			
Task Name	**Cost**	**Q1**	**Q2**	**Q3**	**Q4**	**Q1**	**Q2**	**Q3**	**Q4**
#1 Target identification	$200,000		$200,000						
Previously published data on disease target	$1,000								
New biology that modulates a disease	$199,000								
#2 Target validation	$268,500				$468,500				
Known molecules modulate target	$100,000								
Type of target has a history of success	$1,000								
Genetic confirmation	$80,000								
Availability of known animal models	$7,500								
Low throughput target validation assay that represents biology	$70,000								
Intellectual property of the target	$7,500								
Marketability of the target	$2,500								
#3 Identification of actives	$472,500						$941,000		

14.3.3 Decision Stage #3—Identification of Actives

An *active* is defined as a molecule that shows significant biological activity in a validated screening assay that represents the disease's biology and physiology. By satisfying the advancement criteria listed below for the identification of actives, the project team will begin to define the new composition of matter by linking a chemical structure to the modulation of the target. There are five (or six if invention disclosure occurs at this stage) criteria for evaluation at the identification of the actives decision stage. These are:

- Acquisition of screening reagents.
- Primary HTS assay development and validation.
- Compound library available to screen.
- Actives criteria defined.
- Perform high-throughput screen.
- (Composition of matter invention disclosure).

The advancement criteria supporting the identification of actives can be completed in approximately 12 months in most cases by performing activities in parallel. Table 14.3 illustrates the dependencies and timing associated with a decision to begin activities supporting the confirmation of hits prior to a "go" decision on decision stage #3. The incremental cost associated with decision stage #3 is estimated to be $472,500 (assuming the assay is transferred and validated without difficulty). The accumulated project cost associated with a "no go" decision at this stage is estimated to be $1.46 million. This assumes an at-risk initiation of activities supporting decision stage #4.

14.3.4 Decision Stage #4—Confirmation of Hits

A hit is defined as a consistent activity of a molecule (with confirmed purity and identity) in a biochemical and/or cell-based secondary assay. Additionally, this is the stage at which the project team will make an assessment of the molecular class of each of the hits. There are six (or seven if initial invention disclosure occurs at this stage) criteria for evaluation at the confirmation of hits decision stage. These are:

- Confirmation based on repeat assay, concentration response curve (CRC).
- Secondary assays for specificity, selectivity, and mechanisms.

TABLE 14.3

Identification of Actives

Task Name	Cost	Year 1 Q1	Year 1 Q2	Year 1 Q3	Year 1 Q4	Year 2 Q1	Year 2 Q2	Year 2 Q3	Year 2 Q4	Year 3 Q1	Year 3 Q2	Year 3 Q3	Year 3 Q4
#2 Target validation	$268,500				$468,500								
#3 Identification of actives	$472,500						$941,000						
Acquisition of screening reagents	$100,000												
Primary HTS assay development and validation	$150,000												
Compound library available to screen	$150,000												
Actives criteria defined	$2,500												
Perform high-throughput screen	$70,000												
(Composition of matter invention disclosure)	Variable												
#4 Confirmation of hits	$522,000										$1,463,000		

- Confirmed identity and purity.
- Cell-based assay confirmation of biochemical assay when appropriate.
- Druggability of the chemical class (reactivity, stability, solubility, synthetic feasibility).
- Chemical intellectual property (IP).
- (Composition of matter invention disclosure).

The advancement criteria supporting decision stage #4 can usually be completed in approximately 18 months, depending upon the existence of cell-based assays for confirmation. If the assays need to be developed or validated at the screening lab, we recommend starting that activity at risk concurrent with the CRC and mechanistic assays. Table 14.4 represents the dependencies and timing associated with the decision to begin activities supporting the confirmation of hits prior to a "go" decision on decision stage #3. The incremental cost of confirmation of hits is $522,000. The accumulated project cost at a "no go" decision on decision stage #4 can be as high as $1.8 million if a proceed at risk decision is made on identification of a chemical lead (decision stage #5).

14.3.5 Decision Stage #5—Identification of Chemical Lead

A chemical lead is defined as a synthetically feasible, stable, and drug-like molecule active in primary and secondary assays with acceptable specificity and selectivity for the target. This requires a definition of the structure–activity relationship (SAR) as well as determination of synthetic feasibility and preliminary evidence of in vivo efficacy and target engagement (note: projects at this stage might be eligible for Phase I SBIR). Characteristics of a chemical lead are:

- SAR defined.
- Drugability (preliminary toxicity, hERG, Ames).
- Synthetic feasibility.
- Select mechanistic assays.
- In vitro assessment of drug resistance and efflux potential.
- Evidence of in vivo efficacy of chemical class.
- PK/toxicity of chemical class known based on preliminary toxicity or in silico studies.

In order to decrease the number of compounds that fail in the drug development process, a druggability assessment is often conducted. This assessment is important in transforming a compound from a lead molecule into a drug. For a compound to be considered druggable it should have the potential to bind to a specific target; however, also important is the compound's pharmacokinetic profile regarding absorption, distribution, metabolism, and excretion. Other assays will evaluate the potential toxicity of the compound in screens such as the Ames test and cytotoxicity assay. When compounds are being developed for indications where the predicted patient survival is limited to a few years, it is important to note that a positive result in the cytotoxicity assays would not necessarily limit the development of the compound and other druggability factors (such as the pharmacokinetic profile) would be more relevant for determining the potential for development.

The advancement criteria supporting decision stage #5 will most likely be completed in approximately 12–18 months due to the concurrent activities. We recommend that SAR and druggability assessments begin at risk prior to a "go" on confirmation of hits. Synthetic feasibility and PK assessment will begin at the completion of decision stage #4. The cost of performing the recommended activities to support the identification of a chemical lead is estimated to be $353,300 (Table 14.5). The accumulated project costs at the completion of decision stage #5 are estimated to be $2.1 million including costs associated with at-risk initiation of activities to support decision stage #6.

TABLE 14.4

Confirmation of Hits

Task Name	Cost	Year 2 Q1	Year 2 Q2	Year 2 Q3	Year 2 Q4	Year 3 Q1	Year 3 Q2	Year 3 Q3	Year 3 Q4	Year 4 Q1	Year 4 Q2	Year 4 Q3	Year 4 Q4
#3 Identification of actives	$472,500		$941,000										
#4 Confirmation of hits	$522,000					$1,463,000							
Confirmation based on repeat assay, concentration response curve (CRC)	$50,000												
Secondary assays for specificity, selectivity, and mechanisms	$400,000												
Confirmed identity and purity	$10,000												
Cell-based assay confirmation of biochemical assay when appropriate	$50,000												
Druggability of the chemical class (reactivity, stability, solubility, synthetic feasibility)	$2,000												
Chemical intellectual property (IP) (prior art search, med chemist driven)	$10,000												
(Composition of matter invention disclosure)	Variable												
#5 Identification of chemical lead	$353,300									$1,816,300			

TABLE 14.5
Identification of a Chemical Lead

Task Name	Cost	Year 2				Year 3				Year 4			
		Q1	Q2	Q3	Q4	Q1	Q2	Q3	Q4	Q1	Q2	Q3	Q4
#4 Confirmation of hits	$522,000					$1,463,000							
#5 Identification of chemical lead	$353,300								$1,816,300				
SAR defined	$167,900												
Specificity	$20,000												
Selectivity	$40,000												
Druggability	$107,900												
Solubility	$10,000												
Permeability n = 50	$15,000												
Metabolic stability n = 30 (human, murine, rat)	$40,000												
In vitro toxicology n = 5	$25,000												
hERG (QT prolongation) n = 10	$7,500												
Mini Ames (mutagenicity) n = 3	$5,400												
Cytotoxicity assays n = 3	$5,000												
Synthetic feasibility	$6,500												
Number of steps	$2,500												
Occupational health (starting materials and reagents)	$2,500												
Cost	$1,000												
Availability of starting materials and reagents	$500												
Select mechanistic assays n = 10	$25,000												
No relative drug resistance issues n = 10	$6,000												
Evidence of in vivo efficacy of chemical class (PD study)	$10,000												
PK feasibility of chemical class	$10,000												
Provisional application—composition of matter	$20,000												
#6 Selection of optimized chemical lead	$302,500										$2,118,800		

14.3.6 Decision Stage #6—Selection of Optimized Chemical Lead

An optimized chemical lead is a molecule that will enter IND-enabling GLP studies and GMP supplies will be produced for clinical trials. We will describe the activities that support GLP and GMP development in the next section. This section focuses on the decision process to identify those molecules (note: projects at this stage may be eligible for Phase II SBIR). Criteria for selecting optimized candidates are listed below:

- Acceptable in vivo PK and toxicity.
- Feasible formulation.
- In vivo preclinical efficacy (properly powered).
- Dose range finding (DRF) pilot toxicology.
- Process chemistry assessment of scale-up feasibility.
- Regulatory and marketing assessments.

The advancement criteria supporting decision stage #6 can be completed in approximately 12–15 months. As indicated above, we recommend commencing activities to support the selection of an optimized chemical lead prior to a "go" decision on decision stage #5. In particular, the project team should place emphasis on 6.3 (in vivo preclinical efficacy). A strong lead will have clearly defined pharmacodynamic end stages at the preclinical stage and will set the stage for strong indicators of efficacy at decision stage #11 (clinical proof of concept). The cost of performing the recommended activities to support decision stage #6 is estimated to be $302,500 (Table 14.6). The accumulated project costs at the completion of decision stage #6 are estimated to be $2.4 million, including costs associated with at-risk initiation of activities to support decision stage #7.

14.3.7 Decision Stage #7—Selection of a Development Candidate

A development candidate is a molecule for which the intent is to begin Phase I evaluation. Prior to submission of an IND, the project team must evaluate the likelihood of successfully completing the IND-enabling work that will be required as part of the regulatory application for first in human testing. Prior to decision stage #7, many projects will advance as many as 7–10 molecules. Typically, most pharma and biotech companies will select a single development candidate with one designated backup. Here, we recommend that the anointed "development candidate" be the molecule that rates the best on the six criteria below. In many cases, a pre-IND meeting with the regulatory agency might be considered. A failure to address all of these by any molecule should warrant a "no go" decision by the project team. The following criteria should be minimally met for a development candidate:

- Acceptable PK (with a validated bioanalytical method).
- Demonstrated in vivo efficacy/activity.
- Acceptable safety margin (toxicity in rodents or dogs when appropriate).
- Feasibility of GMP manufacture.
- Acceptable drug interaction profile.
- Well-developed clinical endstages.

The advancement criteria supporting decision stage #7 are estimated to be completed in 12 months but may be compressed to as little as six months. The primary rate limit among the decision criteria is the determination of the safety margin, as this can be affected by the formulation and dosing strategies selected earlier. In this case, the authors have presented a project that includes a seven-day repeat dose in rodents to demonstrate an acceptable safety margin. The incremental costs of activities to support the selection of a development candidate (as shown) are estimated to be approximately $275,000. The accumulated project cost at this stage is approximately $2.4 million to complete decision stages #6, #7, and the FDA Pre-IND meeting (Table 14.7). If the development plan requires a longer toxicology study

TABLE 14.6

Selection of an Optimized Chemical Lead

Task Name	Cost	Year 3 Q1	Year 3 Q2	Year 3 Q3	Year 3 Q4	Year 4 Q1	Year 4 Q2	Year 4 Q3	Year 4 Q4	Year 5 Q1	Year 5 Q2	Year 5 Q3	Year 5 Q4
#5 Identification of chemical lead	$353,300				$1,816,300								
#6 Selection of optimized chemical lead	$302,500						$2,118,800						
Acceptable in vivo PK	$32,500												
Route of administration	$10,000												
Bioavailability	$7,500												
Clearance	$7,500												
Drug distribution	$7,500												
Feasible formulation	$15,000												
In vivo preclinical efficacy (properly powered)	$165,000												
Tumor size and volume	$40,000												
Biomarkers	$25,000												
Survival	$30,000												
Target validation	$30,000												
Dose frequency	$40,000												
Dose range finding (DRF) pilot toxicology	$40,000												
Process chemistry assessment of scale up feasibility	$50,000												
Regulatory and marketing assessments	Variable												
#7 Selection of a development candidate	$275,000								$2,393,800				

TABLE 14.7

Selection of a Development Candidate

Task Name	Cost	Year 4				Year 5			
		Q1	Q2	Q3	Q4	Q1	Q2	Q3	Q4
#6 Selection of optimized chemical lead	$302,500		$2,118,800						
#7 Selection of a development candidate	$275,000				$2,393,800				
Acceptable PK (with a validated bioanalytical method)	$30,000								
Well-developed clinical end stages	$40,000								
Demonstrated in vivo efficacy/activity	$50,000								
Acceptable safety margin (toxicity in rodents or dogs when appropriate)	$125,000								
GMP manufacture feasibility	$25,000								
Acceptable drug interaction profile	$5,000								
#8 Pre-IND meeting with FDA (for non-oncology projects only)	$37,000					$2,430,800			

at this stage, costs can be higher (approximately $190,000 for a 14-day repeat dose study in rats and $225,000 in dogs).

14.3.8 Decision Stage #8—Pre-IND Meeting with the FDA

Pre-IND advice from the FDA may be requested for issues related to the data needed to support the rationale for testing a drug in humans; the design of nonclinical pharmacology, toxicology, and drug activity studies, including design and potential uses of any proposed treatment studies in animal models; data requirements for an IND application; initial drug development plans, and regulatory requirements for demonstrating safety and efficacy. We recommend that this meeting take place after the initiation, but before the completion of tasks to support decision stage #7 (selection of a development candidate). The feedback from the FDA might necessitate adjustments to the project plan. Making these changes prior to candidate selection will save time and money.

Pre-IND preparation will require the following:

- Prepare pre-IND meeting request to the FDA, including specific questions.
- Prepare pre-IND meeting package, which includes adequate information for the FDA to address the specific questions (clinical plan, safety assessments summary, CMC plan, etc.).
- Prepare the team for the pre-IND meeting.
- Conduct pre-IND meeting with the FDA.
- Adjust project plan to address the FDA comments.
- Target product profile.

The advancement criteria supporting decision stage #8 should be completed in 12 months. We recommend preparing the pre-IND meeting request approximately three to six months prior to the selection of a development candidate (provided that the data supporting that decision stage are promising). The cost of performing the recommended activities to support pre-IND preparation #8 is estimated to be $37,000.

14.3.9 Decision Stage #9—Preparation and Submission of an IND Application

The decision to submit an IND application presupposes that all of the components of the application have been addressed. The largest expense associated with the preparation of the IND is related to the CMC activities (manufacture and release of GMP clinical supplies). A "go" decision is contingent upon all of the requirements for the IND having been addressed and that the regulatory agency agrees with the clinical plan. (Note: projects at this stage may be eligible for SBIR BRIDGE awards.) The following criteria should be addressed in addition to addressing comments from the pre-IND meeting:

- Well-developed clinical plan.
- Acceptable clinical dosage form.
- Acceptable preclinical drug safety profile.
- Clear IND regulatory path.
- Human proof of concept (HPOC)/clinical proof of concept (CPOC) plan is acceptable to regulatory agency (pre-IND meeting).
- Reevaluate IP positions.

The advancement criteria supporting decision stage #9 are estimated to be completed in 12 months but might be compressed to as little as six months if necessary. We recommend initiating "at-risk" as long as there is confidence that a qualified development candidate is emerging before completion of decision stage #7 and the plan remains largely unaltered after the pre-IND meeting (decision stage #8). The incremental costs of completing decision stage #9 are estimated to be $780,000. The accumulated project cost at this stage will be approximately $3.2 million (Table 14.8).

TABLE 14.8

Submit IND Application

Task Name	Cost	Year 5 Q1	Q2	Q3	Q4
#8 Pre-IND meeting with FDA (for non-oncology projects only)	$37,000	$2,430,800			
#9 File IND	$780,000		$3,210,800		
Acceptable clinical dosage form	$360,000				
Delivery, reconstitution, practicality	$30,000				
Stability (at least one year)	$80,000				
GMP quality	$250,000				
Acceptable preclinical drug safety profile	$350,000				
Safety index (receptor profiling, safety panels)	$30,000				
Dose response (PK)	$20,000				
Safety pharmacology	$300,000				
Clear IND regulatory path	$30,000				
HPOC/CPOC plan is acceptable to regulatory agency	$40,000				

14.3.10 Decision Stage #10—Human Proof of Concept

Most successful Phase I trials in oncology require 12–21 months for completion, due to very restrictive enrollment criteria in these studies in some cases. There is no "at-risk" initiation of Phase I; therefore, the timeline cannot be shortened in that manner. The most important factors in determining the length of a Phase I study are a logically written clinical protocol and an available patient population. A "go" decision clearly rests on the safety of the drug, but many project teams will decide not to proceed if there is not at least some preliminary indication of efficacy during Phase I. Proceeding to Phase II trials will depend on:

- IND clearance.
- Acceptable maximum tolerated dose (MTD).
- Acceptable dose response (DR).
- Evidence of human pharmacology.
- Healthy volunteer relevance.

We estimate the incremental cost of an oncology Phase I study will be approximately $1 million. This can increase significantly if additional patients are required to demonstrate MTD, DR, pharmacology, and/or efficacy. Our estimate is based on a 25-patient (outpatient) study completed in 18 months. The accumulated project cost at completion of decision stage #10 will be approximately $4.2 million (Table 14.9).

14.3.11 Decision Stage #11—Clinical Proof of Concept

With acceptable dose-ranging and maximum tolerable dose having been defined during Phase I, in Phase II the project team will attempt to statistically demonstrate efficacy. More specifically, the outcome of Phase II should reliably predict the likelihood of success in Phase III randomized trials.

- Meeting the IND objectives.
- Acceptable human PK/PD profile.
- Evidence of human pharmacology.
- Safety and tolerance assessments.

TABLE 14.9

Human Proof of Concept

		Year 5				Year 6				Year 7			
Task Name	**Cost**	**Q1**	**Q2**	**Q3**	**Q4**	**Q1**	**Q2**	**Q3**	**Q4**	**Q1**	**Q2**	**Q3**	**Q4**
#9 File IND	$780,000		$3,210,800										
#10 Human proof of concept	$1,000,000							$4,210,800					
IND/CTA clearance	$242,500												
Acceptable maximum tolerated dose (MTD)	$242,500												
Acceptable dose response (DR)	$242,500												
Evidence of human pharmacology	$242,500												
Healthy volunteer relevance	$30,000												

We estimate the incremental cost of an oncology Phase IIa study will be approximately $5.0 million (Table 14.10). This cost is largely dependent on the number of patients required and the number of centers involved. Our estimate is based on 150 outpatients with studies completed in 24 months. The accumulated project cost at the completion of decision stage #11 will be approximately $9.2 million (Table 14.10).

14.4 Repurposing of Marketed Drugs

Drug repurposing and rediscovery development projects frequently seek to employ the 505(b)(2) drug development strategy. This strategy leverages studies conducted and data generated by the innovator firm that is available in the published literature, in product monographs, or product labeling. Improving the quality of drug development plans will reduce the time of 505(b)(2) development cycles, and reduce the time and effort required by the FDA during the NDA review process. Drug repurposing projects seek a new indication in a different patient population and perhaps a different formulated drug product than what is currently described on the product label. By leveraging existing nonclinical data and clinical safety experience, sponsors have the opportunity to design and execute novel, innovative clinical trials to characterize safety and efficacy in a different patient population. A large database of repurposed drugs is available at http://drugrepurposingportal.com/repurposed-drug-database.php.

The decision stages for drug repurposing are summarized in Table 14.11.

14.4.1 Decision Stage #1: Identification of Actives

For drug repurposing, actives are identified as follows (Table 14.12):

- Acquisition of Active Pharmaceutical Ingredients (API) for screening.
- Primary HTS assay development, validation.
- Actives criteria defined.
- Perform HTS.
- (Submit invention disclosure and consider use patent.)

14.4.2 Decision Stage #2: Confirmation of Hits

Hits are confirmed as follows for a drug repurposing project (Table 14.13):

- Confirmation based on repeat assay, CRC.
- Secondary assays for specificity, selectivity, and mechanisms.
- Cell-based assay confirmation of biochemical assay when appropriate.
- (Submit invention disclosure and consider use patent.)

14.4.3 Decision Stage #3: Gap Analysis/Development Plan

When considering the 505(b)(2) NDA approach, it is important to understand what information is available to support the proposed indication and what additional information might be needed. The development path is dependent upon the proposed indication, change in formulation, route, and dosing regimen. The gap analysis/development plan that is prepared will take this information into account in order to determine what studies might be needed prior to submission of an IND and initiating first-in-man studies. A thorough search of the literature is important in order to capture information available to satisfy the data requirements for the IND. Any gaps identified would need to be filled with studies conducted

TABLE 14.10

Decision Stage #11 in Detail

		Year 6				Year 7				Year 8				Year 9			
Task Name	**Cost**	**Q1**	**Q2**	**Q3**	**Q4**	**Q1**	**Q2**	**Q3**	**Q4**	**Q1**	**Q2**	**Q3**	**Q4**	**Q1**	**Q2**	**Q3**	**Q4**
#10 Human proof of concept	$1,000,000			$4,210,800													
#11 Clinical proof of concept (n = 2)	$5,000,000										$9,210,800						
IND/CTA clearance	$500,000																
Acceptable PK/PD profile	$500,000																
Evidence of pharmacology	$2,500,000																
Efficacy	$1,250,000																
Direct and indirect biomarkers	$1,250,000																
Safety and tolerance assessments	$1,500,000																

(Shaded bars: #10 spans Year 6 Q1–Year 7 Q2; #11 and the tasks below span Year 7 Q3–Year 9 Q2.)

TABLE 14.11

Summary of Decision Stages for Drug Repurposing

		Year 1												Year 2											
Decision Stages	**Cost (M)**	**1**	**2**	**3**	**4**	**5**	**6**	**7**	**8**	**9**	**10**	**11**	**12**	**13**	**14**	**15**	**16**	**17**	**17**	**19**	**20**	**21**	**22**	**23**	**24**
#1 Identification of actives	$500,000		$500,000																						
#2 Confirmation of hits	$205,000				$705,000																				
#3 Initial gap analysis/ development plan	$250,000							$955,000																	
#4 Clinical formulation development	$100,000								$1,055,000																
#5 Preclinical safety data package	$800,000											$1,855,000													
#6 Clinical supplies manufacture	$500,000												$2,355,000												
#7 IND preparation and submission	$500,000														$2,855,000										
#8 Human proof of concept	$1,000,000																			$3,855,000					

TABLE 14.12
Identification of Actives

Decision Stage	Cost	Year 1											
		M1	M2	M3	M4	M5	M6	M7	M8	M9	M10	M11	M12
#1 Identification of actives	$500,000		$500,000										
Acquisition of active pharmaceutical ingredients (API) for screening	Variable												
Primary HTS assay development, validation	Variable												
Actives criteria defined	Variable												
Perform high-throughput screen	Variable												
(Submit invention disclosure and consider use patent)	Variable												
#2 Confirmation of hits	$205,000				$705,000								

TABLE 14.13

Confirmation of Hits

Decision Stage	Cost	Year 1											
		M1	M2	M3	M4	M5	M6	M7	M8	M9	M10	M11	M12
#1 Identification of actives	$500,000		$500,000										
#2 Confirmation of hits	$205,000				$705,000								
Confirmation based on repeat assay, concentration response curve (CRC)	Variable												
Secondary assays for specificity, selectivity, and mechanisms	Variable												
Cell-based assay confirmation of biochemical assay when appropriate	Variable												
(Submit invention disclosure and consider use patent)	Variable												
#3 Initial gap analysis/development plan	$250,000							$955,000					

by the sponsor. A pre-IND meeting with the FDA will allow the sponsor to present their plan to the FDA and gain acceptance prior to submission of the IND and conducting the first-in-man study (Table 14.14).

- CMC program strategy.
- Preclinical program strategy.
- Clinical proof of concept strategy.
- Draft clinical protocol design.
- Pre-IND meeting with the FDA.
- Commercialization/marketing strategy and target product profile.

14.4.4 Decision Stage #4: Clinical Formulation Development

The clinical formulation development will include the following (Table 14.15):

- Prototype development.
- Analytical methods development.
- Prototype stability.
- Prototype selection.
- Clinical supplies release specification.
- (Submit invention disclosure on novel formulation.)

14.4.5 Decision Stage #5: Preclinical Safety Data Package

Preparation of the gap analysis/development plan will identify any additional studies that might be needed to support the development of the compound for the new indication. Based on this assessment, as well as the intended patient population, the types of studies that will be needed to support the clinical program will be determined. It is possible that a pharmacokinetic study evaluating exposure would be an appropriate bridge to the available data in the literature (Table 14.16).

- Preclinical oral formulation development.
- Bioanalytical method development.
- Qualify GLP test article.
- Transfer plasma assay to GLP laboratory.
- ICH S7a (safety pharmacology) and S7b (cardiac tox) core battery of tests.
- Toxicology bridging study.
- PK/PD/tox studies if formulation and route of administration are different.

14.4.6 Decision Stage #6: Clinical Supplies Manufacture

Clinical supplies will need to be manufactured. The list below provides some of the considerations that need to be made for manufacturing clinical supplies (Table 14.17):

- Select cGMP supplier and transfer manufacturing process.
- Cleaning validation development.
- Scale-up lead formulation at GMP facility.
- Clinical label design.
- Manufacture clinical supplies.

TABLE 14.14

Gap Analysis/Development Plan

		Year 1											
Decision Stage	**Cost**	**M1**	**M2**	**M3**	**M4**	**M5**	**M6**	**M7**	**M8**	**M9**	**M10**	**M11**	**M12**
#2 Confirmation of hits	$205,000				$705,000								
#3 Initial gap analysis/development plan	$250,000							$955,000					
CMC program strategy	Variable												
Preclinical program strategy	Variable												
Clinical proof of concept strategy	Variable												
Draft clinical protocol design	Variable												
Pre-IND meeting with FDA	Variable												
Commercialization/marketing strategy and target product profile	Variable												
#4 Clinical formulation development	$100,000								$1,055,000				

TABLE 14.15

Clinical Formulation Development

Decision Stage	Cost	Year 1											
		M1	M2	M3	M4	M5	M6	M7	M8	M9	M10	M11	M12
#3 Final development plan	$250,000							$955,000					
#4 Clinical formulation development	$100,000								$1,055,000				
Prototype development	Variable												
Analytical methods development	Variable												
Prototype stability	Variable												
Prototype selection	Variable												
Clinical supplies release specification	Variable												
(Submit invention disclosure on novel formulation)	Variable												
#5 Preclinical safety data package	$800,000										$1,855,000		

TABLE 14.16

Preclinical Safety Data Package

Decision Stage	Cost	Year 1												Year 2											
		M1	M2	M3	M4	M5	M6	M7	M8	M9	M10	M11	M12	M13	M14	M15	M16	M17	M18	M19	M20	M21	M22	M23	M24
#4 Clinical formulation development	$100,000								$1,055,000																
#5 Preclinical safety data package	$800,000											$1,855,000													
Preclinical oral formulation development	Variable																								
Bioanalytical method development	Variable																								
Qualify GLP test article	Variable																								
Transfer plasma assay to GLP laboratory	Variable																								
ICH S7a (Safety Pharmacology) and S7b (Cardiac Tox) core battery of tests	Variable																								
Toxicology bridging study	Variable																								
PK/PD/Tox studies if formulation and route of administration is different	Variable																								
#6 Clinical supplies manufacture	$500,000												$2,355,000												

TABLE 14.17

Clinical Supplies Manufacture

Decision Stage	Cost	Year 1												Year 2											
		M1	M2	M3	M4	M5	M6	M7	M8	M9	M10	M11	M12	M13	M14	M15	M16	M17	M18	M19	M20	M21	M22	M23	M24
#5 Preclinical safety data package	$800,000										$1,855,000														
#6 Clinical supplies manufacture	$500,000												$2,355,000												
Select cGMP supplier and transfer manufacturing process	Variable																								
Cleaning validation development	Variable																								
Scale-up lead formulation at GMP facility	Variable																								
Clinical label design	Variable																								
Manufacture clinical supplies	Variable																								

14.4.7 Decision Stage #7: IND Preparation and Submission

Following the pre-IND meeting with the FDA, and conducting any additional studies, the IND is prepared in a common technical document format to support the clinical protocol. The IND is prepared in five separate modules that include administrative information, summaries (CMC, nonclinical, clinical), quality data (CMC), nonclinical study reports and literature, and clinical study reports and literature (Table 14.18). Following submission of the IND to the FDA, there is a 30-day review period during which the FDA may ask for additional data or clarity on the information submitted. If after 30 days the FDA has communicated that there is no objection to the proposed clinical study, the IND is considered active and the clinical study can commence.

- Investigator's brochure preparation.
- Protocol preparation and submission to IRB.
- IND preparation and submission.

14.4.8 Decision Stage #8: Human Proof of Concept

Human proof of concept may commence following successful submission of an IND (i.e., an IND that has not been placed on "clinical hold"). The list below provides some information concerning human proof of concept (Table 14.19):

- IND clearance.
- Acceptable MTD.
- Acceptable DR.
- Evidence of human pharmacology.

14.5 Drug Delivery Platform Technology

Historically about 40% of NCEs identified as possessing promise for development, based on drug-like qualities, progress to evaluation in humans. Of those that do make it into clinical trials, about nine out of ten fail. In many cases, innovative drug delivery technology can provide a "second chance" for promising compounds that have consumed precious drug-discovery resources, but were abandoned in early clinical trials due to unfavorable side-effect profiles. For long, the pharmaceutical industry is sitting on a lot of inventions that should be brought to public soon. As one analyst observed, "pharmaceutical companies are sitting on abandoned goldmines that should be reopened and excavated again using the previously underutilized or unavailable picks and shovels developed by the drug delivery industry" (SW Warburg Dillon Read). Although this statement was made more than ten years ago, it continues to apply.

Beyond enablement of new drugs, innovative approaches to drug delivery also hold potential to enhance marketed drugs (e.g., through improvement in convenience, tolerability, safety, and/or efficacy); expand their use (e.g., through broader labeling in the same therapeutic area and/or increased patient acceptance/compliance); or transform them by enabling their suitability for use in other therapeutic areas. These opportunities contribute enormously to the potential for value creation in the drug delivery field. Table 14.20 summarizes the decision stages for the development of drug delivery platform technology.

14.5.1 Decision Stage #1: Clinical Formulation Development

- Prototype development.
- Analytical methods development.
- Prototype stability.
- Prototype selection.
- Clinical supplies release specification.
- (Submit invention disclosure on novel formulation.)

TABLE 14.18

IND Preparation and Submission

		Year 1												Year 2											
Decision Stage	**Cost**	**M1**	**M2**	**M3**	**M4**	**M5**	**M6**	**M7**	**M8**	**M9**	**M10**	**M11**	**M12**	**M13**	**M14**	**M15**	**M16**	**M17**	**M18**	**M19**	**M20**	**M21**	**M22**	**M23**	**M24**
#6 Clinical supplies manufacture	$500,000												$2,355,000												
#7 IND preparation and submission	$500,000														$2,855,000										
Investigator's brochure preparation	Variable																								
Protocol preparation and submission to IRB	Variable																								
IND preparation and submission	Variable																								

TABLE 14.19

Human Proof of Concept

Decision Stage	Cost	Year 2											
		M13	M14	M15	M16	M17	M18	M19	M20	M21	M22	M23	M24
#7 IND preparation and submission	$500,000		$2,855,000										
#8 Human proof of concept	$1,000,000							$3,855,000					
IND clearance	Variable												
Acceptable maximum tolerated dose (MTD)	Variable												
Acceptable dose response (DR)	Variable												
Evidence of human pharmacology	Variable												

TABLE 14.20

Summary of Decision Stages for Drug Delivery Platform Technology

		Year 1				Year 2				Year 3				Year 4				Year 5				Year 6			
Decision Stage	**Cost**	**Q1**	**Q2**	**Q3**	**Q4**	**Q1**	**Q2**	**Q3**	**Q4**	**Q1**	**Q2**	**Q3**	**Q4**	**Q1**	**Q2**	**Q3**	**Q4**	**Q1**	**Q2**	**Q3**	**Q4**	**Q1**	**Q2**	**Q3**	**Q4**
#1 Clinical formulation development	$250,000	$250,000																							
#2 Development plan	$300,000			$550,000																					
#3 Clinical supplies manufacture	$500,000				$1,050,000																				
#4 Preclinical safety data package	$800,000						$1,850,000																		
#5 IND preparation and submission	$500,000										$2,350,000														
#6 Human proof of concept	$1,000,000										$3,350,000														
#7 Clinical proof of concept	$2,500,000															$5,850,000									

See Table 14.21 for a schematic representation of the time and costs associated with development at this stage.

14.5.2 Decision Stage #2: Development Plan

Preparation of a development plan allows the sponsor to evaluate the available information regarding the compound of interest (whether at the development stage or a previously marketed compound) to understand what information might be available to support the proposed indication and what additional information may be needed. The development path is dependent upon the proposed indication, change in formulation, route, and dosing regimen. The development plan that is prepared will take this information into account in order to determine what information or additional studies might be needed prior to submission of an IND and initiating first-in-man studies. A thorough search of the literature is important in order to capture available information to satisfy the data requirements for the IND. Any gaps identified would need to be filled with studies conducted by the sponsor. A pre-IND meeting with the FDA will allow the sponsor to present their plan to the FDA and gain acceptance (de-risk the program) prior to submission of the IND and conducting the first-in-man study (Table 14.22).

- CMC program strategy.
- Preclinical program strategy.
- Clinical proof of concept strategy.
- Draft clinical protocol design.
- Pre-IND meeting with the FDA.

14.5.3 Decision Stage #3: Clinical Supplies Manufacture

- Select cGMP supplier and transfer manufacturing process.
- Cleaning validation development.
- Scale up lead formulation at GMP facility.
- Clinical label design.
- Manufacture clinical supplies.

See Table 14.23 for a schematic representation of the time and costs associated with development at this stage.

14.5.4 Decision Stage #4: Preclinical Safety Package

Preparation of the gap analysis/development plan will identify any additional studies that might be needed to support the development of the new delivery platform for the compound. Based on this assessment, as well as the intended patient population, the types of studies that will be needed to support the clinical program will be determined. It is possible that a pharmacokinetic study evaluating exposure would be an appropriate bridge to the available data in the literature (Table 14.24).

- Preclinical oral formulation development.
- Bioanalytical method development.
- Qualify GLP test article.
- Transfer drug exposure/bioavailability assays to GLP laboratory.
- ICH S7a (safety pharmacology) and S7b (cardiac tox) core battery of tests.
- Toxicology bridging study.

TABLE 14.21
Clinical Formulation Development

Decision Stage	Cost	Year 1 Q1	Year 1 Q2	Year 1 Q3	Year 1 Q4
#1 Clinical formulation development	$250,000		$250,000		
Prototype development	Variable				
Analytical methods development	Variable				
Prototype stability	Variable				
Prototype selection	Variable				
Clinical supplies release specification	Variable				
(Submit invention disclosure on novel formulation)	Variable				
#2 Development plan	$300,000				$550,000

TABLE 14.22
Development Plan

Decision Stage	Cost	Year 1 Q1	Year 1 Q2	Year 1 Q3	Year 1 Q4	Year 2 Q1	Year 2 Q2	Year 2 Q3	Year 2 Q4
#1 Clinical formulation development	$250,000		$250,000						
#2 Development plan	$300,000			$550,000					
CMC program strategy	Variable								
Preclinical program strategy	Variable								
Clinical proof of concept strategy	Variable								
Draft clinical protocol design	Variable								
Pre-IND meeting with FDA	Variable								
#3 Clinical supplies manufacture	$500,000					$1,050,000			

14.5.5 Decision Stage #5: IND Preparation and Submission

Following the pre-IND meeting with the FDA and conducting any additional studies, the IND is prepared in a common technical document format to support the clinical protocol. The IND is prepared in five separate modules, which include administrative information, summaries (CMC, nonclinical, clinical), quality data (CMC), nonclinical study reports and literature, and clinical study reports and literature. Following submission of the IND to the FDA, there is a 30-day review period during which the FDA might ask for additional data or clarity on the information submitted. If after 30 days the FDA has communicated that there is no objection to the proposed clinical study, the IND is considered active and the clinical study can commence (Table 14.25).

- Investigator's brochure preparation.
- Protocol preparation and submission to IRB.
- IND preparation and submission.

14.5.6 Decision Stage #6: Human Proof of Concept

Human proof of concept may commence following successful submission of an IND (i.e., an IND that has not been placed on "clinical hold"). The list below provides some information concerning human proof of concept (Table 14.26):

- IND clearance.
- Acceptable MTD.
- Acceptable DR.
- Evidence of human pharmacology.

TABLE 14.23

Clinical Supplies Manufacture

		Year 1				Year 2				Year 3			
Decision Stage	**Cost**	**Q1**	**Q2**	**Q3**	**Q4**	**Q1**	**Q2**	**Q3**	**Q4**	**Q1**	**Q2**	**Q3**	**Q4**
#2 Development plan	$300,000				$550,000								
#3 Clinical supplies manufacture	$500,000					$1,050,000							
Select cGMP supplier and transfer manufacturing process	Variable												
Cleaning validation development	Variable												
Scale up lead formulation at GMP facility	Variable												
Clinical label design	Variable												
Manufacture clinical supplies	Variable												
#4 Preclinical safety data package	$800,000								$1,850,000				

TABLE 14.24

Preclinical Safety Package

Decision Stage	Cost	Year 1				Year 2				Year 3			
		Q1	Q2	Q3	Q4	Q1	Q2	Q3	Q4	Q1	Q2	Q3	Q4
#3 Clinical supplies manufacture	$500,000					$1,050,000							
#4 Preclinical safety data package	$800,000							$1,850,000					
Preclinical oral formulation development	Variable												
Bioanalytical method development	Variable												
Qualify GLP test article	Variable												
Transfer drug exposure/bioavailability assays to GLP laboratory	Variable												
ICH S7a (Safety Pharmacology) and S7b (Cardiac Tox) core battery of tests	Variable												
Toxicology bridging study	Variable												
#5 IND preparation and submission	$500,000										$2,350,000		

TABLE 14.25
IND Preparation and Submission

		Year 2				Year 3			
Decision Stage	**Cost**	**Q1**	**Q2**	**Q3**	**Q4**	**Q1**	**Q2**	**Q3**	**Q4**
#4 Preclinical safety data package	$800,000			$1,850,000					
#5 IND preparation and submission	$500,000						$2,350,000		
Investigator's brochure preparation	Variable								
Protocol preparation and submission to IRB	Variable								
IND preparation and submission	Variable								

TABLE 14.26
Human Proof of Concept

		Year 3				Year 4			
Decision Stage	**Cost**	**Q1**	**Q2**	**Q3**	**Q4**	**Q1**	**Q2**	**Q3**	**Q4**
#5 IND preparation and submission	$500,000		$2,350,000						
#6 Human proof of concept	$1,000,000				$3,350,000				
IND clearance	Variable								
Acceptable maximum tolerated dose (MTD)	Variable								
Acceptable dose response (DR)	Variable								
Evidence of human pharmacology	Variable								

14.5.7 Decision Stage #7: Clinical Proof of Concept

With acceptable DR and MTD having been defined during Phase I, in Phase II the project team will attempt to statistically demonstrate efficacy. More specifically, the outcome of Phase II should reliably predict the likelihood of success in Phase III randomized trials (Table 14.27).

- IND clearance.
- Acceptable PK/PD profile.
- Efficacy.
- Direct and indirect biomarkers.
- Safety and tolerance assessments.

14.6 Biological Products

The optimal scale-up and the choice of the scale are influenced by several factors in an integrated model. Given in Table 14.28 is a cost estimation model.

The manufacturing process (facility depreciation, raw material costs, quality control, and quality assurance) must match the expected results. As a rule of thumb, the manufacturing expenses should not exceed 15% of the price per dose (vial). Some of the factors influencing the process economy are workforce, chromatographic media, filters and membranes, buffers, other raw materials, number and type of in-process control analyses, and the overall yield. Additional cost comes from complying with environmental requirements. Where organic solvents are used, their disposal is further costly. Waste disposal, particularly the requirement that all material in contact with the genetically modified cells must be properly sterilized and disposed of, adds considerable overheads to the overall production costs.

Economy considerations start with the choice of the expression system, culture conditions, and demand for process robustness; hence this is part of the "design in" strategy recommended. Since a cGMP facility is expensive, outsourcing is highly recommended for new entrants to the biological medicine field. This advice is not merely a cost-saving measure but also offers only logistic solutions. For example, where a

TABLE 14.27

Clinical Proof of Concept

Decision Stage	Cost	Year 3				Year 4				Year 5				Year 6			
		Q1	Q2	Q3	Q4	Q1	Q2	Q3	Q4	Q1	Q2	Q3	Q4	Q1	Q2	Q3	Q4
#6 Human proof of concept	$1,000,000				$3,350,000												
#7 Clinical proof of concept	$2,500,000										$5,850,000						
IND clearance	Variable																
Acceptable PK/PD profile	Variable																
Efficacy	Variable																
Direct and indirect biomarkers	Variable																
Safety and tolerance assessments	Variable																

TABLE 14.28

Input Figures for Cost Calculations

Category	Issue	Index	Comments
General	Expression level	A1	Amount in g/L expressed
	# of batches	A2	
	Process yield	A3	% of purified protein (drug product)
	Dose	A4	mg/dose
	Pack size	A5	mg/vial
	Vials needed	A6	# of vials/dose
Upstream	Facility	B1	Yearly cost ($) of using an upstream component of cGMP facility (including maintenance and workforce)
	Utilization	B2	# months the upstream component is used for the given project
	Culture volume	B3	Volume in liters in a given batch
	Media cost	B4	Price in $/L of culture media
	Utensils	B5	Price in $ for utensils used (e.g., filters, bags, etc.)
Downstream	Facility	C1	Yearly cost ($) for using a downstream component of the cGMP facility (including maintenance and workforce)
	Utilization	C2	# months, the downstream component is used for a given project
	Chromatography steps	C3	Number of chromatography steps
	Binding capacity	C4	Average binding capacity in mg/mL
	Media cost	C5	Chromatography media cost in $/L
	Buffer volume	C7	Total consumption in L (on average 15 column volumes are used/step)
	Buffer cost	C8	$/L
	Utensils	C9	Cost in $ for components used (filters, membranes, bags, etc.)
	Raw materials	C10	Cost in $ for expensive reagents, enzymes, etc.
	Formulation	C11	The cost is $ for the formulation of the drug substance
Fill and Pack	Number of vials	D1	Vials/batch
	Price	D2	Price/vial
	Shipping cost	D3	—?
In-process control	# of analyses	E1	Total number per batch
	Cost of analysis	E2	Average in $/IPC analysis
DS quality control	# of analyses	F1	The total number of drugs substance quality analysis per batch
	Cost	F2	$/analysis
DP Quality control	# of analyses	G1	Total number per batch of the drug product
	Cost	G2	$/analysis
QA release	Cost	H1	$/batch

transgenic animal is involved, few pharmaceutical manufacturers know how to handle animals' farming and comply with good cattle-raising practices. Upstream, downstream, and quality control costs are closely interrelated by variations in-process design and batch sizes versus in-process control and analytical control programs. A robust process will allow for large batches, reduce the workforce's demand, and the number of samples to be analyzed.

The costs of producing a batch of recombinant derived product can be calculated from Table 14.28. It is recommended to use an excel spreadsheet for cost calculations, including specific costs not mentioned in the table.

The cost contributions at various steps are given below. Opportunities should be recognized where costs can be cut, particularly in deciding the magnitude of scale-up. Each step's relative contribution should be the first criterion of selection on which step to be reworked to reduce costs. The relative costs should be considered in terms of long-term impact. For example, a 1% recurring cost can add substantial savings if reduced.

$$\text{Upstream cost} = (\text{B1} \times \text{B2}) / 12 + \text{B3} \times \text{B4} + \text{B5}$$

$$\text{Downstream} = (\text{C1} \times \text{C2}) / 12 = (\text{B3} \times \text{A1} \times \text{C5} \times \text{C3}) / (\text{C4} \times \text{C6} \times 1{,}000) + (\text{C7} \times \text{C8}) + \text{C9} + \text{C10}\,\text{C11}$$

$$\text{Fill and pack} = \text{D1} \times \text{D2} + \text{D3}$$

$$\text{Total cost / batch} = \text{Upstream} + \text{Downstream} + \text{Fill and pack} + \text{E1} \times \text{E2} + \text{F1} \times \text{F2} + \text{G1} \times \text{G2} + \text{H1}$$

$$\text{Yield / batch} = (\text{B3} \times \text{A1} \times \text{A3}) / 100{,}000$$

$$\text{Cost / G} = \text{Total cost / yield(per batch)}$$

$$\text{Cost per vial} = \text{Cost per batch / D1}$$

$$\text{Cost per dose} = (\text{Cost per batch / D1}) \times \text{A6}$$

Based on this model, we can study what components of the entire process can be altered to achieve the best possible production costs.

14.6.1 Batch

- A batch is defined as the cell culture volume processed downstream as a combined amount of material resulting in the drug substance. In continuous cell cultures or transgenic animal technology, the harvest or milk may be pooled in sub-fractions, making it more difficult to define the batch. The batch scheme must provide information about the flow, the harvest procedures, pools, analytical in-process control programs, and intermediary compounds. Also included here are details if several columns are used or where parallel processing or splitting of processing is envisioned. The fact that inclusion bodies can be combined from several fermentation batches and then processed together requires clear identification of starting sub-batches.
- Yield is the composite of each purification step's output. A downstream process comprising such as ten-unit operations with an average recovery of 95% will result in an overall yield of 57%, which is acceptable. However, an average recovery of 80% will result in a total yield of 11%, which is not acceptable in most circumstances. In several cases, more than ten-unit operations are needed to guarantee a safe product making it fair to conclude that one should aim for more than 95% recovery in most if not all unit operations. Some of the most recent trends to alter the molecular structure, e.g., pegylation, have lower yields. Because of the mathematical nature of proportional reduction, small changes in step yields result in dramatic changes; a step yield of 95% where 15 steps are involved gives 46% total yield; the same 15 steps in 75% step yield would give only 1% of the total yield. In most instances, five to ten steps are minimally involved. Therefore, the total yield ranges from 60% to 6% in a 95% to 75% step yield transition.
- Batch size is decided on a variety of considerations; all of them have economic optimization. Large batches require automated facilities but result in a relatively small number of samples to analyze. The cost is inversely proportional to the quantity produced, ranging from about $50/g for insulin, about $15–200/g for monoclonal antibodies, and $1,000+/g for some cytokines. It may be worthwhile for expensive products not to look at production cost optimization as timely entry may be more relevant. Amount needed. A 1,000 L bioreactor with an expression level of 1 g/L produces 1 kg of target protein per reactor volume. A batch or fed-batch culture typically runs for seven days, offering productivity of 100 g/day. A 1,000 L perfusion bioreactor with a 2× flow per 24 hours and an expression level of 1 g/L produces 200 g/day. A transgenic cow expressing 20 g/L milk produces 400 g/day, assuming a volume of 20 L milk per day. In terms of output, the transgenic cow is a far more efficient expression system than the cell culture-based systems and probably less risky. Animal-based expression systems should, therefore, seriously be considered for large-scale operations.

- Batch variations document specifies variability and lack of reproducibility; this may be due to scale-up procedure due to the formation of concentration gradients in large reactors or containers. The risk of batch failure is mainly due to infections; large-scale mammalian cell cultures, having long cell expansion times, including several bioreactors and running over long-time intervals, are associated with higher risk factors than other expression systems. Due to the high cell culture media cost, the economic loss can be substantial.
- Buffer preparation at a large scale requires automation and robotics management, creating an entirely different set of validation requirements and tools, including computer validation (see Section 211.68 [a, b] of FDA CGMP to validate automated systems, mechanized racks, and computers).

14.6.2 Upstream

- Cell cultures offer most opportunities and most problems in scale-up. For example, large-scale animal cell cultures are fundamentally different from conventional microbial fermentation due to mammalian cells' fragility. The cells are easily damaged by mechanical stress making it impossible to use high aeration and agitation; this includes using the newly introduced Wave bioreactors. Fortunately, animal cells grow slowly and at fewer cell densities and do not require the high oxygen inputs typical of microbial cultures. Cell culture scale-up often results in changes in the cell culture supernatant composition, affecting the downstream process. However, except for reactor volume, other parameters like culture medium, pH, temperature, redox potential, osmolality, agitation rate, flow rate, ammonia, glucose, glutamine, lactate concentrations, pCO2, and pO2 remain constant within the prescribed interval limits.
- Expression system selection and eventually, cell line occurs early in the process and is the most important decision. The choice depends on the nature of the target protein (glycosylation, phosphorylation, acylation, size, etc.), expected expression levels, expression system development time, risk of batch failure, safety considerations, the amount needed, and regulatory record
- The expression level varies with the host organism used and the nature of the target protein. Typical expression levels vary widely. In most hosts, these range at less than 1 g/L; *E. coli* generally gives a better yield of 1–4 g/L while mammalian cells when used for antibodies generally produce much higher levels; transgenic animals provide the highest yield of 5–40 g/L; the yield in transgenic plants is uncertain and not widely available for evaluation. The nature and quality of the expressed protein influence the purification yield. Although expression levels of *E. coli* usually are high, expression of the N-terminal extended target protein and the need for in vitro refolding significantly influence the overall process yield. Further, stressed cells tend to express less stable protein resulting in great losses during purification or production of drug substance/product with a shortened lifetime.
- Expression system development time varies widely between various expression systems. However, for most hosts, four to six months are required to develop the system. Once developed, the time to target protein expression depends on the bioreactor system deployed but generally ranges from a few days, e.g., five days for *E. Coli* and other bacteria, two weeks for yeast, four weeks for inset cells, and 2–16 weeks for mammalian cells. The longer development time for transgenic goats and cows (18–24 months) is partly compensated for by the relatively high expression levels and the fast access to target protein once the system has been developed.
- Raw materials vary in price between culture media used for microbial, insect, mammalian cell cultures and commercial-scale fermenter media, the former being the most expensive per liter. Unfortunately, mammalian cell cultures usually offer relatively low expression levels compared to microbial systems, making cultural media a major cost contributor. In an expression system yielding 1,000 g/L with a 40% yield, the contribution of the media cost is about $25/g of protein; when the expression level drops to 10 g/L, the media's cost contribution rises to $2,500/g of protein. Low mammalian cell expression levels adversely affect the process economy.

- Harvesting can be programmed to store inclusion bodies for a longer time (such as two years), and most large-scale operations should validate this storage step.
- Holding times can be long and add cost in commercial production; these are often not considered in developing processes; it is advisable that realistic times should be validated in the initial phases. This aspect is related more to logistics than to science. It takes much longer to empty a 4,000 L tank than to dump a 2 L flask. Often the practical considerations of shift-change (if the process requires more than eight hours) are necessary to design the process. The holding times must be validated.
- Process economy determines the scale-up factor adopted as there is always a certain maximum capacity to which a process can be scaled with economic advantage. A good example of this comes in the manufacturing of insulin, which is produced in quantities of tons rather than grams. If a scale-up process moves from a 100 L fermenter to a 30,000 L liter, the cost is not necessarily proportional due to CAPEX depreciation that may render the scaling less feasible. This comment is contrary to the popular belief that higher volumes sizes of bioreactors are more cost-effective. Also, when outsourcing, it is always a good idea to adjust the process to available bioreactor size as not all CMOs carry all sizes of bioreactors. When processing bacterial cultures, it may be worthwhile to take advantage of pooling inclusion bodies when only smaller size fermenters are available. However, as the batch size decreases, analytical assays' costs increase, so batch size and analytical programs should be carefully balanced.
- Precipitation step scale-up involves only change in the amount of sample and the volume as all volume other parameters like sample pH, conductivity, temperature, concentration, redox potential, holding time, reagent concentration, and precipitation time remain constant within interval limits. The procedure of precipitation also remains identical.

14.6.3 Downstream

- The recombinant technology is associated with several safety issues related to the expression system used, cell banking, fermentation and cell cultures, raw materials used, downstream processing, and unintended introduction of adventitious agents (bacteria, viruses, mycoplasma, prions). The process design should assure the removal of any adventitious agents and other harmful impurities. A rule of thumb says that at least three different chromatographic principles should be used in a biological medicine downstream process. If insect cells, mammalian cells, or transgenic animals have been used, a virus inactivation step and an active virus filtration step should be considered. The adventitious agents and their relation to the expression system used are simply understood as endotoxins, nucleic acids, bioburden, viruses, and prions be an issue in all systems of expression except that viruses and prions are not an issue in microbial systems; prions are also not an issue in other systems except in transgenic animals. The use of raw materials should be carefully investigated. Only raw materials suited for biological medicine processing should be accepted, based on solid documentation on safety and quality
- Column life, when prolonged reduces cost significantly; almost 70% of total production cost goes into downstream processing, mainly in the cost of chromatographic media. Measure taken to prolong column life including longer usage, recharging, etc., must be properly validated and documents. Even though the chromatographic media costs are high, it is wise to select media from other criteria than the price per liter. Service, trouble shooting, linking media, column, and equipment to the same supplier, and regulatory support files may be far more important. The number of failed batches can be reduced by such actions. The major factors influencing chromatographic unit operations' economy are media cost, binding capacity, recovery, column lifetime, linear, flow, and shelf life.
- Chromatography scale-up produces more problems than any other operation in the process. Larger equipment may cause extra-column zone broadening due to different lengths and diameters of outlet pipes, valves, monitor cells, etc. An increase in column diameter may result in a decreased flow rate due to reduced supportive wall force (at constant pressure drop). For

example, a decrease in the flow is observed for a column packed with Sepharose 6 FF when the diameter is increased from 2.6 to 10 cm. The prolonged sample holding times on column may result in precipitation of material resulting in the clotting of pipes, valves, or chromatographic columns. Parameters that are changed proportionally (linear scale-up include sample volume, sample load, column diameter, column area and column volume, flow rate; residence time remains constant (an alternate method would keep residence time constant allow for variations in both column area and height. Parameters that remain constant within the interval limits include sample pH, conductivity, temperature, concentration, redox potential, holding time, bed height, residence time, linear flow rate, binding capacity, back pressure, buffers, equilibration procedure, wash procedure, elution procedure, CIP procedure remain unchanged. Gradients should not be changed linearly but stepwise.

- Filtration step scale-up does not change the limits of the interval or pH, redox potential, temperature, concentration, conductivity, holding time, membrane type, transmembrane pressure, retentate pressure, feed pressure, crossflow velocity, filtrate velocity, wall flux, and the CIP procedures. Parameters that are increased linearly include sample volume and membrane area.

14.6.4 Facility

- Facility costs can be very high with specialized area requirements, specialized workforce required, environment controls and waste disposal needs, etc. A prospective biological medicine marketer would be wise to investigate outsourcing manufacturing, especially if several products are involved that may require separate processing suites. One of the control areas that are often not given full budgeting is monitoring the environment; a 5,000 sq ft facility may cost upwards of $2 million per year only to comply with the monitoring standards. As the regulatory environment is still evolving, the area requirements are likely to change, which may cost substantial redesigning, which is another reason to outsource manufacturing until the market is firmly established. The price per gram of drug substance is significantly reduced by linking process design, scale-up factor, and batch logistics to the facility design, thereby reducing the occupancy time. This requires several set-up levels, one for transfer of technology to pilot scale, from pilot scale to first-stage manufacturing, and from first-stage manufacturing to full-scale manufacturing.
- Cleaning, sanitization, and storage of columns, equipment, and utensils are an integrated part of the manufacturing program. Whereas liberties are routinely taken in small-scale production, these issues can add substantial costs in a poorly designed process and facility and raise contamination risks that may not be acceptable by the regulatory authorities.
- Labor-intensive processes are expensive, and costs may be reduced by reducing unit operations and automation. Each unit operation adds to cost and reduces yield. However, there is a limit to how the number of process steps due to the requirement for effective impurity removal and virus inactivation if insect cells, mammalian cells, or transgenic animals have been used for protein expression. There is an extensive effort to automate systems as generic companies that have reasons to adopt more cost-effective systems enter the market. From robotics to continuous processing systems to wave bioreactors are all efforts to reduce human resource costs. A prospective manufacturer must look at all available and soon-to-be-available alternates in designing the process. However, the US FDA requirements for validating automated processes and computer systems should be implemented as early as possible.
- Environmental issues relate to the disposal of large waste; for example, the use of ammonium sulfate will severely affect the environment in large-scale operations.
- Microbiological quality of the environment during various processing is very important, particularly as the process continues downstream; more intensive control and monitoring are recommended. The environment and areas used for the biological medicines' isolation should also be controlled to minimize microbiological and other foreign contaminants. Biological medicines' typical isolation should be of the same control as the

- Regarding biomaterial disposal, the NIH Guidelines (https://osp.od.nih.gov/wp-content/uploads/NIH_Guidelines.pdf) specifies practices for constructing and handling: 1) recombinant deoxyribonucleic acid (DNA) molecules, and 2) organisms and viruses containing recombinant DNA molecules. In the context of the NIH Guidelines, recombinant DNA molecules are defined as either: 1) molecules that are constructed outside living cells by joining natural or synthetic DNA segments to DNA molecules that can replicate in a living cell, or 2) molecules that result from the replication of those described in 1) above. Synthetic DNA segments that are likely to yield a potentially harmful polynucleotide or polypeptide (e.g., a toxin or a pharmacologically active agent) are considered equivalent to their natural DNA counterpart. If the synthetic DNA segment is not expressed in vivo as a biologically active polynucleotide or polypeptide product, it is exempt from the NIH Guidelines.
- Genomic DNA of plants and bacteria that have acquired a transposable element, even if the latter was donated from a recombinant vector no longer present, are not subject to the NIH Guidelines unless the transposon itself contains recombinant DNA.
- For the manufacturing of biological medicines, the NIH guidance "Experiments Involving More than 10 Liters of Culture" should be followed: https://osp.od.nih.gov/wp-content/uploads/NIH_Guidelines.pdf. Since most recombinant cell lines do not survive outside of a specialized medium, it will not be necessary to perform sanitization of the used medium; however, some companies go through a decontamination process, adding unnecessary cost to the process.

14.6.5 Equipment

- Equipment interaction can determine the choice of chemicals used; sodium chloride is a corrosive agent to stainless steel, whereas sodium acetate is not. These issues should be addressed as early as possible in-process development.
- Utensils are bags, filters, or any other equipment exchanged at regular intervals. It has become common practice to use bags, filters, tubes, etc. to reduce cost and time to cleaning in place procedures. The numberer of steps in a process directly affects the cost and yield; however, reducing the number of steps process can affect robustness and safety and even later costs in additional testing as required by the regulatory authorities. For example, a choice may have to be made to add an adventitious agent removal process to validate the system.

14.6.6 Validation

- Validation of biological processes is an expensive exercise that continues throughout commercial manufacturing operations. Typically, validation steps are initiated when all separation and purification steps are described in detail and presented with flow charts. Adequate descriptions and specifications should be provided for all equipment, columns, reagents, buffers, and expected yields. The FDA defines process validation as: "validation—establishing documented evidence which provides a high degree of assurance that a specific process will consistently produce a product meeting its pre-determined specifications and quality attributes" (FDA 2011). As a result, there is a need to establish comprehensive documentary proof to justify the process and demonstrate that it works consistently. Validation reports for the various key processes would be dependent on the process involved; for example, if an ion-exchange column is used to remove endotoxins, there should be data documenting that this process is consistently effective as done by determining endotoxin levels before and after processing. It is important to monitor the process before, during, and after to determine each key purification step's efficiency. One method commonly used to demonstrate validation is to "spike" the preparation with a known amount of a contaminant and then demonstrate its absence.
- Process design depends on the nature of the target protein, the expression system used, and the demand for safety, robustness, and compliance with cGMP. The qualified raw material must be used to produce a safe product, and the host, process, and product-related impurities

removed. Although variations in-process design may occur, certain general rules apply, such as using at least three chromatographic steps, virus inactivation, and filtration in the process based on insect cells, mammalian cells, or transgenic animals. Target protein stability must be documented throughout processing and upon storage. Process design is a small-scale activity, and in principle, no process should be transferred for scale-up before it is reasonably tested on a small scale. The major process maturity criteria are linked to specifications, robustness, and cGMP compliance. Although drug substance and drug product specifications and their acceptance criteria are not fully defined at this early stage, data from at least three small-scale batches must be provided and tested against available specifications and acceptance criteria. The process must be robust and, to some extent, provide the expected outcome. Knowledge of critical parameters and their interactions is valuable information before scale-up. The process should be tested concerning cGMP to ensure that the process complies with its design and manufacturing procedures. Difficulties should be expected if the expression yield is low, the protein unstable, the purification yield is low, or the process comprises too many steps.

- Equipment change is the most significant aspect of scale-up from laboratory scale to production scale. Not all equipment is available in scalable type. This consideration should be the prime deciding factor in laboratory-scale development. Several suppliers offer a broad line of products in terms of capacity. They are always preferred to single-source suppliers, even if the initial cost is higher to use this equipment. Large scale hardware often has a different design, e.g., pump design may change from the high precision piston, or displacement pumps to rotary, diaphragm, or peristaltic pumps.
- Similarly, low volume multi-port valves are replaced by simple one-way valves, which, combined with large-scale tubing, may substantially expand volumes of equipment accessories and lead to extra dispersion of the target protein molecules. Large-scale equipment is often built of stainless steel and does not withstand high concentrations of sodium chloride. The scale-up issues to consider about large-scale equipment include differences in chromatographic column physics of movement, choice, placement of tubing, valve, reservoir, chemical resistance of construction material, CIP choice, and SIP.
- Process design should be distinguished from process optimization, where factors such as labor, automation, lean management, column lifetime, re-use of utensils, batch planning affect the process economy. The latter issues are dealt with at a later development stage, typically when the process design has been locked.

14.6.7 Testing

- In-process control is less expensive for batch and fed-batch systems compared to continuous cultures. Still, the overall cost may not be too different and is worth considering the FDA's PAT initiative. Milking procedures may result in small-volume bags, increasing the cost for analytical control programs. The insect and mammalian cell end-of-production test comprising sterility, fungi, mycoplasma, and virus testing should be included in the cost calculations
- Analytical assays to test quality may soon become less expensive if manufacturers can skip them as in-processes testing if the process is well developed. This is particularly important as large-scale manufacturing requires larger testing protocols. The FDA guidance on process analytical technology (PAT) at www.fda.gov/media/71012/download is highly relevant. This extended approach, taken during the development phase, includes traditional analytical testing and real-time monitoring of the process parameters and responses. Better monitoring of parameters and responses may result in a reduced analytical in the process control program.
- Safety considerations add to cost significantly. Insect cells, mammalian cells, and transgenic animals can be infected with viruses. Costly virus testing, virus reduction unit operations, and validation programs are needed to ensure product safety. The potential prion infection risk of sheep, goats, and cows is being debated, emphasizing controlled herds.

14.6.8 Quality

- In-process control testing should be minimal, and this is only possible with a well-defined system, which may initially incur higher costs. The trend is to reduce the number of in-process analytical methods and expand on monitoring parameters and responses, thereby keeping strict control of the process in real-time. The number of samples to analyze is inversely related to the batch size; large batches reduce the cost for in-process control.
- Monitoring using online data collection systems is needed to control and adjust parameters critical to processes. This creates a problem because small-scale instruments may not have the same monitoring potential as the large ones (which can be ordered with custom features).
- Quality control testing is required for drug and drug products; reduced test programs should be reconsidered upon scale-up. Some test analyses introduced in an early development phase may be skipped from the batch release program as combined data have confirmed process robustness. The rationale for removing a given analytical assay should be given. The PAT Initiative at the FDA may reduce the testing of products.
- In the process and quality control testing is extensive (see USP, EP, or BP) and expensive because of the nature of tests involved, notwithstanding other validation requirements common to all testing types. The assays used for in-process control can are justified as they provide essential process information during development or the) assays that are used to monitor a given outcome important for in-process control in manufacturing processes. Thus, reducing cost would mean reducing the number of in-process analyses without compromising process control. It is common practice to revise the program as more and more data become available, and the process matures. Another way to reduce costs is to use the process analytical technology (PAT) approach recently suggested by the FDA (www.fda.gov/cder/guidance/5815dft.htm). PAT is a system for designing, analyzing, and controlling manufacturing through timely measurements of critical quality and performance attributes of raw and in-process materials and processes to ensure final product quality. PAT's goal is to understand and control the manufacturing process as quality cannot be tested into products but should be built-in. This approach can be taken during the development phase extending the in-process control program to include traditional analytical testing and real-time monitoring of the process parameters and responses. The PAT framework's desired goal is to design and develop processes that can consistently ensure a predefined quality at the end of the manufacturing process. Such procedures would be consistent with the basic tenet of quality by design and could reduce the risks to quality and regulatory concerns while improving efficiency. A third way to reduce costs is to lower the price per sample by assuring a continuous flow of samples, reducing the time spent on the setup and calibration.
- Quality control testing is performed on both the drug substance (DS) and the drug product (DP) (see BP/EP/USP). The testing typically comprises 10–15 different analytical methods with an average price between $500 and $3,000/sample. If outside laboratories are inducted to provide additional testing, the cost can skyrocket. Animal assays and viral assays can be extremely expensive when outsourced. Yet, outsourcing is still the preferred way of doing these assays to obviate the large cost of maintaining animal houses or viral containment systems and validating the methods.
- Quality assurance systems should assure that the process scale-up does not alter process safety, robustness, or compliance with regulatory demands. If the process is redesigned to scale up, the validity of preclinical data should be considered. Robust systems introduce strict control of unit operation parameters and define parameters in intervals rather than set points. The parameter intervals are tested and justified on a small scale (proven acceptable range), making room to adjust the intervals according to large-scale needs. In the linear scale concept, these parameter intervals are kept constant upon scale-up. Other factors, such as reactor volumes, sample loads, and column diameters, are increased—all in a linear fashion.

14.6.9 Fill

- Formulation fill and pack operations of the API can also be subject to cost reduction depending on the formulation. A lyophilized product will cost more, and if a ready-to-inject formula can be developed, that should be a better choice. The components such as syringes, pen systems, etc., added at this stage add substantially to the cost of the product.

14.6.10 Water

- The quality of water should depend on the intended use of the finished product. For example, CBER requires water for injection (WFI) quality for process water. On the other hand, for in-vitro diagnostics, purified water may suffice. For drugs, the quality of water required depends on the process. Also, because processing usually occurs in cold rooms or at room temperature, the WFI system's self-sanitization to 80° C is lost.
- For economic reasons, some companies manufacture WFI by reverse osmosis rather than by distillation, resulting in contaminated systems because of the nature of processing equipment that is often difficult to sanitize. Any threads or drops in a cold system provide an area where microorganisms can lodge and multiply. Some of the systems employ a terminal sterilizing filter. However, the primary concern is endotoxins, and the terminal filter may merely serve to mask the true quality of the WFI used. The limitations of relying on a 0.1 ml sample of WFI for endotoxins from a system should also be recognized. As with other WFI systems, if cold WFI water is needed, point-of-use heat exchangers can be used.
- Buffers can be manufactured as sterile, non-pyrogenic solutions and stored in sterile containers. Some of the smaller facilities have purchased commercial sterile, non-pyrogenic buffer solutions.
- The product or storage of non-sterile water that may be of reagent grade or used as a buffer should be evaluated from both a stability and microbiological aspect.

14.6.11 Facility Design

Figure 14.1 shows a typical layout for a biological medicine manufacturing unit. The manufacturing layout of biological products is determined by two major factors: the size of production and the type of production; in most cases, the conditions of containment described above and the need to process products under cleanroom conditions are like the processing of sterile products otherwise. As a rule of thumb, the environment should be comparable to the preparation room environment for sterile products. There are four major types of work performed in biological product manufacturing, and given below are the requirements for each of these phases:

- Master cell bank and working cell bank: A dedicated room is to be made available for each GMC; this room includes a cold storage system (often a liquid nitrogen system) and a cold (–70° C) cabinet. The cells in the MCB are used to create WCB, and both are kept under high security. It is recommended that this be a vaulted area with class a 100,000 environment; generally, a 100–200 square foot area would suffice for this purpose. Some manufacturers divide the room into two, one for MCB and one for WCB, with a restricted entrance. In some designs, a direct transfer from WCB to the inoculum/culture room (see figure) is allowed through a transfer window under negative pressure. However, this practice is questioned based on the need to maintain a certain area classification; thus, the MCB/WCB is considered as supply center at the time of use, processed through materials dispensing. In all instances, a duplicate MCB shall be maintained off-site from the immediate manufacturing area. These rooms should have a backup supply of electricity to assure no power breakdown losses and alarms to record temperature variations in the cabinets storing the GMCs, an el. This electronic recording device transmitting the temperature at which the GMCs are stored should be installed. The room should also

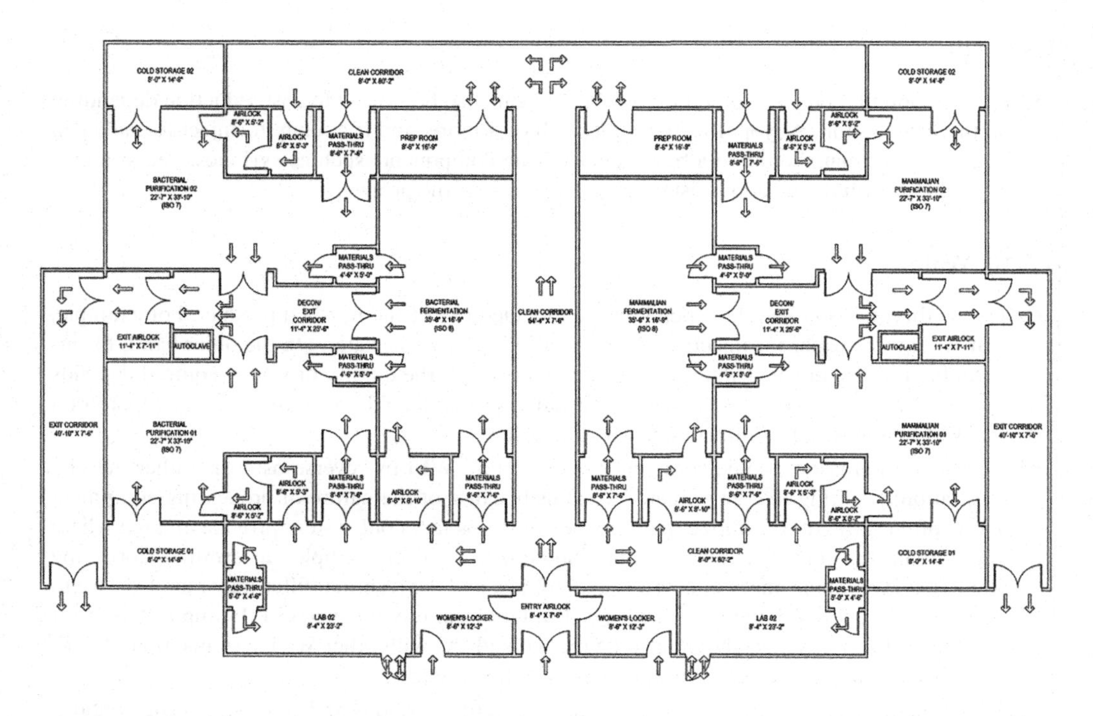

FIGURE 14.1 Typical layout of a recombinant manufacturing facility.

be equipped with an automated pressure differential; the room should be maintained negative concerning the corridor. This room is dedicated to each GMC; the reason is to avoid mixing up cultures, access restrictions to different personnel, and the storage requirements.

- Inoculum room: This is the first room where the culture tubes are opened to make WB, or for making the inoculum for fermentation should be a class 10,000 room. If the fermentation system used is a closed inline system, this room will also have a 4–8 L fermenter to make the starter culture; the culture will then be directly transferred to larger-sized fermenters. Where roller bottles are used, this room will serve as the staging room to prepare the culture for inoculation into the bottles, which would be done in another room because of the operation's size. The culture is handled under a biosafety laminar flow hood (biosafety hoods prevent operator exposure). The room should have a 10,000 classification with class 100 under the laminar flow hood. Generally, this room will be connected to the fermentation area, the recovery area, and the roller bottle preparation area, preferably through a negative pressure passing carousel. The room should be the smallest size possible (100–200 square feet).
- Fermentation room: This is generally the largest room of the facility or may comprise a series of rooms depending on production size. Where larger fermenters such as 25,000 L sizes are involved, this may take a three-stage fermenting. A facility of this size would likely be a 20,000+ square foot facility that may comprise several floors to accommodate large fermenters. However, for many biological medicines of low dosing, fermenters of 500–2,000 L should be sufficient, and these can be accommodated on a single floor basis. The area classification for this room is 100,000 unless a complete closed system is used (recommended) wherein general pharmaceutical-grade classification (unclassified) may be used.
- Recovery room: The fermentation (either from fermenters or from roller bottles) is brought to this room for the first processing stage. Where inclusion bodies are involved (such as in the use of bacterial cultures), this room will be cold centrifuge and cell disrupters; for the mammalian culture systems where the protein is secreted, this will be the first stage reduction of volume through filtration. This room is also used to store the product where refolding is generally

involved in the 2–8° C environment (provided as walk-in refrigerators). This area classification of this room remains 100,000. A room of about 500 square feet is required for this purpose.

- Downstream processing room: This is the second 10,000 classification room with large square footage under laminar flow hoods for the purification process. It is noteworthy that dedicated contact equipment (columns, vessels, etc.) is required for each product. A room of about 1,000 square feet is required as a minimum; the room's size will depend on the volume of production and the steps involved; in some instances, this may take more than 5,000 square feet where large-scale filtration equipment is involved and may comprise several floors. Some manufacturers do their downstream processing in different facilities; in such instances, there should be proper SOPs describing fermentation product packaging and transportation. Also, for some biological products, such practice is subject to extensive validation, such as biosimilars.
- Media and buffer preparation rooms: Each process requires a specific buffer and media; depending on the size, the operation's size can be substantial. For example, when using large fermenters (1,000 L or up), it may be advisable to switch to closed systems of media preparation and transfer to fermenters; however, for most medium and small-scale operations, a large media preparation room is required (1,500+ square feet) with 10,000-classification and work in class 100 hood; the media prepared is then transferred to the storage area and issued a specification code; the same applies to buffers used in downstream processing. Buffers should be prepared in a separate room and transported in closed containers to the storage area before dispensing.
- Storage rooms: Incoming material is stored in special environment-controlled areas; large refrigerated space is required for many components, including media and buffer. This room is also a 100,000-classification room. A part of the room is dedicated to staging supplies at the time of batch issues for production, wherein material will be gathered from the WCB, media, and buffer rooms.
- Finished product storage room: The room's size depends on the dosing unit size but generally, it is a relatively small room, about 100 square feet, where the concentrate is stored at refrigerated temperature. The classification is the same as the general pharmaceutical unclassified area since the product is now sealed in its primary and secondary packaging.

14.6.12 Cleaning

Validation of the cleaning procedures for the processing of equipment, including columns, should be carried out. This is especially critical for a multi-product facility. The manufacturer should have determined the degree of effectiveness of the cleaning procedure for each biological medicine or intermediate used in that piece of equipment. Validation data should verify that the cleaning process will reduce the specific residues to an acceptable level. However, it may not be possible to remove absolutely every trace of material, even with a reasonable number of cleaning cycles. The permissible residue level, generally expressed in parts per million (ppm), should be justified by the manufacturer. Cleaning should remove endotoxins, bacteria, toxic elements, and contaminating proteins while not adversely affecting the column's performance. There should be a written equipment cleaning procedure that provides details of what should be done and the materials to be utilized. Some manufacturers list the specific solvent for each biological medicine and intermediate. For stationary vessels, often clean-in-place (CIP) is used. In these instances, necessary diagrams should be drawn to identify specific parts (e.g., valves, etc.) that are part of the cleaning protocol.

After cleaning, there should be some routine testing to ensure that the surface has been cleaned to the validated level. One common method is the analysis of the final rinse water or solvent for the cleaning agents' presence last used in that piece of equipment. There should always be a direct determination of the residual substance.

The efficiency of the cleaning system would depend, to a large degree, on the robustness of the analytical system used to characterize the cleaning endpoints. The modern analytical apparatus's sensitivity has lowered some detection thresholds below parts per million (ppm), even down to parts per billion (ppb). The residue limits established for each piece of apparatus should be practical, achievable, and verifiable.

There should be a rationale for establishing certain levels that must be documented to prove their scientific merit. Another factor to consider is the possible non-uniform distribution of the residue on a piece of equipment. The actual average residue concentration may be more than the level detected.

14.6.13 Filling and Finishing

The products of biotechnology are proteins and peptides that are relatively unstable molecules compared to most organic pharmaceuticals. Most biotechnology processes involve transferring proteins from one stabilizing or solubilizing buffer to another during the purification process. Ultimately, the protein is exchanged into its final solution dosage form, where long-term stability is achieved. These products often require lyophilization to achieve long-term stability because of the potential for degradation by various mechanisms, including deamidation, aggregation, oxidation, and possible proteolysis by trace levels of host cell proteases. The protein's final dosage form usually contains stabilizing compounds that result in the optimal pH and solution conditions necessary for long-term product stability and the desired properties for the product (tonicity). These compounds include proteins, polyhydric alcohols, amino acids, carbohydrates, bulking agents, inorganic salts, and nonionic surfactants. Also, these excipients may be required for stable lyophilized cake formation. There are special requirements for lyophilized products, such as the control of moisture levels, that are generally defined in the individual USP monograph, which may be important to product stability. Significantly, the assessment of protein stability usually requires multiple analytical methods, each of which may be used to assess a specific mode of protein degradation. The use of accelerated stability studies to predict protein formulations' shelf life is often complicated by the effects of temperature on protein conformation, resulting in non-Arrhenius behavior. Thus, reliance on real-time, recommended storage condition stability studies is often required for establishing the expiration dating of biotechnology-derived products.

Biological medicines are not terminally sterilized and must be manufactured by aseptic processing. The presence of process-related contaminants in a product or device is chiefly a safety issue. The sources of contaminants are primarily the cell-substrate (DNA, host cell proteins, and other cellular constituents, viruses), the media (proteins, sera, and additives), and the purification process (process-related chemicals and product-related impurities).

Because of stability considerations, most biological medicines are either refrigerated or lyophilized. Low temperatures and low moisture content are also deterrents to microbiological proliferation. To validate the aseptic processing of the non-preserved single dose biological medicine (that is aseptically filled) stored at room temperature as a solution, the limitations of a 0.1% media fill contamination rate should be recognized.

Media fill data and validation of the aseptic manufacturing process should be well documented. Some biological medicines may not be very stable and may require gentle mixing and processing. Whereas double filtrations are relatively common for aseptically filled parenteral single filtration at low pressures is usually performed for biological medicines. It is for this reason that manufacturing directions be specific, with maximum filtration pressures given.

The environment and accessibility for the batching of non-sterile biological medicines should be controlled. Because many of these products lack preservatives, inherent bacteriostatic r fungistatic activity, and bioburden before sterilization should be low. This bioburden should be determined before sterilization of these bulk solutions before filling. The batching or compounding of these bulk solutions should be controlled to prevent any potential increase in microbiological levels that may occur up to the time that the bulk solutions are filtered (sterilized). One concern with any microbiological level is the possible increase in endotoxins that may develop. Good practice for compounding these products would also include batching in a controlled environment and sealed tanks, particularly if the solution is to be stored before sterilization. Good practice would also include limitations on the length of manufacturing time between formulation and sterilization.

In-process testing is an essential part of quality control and ensures that an operation's actual, real-time performance is acceptable. Examples of in-process controls are stream parameters, chromatography profiles, protein species, protein concentrations, bioactivity, bioburden, and endotoxin levels. This set of in-process controls and the selection of acceptance criteria require coordination with the validation program results.

The filling of biological medicines into ampoules or vials presents many of the same problems as with the processing of conventional products. In established companies, these issues are addressed using adequate documentation; however, for the new biological medicines facility, attempting to develop and prove clinical effectiveness and safety and validate sterile operations, equipment, and systems, can be a lengthy process, particularly if requirements are not clearly understood.

The batch size, at least when initially produced, likely will be small. Because of the small batch size, filling lines may not be as automated as other products typically filled in larger quantities. Thus, more people are filling these products, particularly at some of the smaller, newer companies. This can bring quality inconsistencies. During filling, problems include inadequate attire; deficient environmental monitoring programs; hand-stoppering of vials, particularly those that are lyophilized, and failure to validate some of the basic sterilization processes. Because of people's active involvement in filling and aseptic manipulations, the number of persons involved in these operations should be minimized. An environmental program should include an evaluation of microbiological samples taken from people working in aseptic processing areas.

Another concern about product stability is inert gas's use to displace oxygen during processing and filling the solution. As with other products that may be sensitive to oxidation, the solution's dissolved oxygen levels should be established. Likewise, the filling operation's validation should include parameters such as line speed and location of filling syringes concerning closure to assure minimal exposure to air (oxygen) for oxygen-sensitive products. In the absence of inert gas displacement, the manufacturer should demonstrate that the product is not affected by oxygen.

Typically, vials to be lyophilized are partially stoppered by a machine. Where an operator places the stopper manually, serious problems can arise. Another major concern with the filling operation of a lyophilized product is the assurance of fill volumes. A low fill would represent a sub potency in the vial. Unlike a powder or liquid fill, a low fill would not be readily apparent after lyophilization, particularly for a product where the active ingredient may be only a milligram. Because of the clinical significance, sub-potency in a vial potentially can be a very serious situation, clinically.

14.7 Testing

The following tests are applicable for in-process, bulk, and product testing. The tests that are needed will depend on the process and the intended use of the product.

- Quality.
  - Color/appearance/clarity
  - Particulate analysis
  - pH determination
  - Moisture content
  - Host cell DNA
- Identity: A single test for identity may not be sufficient. Confirmation is needed that the methods employed are validated.
  - Peptide mapping (reduced/non-reduced)
  - Gel electrophoresis
  - SDS PAGE
  - Isoelectric focusing (IEF)
  - Immunoelectrophoresis
  - Two-dimensional electrophoresis
  - Capillary electrophoresis

    - HPLC (chromatographic retention)
    - Immunoassay
    - ELISA
    - Western blot
    - Radioimmunoassay
    - Amino acid analysis
    - Amino acid sequencing
    - Mass spectroscopy
    - Molecular weight (SDS PAGE)
    - Carbohydrate composition analysis (glycosylation)
- Protein concentration/content.
- Tests that may be encountered:
    - Protein quantitation
    - Lowry
    - Biuret method
    - UV spectrophotometry
    - HPLC
    - Amino acid analysis
    - Partial sequence analysis
- Purity: "Purity" means relative freedom from the extraneous matter in the finished product, whether harmful to the recipient or deleterious to the product. Purity includes, but is not limited to, relative freedom from residual moisture or other volatile substances and pyrogenic substances. Protein impurities are the most common contaminants. These may arise from the fermentation process, media, or the host organism. Endogenous retroviruses may be present in hybridomas used for monoclonal antibody production. Specific testing for these constituents is imperative in vivo products. Removal of extraneous antigenic proteins is essential to assure the safety and effectiveness of the product.
    - Tests for protein impurities:
        - Electrophoresis
            - SDS PAGE
            - IEF
        - Dimensional electrophoresis
        - Peptide mapping
        - Multi antigen ELISA
    - HPLC; size-exclusion HPLC; reverse-phase HPLC
    - Tests for non-protein impurities:
        - Endotoxin testing
        - USP rabbit pyrogen test
        - Limulus amebocyte lysate (LAL) E
        - Endogenous pyrogen assay
- Pyrogen contamination: Pyrogenicity testing should be conducted by injecting rabbits with the final product or by the limulus amebocyte lysate (LAL) assay. The same criteria used for acceptance of the natural product should be used for the biotech product. The presence of endotoxins in some in vitro diagnostic products may interfere with the performance of the device. Also, it is essential that in vivo, products be tested for pyrogens. Certain biological pharmaceuticals are pyrogenic in humans despite having passed the LAL test and the rabbit pyrogen test. This phenomenon may be due to materials that appear to be pyrogenic only in humans. An endogenous

pyrogen assay is used to predict whether human subjects will experience a pyrogenic response. Human blood mononuclear cells are cultured in vitro with the final product, and the cell culture fluid is injected into rabbits. Fever in the rabbits indicates the product contains a substance that may be pyrogenic in humans.

- USP rabbit pyrogen test
- Limulus amebocyte lysate (LAL)
- Endogenous pyrogen assay

- Viral contamination: Tests for viral contamination should be appropriate to the cell-substrate and culture conditions employed. The absence of detectable adventitious viruses contaminating the final product should be demonstrated.
    - The cytopathic effect in several cell types
    - Hemadsorptions embryonated egg testing
    - Polymerase chain reaction (PCR)
    - Viral antigen and antibody immunoassay
    - Mouse antibody production (MAP)
- Nucleic acid contamination: Concerns about nucleic acid impurities arise from the possibility of cellular transformation events in a recipient. Removal of nucleic acid at each step in the purification process may be demonstrated in pilot experiments by examining the extent of eliminating added host cell DNA. Such an analysis would provide the theoretical extent of the removal of nucleic acid during purification. Direct analyses of nucleic acid in several production lots of the final product should be performed by hybridization analysis of immobilized contaminating nucleic acid utilizing appropriate probes, such as nick-translated host cell and vector DNA. Theoretical concerns regarding transforming DNA derived from the cell-substrate rate will be minimized by the general reduction of contaminating nucleic acid.
    - DNA hybridization (dot blot)
    - Polymerase chain reaction (PCR)
- Protein contamination.
    - SDS PAGE
    - PLC
    - IEF
- Foreign protein contamination.
    - Immunoassays
    - Radio immunoassays
    - ELISA
    - Western blot
    - SDS PAGE
    - Two-dimensional electrophoresis
- Microbial contamination: Appropriate tests should be conducted for microbial contamination that demonstrates the absence of detectable bacteria (aerobes and anaerobes), fungi, yeast, and mycoplasma applicable.
    - USP sterility test
    - Heterotrophic plate count and total yeasts and molds
    - Total plate count
    - Mycoplasma test
    - LAL/pyrogen
- Chemical contaminants: Other sources of contamination must be considered, e.g., allergens, petroleum oils, residual solvents, cleaning materials, column leachable materials, etc.

- Potency (activity): "Potency" is interpreted to mean the specific ability or capacity of the product, as indicated by appropriate laboratory tests or by adequately controlled clinical data obtained through the administration of the product in the manner intended to produce a given result. Tests for potency should consist of either in vitro or in vivo tests, or both, specifically designed for each product to indicate its potency. A reference preparation for the biological activity should be established and used to determine the bioactivity of there a product's activity; in-house biological potency standards should be cross-referenced against international (World Health Organization [WHO], National Institute of Biological Standards and Control [NIBSC]) or national (National Institutes of Health [NIH], National Cancer Institute [NCI], Food and Drug Administration [FDA]) reference standard preparations, or USP standards. Validated methods of potency determination include:
  - Whole animal bioassays
  - Cell culture bioassays
  - Biochemical/biophysical assays
  - Receptor-based immunoassays
  - Potency limits:
    - Identification of agents that may adversely affect potency
    - Evaluation of functional activity and antigen/antibody specificity
    - Various immunodiffusion methods (single/double)
    - Immunoblotting/radio- or enzyme-linked immunoassays
    - HPLC-validated to correlate certain peaks the to biological activity
- Stability: "Stability" is the capacity of a product to remain within specifications established to ensure its identity, strength, quality, purity, safety, and effectiveness as a function of time. Studies to support the proposed dating period should be performed on the final product. Real-time stability data would be essential to support the proposed dating period. Testing might include the stability of potency, pH, clarity, color, particulates, physiochemical stability, moisture, and preservatives. Accelerated stability testing data may be used as supportive data. Accelerated testing or stress tests are studies designed to increase the ratio of chemical or physical degradation of a substance or product using exaggerated storage conditions. The purpose is to determine kinetic parameters to predict the tentative expiration dating period. The product's stress testing is frequently used to identify potential problems encountered during storage and transportation and to vide an estimate of the expiration dating period. This should include a study of the effects of temperature fluctuations as appropriate for shipping and storage conditions. These tests should establish a valid dating period under realistic field conditions with the containers and closures intended for the marketed product. Some relatively fragile biotechnologically derived proteins may require gentle mixing and processing and only a single filtration at low pressure. The manufacturing directions must be specific with maximum filtration pressures given to maintain stability in the final product. Products containing preservatives to control microbial contamination should have the preservative content monitored. This can be accomplished by performing microbial challenge tests (i.e., USP antimicrobial preservative effectiveness test) or by performing chemical assays for the preservative. Areas that should be addressed are:
  - Effective monitoring of the stability test environment (i.e., light, temperature, humidity, residual moisture)
  - Container/closure system used for bulk storage (i.e., extractables, chemical modification of the protein, change in stopper formulations that may change extractable profile)
  - Identify materials that would cause product instability and test for the presence of aggregation, denaturation, fragmentation, deamination, photolysis, and oxidation
  - Tests to determine aggregates or degradation products:
    - SDS PAGE
    - IEF

- HPLC
- Ion exchange chromatography
- Gel filtration
- Peptide mapping
- Spectrophotometric methods
- Potency assays
- Performance testing
- Two-dimensional electrophoresis

- Batch-to-batch consistency: The basic criterion for determining that a manufacturer is producing a standardized and reliable product is the demonstration of lot-to-lot consistency concerning certain predetermined release specifications.
  - Uniformity: Identity, purity, functional activity
  - Stability: Acceptable performance during shelf life, precision, sensitivity, specificity. Like other small molecules, protein drugs are subject to demonstrating stability (providing a predetermined minimum potency) to the time of use. Also, a safety profile since the degradation products of protein drugs can be immunogenic, compared to small molecules where the concern is mainly the creation of toxic molecules. Biological medicines' stability studies are conducted at three levels: pre-formulation, formulation development, and formal GMP studies. The pre-formulation studies determine the basic stability properties of a bulk protein or peptide. The accelerated studies at this stage are primarily intended to establish stability-indicating assays and other analytic methods. The formulation development studies are intended for the candidate formulation and encompass large studies that evaluate the effects of excipients, container/closure systems, and, where lyophilized, a study of myriad factors that can alter products' characteristics. The data generated in the formulation development studies is used to select the final formulation and design the studies that follow formal GMP studies. The formal stability studies are used to support clinical use, IND, and then through a biological license application (submitted to CDER; effective June 2003, biological medicines are now handled by CDER). When preparing supplies for the clinical use, it is important to know that there is no need to demonstrate shelf-life for the commercial dosage form and only stability demonstration is required during the testing phase, such as six months; many manufacturers used the frozen product to assure adequate stability; this may create a logistics problem of assuring that the clinical sites can store the produce frozen. Products that may be adversely affected by freezing will not be subject to this method of reducing clinical startup time. Also, at this stage of initial clinical testing under an IND, the test methods need not be fully validated or having demonstrated robustness; if reproducibility and repeatability are demonstrated, this should be acceptable to FDA. The formal GMP studies monitor commercial lots, and clear ICH guidelines are available to follow these studies' protocols (see ICH Stability Guidelines for Biologics, www.fda.gov/media/71441/download)
- Testing control: A quality control program for the drug substance and drug product must be defined, and the acceptance criteria for each analysis. The setting of acceptance criteria is an ongoing activity throughout development (and scale-up) as more and more data become available. A batch is released, provided all analytical results are within the specified ranges. A high acceptance rate should be expected if the process is robust and in compliance, implying that both the regulatory authorities and the manufacturer often share identical views. The process designer must carefully consider the issues mentioned above when designing the purification process (the design principle). Much of the design can be carried out before entering the laboratory due to the restrictions governing biological medicine processing. The pre-design phase is called process modeling, thus preceding the experimental design phase for optimization and testing, which takes place in the laboratory. In general, quality control systems for biotechnology-derived products are very similar to those quality control systems

routinely employed for traditional pharmaceutical products in such areas as raw material testing and release, manufacturing and process control documentation, and aseptic processing. Biotechnology-derived product quality control systems incorporate some of the same philosophies applied to the analysis of low molecular weight pharmaceutical products. These include using chemical reference standards and validated methods to evaluate a broad spectrum of known and potential product impurities and potential breakdown products. The quality control systems for biotechnology-derived products are generally analogous to those established for traditional biologicals concerning determining product sterility, product safety in experimental animals, and product potency. The fundamental difference between quality control systems for biotechnology-derived products and traditional pharmaceuticals is in the types of methods used to determine product identity, consistency, purity, and impurity profiling. Furthermore, in biotechnology quality control, it is frequently necessary to use a combination of final product and validated in-process testing and process validation to ensure the removal of undesired real or potential impurities to the levels suggested by regulatory agencies. Biotechnology-derived products generally require a detailed characterization of the production organism (cell), a complete assessment of the means of cell growth/propagation, and an explicit analysis of the final product recovery process. The complexity of the quality control systems for biotechnology-derived products is related to both the size and structural characteristics of the product and the manufacturing process. The laboratory controls are like what is expected in normal cGMP/GLP compliance for all pharmaceutical products with special consideration given to unique materials and their handling:

- Training: Laboratory personnel should be adequately trained for the jobs they are performing
- Equipment maintenance/calibration/monitoring: Documentation and scheduling for maintenance, calibration, and monitoring of laboratory equipment involved in the measurement, testing, and storage of raw materials, product samples, and reference reagents
- Validation: All laboratory methods should be validated with the equipment and reagents specified in the test methods. Changes in vendor and specifications of major equipment/reagents would require revalidation. Raw data should support validation parameters in submitted applications
- Standard/reference material: Reference standards should be well characterized and documented, properly stored, secured, and utilized during testing
- Storage of labile components: Laboratory cultures and reagents, such as enzymes, antibodies, test reagents, etc., may degrade if not held under proper storage conditions.
- Laboratory SOPs: Procedures should be written, applicable, and followed. Quality control samples should be properly segregated and stored

14.8 Documentation Process

The development program comprises various activities comprising project planning, cell banking, process development, analytical procedures, scale-up, manufacture, stability studies, preparation of reference materials, and quality assurance. The work will ultimately lead to a process for the manufacture and control of the licensed product. To obtain a license, extensive documentation must be provided (new drug application, biological license application). However, much of the work carried out during development and scale-up is not included in the said applications. It is up to the project owner to provide the development documentation upon inspection from regulatory authorities. The statement "if it is not documented, it has not been carried out" should be taken rigorously.

A major part of the documentation required can be planned (e.g., cell banking reports, unit operation descriptions, development reports, analytical method descriptions, batch records). Other reports (e.g., summary reports) are written along with the experimental work. Although such reports do not describe the final work, they are very useful for informing the coming users about the rationale for decision-making. It is therefore recommended to include summary reports in the tech transfer package.

The drug development program produces hundreds or even thousands of documents written by different people from different departments and often from different companies. Any of these documents may be needed at a later stage, and it is necessary to set up an efficient documentation system to assure document tracking. An important part of the tracking procedure is to ensure efficient authentication of the document comprising information of author, date, version, company, facility, etc.

14.8.1 Process Analytical Technology (PAT)

Over the past few years, several technical, regulatory, and business interests have converged, generating breakthrough possibilities in the growth and execution of pharmaceutical production processes. The PAT tools are incorporated to enable ongoing process monitoring and design, track, analyze, and regulate the outcomes from the outset of the manufacturing process. This timely assessment helps high-quality drug product to be produced that always meets its specifications. PAT tools can be applied to raw materials, in-process materials, and the overall process.

The FDA's emphasis on PAT for upstream bioprocesses with a particular focus on monoclonal antibodies is widely mentioned at a regulatory level. Cell culture presents itself as a suitable opportunity for PAT tools to be explored. This is mostly due to the post-translational modifications of the proteins that occur with these cells in the production bioreactor. These modifications can significantly affect product quality, potency, and stability. Some of these quality attributes critical to the final product are tested at the time of release using offline HPLC, MS methods.

But with a more in-depth knowledge process over the last few years, several studies and experimental data have demonstrated that the upstream process conditions cause product variations in a typical process used to manufacture mAbs. The cell culture process parameters also impact the downstream purification process. Thus, monitoring process conditions and the critical quality attributes (glycosylation, charge variants, etc.) in real-time during the upstream bioprocessing lead to establishing a control strategy for these variations by early detection rather than at the time of lot release. An offline biochemical analyzer for key nutrients and metabolites is part of the bioreactor monitoring process. However, recently there is a greater emphasis on integration to use this direct measurement of analytics (inline, online) in the bioreactor on a real-time basis. This integration leads to an optimized and well-controlled feeding strategy for precise monitoring of the process. Monitoring nutrients in real-time provides the capacity for feed-forward control. The key nutrients identified to be critical to culture performance can be maintained in range throughout the process. The inline monitoring also reduces operator variability due to sample preparation for measurements, savings on time and effort, and, most importantly, on additional volume lost due to sampling.

Like the inline biochemical analyzer, spectroscopy-based technology is used for inline monitoring of viable cell density. While automated cell counters have mostly replaced the traditional microscopy measurements, the relatively newer inline spectroscopy eliminates the drawbacks of the trypan blue dye cell counting method, particularly when cell clumping at higher cell densities. In the spectroscopy method of measurement, cells' ability to store electric charge and act as capacitors under an electric field is used. The measured capacitance is proportional to the viable cell density in the bioreactor. Radio-frequency impedance is also another tool that is used for cell density measurements. Coupling the inline measurement to the real-time nutrient analysis further tightens the feed-forward control strategy to support and maintain high cell densities without nutrient limitation or to lower cell viability. Thus, online biomass measurement, substrate measurement, and even at-line product measurements are significant PAT advances.

Near-Infrared spectroscopy and Raman spectroscopy are useful tools for real-time monitoring of cell culture parameters wherein constant information on pH, DO, and other various metabolites are provided without the need for any manual sampling. PAT methods are increasing in their use for upstream bioprocessing and are being extended to provide more specific analytical techniques to assist in protein quality assessment. The uncertainty in product variability is minimized to create an efficient process by taking these metrics into real-time and developing effective feedback/feed-forward control. These analytical tools also lead to minimal intervention reducing the risk of contamination.

Another key area for PAT advancements includes real-time release without depending on end-product testing that is typically performed. With new dosage forms, smaller patient populations, and other modalities on the rise, real-time testing and release are highly desirable. Smaller manufacturing platforms make on-site manufacturing at hospitals and public health areas a possibility. The focus lies not only on the outcomes but also on the relationship between the various subsystems requiring evaluation. For example, while real-time monitoring will show deviations and predict a specific batch's outcome, the analytics is made a step further to compare the performance with other batches and determine what measures are required to improve the process and minimize errors.

PAT tools implementation is not as widespread in biopharma as the chemical or, in general, the pharmaceutical industry. Even within the biological medicine industry, the implementation seems more common on the upstream than the downstream. Downstream processes can benefit significantly from the integration of MS tools. However, the cumbersome instrumentation and the bulkiness make it a challenge. Some of the key reasons that limit the adoption of PAT include the cost, a lack of clear understanding of the technology barriers, and finally, to an extent, the regulatory expectations or even the lack of incentives.

There is a dire need for specialized expertise on integrating these sensors, program the feedback or feed-forward control loops, particularly validation when applied to a GMP manufacturing environment. These challenges are a significant barrier to PAT adoption, especially to small and medium-sized manufacturers and even some contract manufacturing organizations. One way to encourage these analytical tools will have to come from the CMOs.

14.8.2 Automation

Automation is critical in the control, collection, and use of data. To maximize automation, equipment, data collection must be integrated effectively with the process and facilitate technology transfer and scale-up. To ensure process data and process analysis, consolidation into a single automation platform will support both early-stage and late-stage process development in addition to being easy for compliance. The biopharma industry is behind in adopting innovative methods (cloud computing, Internet of Things) compared to other industries. However, these novel approaches with additional risks, coordination between the various functional groups, handling raw materials and waste materials, processes, and the unit operations that make up the process are key to successful and efficient production automation. The automation platforms should be capable of integrating with bioreactors, purification systems, and mixers from other vendors. The integration helps improve data management, increase unit operation integration, and provide comprehensive control.

In-process analysis plays an essential part in the process and can be streamlined and implemented. These analytics can include valuable data, including raw materials (e.g., cell culture media, resin), processes bioreactor and capture phases, and drug ingredients. The advances in peripherals such as sensors, valves, pumps designed with additional feedback, and intelligence are also part of future automation possibilities.

Automation requires the collection and archiving of the data to create an operational model. These advances go hand in hand with the bioprocess software that allows the customized use of data, for example, creating feedback control loops. Data are useful only if these can be interpreted and made meaningful. Automation is a critical driver in connecting the various new technologies and tools to a bioprocess and enhancing a simple facility towards a smart facility. Even regulatory agencies recognize the value and potential of data; it works towards identifying key issues, address them, and optimize the production process.

The key to a successful process is to incorporate integrated automation and digital infrastructure that suits the manufacturer's capabilities and needs. Investments in integrated systems and automation solutions should be simplified to encourage industry-wide adoption.

Automation is a critical feature in single-use technology; however, there is a presumption that these components and modules may lack the accuracy and sensitivity associated with traditional systems. This perception may have been true a decade ago, but the technological advancements made within the single-use technology have only improved and increased process efficiency and productivity. An excellent example of combining single-use technology and automation effectively is the biomanufacturing platform, FlexFactory, offered by Cytiva Life Sciences. The various unit operations in this platform are connected via single-use tubing sets that operate on various automation schemes, increasing flexibility and productivity. Cytiva Life Sciences has been able to use this platform (FlexFactory) to build its turnkey modular facility solution. Using manufacturing execution systems (MES) and enterprise resource planning (ERP) to interface with automation will help establish the management infrastructure and maximize manufacturing efficiency. The data feed can be initiated at the start of the production process with raw materials being used in the upstream process and move along throughout the process, including data from purification and filtration steps. For example, Wonderware and DeltaV™ with the FlexFactory platform help ensure broad compatibility with the leading MES and ERP systems. These kinds of interfaces and facility advances build process optimization that boosts productivity and reduces the inherent risks of biomanufacturing, provided the fully integrated framework offers high levels of accuracy, monitoring, and execution.

14.9 Predictions

The next-generation technologies, methods, and planning will offer greater efficiency, improved resilience, and decrease costs, all of which are important for the sustained growth of the biological medicine industry. Process intensification, continuous manufacturing, and single-use technologies are the approaches that are fast entering the manufacturing plans. The potential to increase productivity, reduce manufacturing footprint, further improve the facility utilization and, most importantly, accelerate timelines for milestones in the development cycle and fast to market is achievable with discreet use of these approaches. Process intensification upstream can help deliver high titers but can undoubtedly lead to bottlenecks downstream, and hence strategically using these tools is key to process efficiency.

With mAb production processes continuing to evolve, it is essential to develop a platform process strategy with some flexibility built to accommodate similar products manufactured using the same host cell type, similar upstream and downstream processes. Facility utilization is maximized, but the platform process should not forego additional innovations and new technology adaptation. Achieving a balance in adopting changes is required to handle better the changing needs and demands of the market needs, adding more products in the pipelines while continuing to be part of innovation and targeted improvements that emphasize simplification and intensification.

The manufacturing infrastructure should be designed to easily switch between multiple products to ensure that capital investment is depreciated efficiently. The ability to switch to multiple products without long downtime leads to better asset utilization.

The opportunities for process intensification should be used at every stage to increase upstream productivity with improved cell line, using a concentrated fed-batch process, optimizing current processes with new media, or resins evaluation, simplifying operation by eliminating no-value activities and carefully using data analytics to build intelligence into the process via inline monitoring, real-time release.

The use of continuous processing, single-use technology, modular yet flexible facilities, adherence to compliance, data integration via automation, and PAT are essential tools for connecting and realizing the full benefit and capabilities of operating an efficient facility.

A modular facility design of the future will be entirely different from the current trends. It will reduce operating costs, allow faster turnaround, and, most importantly, making affordable medicine a reality.

Both process intensification and hybrid continuous manufacturing are dominating the biomanufacturing industry. High volume cell density reduces seed train duration or using the perfusion process for seed bioreactor, operating the production process as a concentrated fed-batch process are methods that are being accepted and evaluated for feasibility at a large scale. These approaches and designs help create flexibility to optimize the use of operating space. Selecting reliable suppliers to support this implementation is critical and essential to developing a supplier relationship that ensures dependable, consistent, and affordable services are provided.

Understanding the implications, advantages, and disadvantages of each of the future possibilities will play a critical role in their successful implementation that will lead to a drastic reduction in the footprint of a production floor operation, reducing cost and capital, and ultimately increasing the speed to reach the patient market space. Improvements made on the process front will have to be realized down to the cell level, e.g., if a manufacturer uses perfusion technology for higher titers, then the cell line should be capable of withstanding longer run times and must demonstrate genetic stability without compromising on the product quality for the entirety of the production process. These measures, along with improved approaches to pipeline development, cost savings, and more scalable and agile production, are all important to meet the biological industry's evolving demands. The realizations that the key drivers will soon be fully integrated lead to the automated process starting with cell culture and progressing to product formulation seamlessly.

14.10 Conclusion

Cost-effective drug development requires the adoption of advanced technologies such as genomics, metabolomics, cloud computing, novel assay methods, and creative clinical testing models. These technologies develop fast, and a future perspective view is essential for all developers, particularly the small entities. The development costs projected in this chapter apply mostly to smaller companies; large pharma costs are several times higher, and it is for this reason that most smaller companies succeed in developing drugs faster, and big pharma is always welcoming these discoveries. While we have developed around 1,700 new molecular entities, there remain endless opportunities for new drug discovery to explore.

ADDITIONAL READING

Aarons L, Karlsson MO, Mentré F, et al. Role of modelling and simulation in phase I drug development. *Eur J Pharm Sci.* 2001;13(2):115–122.

Adams CP, Brantner VV. Estimating the cost of new drug development: is it really 802 million dollars? *Health Aff* (Millwood). 2006;25(2):420–428.

Alfaro CL. Emerging role of drug interaction studies in drug development: the good, the bad, and the unknown. *Psychopharmacol Bull.* 2001;35(4):80–93.

Alhenc-Gelas F, Parmentier L, Bisagni A. Pharmacogenetic and pharmacogenomic studies. Impact on drug discovery and drug development. *Therapie.* 2003;58(3):275–282.

Au R. The paradigm shift to an "open" model in drug development. *Appl Transl Genom.* 2014;3(4):86–89.

Bajaj JS. Drug development in India. *Indian J Physiol Pharmacol.* 1981;25(2):95–104.

Baras AI, Baras AS, Schulman KA. Drug development risk and the cost of capital. *Nat Rev Drug Discov.* 2012;11(5):347–348.

Benedetti A, Khoo J, Sharma S, Facco P, Barolo M, Zomer S. Data analytics on raw material properties to accelerate pharmaceutical drug development. *Int J Pharm.* 2019;563:122–134.

Beyoğlu D, Idle JR. Metabolomics and its potential in drug development. *Biochem Pharmacol.* 2013;85(1):12–20.

Bhattacharya I, Heatherington A, Barton J. Applying the best of oncology drug development paradigms to the non-malignant space. *Drug Discov Today.* 2016;21(12):1869–1872.

Boyd RA, Lalonde RL. Nontraditional approaches to first-in-human studies to increase efficiency of drug development: will microdose studies make a significant impact? *Clin Pharmacol Ther.* 2007;81(1):24–26.

Brazell C, Freeman A, Mosteller M. Maximizing the value of medicines by including pharmacogenetic research in drug development and surveillance. *Br J Clin Pharmacol.* 2002;53(3):224–231.

Brodniewicz T, Grynkiewicz G. Preclinical drug development. *Acta Pol Pharm.* 2010;67(6):578–585.

Carlson B. Aptamers: the new frontier in drug development? *Biotechnol Health.* 2007;4(2):31–36.

Casty FE, Wieman MS. Drug development in the 21st century: the synergy of public, private, and international collaboration. *Ther Innov Regul Sci.* 2013;47(3):375–383.

Clegg LE, Mac Gabhann F. Molecular mechanism matters: benefits of mechanistic computational models for drug development. *Pharmacol Res.* 2015;99:149–154.

Coates S, Pohl O, Gotteland JP, Täubel J, Lorch U. Efficient design of integrated and adaptively interlinked protocols for early-phase drug development programs. *Ther Innov Regul Sci.* 2020;54(1):184–194.

Cockburn IM, Henderson RM. Scale and scope in drug development: unpacking the advantages of size in pharmaceutical research. *J Health Econ.* 2001;20(6):1033–1057.

Cohen JP, Sturgeon G, Cohen A. Measuring progress in neglected disease drug development. *Clin Ther.* 2014;36(7):1037–1042.

Collier R. Drug development cost estimates hard to swallow. *CMAJ.* 2009;180(3):279–280.

Cook J, Hunter G, Vernon JA. The future costs, risks and rewards of drug development: the economics of pharmacogenomics. *Pharmacoeconomics.* 2009;27(5):355–363.

Data JL, Willke RJ, Barnes JR, DiRoma PJ. Re-engineering drug development: integrating pharmacoeconomic research into the drug development process. *Psychopharmacol Bull.* 1995;31(1):67–73.

Desai N, Edwards AJ, Ernest TB, Tuleu C, Orlu M. 'Big Data' informed drug development: a case for acceptability. *Drug Discov Today.* 2021:26(4):865–869.

DiMasi JA. The value of improving the productivity of the drug development process: faster times and better decisions. *Pharmacoeconomics.* 2002;20 Suppl 3:1–10.

DiMasi JA, Grabowski HG, Hansen RW. The cost of drug development. *N Engl J Med.* 2015;372(20):1972.

DiMasi JA, Hansen RW, Grabowski HG. The price of innovation: new estimates of drug development costs. *J Health Econ.* 2003;22(2):151–185.

Dondapati SK, Stech M, Zemella A, Kubick S. Cell-free protein synthesis: a promising option for future drug development. *BioDrugs.* 2020;34(3):327–348.

Drews J, Ryser S. The role of innovation in drug development. *Nat Biotechnol.* 1997;15(13):1318–1319.

Dunne M. Antiretroviral drug development: the challenge of cost and access. *AIDS.* 2007;21 Suppl 4:S73–S79.

Dunyak J, Mitchell P, Hamrén B, et al. Integrating dose estimation into a decision-making framework for model-based drug development. *Pharm Stat.* 2018;17(2):155–168.

Duttagupta S. Outcomes research and drug development. *Perspect Clin Res.* 2010;1(3):104–105.

FDA. Guidance for Industry. 2011. Retrieved from: https://www.fda.gov/files/drugs/published/Process-Validation--General-Principles-and-Practices.pdf

Fermini B, Coyne ST, Coyne KP. Clinical trials in a dish: a perspective on the coming revolution in drug development. *SLAS Discov.* 2018;23(8):765–776.

Frank RG. New estimates of drug development costs. *J Health Econ.* 2003;22(2):325–330.

Frohlich ED. New drug development and the health care crisis. *Hypertension.* 1994;24(5):529–530.

Fuhr U, Weiss M, Kroemer HK, et al. Systematic screening for pharmacokinetic interactions during drug development. *Int J Clin Pharmacol Ther.* 1996;34(4):139–151.

Gant TW. Application of toxicogenomics in drug development. *Drug News Perspect.* 2003;16(4):217–221.

Getz K. Improving protocol design feasibility to drive drug development economics and performance. *Int J Environ Res Public Health.* 2014;11(5):5069–5080.

Ginsburg GS, Konstance RP, Allsbrook JS, Schulman KA. Implications of pharmacogenomics for drug development and clinical practice. *Arch Intern Med.* 2005;165(20):2331–2336.

Glickman SW, Rasiel EB, Hamilton CD, Kubataev A, Schulman KA. Medicine: a portfolio model of drug development for tuberculosis. *Science.* 2006;311(5765):1246–1247.

Goozner M. A much-needed corrective on drug development costs. *JAMA Intern Med.* 2017;177(11):1575–1576.

Hill-McManus D, Marshall S, Liu J, Willke RJ, Hughes DA. Linked pharmacometric-pharmacoeconomic modeling and simulation in clinical drug development. *Clin Pharmacol Ther.* 2021 Jul;110(1):49–63.

Hirsch IB, Martinez J, Dorsey ER, et al. Incorporating site-less clinical trials into drug development: a framework for action. *Clin Ther.* 2017;39(5):1064–1076.

Howie LJ, Hirsch BR, Abernethy AP. A comparison of FDA and EMA drug approval: implications for drug development and cost of care. *Oncology* (Williston Park). 2013;27(12):1195, 1198–1200, 1202 passim.

Hughes DA, Walley T. Economic evaluations during early (phase II) drug development: a role for clinical trial simulations? *Pharmacoeconomics.* 2001;19(11):1069–1077.

Hunt CA, Guzy S, Weiner DL. A forecasting approach to accelerate drug development. *Stat Med.* 1998;17(15–16):1725–1740; discussion 1741–1743.

Jacobson-Kram D, Mills G. Leveraging exploratory investigational new drug studies to accelerate drug development. *Clin Cancer Res.* 2008;14(12):3670–3674.

Jayasundara K, Hollis A, Krahn M, Mamdani M, Hoch JS, Grootendorst P. Estimating the clinical cost of drug development for orphan versus non-orphan drugs. *Orphanet J Rare Dis.* 2019;14(1):12.

Jönsson B. Bringing in health technology assessment and cost-effectiveness considerations at an early stage of drug development. *Mol Oncol.* 2015;9(5):1025–1033.

Joshi HN. Drug development and imperfect design. *Int J Pharm.* 2007;343(1–2):1–3.

Kaufman L, Gore K, Zandee JC. Data standardization, pharmaceutical drug development, and the 3Rs. *ILAR J.* 2016;57(2):109–119.

Kesselheim AS, Wang B, Avorn J. Defining "innovativeness" in drug development: a systematic review. *Clin Pharmacol Ther.* 2013;94(3):336–348.

Khor TO, Ibrahim S, Kong AN. Toxicogenomics in drug discovery and drug development: potential applications and future challenges. *Pharm Res.* 2006;23(8):1659–1664.

Knight-Schrijver VR, Chelliah V, Cucurull-Sanchez L, Le Novère N. The promises of quantitative systems pharmacology modelling for drug development. *Comput Struct Biotechnol J.* 2016;14:363–370.

Kola I. The state of innovation in drug development. *Clin Pharmacol Ther.* 2008;83(2):227–230.

Kuhlmann J. Alternative strategies in drug development: clinical pharmacological aspects. *Int J Clin Pharmacol Ther.* 1999;37(12):575–583.

Kumar B, Prakash A, Ruhela RK, Medhi B. Potential of metabolomics in preclinical and clinical drug development. *Pharmacol Rep.* 2014;66(6):956–963.

Lakkis MM, DeCristofaro MF, Ahr HJ, Mansfield TA. Application of toxicogenomics to drug development. *Expert Rev Mol Diagn.* 2002;2(4):337–345.

Lara Gongora AB, Carvalho Oliveira LJ, Jardim DL. Impact of the biomarker enrichment strategy in drug development. *Expert Rev Mol Diagn.* 2020;20(6):611–618.

Lathia CD. Biomarkers and surrogate endpoints: how and when might they impact drug development? *Dis Markers.* 2002;18(2):83–90.

Lee H. Genetically engineered mouse models for drug development and preclinical trials. *Biomol Ther* (Seoul). 2014;22(4):267–274.

Lendrem DW, Lendrem BC. Torching the Haystack: modelling fast-fail strategies in drug development. *Drug Discov Today.* 2013;18(7–8):331–336.

Lieberman R, McMichael J. Role of pharmacokinetic-pharmacodynamic principles in rational and cost-effective drug development. *Ther Drug Monit.* 1996;18(4):423–428.

Liebman MN. Biomedical informatics: the future for drug development. *Drug Discov Today.* 2002;7(20 Suppl) Suppl:S197–S203.

Lindsley CW. New statistics on the cost of new drug development and the trouble with CNS drugs. *ACS Chem Neurosci.* 2014;5(12):1142.

Lockhart MM, Babar ZU, Garg S. New Zealand's drug development industry--strengths and opportunities. *N Z Med J.* 2010;123(1317):52–58.

Mahajan R, Gupta K. Food and drug administration's critical path initiative and innovations in drug development paradigm: challenges, progress, and controversies. *J Pharm Bioallied Sci.* 2010;2(4): 307–313.

Mandema JW, Gibbs M, Boyd RA, Wada DR, Pfister M. Model-based meta-analysis for comparative efficacy and safety: application in drug development and beyond. *Clin Pharmacol Ther.* 2011;90(6):766–769.

Mason M, Levenson J, Quillin J. Direct-to-consumer genetic testing and orphan drug development. *Genet Test Mol Biomarkers.* 2017;21(8):456–463.

Mattes JA. Patent laws: could changes enhance drug development ment? *Arch Gen Psychiatry.* 1997;54(10):970.

Maxmen A. Busting the billion-dollar myth: how to slash the cost of drug development. *Nature.* 2016;536(7617):388–390.

Meekings KN, Williams CS, Arrowsmith JE. Orphan drug development: an economically viable strategy for biopharma R&D. *Drug Discov Today.* 2012;17(13–14):660–664.

Melethil S. Patent issues in drug development: perspectives of a pharmaceutical scientist-attorney. *AAPS J.* 2005;7(3):E723–E728.

Michelle A, Nathan PC, Viswanath D, Zhuyin L, Sitta GS. All considerations for early phase drug discovery, in assay guidance manual [https://www.ncbi.nlm.nih.gov/books/NBK53196/]. Licensed under a Creative Commons Attribution-NonCommercial-ShareAlike 3.0 Unported license (CC BY-NC-SA 3.0)

Mikami T, Aoki M, Kimura T. The application of mass spectrometry to proteomics and metabolomics in biomarker discovery and drug development. *Curr Mol Pharmacol.* 2012;5(2):301–316.

Moghadam BT, Alvarsson J, Holm M, Eklund M, Carlsson L, Spjuth O. Scaling predictive modeling in drug development with cloud computing. *J Chem Inf Model.* 2015;55(1):19–25.

Morgan S, Grootendorst P, Lexchin J, Cunningham C, Greyson D. The cost of drug development: a systematic review. *Health Policy.* 2011;100(1):4–17.

Mould DR. Model-based meta-analysis: an important tool for making quantitative decisions during drug development. *Clin Pharmacol Ther.* 2012;92(3):283–286.

Mudd SR, Comley RA, Bergstrom M, et al. Molecular imaging in oncology drug development. *Drug Discov Today.* 2017;22(1):140–147.

Murphy MP. Current pharmacogenomic approaches to clinical drug development. *Pharmacogenomics.* 2000;1(2):115–123.
Naci H, Carter AW, Mossialos E. Why the drug development pipeline is not delivering better medicines. *BMJ.* 2015;351:h5542.
Nakayama N, Bando Y, Fukuda T, et al. Developments of mass spectrometry-based technologies for effective drug development linked with clinical proteomes. *Drug Metab Pharmacokinet.* 2016;31(1):3–11.
Nation RL. Chirality in new drug development. Clinical pharmacokinetic considerations. *Clin Pharmacokinet.* 1994;27(4):249–255.
Niblack JF. Why are drug development programs growing in size and cost? A view from industry. *Food Drug Law J.* 1997;52(2):151–154.
Nordsletten DA, Yankama B, Umeton R, Ayyadurai VA, Dewey CF. Multiscale mathematical modeling to support drug development. *IEEE Trans Biomed Eng.* 2011;58(12):3508–3512.
Norman P. Predictive toxicology in drug development. *Drug News Perspect.* 2003;16(4):254–256.
Orloff J, Douglas F, Pinheiro J, et al. The future of drug development: advancing clinical trial design. *Nat Rev Drug Discov.* 2009;8(12):949–957.
Pastores GM, Gupta P. Orphan drug development. *Pediatr Endocrinol Rev.* 2013;11 Suppl 1:64–67.
Portela C. Clinical needs as a starting point for different strategies in computational drug development. *Drug Res* (Stuttg). 2019;69(8):458–466.
Poste G, Carbone DP, Parkinson DR, Verweij J, Hewitt SM, Jessup JM. Leveling the playing field: bringing development of biomarkers and molecular diagnostics up to the standards for drug development. *Clin Cancer Res.* 2012;18(6):1515–1523.
Preskorn SH. CNS drug development: part III: future directions. *J Psychiatr Pract.* 2011;17(1):49–52.
Rahmoune H, Martins-de-Souza D, Guest PC. Application of proteomic approaches to accelerate drug development for psychiatric disorders. *Adv Exp Med Biol.* 2017;974:69–84.
Rajman I. PK/PD modelling and simulations: utility in drug development. *Drug Discov Today.* 2008;13(7–8):341–346.
Ramamoorthi R, Graef KM, Dent J. Repurposing pharma assets: an accelerated mechanism for strengthening the schistosomiasis drug development pipeline. *Future Med Chem.* 2015;7(6):727–735.
Rashid MBMA. Artificial intelligence effecting a paradigm shift in drug development. *SLAS Technol.* 2020:2472630320956931.
Rawlins MD. Cutting the cost of drug development? *Nat Rev Drug Discov.* 2004;3(4):360–364.
Reynolds KS. Acceleration of drug development: a collaboration of many stakeholders. *Clin Pharmacol Ther.* 2013;93(6):455–459.
Ross BD. High-field MRS in clinical drug development. *Expert Opin Drug Discov.* 2013;8(7):849–863.
Rumore MM. The decline in new drug development. *Am Pharm.* 1992;NS32(4):73–78.
Safir MC, Bhavnani SM, Slover CM, Ambrose PG, Rubino CM. Antibacterial drug development: a new approach is needed for the field to survive and thrive. *Antibiotics* (Basel). 2020;9(7):412.
Samara E, Granneman R. Role of population pharmacokinetics in drug development. A pharmaceutical industry perspective. *Clin Pharmacokinet.* 1997;32(4):294–312.
Sasaki RR, McGibbon G, Lee MS, Murray CL, Pharr B. New perspectives and lessons learned in the identification of impurities in drug development. *Drug Discov Today.* 2014;19(11):1691–1695.
Sertkaya A, Jessup A, Wong HH. Promoting antibacterial drug development: select policies and challenges. *Appl Health Econ Health Policy.* 2017;15(1):113–118.
Seymour M. The best model for humans is human -- how to accelerate early drug development safely. *Altern Lab Anim.* 2009;37 Suppl 1:61–65.
Shanti A, Teo J, Stefanini C. In vitro immune organs-on-chip for drug development: a review. *Pharmaceutics.* 2018;10(4):278.
Shaw DL. Is open science the future of drug development? *Yale J Biol Med.* 2017;90(1):147–151.
Somberg JC. Drug development costs. *J Clin Pharmacol.* 1987;27(5):335.
Song Y, Dhodda R, Zhang J, Sydor J. A high efficiency, high quality and low cost internal regulated bioanalytical laboratory to support drug development needs. *Bioanalysis.* 2014;6(10):1295–1309.
Srinivasan M, White A, Chaturvedula A, et al. Incorporating pharmacometrics into pharmacoeconomic models: applications from drug development. *Pharmacoeconomics.* 2020;38(10):1031–1042.
Stahel R, Bogaerts J, Ciardiello F, et al. Optimising translational oncology in clinical practice: strategies to accelerate progress in drug development. *Cancer Treat Rev.* 2015;41(2):129–135.

Subbaraman N. Flawed arithmetic on drug development costs. *Nat Biotechnol.* 2011;29(5):381.

Sultana SR, Marshall S, Davis J, Littman BH. Experiences with dose finding in patients in early drug development: the use of biomarkers in early decision making. *Ernst Schering Res Found Workshop.* 2007;(59):65–79.

Suryawanshi S, Zhang L, Pfister M, Meibohm B. The current role of model-based drug development. *Expert Opin Drug Discov.* 2010;5(4):311–321.

Turner SM, Hellerstein MK. Emerging applications of kinetic biomarkers in preclinical and clinical drug development. *Curr Opin Drug Discov Devel.* 2005;8(1):115–126.

Uteng M, Urban L, Brees D, et al. Safety differentiation: emerging competitive edge in drug development. *Drug Discov Today.* 2019;24(1):285–292.

van der Laan S, Salvetat N, Weissmann D, Molina F. Emerging RNA editing biomarkers will foster drug development. *Drug Discov Today.* 2017;22(7):1056–1063.

Van Walle I, Gansemans Y, Parren PW, Stas P, Lasters I. Immunogenicity screening in protein drug development. *Expert Opin Biol Ther.* 2007;7(3):405–418.

Venditti JM. Preclinical drug development: rationale and methods. *Semin Oncol.* 1981;8(4):349–361.

Vernon JA, Golec JH, Dimasi JA. Drug development costs when financial risk is measured using the Fama-French three-factor model. *Health Econ.* 2010;19(8):1002–1005.

Wagner HN. Nonimaging detectors in drug development and approval. *J Clin Pharmacol.* 2001;41(S7):125S–126S.

Wang YI, Oleaga C, Long CJ, et al. Self-contained, low-cost body-on-a-chip systems for drug development. *Exp Biol Med* (Maywood). 2017;242(17):1701–1713.

Webb TR. Improving the efficiency of the drug development by expanding the scope of the role of medicinal chemists in drug discovery. *ACS Med Chem Lett.* 2018;9(12):1153–1155.

Wei AH. Accelerating early drug development: come on down under! *Ann Oncol.* 2017;28(7):1655–1657.

Wen Y, Yang ST. The future of microfluidic assays in drug development. *Expert Opin Drug Discov.* 2008;3(10):1237–1253.

Yamane N, Igarashi A, Kusama M, Maeda K, Ikeda T, Sugiyama Y. Cost-effectiveness analysis of microdose clinical trials in drug development. *Drug Metab Pharmacokinet.* 2013;28(3):187–195.

Yan EC, Chen L. A cost-related approach for evaluating drug development programs. *Stat Med.* 2004;23(18):2863–2873.

Young D. Letting the genome out of the bottle: prospects for new drug development. *Ann N Y Acad Sci.* 2001;953:146–150.

Zhang W, Wang J, Menon S. Advancing cancer drug development through precision medicine and innovative designs. *J Biopharm Stat.* 2018;28(2):229–244.

Zhao M, Yang CC. Drug repositioning to accelerate drug development using social media data: computational study on Parkinson disease. *J Med Internet Res.* 2018;20(10):e271.

15

Intellectual Property

EVERYTHING THAT CAN BE INVENTED HAS BEEN INVENTED.

—Charles H Duell, United States Patent Office Director, telling President McKinley to abolish the office in 1899

15.1 Background

Intellectual property is a major consideration in the new drug discovery platform. The high cost of development can only be rationalized if the companies could recoup their investment. Therefore, understanding what intellectual property entails is additionally important in developing new technologies around the protected inventions. Unfortunately, most scientists are generally not familiar with the nuances of intellectual property laws.

Intellectual property is the lifeline of every industry; it is a lot more than the patents (Figure 15.1), but the focus pertinent to the reader of this chapter is the patenting process associated with new drug development.

As the new drug discoveries become more complex like the biological medicines, patents' scope expands fast from the molecular entity to its manufacturing process and the delivery systems. Most research entities continuously develop the freedom to operate landscape requiring close collaboration between the legal teams and the scientists. Still, litigation is widespread in this industry. This chapter focuses on how scientists can collaborate with the legal teams and, in most cases, themselves suggest innovative steps to strengthen the value of their discoveries.

Fine points about the vocabulary used in a patent application and the legal language are essential to understand. All types of patents, differences in the international patent laws, and a detailed description of patents related to a new class of drugs are presented in this chapter.

15.2 About Patents

The term "patent" is derived from "letters patent," an open letter by which a sovereign entity conferred a special privilege or right on the subject. The first recorded patent was granted to Filippo Brunelleschi in 1421 in Florence, Italy, for an industrial invention. Since then, countries have set their own rules to grant patents, including the duration, types of patents, and filing rules.

An invention is a government-granted property right (an owned object of property that comes into existence the moment it is invented) for an innovation. For a limited period, a US patent allows inventors to "exclude anyone from creating, using, offering for sale, or selling their invention within the United States or importing their invention into the United States" (https://www.uspto.gov/web/offices/pac/mpep/s301.html).

There are two types of exclusivities available. One is from a patent granted. The other applies in the US is the regulatory exclusivity of 12 years since the launch date for biological drugs and five years for chemical drugs, regardless of the patent protection.

A new drug entity is generally protectable as a new chemical structure, a new synthesis or manufacture method, and new use. In chemical entities, the manufacturing method is usually not exclusive as other

DOI: 10.1201/9781003146933-15

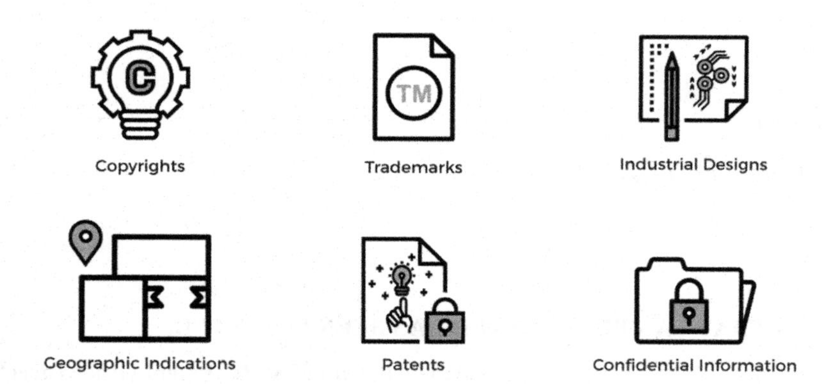

FIGURE 15.1 Types of intellectual properties. Source: www.dreamstime.com/types-intellectual-property-eight-types-intellectual-property-image126810421.

methods can synthesize a product. Still, in complex drugs, the manufacturing process can be protected by various patents, including the upstream parameters, downstream processes, and further purification.

Table 15.1 lists the 51,566 patents protecting biological drugs in the order of the number of patents protecting each entity. This database will serve as a starting point for deciding which product to develop and comes in handy when creating a freedom-to-operate document for the approved biological products.

15.3 Patent Landscape

A patent is awarded in various legal jurisdictions based on various considerations, but most commonly, it defines the boundary lines of invention, novelty, non-obviousness, and utility. Intellectual property includes additional elements.

As of May 2020, there were more than ten million patents issued in the US. The first US patent was issued in 1790 (three that year), and it was not until 1836 that the first patent was issued to a foreigner. The rate of patent rejections is highly variable based upon technology and, interestingly, whether the inventor is a US citizen (Table 15.2).

The global filing of patents is shown in Figure 15.2 from 2004 to 2018, as reported by 160 patent offices worldwide.

Table 15.3 lists links to patent search resources around the world. There are over 160 patent offices around the world.

15.4 Patent Laws

Patents give the patent holder the right to prevent others from making, using, selling, or importing a patented invention for a set period in the United States (or the nation of the patent) (generally, twenty years from the date a patent application was filed). A person who does so without the patent holder's consent infringes the patent and may be subject to monetary damages and other legal remedies. Patent exclusivity encourages innovation by allowing the patent holder to recuperate any costs invested during research and development. Patentees may also benefit from exclusivity since it shields them from the competition, allowing them to charge higher-than-competitive prices for patent-protected items. Pharmaceuticals, which are expensive to create yet quickly imitated once on the market, require patent incentives.

Beyond the active ingredient, pharmaceutical patents can cover a wide range of aspects of medication or biologics. Among the claims made by such "secondary patents" are:

- Techniques of employing the pharmaceutical (e.g., to treat a certain ailment); methods of manufacturing or technologies utilized to create the pharmaceutical; methods or technologies for administering the pharmaceutical; or additional compounds connected to the active ingredient, such as intermediaries.

TABLE 15.1

Patents Protecting Biological Medicines

Biological Drug	Number of Patents
Parathyroid hormone	3396
Interferon alfa-2b	3168
Peanut	3139
Gonadotropin, chorionic	3099
Somatropin	2605
Urokinase	2436
Botulism antitoxin heptavalent	1757
Bevacizumab	1712
Albumin human	1702
Hyaluronidase	1588
Rituximab	1390
Hyaluronidase	1330
Zoster vaccine live	1170
Histamine	1151
Alemtuzumab	972
Albumin human	847
Panitumumab	837
Trastuzumab	828
Filgrastim	816
Adalimumab	796
Collagenase	782
Trastuzumab	750
Hyaluronidase-oysk	720
Darbepoetin alfa	700
Etanercept	598
Insulin human	592
Asparaginase	583
Cetuximab	552
Epoetin alfa	518
Insulin recombinant human	504
Nivolumab	399
Bacillus anthracis	369
Infliximab	338
Pancrelipase amylase,	315
Protease	315
Anakinra	303
Immunoglobulin g	282
Peginterferon alfa-2b	264
Aprotinin	254
Tocilizumab	253
Alteplase	243
Interferon beta-1a	238
Palivizumab	236
Sargramostim	230
Basiliximab	222
Insulin aspart	207
Insulin lispro	195

TABLE 15.1 (CONTINUED)

Patents Protecting Biological Medicines

Biological Drug	Number of Patents
Onabotulinumtoxina	190
Ipilimumab	185
Denosumab	184
Abciximab	179
Insulin glargine	178
Pertuzumab	175
Golimumab	173
Human immunoglobulin g	165
Natalizumab	163
Ranibizumab	158
Daclizumab	154
Ibritumomab tiuxetan	137
Aldesleukin	134
Belimumab	129
Ustekinumab	129
Chymopapain	128
Hemin	113
Pembrolizumab	112
Ofatumumab	111
Gemtuzumab ozogamicin	108
Lixisenatide	108
Omalizumab	108
Bacillus calmette-guerin	101
Pegfilgrastim	94
Pegaspargase	89
Denileukin diftitox	84
Influenza virus vaccine	84
Aflibercept	80
Atezolizumab	80
Interferon beta-1b	79
Brentuximab vedotin	78
Eculizumab	75
Immune globulin	74
Peginterferon alfa-2a	74
Ramucirumab	72
Certolizumab pegol	70
Pancrelipase	70
Abatacept	68
Mepolizumab	66
Follitropin alfa/beta	60
Insulin degludec	60
Pegvisomant	60
Avelumab	56
Dulaglutide	56
Botulinum toxin type b	52
Albiglutide	51
Tenecteplase	49

(Continued)

TABLE 15.1 (CONTINUED)
Patents Protecting Biological Medicines

Biological Drug	Number of Patents
Imiglucerase	48
Rasburicase	48
Sipuleucel-t	46
Ocrelizumab	45
Reteplase	44
Insulin detemir	42
Interferon gamma-1b	39
Palifermin	39
Elotuzumab	38
Menotropins fsh 1h	37
Fibrinogen human	33
Fibrinogen human	33
Hepatitis b vaccine recombinant	33
Durvalumab	32
Urofollitropin	32
Insulin lispro recombinant	31
Rabies vaccine	30
Ado-trastuzumab emtansine	28
Daratumumab	28
Obinutuzumab	28
Canakinumab	27
Agalsidase beta	26
Alirocumab	26
Thrombin human	26
Insulin aspart recombinant	25
Insulin detemir recombinant	25
Menotropins	25
Necitumumab	25
Dermatophagoides farinae	24
Siltuximab	24
Thyrotropin alfa	24
Bacillus calmette-guerin substrain tice live antigen	23
Rilonacept	23
Dermatophagoides pteronyssinus	22
Reslizumab	21
Autologous cultured chondrocytes	20
Romiplostim	20
Becaplermin	19
Belatacept	19
Blinatumomab	19
Evolocumab	19
Vedolizumab	19
Antihemophilic factor recombinant	18
Laronidase	18
Sarilumab	18
Anti-inhibitor coagulant complex	16

TABLE 15.1 (CONTINUED)
Patents Protecting Biological Medicines

Biological Drug	Number of Patents
Antihemophilic factor human	16
Inotuzumab ozogamicin	16
Interferon alfa-n3	16
Secukinumab	16
Benralizumab	15
Hepatitis a vaccine	15
Insulin glulisine recombinant	15
Metreleptin	15
Abobotulinumtoxina	14
Ambrosia artemisiifolia	14
Histamine phosphate	14
Human papillomavirus quadrivalent types 6, 11, 16, and 18 vaccine, recombinant	14
Incobotulinumtoxina	14
Dupilumab	13
Corticorelin ovine triflutate	12
Immune globulin intravenous human	11
Capromab pendetide	10
Collagenase clostridium histolyticum	10
Dornase alfa	10
Ixekizumab	10
Pneumococcal vaccine polyvalent	10
Tuberculin purified protein derivative	10
Ziv-aflibercept	10
Antihemophilic factor recombinant	9
Olaratumab	9
Raxibacumab	9
Antihemophilic factor human	8
Asfotase alfa	8
Beractant	8
Immune globulin human	8
Ocriplasmin	8
Salmonella typhi ty21a	8
Anti-thymocyte globulin rabbit	7
Antihemophilic factor/von Willebrand factor complex human	7
Brodalumab	7
Cat hair	7
Factor ix complex	7
Galsulfase	7
Choriogonadotropin alfa	6
Dinutuximab	6
Human c1-esterase inhibitor	6
Latrodectus mactans	6

(Continued)

TABLE 15.1 (CONTINUED)

Patents Protecting Biological Medicines

Biological Drug	Number of Patents
Sacrosidase	6
Varicella virus vaccine live	6
Velaglucerase alfa	6
von Willebrand factor recombinant	6
Antithrombin iii human	5
Somatropin [rdna origin]	5
Alglucosidase alfa	4
Antihemophilic factor, recombinant	4
Calfactant	4
Desirudin recombinant	4
Ecallantide	4
Equine thymocyte immune globulin	4
Hepatitis a vaccine, inactivated	4
Idursulfase	4
Isatuximab-irfc	4
Methoxy polyethylene glycol-epoetin beta	4
Peginterferon beta-1a	4
Poractant alfa	4
Rho d immune globulin	4
Smallpox vaccinia vaccine, live	4
Talimogene laherparepvec	4
Coagulation factor ix recombinant	3
Fremanezumab-vfrm	3
House dust mite, dermatophagoides pteronyssinus	3
Human plasma proteins	3
Imciromab pentetate	3
Mecasermin rinfabate recombinant	3
Plasma protein fraction human	3
Ravulizumab-cwvz	3
Sebelipase alfa	3
Taliglucerase alfa	3
Technetium tc-99m albumin colloid kit	3
Asparaginase erwinia chrysanthemi	2
Bezlotoxumab	2
Clostridium tetani toxoid antigen formaldehyde inactivated,	2
Diphtheria and tetanus toxoids and acellular pertussis adsorbed and inactivated poliovirus vaccine	2

TABLE 15.1 (CONTINUED)

Patents Protecting Biological Medicines

Biological Drug	Number of Patents
Diphtheria and tetanus toxoids and acellular pertussis adsorbed, hepatitis b recombinant and inactivated poliovirus vaccine combined	2
Diphtheria and tetanus toxoids and acellular pertussis vaccine adsorbed	2
Guselkumab	2
Hepatitis a and hepatitis b recombinant vaccine	2
Idarucizumab	2
Immune globulin infusion human	2
Insulin glargine recombinant	2
Lixisenatide	2
Insulin recombinant human	
Insulin susp isophane recombinant human	2
Isatuximab	2
Meningococcal group b vaccine	2
Neisseria meningitidis group a capsular polysaccharide diphtheria toxoid conjugate antigen	2
Ovine digoxin immune fab	2
Pneumococcal 13-valent conjugate vaccine	2
Rotavirus vaccine, live, oral	2
Coagulation factor ix recombinant human	1
Coagulation factor viia recombinant	1
Elosulfase alfa	1
Human fibrinogen, human thrombin	1
Human papillomavirus 9-valent vaccine, recombinant	1
Influenza vaccine, adjuvanted	1
Insulin aspart	1
Insulin degludec	1
Liraglutide	1
Obiltoxaximab	1
Pegademase bovine	1
Polatuzumab vedotin-piiq	1
Poliovirus type 1 antigen	1

TABLE 15.2

Total Patent Applications and Awarded Patents by the USPTO from 1790 to 2019

Type of Application	Total Filed	Percentage Approved
Utility	19,774,364	53%
Design	870,770	69%
Plant	35,161	89%
All	21,064,418	54%
Foreigners	4,051,671	35%

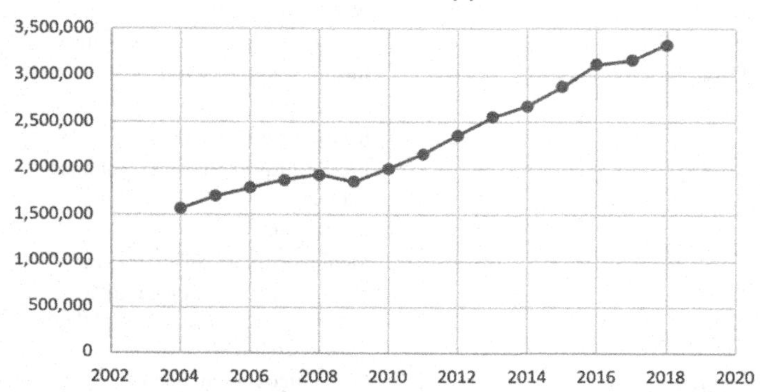

FIGURE 15.2 Yearly global patent filing 2004–2017.

TABLE 15.3

Patent Search Resources

US	www.uspto.gov
India	www.ipindia.nic.in/
Europe	www.european-patent-office.org
Japan	www.jpo.go.jp/
Korea	www.kipo.go.kr
Italy	www.info-brevetti.org/
Canada	http://strategis.ic.gc.ca/sc_mrksv/cipo/
Australia	www.ipaustralia.gov.au/
African Region	www.aripo.wipo.net/
New Zealand	www.iponz.govt.nz/
Singapore	www.ipos.gov.sg/
UK	www.ukpats.org.uk
WIPO	www.wipo.int/patentscope/en/
PCT: Patent Cooperative Treaty	www.wto.org/english/tratop_e/trips_e/trips_e.htm www.pctlearningcenter.org/
Public Patent Foundation	www.pubpat.org/index.html
Intellectual Property Owners Association	www.ipo.org/
Global: Espacenet	https://worldwide.espacenet.com/patent/
China	http://english.sipo.gov.cn
Trilateral: US, Japan, EU	www.trilateral.net/index
ASEAN	www.aseanip.org

15.4.1 Pharmaceutical Patenting Practices

From the patent holders' perspective, the practices described below are appropriate uses of their patents' legal rights. However, critics view these practices as harmful strategies that exploit the patent system in ways that Congress did not intend.

- Evergreening, also known as patent "layering" or "life-cycle management," is a process in which drug companies purportedly try to extend their patent monopolies on medications by getting new patents as old ones expire. Because diverse pharmaceutical products are patentable, a single pharmaceutical product can be protected by hundreds of patents. According to critics of evergreening, secondary patents are generally for small modifications or auxiliary parts of a pharmaceutical product and effectively extend patent protection of the original product beyond Congress's term. Defenders argue that any extra patents must include significant inventions and enhancements to existing items and that so-called secondary patents must pass the same patentability and inspection procedures as any other patent.
- The process by which a brand manufacturer leverages its current dominating market position to urge doctors, pharmacists, and customers to "jump" from one drug with soon-expiring patents to a newer version of the same (or similar) drug with later-expiring patents is known as "product hopping." An extended-release form, a new dosage, a changed mode of administration (e.g., capsules to tablets), or a slight chemical modification could all be part of the new edition of the medication. The brand maker may use a marketing campaign and discounts and rebates to encourage the shift. Product hopping usually takes one of two forms: a "hard switch," in which the brand removes the original product from the market, or a "soft switch," The brand leaves the original product on the market. Product hopping opponents argue that the new product usually provides little or no clinical benefit. The adjustment is made solely to avoid generic competition by removing the original product's market before the predicted generic entrance date. Manufacturers have legitimate motivations to develop and patent new items, according to their defenders. Clinical advantages are frequently found in novel products (for example, fewer side effects or better patient compliance).
- "Patent thickets," as the phrase suggests, refers to a brand manufacturer's strategy of acquiring many patents relating to a single product, preventing competitors from entering the market or making it too expensive and hazardous to do so. Manufacturers got an average of 71 patents on each drug, according to a recent survey of the top 12 drugs by gross US sales. When it comes to biologics, concerns about patent thickets are more widespread than with small-molecule chemical medications. This may be due, at least in part, to the complexity of producing a medicine using living cells, which provides many options for patenting novel techniques or patenting the use of a different medium for cell growth or a dosage change. Critics argue that patent thickets are created by patenting minor or secondary improvements, which effectively delays competition because generics or biosimilars must challenge or design around each patent, which can be costly or complex. The patents on these products, according to their proponents, illustrate the types of advances that the patent rules were intended to encourage. During the patent examination procedure, each patent was found to be legitimate.
- "Pay-for-delay" settlements occur when generic (or biosimilar) manufacturers submit shortened applications for products covered by certain unexpired patents, and brand manufacturers may commence patent litigation under Hatch-Waxman and the BPCIA procedures. Some brand manufacturers have paid (or otherwise compensated) generic producers in exchange for the generic manufacturers agreeing to postpone the market launch. The Supreme Court has ruled that this method, known as "reverse payment" or "pay-for-delay," maybe a legal exercise of patent exclusivity in some cases but may violate antitrust laws in others. Pay-for-delay agreements, according to critics, are used by brand manufacturers to safeguard weak patents from invalidation; yet, because pay-for-delay agreements end the litigation, patent validity and infringement problems remain unanswered. As a result, critics argue that pay-for-delay harms competition by allowing the brand manufacturer to 1) avoid the danger of having its patents invalidated,

2) postpone generic competition from entering the market, and 3) effectively extend its exclusive right to market the listed drug. Defenders argue that settlements are a reasonable means to decrease the cost and risk of litigation, pointing out that the vast majority of claims are settled in all areas of law. Furthermore, defenders claim that the case might end with the brand maker winning, thereby barring competition until the patent period expires. Defenders argue that settling the case ensures generic entry before the patent period expires.

- Combinations of these techniques can be used. Although these tactics are described separately, opponents argue that they are sometimes utilized together. Some brand manufacturers, for example, may use a pay-for-delay settlement to postpone generic entry by combining product hopping with pay-for-delay settlements. On the other hand, the brand manufacturer shifts the market to a new product that is protected by patent exclusivity.

15.5 Types of Patents

Utility patents are for a new method, composition, or device. Design patents are for the new ornamental design of an article of manufacture. Finally, plant patents provide patent protection for any asexually reproduced distinct and new variety of plants.

Patents for utility and plant inventions are normally issued for 20 years, beginning on the date of grant and ending 20 years after the application was filed. Therefore, you must pay the relevant maintenance costs promptly.

Design patents are valid for 14 years from the date of grant. Thus, design patents do not require any ongoing maintenance expenses.

The patent is personal property: it can be sold, assigned, or transferred as determined by the owner. Of course, there can be disputes, in which case the authority or jurisdiction concerned has to mediate and investigate infringement. If infringement is found, a determination must be made to grant penalties to the violator and award damages to the rightful owner.

In the 1990s, the establishment of the World Trade Organization set forth a common minimum set of rights that should be granted to all patent owners by governments and 20 years (from the date the application was filed) as the term of the patent.

15.5.1 Utility Model in the EU

A utility model is a type of intellectual property protection that protects inventions and is similar to a patent. Many countries have this type of right, although the United States, the United Kingdom, and Canada, for example, do not. A utility model is comparable to a patent, except it is usually less expensive to obtain and maintain. It has a shorter term (generally six to 15 years), shorter grant lag, and less stringent patentability requirements. It is only available for inventions in certain technology fields and/or only for products in some countries. Utility models can be described as second-class patents.

While no international convention mandates the protection of utility models (unlike copyright, trademarks, or patents) and they are not covered by the TRIPS agreement, they are covered by the Paris Convention for the Protection of Industrial Property, which means that countries that do protect utility models must adhere to rules like national treatment and priority. Utility models are also available through the Patent Cooperation Treaty (PCT) system of international patent applications (in countries that have a utility model system).

A utility model is a statutory exclusive right granted for a short time (the "term") in exchange for an inventor providing enough teaching of his or her invention to allow a person of ordinary ability in the relevant art to perform it. Utility model laws offer rights comparable to patent laws, although they are better suited to "incremental inventions." Specifically, a utility model is a "right to restrict others from commercially using a protected invention without the authorization of the right holder(s) for a specified length of time" (https://ec.europa.eu/growth/industry/policy/intellectual-property/patents/utility-models_en).

The "utility model" is defined by terms like "petty patent," "innovation patent," "short-term patents," "minor patent," and "little patent," among others. The German and Austrian utility model is known as the "Gebrauchsmuster," which impacted countries like Japan.

The invention must be novel in most nations with utility model legislation. Many patent or utility model offices, on the other hand, do not conduct a substantive review and instead just grant the utility model after verifying that utility model applications meet formal requirements. The awarding process for a utility model is frequently referred to as "utility model registration." Furthermore, some countries restrict certain subject matters from the protection of utility models. Methods (i.e., procedures), chemical compounds, plants, and animals, for example, are not protected as utility models in some nations.

An invention can also be protected in the EU under utility models that have:

- Registered territorial IP right.
- Available in a limited number of countries.
- No central filing in Europe.
- Protection for up to ten years.
- Search report in some countries only.
- Registered and published after a few months.
- Generally, no substantive examination (novelty, inventiveness, industrial applicability).
- Reviewed only in invalidation or infringement proceedings.

The means of protecting the utility model include:

Contractual

- Restrictive covenants in employment contracts.
- Non-disclosure agreements.

Practical

- Limited access to information.
- "Need to know."
- Encryption of data.
- Monitored entry to installations.

15.5.2 Provisional Application

In the US, one can take the option of filing a Provisional Application for Patent. The provisional application discloses detailed information about the invention, but not to the regular application's depth. You must file a regular patent application on the invention of your provisional application within one year.

The provisional application establishes a registration date for your invention earlier than the ultimate date of patent issue after filing the regular application. In no way does the provisional resemble a regular utility patent, as it expires in a year, cannot be searched, and "it does not start a 20-year patent term running" (https://www.uspto.gov/patents/basics/types-patent-applications/provisional-application-patent).

Provisional applications are usually filed for reasons of urgency to establish priority. However, sometimes there are many good reasons not to file a provisional application, such as higher overall costs and the extra time delay before the patent is granted (prosecution will begin only on the utility application). In addition, US patent laws have been amended to allow upgrading of the provisional application into a utility patent application.

An alternative means of proving that you were the first to think of the idea is a disclosure document. A disclosure document is "evidence of conception" of an idea or an invention. In no way does it substitute for a provisional application or a regular utility patent application. For a fee of $10, it enables the applicant to have a recorded proof of date of conception provided the regular patent application follows it up within two years of receipt of the disclosure document at the USPTO. Unlike a provisional application,

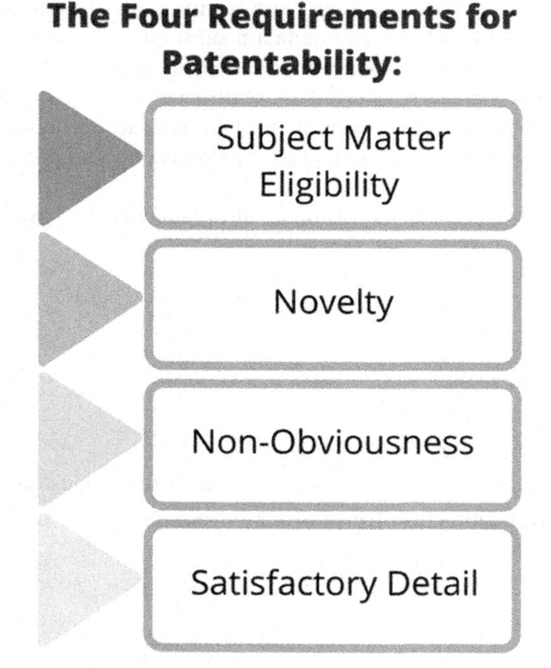

The Four Requirements for Patentability:
Subject Matter Eligibility
Novelty
Non-Obviousness
Satisfactory Detail

FIGURE 15.3 Elements of patentability.

the disclosure document's date cannot be considered an effective filing date. Because the provisional application provides an earlier filing date, most intellectual property offices recommend filing the provisional application and not bothering with the disclosure document (Figure 15.3).

15.6 Nonobviousness

Under European patent law, the term "inventive step" is commonly used, whereas, in American patent law, the term "non-obviousness" is commonly employed. The innovative step and non-obviousness represent a basic patentability condition found in most patent laws, which states that an invention must be sufficiently inventive—non-obvious—to be patented. "[The] non-obviousness principle examines whether the invention is an acceptable distance beyond or above state of the art," to put it another way (https://www.uspto.gov/web/offices/pac/mpep/s2141.html). The purpose of the inventive step, or non-obviousness, is to avoid granting patents for inventions that are merely the result of "normal product design and development," to strike a proper balance between the patent system's incentive, which is to encourage innovation, and its social cost, which is to confer temporary monopolies. As a result, the non-obviousness bar serves as a barometer of what society considers to be a valuable finding.

"If a concept is so clear that people in the area would develop it without much effort," according to the inducement theory, "then the incentives offered by the patent system may be unneeded to generate the idea." As a result, "some ways of weeding out those inventions that would not be revealed or conceived but for the inducement of a patent" are required (https://www.yalelawjournal.org/pdf/974_sp3xq85q.pdf).

The Teaching, Suggestion, and Motivation (TSM) test is more like the requirement for novelty than for non-obviousness. Examples of what is obvious and what is non-obvious are provided in Table 15.4. References indicate the legal suits that present the argument.

TABLE 15.4
Comparison of Obvious and Non-Obvious Determination in Patentability

Obvious	Non-Obvious
A mere change in the form or proportions (Evans, 1822)	Change in the "principle of the machine" (Evans, 1822)
Change of a material for a known material without changing function even if a lower cost result (Hotchkiss, 1851)	Unusual or surprising consequences (Great Atlantic, 1950)
Only unites old elements with no change in their respective functions (Great Atlantic, 1950)	Only when the whole in some way exceeds the sum of its parts is the accumulation of old devices patentable (Great Atlantic, 1950)
When a patent claims a structure already known in the prior art that is altered by the mere substitution of one element for another known in the field, the combination must do more than yield a predictable result (Adams, 1966)	Non-predictable results from a substitution/combination (reversed Adams)
[T]he two [pre-existing elements] in combination did no more than they would in separate, sequential operation (*Anderson's-Black Rock, Inc. v. Pavement Salvage Co.* [1969])	Synergism from a combination (reversed Adams)
Prior art suggests a mere possibility of such a solution even if it does not say the exact ranges (TSM)	Skepticism or disbelief before the invention (Environmental Designs, 1983). Failure of others (Graham, 1966)
The claimed solution is not used in practice, and the lawsuit is brought by a patent troll	Copying, praise, unexpected results, and industry acceptance (Allen Archery, 1987). Commercial success (Graham, 1966).
Combining prior art elements according to known methods to yield predictable results (KSR, 2007)	Non-predictable result(s) even if the combination involves known elements and methods, and better yet, if an element or a method is new
Simple substitution of one known element for another to obtain predictable results (KSR, 2007)	Non-predictable result(s) of a substitution
Use of known techniques to improve similar devices (methods or products) in the same way (KSR, 2007)	Use of a technique to improve dissimilar devices (methods, products) even if the technique is known in another field
"Obvious to try": choosing from a finite number of identified, predictable solutions, with a reasonable expectation of success (KSR, 2007)	If the solution is unpredictable and found experimentally, and better yet, if the very existence of a solution (suitable range) is unpredictable
Known work in one field of endeavor may prompt variations of it for use in either the same field or a different one based on design incentives or other market forces if the variations are predictable to ordinary skill in the art (KSR, 2007)	Use of a technique, even if known in another field, to improve dissimilar devices (methods, products) if "the actual application is beyond his or her skill" (KSR, 2007) i.e., variations are unpredictable
When a work is available in one field of endeavor, design incentives and other market forces can prompt variations, either in the same field or a different one. If a person of ordinary skill can implement a predictable variation, § 103 likely bars its patentability (*Sakraida v. AG Pro, Inc.* [1976])	Long felt but unsolved needs (Graham, 1966) unless these needs are solved by a newly publicly disclosed method (with a predictable claim range)
If a technique has been used to improve one device, and a PHOSITA would recognize that it would improve similar devices in the same way, using the technique is obvious	Unless [the technique's] actual application is beyond [PHOSITA's] skill (*Sakraida v. Ag Pro, Inc.* [1976])
Although "doubtless a matter of great convenience, producing a desired result in a cheaper and faster way, and enjoying commercial success," the claimed system "did not produce a new or different function" and therefore was not patentable (*Sakraida v. Ag Pro, Inc.* [1976])	Commercial success (Graham, 1966)
There is no change in the respective functions of the combination elements; this particular use of the assembly of old elements would be obvious to any person skilled in the art of mechanical application (*Sakraida v. Ag Pro, Inc.* [1976])	Commercial success (Graham, 1966)

(*Continued*)

TABLE 15.4 (CONTINUED)

Comparison of Obvious and Non-Obvious Determination in Patentability

Obvious	Non-Obvious
There is no change in the respective functions of the combination elements; this particular use of the assembly of old elements would be obvious to any person skilled in the art of mechanical application (*Sakraida v. Ag Pro, Inc.* [1976])	The elapsed time between the prior art and the patent's filing date (*Leo Pharm. Prods., Ltd. v. Rea*, 726 f.3d 1346, 1350 [Fed. Cir. 2013])
Some teaching, suggestion, or motivation in the prior art would have led one of ordinary skill to modify the prior art reference or combine prior art reference teachings to arrive at the claimed invention (KSR, 2007)	The prior art teaches away from the claimed solution
Commercial success by itself is not sufficient (*Sakraida v. Ag Pro, Inc.* [1976])	Commercial success (Graham, 1966)
(Near) simultaneous invention by two or more independent inventors	Long felt the need for a solution to a real problem that has been recognized in the prior art or the industry (Graham, 1966)

Source: Inventive Step and Non-Obviousness. *Wikipedia*. https://en.wikipedia.org/wiki/Inventive_step_and_non-obviousness.

Congress took matters into its own hands and enacted the Patent Act of 1952, 35 USC Section 103, to reduce the impact of non-obviousness on patentability, eliminate the flash of the genius test, and provide a more fair and practical way to determine whether the invention disclosure deserves a patent monopoly:

> A patent may not be obtained through the invention is not identically disclosed or described as outlined in section 102 (Novelty requirement) of this title, if the differences between the subject matter sought to be patented and the prior art is such that the subject matter would have been obvious at the time the invention was made to a person having ordinary skill in the art to which said subject matter pertains. However, patentability shall not be negated by the way the invention was made.

The final statement regarding the matter was included to counteract the genius test's flash. The Patent Act of 1952 introduced 35 USC 103, essentially codifying non-obviousness as a condition for proving that an idea is patentable. The section essentially demands a comparison of the subject matter sought to be patented and the previous art to establish whether the patent's subject matter would have been obvious to a person of ordinary skill in the art, AKA PHOSITA, at the time of the invention. (Similar criteria have been enacted and are in use in many other nations.) Clark argued that by codifying and clarifying the common law surrounding the Patent Act, Congress meant to codify and explain the requirement of non-obviousness. However, because PHOSITA does not exist, this test proved confusing and of little use in reality.

The concept of nonlinearity is also extended to the definition of innovation or novelty. The US patent laws define that if a claimed invention is obvious, then it is not novel; the example is given above regarding the mixture of antibiotics tells that a patent can be claimed if the MIC is either higher or lower, an outcome not anticipated.

The non-obviousness test extends to inherent properties; for example, if a natural product is used to treat a certain disease, any chemical extracted would not be patentable since it merely represents its inherent character.

Non-obviousness is a non-linearity; inventions must be unanticipated, meaning that linear thinking should not identify them. This teaching of non-obviousness is critical for scientists entering the field of developing innovations, not necessarily acquiring a patent but expanding their vision to a different set of possibilities.

15.7 Patent Management

15.7.1 Broad Coverage

A single biological product can be protected by numerous patents claiming subject matter ranging from nucleic acid and amino acid sequences, expression vectors, cell-based expression systems, upstream and downstream methods for producing and purifying the drug substance, optimized formulations developed to stabilize the drug product, devices used for administration, general methods of use, indication-specific methods of use, functional assays developed to release the drug product for sale, elucidate the method of action and analytical or diagnostic assays. Given the patentable subject matter scope, it is not uncommon to identify anywhere from 50 to more than 100 patent filings relevant to a single biological product. For example, Table 15.5 highlights the possible patent claims available in the case of an antibody product.

15.7.2 Submarine Patents

A complex scheme of cross-licensing and conflicting patent applications filed before 1995 has created the possibility of submarine patents that emerge just when the first composition of matter patent is ready to expire. Two such examples are interferon-alpha and etanercept, both of which will enjoy decades of exclusivity in total defiance of the patent law's spirit. They were able to exploit a weakness in the patenting system in the US; the laws have been changed since the term of the patent is now 20 years from the date of the first filing and *not* 17 years from the date of issuance of the submarine patents exploit. This threat is not available outside of the US. There is no way to go around these patents.

TABLE 15.5
Possible Patent Claims for Antibody Products

Antibody Product	Possible Patent Claims
Amino acid sequence	Amino acid sequence of: Complete heavy and light chains Heavy and light chain variable regions CDR regions Modifications made to the framework, CDR, or Fc regions
Nucleic acid sequence	Nucleic acid sequences encoding any or all of the above-listed amino acid sequences
Expression vector	Every individual element and/or combination of the vector elements are used to express the sequence in a suitable host cell, including promoter, enhancer, other regulatory sequences, and selection marker
Expression system	Host cells engineered to express the product
Culture conditions	Media components Culture method/feed media Optimized culture conditions
Purification	Chromatography Methods claiming the use of particular resins alone or in series Optimized conditions Compositions having a defined level of purity or homogeneity
Formulation	Pharmaceutical compositions comprising the drug product
Device	Device for administration and use thereof
Methods of use	Broad mechanism-based methods of use Disease-specific methods of use Indication-specific treatment regimens corresponding to the product label
Diagnostic methods and kits	Methods and/or kits used to identify select patents which are more or less likely to respond to treatment
Analytical methods	Assays developed to monitor the quality or purity of the product
Platform technology	Platform technologies and assays used to discover or optimize the structural and/or functional features of the product or processes used to manufacture or purify the product

15.7.3 System Expression Patents

There are patents like the Cabilly patents covering the basic expression technology; these are more like generic patents. In this specific case, unless the product happens to be produced by Genentech, a biosimilar developer can get a license. This patent expired in 2017. There is no way to go around these patents.

15.7.4 Process Patents of Originator

While most of the attention is diverted to patents' composition, the process patents can be the biggest challenge. This threat has come to the surface as the large market cap products like adalimumab and etanercept have come close to expiry. While many of these patents will be challenged and some may be taken down, the detail with which these patents carve out a protected territory is amazing. For example, in the etanercept case, you have to prove that the composition of amino acids during upstream manufacturing does not match the claimed distribution; the amino acid composition is not monitored in most upstream processes anyway. These patents' scope can include the choice of media, upstream conditions, pH and composition of buffers, downstream purification columns and order of their use, and even a higher purity claim.

Given many bioprocessing patents, both by the originator and third parties, it has already become very difficult and scientifically challenging to frame a suitable manufacturing process. The problems relating to this aspect can be appreciated from such patents that dictate that the composition of amino acids during the upstream processing must be within specific ranges; ironically, this is not a common test. Even the composition of media is often not known to the developer. However, once such patents have been issued, it becomes incumbent on the developer to study this facet.

15.7.5 Third-Party Process Patents

While the challenge of going around the originator process patents can be demanding, there are possibilities of third-party patents that may either apply to a specific product or a class of product. Generally, a biosimilar developer would create a manufacturing pathway to go around the originator patent and then make an extensive search of third-party patents.

15.7.6 Formulation Composition

Early developers of biological products ignored these patents' value, but now we see formulation patents intended to raise the barrier of demonstrating similarity. While the intent of developing these patents was to keep the biosimilar developers out of the market, if the agencies require Q/Q products, this has not worked out. So instead, the agencies, realizing this, would allow alternate formulations.

15.7.7 Lifecycle Formulation Projections

A recent trend seen is a change of formulation as the patent on the composition of matter come close to expiry; for example, switching from a lyophilized formulation to a solution or adopting a high concentration subcutaneous formulation instead of an intravenous solution (as has happened with some anticancer drugs where the time to administer is significantly reduced using subcutaneous formulation) brings a greater challenge to biosimilar developer to develop an intravenous formulation or a subcutaneous formulation that is now covered under a new patent? The originator plans to switch its patients to a more friendly formulation, which may be a formidable marketing challenge. However, unless the new formulation has been marketed, it becomes a challenge for the biosimilar product developer to secure reference samples to compare its product against, provided it was possible to go around any intellectual property challenges.

15.7.8 Alternate Offering

While the originator product may have been launched in a limited presentation, these might change over time, often to create a useful diversity; for example, prefilled syringes or injectors in place of vials change the marketing and distribution landscape in light of the reimbursement complexities.

Dosing and indications: While the early developers of biological drugs ignored the power of creating patents around specific use of these products, including indications, this is now the trend, and just about every big molecule as it comes closer to expiry will be spread with multiple patents that include specific dose, condition of use and even dosing schedule. A case example is a patent held by Abbvie for administering exactly 40 mg of adalimumab exactly every other week. Such patents are intended to block biosimilar developers from developing a similar product in use and hoping that the regulatory agencies would not allow alternate dosing or indications. However, the regulatory agencies, realizing this threat, have opened up to alternate suggestions. These can be, however, very difficult to overcome. Ironically, many of these patents have surfaced recently, giving shock to major developers of biosimilar products that may have already gone through expensive clinical trials only to find that they will not be able to launch these at the end of the trial products. Thus, a biosimilar developer needs not to examine the existing intellectual property but what may be forthcoming.

15.7.9 Delivery Devices

The originator may have many patents on the delivery device since all of these devices are specific to the product, even when supplied by device manufacturing companies selling such devices to multiple users. Thus, device selection can have a significant impact on the marketability of a biosimilar product.

15.7.10 Unpatentable Inventions

Unmodified pre-existing articles of nature cannot be patented. For example, you cannot patent an unmodified natural chemical, gene, protein, or animal or plant species. However, you can patent a modified form of an article of nature if the modification serves a useful purpose. For example, you can patent the use of existing articles of nature in devices, compounds, or diagnostic kits useful.

In summary, one should craft patent claims around the non-obvious practical use of a gene or protein, or its modified form, instead of patenting the gene or protein itself as a composition of matter.

One cannot patent laws of nature, physical phenomena, abstract ideas, literary, dramatic, musical, and artistic works. However, these can be copied write-protected. In addition, you cannot patent inventions that are considered not useful or physically impossible by the USPTO (for example, perpetual motion machines) or considered offensive to public morality.

Section 101 of the Patent Act defines the subject matter that can be patented as any process, machine, manufacturing, or composition of matter (the "congressional categories"). However, courts have recognized that some inventions do not fit into one of the four legislative categories for ages. Abstract conceptions, natural phenomena, and natural rules (the "judicial exceptions") are examples of such innovations.

Since 2012, the Supreme Court has issued three significant judgments prohibiting the patenting of certain sorts of inventions. First, in *Mayo v. Prometheus*, patents on medical diagnosis and analysis were outlawed. Then, in *Association for Molecular Pathology v. Myriad Genetics* (AKA *Myriad Genetics*), patents for manufactured DNA specified by a natural nucleic acid sequence were prohibited. Finally, the Alice ruling prohibited patents on computer hardware and software that are defined by their usage in financial transactions or other "abstract notions." While many anti-patent factions (particularly Silicon Valley and the generic medication sector) have applauded these verdicts (together known as the "Alice" decisions), institutions that rely on innovation, such as research universities, single inventors, and biotechnology corporations, have slammed them. The Alice trifecta also overturns almost a century of opposite judicial history, puts the US out of line with international patenting practices, and violates TRIPS Section 5 Article 27 Part 3. Congress has finally proposed legislation to solve the Alice trifecta, but as of this writing, nothing has come to fruition.

Molecular profiling and individualized therapy are providing new insights into disease treatment while at the same time providing new technologies and therapies. Although the concept of genomic and proteomic analysis is not new, the wealth of patentable information gleaned from these molecular insights is constantly challenging current health and patent laws.

Innovations in software, medical treatments, and business methods are vital to any country's economic health, and it is commonly agreed that continued investment in these disciplines demands adequate remuneration for the innovators. However, it is commonly understood that issuing patents for such discoveries requires careful consideration, and many governments are still debating how to handle such requests.

15.7.11 Software Patents

The general theory in the United States is that a software invention is patentable provided it fits two criteria:

It's one-of-a-kind, which means it's something new.

It's related to a machine, in the sense that the sort of hardware platform on which the software runs is defined, ensuring that a patent isn't given for the description of an abstract process but rather for something that necessitates a certain type of physical hardware. (As we'll see, this is a little more open-ended than the machine requirements in other countries.)

However, there are three forms of software that aren't patentable:

An algorithm, for starters, cannot be patented.

It is impossible to copyright a scientific law.

Patenting an abstract concept is impossible.

In the European Union, software is not patentable on its own. It can only be patented as a "computer-implemented invention," which is defined as a software program that performs some innovative and valuable function within a patented hardware device.

Countries like Japan, India, and South Korea often follow the EU's lead, allowing software to be patented only if it is a component of a hardware invention. China has traditionally had the same attitude on software patents, while newly disclosed patent examination rules suggest the country is warming to the idea of patenting software as a separate entity. For example, China's State Intellectual Property Office (SIPO) guidelines announced earlier this year now allow for the patenting of both a (storage) medium and a computer program technique. Some experts believe that the two aspects—storage devices and software—may be patentable individually.

15.7.12 Medical Method Patents

In the United States, a medical method is patentable if it fits three criteria:

Specificity: It is specific enough to identify its limitations.

It has a practical application as a method of treating a specific condition using a specific medicine.

It has a central transformative effect, which means it fundamentally alters the nature of the target.

If a medical technique patent application is new and innovative and isn't a kind of surgery, therapy, or diagnostics, the EPO will accept it. As previously stated, refusing patents for surgical, therapeutic, and diagnostic processes is meant to relieve clinicians of the fear of inadvertently infringing on someone's patent while treating a patient.

Japan has a similar principle to the EPO, allowing medical patents as long as they do not interfere with the work of practicing physicians. Since 1992, China has authorized pharmaceutical patents. Surprisingly, Chinese examiners do not search for a patent claim to fit a set of permitted conditions when it comes to medical treatments. Instead, they maintain a list of all the medical treatments that are not patentable. South Korea doesn't grant medical technique patents, and neither does India, which disqualifies "any procedure for the medicinal, surgical, curative, prophylactic, diagnostic, therapeutic, or other treatment of human beings or any process for a similar animal therapy that renders them disease-free."

15.8 Patent Classification

15.8.1 Class 435

The US Patent Office Classification 435 (Chemistry: Molecular Biology and Microbiology; www.uspto.gov/web/offices/ac/ido/oeip/taf/def/435.htm) includes the following subcategories related to therapeutic proteins. The search at the USPTO can be made in advanced search mode using CCL/"435/69.6" for searching blood proteins; CCL/"435/69.5" for lymphokines; CCL/"435/69.2" for interleukins; and CCL/"435/69.51" for interferons.

- 69.1: Recombinant DNA technique included in the method of making a protein or polypeptide
- 69.2: Enzyme inhibitors or activators
- 69.3: Antigens
- 69.4: Hormones and fragments thereof
- 69.5: Lymphokines or monokines
- 69.5: Interferons
- 6.52: Interleukins
- 69.6: Blood proteins
- 69.7: Fusion proteins or polypeptides
- 69.8: Signal sequence (e.g., beta-galactosidase, etc.)
- 69.9: Yeast derived

A search under CCL/"435/69.1" yields 16,245 (July 2020) patents, including the earliest patents wherein insulin was produced by genetically modified fungi from the University of Minnesota and the two classic patents from Stanford Columbia. (The last two patents are reproduced here in their entirety.) (See U.S. Patent and Trademark Office 2011.)

15.8.2 Class 424

The definition of Class 424 (Drug, Bio-Affecting and Body Treating; www.uspto.gov/web/offices/ac/ido/oeip/taf/def/424.htm]) contains controlling statements on the class lines.

93.2 Genetically modified micro-organism, cell, or virus (e.g., transformed, fused, hybrid, etc.): This subclass is indented under subclass

93.1 Subject matter involving a micro-organism, cell, or virus which (a) is a product of recombination, transformation, or transfection with a vector or a foreign or exogenous gene or (b) is a product of homologous recombination if it is directed rather than spontaneous or (c) is a product of fused or hybrid cell formation. (1) Note. Examples of subject matter included in this and the indented subclass are compositions containing micro-organisms, cells, or viruses resulting from (a) a process in which the cellular matter of two or more fusing partners is combined, producing a cell which initially contains the genes of both fusing partners or (b) a process in which a cell is treated with an immortalizing agent which results in a cell which proliferates in long term culture or (c) a process involving recombinant DNA methodology. (2) Note. Excluded from this subclass are products of unidentified or non-induced mutations, microbial conjugation products wherein specific genetic material is not identified and controlled, and products of natural, spontaneous, or arbitrary conjugation recombination events. These products are not considered genetically modified for this subclass and will be classified as unmodified microorganisms, cells, or viruses.

93.21 Eukaryotic cell: This subclass is indented under subclass 93.2. Subject matter involving a eukaryotic cell, such as an animal cell, plant cell, fungus, protozoa, or higher algae, has been genetically modified. (1) Note. A eukaryotic cell has a nucleus defined by a nuclear membrane wherein the nucleus contains chromosomes that comprise the cell's genome.

93.3 Intentional mixture of two or more microorganisms, cells, or viruses of different genera: This subclass is indented under subclass 93.1. Subject matter involving a mixture consisting of two or more different microbial, cellular, or viral genera. (1) Note. A mixture of E. coli and Pseudomonas or a mixture of Aspergillus and Bacillus would be considered proper for this subclass. In contrast, a mixture of Bacillus cereus and Bacillus brevis would be classified under Bacillus rather than in this subclass since they are both in the genus Bacillus. (2) Note. Rumen, intestinal, vaginal, etc., microflora mixtures are mixtures appropriate for this subclass unless mixture constituents are disclosed and are contrary to the subclass definition.

133.1 Structurally modified antibody, immunoglobulin, or fragment thereof (e.g., chimeric, humanized, CDR-grafted, mutated, etc.): This subclass is indented under subclass 130.1. Subject matter involving an antibody, immunoglobulin, or fragment thereof that is purposely altered concerning its amino acid sequence or glycosylation or concerning its composition of heavy and light chains of immunoglobulin regions or domains, as compared with that found in nature; or wherein the antibody, immunoglobulin, or fragment thereof is part of a larger, synthetic protein. (1) Note. Structurally modified antibodies may be made by chemical alteration or recombination of existing antibodies or various cloning techniques involving recombinant DNA or hybridoma technology. (2) Note. Structurally modified antibodies may be chimeric (i.e., comprising amino acid sequences derived from two or more nonidentical immunoglobulin molecules, such as interspecies combinations, etc.). (3) Note. Structurally modified antibodies may have domain deletions or substitutions (e.g., deletions of particular constant-region domains or substitutions of constant-region domains from other classes of immunoglobulins). (4) Note. Structurally modified antibodies may have deletions of particular glycosylated amino acids or may have their glycosylation otherwise altered, altering their function. (5) Note. While expression of cloned antibody genes in cells of species other than from which they originated may result in altered glycosylation of the product, compared with that found in nature, this subclass and indented subclasses are not meant to encompass such antibodies or fragments thereof unless such cloning is a deliberate attempt to alter their glycosylation. However, such antibodies or fragments may still be classified here or in indented subclasses if structurally modified in other ways (e.g., if they are single chains, etc.). (6) Note. It is suggested that the patents of this subclass and indented subclasses be cross-referenced to the appropriate subclass(es) that provide for the binding specificities of these antibodies if disclosed.

141.1 Monoclonal antibody or fragment thereof (i.e., produced by any cloning technology): This subclass is indented under subclass 130.1. Subject matter involving an antibody or fragment thereof produced by a clone of cells or cell line, which clone of cells or cell line is derived from a single antibody-producing cell or antibody-fragment-producing cell, wherein said antibody or fragment thereof is identical to all other antibodies or fragments thereof produced by that clone of cells or cell line. (1) Note. This and the indented subclasses provide for bio-affecting and body-treating compositions of antibodies or fragments thereof as well as bio-affecting and body-treating methods of using said compositions said antibodies, or said fragments, which antibodies or antibody fragments are produced by any cloning technology that yields identical molecules (e.g., hybridoma technology, recombinant DNA technology, etc.). (2) Note. Monoclonal antibodies, per se, are considered compounds and are provided for elsewhere. See the search notes below. (3) Note. Monoclonal antibodies are sometimes termed monoclonal receptors or immunological binding partners.

1.49 and 1.53, for methods of using radiolabeled monoclonal antibodies or compositions thereof for bio-affecting or body-treating purposes and said compositions, per se.

9.1 for using monoclonal antibodies or compositions for in vivo testing or diagnosis and said compositions, per se.

178.1 for bio-affecting or body-treating methods of using monoclonal antibodies or fragments thereof that are conjugated to or complexed with non-immunoglobulin material; bio-affecting or body-treating methods of using compositions of monoclonal antibodies or fragments thereof, which monoclonal antibodies or fragments thereof are conjugated to or complexed with non-immunoglobulin material; and said compositions, per se.

199.1 Recombinant virus encoding one or more heterologous proteins or fragments thereof: This subclass is indented under subclass 184.1. Subject matter involving a virus into whose genome is integrated one or more nucleic acid sequences encoding one or more heterologous proteins or fragments thereof. (1) Note. A heterologous protein is one derived from another species (e.g., another viral species). (2) Note. Such genetically modified viruses may be used as multivalent vaccines.

200.1 Recombinant or stably transformed bacterium encoding one or more heterologous proteins or fragments thereof: This subclass is indented under subclass 184.1. Subject matter involving a bacterium whose genome is integrated one or more nucleic acid sequences encoding one or more heterologous proteins or fragments thereof; or involving a bacterium that carries stable, replicative plasmids that include one or more nucleic acid sequences encoding one or more heterologous proteins or fragments thereof.

(1) Note. A heterologous protein is one derived from another species (e.g., another bacterial species).
(2) Note. Such genetically modified bacteria may be used as multivalent vaccines.

201.1 Combination of viral and bacterial antigens (e.g., multivalent viral and bacterial vaccine, etc.) This subclass is indented under subclass 184.1. Subject matter involves a combination of viral and bacterial antigens, such as those found in a multivalent viral and bacterial vaccine.

202.1 Combination of antigens from multiple viral species (e.g., multivalent viral vaccine, etc.): This subclass is indented under subclass 184.1. Subject matter involving a combination of antigens from multiple viral species, such as that found in a multivalent viral vaccine. (1) Note. A combination of antigens from multiple viral species' variants should be classified with that viral species.

203.1 Combination of antigens from multiple bacterial species (e.g., multivalent bacterial vaccine, etc.): This subclass is indented under subclass 184.1. The subject matter involves combining antigens from multiple bacterial species found in a multivalent bacterial vaccine. (1) Note. A combination of antigens from multiple bacterial species variants should be classified with that bacterial species.

15.8.3 Class 801

This subclass, 801 (Involving Antibody or Fragment Thereof Produced by Recombinant DNA Technology; www.uspto.gov/web/offices/ac/ido/oeip/taf/def/801.htm) is indented under the class definition: subject matter involving an antibody or fragment thereof produced by recombinant DNA technology.

Another field of recombinant DNA technology relates to producing a specific protein produced by a transformed microorganism. The structure (amino-acid sequence) may be known or isolated in a pure state but whose structure is not yet elucidated, or a product known only by its activity in some impure mixture. In the last of these cases, the product can be claimed per se as a new compound characterized by its structure (which will generally be known once the gene has been obtained and sequenced). The gene itself, or at least the cDNA coding for the protein, can also be claimed.

Where the product has previously been obtained in the pure state, a per se claim is no longer possible. However, the invention can still be claimed in various ways to cover the product whenever made by recombinant DNA techniques. In the European Patent Office, for example, the patentee could claim the isolated gene for the product, a vector containing the gene, the host cell transformed with the vector, the process for obtaining any of these, and finally, the process for obtaining the end-product, which would be infringed by sale of the product obtained by that process. In addition, it may be possible to claim the unglycosylated protein per se even when the natural glycosylated form is known. In the United Kingdom, it is possible to go further and claim, for example, "human tissue plasminogen activator as produced by recombinant DNA technology."

A claim to a recombinant product defined by one specific amino acid sequence is likely to give a scope of protection that is too narrow since any natural protein; there are some regions in which it is possible to change one or two amino acids without affecting the function of the protein and other regions where any change in the exact amino acid sequence will alter or destroy the activity. Thus, although porcine and bovine insulin differs slightly from human insulin, they have essentially the same activity in humans. To solve this problem, claims are drafted for proteins that have a certain degree of homology with the defined amino acid sequence or that may have a certain number of possible amino acid deletions, additions, or substitutions (some of which have been so broad as to claim practically all possible proteins). However, such a claim must necessarily cover many useless products because a change of one amino acid may cause a complete loss of activity and is likely to be invalid for this reason. A better claim combines such a possibility of structural variation with a requirement that the product must have a certain defined activity. Wishfully, the courts need to interpret a claim to a specific protein structure as covering also minor variations such as might be expected to occur in nature, which does not alter the claimed product's properties.

The claims to DNA sequences may be placed in four categories of increasing breadth:

- A "picture" claim to one specific DNA sequence.
- Including other DNA sequences coding for the same protein (genetic code redundancy).

- Including DNA sequences coding for modified proteins having the same function.
- Including DNA sequences coding for significantly modified proteins, some of which may not be functional, including noncoding DNA sequences.

15.9 Biological Patents

In terms of bioethics, gene patenting is a contentious subject. Concerns concerning genetic patenting have been expressed in three ways. For starters, some argue that patenting genetic material is wrong since it regards life as a commodity. Second, some argue that living materials are found in nature and hence cannot be copyrighted. Finally, the fear of allowing patents on genetic material will undermine people and other animals' dignity by subjecting their genes to ownership by other people. The World Trade Organization (WTO) is required by agreements like the Agreement on Trade-Related Aspects of Intellectual Property Rights (TRIPS) to have intellectual property protection laws in place for most biological innovation, making it unlikely that many countries will outright prohibit gene patents.

A major ethical issue involving gene patents is how the patents are used post-issuance. One major issue is that using patented materials and methods will be prohibitively expensive or even impossible due to constraints imposed by the patent owner. Additionally, given the large markets for these products, the innovators create a firewall around their composition patent to continue to reap benefits far beyond the initial exclusivity; this violates the basic ethical considerations when patents are issued so that once the patents expire, mankind can benefit from it.

Australia accepts the validity of patents on naturally occurring DNA sequences.

In the United States, natural biological substances themselves can be patented (apart from any associated process or usage) if they are sufficiently "isolated" from their naturally occurring states. Historical examples of such patents include those on adrenaline, insulin, vitamin B12, and various genes. The United States Supreme Court, on the other hand, comes to the opposite conclusion. According to the European Patent Organization, natural biological products, including gene sequences, can be patented if they are "isolated from [their] natural environment or created through a technical procedure" (https://www.epo.org/law-practice/legal-texts/html/guidelines/e/g_ii_5_2.htm). However, in a landmark decision in June 2013, the United States Supreme Court ruled that naturally occurring DNA sequences are not patentable.

According to the European Patent Office, European patents cannot be granted for techniques that involve the killing of human embryos.

In 1980 the Supreme Court held in *Diamond v. Chakrabarty* (447 US 330; 1980) voted that inventions involving living organisms altered by man were entitled to patent law protection. The Court's interpretation of the breadth of section 101 provided the nascent biotechnology industry with precisely the type of stimulus necessary to launch and drive a furious and exciting period of development.

As with all inventions, the claims define the scope of enforceable rights possessed by a patentee in biotechnology patents. Deficiencies in drafting the broadest possible claim scope can become a serious stumbling block for the patentee attempting to enforce its rights. Given the important role, claims play in the interpretation, and effective use of patent rights, how claims function to protect biotechnology inventions in the field of biotechnology merits discussion. Consider a situation where a broad yet poorly drafted patent claim is invalidated due to formalistic deficiencies; the patentee is left with a scope of protection not much broader than the actual species of protein developed. When this occurs, competitors may easily make insignificant changes and escape the literal scope of the claims. The Federal Circuit has emphasized that the claims' function is to measure the enforceable scope of patent protection. This function must be preserved to ensure that patents continue to stimulate further innovation.

However, the equivalents' doctrine provides an equitable framework to prevent the accused infringer from making minor changes to escape the claim. Thus, it seems appropriate that a patentee holding unduly narrowed patent claims to a protein should be able to bypass the restrictions imposed by the literal scope of patent claims in extraordinary situations to protect him from "the unscrupulous copyist" who makes "unimportant and insubstantial changes and substitutions in the patent which, though adding nothing, would be enough to take the copied matter outside the claim, and hence outside the reach of the law" (*Graver Tank*, 339 US at 607).

Before 1995, the expiration date of these various aspects of the biotech invention could be years apart. However, with the change in US patent law, most patents expire 20 years from the date they are filed unless they receive an extension due to a patent office delay or a regulatory delay or receive a pediatric exclusivity extension.

15.9.1 Biological Products

Biological products can obtain market exclusivity from a combination of three primary sources: 1) regulatory exclusivities, 2) patents, and 3) trade secrets or proprietary information. Regulatory Exclusivities and Patents protect a product's market for a defined period. The BPCIA provides 12 years of regulatory exclusivity to innovative biologic products approved by filing a full BLA. Generally speaking, United States patents have a "20-year term" that begins on the date the patent issues and ends on the date that is 20 years from the earliest priority date the application was filed. (There is an exception to the "20-year term," which applies to patents that were in force on June 8, 1995, or that issued from an application that was filed before June 8, 1995. Patents within this category have a greater term than the "20-year term," or 17 years from the patent grant date [35 USC 154 {c}].) However, some of the baseline periods of exclusivities defined in the statutory provision can be extended for additional periods by pediatric exclusivities, patent term extension, and patent term adjustments.

Regulatory exclusivities provide market protection to innovative products regardless of whether the products have patent protection. In the absence of patent protection, a generic drug can immediately enter the market upon the expiration of the regulatory exclusivity period. Therefore, creating and managing a strong patent portfolio is crucial for the business model for biological medicine companies.

Patents can issue at any point during the development cycle of a drug product. For example, some patents claiming the drug substance itself may issue before or during the NDA or BLA filing. Other patents, such as a patent that claims the commercial formulation or the use of a customized delivery device, or a detailed treatment regimen, will likely issue much later after human clinical testing is completed. Also, life cycle management practices will occasionally give rise to submarine patents that provide an unexpected patent exclusivity extension.

A submarine patent is a term used to refer to a patent filed before the change in the law in 1995 but issues years later due to a delay, such as an interference proceeding. The patent application remains secret in the patent office because it was filed before publishing the application and then suddenly surfaces, hence submarine. The result is a patent that issues years after the technology has advanced, and the patent receives a term of 17 years from the issue because it is issued under the rules of the previous statute.

Furthermore, innovation is an inherent feature of product development. Later discovered inventions, such as an optimized purification process or method of use, could provide additional patent exclusivity in the form of a late issuing patent. Therefore, the regulatory market and the patent exclusivities may, or may not, run concurrently.

Trade secret laws can vary from state to state but share the unifying characteristics of requiring that the information is of economic value to the owner. The owner establishes and maintains reasonable efforts to protect the information from public disclosure.

Typically, subject matter that a biological medicine manufacturer considers proprietary trade secrets is not included in their patent disclosures, subject to publication.

Trade secret protection is not limited by any defined statutory period and can provide companies with a competitive advantage for as long as the information remains confidential. For example, the biologic manufacturer could keep information about critical process controls used during manufacturing or downstream bioprocess steps to produce the reference product. As long as the information remains confidential, the trade secret/proprietary information will confer the manufacturer a competitive advantage. Manufacturing process controls are developed and established for each product/process and play an integral role in defining the biological drug product's quality and purity.

15.9.2 Monoclonal Antibody Technology

Biotechnology products are also derived from the immune system's workings responsible for producing white blood cells, or lymphocytes. These cells originate as stem cells in the bone marrow and differentiate and mature either in the bone marrow to B-lymphocytes (B cells) or in the thymus gland to T-lymphocytes (T cells). The B cells' main task is to produce antibodies in response to exposure to the foreign substance through interaction on B cells' surface receptors. Upon activation, the activated B cell undergoes rapid division and develops into a clone of identical plasma cells, all of which secrete antibody molecules with the same specificity to the antigen as did the original B cell. The antibodies thus produced (immunoglobulins or Ig molecules) are complex proteins with the letter Y's approximate shape with binding sites in its branches for a particular antigen. The antibodies react with antigen molecules and form a cross-linked, insoluble structure, removing the antigen from circulation. The antigen is located on the surface of a foreign cell like a bacterium. The antibodies bind to the surface (opsonization), rendering the cell ready for destruction by macrophages or other immune system components.

Antibodies isolated from human blood, particularly in immunoglobulin-G (IgG or gamma-globulin), have been used therapeutically for a long time, such as providing immunity against viral infections; the potency will depend on how recent the donor had experienced the infection. Antibodies are also a powerful tool in diagnosing disease and also in the identification of biological organisms. Initial inventions could not characterize the sequence of the amino acid in the antibody molecules. The hybridoma lines were deposited as part of patent application disclosure; later, as more refined methods became available, the sequencing of the antibodies was submitted instead of or in addition to cell line deposits. Characterization of amino acid sequencing of antibodies also allowed the use of recombinant DNA technologies to produce antibodies. Recombinant DNA's use addressed another problem with the therapeutic use of monoclonal antibodies where mouse proteins, upon repeated administration, reacted with the patient's immune system, reducing their effectiveness or even causing a harmful allergic reaction. Antibodies are produced by recombinant (rDNA) methods using chimeric MAbs in which the variable regions (the arms of the Y) remain murine, but the constant regions (the base of the Y) are replaced with the constant regions of a human antibody. Another advancement in the technology came when there was a replacement of all but the actual hypervariable regions, which give the specificity to give a humanized antibody.

More advances in technology allowed the use of fragments of antibody genes to be expressed on a carrier's surface, such as a bacteriophage enabling fragments coding for hypervariable regions of the desired specificity for selection and incorporation into genes to be expressed to give fully human monoclonal antibodies. This made the technology for chimeric and humanized antibodies obsolete by the time the first of these products came on the market. The phage display technique can also be used to find large or small molecules that bind to a particular structure, for example, a receptor or its ligand. Antibodies having certain specificities are also used as catalysts by holding two reagent molecules together in the correct configuration to proceed.

A monoclonal antibody product can be protected by claims to the nucleic acid encoding the antibody protein, and the vector constructs, the cell line harboring the vector that expresses the protein, the method of harvesting the antibody from the cell line, the method of purifying the protein from the cell line components, the formulation that the antibody is administered in, the device the antibody is administered with, any diagnostic testing or analytical testing methods, and the method of using the antibody to treat a given disease or condition.

15.9.3 Antisense Technology

If the genetic coding of a gene that plays a role in sickness is discovered, it could be used to selectively stop it. Double-helical DNA makes up genes. The genetic code in that region of DNA is replicated out as a single strand of RNA termed messenger RNA when a gene is turned on. Because it may be translated into a string of amino acids to make a protein, messenger RNA is referred to as a "sense" sequence. The "antisense" strand is the opposite of a DNA double helix (against T, T opposite A, C opposite G, G opposite C). Short antisense DNAs can be made to work as drugs by attaching to messenger RNAs from disease genes, thanks to the antisense coding sequence of the disease gene. However, the disease-causing protein cannot be produced because the genetic code in the RNA cannot be read.

Generally, a fragment of 20 bases length will be specific for one particular gene and therefore not interfere with the expression of other genes. However, several difficulties arise in developing antisense drugs that range from the instability of single-stranded DNA in vivo to finding suitable delivery systems. The stability problem may be overcome by chemical modification of the DNA chain's backbone, such as replacing the phosphate groups with hydrolyzed groups less easily, and these modifications can be patented.

15.9.4 Transgenic Plants

Unlike animal cells, plant cells have an external cell wall that is difficult to penetrate when introducing genetic material. It is also difficult for the vector to move around in the cell because of the cellular environment. Novel techniques like placing DNA molecules on the surface of micronized glass beads physically shot into cells are thus used. Once transformed, the plants can be bred in the normal process. Transgenic plants' purpose is to produce higher yields, improved nutritional quality, and lower production costs.

15.10 Freedom to Operate

Freedom-to-operate (FTO) opinions provide a detailed analysis of each of the patents and patent applications deemed relevant to the making, using, or selling of a product, in this case, a biological medicine product. The opinion provides a discussion of each patent/application, and whether it is infringed, invalid, and/or will expire before the product launch. It serves several functions for the biological medicine applicant. The more traditional function is to provide a well-reasoned opinion that will prevent an assessment of treble damages should a court decide that the biological medicine product does infringe a patent. But, more importantly, here, it provides a strategic landscape for designing around any patents that may be infringed as well as providing the lists of patents that will likely be asserted by the innovator or, as the statute refers to it, the Reference Product Sponsor (RPS) during the patent exchange phase.

The composition of matter includes the gene sequence responsible for expressing the product; these patents cannot go around. Fortunately, most of these are expiring, and while there is significant diversity in the dates when these patents expire, there is definite data available to assess these. A difference of two to four years across various major markets is not unusual; therefore, the date of composition matter would determine the domicile of manufacturing for the first launch.

A person tasked with determining when a biological medicine manufacturer will have freedom to operate will have to undertake a multi-faceted approach to identifying all relevant patents and patent applications. First, to identify all relevant patents/applications, one will have to prepare a search terms list. At a minimum, these should include a list of the different parties that contributed to the product's discovery and development and a list of alternative names used to refer to the biologic during the development process.

The fact that biological products tend to have a complicated lineage that often involves the participation of multiple parties means that it is likely that multiple parties could own patents that cover a single product. This is because it is common for the initial discovery of a molecular target or lead molecule to be performed by a university or innovative biotech company that subsequently decides to license, sell or work collaboratively with a pharmaceutical company to develop the candidate molecule biologic product. Since innovation will continue throughout the drug development process, anyone, or all of the parties involved in the drug development process, could own patents relevant to the product.

Once the amino acid sequence is identified, it can be used to search sequence databases for patents claiming the amino acid sequence used to express the biologic product. A public sequence database available for such searches is BLAST, which stands for Basic Local Alignment Search Tool (http://blast.ncbi.nlm.nih.gov/Blast.cgi). Alternatively, several paid databases, such as GenomeQuest, and search firms, will search for the applicant.

Once the search terms are identified, one must do extensive searching in a patent database. Several publicly available databases, including the USPTO and EPO, do not allow for numerous open-ended operators. Therefore, they are more difficult to search than paid databases, which tend to have more robust search capabilities. In addition to searching for product-specific patents/applications, one must also search for general methods related to the biologic's production, such as media and conditions for growing the cell line and expressing and purifying proteins monoclonal antibodies. One example of a general method patent for monoclonal antibody expression was issued to Genentech (http://patft.uspto.gov/netahtml/PTO/srchnum.htm, enter 6331415). Unfortunately, this patent also happens to be a submarine patent referred to as Cabilly II. After a long-winded prosecution involving interference proceedings and re-examination, US Patent 6,331,415 was eventually granted in 2001. This patent expired on December 18, 2018, receiving benefits for 17 years from issue, although it has a priority claim dating back to 1983. Claim 1 of this patent broadly covers a process for producing an antibody molecule comprising at least the variable domains of the heavy and light chains in a single host cell.

There will be hundreds, if not thousands, of patents to screen through once the search terms are entered into the chosen database. The search results must be narrowed down to those patents most relevant to the biological medicine applicant's cell line, media, production process, bioreactor technology, purification process, formulation, and assays. Those patents closest to these must be analyzed on a claim-by-claim basis to determine whether the biological medicine applicant has the freedom to operate in the market. This analysis is what makes up the final FTO opinion.

In addition to identifying the final set of patents to be analyzed, the person preparing the opinion will need to determine each patent's expiration date. As discussed above, this includes determining the relevant filing date of the claims at issue, the amount of patent term adjustment awarded for delay by the USPTO, the effect of any terminal disclaimers filed by the patentee, the amount of patent term extension awarded for regulatory approval delays (if any), and whether the maintenance fees have been timely paid. Some patents may become irrelevant to the analysis by knowing the expiration date as they may expire before the biological medicine product's expected launch date.

The FTO opinion should analyze each claim and whether the current processes, product, or treatment indications will infringe the patent. For patent applications, as opposed to patents that may be identified, one must look at the most recent set of claims to determine the likelihood of infringement as the claims read at that time and analyze the likelihood the patent will issue. For example, suppose the patent application is considered likely to be infringed. In that case, this application will need to be put on a watch list to follow the prosecution during the biological medicine product development.

Once the FTO opinion is drafted, the biological medicine applicant must develop a strategy for moving forward if patents will not expire before launch and are likely to be considered infringing. For example, suppose the patent claims cannot be designed around because, e.g., it would be too costly, require too much time or render the product non-biological medicine. In that case, the options include challenging the patent or requesting a license from the patent holder. If the decision is to challenge the patent, an invalidity opinion should be drafted. This opinion can be used to craft a post-grant challenge of the patent. Alternatively, the invalidity opinion can be held as a bargaining tool during the patent exchange phase of the BPCIA statute requirements.

There are three post-grant methods for challenging a patent in the USPTO. These include *ex parte* reexamination, *inter partes* review, and post-grant review. There are pros and cons to each choice. *Ex parte* reexamination is the least expensive and does not require that the challenger be identified. However, the challenger cannot participate in the process once the initial challenge is filed. Instead, the patent examining corps conduct the reexamination. This process takes about two years.

The strategy to manage the lifecycle of the product begins very early. It requires an extensive and intensive strategy of creating intellectual property as the product goes through various stages of development and regulatory approvals. For example, as various clinical trials prove successful, applications are filed for specific treatment and at a specific dose. The patents keep emerging, particularly closer to the dates when the composition or gene sequence patents appear expiring. The originators are betting that the boundaries created around the manufacturing, formulation, and use of these products will deter developers of biological medicines from entering the market. They are also betting that the changes needed to the product design will be so broad that the regulator may consider them no longer as biological medicines.

15.11 Conclusion

Intellectual property creation and protection are essential to innovation. Over time, patents have become very sophisticated, and securing these protections requires a team effort involving the scientists at every step of discovery and improvements of systems. While the scientists are not expected to know the nuances of the law of patents, a basic understanding of what constitutes an invention is important to ensure that inventions are not lost, but at the same time, inventions of others are not infringed. Understanding the patenting process also introduces a remarkable treasure of information buried in the patents that scientists must read; this chapter provides the tools to the scientists to engage fully with the legal teams.

ADDITIONAL READING

Arya R, Bhutkar S, Dhulap S, Hirwani RR. Patent analysis as a tool for research planning: study on natural based therapeutics against cancer stem cells. *Recent Pat Anticancer Drug Discov.* 2015;10(1):72–86.

Berger G. Pharmaceutical patent landscape for cancer immunotherapy: an interview with Gilles Berger. *Pharm Pat Anal.* 2019;8(5):163–164.

Dhulap S, Kulkarni M. Nonobviousness of pharmaceutical inventions: implications for patent prosecution and litigation. *Pharm Pat Anal.* 2019;8(4):91–107.

Dolgin E. Patent-free pact pushes the boundaries of precompetitive research. *Nat Med.* 2014;20(6):564–565.

Edlin C. The importance of patent sharing in neglected disease drug discovery. *Future Med Chem.* 2011;3(11):1331–1334.

Gaudry KS. Uncharted territories of the patent-restoration due-diligence challenge. *Food Drug Law J.* 2011;66(1):121–138, iii.

Grabowski HG, Moe JL. Impact of economic, regulatory, and patent policies on innovation in cancer chemoprevention. *Cancer Prev Res (Phila).* 2008;1(2):84–90.

Grandjean N, Charpiot B, Pena CA, Peitsch MC. Competitive intelligence and patent analysis in drug discovery. *Drug Discov Today Technol.* 2005;2(3):211–215.

Guerin L, Wickham M. Patent watch: Australia's highest court decides isolated nucleic acids are not patent eligible. *Nat Rev Drug Discov.* 2015;14(12):813.

Gupta H, Kumar S, Roy SK, Gaud RS. Patent protection strategies. *J Pharm Bioallied Sci.* 2010;2(1):2–7.

Hattori K, Wakabayashi H, Tamaki K. Predicting key example compounds in competitors' patent applications using structural information alone. *J Chem Inf Model.* 2008;48(1):135–142.

Hervey M. Harnessing AI in drug discovery without losing patent protection. *Drug Discov Today.* 2020;25(6):949–950.

Higgins MJ, Graham SJ. Intellectual property. Balancing innovation and access: patent challenges tip the scales. *Science.* 2009;326(5951):370–371.

Hutson S. Pharma 'patent trolls' remain mostly the stuff of myth. *Nat Med.* 2009;15(11):1240.

Kapczynski A, Kesselheim AS. 'Government patent use: a legal approach to reducing drug spending. *Health Aff (Millwood).* 2016;35(5):791–797.

Kesselheim AS, Avorn J. Using patent data to assess the value of pharmaceutical innovation. *J Law Med Ethics.* 2009;37(2):176–183.

Kettle JG, Cassar DJ. Covalent inhibitors of the GTPase KRAS. *Expert Opin Ther Pat.* 2020;30(2):103–120.

Kleczkowska P, Kowalczyk A, Lesniak A, Bujalska-Zadrozny M. The discovery and development of drug combinations for the treatment of various diseases from patent literature (1980-present). *Curr Top Med Chem.* 2017;17(8):875–894.

López Tricas JM. [Patent expiry for profitable drugs]. *Farm Hosp.* 2012;36(1):1–2.

McGee JE, Roy A. Patent review. *Comb Chem High Throughput Screen.* 2011;14(10):926–928.

Melethil S. Patent issues in drug development: perspectives of a pharmaceutical scientist-attorney. *AAPS J.* 2005;7(3):E723–E728.

Noonan K. Patent watch: diagnostic patents at risk after Federal Circuit decisions. *Nat Rev Drug Discov.* 2016;15(6):377.

Saotome C, Nakaya Y, Abe S. Patent production is a prerequisite for successful exit of a biopharmaceutical company. *Drug Discov Today.* 2016;21(3):406–409.

Satchell J, Stark A. Experimental evidence to support a patent application: are in silico data enough? *Future Med Chem.* 2011;3(9):1089–1092.

Sebastian TE, Yerram CB, Saberwal G. Patent holdings of US biotherapeutic companies in major markets. *Drug Discov Today.* 2009;14(9–10):442–445.

Senger S. Assessment of the significance of patent-derived information for the early identification of compound-target interaction hypotheses. *J Cheminform.* 2017;9(1):26.

Sherkow JS. Patent law's reproducibility paradox. *Duke Law J.* 2017;66(4):845–911.

Song CH. Creating commercial value from patents: the interplay between patent protection and patent information management. *Pharm Pat Anal.* 2016;5(6):361–365.

U.S. Patent and Trademark Office. Class 424. 2000. Retrieved from: https://www.uspto.gov/web/offices/ac/ido/oeip/taf/def/424.htm

Waters H. Patent-sharing scheme for neglected diseases may have catch. *Nat Med.* 2011;17(12):1529.

Webber PM. A guide to drug discovery. Protecting your inventions: the patent system. *Nat Rev Drug Discov.* 2003;2(10):823–830.

Yamanaka T, Kano S. Mapping lifecycle management activities for blockbuster drugs in Japan based on drug approvals and patent term extensions. *Drug Discov Today.* 2016;21(2):306–314.

Yamanaka T, Kano S. Patent term extension systems differentiate Japanese and US drug lifecycle management. *Drug Discov Today.* 2016;21(1):111–117.

Yang K, Deangelis RA, Reed JE, Ricklin D, Lambris JD. Complement in action: an analysis of patent trends from 1976 through 2011. *Adv Exp Med Biol.* 2013;735:301–313.

Zaman K. An important addition to the 'recent patent' journal series. *Recent Pat Endocr Metab Immune Drug Discov.* 2012;6(1):1–3.

Index

A

Accrufer (ferric maltol), 44
"Active" targeted nanomedicine, 208
Adakveo (crizanlizumab-tmca), 43
Adcetris (brentuximab vedotin), 55
Additive manufacturing, xxxi–xxxii
Addyi (flibanserin), 49
Adempas (riociguat), 52
Adeno-associated virus (AAV), 382
Adjuvants, 431
Adlyxin (lixisenatide), 48
Advanced manufacturing, xxxii–xxxiii
Advanced therapy medicinal products (ATMPs), 31
Aemcolo (rifamycin), 45
Aimovig (erenumab-aooe), 46
Ajovy (fremanezumab-vfrm), 45
Aklief (trifarotene), 43
Akynzeo (fosnetupitant and palonosetron), 46
Akynzeo (netupitant and palonosetron), 51
Alecensa (alectinib), 49
Aliqopa (copanlisib), 47
Alkaloids, 451
Alpha helix, 256
Altair Knowledge Studio, 86
Alunbrig (brigatinib), 47
Amyvid (Florbetapir F 18), 54
Angiotensin-converting enzyme 2 (ACE2), 432
Annovera (segesterone acetate and ethinyl estradiol vaginal system), 45
Anoro Ellipta, 52
Anthim (obiltoxaximab), 48
Antibiotics
  genomic approaches, 238–240
  phage therapy, 244–246
  post-genomics
    metabolomics to meta-omics, 242–244
    transcriptomics, proteomics, and lipidomics, 241–242
  reverse genomics, 240–241
  semi-synthesis, 236
  synthetic routes, 237–238
Antibody therapeutic proteins
  affimer proteins, 268–269
  affinity maturation, 271–272
  antibody cocktail treatments, 274
  antibody–drug conjugates, 275
  antigenized antibodies, 272
  bispecific antibodies (BsAbs), 269–270
  crystallizable fragment (Fc), 273
  development of, 275–277
  diffusion within cells, 274
  drug/toxin conjugation, 272–273
  exogenous methods
    mouse hybridoma, 278–280
    surface display libraries, 280–287
    transgenic mice, 280
  fab fragments and single-chain antibodies, 270
  humanized and chimeric mAbs, 270–271
  IgG1 fusion proteins, 272
  mode of action, 266–267
  multi-specific antibodies (MsAbs), 270
  nave antibody repertoire, 273
  precision medicine, 274
  recombinant antibodies, 267–268
  structural protein scaffolds, 268–269
  synthetic antibodies, 268
Aptiom (eslicarbazepine acetate), 52
Arabian medicine, 25
Arcapta Neohaler, 55
Aristada (aripiprazole lauroxil), 49
Artesunate (artesunate), 42
Artificial intelligence (AI), 20, xxxiii
  AI-based tools, 73
  application, 72, 82–83
  biomarkers, 81
  biomedical, clinical and patient data, 80
  in biomedical data, 69
  CADD, 82
  COVID-19 pandemic, 70
  deep learning, 69, 70
  drug discovery and development
    application of, 76
    automation, 79
    biological "target," 78–79
    biomarkers, 79
    clinical trials, 79
    computer-aided synthesis planning (CASP), 77
    multiparameter optimization, 77
    quantitative structure–activity relationship (QSAR) approach, 77
    robotics, 79
    therapeutic candidates, 79
  drug repurposing, 80
  drug target identification and validation, 80
  genome research, 81
  high-throughput screening, 81–82
  machine learning, 69, 70
  manufacturing process improvement, 81
  medical research, 73
  neural networks, 69, 70
  preclinical candidates screening, 80
  target-based and phenotypic drug discovery, 80
  tools, 83–86
Asimov, Isaac, 7
Asparlas (calaspargase pegol-mknl), 44
Aspirin, 26
At-risk initiation, 471

Aubagio (teriflunomide), 53
Austedo (deutetrabenazine), 47
Autoimmune disorders, 24
Automated machine learning (autoML), 84
Automation, 524–525, xxxiii
Avycaz (ceftazidime-avibactam), 50
Axumin (fluciclovine F 18), 48
AYUSH, 447
Ayvakit (avapritinib), 43

B

Balversa (erdafitinib), 44
Barhemsys (amisulpride), 43
Batch-to-batch consistency, 521
Bavencio (avelumab), 48
Baxdela (delafloxacin), 47
Bayes' theorem, xxxiii
  aging paradigm, 12
  artificial intelligence and machine learning, 11
  to COVID-19, 11
  to drug discovery, 13
  Kuhn's methodological ideas, 12
  paradigm shift
    crisis, 14–15
    normal science, 14
    pre-science, 14
    revolution, 15
  statistical problems, 11
Beleodaq (belinostat), 51
Belsomra (suvorexant), 51
Belviq (lorcaserin hydrochloride), 54
Benlysta (belimumab), 56
Benznidazole, 47
Beovu (brolucizumab–dbll), 43
Besponsa (inotuzumab ozogamicin), 47
Beta-sheet, 256
Bevyxxa (betrixaban), 47
Big data and analytics, xxxiii
Biktarvy (bictegravir, embitcitabine, tenofovir alafenamide), 46
Biocatalyst, xxxiii–xxxiv
Bioinformatics, xxxiv
  Human Genome Project, 71
  model-based product development, 72
  proteomics, 71
Biological manufacturing, xxxiv–xxxv
Biological patents
  antisense technology, 552–553
  biological products, 551
  monoclonal antibody technology, 552
  transgenic plants, 553
Biological products, 405
  batch, 505–506
  cleaning, 515–516
  cost contributions, 505
  downstream, 508–509
  economy considerations, 503
  equipment, 510
  facility, 509–510
  facility design, 513–515
  filling and finishing, 516–517
  formulation fill, 513
  manufacturing process, 503
  quality, 512
  robust process, 505
  testing, 511
  upstream, 507–508
  validation, 510–511
  water, 513
Biological sequences, 74
Biomarkers
  artificial intelligence (AI), 81
  BEST, 136
  Biomarker Qualification Program, 137
  clinical trial design, 133
  drug discovery and development, 79
  FDA-approved markers, 134
  genomic, proteomic, and metabolomic technologies, 135
  imaging techniques, 136
  PD biomarkers, 137
  personalized medicine, 135–136
  predictions, of human responses, 136
  quantitative predictions, 135
  robust clinical study, 133
  surrogate endpoints, 136
Biomedicines, 30
Bioreactor cycle, 311–312
Blenrep (belantamab mafodotin-blmf), 42
Blincyto (blinatumomab), 51
Blockchain, xxxv
Bosulif (bosutinib), 54
Botanical products, 439
  approval rules in different countries, 449–451
  chemistry, manufacturing, and control (CMC) requirements, 455–462
  complimentary medicines (*see* Complimentary medicines)
  efficacy and safety, 454
  human use, 454–455
  pharmacologically active phytochemical, 451–452
  regulation and legislation of, 448
  specifications, 452–453
  standardization, 453–454
  standardized botanical preparation, 452
  therapeutic efficacy, 448
The Botanical Review Team (BRT), 448
Braftovi (encorafenib), 46
Brain-on-a-chip systems, 129–130
Braschi, Giannina, 7
Breo Ellipta, 52
Bridion (sugammadex), 49
Brightics AI, 85
Brin, David, 6
Brineura (cerliponase alfa), 47
Brintellix (vortioxetine), 52
Briviact (brivaracetam), 48
Brukinsa (zanubrutinib), 43
Brunner, John, 7
Butler, Octavia E., 7
Byfavo (remimazolam), 42

C

Cablivi (caplacizumab-yhdp), 44
Calquence (acalabrutinib), 47
Cancer, 207–211
Capacity building, xxxv
Caplyta (lumateperone tosylate), 43
Caprelsa (vandetanib), 55
CAR-T techniques, 381
CAR-T therapy, xxxv
Cell culture operations, 309–311
Cell line development, 307–308
Cell therapy, xxxv–xxxvi
 allogenic cell therapy, 403–404
 blood transfusion, 401
 CAR-T therapy, 402–403
 cell banking system procedures, 407
 cell culture procedures, 406–407
 cell elimination strategies, 383
 cellular gene therapy products
  adventitious agent testing, 408
  cell identity, 408
  frozen cell banks, 409
  general safety test, 408
  potency, 408
  purity, 408
  viability, 408
 collection of cells, 405–406
 embryonic stem cell nuclear transfer (ntESCs), 385
 embryonic stem cells, 384, 385, 402
 epithelial cells, 385, 402
 hematopoietic stem cells (HSCs), 402
 immune cell treatment, 402
 immunotherapy, 385
 materials, during manufacturing, 407–408
 multipotent cells (MSCs), 382, 385
 nervous stem cells (NSCs), 385, 402
 parthenogenetic (pES), 385, 402
 pluripotent stem cells, 384, 402
 radioisotopes/toxins to cell preparations, 409
 red blood cell, 384
 somatic cell gene therapy, 384
 somatic cell therapy, 401
 therapeutic transgenes, 386
 tissue typing, 406
Cerdelga (eliglustat), 51
Cerianna (fluoroestrdiol F18), 42
Chemical contaminants, 519
Chemical entities, 531
Chemical lead compound, 471
Cholbam (cholic acid), 50
Choline C 11 Injection, 53
Cinqair (reslizumab), 48
Clancy, Tom, 6
Cognitive science, 20
Cometriq (cabozantinib), 53
Commercialization stage, 471
Complimentary medicines
 development innovations, 441–442
 genomics and biomarkers, 442–444
 metabolomics and metabonomics, 445–446
 proteomics, 444–445
 target identification of label-free botanical products, 445
The Condition of Muzak, 8
Continuous manufacturing, xxxvi
 advantages of intensification, 333
 commercial-scale and formulations, 334
 continuous chromatography systems
  periodic countercurrent chromatography (PCC), 337
  simulated moving bed (SMB) chromatography, 337
  straight through processing (STP), 336
 hybrid approach, 336
 process intensification, 333
 process monitoring and data acquisition, 334
 product quality, 333
Controlled Substances Act, 28
Controls, xxxvi–xxxvii
Copiktra (duvelisib), 45
Corlanor (ivabradine), 50
Cosentyx (secukinumab), 50
Cotellic (cobimetinib), 49
Counter-screen, 471
COVID-19, 17
 vaccine, 421, 432–433
Cresemba (isavuconazonium sulfate), 50
CRISPR, xxxvii
Crysvita (burosumab-twza), 46
Cumulative cost, 471
Cyramza (ramucirumab), 51

D

Daklinza (daclatasvir), 49
Daliresp (roflumilast), 56
Dalvance (dalbavancin), 51
Danyelza (naxitamab-gqgk), 41
Darzalex (daratumumab), 49
Data harmonization, 75–76, xxxvii
Dataism, 1
Datscan (ioflupane i-123), 56
Daurismo (glasdegib), 45
Dayvigo (lemborexant), 43
Decision stage, 471
DeepDTnet, 87, 88
Deep learning, 86
 biological sequences, 74
 feedforward neural network (FNN), 73, 74
 graph representation learning, 74
Deep learning architecture, xxxvii–xxxviii
DeepMind, 70
Defitelio (defibrotide sodium), 49
Delphi method, 3
Dendrimers, xxxviii
de Nostredame, Michel, 6
Detectnet (copper Cu 64 dotatate injection), 42
Diabetes, 207
Diacomit (stiripentol), 45
Dick, Philip K, 8
Dificid (fidaxomicin), 55
Digital clinical trials, xxxviii

Digital control, xxxviii
Digital health, xxxix
Digital health companies, 34
Digital technology, 73
Disease stratification, 37
DNA transfection, 430
DNA vaccine
  advantages of, 433
  adverse effects, 435
  antibody responses, 436–437
  delivery, 435–436
  and gene therapy, 433
  making of, 434
  for veterinary use, 433
Documentation process
  automation, 524–525
  process analytical technology (PAT), 523–524
Dojolvi (triheptanoin), 42
Doptelet (avatrombopag), 46
Dotarem (gadoterate meglumine), 53
Drug absorption, 346
Drug delivery platform technology
  clinical formulation development, 495, 499, 500
  clinical proof of concept, 503, 504
  clinical supplies manufacture, 499, 501
  development plan, 499, 500
  human proof of concept, 500, 503
  IND preparation and submission, 500, 503
  preclinical safety package, 499, 502
Drug development assays
  assay optimization, 143–144
  batch testing
    analytical gel filtration, 153
    commercial enzymes, 154
    co-purification of contaminating enzymes, 154
    crude enzyme preparations, 154
    Edman sequencing, 154
    identity and mass purity, 152
    mass spectrometry (MS), 153
    mock parallel purification, 154–155
    peptide mass finger printing, 154
    reversal of enzyme activity, 155
    reversed-phase HPLC (RP-HPLC), 153
    SDS-PAGE, 153
    Western blot, with specific antibody, 153
    whole mass for protein, 153
  critical path, 146
  cross-validation, 146
  ELISA-type assays (*see* ELISA-type assays)
  enzymatic contamination
    signs of, 151–152
    solutions for, 152
  enzymatic purity
    hill slope, 157–159
    IC50 values, 157
    inhibitor-based studies, 156–157
  enzyme impurities
    enzyme concentration, 156
    format selection, 156
    substrate Km, 155–156
    substrate selectivity, 155
  filtration assays, 149–150
  in-study validation, 146
  pharmacokinetics and drug metabolism
    CYP450 inhibition profiling, 187
    hepatic microsome stability, 184–185
    lipophilicity, 183–184
    permeability, 188
    plasma protein binding, 185–186
    plasma stability, 185
    screening cytotoxicity and hepatotoxicity test, 186–187
    solubility, 184
    two-tier approach, flowchart of, 183
  pre-study validation, 145–146
  scintillation proximity assays (SPA), 147–149
  substrate-based studies
    comparison studies, 160
    enzyme source, 160
    format comparison, 160
    substrate Km determination, 159
    substrate selectivity studies, 159–160
  and validation, 144–145
  in vitro toxicity and drug efficacy testing, 177
  in vivo assay validation
    cross-validation, 179
    flowchart for, 178
    in-study validation, 179
    pre-study validation, 179
    procedures, 180–182
    resources, 179–180
Drug development strategies, 439
Drug discovery
  clinical trials
    advance innovative trial designs, 132
    biomarkers, 133–137
    disease- or indication-specific trial designs, 132–133
    patient preferences, 133
    patient responses, 132
    streamlining and automating clinical trials, 133
  DNA libraries, 126–128
  high-throughput screening (HTS)
    evolving technologies in, 93
    factors hindering drug discovery, 93
    fragment-based screening, 95
    gene-based testing, 95–97
    induced neurons (iNs), 92
    ligandomics, 95
    modeling, 94–95
    phenotypic screening, 94
    target-based HTS, 92
    target identification, 97–112
  IND exploratory research strategy, 137–139
  Lipinski's rule of five (RO5), 118–121
  microphysiometry
    brain-on-a-chip systems, 129–130
    heart-on-a-chip, 130
    human-on-a-chip, 131
    kidney-on-a-chip, 130
    lung-on-a-chip, 130

microfluidics, 129
nephron-on-a-chip, 130–131
organs-on-a-chip (OOC), 129
skin-on-a-chip, 131
vessel-on-a-chip, 131
modern, multifaceted approach to, 92
Noble prizes award for, 32–34
140 years of, 35
online resources on, 99–106
optimization of, 91
orphan drugs, 140–141
PK–PD relationship, 115–118
repurposing, 139–140
safety testing
animal models, 122–123
cell models, 122
neurotoxicity, 122
replacing animal testing, 123–124
safety risks, 121
in silico approaches, 121
validation, 122
structural biology
cryo-electron microscopy (CryoEM), 114
cryoEM, 114
experimental data, 114
liquid chromatography technologies, 112
mass spectrometry, 113
multiple anomalous dispersion (MAD) methods, 113
protein complexes, 114
protein crystallography, 113
protein fusion partners, 112
protein structure, 113
SDS-PAGE gels, 112
synthetic biology, 124–125
timeline of, 91, 92
Drug repurposing
clinical formulation development, 490, 492
clinical supplies manufacture, 490, 494
confirmation of hits, 485, 489
gap analysis/development plan, 485, 490, 491
human proof of concept, 495, 497
identification of actives, 485, 488
IND preparation and submission, 495, 496
preclinical safety data package, 490, 493
Drug research, 26
Duavee (conjugated estrogens/bazedoxifene), 52
Duchenne muscular dystrophy, 40
Dupixent (dupilumab), 47
Durham-Humphrey Amendment, 27

E

Earth, 6
Ebanga (ansuvimab-zykl), 41
Edarbi (azilsartan medoxomil), 56
Edurant (rilpivirine), 55
Egyptian medicine, 25
Elelyso (taliglucerase alfa), 54
Eliquis (apixaban), 53
ELISA-type assays
AlphaScreen Format
isothermal calorimetry (ITC), 175–176
nuclear magnetic resonance (NMR), 175
optical biosensors, 175
sedimentation analysis, 176
X-ray crystallography, 176
antibody and enzyme-based detection, 167
assay design and development, 168–169
fluorescence/Förster resonance energy transfer (FRET), 172–173
fluorescence polarization/anisotropy, 169–172
general considerations, 167–168
time-resolved (TR) FRET, 172–173
Elzonris (tagraxofusp-erzs), 44
Emflaza (deflazacort), 48
Emgality (galcanezumab-gnlm), 45
Empliciti (elotuzumab), 49
The English Assassin: A Romance of Entropy, 8
Enhertu (fam-trastuzumab deruxtecan-nxki), 43
Enspryng (satralizumab-mwge), 42
Entresto (sacubitril/valsartan), 50
Entyvio (vedolizumab), 51
Enzymatic purity, 151
Enzyme identity, 150–151
Epclusa (sofosbuvir and velpatasvir), 48
Epidioloex (cannabidiol), 46
Eradicable diseases
cysticercosis, 233
guinea worm disease, 232
lymphatic filariasis, 232
malaria, 234
measles, mumps, and rubella, 232–233
onchocerciasis, 233
polio, 232
trachoma, 233
yaws, 233
Erivedge (vismodegib), 54
Erleada (apalutamide), 46
Erwinaze (asparaginase *Erwinia chrysanthemi*), 55
Esbriet (pirfenidone), 51
Eucrisa (crisaborole), 48
European Collection of Cell Cultures, 338
European Medicines Agency (EMA), 421
Evenity (romosozumab-aqqg), 44
Evrysdi (risdiplam), 42
ExEm Foam (air polymer-type A), 43
Exondys 51 (eteplirsen), 48
Extended reality (XR), xxxix
Extracellular RNA, 427
Extracellular tumor (ECF) fluid, 208
Eylea (aflibercept), 55

F

Fahrenheit 451, 6
Farxiga (dapaglifozin), 52
Farydak (panobinostat), 50
Fasenra (benralizumab), 47
FD&C Act, 27
Federal Food, Medicine, and Cosmetic Act, 28
Feedforward neural network (FNN), 73, 74

Ferriprox (deferiprone), 55
Fetroja (cefiderocol), 43
Firazyr (icatibant), 55
Firdapse (amifampridine), 41
Flexible production, xxxix–xl
Fluorodopa F 18, 43
Food and Agriculture Organization, 446
Food and Drug Act, 26
Forecasting, 3
Freedom-to-operate (FTO), 553–554
From the Earth to the Moon, 6
Fulyzaq (crofelemer), 53
Fumigation agents, 460
Futility, 6
Fycompa (perampanel), 53

G

Ga-68-DOTATOC, 43
Gadavist (gadobutrol), 56
Galafold (migalastat), 45
Gallium 68 PSMA-11, 41
Gamifant (emapalumab-lzsgemapalumab-lzsg), 45
Gastrointestinal tract's enzyme degradation, 346
Gattex (teduglutide), 53
Gavreto (pralsetinib), 42
Gazyva (obinutuzumab), 52
Gemtesa (viberon), 41
GenBank(R), 337
Gene therapy, xl
  adenoviral vectors
    adeno-associated virus, 413
    gene delivery systems, 413
    measurement of particles *vs.* infectious units, 412–413
    replication-competent adenovirus, 413
  CRISPR-Cas system, 395–397
  DNA-based medicines, 381
  DNA-based therapeutics, 397
  downstream manufacturing, 388–391
  electroporation, passive delivery, and ballistic delivery, 383
  gene editing, 382, 392–393, 395
  gene silencing, 383
  gene transfer technologies
    approved products, 399, 400
    mechanical and electrical techniques, 398
    vector-assisted delivery systems, 398–399
  genome translation and transcription process, 382
  in vivo gene therapy, 384
  lifetime treatment, 381
  multipotent cells, 382
  reclinical evaluation of, 414–416
  reprogramming, 383
  risks of, 391–392
  somatic cell gene therapy, 384
  techniques, 393–395
  therapeutic transgenes, 386
  tissue culture, 381
  types of, 382
  vectors for
    adventitious agents, 410–411
    lot-to-lot release testing and specifications, 410
    manufacturing, 386–388
    master viral banks, 409–410
    modifications in, 413–414
    plasmid vector products, 411
    retroviral vector products, 411–412
    vector construction and characterization, 409
    vector production system, 409
    viral infection, 383
Genome sequencing power, xl
Genomic biomarkers, xl
Genvoya, 49
Giapreza (angiotensin II), 46
Gilotrif (afatinib), 52
Givlaari (givosiran), 43
Glycosides, 451–452
The Golden Man, 8
Gold nanoparticles, 195
Greek medicine, 25
Green Revolution, 17

H

Harvoni (ledipasvir/sofosbuvir), 51
Healing therapies, 38
Heart-on-a-chip, 130
Hemlibra (emicizumab), 47
Hepatitis C, 231
Herbert, Frank, 8
Hetlioz (tasimelteon), 52
High cell density cryopreservation, 309
High-throughput screening (HTS), 13, xl–xli
  defined, 471
  enzymatic assays for
    detection system linearity, 162
    enzyme reaction progress curve, 163
    IC50 for inhibitors, 165–166
    initial velocity, 161–162
    Km and Vmax, measurement of, 163–165
    optimization experiments, 166–167
  evolving technologies in, 93
  factors hindering drug discovery, 93
  fragment-based screening, 95
  gene-based testing, 95–97
  induced neurons (iNs), 92
  ligandomics, 95
  modeling, 94–95
  phenotypic screening, 94
  target-based HTS, 92
  target identification, 97–112
Horizant (gabapentin enacarbil), 55
Human Genome Initiative, 29
Human Genome Project, 29
Human interactome, xli
Humanism, 1
Humanity, 2
Human-on-a-chip, 131
Hunter, John, 25
Huxley, Aldous, 5
Hybridoma Databank (HDB), 338

I

IBD drugs, 207
IBM, 84–85
Ibrance (palbociclib), 50
Ibsrela (tenapanor), 43
Iclusig (ponatinib), 53
Idhifa (enasidenib), 47
Ilumya (tildrakizumab), 46
Imbruvica (ibrutinib), 52
Imcivree (setmelanotide), 41
Imfinzi (durvalumab), 47
IMGT/mAb-DB, 338
Immunogenicity
 adaptive system, 290–291
 immunogenicity testing, 289–290
 innate system, 290
 protein immunogenicity, 288–289
Impavido (miltefosine), 51
Incivek (telaprevir), 55
Incremental cost, 471
Indian medicine, 25
Individualized treatment, 37
Industrial biotech, xli
Ingrezza (valbenazine), 47
Inlyta (axitinib), 54
Inmazeb (atoltivimab, maftivimab, and odesivimab-ebgn), 42
Innovative drug discovery, 439
Inorganic impurities, 460
Inqovi (decitabine and cedazuridine), 42
Inrebic (fedratinib), 44
Instant monitoring, 36
Intellectual property, 532
International Regulatory Cooperation for Botanical Products, 447
Invokana (canagliflozin), 52
Ipecacuanha, 26
Isturisa (osilodrostat), 42
It Can't Happen Here, 6

J

Jakafi (ruxolitinib), 55
Jardiance (empagliflozin), 51
Jenner, Edward, 25
Jetrea (ocriplasmin), 53
Jeuveau (prabotulinumtoxinA-xvfs), 44
Jublia (efinaconazole), 51
Juxtapid (lomitapide), 53

K

Kadcyla (ado-trastuzumab emtansine), 53
Kalydeco (ivacaftor), 54
Kanuma (sebelipase alfa), 49
Kefauver-Harris Amendment, 28
Kengreal (cangrelor), 50
Kerydin (tavaborole), 51
Kevzara (sarilumab), 47
Keytruda (pembrolizumab), 51
Kidney-on-a-chip, 130
Kisqali (ribociclib), 48
Klisyri tirbanibulin, 41
KNIME Analytics Platform, 85
Koselugo (selumetinib), 42
Krintafel (tafenoquine), 46
Kybella (deoxycholic acid), 50
Kynamro (mipomersen sodium), 53
Kyprolis (carfilzomib), 54

L

Lampit (nifurtimox), 42
Lartruvo (olaratumab), 48
The Left Hand of Darkness, 8
Lenvima (lenvatinib), 50
Les Prophéties, 6
Lewis, Sinclair, 6
Library, 471
Libtayo (cemiplimab-rwlc), 45
Ligandomics, xli–xlii
Linzess (linaclotide), 54
Lipinski's rule of five (RO5), 118–121
Lipopolyplexes (LPPs), 429
Liposomes, xlii
Living entities, 307
Lokelma (sodium zirconium cyclosilicate), 46
Long-term diseases, 34
Lonsurf (trifluridine and tipiracil), 49
Lorbrena (lorlatinib), 45
The Lord of the Rings, 7
Lorenz attractor, 10
Lucemyra (lofexidine hydrochloride), 46
Lumason (sulfur hexafluoride lipid microsphere), 51
Lumoxiti (moxetumomab pasudotox-tdfk), 45
Lung-on-a-chip, 130
Lutathera (lutetium Lu 177 dotatate), 46
Luzu (luliconozole), 52
Lymphoseek (technetium Tc 99m tilmanocept), 53
Lynparza (olaparib), 50
Lyosphere, xlii

M

Machine learning, xxxiii
 deep learning (*see* Deep learning)
 elements of, 69, 70
Macrilen (macimorelin acetate), 46
Margenza margetuximab (anti-HER2 mAb), 41
Mass purity, 151
Mavyret (glecaprevir and pibrentasvir), 47
Mayzent (siponimod), 44
McCloud, Scott, 8
Media, 308–309
Medicine development, 28–29
Mekinist (trametinib), 52
Mektovi (binimetinib), 46
Mepsevii (vestronidase alfa-vjbk), 47
Mesoscales, 19
Mesoscience, xlii–xliii
Messenger RNA (mRNA), 41

Metabolomics, xliii
Metabonomics, xliii
MHC class I and II, xliii
Microbial contamination, 519
Microbial limits, 460
Microbiome, 37
  biomarkers, 248
  drug metabolism, 247
  drug toxicity, 247–248
  impact on health, 246–247
Microfluidics, 129, xliii–xliv
Microphysiometry, xliv
  brain-on-a-chip systems, 129–130
  heart-on-a-chip, 130
  human-on-a-chip, 131
  kidney-on-a-chip, 130
  lung-on-a-chip, 130
  microfluidics, 129
  nephron-on-a-chip, 130–131
  organs-on-a-chip (OOC), 129
  skin-on-a-chip, 131
  vessel-on-a-chip, 131
Microwave, xliv
Modeling systems
  Bayesian framework, 8
  Bayes' theorem (*see* Bayes' theorem)
  in consecutive refinements, 8
  differential equation, 9
  double pendulum, 10
  Lorenz attractor, 10
  nonlinear dynamical equations, 9
  regime transitions, 19
  research domains, 19
  scientific approach, 9
Model operations (Modelops), 84
Moderna COVID-19 vaccine, 430
Modern medicine, 439
Molecular entities, 41–56
Monjuvi (tafasitamab-cxix), 42
Monoclonal Antibody Index, 338
Moorcock, Michael, 8
Motegrity (prucalopride), 44
Movantik (naloxegol), 51
Moxidectin (moxidectin), 46
mRNA vaccine, 381, xliv
  acquired immunity, 423
  antigen expression, 423
  applications of, 423
  autoimmunity type I interferon responses, 426
  candidate vaccine antigen sequences, 427
  contaminants in, 423
  COVID-19 vaccine, 432–433
  formulation and delivery, 429–432
  GMP production of, 428
  in vitro transcribed (IVT) mRNA, 427
  lineaRx PCR-based production of, 428
  major histocompatibility complex (MHC), 425, 426
  mechanism of action of, 424
  MHC molecules' function, 423
  plasmid DNA, 427, 428
  rolling circle amplification (RCA), 428
  T cells'proliferation, 423
  viral replicon particles (VRPs), 424
Mulpleta (lusutrombopag), 45
Multi-host diseases, 231
Multimodal PaML (Predictive Analysis and Machine Learning) Tools, 83
Myalept (metreleptin for injection), 51
Mycotoxins, 460
Myrbetriq (mirabegron), 54

N

Nanomaterials, 195
Nanomedicine, xliv
Nanomedicine elements, 196
Nanoparticles, xlv
  carriers, 207
  clearance of, 210
  delivery routes, 196–199
  dendrimers, 200
  diagnostics, 206
  fullerenes, 204
  liposomes, 196–200
  metal particles, 203
  pharmaceutical industry, 196
  polymers, 200–203
  quantum dots, 203–204
  theranostics, 204–206
  types of, 196
Nanotechnology-based products, 208
Nanotechnology revolution, 17
Narrative of Arthur Gordon Pym of Nantucket, 7
Narrative technique, 8
The National Nanotechnology Initiative, 195
Natpara (parathyroid hormone), 50
Natroba (spinosad), 56
Nephron-on-a-chip, 130–131
Nerlynx (neratinib maleate), 47
Nesina (alogliptin), 53
NETSPOT (gallium Ga 68 dotatate), 48
Network medicine, xlv
Network proximity, xlv
Neuraceq (florbetaben F 18 injection), 51
Neurological diseases, xlv–xlvi
Neurological disorder NMEs, 40
Neutroval (tbo-filgrastim), 54
New chemical entity (NCE), 26
  clinical proof of concept, 483, 486
  confirmation of hits, 474, 475, 477
  defined, 471
  development candidate, 479, 481, 482
  human proof of concept, 483, 484
  identification of actives, 474, 476
  identification of chemical lead, 476, 478
  IND application, 482–483
  Pre-IND Meeting with FDA, 482
  selection of optimized chemical lead, 479, 480
  target identification, 472, 474
  target validation, 472, 474
New molecular entities (NMEs), 38
Nexletol (bempedoic acid), 43

NIH genetic sequence database, 337–338
Ninlaro (ixazomib), 49
Noble prizes award, for work-related drug discovery, 32–34
Non-antibody therapeutic proteins
  enzymes, 264
  hormone peptide drugs, 262–263
  human bone formation protein, 264
  human cytokines, 263
  human hematopoietic factor, 263
  human plasma protein factor, 263
Non-injectable drug administration, 347
Nonlinearity, xlvi
Nonlinear narrative, 8
Nonobviousness, 540–542, xlvi
Nonreplicating transcript, 424
Non-viral delivery methods, 430
Northera (droxidopa), 51
Nourianz (istradefylline), 43
Nubeqa (darolutamide), 44
Nucala (mepolizumab), 49
Nucleic acid contamination, 519
Nucleoside modification, xlvi
Nucleotide vaccines, 421
Nulojix (belatacept), 55
Nuplazid (pimavanserin), 48
Nurtec ODT (rimegepant), 42
Nuzyra (omadacycline), 45

O

Ocaliva (obeticholic acid), 48
Ocrevus (ocrelizumab), 47
Ocular drug delivery, 199
Odomzo (sonidegib), 50
Ofev (nintedanib), 51
Off-target activity, 471
Olinvyk (oliceridine), 42
Olumiant (baricitinib), 46
Olysio (simeprevir), 52
Omegaven (fish oil triglycerides), 45
Omontys (peginesatide), 54
Ongentys (opicapone), 42
Online monitoring, 333
Onpattro (patisiran), 45
Opdivo (nivolumab), 50
Opsumit (macitentan), 52
Orbactiv (oritavancin), 51
Organs-on-a-chip (OOC), 129, xlvi
Orgovyx relugolix, 41
Orilissa (elagolix sodium), 45
Orkambi, 50
Orladeyo berotralstat, 41
Orphan drugs, 140–141
Orthogonal assay, 471, xlvii
Orwell, George, 5
Osphena (ospemifene), 53
Otezla (apremilast), 51
Oxbryta (voxelotor), 43
Oxervate (cenegermin-bkbj), 45
Oxlumo (lumasiran), 41
Ozempic (semaglutide), 46

P

Packaging, xlvii
Padcev (enfortumab vedotin-ejfv), 43
PaML, 85
Paradigm shift, xlvii
Parsabiv (etelcalcetide), 48
Particle size, 460
Passive immunization, xlvii
Pasteur, Louis, 25, 231
Patent
  alternate offering, 544–545
  applications and awarded patents, 536
  biological patents, 550–553
  claims for antibody products, 543
  classification, 546–551
  defined, 532
  delivery devices, 545
  formulation composition, 544
  lifecycle formulation projections, 544
  medical method patents, 546
  patents protecting biological medicines, 533
  pharmaceutical patenting practices, 537–538
  process patents of originator, 544
  software patents, 546
  submarine patents, 543
  system expression patents, 544
  third-party process patents, 544
  types of, 538–540
  unpatentable inventions, 545–546
Pathogen-associated molecular pattern (PAMP), xlviii
Pemazyre (pemigatinib), 42
Peripheral nervous system, 20
Perjeta (pertuzumab), 54
Personal genomics, xlviii
Personalized medications, 35
Pesticides, 460
Pfizer-BioNTech COVID-19 vaccine, 429
Phage therapy, xlviii
Pharmaceuticals, 23, 37–38
Pharmacokinetics, of therapeutic proteins
  absorption, 293–295
  distribution, 295
  elimination, 295–297
  formulation and immunogenicity factors, 293
  protein modification
    albumin–protein fusions, 297
    Fc fusion, 298
  protein pegylation, 298
  unnatural construction, 298–300
Picato (ingenol mebutate), 54
Pifeltro (doravirine), 45
Pinsker, Sarah, 5
Piqray (alpelisib), 44
Pizensy (lactitol), 43
Plasmid DNA, 31
Plegridy (peginterferon beta-1a), 51
Poe, Edgar Allan, 7
Polivy (polatuzumab vedotin-piiq), 44
Polymerase-chain-reaction (PCR)-produced linear DNA, 427
Polymers, 199

Polyphenols, 452
Pomalyst (pomalidomide), 53
Portrazza (necitumumab), 49
Poteligeo (mogamulizumab-kpkc), 45
Potency, 520
Potiga (ezogabine), 55
Praluent (alirocumab), 50
Praxbind (idarucizumab), 49
Predictions, 525–526
  crystal structure, at atomic level, 5
  defined, 3
  divination, 5
  early detection and, 36
  forecasting, 3
  function parameters, 4
  in mathematics, 4–5
  in novel, 7
  regression analysis, 4
  repeatable experiments/observational studies, 4
  solar cycle predictions, 4
  statistical inference, 3
  vision and prophecy, 5
Prepopik, 54
Pretomanid (PA-824), 44
Prevymis (letermovir), 47
Primary assay, 471
Process analytical technology (PAT), 523–524, xlvii
Process data analytics, xlviii–xlix
Process intensification, xlix
Process optimizations
  bioreactor cycle, 311–312
  cell culture operations, 309–311
  cell line development, 307–308
  high cell density cryopreservation, 309
  media, 308–309
Protein Data Bank (PDB), 338
Protein folding, 23
Protein structure and properties
  association and aggregation, 261
  post-translational modification (PTM), 257–260
  primary structure, 252–255
  quaternary structure, 257
  secondary structure, 256
  tertiary structure, 256–257
Proteomics, xlix
Public Health Service Act, 28
Purity, 518
Pyrogen contamination, 518–519

Q

Qinlock (ripretinib), 42
Qualified task, 471
Quantified extracts, 456
Quantum dots (QDs), xlix
Quinine, 26

R

RapidMiner, 85
Rapid scale-up, xlix–l
Rapivab (peramivir), 50
Rare diseases, 1
raxibacumab (raxibacumab), 53
Reblozyl (luspatercept–aamt), 43
Recarbrio (imipenem, cilastatin, and relebactam), 44
Regression analysis, 4
Regulatory approvals, 469
Repatha (evolocumab), 49
Retevmo (selpercatinib), 42
Revcovi (elapegademase-lvlr), 45
Rexulti (brexpiprazole), 50
Reyvow (lasmiditan), 43
Rhopressa (netarsudil), 46
Rinvoq (upadacitinib), 44
RNA vaccinology, 431
Robertson, Morgan, 6
Roman medicine, 25
Roosevelt, Franklin D., 27
Roosevelt, Theodore, 26
Rozlytrek (entrectinib), 44
Rubraca (rucaparib), 48
Rukobia (fostemsavir), 42
Rule of five (RO5), 118–121
Rydapt (midostaurin), 47

S

Sarclisa (isatuximab), 42
saRNA pharmacokinetics, 430
saRNA vaccines, 430
SARS-CoV-2, 432
Savaysa (edoxaban), 50
Scenesse (afamelanotide), 43
Secondary assay, 471–472
Secreted mucin-type glycoproteins, 347
Selectivity, 109
Sennae folium, 456
Serendipity, 23
Seysara (sarecycline), 45
Signifor (pasereotide), 53
Siliq (brodalumab), 48
Single-use technology (SUT)
  advantages, 315
  biomass sensors, 320
  biopharmaceutical manufacturing, 313
  cGMP concern, 312
  connectors, 322–323
  containers and mixing systems, 313
  disposable bioreactors, 318
  disposable filters, 312
  disposable sensors, 318
  downstream processing
    cell harvest, 325–326
    fill finish operations, 329
    general filtration applications, 328–329
    material selection, 331
    polymers and additives, 330–331
    purification, 326–327
    regulatory, 332–333
    testing, 331–332
    UF/DF and TFF, 328

virus removal, 327–328
drums, containers, and tank liners, 313–315
electrochemical sensors, 320
manufacturing location, 312
optical sensors, 319–320
pressure sensors, 320–321
process analytical technology (PAT), 318
pumps, 323–324
sampling, 324–325
sampling systems, 321–322
single-use bioreactors (SUBS), 315–318
tube welder and sealers, 324
tubing, 323
Sirturo (bedaquiline), 53
Sivextro, 51
Skin-on-a-chip, 131
Skyrizi (risankizumab-rzaa), 44
Smart Flexware systems, 312
Sogroya (somapacitan-beco), 42
Solosec (secnidazole), 47
Somatic cell therapy, 381
Sovaldi (sofosbuvir), 52
Spinraza (nusinersen), 48
S protein, 433
Stability, 520–521
Standardized extracts, 456
Stand on Zanzibar, 7
Steglatro (ertugliflozin), 46
Stendra (avanafil), 54
Stivarga (regorafenib), 53
Stratum cornea, 199
Strensiq (asfotase alfa), 49
Stribild, 54
Striverdi Respimat (olodaterol), 51
Structural biology, l
Sultana's Dream, 7
Sunosi (solriamfetol), 44
Surfaxin (lucinactant), 54
Swift, Jonathan, 6
Sylvant (siltuximab), 51
Symdeko (tezacaftor; ivacaftor), 46
Symproic (naldemedine), 48
Synribo (omacetaxine mepesuccinate), 53
Synthetic biology, l–li
Systems pharmacology, li

T

Tabrecta (capmatinib), 42
Tafinlar (dabrafenib), 52
Tagrisso (osimertinib), 49
Takhzyro (lanadelumab), 45
Taltz (ixekizumab), 48
Talzenna (talazoparib), 45
Tanzeum (albiglutide), 51
Targeted delivery, li
Target identification
cell-based models, 110–111
drug interactions, 97
historical drug targets, 98
hit identification, 98, 107–109
Mendelian randomization in, 98
target validation and efficacy, 109–110
in vivo testing, 111–112
Tauvid (flortaucipir F18), 42
Tavalisse (fostamatinib), 46
Tazverik (tazemetostat), 43
Tecentriq (atezolizumab), 48
Tecfidera (dimethyl fumarate), 52
Technology evolution, 2
Tegsedi (inotersen), 45
Tepezza (teprotumumab-trbw), 43
Terpenes, 452
Testing control, 521–522
Tetracycline, 448
Theory of chaos, 10
Theranostics, li
Therapeutic proteins' development systems
administration route selection, 345
alteplase recombinant injection, 366
coagulation factor VIIa (recombinant) injection, 365
daclizumab for injection, 365
delivery routes
intravenous, 353
nasal, 356
ocular, 358–359
oral, 355
pulmonary, 357–358
rectal, 359
subcutaneous, 353–355
transdermal, 356–357
formulation technologies
higher concentration formulations, 361–363
hydrogels and in situ forming gels, 359–360
liposome, 360–361
nanoparticles, 360
infliximab for injection, 365
interferon alfa-2a injection, 363
interferon Alfacon-1 injection, 364
interferon alfa-n3 injection, 364
interferon beta-1a injection, 364
interferon beta-1b, 364
interferon gamma-1b injection, 365
interleukin injection (IL-2), 363
Oprelvekin injection, 363
physicochemical properties, 345, 367–374
practicality and probability factors, 345
reteplase recombinant, 366
routes of administration
excipients and properties, 347–349
liquid formulations, 351–352
lyophilized formulations, 352–353
pH, 349
protectants, 350–351
selection, 346–347
stabilizers, 351
surface tension, 350
tonicity, 350
structural features of proteins, 345
3D printing, 38, xxxi
TIBco Data Science, 85
Tibsovo (ivosidenib), 46

TissueBlue (Brilliant Blue G Ophthalmic Solution), 43
Tivicay (dolutegravir), 52
TNF receptor fusion protein, 38
TPOXX (tecovirimat), 46
Traditional Chinese medicine (TCM), 24
Tradjenta (linagliptin), 55
Tremfya (guselkumab), 47
Tresiba (insulin degludec injection), 49
Trikafta (elexacaftor/ivacaftor/tezacaftor), 43
Trodelvy (sacituzumab govitecan-hziy), 42
Trogarzo (ibalizumab-uiyk), 46
Trulicity (dulaglutide), 51
Tudorza Pressair (aclidinium bromide), 54
Tukysa (tucatinib), 42
Turalio (pexidartinib), 44
21st-Century Cures Act, xxxi
Tymlos (abaloparatide), 47

U

Ubrelvy (ubrogepant), 43
Ultomiris (ravulizumab), 44
Unituxin (dinutuximab), 50
Uplizna (inebilizumab-cdon), 42
Uptravi (selexipag), 49

V

Vabomere (meropenem and vaborbactam), 47
Vaccine, 36–37
  comparison of, 422
  DNA vaccine (*see* DNA vaccine)
  inactivated vaccines, 234
  live-attenuated vaccines, 234
  mRNA vaccine (*see* mRNA vaccine)
  nucleic acid vaccines, 234–235
  subunit, recombinant, polysaccharide, and conjugate vaccines, 234
  toxoid vaccines, 234
  types of, 422
Varubi (rolapitant), 49
Veklury (remdesivir), 42
Veltassa, 49
Venclexta (venetoclax), 48
Verzenio (abemaciclib), 47
Vessel-on-a-chip, 131
Viberzi (eluxadoline), 50
Victrelis (boceprevir), 55
Viibryd (vilazodone hydrochloride), 56
Viltepso (viltolarsen), 42
Vimizim (elosulfase alfa), 52
Viral contamination, 307, 519
Viral replicon particles (VRPs), 424
Visible neural networks, 74
Vitrakvi (larotrectinib), 45
Viya, 85
Vizamyl (flutemetamol F 18 injection), 52
Vizimpro (dacomitinib), 45
Voraxaze (glucarpidase), 54
Vosevi (sofosbuvir, velpatasvir and voxilaprevir), 47
Vraylar (cariprazine), 49
Vyepti (eptinezumab-jjmr), 43
Vyleesi (bremelanotide), 46
Vyndaqel (tafamidis meglumine), 44
Vyondys 53 (golodirsen), 43
Vyzulta (latanoprostene bunod ophthalmic solution), 47

W

Wakix (pitolisant), 44
Water content, 460
Wells, HG, 7
Winlevi (clascoterone), 42
Withering, William, 25
World Health Organization, 447

X

Xadago (safinamide), 48
Xalkori (crizotinib), 55
Xarelto (rivaroxaban), 55
Xcopri (cenobamate), 43
Xeglyze (abametapir), 42
Xeljanz (tofacitinib), 53
Xenleta (lefamulin), 43
Xepi (ozenoxacin), 46
Xerava (eravacycline), 45
Xermelo (telotristat ethyl), 48
Xiidra (lifitegrast ophthalmic solution), 48
Xofigo (radium Ra 223 dichloride), 52
Xofluza (baloxavir marboxil), 45
Xospata (gilteritinib), 44
Xpovio (selinexor), 44
Xtandi (enzalutamide), 54
Xtoro (finafloxacin otic suspension), 50
Xuriden (uridine triacetate), 49

Y

Yervoy (ipilimumab), 55
Yondelis (trabectedin), 49
Yupelri (revefenacin), 45

Z

Zaltrap (ziv-aflibercept), 54
Zejula (niraparib), 48
Zelboraf (vemurafenib), 55
Zemdri (plazomicin), 46
Zepatier (elbasvir and grazoprevir), 48
Zeposia (ozanimod), 42
Zepzelca (lurbinectedin), 42
Zerbaxa (ceftolozane/tazobactam), 50
Zinbryta (daclizumab), 48
Zinplava (bezlotoxumab), 48
Zioptan (tafluprost), 54
Zokinvy (lonafarnib), 42
Zontivity (vorapaxar), 51
Zulresso (brexanolone), 44
Zurampic (lesinurad), 49
Zydelig (idelalisib), 51
Zykadia (ceritinib), 51
Zytiga (abiraterone acetate), 55

Printed in the United States
by Baker & Taylor Publisher Services